Magnetic Resonance Imaging:
Physical Principles and Sequence Design

Second Edition

Robert W. Brown, Ph.D.

Institute Professor and Distinguished University Professor
Case Western Reserve University, Cleveland, Ohio, USA

Yu-Chung N. Cheng, Ph.D.

Associate Professor of Radiology
Wayne State University, Detroit, Michigan, USA

E. Mark Haacke, Ph.D.

Professor of Radiology, Wayne State University, Detroit, Michigan, USA
Professor of Physics, Case Western Reserve University, Cleveland, Ohio, USA
Adjunct Professor of Radiology, Loma Linda University, Loma Linda, California, USA
Adjunct Professor of Radiology, McMaster University, Hamilton, Ontario, Canada
Distinguished Foreign Professor, Northeastern University, Shenyang, Liaoning, China

Michael R. Thompson, Ph.D.

Principal Scientist, Toshiba Medical Research Institute
Cleveland, Ohio, USA

Ramesh Venkatesan, D.Sc.

Manager, MR Applications Engineering
Wipro GE Healthcare Pvt. Ltd., Bangalore, Karnataka, India

WILEY Blackwell

Library of Congress Cataloging-in-Publication Data

Brown, Robert W., 1941– author.
  Magnetic resonance imaging : physical principles and sequence design / Robert W. Brown,
Yu-Chung N. Cheng, E. Mark Haacke, Michael R. Thompson, Ramesh Venkatesan. – Second edition.
     p. ; cm.
  Preceded by Magnetic resonance imaging : physical principles and sequence design /
E. Mark Haacke ... [et al.]. c1999.
  Includes bibliographical references and index.
  ISBN 978-0-471-72085-0 (cloth)
I. Cheng, Yu-Chung N., author. II. Haacke, E. Mark., author. III. Thompson, Michael R., author.
IV. Venkatesan, Ramesh., author. V. Title.
  [DNLM: 1. Magnetic Resonance Imaging. 2. Physical Phenomena. WN 185]
  RC78.7.N83
  616.07′548–dc23
                                                                         2014000051

Cover design by Wiley

Printed and bound in Malaysia by Vivar Printing Sdn Bhd

1 2014

Contents

8 Introductory Signal Acquisition Methods: Free Induction Decay, Spin Echoes, Inversion Recovery, and Spectroscopy $\qquad$ 113

9 One-Dimensional Fourier Imaging, k-Space, and Gradient Echoes $\qquad$ 141

Foreword to the Second Edition

Jeffrey L. Duerk

Almost 30 years ago, while a graduate student at Case Western Reserve University, I enrolled in a new course: The Physics of Magnetic Resonance Imaging (PHYS 431) that was being offered by Professors Mark Haacke and Robert Brown. Whole-body MR imaging systems had just emerged on the marketplace and the go-go days of MRI were upon us as numerous companies were dramatically ramping up their research and development efforts in this emerging, yet unproven field. In Cleveland alone, there was Picker International (now Philips Medical Systems) and Technicare (now GE); there were almost 20 MR systems in hospitals and at the manufacturers' facilities. The worldwide need for scientists and engineers with excellent preparation in the underlying physics of MR, signal detection, k-space, and a variety of pulse sequences was clear. Ultimately, over the next few years, PHYS 431 class notes were organized into sections, then chapters, and, eventually, 'the green bible' as we know this book today. Within a few years, it was translated into Chinese. For many, the book has served not only as a textbook, but as a sustaining reference on numerous aspects of NMR and MR imaging. Today, 'Haacke, Brown, Thompson and Venkatesan' has reached 2000 citations and counting.

For me, in the intervening 30 years, I went from a student to an industry-based researcher who still remembers fondly those go-go days, the advances and friendships formed, and the definitive impact that MRI provided in patient care. Upon returning to academia, I have seen my own students cut their teeth on this book, move to industry and academic positions, and go on to adopt it in their own courses. This has been repeated across universities, programs, and institutions around the world. The impact of this seminal teaching book is hard to calculate. Like Abragam before it, the book has achieved its authors' goals of sustainable impact and becoming a classic in the field.

Like all things, the field has changed dramatically since its original publication. Scan times of 25 minutes are now replaced by those of 25 milliseconds, or so, using novel sequences, novel trajectories, and constrained reconstruction. Field strengths of $0.15\,\mathrm{T}$, $0.3\,\mathrm{T}$, and $0.5\,\mathrm{T}$ are replaced by the now more common field strengths of $1.5\,\mathrm{T}$ and $3.0\,\mathrm{T}$, with $7.0\,\mathrm{T}$, $9.4\,\mathrm{T}$, and higher either solidly established or emerging on the horizon. Gradient strengths have increased from the lowly $3\,\mathrm{mT/m}$ 30 years ago to $40\,\mathrm{mT/m}$ on many systems today and soon some systems will have the capability of $80\,\mathrm{mT/m}$. Topics that have emerged today were not fully formed at the time of the first edition, and, hence, this version is not only greatly anticipated but also fulfills the promise of the original version in providing solid practical and rigorous theoretical underpinnings, and relevant challenging homework questions. Topics like parallel imaging via RF receive coils arrays and numerous other technical insights highlight the additions. The challenge, of course, is how to keep a 'classic' a classic in such a dynamic and rapidly evolving field as MR imaging. As with the early versions, I tip my hat to the authors for their selection of topics and also their patience in allowing 'hot' fields to reach an appropriate level of sustainability and impact before inclusion here.

On behalf of others like me, who grew up (and continue) using 'the green bible,' I want to extend my congratulations and thanks to the authors for this new edition. I anxiously await not only the next generation of discoveries it facilitates but also the next generation of scientists it supports. Well done!

Jeffrey L. Duerk, Ph.D.
Dean, Case Western Reserve University School of Engineering
Leonard Case Professor
Professor, Biomedical Engineering & Radiology
Case Western Reserve University
Cleveland, OH

June 11, 2013

Hiroyuki Fujita

Studying the second edition of this textbook on MRI physics has connected marvelous memories: my beginning graduate school experience, many early and long-lasting friendships, internships and major responsibilities with leading OEMs, returning to direct physics research at my alma mater, and then incubating and growing an MRI manufacturing company, Quality Electrodynamics. QED's success has led to such recognitions as a Presidential and First Lady's guest of honor at the 2012 State of the Union Address and a 2013 Presidential Award for Export. From my own education to the training of my team to the business awards, this big green book started and buttressed it all.

I can echo Professor Jeff Duerk's words about his start in MRI because I too began by enrolling in PHYS 431, but a decade later. By the 1990s, this 'Physics of Imaging' had become a standard CWRU course for a graduate imaging track in both the physics and the biomedical engineering departments. The notes from this course became the primary teaching tool in MRI, which I refer to here as the big green book. Professor Mark Haacke introduced me to MR imaging before he left Case Western Reserve University to start his own company and research institute. Immediately after this, I began my Ph.D. with Professor Robert Brown in hardware design, a key move in view of QED's rf coil products. Thus began a series of prideful career-long collaborations with Professor Brown that continues to this day.

The big green book provided a foundation for all the CWRU graduate students I knew in MRI. My good friends, Mike Thompson and Norman Cheng, have been promoted from beginning students to achieving co-authorship. Like myself, they studied the course material, and went on to be teaching assistants, lecturers, and faculty. We could see the influence of the venerable physics textbooks such as Jackson's *Classical Electrodynamics* (which influenced the QED name as well!) and Kittel's just-in-time *Thermal Physics* homework. It is satisfying to notice how the 'critical thinking' goals that are so much in the current educational news — connecting new work to old, applying theory to practice, taking a first step even if the second is not yet clear, finding alternatives if one path fails, looking at whether a solution makes sense, and learning to collaborate — are strongly reflected in this textbook's many problems and the lead-up to them. I am currently serving on the U.S. Manufacturing Council committee tasked with advising the Secretary of Commerce. Science education is recognized as having ever-increasing significance when discussing national policies necessary to improve the current and future workforce in America. I feel that the big green book is emblematic as a key tool in connecting physics and math to imaging science, biology, and chemistry, and preparing the student for an important high-tech career. This is a real teaching tool well received by many generations of CWRU students.

The rf material added in the second edition, especially in the new Chapter 28 on parallel imaging, is really welcome. Over the past decade, my industrial colleagues and I have constantly referenced this textbook and its chapters on signal-to-noise and contrast analysis, sequence parameters, and especially rf software and hardware topics. The green book is evident on many shelves of our company and, wherever we visit, we often observe that it is so beat-up a new edition is really needed. It is not just the expanded rf treatment that will stimulate folks to replace their (dilapidated) first editions.

As the writer of a foreword in this new edition, I perhaps have the responsibility to revisit the original words by Professor Felix Wehrli to report on what has been added. The book continues to be most appropriate for the physics and engineering graduate and advanced undergraduate classes, with the first two years of math and science in typical technical university curricula as sufficient prerequisites. On the face of it, this second edition is not changed terribly much, with one chapter added to the original twenty-seven. Besides new material in Chapters 17 and 28, however, there seem to be countless improvements found throughout the text and, particularly, the problems. With the new material taking us to a 1000-page book, the authors can be forgiven the omission of some topics such as diffusion tensor weighted imaging. I do know in practice they tend to emphasize hardware better by teaching the material in Chapter 27 earlier in the semester, and I suggest other instructors adopting this text do the same. In my world one can understand why I believe this is a very good suggestion.

Professor Wehrli spoke of 'exceptional didactic skill' and predicted '*Magnetic Resonance Imaging: Physical Principles and Sequence Design* is likely to become the daily companion of the MRI scientist and a reference standard for years to come.' I believe his prediction came true. Over the past decade, the book has exceeded 5,000 printed copies and been cited thousands of times, more than those from a number of standard physics textbooks. Its sales have stayed constant right up to the present time. I expect that the new edition will, in the words of Professor Duerk, keep this classic a classic in the coming decade. With my close connections to the authors, customers and contacts in industry and academia often ask me if I know anything about any new edition. After 14 years, I'm thrilled to tell them the second edition is finally here!

Hiroyuki Fujita, Ph.D.
Quality Electrodynamics LLC
Mayfield Village, OH

June 28, 2013

Foreword to the First Edition

Jeffrey L. Duerk

I heard my first lecture on an emerging field in medical imaging known as Nuclear Magnetic Resonance Imaging in 1983 as an electrical engineering graduate student at The Ohio State University. I was captivated and soon moved to Cleveland, a city then considered by many to be a United States center for the development of MR imaging and where both Picker International and Technicare were located a few miles apart. After studying many manuscripts, books and 'primers,' I enrolled in a new Physics and Biomedical Engineering course at Case Western Reserve University denoted by PHYS/EBME 431: The Physics of Medical Imaging, taught by Prof. E. Mark Haacke. In large part, the present book has grown and evolved from the class notes and lectures from this course's offering over the years.

The power of Magnetic Resonance Imaging (MRI) in the diagnostic arena of patient care is unquestionable. A multitude of books exist to assist in the training/teaching of clinicians responsible for interpreting MR images. Since joining the faculty of Case Western Reserve University almost a decade ago, I have been asked by graduate students, new industry hires, and fellow professors (from both CWRU and institutions throughout the world), if there was a book I could recommend which would provide sufficient depth in physics and MR imaging principles to serve as either a textbook or a complete tutorial for basic scientists. In my opinion, there were none which could provide the basic scientist with the tools to understand well the physics of MRI and also understand the engineering challenges necessary to develop the actual acquisitions (known as pulse sequences) which ultimately lead to the images. While there were no single sources available, I implored all to be patient. Today, I believe that patience has been rewarded as the book has arrived.

While much has changed in the field since my introduction to it in the early 1980's (e.g., the 'N' in NMR Imaging and the company Technicare are both gone), the power of this book is that many central concepts in MRI are rather more permanent, and their coverage here is superb. The influence by such notable predecessors as Abragam, Slichter, and Ernst is, at times, unmistakable. Mostly, the personal descriptive and analytical teaching style of Drs. Haacke, Brown, Thompson and Venkatesan builds an understanding of new concepts while clarifying old ones from the solid foundation provided earlier in the text. Another particular advantage of this book is that the notation is consistent, and located in a single reference; the readers do not have to overcome notational differences among our predecessors or difficulties in separating fundamental concepts from advanced material. Importantly, virtually every homework problem in the text has been designed to emphasize a central concept crucial to MRI. When I page through the book, I am often able to find the same derivations in the homework questions as in my log-books from the early part of my career in MRI. Insights from the authors are present throughout the text as well as within the problems; they provide those less experienced with glimpses (which later become illuminating flashes (no pun intended)) into how MR physics and sequences work and how they can be taken advantage of in the application to new ideas.

While I have been a co-instructor for EBME/PHYS 431 for a number of years and have used drafts of this book as the textbook, by now it bears little resemblance to the class notes of the initial offering in 1985. For that matter, the field of MRI has exploded with new techniques, new applications and far greater understanding and analysis of the innumerable aspects of the MRI hardware and software on image quality. I have benefited from my long friendships with Drs. Haacke and Brown, and the more recent ones with Drs. Thompson and Venkatesan. If you were to walk into the CWRU MRI Laboratory today, you would find no less than five drafts of this book on the shelves. The greatest tribute to these authors in their efforts to compile an important comprehensive treatise on the physics of MRI and MR sequence design can be heard in our research group's discussions of new imaging techniques (and likely those in the future at other institutions world-wide) when someone beckons 'Grab 'Haacke and Brown'!'

Jeffrey L. Duerk, Ph.D.
Director, Physics Research
Associate Professor-Departments of Radiology and Biomedical Engineering
Case Western Reserve University
Cleveland, OH

January 20, 1999

Felix W. Wehrli

Haacke et al.'s new book spans a significant portion of proton MRI concerned with the design of MRI pulse sequences and image phenomenology. The work, designed for the physicist and engineer, is organized in twenty-seven chapters. The first eight chapters deal with the fundamentals of nuclear magnetic resonance, most of which is based on the classical Bloch formalism, except for a two chapter excursion into quantum mechanics. This portion of the book covers the basic NMR phenomena, and the concepts of signal detection and data acquisition. Chapters 9 and 10 introduce the spatial encoding principles, beginning with one-dimensional Fourier imaging and its logical extension to a second and third spatial dimension. Chapter 11 treats continuous and discrete Fourier transforms, followed in Chapters 12 and 13 by sampling principles, filtering and a discussion of resolution. Chapter 14 may be regarded as the opening section of the book's second part exploring more advanced concepts, beginning with treatment of non-Cartesian imaging and reconstruction. In Chapter 15, the properties of signal-to-noise are dealt with in detail including a discussion of the important scaling laws, followed, in Chapter 16 by a return to a more advanced treatment of rf pulses, along with such concepts as spatially varying rf excitation and spin-tagging. Chapter 17 is dedicated to the various currently practiced methods for water-fat separation, and in Chapters 18 and 19, the authors delve into the ever-growing area of fast imaging techniques. Chapter 18 is entirely dedicated to steady-state gradient-echo imaging methods to which the authors have themselves contributed a great deal since the inception of whole-body MRI. Chapters 19 and 20 address echo train methods focusing on EPI, T_2^* dephasing effects and the resulting artifacts, ranging from intravoxel phase dispersion to spatial distortion. Chapter 21 is a brief introduction to the physics underlying diffusion-weighted imaging and pertinent measurement techniques. Chapter 22 treats the quantification of the fundamental intrinsic parameters, spin density, T_1 and T_2. Chapters 23 and 24 deal with the manifestions of motion and flow in terms of the resulting artifacts and their remedies, followed by a broad coverage of the major angiographic and flow quantification methods. The topic of Chapter 25 is induced magnetism and its various manifestations, including a discussion of its most significant application — brain functional MRI exploiting the BOLD phenomenon. In Chapter 26, the authors return to pulse sequence design, reviewing the design criteria for the most important pulse sequences and discussing potential artifacts. The final Chapter 27, at last, discusses hardware in terms of magnets, rf coils and gradients.

This book is the result of a monumental five-year effort by Dr. Haacke and his coauthors to generate a high-level, comprehensive graduate and post-graduate level didactic text on the physics and engineering aspects of MRI. The work clearly targets the methodology of bulk proton imaging, deliberately ignoring chemical shift resolved imaging or treatment of biophysical aspects such as the mechanisms of relaxation in tissues. Understanding the book requires college-level vector calculus. However, many of the basic tools, such as Fourier transforms and the fundamentals of electromagnetism, are elaborated upon either in dedicated chapters or appendices. The problems interspersed in the text of all chapters are a major asset and will be appreciated by student and teacher alike.

There is no doubt that the authors have succeeded in their effort to create a textbook that finally fills a need which has persisted for years. Haacke et al.'s book is, in the reviewer's assessment, the most authoritative new text on the subject, likely to become an essential tool for anyone actively working on MRI data acquisition and reconstruction techniques, but also for those with a desire to understand MR at a more than superficial level. The work is a rare synthesis of the authors' grasp of the subject, and their extensive practical experience, which they share with the reader through exceptional didactic skill.

The book has few flaws worth mention at all. First, not all chapters provide equal coverage of a targeted topic in that the book often emphasizes areas in which the authors have excelled themselves and thus are particularly experienced. Such a personal slant, of course, is very much in the nature of a treatise written by a single group of authors. On the other hand, the coherence in terms of depth of treatment, quality of illustrations and style, offered here, is never achievable with edited books. A case in point of author-weighted subject treatment is fast imaging, which is heavy on steady-state imaging. The following chapter on echo-train imaging almost exclusively deals with EPI and only secondarily with RARE and its various embodiments. Likewise, diffusion is treated only at its most fundamental level with little mention of anisotropic or restricted diffusion, or diffusion tensor imaging. Though the suggested reading list is helpful, a division into historic articles and those more easily accessible to the student would have been helpful since many of the historic papers cited would have to be retrieved from the library's storage rooms provided they are available at all. Finally, an introduction to the imaging hardware earlier (rather than as the last chapter) would help the novice bridging the gap between theory and instrumentation. None of the above, however, should detract from the book's high quality and practical usefulness.

In summary, the authors need to be congratulated on a superb product; a text vital to those concerned with MRI at a rigorous level. *Magnetic Resonance Imaging: Physical Principles and Sequence Design* is likely to become the daily companion of the MRI scientist and a reference standard for years to come.

Felix W. Wehrli, Ph.D.
Professor of Radiologic Science and Biophysics
Editor-in-Chief, *Magnetic Resonance in Medicine*

February 9, 1999

This book is dedicated to our parents:

William James Brown
Florence Elizabeth Brown

Shih-Tai Cheng
Tuan-Yu Cheng

Helena Doris Haacke
Ewart Mortimer Haacke

Robert Thompson
Mary Christina Thompson

Ramasubramaniam Venkatesan
Saroja Venkatesan

Preface to the Second Edition

In the second edition of this book, we have made more improvements and corrections in texts, equations, and homework problems than we can count, enhanced some chapters with new material, added a sizable new chapter, and updated a number of figures in various chapters. In particular, this includes a proof of the equal numbers in discrete Fourier transform pairs in Sec. 12.2.4, the correct interpretation of the T_2^* filter effect on resolution in Sec. 13.5, revised materials throughout Ch. 16, new material on off-resonance excitation principles in Sec. 17.2.2, optimizing contrast in short-T_R steady-state incoherent imaging in Sec. 18.1.2, a special discussion relating the 2D DFT with a 1D DFT as originally proposed by Professor Peter Mansfield in the 1970s in Sec. 19.9, a rigorous derivation of reducing a 3D dataset to 2D in Sec. 20.3.5, and an introduction to parallel imaging in Ch. 28.

Over the past decade, we indeed followed up our statement of motivation made in the preface to the first edition by teaching hundreds of graduate students and advanced undergraduate students at our home universities. We are aware of many other classes at other universities where the first edition of this book played an important role. MRI education continues to be our primary goal, but we have been gratified by the book's value as a research reference. Limitations remain and, alas, important topics are still missing. There are certain other MRI books that have since appeared and to which we enthusiastically refer the interested reader; we have added them to our suggested readings. To address missing topics, newly emerging topics, and amendments and corrections to the second edition, we have set up a website for students, teachers, and researchers. We are posting the many exam problems and optional homework examples developed in our years of teaching and we offer contacts with lecturers to compare solutions. However, students should try to solve these problems by themselves!

Preface to the First Edition

The principal motivation for this book is to create a self-contained text that could be used to teach the basics of magnetic resonance imaging to both graduate students and advanced undergraduate students. Although this is not a complete research treatise on MRI, it may also serve as a useful reference text for those experienced in the field. Time and page limitations have made it impossible to include detailed discussions of exchange processes, rf penetration, k-t space, perfusion, and parametric reconstruction methods, to name a few important topics omitted. MR simulations, interactive MRI, and distance learning are other important issues that may be addressed in an expanded web-based companion volume in the future. We hope that the present text is a useful complement to the many technical details available on coil concepts in the MR technology book by Chen and Hoult and on diffusion in the microscopic imaging book by Callaghan.

To varying degrees, the chapters contain discussions of the technical details, homework problems, sequence concepts, and the resulting images. Key points are often highlighted by italicized text and single quotation marks usually signify the introduction of MR nomenclature or stylized language. Representative references appear at the end of each chapter, but only general review or introductory articles, or selected papers with which we are especially familiar, are referenced. It is beyond the scope of this book to make any attempt to present a complete bibliography.

The first fifteen chapters of the text are introductory in nature and could perhaps serve as a one-semester course. After the brief preview given in chapter one, they wend their way from the basic dynamics of nuclear magnetic moments, to the concepts of imaging, and later to the effects of reconstruction type, contrast and noise. The next eleven chapters represent the bulk of the imaging applications addressed; they could either be covered in a second semester or the basic concepts of each could be interspersed with those of the earlier chapters comprising a faster paced single-semester course (which has been our tendency). The eleven chapters begin with brief excursions into the areas of rf pulse design and chemical shift imaging, and are followed by detailed discussions on fast imaging, magnetic field inhomogeneity effects, motion, flow, diffusion, sequence design and artifacts. A unified discussion of the rf, gradient and main magnet coils is contained in the last chapter. Alternatively, we do find appealing the assimilation of coil hardware issues with material in earlier chapters where appropriate. The appendices contain review material for basic electromagnetism and statistics as well as a list of acquisition parameters for the images in the book.

Acknowledgments

In the second edition of this book, we add to the previous acknowledgment by showing our appreciation to the following people. For the new material in Ch. 17 on off-resonance excitation principles, we thank Yongquan Ye; for the new material in Ch. 18 on optimizing contrast in short-T_R steady-state incoherent imaging, we thank Jaladhar Neelavalli; for the efficient 1D analogue to the 2D DFT as applied to echo planar imaging in Ch. 19 we thank Yingbiao Xu; for general help with the book, we thank Prithvi Gopinath and Yashwanth Katkuri; for detailed help with Ch. 28 on parallel imaging, we thank Charles Poole, Yong Wu, and Zhen Yao; and for the replacement figures, we thank Saifeng Liu. Finally, we note Tim Eagan's contributions from his years as a lecturer in our course and Mark Griswold for his encouragement and discussions, and we acknowledge former and present students who gave us recent feedback: Tanvir Baig, Lisa Bauer, Xin Chen, Tesfaye Kidane, Xingxian Shou, and Victor Taracila.

Acknowledgments to the First Edition

Much like all major technologies, the development of magnetic resonance imaging has been a step-by-step process, building over many years on the ideas and experience of innumerable researchers in the field. The development of this book has itself been based not only on many years of our teaching magnetic resonance imaging (we are well into our second decade), but also on the efforts of numerous colleagues and collaborators, both faculty and students. Sometimes, a particular discussion or imaging result or insight has been directly due to the efforts of a single M.S. or Ph.D. student. To all those who have directly or indirectly contributed, we are indebted. Specifically, we thank the following people for reading different parts of the text and reviewing specific chapters: Gabriele Beck, Andreas Brenner, James Brookeman, Mark Conradi, Lawrence Crooks, Thomas Dixon, Jeff Duerk, Jens Frahm, Gary Glover, Jürgen Hennig, Christopher Hess, Steve Izen, Permi Jhooti, Stephan Kannengeiser, Peter Kingsley, Uwe Klose, Zhi-Pei Liang, Michal Lijowski, Robert Ogg, John Pauly, Jean Tkach, Yi Wang, Felix Wehrli, Robert Weiskoff, Eric Wong and Ian Young. We also owe our gratitude to the following people for assisting in either the collection or processing of the data for images shown in the text: Azim Celik, Xiaoping Ding, Karthikeyan Kuppusamy, Debiao Li, Weili Lin, Yi Wang and Yingjian Yu. Special thanks are also due to Peter Kingsley for reading many of the early versions of numerous chapters, to Marinus T. Vlaardingerbroek and Jacques den Boer for incorporating some of the nomenclature into their own book on MRI, and particularly to Norman Cheng for his participation in the entire process of scrutinizing the text, solving problems, and facilitating the final editing of the book. The following students and fellow researchers need special mention for their feedback and corrections on several specific aspects of different chapters: Hongyu An, Markus Barth, Hiro Fujita, Pilar Herrero, Frank Hoogenraad, Renate Jerecic, Shantanu Kaushikkar, Weigi Kong, Song Lai, Jingzhi Liu, Jürgen Reichenbach, Jacob Willig, Yingbiao Xu and Anne Marie Yunker. Finally, our thanks to Jan Lindley for her secretarial support during the last two years of this project.

During our own tenure in this field, we have personally benefited from our involvement with both Siemens Medical Systems (Erlangen, Germany) and Picker International (Cleveland, Ohio). Many of the imaging methods have been developed thanks to a collaborative agreement with Siemens. All images presented in this text were acquired with a 1.5 T Siemens VISION scanner. We would like to thank the following people in Siemens for their support over the years: Richard Hausmann, Randall Kroeker, Gerhard Laub, Gerald Lenz, Wilfried Loeffler, Hermann Requardt, Erich Reinhardt and Franz Schmitt. We would also like to thank Gordon DeMeester, Surya Mohapatra, Michael Morich and John Patrick at Picker for longstanding support and collaboration.

Although we have played the role of teacher in giving this course, we have benefited from the entire educational experience of preparing this book. We are grateful to the many students and colleagues who have taught us in this process over and above those mentioned so far. These include: Michael Martens, Todd Parrish, Cynthia Paschal, Labros Petropoulos, Shmaryu Shvartsman, Jean Tkach, Piotr Wielopolski and Fredy Zypman.

The mistakes that remain are, of course, our responsibility alone. For these errors, we apologize in advance. We invite you to share your thoughts and to provide suggestions for improvements in the text. In this way, we can establish an updated list of corrections and additions, taking full advantage of the exciting new manner in which educational issues, open problems, and databases in MRI may now be addressed via the internet.

On a more personal note, we are most happy to finally have this chance to thank our families and friends who have supported and sustained the writing efforts over the last five years. Their patience and encouragement were crucial to the book's completion.

Chapter 1

Magnetic Resonance Imaging: A Preview

Chapter Contents

Introduction

The primary purpose of this chapter is to provide a succinct overview of the basic principles involved in the process of using nuclear magnetic resonance for imaging. This overview is in the form of a list of results, without derivation, in order to provide a story line and goals for the reader to follow in the detailed treatment of this material in the coming chapters.

The chapter begins with an explanation of the name, 'magnetic resonance imaging,' or MRI, followed by a short and inadequate history[1] of some of the developments that led to the discovery of key imaging concepts. The third, and largest, section is a preview of the subsequent twenty-seven chapters. Finally, some relevant reference texts and articles are listed in the Suggested Reading at the end of the chapter.

1.1 Magnetic Resonance Imaging: The Name

Magnetic resonance imaging is a relatively new discipline in the realm of applied sciences. A main thrust has come from the imaging of soft tissues in the human body and metabolic processes therein, such that it occupies a strong position in biomedical science applications.

---

[1] A great deal of the history of nuclear magnetic resonance and MRI is presented in volume one of the *Encyclopedia of Nuclear Magnetic Resonance*, which is listed in the historical/review references.

MRI is a powerful imaging modality because of its flexibility and sensitivity to a broad range of tissue properties. One of the original reasons for the excitement about MRI was, and continues to be, its relative safety, where the 'noninvasive' nature of the magnetic fields employed makes it possible to diagnose conditions of people of almost any age. Today MRI also offers great promise in understanding much more about the human body, both its form and its function.

MRI stems from the application of nuclear magnetic resonance (NMR) to radiological imaging. The adjective 'magnetic' refers to the use of an assortment of magnetic fields and 'resonance' refers to the need to match the (radio)frequency of an oscillating magnetic field to the 'precessional' frequency of the spin of some nucleus (hence the 'nuclear') in a tissue molecule. It might be more accurate to refer to this field as NMRI rather than MRI, but there is widespread concern over any phrase containing the word 'nuclear.' Although the nuclear component simply refers to a benign role of the 'spin' of the nucleus in the process, the word has been suppressed and the public and the profession have embraced the MRI acronym.

1.2   The Origin of Magnetic Resonance Imaging

To describe the history of any technological advance in a given field is a very difficult and sensitive issue; to offer a brief and incomplete account is fraught with peril. Still, the beginning student may be aided and inspired by even a short historical discussion. It may be said that MRI had its beginnings in 1973 with the seminal papers by Lauterbur and Mansfield. It was already well known that the intrinsic angular momentum (or 'spin') of a hydrogen nucleus (the proton) in a magnetic field precesses about that field at the 'Larmor frequency' which, in turn, depends linearly on the magnitude of the field itself. Their idea was very simple. If a spatially varying magnetic field is introduced across the object, the Larmor frequencies are also spatially varying. They proposed and showed that the different frequency components of the signal could be separated to give spatial information about the object. This key point of spatially encoding the data opened the door to MR imaging. Others also recognized the importance of this area, with early attention brought to tumor detection by Damadian.

Something may be learned here by the beginning student. Often the basic step toward new developments, which may become quite complicated as a whole, is a simple connecting idea. The concept of using a magnetic field gradient was one such 'aha' that captured the essence of MRI as it is practiced today, much like the coupling of the nuclear spin of the proton to the magnetic field was the key to the early experiments by both Bloch's group and Purcell's group in their pioneering work in NMR.

The concept of nuclear magnetic resonance had its underpinnings with the discovery of the spin nature of the proton. Leaning on the work of Stern and Gerlach from the early 1920's, Rabi and coworkers pursued the spin of the proton and its interaction with a magnetic field in the 1930's. With this foundation in hand in 1946, Bloch and Purcell extended these early quantum mechanical concepts to a measurement of an effect of the precession of the spins around a magnetic field. Not only did these gentlemen successfully measure a precessional signal from a water sample and a paraffin sample, respectively, but they explained precociously many of the experimental and theoretical details that we continue to draw from still today. For this work, they shared the Nobel prize in physics in 1952.

1.3 A Brief Overview of MRI Concepts

In this section, we attempt to introduce and list for the reader the basic elements that make MRI possible. The derivations, explanations and related details of these results are covered principally in Chs. 2–15. Although the later chapters, Chs. 16–28, are focused on advanced applications and concepts, additional related results are presented there as well.

1.3.1 Fundamental Interaction of a Proton Spin with the Magnetic Field

We have alluded to the idea that MRI is based on the interaction of a nuclear spin with an external magnetic field, $\vec{B}_0$. The dominant nucleus in MRI is the proton in hydrogen and its interaction with the external field results in the precession of the proton spin about the field direction (see Fig. 1.1). Imaging of humans rests on the ability to manipulate, with a combination of magnetic fields, and then detect, the bulk precession of the hydrogen spins in water, fat and other organic molecules.

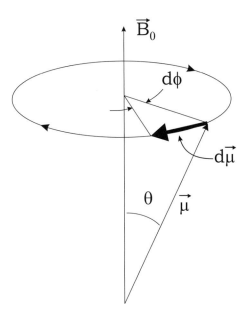

Fig. 1.1: By definition, precession is the circular motion of the axis of rotation of a spinning body about another fixed axis caused by the application of a torque in the direction of the precession. The interaction of the proton's spin with the magnetic field produces the torque, causing it to precess about $\vec{B}_0$ as the fixed axis. When looking down from above the vector $\vec{B}_0$, the precession of the magnetic moment vector $\vec{\mu}$, which is proportional to the spin vector, is clockwise. For the customary counterclockwise definition of polar angles, the differential $d\phi$ shown is negative.

The basic motion of the proton spin may be understood by imagining it as a spinning gyroscope that is also electrically charged. It thus possesses an effective loop of electric current around the same axis about which it is spinning. This effective current loop is capable of interacting with external magnetic fields as well as producing its own magnetic field. We describe the strength with which the loop interacts with an external field, as well as the strength with which the loop produces its own field, in terms of the same 'magnetic dipole moment' vector $\vec{\mu}$. The direction of this vector is nothing other than the spin axis itself and, like a compass needle, the magnetic moment vector will tend to align itself along any external static magnetic field, $\vec{B}_0$. This is like the initial tendency of a gyroscope to fall in the direction of gravity. However, the tendencies are complicated by the spin in exactly the same way as is the gyroscopic motion. Instead of 'falling' along the field direction, the magnetic moment vector, like the spinning gyroscope, will precess around the field direction. In Ch. 2, we find that the precession angular frequency for the proton magnetic moment vector (and for the spin axis as well) is given by

$$\omega_0 = \gamma B_0 \tag{1.1}$$

where γ is a constant called the gyromagnetic ratio. In water, the hydrogen proton has a γ value of roughly 2.68×10^8 rad/s/tesla (so that $\gamma\!\!\!/ \equiv \gamma/(2\pi)$ is 42.6 MHz/tesla). For a 2 T field, for example, the spins precess at a radiofrequency of 85.2 MHz, just below the FM range for radio broadcasting. (We use SI units throughout the text.) This precession frequency is referred to as the Larmor frequency and (1.1) is referred to as the Larmor equation.

1.3.2   Equilibrium Alignment of Spin

The magnetic moment vector for a typical proton is prevented from relaxing fully to an alignment along the external magnetic field because of thermal energy associated with the absolute temperature T. From the discussions in Chs. 5 and 6, we can compare the magnetic field interaction with the average thermal energy kT, where k is the Boltzmann's constant. At human body temperatures, the thermal energy is millions of times larger than the quantum energy difference for parallel alignment (lower energy) versus anti-parallel alignment (higher energy). For a proton with only two quantum spin states, these are the only two possible alignments. Significantly, the frequency in the quantum energy difference, $\hbar\omega_0$, is nothing other than the Larmor precession frequency (1.1) where $\hbar \equiv h/(2\pi)$ in terms of Planck's quantum constant h.

The extreme smallness of the quantum spin energy compared with the thermal energy means that the fraction $\hbar\omega_0/(kT) \ll 1$. In that case, the Boltzmann probability discussion in Ch. 6 demonstrates why the number of spins parallel to the magnetic field exceeding the number anti-parallel to that field, the 'spin excess,' is also very small. Specifically, the spin excess is suppressed by a factor involving that fraction:

$$\text{spin excess} \simeq N\frac{\hbar\omega_0}{2kT} \tag{1.2}$$

where N is the total number of spins present in the sample. In Prob. 1.1, it is found that the spin excess is only one in a million spins even for a magnetic field strength as large as 0.3 T.

Since the spin excess is millions of times smaller than the total number of proton spins, it might be guessed that no significant signal would be detected at room temperature. However, there are Avogadro numbers of protons in a few grams of tissue. Consider the average magnetic dipole density, or 'longitudinal equilibrium magnetization' M_0 for the component of the magnetic moment vector along the external field direction. For a sample with ρ_0 defined as the number of protons per unit volume (or the 'spin density'), the longitudinal equilibrium magnetization is found in Ch. 6 to be given by the proton magnetic moment component $\gamma\hbar/2$ multiplied by the relative spin excess (1.2) times the spin density. Noting (1.1), it is thus given by

$$M_0 \quad = \quad \frac{\rho_0\gamma^2\hbar^2}{4kT}B_0 \qquad (1.3)$$

This equilibrium value, while limited by the spin excess, leads to measurable NMR effects to be described next.

Problem 1.1

Using $\hbar = 1.05 \times 10^{-34}$ joule·s, $k = 1.38 \times 10^{-23}$ joule/K and $T = 300\,\text{K}$, find the spin excess as a fraction of N for protons at 0.3 tesla.

1.3.3 Detecting the Magnetization of the System

Even in a macroscopic body, a bulk nonvanishing spin excess is not enough to guarantee a detectable signal. In a classical picture (which is derived from the quantum underpinnings in Ch. 5), the magnetization vector (the magnetic moment vector density due to the spin population) must be tipped away from the external field direction in order to initiate precession. The magnetization corresponding to the aggregate proton spins will therefore produce a changing magnetic flux in any nearby 'receive' coil (Ch. 7) as it precesses around the external magnetic field. To accomplish this, as discussed in Chs. 3 and 4, the magnetization can be rotated away from its alignment along the B_0 axis (i.e., from its longitudinal direction) by applying a radiofrequency (rf) magnetic field for a short time (an rf 'pulse'). This rf pulse is produced from another nearby 'transmit' coil (which may be the same as the receive coil, provided its radiofrequency is tuned to the Larmor frequency; see Fig. 1.2). This is the resonance condition in MRI described earlier and it ensures that the precessing spin gets a continuously synchronized push (rotation) away from the longitudinal direction (the z-axis, say).

Suppose that $\vec{M}$ has been rotated by an rf pulse to a direction orthogonal to $\vec{B}_0 = B_0\hat{z}$. (The rf pulse that tips all the original longitudinal magnetization, or z-magnetization, through an angle of 90° into the transverse, or x-y, plane is called a $\pi/2$-pulse.) The resulting 'transverse magnetization' has magnitude M_0 and begins to precess clockwise in the x-y plane. Its rectangular components have sinusoidal time dependence with frequency given by the Larmor frequency. As defined in Ch. 4, the complex magnetization is

$$M_+(t) \equiv M_x(t) + iM_y(t) = M_0 e^{-i\omega_0 t + i\phi_0} \qquad (1.4)$$

in terms of the magnitude and the (polar angle) phase. This shows an important connection between the time-dependence of the complex phase and the rotation of the magnetization. *The phase angle gives the direction in the x-y plane of the two-dimensional transverse magnetization vector.* The initial phase ϕ_0 is determined by the choice of rotational axis for the initial rotation into the transverse plane. For the example in Fig. 1.2, $\phi_0 = \pi/2$.

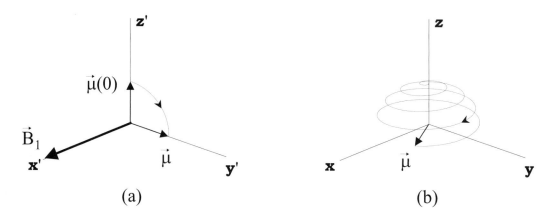

(a)   (b)

Fig. 1.2: Illustration from Ch. 3 of the effect of an rf pulse on an individual magnetic moment $\vec{\mu}$. (a) In a frame rotating about $\vec{B}_0$ (which is along $\hat{z}$, say) at the Larmor frequency (with coordinates x', y' and $z' = z$), there is no observed precession about $\vec{B}_0$. Upon application of an rf magnetic field pulse applied along $\hat{x}'$, the magnetic moment is rotated about $\hat{x}'$ at a rate corresponding to the frequency $\omega_1 = \gamma B_1$ determined by the amplitude of the rf field, B_1. A $\pi/2$ flip relative to its starting position along $\hat{z}'$ is achieved in a time τ_{rf} provided that $\omega_1 \tau_{rf} = \pi/2$. (b) The behavior of the same magnetic moment rotation is observed to be more complicated in the fixed laboratory frame. This picture has been constructed for the case $\omega_1 = 0.06\omega_0$. In actual MR applications, the frequency ω_1 would be much smaller in relation to ω_0, but then the spiraling would be too dense to illustrate.

The signal analyzed in Ch. 7 corresponds to the voltage induced in a receive coil from the time-varying magnetic flux that, in turn, is produced by a rotating magnetization. The inductive coupling of the receive coil to the magnetization may be described, according to a reciprocity principle, as equivalent to a constant flux, produced by a unit current flowing around the receive coil, that penetrates the precessing magnetization of the sample. The voltage, or electromotive force (*emf*), induced in the receive coil is given by

$$ emf = -\frac{d}{dt} \int d^3r \, \vec{M}(\vec{r}, t) \cdot \vec{\mathcal{B}}^{receive}(\vec{r}) \tag{1.5} $$

where $\vec{\mathcal{B}}^{receive}$ is the magnetic field produced by the receive coil per unit current. Ignoring any spatial variations and noting that the time derivative of the phase in the transverse magnetization (1.4) dominates the time derivative in (1.5), the *emf* is proportional to $\omega_0 M_0$. (In other words, the dominant time dependence is due to precession.) From (1.3) and (1.1), it follows that the signal from an MR experiment will depend on the square of the static magnetic field B_0

$$ \text{signal} \propto \frac{\gamma^3 B_0^2 \rho_0}{T} \tag{1.6} $$

The interest in higher fields stems from the growth of the signal with field strength; we return later in the preview to address the field dependence of the signal-to-noise ratio.

1.3.4 Magnetic Resonance Spectroscopy

Hydrogen protons in different molecules are immersed in slightly different magnetic environments, even in the presence of identical external magnetic fields. That is, different chemical compounds have slightly different local magnetic fields which means that the local Larmor frequency is 'chemically shifted' to different values $\omega_0(j)$ depending upon the molecular species type j. Chemical shift imaging is discussed in Chs. 8, 10, and 17.

Chemical shift imaging may be considered as adding another dimension, corresponding to the frequency range of different species. Each species will have its own contribution to the total signal. For instance, the transverse magnetization (1.4) gives a signal

$$\text{signal} \propto \sum_j M_0(j)\omega_0(j)e^{-i\omega_0(j)t+i\phi_0(j)} \tag{1.7}$$

Here, the time derivative of the phase in (1.4) again yielded the factors $\omega_0(j)$ in the leading terms.

The goal in magnetic field spectroscopy is to find the relative (spectral) amplitudes of the different frequency components, $M_0(j)$, in (1.7), whose spin densities $\rho_0(j)$ would enter via (1.3). This may be analyzed utilizing a Fourier transform to map the time domain back into a frequency domain. The goal in chemical shift imaging is the spatial disentangling of the signals of different tissue (spectral) components, such as water and fat.

1.3.5 Magnetic Resonance Imaging

The goal of imaging is to correlate a series of signal measurements with the spatial locations of the various sources. When all protons are represented by just one chemical species such as water, then the above spectroscopic analysis simply gives the total signal from all spins regardless of their spatial location in the static magnetic field, as long as that field is uniform. We now utilize the fact that the addition of a *spatially changing magnetic field across the sample produces a signal with spatially varying frequency components* according to

$$\omega(x) = \gamma B(x) \tag{1.8}$$

where x denotes the spatial coordinate along the direction of the gradient of the field. This means that the spectral components now represent spatial information and, in turn, leads to the possibility that the signal could be 'inverted' and the physical object could be reconstructed (Chs. 9 and 14) or 'imaged.'

The inversion of the signal is greatly facilitated through a connection to Fourier transforms (Chs. 9, 10, and 11). By constructing an additional coil (a linear gradient coil) that changes the original field $\vec{B}_0$ linearly in some direction, the phase in (1.4) becomes linear in the coordinates of that direction, so that the mapping back and forth between signal space and the image position space may be carried out with a Fourier transform. With more gradient coils, data reconstruction by inverse Fourier transformation can be carried in more spatial dimensions. Two- and three-dimensional 'imaging' in MRI is elegantly realized with this powerful mathematical tool (Ch. 10).

In particular, the application of a finite bandwidth rf excitation centered at the Larmor frequency of the combined static field plus a gradient field leads to the excitation of a layer, or slice, of spins orthogonal to that gradient with slice thickness TH, say (see Fig. 1.3). By employing different configurations of gradient coils, the choice of gradient direction is completely flexible, a powerful procedure allowing slices to be acquired in any orientation. No physical rotation of the sample is required.

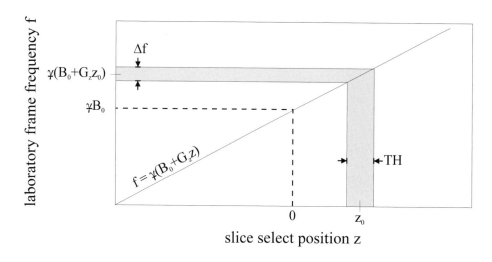

Fig. 1.3: The precession frequency $(f = \omega/(2\pi))$ in the laboratory frame is a function of position along the slice select axis. The original static field B_0 has been supplemented with a field with constant gradient G_z in the z-direction. The central frequency and spectral bandwidth of the rf pulse $(\Delta f \equiv BW_{rf}$, the shaded horizontal strip) are such that the slice of thickness $\Delta z \equiv TH$ (the shaded vertical strip) is uniformly 'excited' (i.e., all spins in the slice have the resonance condition satisfied). The fact that the slice is offset from the origin in the z-direction by z_0 implies that the center frequency of the rf pulse must be offset from the static Larmor frequency $f_0 = \gamma B_0$ by $\gamma G_z z_0$ as has been shown along the frequency axis.

1.3.6   Relaxation Times

An important factor in the strength of the signal has been omitted in the above discussions and must be considered. It is the 'spin-lattice' decay or relaxation of the signal due to the interactions of the spins with their surroundings. After the magnetization has been rotated into the transverse plane, it will tend to grow back along the direction of the static field $\vec{B}_0$, chosen here to be $\hat{z}$. This rate of regrowth can be characterized by a time constant T_1 called the longitudinal relaxation time and arises from the interaction between the spins and the atomic neighborhood. The magnetization time evolution is described by the solutions given in Ch. 4 for the famous Bloch equations which incorporate both relaxation and precession effects. For an initial situation where $M_z(0) = 0$ (for example, the condition achieved following the application of a $\pi/2$-pulse), the subsequent regrowth of M_z is given by

$$M_z(t) = M_0(1 - e^{-t/T_1}) \tag{1.9}$$

If the data are sampled following the application of another rf $\pi/2$-pulse at a time τ short compared to T_1, the longitudinal magnetization $M_z(\tau)$ is suppressed according to (1.9). Therefore, any transverse magnetization obtained by an rf rotation of $M_z(\tau)$ into the transverse plane will also be suppressed.

With the recognition of another relaxation effect, a more realistic assessment of the MRI signal may be achieved. The 'dephasing' of clusters of spins represents a 'spin-spin' decay of the transverse magnetization before data sampling can occur. Consider an experiment (Ch. 8) where a $\pi/2$ rf pulse is applied at interval time T_R where any previous transverse magnetization has decayed away due to the spin-spin effect and only the longitudinal magnetization corresponding to (1.9) remains to be rotated into the transverse plane. If the signal data are instantaneous sampled at a time T_E ('echo time,' see below for an explanation of this nomenclature) following the rf pulse, the signal is proportional to the magnitude of the transverse magnetization given by

$$M_\perp(T_E) = M_0(1 - e^{-T_R/T_1})e^{-T_E/T_2} \tag{1.10}$$

In (1.10), the term e^{-T_E/T_2} represents the spin-spin decay factor characterized by the time constant T_2; it is caused by a loss of coherence between different spins (this is more commonly referred to as dephasing of spins). Their phases disperse due to variations in the local precessional frequencies.

In general, signals would suffer additional suppression due to dephasing from external field inhomogeneities (T_2 would be replaced by a smaller relaxation time $T_2^* < T_2$). But a 'rephasing' or 'echoing' of this source of dispersion has been assumed in (1.10) such that the additional suppression has been avoided. This can be achieved by an additional rf pulse application, where the basic idea is to flip all the spins 180° in the transverse plane. The dephasing is reversed and the refocusing of any external field dispersion occurs at the echo time T_E.

The three tissue parameters (the spin density and the two relaxation times, T_1 and T_2) play principal roles throughout the book. Their specific measurements using MR techniques are the subject of Ch. 22.

1.3.7 Resolution and Contrast

An interesting aspect of MRI is the fact that resolution (the size of the spatial features that can be distinguished) does not depend upon the wavelength of the input rf field. Radio-frequencies generally have wavelengths on the order of meters, yet resolution in an MR image is on the order of millimeters. In fact, the inherent resolution in MR is a function of the way the signal and noise are sampled and filtered (see Chs. 12, 13, and 15) and it is ultimately limited only by the diffusion (Ch. 21) of the protons through the tissue and the local magnetic field nonuniformities around the proton.

The success of MRI goes beyond resolution and is understood by recognizing its large number of useful variables. MRI can be used to differentiate between materials because of its sensitivity to proton densities, relaxation times, temperature, proton motion, the chemical shift in the Larmor frequencies, and tissue heterogeneity, as examples. This large set of variables permits images to be generated with different levels of contrast based upon the desired usage. Therefore, MRI is more versatile than those imaging techniques restricted to only one type of contrast.

Contrast-to-noise and contrast mechanisms are first described in Ch. 15 but important aspects of image contrast already can be understood from (1.10). Examining the behavior of the exponentials, we see that for long T_R (relative to T_1) and short T_E (relative to T_2), the image will be sensitive only to the tissue spin density (Fig. 1.4a). For $T_E \simeq T_2$ and long T_R, the image is weighted by both spin density and T_2 (Fig. 1.4b) and the contrast between tissues with different T_2 is enhanced. Often the spin density-weighted images and T_2-weighted images exhibit similar contrast features, the latter enhancing the former. Lastly, for $T_R \leq T_1$, and short T_E, the image is weighted by both spin density and T_1 (Fig. 1.4c).

1.3.8   Magnetic Field Strength

The interest in higher fields stems from the fact that the signal-to-noise ratio (SNR is the subject of Ch. 15) increases with field strength. While machines providing lower fields (less than 0.5 T) are less expensive, they produce lower SNR, as compared to mid fields (0.5 T to 1.0 T) and high fields (higher than 1.0 T). The signal (1.6) exhibits quadratic growth with B_0 but this is partially offset by the fact that the noise has linear B_0 dependence at high fields. In the range from 0.5 T to 7.0 T,[2] the implied linear growth of SNR with field strength has been experimentally validated in human experiments.

There also has been concern about rf heating and nonuniform rf fields, where wavelengths finally play a role, as higher fields are considered. (Table 1.1 shows a comparison of free-space wavelengths for the different frequency ranges of familiar electromagnetic wave categories.) However, we have noted that the field strength of 1.0 T corresponds to 42.6 MHz, and this implies a rather long seven-meter free-space wavelength for imaging protons. Hence the rf field wavelengths for higher magnetic fields fall below 1 m only above 7.0 T. On the other hand, in humans, the relative electrical permittivity ϵ_r is about 50 near 1 T to 2 T, and the interior wavelengths are therefore reduced by a factor of $1/\sqrt{\epsilon_r}$ inside the body. This reduces the effective wavelength to about 1 m at 1 T for *in vivo* imaging and rf field nonuniformity must be considered at higher B_0 values.

More detailed rf pulse considerations are the subject of Ch. 16. The design issues for the coils producing the static field, the gradient fields and the rf fields are discussed in Ch. 27.

Problem 1.2

Find the frequency and free-space wavelength associated with the rf field required for proton magnetic resonance at each of the different B_0 values of a) 0.04 T, b) 0.2 T, c) 1.5 T, and d) 8 T.

---

[2]There are 9.4 T and 11 T units now in operation, but only limited data are available pertaining to this issue.

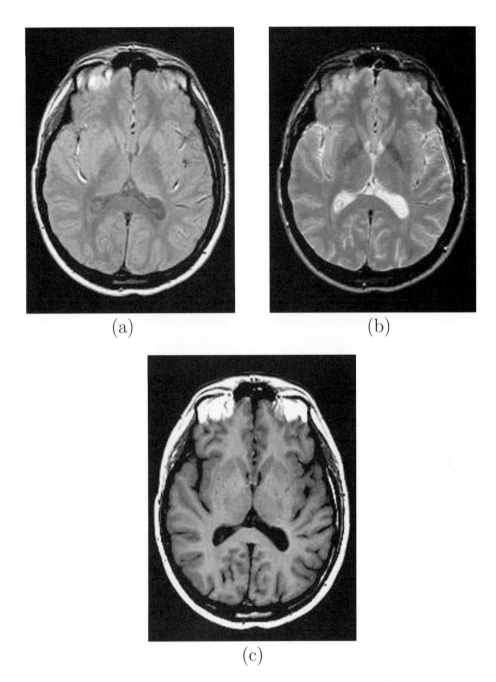

Fig. 1.4: Images of the human head with different forms of contrast: (a) a spin density-weighted image, (b) a T_2-weighted image, and (c) a T_1-weighted image. These different acquisitions can be seen to create different contrasts between white matter, gray matter, and cerebrospinal fluid. They all reveal excellent anatomic detail.

Category	Subcategory	Frequency (MHz)	Field strength (T)	Wavelength (m)
radio waves	LF (long wave)	0.03–0.3	7×10^{-4}–7×10^{-3}	10^4–10^3
	MF (medium wave)	0.3–3	7×10^{-3}–0.07	10^3–10^2
	AM radio (MF)	0.52–1.71	0.012–0.04	577–175
	HF (short wave)	3–30	0.07–0.7	10^2–10
	VHF	30–300	0.7–7	10–1
	FM radio (VHF)	87.5–108	2.05–2.54	3.43–2.78
	UHF	300–3×10^3	7–70	1–0.1
	SHF	3×10^3–3×10^4	70–700	0.1–0.01
microwaves		10^4–3×10^5	235–7×10^3	0.03–10^{-3}

Table 1.1: Range of radio and microwave frequencies from Wikipedia® at en.wikipedia.org. Under the subcategory heading, the letter F refers to frequency. The letters L, M, H, V, U, and S in front of the letter F refer to low, medium, high, very, ultra, and super, respectively. Associated free-space wavelengths and NMR field strengths for protons are given here.

1.3.9   Key Developments in Magnetic Resonance

An important mechanism in MRI is the 'echoing' capability discussed earlier for the recovery of some of the signal lost to transverse relaxation. (We should also mention 'gradient echoes' where dephasing brought about by the external gradient field itself is countered by reversing the gradient direction during its application.) When Hahn formulated the 'spin echo' concept, it was through an application of multiple rf pulses. This concept made it possible to collect data in what would otherwise be considered poor experimental conditions (inhomogeneous magnetic fields) where little signal would remain. What he had found initially to be a spurious signal later became a workhorse in NMR and in clinical MRI where disease states are often clearly diagnosed in T_2-weighted images (see Fig. 1.4b).

In a somewhat related manner, what presents itself as an unexpected and even bothersome image inaccuracy, or an 'artifact,' may end up opening new doors and even a new direction of research. Two examples of this include MR angiography (the study of blood vessels using MRI) and MR brain functional imaging. The first example came about because of a thrust to eliminate flow and motional blurring. In so doing, early researchers came up with the concept of flow compensation. Eliminating the artifacts in this way led to the very pleasant surprise of enhanced images of blood vessels; thus began the subfield of MR angiography. The phenomena of blood flow and heart and lung motion and the methods for obtaining their images are detailed in Chs. 23 and 24.

The second example occurred when the loss of signal due to the magnetic susceptibility of a contrast agent was so large, it led to a dramatic loss of signal on its first pass through the brain. It was soon realized that veins also had a different susceptibility than the rest of the brain and, hence, veins could be recognized by their phase alone or the signal loss they caused at long echo times. When blood flow changes, so does the blood deoxyhemoglobin concentration and, therefore, the blood susceptibility and its effect on the signal also change. Evidently, blood flow changes occur when the brain activates, which, in turn, leads to signal changes. Today, we can measure these changes in a matter of seconds; i.e., in that sense, we can detect the brain function. This is the basis of MR brain functional imaging known as fMRI and has led to a major focus in the fields of neuroscience and neuroradiology. It is discussed in Ch. 25.

Besides artifacts, there were other reasons to improve the MR methodology. The original spin echo scans took a long time to acquire and could not offer dynamic imaging to study, for example, the beating heart. To speed up data acquisition, researchers took advantage of fast 'gradient echo' imaging methods, where no extra refocusing rf pulses are applied. The flexibility of these methods led to reductions of scan times from minutes to seconds (see Ch. 18) and to fewer flow artifacts. The 'echo planar' methods, which could acquire data in a fraction of a second (see Ch. 19), were developed around a train of gradient echoes following either a single rf pulse or a second refocusing spin echo acquisition. Further improvements in speed are possible today via 'parallel imaging,' a method based on the simultaneous use of multiple rf coils in order to replace a portion of the data acquired through changes in the gradient field (see Ch. 28). All of these methods have direct implications for high-resolution MR angiography and functional brain imaging as well as for cardiac MRI.

Irrespective of the method, inhomogeneities in the external magnetic field still lead to image distortion (see Ch. 20). These are less of a problem today because of improvements in main magnet design (see Ch. 27), but some inhomogeneity effects remain that are caused by eddy currents generated within the magnet structure and by the local fields in the body itself (see Ch. 25). These remnant effects are being addressed today with improved sequence designs (see Ch. 26) and better processing concepts.

We turn now to the details and the exposition of these and other key MRI concepts in the coming chapters. It is hoped that the discussions throughout this book will elucidate the brief remarks in this overview.

Suggested Reading

Certain references that offer a good background for this opening chapter are given next. More general references are listed later.

- F. Bloch. Nuclear induction. *Phys. Rev.*, 70: 460, 1946.

- R. Damadian. Tumor detection by nuclear magnetic resonance. *Science*, 171: 1151, 1971.

- W. Gerlach and O. Stern. Ueber die Richtungsquantelung im Magnetfeld. *Ann. Phys.*, 74: 673, 1924.

- E. L. Hahn. Spin echoes. *Phys. Rev.*, 80: 580, 1950.

- P. C. Lauterbur. Image formation by induced local interactions: Examples employing NMR. *Nature*, 242: 190, 1973.

- P. Mansfield and P. K. Grannell. NMR 'diffraction' in solids? *J. Phys. C: Solid State Phys.*, 6: L422, 1973.

- E. M. Purcell, H. C. Torrey and R. V. Pound. Resonance absorption by nuclear magnetic moments in a solid. *Phys. Rev.*, 69: 37, 1946.

- I. I. Rabi, J. R. Zacharias, S. Millman and P. Kusch. A new method of measuring nuclear magnetic moments. *Phys. Rev.*, 53: 318, 1938.

There are a number of texts and articles on magnetic resonance. We have grouped these according to (1) primary technical references, which contain a great deal of relevant information to this text, (2) secondary references, both technical and clinical which also contain much useful information, (3) tertiary references, which will broaden the reader's perspective on MR in general, and (4) some interesting review articles and texts to add overview and historical perspectives.

Primary Technical References

- A. Abragam. *The Principles of Nuclear Magnetism.* Clarendon Press, Oxford, 1983.

- M. A. Bernstein, K. F. King and X. J. Zhou. *Handbook of MRI Pulse Sequences.* Elsevier Academic Press, Burlington, 2004.

- P. T. Callaghan. *Principles of Nuclear Magnetic Resonance Microscopy.* Oxford, New York, 1991.

- C.-N. Chen and D. I. Hoult. *Biomedical Magnetic Resonance Technology.* Bristol, Philadelphia, 1989.

- E. Fukushima and S. B. W. Roeder. *Experimental Pulse NMR: A Nuts and Bolts Approach.* Westview Press, Boulder, 1993.

- P. Mansfield and P. G. Morris. *NMR Imaging in Biomedicine. Supplement 2, Advances in Magnetic Resonance.* Ed. J. S. Waugh, Academic Press, New York, 1982.

- P. G. Morris. *Nuclear Magnetic Resonance Imaging in Medicine and Biology.* Oxford, New York, 1986.

- A. M. Parikh. *Magnetic Resonance Imaging Techniques.* Elsevier, New York, 1992.

- M. T. Vlaardingerbroek and J. A. den Boer. *Magnetic Resonance Imaging: Theory and Practice.* Springer Verlag, 3rd ed., Berlin, 2010.

- Z. P. Liang and P. C. Lauterbur. *Principles of Magnetic Resonance Imaging: A Signal Processing Perspective.* IEEE Press, New York, 1999.

Secondary Technical and Clinical References

- E. R. Andrew. *Nuclear Magnetic Resonance.* Cambridge University Press, New York, 1955.

- M. A. Brown and R. C. Semelka. *MRI: Basic Principles and Applications.* Wiley-Blackwell, Hoboken, 2010.

- R. R. Edelman, J. R. Hesselink and M. B. Zlatkin. *MRI: Clinical Magnetic Resonance Imaging.* Saunders, 3rd ed., Philadelphia, 2005.

- D. G. Gadian. *Nuclear Magnetic Resonance and Its Applications to Living Systems.* Oxford, 2nd ed., New York, 1995.

- E. M. Haacke and J. R. Reichenbach (Eds.). *Susceptibility Weighted Imaging in MRI: Basic Concepts and Clinical Applications.* Wiley-Blackwell, Hoboken, 2011.

- R. H. Hashemi, W. G. Bradley and C. J. Lisanti. *MRI: The Basics.* Lippincott Williams & Wilkins, 3rd ed., Philadelphia, 2010.

- J. M. Jin. *Electromagnetic Analysis and Design in Magnetic Resonance Imaging.* CRC Press, Boca Raton, 1998.

- J. E. Potchen, E. M. Haacke, J. E. Siebert and A. Gottschalk. *Magnetic Resonance Angiography: Concepts & Applications.* Mosby, St. Louis, 1993.

- R. T. Schumacher. *Introduction to Magnetic Resonance.* W. A. Benjamin, Inc., New York, 1970.

- C. P. Slichter. *Principles of Magnetic Resonance.* Springer Verlag, 3rd ed., New York, 2010.

- D. D. Stark and W. G. Bradley, Jr. *Magnetic Resonance Imaging.* Mosby Year Book, 3rd ed., St. Louis, 1999.

- P. Tofts (Ed.). *Quantitative MRI of the Brain: Measuring Changes Caused by Disease.* John Wiley and Sons Ltd., Chichester, 2003.

- F. W. Wehrli. *Fast Scan Magnetic Resonance: Principles and Applications.* Raven Press, New York, 1990.

- C. Westbrook, C. K. Roth and J. Talbot. *MRI in Practice.* Wiley-Blackwell, Chichester, 2011.

Tertiary References

- A. Bax. *Two-Dimensional Nuclear Magnetic Resonance in Liquids.* Delft University Press, Delft, 1982.

- P. T. Beall, S. R. Amtey and S. R. Kasturi. *NMR Data Handbook for Biomedical Applications.* Pergamon Press, New York, 1984.

- J. D. de Certaines, W. M. M. J. Bovée and F. Podo (Eds.). *Magnetic Resonance Spectroscopy in Biology and Medicine: Functional and Pathological Tissue Characterization.* Pergamon Press, Oxford, 1992.

- R. R. Ernst, G. Bodenhausen and A. Wokaun. *Principles of Nuclear Magnetic Resonance in One and Two Dimensions.* Oxford, New York, 1987.

- M. H. Levitt. *Spin Dynamics: Basics of Nuclear Magnetic Resonance.* John Wiley and Sons Ltd., Chichester, 2008.

- W. W. Paudler. *Nuclear Magnetic Resonance: General Concepts and Applications.* Wiley, New York, 1987.

- C. P. Poole. *Theory of Magnetic Resonance.* Wiley, New York, 1987.

- N. Salibi and M. A. Brown. *Clinical MR Spectroscopy: First Principles.* Wiley-Liss, New York, 1998.

Historical/Review References

- D. M. S. Bagguley (Ed.). *Pulsed Magnetic Resonance: NMR, ESR, and Optics: A Recognition of E. L. Hahn.* Oxford Science, Oxford, 1992.

- B. Blümich and W. Kuhn (Eds.). *Magnetic Resonance Microscopy: Methods and Applications in Materials Science, Agriculture and Biomedicine.* VCH, Weinheim, 1992.

- G. M. Grant and R. K. Harris (Eds.). *Encyclopedia of Nuclear Magnetic Resonance, Volume 1, Historical Perspectives.* John Wiley and Sons, Chichester, 1996.

- W. S. Hinshaw and A. H. Lent. An introduction to NMR imaging: From the Bloch equation to the imaging equation. *Proc. IEEE*, 71: 338, 1983.

- I. L. Pykett, J. H. Newhouse, F. S. Buonanno, T. J. Brady, M. R. Goldman, J. P. Kistler and G. M. Pohost. Principles of nuclear magnetic resonance imaging. *Radiology*, 143: 157, 1982.

- I. L. Pykett, J. H. Newhouse, F. S. Buonanno, T. J. Brady, M. R. Goldman, J. P. Kistler and G. M. Pohost. Principles of nuclear magnetic resonance imaging. *Radiology*, 143: 157, 1982.

Chapter 2

Classical Response of a Single Nucleus to a Magnetic Field

Chapter Contents

Summary: The concept of a magnetic moment is described. The classical equations of motion for the magnetic moment in the presence of an external field are developed. Solutions for static fields are found and their connection to gyroscopic precession is made.

Introduction

Magnetic resonance imaging (MRI) works because we can observe the way the protons in the human body respond to external magnetic fields. The MRI experiment is really a combination of a two-step process where, in the first stage, the proton 'spin' orientation is manipulated by an assortment of applied magnetic fields. In the second stage, changes in orientation can be measured through the interaction of the proton's magnetic field with a coil detector. Although each proton field is minuscule, a significant signal can be measured resulting from the sum of all fields of all affected protons of the body.

In this chapter, and the next, the focus is on the basic element of the first stage, a single proton's response to an external field, ignoring the interactions of each proton with its surroundings. These important interactions are deferred to the fourth chapter, where we shall include their effects in the equations of motion.

Extensive use is made of a classical picture where the proton is viewed as a tiny spinning charge with an attendant circulating electric current. Indeed, much of MRI theory can be understood classically, although in Ch. 5 we will show how to derive the principal results of this chapter in the more fundamental quantum mechanical framework.

2.1   Magnetic Moment in the Presence of a Magnetic Field

In this section, we briefly review the magnetic force, magnetic moment given by a current loop, torque due to the force, and its relation to the magnetic moment and field. We also provide another example of the torque for a magnetic dipole in an external field. The torque is related to the change of angular momentum as discussed in Sec. 2.2 where it serves as a building block of the Bloch equation.

2.1.1   Torque on a Current Loop in a Magnetic Field

We begin with a study of magnetic forces on current-carrying conductors, in order to introduce the interaction of a proton with an external magnetic field. A circular loop of current I and area A is pictured with two different orientations in Fig. 2.1. If an external magnetic field $\vec{B}$ is turned on, the loop will feel a differential force on each of its differential segments $d\vec{\ell}$ given by the basic Lorentz force law (see Appendix A),

$$d\vec{F} = I d\vec{\ell} \times \vec{B} \qquad (2.1)$$

This cross product implies that the differential force is perpendicular to the plane defined by two vectors: the current segment and the magnetic field evaluated at that segment. It is in the direction that a right hand screw, perpendicular to the plane, advances when rotated from the current segment vector to the magnetic field vector.

   The total force on the circular loop, and indeed on any closed loop, due to a uniform (constant over space) external magnetic field is zero. As an example, the symmetrical vector sum of the differential forces on either current loop in Fig. 2.1 clearly vanishes for any loop orientation. To prove it in general, the result follows from an integral over (2.1), where I and $\vec{B}$ can be taken outside the integral, since $\oint d\vec{\ell} = 0$ for an integration around any closed path. Now zero total force means zero change in the total momentum $\vec{p}$, from Newton's law,

$$\vec{F} = \frac{d\vec{p}}{dt} \qquad (2.2)$$

Therefore, a current loop initially at rest in a spatially constant magnetic field stays at rest. (For the present, we also assume the field is constant in time.) But this is not the whole story. A current loop can be rotated by the field, depending on the loop's orientation.

   Rotations can arise from forces applied off center, even when the vector sum of all forces cancels out. The vector quantity used to describe the rotation of an object is torque ($\vec{N}$).[1] If the sum of the differential torque contributions,

$$d\vec{N} = \vec{r} \times d\vec{F} \qquad (2.3)$$

is nonzero, the current loop can be expected to rotate, instantaneously, at least, about the axis along $d\vec{N}$. In (2.3), $\vec{r}$ is the position vector from, say, the center of the loop to the point of application of the differential force.

---

[1]Discussions of torque can be found in most introductory physics textbooks.

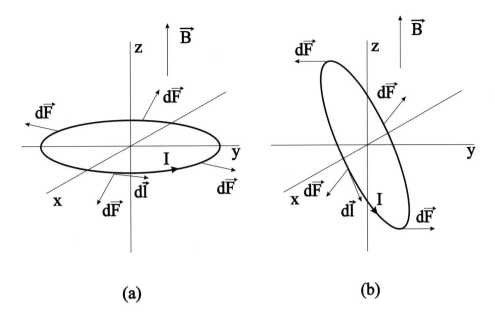

Fig. 2.1: Circular current loop depicted in two different orientations relative to a uniform magnetic field. The forces on representative differential current segments are shown (one $d\vec{\ell}$ is explicitly shown in each case). The first (a) shows the current plane perpendicular to the field where there is no net twist (torque); the second (b) shows the current plane at an arbitrary angle to the field where there is a nonzero torque.

Problem 2.1

If the total force on a current loop (or any system, for that matter) is zero ($\oint d\vec{F} = 0$), show that the total torque $\vec{N} = \oint \vec{r} \times d\vec{F}$ is independent of the choice of origin. Hint: Change to a primed coordinate system where $\vec{r} = \vec{r'} + \vec{r}_0$, with an arbitrary shift $\vec{r}_0$.

In the special case where the plane of the circular loop is perpendicular to a constant magnetic field, Fig. 2.1a, each $\vec{r}$ is parallel to its $d\vec{F}$ so each differential torque is zero. But in the general case, Fig. 2.1b, where the plane is at some arbitrary angle to that field, it is evident that there is a net torque rotating the loop back into the perpendicular plane. We come back to what the proton actually does in response to a similar torque, after a discussion of a basic torque formula.

The formula for the net torque on any current distribution, which is exact in a constant magnetic field, is given in terms of the 'magnetic dipole moment' or simply 'magnetic moment' $\vec{\mu}$:

$$\vec{N} = \vec{\mu} \times \vec{B} \qquad (2.4)$$

with $\vec{\mu}$ itself to be discussed shortly. This cross product can be taken with respect to any point, but because the net force is zero, the net torque vector is independent of the origin chosen (see the previous problem). In place of a general argument for (2.4),[2] we present a

---

[2]See Appendix A for further remarks and references.

specific calculation of the torque on a circular loop. This serves as an example of how a loop magnetic moment arises in electromagnetic formulas, and the result can be used to verify the form (2.4). But first a formula for the magnetic moment of a current loop is needed.

To prescribe the magnetic moment for a planar loop, imagine a right-hand screw piercing the interior of the loop, and perpendicular to the plane of the loop. Define a unit vector $\hat{n}$ to point along the direction the screw advances, if the screw is rotated in the same sense as the current flows. The magnetic moment vector for planar loops is given by

$$\vec{\mu} = IA\,\hat{n} \tag{2.5}$$

where A is the area of the loop interior. A sample planar moment is illustrated in Fig. 2.2, along with an alternative description of the right-hand rule.

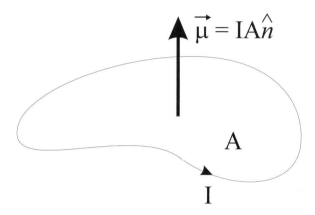

Fig. 2.2: A loop with current I lying in a plane. The perpendicular unit vector $\hat{n}$ points up from the side where the area A is on our left if we were to walk along the current path in the direction of current flow. The magnetic moment for the loop is $IA\hat{n}$.

The torque due to a constant magnetic field is to be calculated for a circular loop with radius R and current I centered in the x-y plane. Let the field lie in the y-z plane and have magnitude B. The differential torque on $d\vec{\ell}$ can be written quite generally as

$$d\vec{N} = \vec{r} \times (Id\vec{\ell} \times \vec{B}) = Id\vec{\ell}\,(\vec{B} \cdot \vec{r}) - I\vec{B}\,(d\vec{\ell} \cdot \vec{r}) \tag{2.6}$$

Use has been made of the double cross-product formula[3] after combining (2.1) and (2.3). The torque can be calculated with respect to the origin (we have seen that torque on a closed current loop is independent of this choice). The magnetic field and the cylindrical unit vectors shown in Fig. 2.3a are

$$\begin{aligned}
\vec{B} &= B(\cos\theta\,\hat{z} + \sin\theta\,\hat{y}) \\
\hat{\rho} &= \cos\phi\,\hat{x} + \sin\phi\,\hat{y} \\
\hat{\phi} &= -\sin\phi\,\hat{x} + \cos\phi\,\hat{y}
\end{aligned} \tag{2.7}$$

---

[3]The 'BAC-CAB' rule is $\vec{A} \times (\vec{B} \times \vec{C}) = \vec{B}(\vec{A} \cdot \vec{C}) - \vec{C}(\vec{A} \cdot \vec{B})$.

where the angles are also illustrated in that figure. With $d\vec{\ell} = Rd\phi\,\hat{\phi}$ and $\vec{r} = R\,\hat{\rho}$, the second scalar product in (2.6) is zero, and a reduction of the first scalar product using (2.7) yields

$$d\vec{N} = IBR^2\sin\theta\,\sin\phi\,\hat{\phi}\,d\phi \qquad (2.8)$$

An integration of (2.8) over the polar angle ϕ, with $\hat{\phi}$ from (2.7), gives the total torque. There is no net y-component because $\int_0^{2\pi} d\phi\sin\phi\cos\phi = 0$. The integral $\int_0^{2\pi} d\phi\sin^2\phi = \pi$ is needed[4] for the calculation of the net x-component, leading to

$$\vec{N} = -I\pi R^2 B\sin\theta\,\hat{x} \qquad (2.9)$$

Equation (2.9) is exactly $\vec{\mu}\times\vec{B}$ in view of the fact that the magnetic dipole moment for the circular loop of Fig. 2.3a is

$$\vec{\mu} = I\pi R^2\hat{z} \qquad (2.10)$$

The reader is invited to investigate, in similar fashion, both the force and the torque for the example of a rectangular loop in Prob. 2.2.

Exact for constant fields, the torque formula (2.4) is also very accurate for small loops in a spatially varying field. The only requirement is that the loop scale (say, its diameter D) must be much less than the typical distances over which the field changes. (For example, $|\Delta B| \simeq |\partial B/\partial x|D \ll |B|$.) Corrections would arise from, for example, 'higher moments' such as electric quadrupole moments. In the case of a proton, however, the electric quadrupole moment, and all other higher moments, are zero.

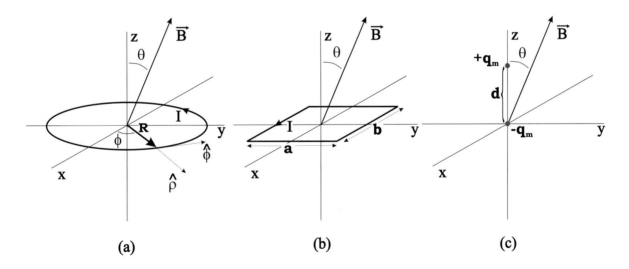

(a)   (b)   (c)

Fig. 2.3: Circular (a) and rectangular (b) current loops lying in the x-y plane and a magnetic-charge pair along the z-axis (c), all experiencing a constant magnetic field. In each case, the field lies in the z-y plane.

---

[4]Such integrals lead to a rule of thumb: The average value of $\sin^2\phi$ or $\cos^2\phi$ over any multiple of $\pi/2$ is $1/2$.

Problem 2.2

Consider the constant magnetic field in the z-y plane at an angle θ with the z-axis as shown in Fig. 2.3b. A current I flows in a rectangular loop with sides a and b lying in the x-y plane.

a) Show that the differential forces on the four respective current legs have the forms $IB(-\cos\theta\hat{y} + \sin\theta\hat{z})\,|dx|$, $-IB(\sin\theta\hat{z} - \cos\theta\hat{y})\,|dx|$, $IB\cos\theta\hat{x}\,|dy|$, and $-IB\cos\theta\hat{x}\,|dy|$.

b) Show that, after integration, the total force on the loop is zero.

c) Show that the differential torques on the four respective current legs relative to the center of the loop have the forms $[x\hat{x} - \frac{a}{2}\hat{y}] \times [IB(-\cos\theta\hat{y}+\sin\theta\hat{z})\,|dx|]$, $[x\hat{x}+\frac{a}{2}\hat{y}] \times [-IB(\sin\theta\hat{z}-\cos\theta\hat{y})\,|dx|]$, $[\frac{b}{2}\hat{x}+y\hat{y}] \times [IB\cos\theta\hat{x}\,|dy|]$, and $[-\frac{b}{2}\hat{x}+y\hat{y}] \times [-IB\cos\theta\hat{x}\,|dy|]$.

d) Show that the integration of the results in (c) is simplified by the vanishing of certain integrands odd in x or y, leading to a net torque on the loop given by $-IBab\sin\theta\hat{x}$. Again, the double cross product formula could have been used to bypass the force calculation, in achieving this result.

e) Find the magnetic moment vector for this loop from (2.5) and show that the total torque found in (d) agrees with the formula (2.4).

2.1.2   Magnet Toy Model

A magnetic dipole moment can be viewed as a pair of magnetic charges with equal magnitudes and opposite signs, in analogy with the way electric charges lead to electric dipole moments. The word 'dipole' has its origin in this model, which is an acceptable alternative to the current loop picture as long as we use it to investigate only the field outside the moment structure. The field inside for the charge pair is different than that for the current loop. It should also be noted that magnetic monopoles have yet to be observed in nature.

The magnetic moment in Fig. 2.3c resembles a bar magnet with the positive and negative magnetic charges playing the role of the north and south poles, respectively. The analogy to an electric dipole moment (Appendix A) implies that the magnetic moment vector is

$$\vec{\mu}_m = \hat{n}q_m d \tag{2.11}$$

where d is the distance between the magnetic charges, and $\hat{n}$ points along the line directed from the negative charge $-q_m$ to the positive charge q_m. We wish to check that the net torque on the pair of magnetic charges has the expected form (2.4).

The force on a magnetic charge q_m due to a magnetic field is like that on an electric charge due to an electric field. It is

$$\vec{F}_m = q_m\vec{B} \tag{2.12}$$

Since the total force is zero, for convenience we can choose the torque reference point to lie on the negative charge (the origin in Fig. 2.3c). With respect to that point, the net torque is that due to the force on the charge at $z = d$,

$$\vec{N}_m = (\hat{z}d) \times (q_m \vec{B}) \tag{2.13}$$

Expression (2.13) obviously agrees with (2.4) and implies a rotation of the magnetic-charge dipole toward the field direction. The torque equation (2.4) is the starting point for future classical discussions of the magnetic-moment behavior in the presence of a magnetic field. It applies as well to fields that vary in space and time.

2.2   Magnetic Moment with Spin: Equation of Motion

The lesson so far is that a magnetic moment, such as that corresponding to a current loop or a bar magnet, will try to line up along the direction of an external magnetic field. This is much as a falling pendulum tries to align itself with the direction of gravity.[5] If the moment is associated with an angular momentum (a 'spinning'), then the motion is changed. To see what the new motion is, we introduce in this section the general differential equation for angular momentum in the presence of external torque and the atomic relation between intrinsic angular momenta and magnetic moments. The resulting differential equation is solved for a special case in Sec. 2.3.

2.2.1   Torque and Angular Momentum

Nonzero total torque on a system implies that the system's total angular momentum $\vec{J}$ must change according to

$$\frac{d\vec{J}}{dt} = \vec{N} \tag{2.14}$$

This equation, discussed in most introductory mechanics textbooks, can be derived, as a problem, for a single point mass.

Problem 2.3

Consider a point mass m moving at velocity $\vec{v}(t)$ with position $\vec{r}(t)$ defined by some origin. Its angular momentum relative to that origin is therefore $\vec{J} = \vec{r} \times \vec{p}$ with $\vec{p} = m\vec{v}$. Derive (2.14) by taking the time derivative of this angular momentum. Note (2.2) and (2.3).

The generality of (2.14) follows by considering a system as a limit of many point particles. The total angular momentum is the corresponding limit of

$$\vec{J} = \sum_i \vec{r}_i \times \vec{p}_i \tag{2.15}$$

with respect to some origin.

---
[5]We return to a related gravitational analogy in Sec. 2.3.

2.2.2   Angular Momentum of the Proton

We next formulate the connection between the proton intrinsic angular momentum (or what is often referred to as its 'spin') and its moment. The connections for other nuclear particles are also of interest.

The proton spin can be thought of as leading to a circulating electric current, and, hence, an associated magnetic moment. The direct relationship between the magnetic moment and the spin angular momentum vector is found from experiment,

$$\vec{\mu} = \gamma \vec{J} \tag{2.16}$$

The proportionality constant in (2.16) is called the gyromagnetic (or magnetogyric) ratio and depends on the particle or nucleus. For the proton, it is found to be[6]

$$\gamma = 2.675 \times 10^8 \text{ rad/s/T} \tag{2.17}$$

or, what may be referred to as 'gamma-bar,'

$$\gamma\!\!\!\!- \equiv \frac{\gamma}{2\pi} = 42.58 \text{ MHz/T} \tag{2.18}$$

where T is the tesla unit of magnetic field and is equal to 10,000 gauss (G). Of all the numbers in MR, $\gamma\!\!\!\!-$ is probably the one most often used in back-of-the-envelope calculations. From (2.16) we are justified, in any discussion, to refer either to spin, or to the magnetic dipole moment, since they track each other.

It is useful to compare the experimental values for the gyromagnetic ratios with a formula for a simply structured system. Consider a point particle with charge q, mass m, and speed v going in a circle of radius r. A calculation carried out in the following problem yields the result for the gyromagnetic ratio of a point particle

$$\gamma \text{ (point charge in circular motion)} = \frac{q}{2m} \tag{2.19}$$

This is not an accurate formula for the nuclear particles of interest, but it does help us understand the differences due to mass.

The simple result (2.19) also arises as a coefficient in basic magnetic moment quantities. In Ch. 5, we will introduce the quantum unit of angular momentum $\hbar \equiv h/2\pi$ (also referred to as 'h-bar') where h is Planck's constant. For the charge e and mass m_e of the electron, the basic magnetic moment unit is the Bohr magneton

$$\mu_B \equiv \frac{e\hbar}{2m_e} = 9.27 \times 10^{-24} \text{ A} \cdot \text{m}^2 \tag{2.20}$$

For the same charge but with a proton mass, the nuclear magneton is

$$\mu_n \equiv \frac{e\hbar}{2m_p} = 5.05 \times 10^{-27} \text{ A} \cdot \text{m}^2 \tag{2.21}$$

---

[6]To this accuracy, the measured value for a proton bound in H_2O is the same as that for a free proton.

Problem 2.4

---

a) Show that the angular momentum $\vec{r} \times \vec{p}$ of the circulating particle with respect to the center is $mrv\hat{n}$ where $\hat{n}$ is a unit vector perpendicular to the plane of the circle. Here, $\hat{n}$ points in a direction given by the right-hand rule applied to the particle's motion.

b) Show that the magnetic moment associated with the motion of the point charge is $qvr/2$ and thus that the gyromagnetic ratio is given by (2.19).

c) Evaluate numerically the gyromagnetic ratio γ (2.19), choosing the same mass (1.67×10^{-27} kg) and charge (1.60×10^{-19} C) as for a proton. The difference between your answer and (2.17) is due to the more complicated motion of the proton constituents, the 'quarks.' For related reasons, a neutron has a nonvanishing magnetic moment despite its zero overall charge.

2.2.3 Electrons and Other Elements

From the mass dependence discussed in Sec. 2.2.2 (see also Prob. 2.4), it is not surprising that the γ factors can vary from one particle to another, if only because their masses may differ. Indeed, the electron γ factor is expected to be much larger than that for the proton in view of the inverse mass dependence. The difference between the observed ratio

$$\frac{|\gamma_e|}{\gamma_p} = 658 \tag{2.22}$$

and the measured mass ratio $m_p/m_e = 1836$ (the electron mass is 9.11×10^{-31} kg) is due to the difference in the structure of the two particles. The electron has no apparent size, while the proton has a size on the order of 1 fermi (10^{-15} m) and is a complex composite of quarks. They do, however, have exactly the same spin.

Why do we not use electron imaging for tesla-level magnetic fields? The principal reason is the striking difference in the frequency with which a magnetic moment precesses about a static magnetic field, and which will be discussed in Sec. 2.3. The precession frequency is proportional to the gyromagnetic ratio and, with the difference shown in (2.22), it is much larger for the electron. In the standard MRI experiment, an additional, oscillating magnetic field is required,[7] whose frequency is matched with the precession frequency. For static fields in the tesla range, a radiofrequency field in the microwave spectrum is thus needed for electron experiments. However, too much energy would be deposited in human bodies, if electron spins were 'excited' by these rf fields. Although lowering the frequency by reducing the static field strength is an alternative, the relatively small concentration of free or unpaired electrons inside normal human subjects leads to a much lower signal-to-noise ratio.

For nuclei, the first requirement is nonzero intrinsic angular momentum (total 'spin'). It might be guessed, incorrectly, that magnetic moments of heavier nuclei would be rather

---

[7]The additional field is detailed in the next chapter.

smaller, roughly by the inverse ratio of their total masses to the proton mass, than that for a proton. In reality, they usually are not very much smaller, nor are they ever very much larger. Only the 'outer shell' nucleons contribute to the total angular momentum of heavier nuclei; the total nuclear mass is not relevant to the determination of the γ factor. In general, protons and, separately, neutrons pair up as much as possible inside of a nucleus, with their spins and orbital motions canceling.

Consider the different nuclear cases. Each 'even-even' nucleus (even numbers of protons and even numbers of neutrons) has zero total angular momentum, and, hence, zero magnetic moment. For this reason, we cannot image the ^{16}O and ^{12}C in our bodies with the MR techniques under discussion. The magnetic moment of an even-odd nucleus can be approximately understood in terms of the single unpaired nucleon, but admixtures of states differing in the configurations of the other nucleons must sometimes be taken into account. The unpaired proton and neutron in odd-odd nuclei are not in the same orbital state and do not conspire to give zero spin, in general. For example, nitrogen has twice the spin of hydrogen, and a nonvanishing magnetic moment.

The γ factors in (2.16) for nuclei with nonzero angular momentum are consequently within an order of magnitude or so of that for the proton. The relation to the nuclear magnetic moment does involve the nuclear spin I_N

$$\gamma = \frac{\mu}{I_N} \tag{2.23}$$

The gyromagnetic ratios are determined by measurements, and their values are often rather smaller than that for the proton.

Smaller values for γ are not the only reason, however, that imaging of elements other than hydrogen is difficult in the human body. The problem is usually one of low concentration. Still, sodium (^{23}Na) and phosphorus (^{31}P) are of imaging interest in view of their nonvanishing magnetic moments (their spins are '3/2' and '1/2' in quantum units $\hbar$ in terms of which the proton has spin '1/2,' see Ch. 5). Their relative γ factors, spin, and concentration are listed together with other nuclei of interest in Table 2.1.

2.2.4   Equation of Motion

Using both the relation (2.16) between the spin and the magnetic moment and the expression (2.4) for torque on a magnetic moment due to an external magnetic field $\vec{B}$, we find that (2.14) reduces to

$$\frac{d\vec{\mu}}{dt} = \gamma \vec{\mu} \times \vec{B} \tag{2.24}$$

This fundamental equation of motion is at the heart of the rotations and precessions that we shall frequently discuss. It is a simple version of the Bloch equation to be presented in Ch. 4. Important corrections arise from the interactions of spins with their surroundings, processes which are referred to as 'relaxation' phenomena.

Nucleus	Spin	Magnetic moment	γ	Abundance in human body
hydrogen ^{1}H	1/2	2.7928	42.58	88 M
sodium ^{23}Na	3/2	2.2175	11.27	80 mM
phosphorus ^{31}P	1/2	1.1316	17.25	75 mM
oxygen ^{17}O	5/2	−1.8938	−5.77	17 mM
fluorine ^{19}F	1/2	2.6289	40.08	4 μM

Table 2.1: List of selected nuclear species with their spins (in units of $\hbar$ where the proton has spin 1/2), their associated magnetic moments in units of a nuclear magneton μ_n (2.21), gyromagnetic ratios γ (in units of MHz/T), and their relative body abundances (1 M = 1 molar = 1 mole/liter). For comparison, the hydrogen (^{1}H) molarity of water is 110 M, and brain gray matter, for example, has a water content of 80% leading to an abundance of 88 M. The quoted body abundances will vary from tissue to tissue. Certain common elements are omitted, such as ^{12}C and ^{16}O, because their nuclear spins (and hence their nuclear magnetic moments) are zero. A negative sign for the moment and gyromagnetic ratio refers to the fact that the magnetic moment is anti-parallel to the angular momentum vector.

Problem 2.5

Demonstrate that (2.24) implies $d\mu/dt = 0$. Hint: Form a scalar (dot) product of both sides of (2.24) with $\vec{\mu}$.

2.3 Precession Solution: Phase

The differential equation (2.24) for a static field is readily solved, and the corresponding precessional motion is important to the MR application. Different approaches to this solution are described below. A comparison with a well-known gravitational analogy is briefly discussed before the magnetic moment case is detailed.

2.3.1 Precession via the Gyroscope Analogy

If instead of a pendulum we consider an object spinning along its axis, a gyroscope or spinning top, experience tells us that it does not fall but rather precesses around the gravity axis. The precession in Fig. 2.4a is the result of a gravitational torque perpendicular to the spin axis. Exactly analogous precession takes place for a spinning magnetic moment experiencing torque from a constant external magnetic field. However, the torque,[8] and hence the precession, are in the opposite direction. Compare the figure to Fig. 2.5.

---

[8]The pendulum tends to fall down toward the gravity direction, while the magnetic moment, in the absence of the spin effect, tends to swing up toward the magnetic field direction.

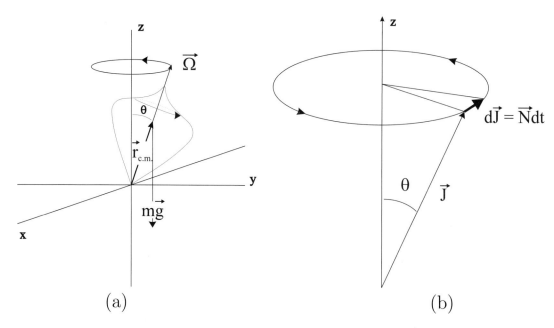

Fig. 2.4: (a) A symmetrical spinning top with spin angular velocity $\vec{\Omega}$ and mass m precessing in a constant gravitational field. (b) The corresponding angular momentum diagram showing how the gravitational torque leads to precession. The precession is in the opposite sense to that for a magnetic moment immersed in a magnetic field pointing in the positive z-direction (see Fig. 2.5).

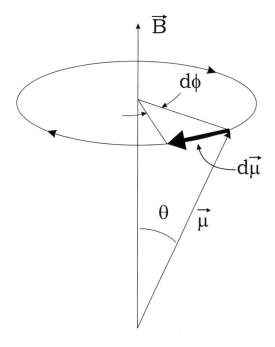

Fig. 2.5: Clockwise precession of a proton's spin about a magnetic field. As shown, the differential $d\phi$ is negative.

There is a direct correspondence between the equations for a magnetic moment and a spinning top immersed in constant vertical magnetic and gravitational fields, respectively. It is easy to show that the force on a rigid body like a top due to a uniform gravitational pull on all of its parts is equivalent to a total force mg applied at its center of mass (c.m.). The resultant torque with respect to the bottom support pivot is $\vec{r}_{c.m.} \times (-mg\hat{z})$ where $\vec{r}_{c.m.}$ is the position of the c.m. relative to the pivot. The torque is in the direction of increasing azimuthal angle in Fig. 2.4b, and, as it will be proven when the corresponding magnetic-moment case is solved later, the top precesses along a cone at constant θ.

The torque expressions $\gamma B \vec{\mu} \times \hat{z}$ and $-mgr\vec{r}_{c.m.} \times \hat{z}$ map into one another for $\vec{\mu}$ parallel to $\vec{r}_{c.m.}$. Furthermore, the angular momentum for a symmetrical rigid body is $I\vec{\Omega}$ with I the moment of inertia and $\vec{\Omega}$ the angular velocity vector pointing along the spin axis. This, too, is parallel to the angular momentum associated with $\vec{\mu}$. The equation $d\vec{J}/dt = \vec{N}$ looks the same for both.

More general top trajectories, including nutations which follow an initial downward 'shove,' have counterparts (and some differences) in the magnetic moment case. This is especially true when time-dependent magnetic fields are considered in Ch. 3.

2.3.2 Geometrical Representation

Some general remarks can be made about the motion predicted by the 'magnetic torque' (2.24). When the time rate of change of a vector is proportional to a cross product involving that vector, we immediately see its magnitude $\mu = |\vec{\mu}|$ is unchanged.

The magnitude may be fixed but the direction is changing. The instantaneous change in the magnetic moment direction is equivalent to an instantaneous left-handed rotation about $\vec{B}$, the other vector in the cross product. To see the rotation and get the instantaneous rotation frequency, consider Fig. 2.5. The differential change in the moment in time dt is $d\vec{\mu} = \gamma\vec{\mu} \times \vec{B}dt$, which is perpendicular to the plane defined by $\vec{\mu}$ and $\vec{B}$. This pushes the tip $\vec{\mu}$ (when viewing from 'above' with $\vec{B}$ pointing at the viewer) on a clockwise precession around a circular path. The tip would stay on that same circle if $\vec{B}$ were constant in time. If $d\phi$ is the angle subtended by $d\vec{\mu}$, and θ is the angle between $\vec{\mu}$ and $\vec{B}$, the geometry of Fig. 2.5 indicates that

$$|d\vec{\mu}| = \mu \sin\theta |d\phi| \tag{2.25}$$

On the other hand,

$$|d\vec{\mu}| = \gamma |\vec{\mu} \times \vec{B}|dt = \gamma \mu B \sin\theta dt \tag{2.26}$$

A comparison gives $\gamma B|dt| = |d\phi|$ with $B \equiv |\vec{B}|$, giving the well-known Larmor precession formula,

$$\omega \equiv \left|\frac{d\phi}{dt}\right| = \gamma B \tag{2.27}$$

along an instantaneous axis defined by a left-handed screw rotation about $\vec{B}$. That is,

$$\frac{d\phi}{dt} = -\omega \tag{2.28}$$

so that the angular velocity vector is[9]

$$\vec{\omega} = -\omega\hat{z} \tag{2.29}$$

If the field is along the z-axis and constant in time, $\vec{B} = B_0\hat{z}$, the solution of (2.28) is

$$\phi = -\omega_0 t + \phi_0 \qquad \text{(constant field case)} \tag{2.30}$$

where ϕ_0 is the initial angle. Again, notice the minus sign (ϕ is the usual azimuthal angle defined in right-handed fashion around the z-axis); (2.30) shows constant left-handed precession around the field direction. From now on, we define the Larmor frequency for the constant field case to be

$$\omega_L(\text{constant field}) \equiv \omega_0 \equiv \gamma B_0 \tag{2.31}$$

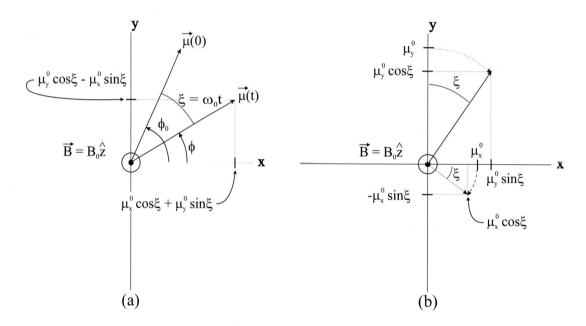

(a)   (b)

Fig. 2.6: The vector $\vec{\mu}(t)$ is obtained by the clockwise rotation of $\vec{\mu}(0)$ through an angle $\xi = \omega_0 t$ about the z-axis ($\phi = -\xi + \phi_0$). The Cartesian coordinates of $\vec{\mu}(t)$, shown in (a), can be found by rotating the individual components of $\vec{\mu}(0)$, as shown in (b). Note that $\mu_x^0 \equiv \mu_x(0)$, $\mu_y^0 \equiv \mu_y(0)$. The z-component of the vector is not changed; only the transverse components are shown in the figures. The clockwise rotation corresponds to magnetic-moment precession about the static field $B_0\hat{z}$.

2.3.3   Cartesian Representation

What about a formula for $\vec{\mu}(t)$ in terms of Cartesian axes? As an alternative to working with (2.30), it is possible to use the rotation picture developed above and trigonometry to

---

[9]We shall use the convention that angular frequencies are positive. The rotation sense can be indicated by specifying the angular velocity vector, about whose direction the rotation is right-handed. Therefore, the rotation indicated by (2.28) is *left-handed* with respect to the *positive z*-axis.

derive the answer for $\vec{B} = B_0 \hat{z}$. Note first that the z-component of the magnetic moment is unchanged during the rotation. In Fig. 2.6, the new x- and y-components resulting from the separate rotations of the two vectors $\mu_x(0)\hat{x}$ and $\mu_y(0)\hat{y}$ are shown. Adding these, we can obtain formulas for the total x and y components of $\vec{\mu}$. The combined answer in terms of their initial values has the rotation form

$$\vec{\mu}(t) = \mu_x(t)\hat{x} + \mu_y(t)\hat{y} + \mu_z(t)\hat{z} \tag{2.32}$$

with

$$\begin{aligned} \mu_x(t) &= \mu_x(0)\cos\omega_0 t + \mu_y(0)\sin\omega_0 t \\ \mu_y(t) &= \mu_y(0)\cos\omega_0 t - \mu_x(0)\sin\omega_0 t \\ \mu_z(t) &= \mu_z(0) \end{aligned} \tag{2.33}$$

Problem 2.6

It will be useful in later discussions to have the answer (2.33) rederived as a solution to the differential equation (2.24).

a) For $\vec{B} = B_0 \hat{z}$, show that the vector differential equation (2.24) decomposes into the three Cartesian equations

$$\begin{aligned} \frac{d\mu_x}{dt} &= \gamma \mu_y B_0 = \omega_0 \mu_y \\ \frac{d\mu_y}{dt} &= -\gamma \mu_x B_0 = -\omega_0 \mu_x \\ \frac{d\mu_z}{dt} &= 0 \end{aligned} \tag{2.34}$$

b) By taking additional derivatives, show that the first two equations in (2.34) can be decoupled to give

$$\begin{aligned} \frac{d^2\mu_x}{dt^2} &= -\omega_0^2 \mu_x \\ \frac{d^2\mu_y}{dt^2} &= -\omega_0^2 \mu_y \end{aligned} \tag{2.35}$$

These decoupled second-order differential equations have familiar solutions of the general form $C_1 \cos\omega_0 t + C_2 \sin\omega_0 t$.

c) By putting the general solutions back into the first-order differential equations (2.34), and by assuming the initial conditions used previously, show that you recover (2.33).

2.3.4   Matrix Representation

It is useful to unite (2.32) and (2.33) in matrix notation.

$$\vec{\mu}(t) = R_z(\omega_0 t)\vec{\mu}(0) \tag{2.36}$$

Here we mix notation a bit, and view vectors as column matrices. For example,

$$\vec{\mu}(t) = \begin{pmatrix} \mu_x(t) \\ \mu_y(t) \\ \mu_z(t) \end{pmatrix} \tag{2.37}$$

$R_z(\theta)$ in (2.36) corresponds to a clockwise rotation of vectors through an angle θ about the z-axis and can be represented by the matrix

$$R_z(\theta) = \begin{pmatrix} \cos\theta & \sin\theta & 0 \\ -\sin\theta & \cos\theta & 0 \\ 0 & 0 & 1 \end{pmatrix} \tag{2.38}$$

This is yet another mathematical representation of the physical picture of the magnetic moment precessing at a constant angular frequency around a constant magnetic field.

Problem 2.7

Show that, if (2.38) is substituted into (2.36), then (2.32) and (2.33) are recovered, assuming $\theta = \omega_0 t$.

2.3.5   Complex Representations and Phase

The fact that the principal action of the proton spin in a constant magnetic field is a rotation in the two-dimensional transverse plane suggests that a complex number representation will be useful. The two degrees of freedom, μ_x and μ_y, can be given in terms of the real and imaginary parts of

$$\mu_+(t) = \mu_x(t) + i\mu_y(t) \tag{2.39}$$

The addition of the first differential equation plus i times the second in (2.34) yields

$$\frac{d\mu_+}{dt} = -i\omega_0 \mu_+ \tag{2.40}$$

The solution of (2.40) is perhaps the easiest of all,

$$\mu_+(t) = \mu_+(0)e^{-i\omega_0 t} \tag{2.41}$$

In (2.41), $e^{-i\omega_0 t}$ represents a clockwise rotation in the complex plane, or equivalently, about $\hat{z}$, consistent with the precession picture drawn earlier. It is seen that *phase directly relates to position and is of utmost importance in the description of spin motion.*

Problem 2.8

Show that the real and imaginary parts of (2.41) agree with the first two solutions in (2.33).

In view of the importance of phase, it is useful to introduce a standard phase notation. In general, the complex number $\mu_+(t)$ can be written in terms of its magnitude and phase

$$\mu_+(t) = |\mu_+(t)|e^{i\phi(t)} \tag{2.42}$$

The solution (2.41) has constant magnitude

$$|\mu_+(t)| = |\mu_+(0)| \tag{2.43}$$

Thus that solution can be re-expressed as

$$\mu_+(t) = |\mu_+(0)|e^{i\phi_0(t)} \tag{2.44}$$

where the phase is

$$\phi_0(t) = -\omega_0 t + \phi_0(0) \tag{2.45}$$

The adaptation of the static-field phase (2.45) to include the effects of other fields is a primary subject in Ch. 20.

Suggested Reading

For a review of some of the basic physics concepts, the following three texts are useful:

- H. Goldstein. *Classical Mechanics: Pearson New International Edition.* Pearson, 3rd ed., London, 2014.

- D. Halliday, R. Resnick and K. S. Krane. *Physics.* John Wiley and Sons, New York, 1992.

- J. D. Jackson. *Classical Electrodynamics.* John Wiley and Sons, 3rd ed., Hoboken, 1999.

For a more comprehensive list of active NMR elements (i.e., those with nonzero spin), see, for example:

- P. T. Beall, S. R. Amtey and S. R. Kasturi. *NMR Data Handbook for Biomedical Applications.* Pergamon Press, New York, 1984.

Chapter 3

Rotating Reference Frames and Resonance

Chapter Contents

Summary: The combined effect of two perpendicular fields, one a static field and the other a much smaller rf field, is considered. The motion of a magnetic moment immersed in these fields is analyzed by the use of a rotating reference frame defined in terms of the frequency of the harmonic field. It is shown that the magnetic moment is most efficiently rotated away from the static-field direction when the frequency of the rf field matches the Larmor precessional frequency, a resonance condition.

Introduction

We have seen that, at any given point in time, the interaction of a classical magnetic moment with an external magnetic field is equivalent to an instantaneous rotation of the moment about the field. For a static field, the rotation is a constant precession about the fixed field axis. In the present chapter, we wish to consider the effect of adding other magnetic fields. We are most interested in the combination of a radiofrequency (rf) field perpendicular to a much larger constant field.

The interest in the additional field stems from a new application of the lesson from the last chapter. The act of turning on a perpendicular field for some period of time should tip any magnetic moment, initially aligned along the original static field, away from that direction. Such rotations leave the classical moment precessing at an angle[1] around the

---

[1]The more fundamental quantum picture allows only two spin states for any measurements along the static direction, either parallel or anti-parallel. The use of a classical picture of a moment or spin precessing at some angle is still appropriate in MR, as explained in Ch. 5.

original static field. Even very weak rf fields can be used, as we shall see, to rotate an initially aligned spin into the plane transverse to the static field, or, for that matter, to any angle away from its initial alignment. It is to be shown in this chapter that the key is to tune the radiofrequency to the Larmor frequency. The rotation will be most effective when this 'resonance condition' is satisfied.[2]

The rf field described above is the so-called 'transmit' field; it is produced by a coil system separate from the static field source. The precessing (or 'excited') protons produce their own rf field at the Larmor frequency. The rf field produced by the protons can be detected by the transmit system, or by an altogether different rf coil system. See Chs. 7 and 27.

3.1   Rotating Reference Frames

Suppose we are making magnetic moment measurements in a reference frame rotating at the Larmor precession frequency. Such frames rotate clockwise around the z-axis as seen from above the origin ($z > 0$) in a laboratory frame with a constant magnetic field pointing in the positive z-direction. See Fig. 3.1. From our rotating perspective, the spin axis is not moving at all. This reference frame has proven to be very useful in describing MRI experiments, and a mathematical framework is given for it below.

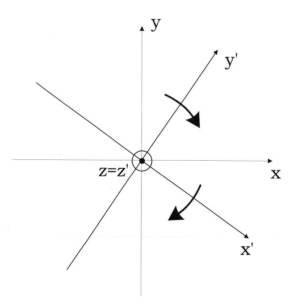

Fig. 3.1: The sense of the rotation of a primed reference frame in which a magnetic moment is at rest. The primed frame rotates clockwise around the $z = z'$ axis for a static magnetic field pointing in the $+\hat{z}$ direction according to a laboratory observer positioned above ($z > 0$) the x-y plane. The rotation frequency is the Larmor precession frequency (2.31).

---

[2]Adding a static perpendicular field, on the other hand, to the original static field would not yield the same kind of rotation. According to the solutions worked out in Ch. 2, it instead leads to a precession about the new, resultant field direction.

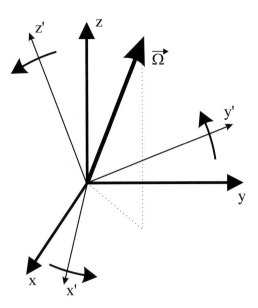

Fig. 3.2: The primed reference frame rotating according to a general angular velocity $\vec{\Omega}$ relative to the unprimed reference frame. The rotation is counterclockwise around $\vec{\Omega}$.

In Fig. 3.2, a laboratory (fixed) reference frame, denoted by the unprimed Cartesian coordinates (x, y, z) and their associated unit vectors, is compared to another frame denoted by primed quantities (x', y', z'), which is rotating about an arbitrary axis with respect to the fixed frame. The instantaneous rotation of this frame is defined by a rotational angular velocity vector $\vec{\Omega}$. The direction of this vector is the axis around which the primed frame is being rotated and its magnitude is the angular speed of rotation in radians per second. The angular velocity may be changing with time, $\vec{\Omega} = \vec{\Omega}(t)$. We go on to consider some vector $\vec{C}$ fixed (at rest) in the rotating frame, whence it must be rotating in the laboratory.

Any vector $\vec{C}$ instantaneously rotated by $\vec{\Omega}$ has its time rate of change with respect to the laboratory frame coordinates given by

$$\frac{d\vec{C}}{dt} = \vec{\Omega} \times \vec{C} \tag{3.1}$$

One way to see (3.1) is to rewrite $\vec{C}$ in terms of its components parallel and perpendicular to $\vec{\Omega}$

$$\vec{C}(t) = \vec{C}_{\parallel} + \vec{C}_{\perp} \tag{3.2}$$

The parallel component is unchanged

$$d\vec{C}_{\parallel} = 0 \tag{3.3}$$

The perpendicular component has a differential change whose magnitude can be calculated just as the differential arc length $d\mu$ was in Fig. 2.5. This step is left as an exercise for the reader. The combination of (3.2), (3.3), and the next equation, (3.4), yields (3.1).

Problem 3.1

Reversing the argument given in the discussion of Sec. 2.3 and defining the unit vector $\hat{n}$ parallel to $\vec{\Omega} \times \vec{C}$, show that

$$d\vec{C}_\perp = \Omega dt |\vec{C}_\perp| \hat{n} = \vec{\Omega} \times \vec{C} dt \tag{3.4}$$

Now replace $\vec{C}$ by a more general vector function $\vec{V}$ not necessarily at rest in the rotating reference frame. In general, $\vec{V}$ is time dependent in both frames, and its respective Cartesian components in the two frames remain different because of the rotation. In the unprimed (inertial) frame where the unit vectors are fixed in time:

$$\vec{V}(t) = V_x(t)\hat{x} + V_y(t)\hat{y} + V_z(t)\hat{z} \tag{3.5}$$

In the primed frame, define the components of $\vec{V}$ with respect to the primed unit vectors,

$$\vec{V}'(t) = \vec{V}(t) = V_{x'}(t)\hat{x}'(t) + V_{y'}(t)\hat{y}'(t) + V_{z'}(t)\hat{z}'(t) \tag{3.6}$$

There is no need to distinguish between $\vec{V}'$ and $\vec{V}$ since they refer to the same vector. The primed unit vectors are rotating relative to the unprimed, so they are time dependent.

Either (3.5) or (3.6) can be used to represent $\vec{V}(t)$, and to compute its time derivative. The two ways must give the same answer, i.e.,

$$
\begin{aligned}
\frac{dV_x}{dt}&\hat{x} + \frac{dV_y}{dt}\hat{y} + \frac{dV_z}{dt}\hat{z} \\
&= \frac{dV_{x'}}{dt}\hat{x}'(t) + \frac{dV_{y'}}{dt}\hat{y}'(t) + \frac{dV_{z'}}{dt}\hat{z}'(t) + V_{x'}\frac{d\hat{x}'(t)}{dt} + V_{y'}\frac{d\hat{y}'(t)}{dt} + V_{z'}\frac{d\hat{z}'(t)}{dt}
\end{aligned}
\tag{3.7}
$$

The unit vectors $\hat{x}'$, $\hat{y}'$, $\hat{z}'$ are examples of the $\vec{C}$ vectors discussed above. For instance,

$$\frac{d\hat{x}'}{dt} = \vec{\Omega} \times \hat{x}' \tag{3.8}$$

The time derivative of (3.5) thus can be written in convective form as

$$\frac{d\vec{V}}{dt} = \left(\frac{d\vec{V}}{dt}\right)' + \vec{\Omega} \times \vec{V} \tag{3.9}$$

where the primed derivative is defined as

$$\left(\frac{d\vec{V}}{dt}\right)' \equiv \frac{dV_{x'}(t)}{dt}\hat{x}'(t) + \frac{dV_{y'}(t)}{dt}\hat{y}'(t) + \frac{dV_{z'}(t)}{dt}\hat{z}'(t) \tag{3.10}$$

This derivative represents the rate of change of the vector quantity with respect to the rotating reference frame.

Consider $\vec{\mu}$ as the vector quantity $\vec{V}(t)$ in (3.9)

$$\frac{d\vec{\mu}}{dt} = \left(\frac{d\vec{\mu}}{dt}\right)' + \vec{\Omega} \times \vec{\mu} \tag{3.11}$$

On the other hand, (2.24) is

$$\frac{d\vec{\mu}}{dt} = \gamma\vec{\mu} \times \vec{B} \tag{3.12}$$

From a comparison of (3.11) and (3.12), we can bank on the primed rate to be

$$\left(\frac{d\vec{\mu}}{dt}\right)' = \gamma\vec{\mu} \times \vec{B}_{eff} \tag{3.13}$$

where the 'effective magnetic field' in the rotating frame is

$$\vec{B}_{eff} = \vec{B} + \frac{\vec{\Omega}}{\gamma} \tag{3.14}$$

The effective magnetic field is useful in the determination of the precessional motion, and *a key concept in the magnetic moment analysis in general.* In the primed (rotating) frame, $\vec{\mu}$ is observed to have motion equivalent to the instantaneous rotation due to a 'total' magnetic field given by (3.14). This effective field is the superposition of the external magnetic field plus a fictitious magnetic field whose magnitude is $|\vec{\Omega}|/\gamma$ and whose direction is the same as that of the vector $\vec{\Omega}$. The rotational motion around $\vec{B}_{eff}$ is the by now familiar clockwise or left-handed precession (for an instant, at least) looking backwards along its direction.

The freedom to choose the primed frame leads to a rapid rederivation of the solution found for the constant magnetic field problem. Take $\vec{\Omega}/\gamma = -\vec{B}$. Then $(d\vec{\mu}/dt)' = 0$ from (3.13), so $\vec{\mu}$ is constant in the primed frame. For the example where $\vec{B} = B_0\hat{z}$, it means $\vec{\mu}$ rotates in the unprimed frame at a fixed angle with respect to the z-axis, and at fixed angular velocity $\vec{\Omega} = -\gamma B_0\hat{z}$ (that is, left-handedly or clockwise around z). This implies the solution (2.41) or (2.45).

3.2 The Rotating Frame for an RF Field

Consider a proton spin aligned along $B_0\hat{z}$. An rf magnetic field $\vec{B}_1$ is added to 'tip' the spin away from $\hat{z}$.[3] According to (3.13), $\vec{B}_1$ must have components in the x or y direction (i.e., 'transverse' or 'perpendicular' components) in order to rotate $\vec{\mu}$ away from the z-axis. The Larmor frequency, to which the applied transmit field's frequency should be matched, generally lies in the rf range for conventional MRI (see Ch. 2). Recall that this field is referred to as the transmit rf field.

---

[3]Throughout the book, this will often be referred to as a spin flip, in view of the common usage of phrases like 'flip angle.' The terminology is motivated by the quantum picture (see Ch. 5) where, as we have stated in an earlier footnote, the proton has only 'spin-up' or 'spin-down.' Nevertheless, a classical picture of continuous spin rotations remains adequate for the present discussion.

3.2.1   Polarization

In the present context, 'polarization' refers to the direction of the magnetic field,[4] so a sinusoidal field linearly polarized along the x-axis is

$$\vec{B}_1^{lin} = b_1^{lin} \cos \omega t \, \hat{x} \tag{3.15}$$

There is additional time dependence in the amplitude b_1^{lin} representing the need to turn the field on and off. For the present, however, we ignore such time dependence, since, in practice, b_1^{lin} varies only over times much larger than the rf laboratory period $2\pi/\omega$.

The usefulness of a rotating reference frame in the analysis of the static field is incentive to consider such frames for the combined static plus rf fields. The motivation can be made more compelling by the following picture: Imagine a spin precessing at a small angle around the static field direction. To tip this spin down to a larger angle, an additional field should be synchronized to push the spin down at a given position every time the spin comes back around in its precession to this same position. (This is much like timing the pushing of a child on a swing; it serves as a useful analog here and for the resonance condition discussed in the next section.) In the reference frame language, it is necessary to have some transverse component of the B_1 field at rest (constant), or nearly so, in the rotating reference frame.

Let us in fact define the rotating reference frame using the laboratory frequency ω of the rf field, instead of ω_0.[5] Take the primed frame to be that frame undergoing negative (clockwise) rotation, with respect to the laboratory frame, around the z-axis with angular frequency ω. The corresponding angular velocity is

$$\vec{\Omega} = -\omega \hat{z} \tag{3.16}$$

The unit vector $\hat{x}'$ rotates clockwise, with time, in the negative ϕ direction.

$$\hat{x}' = \hat{x} \cos \omega t - \hat{y} \sin \omega t = R_z(\omega t)\hat{x} \tag{3.17}$$

assuming $\hat{x}'(0) = \hat{x}(0)$. Similarly,

$$\hat{y}' = \hat{x} \sin \omega t + \hat{y} \cos \omega t = R_z(\omega t)\hat{y} \tag{3.18}$$

The $\vec{B}_1$ field can be expressed in terms of the primed basis. The inversion of (3.17) and (3.18) is

$$\hat{x} = \hat{x}' \cos \omega t + \hat{y}' \sin \omega t = R_z(-\omega t)\hat{x}' \tag{3.19}$$

$$\hat{y} = -\hat{x}' \sin \omega t + \hat{y}' \cos \omega t = R_z(-\omega t)\hat{y}' \tag{3.20}$$

equivalent, as noted, to the rotation of the primed unit vectors by $R_z(-\omega t)$ in the positive ϕ-direction. From double-angle trigonometric formulas, (3.15) and (3.19) lead to

$$\vec{B}_1^{lin} = \frac{1}{2} b_1^{lin} [\hat{x}'(1 + \cos 2\omega t) + \hat{y}' \sin 2\omega t] \tag{3.21}$$

---

[4]In most electromagnetic discussions, polarization refers to the electric field direction.

[5]This is more natural. The Larmor frequency changes from particle species to species, and it varies with the magnetic field strength. The frequency ω, on the other hand, is under experimental control.

Equation (3.21) displays a constant term plus two oscillating terms whose effects average to zero over times that are half multiples of the rf period or, more relevantly, for all times large compared to the rf period. The definition for an average over a time interval T is given by

$$< f(t) > \equiv \frac{1}{T} \int_0^T dt \, f(t) \tag{3.22}$$

With the details left as a problem for the reader, the primed-frame time averaged value of (3.21) is

$$< \vec{B}_1^{lin} >_{\text{primed}} = \frac{1}{2} b_1^{lin} \hat{x}' \tag{3.23}$$

for constant b_1^{lin}.

Problem 3.2

Show that the average (3.22) over time interval T for $f(t) = \sin(n\omega t)$ or $f(t) = \cos(n\omega t)$ for any positive integer n is zero when

    a) $T = 2m\pi/\omega$ for any positive integer m (or $T = m\pi/\omega$ for even n)

or when the following limit is taken

    b) $T \gg 2\pi/\omega$

The reduced amplitude $\frac{1}{2} b_1^{lin}$ in (3.23) is noteworthy. *It implies that only half of the original linearly polarized field (3.15) amplitude is available in the rotating reference frame for tipping the spin.* Also, (3.23) is still valid for a time dependent $b_1^{lin}(t)$, provided it changes only over time scales much larger than the rf period $2\pi/\omega$. It has been noted earlier that such scales are consistent with MR applications. In that case, $b_1^{lin}(t)$ can be considered to be a constant in the integration for time averaging.

3.2.2 Quadrature

We can construct an efficient rf field where the original laboratory amplitude is the same as the amplitude in the rotating reference frame. A 'left-circularly polarized' rf field that is constant in the rotating frame defined by (3.16) is obtained by a superposition. Adding two linearly polarized rf fields with the same frequency and peak amplitude, but perpendicular to each other and 90° out of phase (with respect to time dependence), gives

$$\vec{B}_1^{cir} = B_1(\hat{x} \cos \omega t - \hat{y} \sin \omega t) \tag{3.24}$$

The combination of unit vectors in (3.24) is nothing other than $\hat{x}'$, so that equivalently

$$\vec{B}_1^{cir} = B_1 \hat{x}' \tag{3.25}$$

It is obvious that the field (3.25) is 'at rest' in the frame (3.16). Importantly, the (generally time dependent) amplitude $B_1(t)$ is the full rotating frame amplitude available for spin flipping. In the discussion of Ch. 27, it will be seen that less power is required from the rf coil amplifier to produce a given spin flip with left-circularly polarized fields than with linearly polarized fields. This advantage is related to the factor of one-half found in (3.23). The 90° phase difference between the x and y coordinates of the laboratory field (3.24) has led to calling (3.25) a 'quadrature' field. Because of the power advantage, and other factors concerning signal-to-noise and the need for rf spatial homogeneity, such rotating fields are commonly used in MR.

3.3   Resonance Condition and the RF Pulse

The equation of motion (3.13) in the rotating reference frame for a spin immersed in the combination of the constant field $\vec{B}_0 = B_0\hat{z}$ and the left-circularly polarized field (3.25) is

$$
\begin{aligned}
\left(\frac{d\vec{\mu}}{dt}\right)' &= \vec{\mu} \times [\hat{z}'(\omega_0 - \omega) + \hat{x}'\omega_1] \\
&= \gamma\vec{\mu} \times \vec{B}_{eff}
\end{aligned} \tag{3.26}
$$

setting $\hat{z}' = \hat{z}$ for the rotation (3.16). Appearing in (3.26) are the Larmor frequency $\omega_0 \equiv \gamma B_0$, the rf laboratory frequency ω, and the spin-precession frequency ω_1 generated by the circularly polarized rf field (3.24),

$$
\omega_1 \equiv \gamma B_1 \tag{3.27}
$$

The effective magnetic field is

$$
\vec{B}_{eff} \equiv [\hat{z}'(\omega_0 - \omega) + \hat{x}'\omega_1]/\gamma \tag{3.28}
$$

Equation (3.26) in the primed coordinates is an important result. In general, it states that there is left-handed (clockwise) precession in the primed frame around the axis defined by $\vec{B}_{eff}$. Leaving a more general precession discussion to Sec. 3.3.4, we focus now on a special rotating reference frame, where the applied rf frequency ω matches the Larmor frequency ω_0. The first term is then eliminated in (3.28), leading to *the cornerstone equation of motion*

$$
\left(\frac{d\vec{\mu}}{dt}\right)' = \omega_1\vec{\mu} \times \hat{x}' \qquad (\text{when } \omega = \omega_0) \tag{3.29}
$$

There is then only a precession about the $\hat{x}'$ axis with the precessional frequency ω_1 given in (3.29). The stipulation for a given static uniform field B_0 is that

$$
\omega = \omega_0 \qquad (\text{on-resonance condition}) \tag{3.30}
$$

the origin of the 'resonance' reference in the acronyms NMR and MRI. Under this condition, the B_1 field is maximally synchronized to tip the spin around the x'-axis.

3.3.1 Flip-Angle Formula and Illustration

A B_1 field applied on-resonance for a finite time is called an 'rf pulse.' Suppose the rf field is turned on (quickly) to a constant value $B_1\hat{x}'$ for a time interval τ and then it is just as rapidly turned off. From the precession lessons of Ch. 2 (or from the explicit solutions of the next subsection), (3.29) implies that the spin rotates through the angle

$$\Delta\theta = \gamma B_1 \tau \qquad (3.31)$$

around $\hat{x}'$. For example, the size of B_1 required for a $90°$ flip angle over $1.0\,\mathrm{ms}$ is $5.9\,\mu\,\mathrm{T}$ ($0.059\,\mathrm{G}$) for protons. Despite the simplicity, this computation is given as a problem, in view of its importance to MR analysis.

An illustration of various spin trajectories is helpful in highlighting the effectiveness of being on-resonance for tipping spins. Trajectories in the primed and unprimed frames for both off-resonance and on-resonance conditions are shown in Fig. 3.3. The pictures are generated from the solutions of Sec. 2.3 which are easily adapted to a constant $B_1\hat{x}'$ in the rotating frame. (See the following subsection for both constant and time dependent adaptations.) The pure on-resonance rotation about the x' axis is observed in Fig. 3.3a. The corresponding spiraling down found in the laboratory is shown in Fig. 3.3b. The off-resonance motion in the primed frame (Fig. 3.3c) shows the expected precession about the total field. In Fig. 3.3d, the laboratory picture is that of a superposition of this precession on top of the rotation of the primed frame. On-resonance, even a weak rf field would readily rotate the spin down into the transverse plane. By contrast, the farther off-resonance a spin

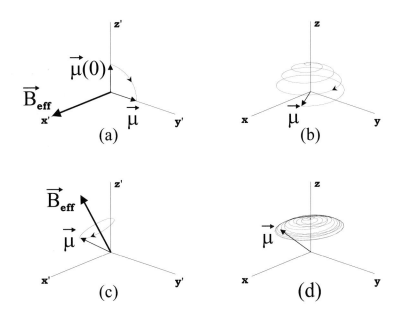

Fig. 3.3: An on-resonance $\pi/2$ spin flip as viewed in the primed (a) and unprimed (b) frames for $\omega = \omega_0$ and $\omega_1 = 0.06\,\omega_0$. An off-resonance trajectory as viewed in the primed (c) and unprimed (d) frames corresponds to the offset value, $\omega = 0.85\,\omega_0$, with $\omega_1 = 0.06\,\omega_0$. In MR applications, the frequency ω_1 would be much smaller in relation to the rf frequency, but the spiraling would then be much too dense to illustrate. See Prob. 3.3.

becomes, the closer the effective field is to the static field, and the less the spin is tipped from the vertical.

Problem 3.3

In many MR experiments it is necessary to flip a spin, which is initially along the z-axis, into the x'-y' plane by using an appropriate rf pulse. This is referred to as a '90°' or '$\pi/2$' pulse. If the desired rf pulse time interval is 1.0 ms, what B_1 magnitude in μT (1 T = 10,000 G) is required for

  a) a proton spin? (answer given above)

  b) an electron spin? (See (2.22).)

  c) How many Larmor precession cycles take place in the laboratory frame, for $B_0 = 1.0$ T, during the $\pi/2$ flip of the proton spin in (a)? See Fig. 3.3.

3.3.2   RF Solutions

The fact that the magnetic resonance effect is more easily understood in the corresponding rotating reference frame is also reflected by the manner in which an analytical solution is found for the motion of the magnetic moment. In the rotating frame, let the rf field be constant along $\hat{x}'$,

$$\vec{B}_1 = B_1 \hat{x}' \tag{3.32}$$

The total effective field (3.28) on-resonance is thus given by (3.32). The magnetic moment vector motion is found by transcribing the solution (2.33) according to the substitutions $z \to x'$, $y \to z'$, $x \to y'$

$$
\begin{aligned}
\mu_{x'}(t) &= \mu_{x'}(0) \\
\mu_{y'}(t) &= \mu_{y'}(0)\cos\phi_1(t) + \mu_{z'}(0)\sin\phi_1(t) \\
\mu_{z'}(t) &= -\mu_{y'}(0)\sin\phi_1(t) + \mu_{z'}(0)\cos\phi_1(t)
\end{aligned}
\tag{3.33}
$$

with

$$\phi_1(t) = \omega_1 t \tag{3.34}$$

in terms of the precession frequency, $\omega_1 \equiv \gamma B_1$, and the rotating frame components of the initial vector value, $\vec{\mu}(0)$. The solution may be rewritten as a rotation matrix operation.

$$\vec{\mu}(t) = R_{x'}(\phi_1(t))\vec{\mu}(0) \tag{3.35}$$

using

$$
R_{x'}(\theta) = \begin{pmatrix} 1 & 0 & 0 \\ 0 & \cos\theta & \sin\theta \\ 0 & -\sin\theta & \cos\theta \end{pmatrix}
\tag{3.36}
$$

The general time-dependent case (with arbitrary initial time t_0) is solved by the substitution $\phi_1 \to \phi_1(t)$ and $\vec{\mu}(0) \to \vec{\mu}(t_0)$ where

$$\phi_1(t) = \int_{t_0}^{t} dt' \omega_1(t') \tag{3.37}$$

in which

$$\omega_1(t) = \gamma B_1(t) \tag{3.38}$$

This is required for rf pulses of finite time duration and more general temporal envelopes. A sequence of such rf pulses can be modeled by products of rotations. For example, the (clockwise) rotation through an angle θ_1 around $\hat{x}'$ (due to the application of (3.32) for a finite time interval) followed by the rotation through θ_2 around $\hat{y}'$ (applying $B_{1y'}(t)\hat{y}'$ for some later, non-overlapping, time interval) yields

$$\vec{\mu}(t) = R_{y'}(\theta_2) R_{x'}(\theta_1) \vec{\mu}(t_0) \tag{3.39}$$

with

$$R_{y'}(\theta) = \begin{pmatrix} \cos\theta & 0 & -\sin\theta \\ 0 & 1 & 0 \\ \sin\theta & 0 & \cos\theta \end{pmatrix} \tag{3.40}$$

Problem 3.4

A static field points uniformly along the positive z-axis. A classical spinning particle, with positive gyromagnetic ratio γ and fixed magnetic moment magnitude μ, has its spin initially in the direction of the static field. A circularly polarized rf field points along the $\hat{y}'$ axis with time-dependent amplitude $B_{1y'}(t)$ (e.g., the rf field may be turned off at a later time) applied on-resonance starting at $t = 0$.

a) Give expressions analogous to (3.33) for all three magnetic-moment vector components in the rotating (prime) reference frame for time $t > 0$. Your answer will be in terms of a definite integral.

b) Show that the equation of motion (2.24) is satisfied by your answers in (a) for $\vec{B} \to B_{1y'}\hat{y}'$.

c) Find the generalization of (2.35) needed for this time-dependent case.

3.3.3 Different Polarization Bases

In going from a linearly polarized rf field to a circularly polarized rf field, it is natural to replace the 2D Cartesian basis ($\hat{x}$ and $\hat{y}$, say) by a complete basis made up of the left-circular (or left-circulating) unit vector

$$\hat{x}^{left} = \hat{x} \cos\omega t - \hat{y} \sin\omega t = \hat{x}' \tag{3.41}$$

and the right-circular (right-circulating) unit vector

$$\hat{x}^{right} = \hat{x}\,\cos\omega t + \hat{y}\,\sin\omega t \tag{3.42}$$

It has been seen that the rf field $\vec{B}_1^{left} \propto \hat{x}^{left}$ is maximally effective in tipping the spin around the x'-axis. A right-circularly polarized field $\vec{B}_1^{right} \propto \hat{x}^{right}$ is completely ineffective, according to the problem which follows. The right-circular field would be appropriate, on the other hand, for a reference frame rotating in right-handed fashion (counterclockwise) with frequency ω about the z-axis.

Problem 3.5

Show that

$$\hat{x}^{right} = \hat{x}'\,\cos 2\omega t + \hat{y}'\,\sin 2\omega t \tag{3.43}$$

using steps like those used in deriving (3.21). Its time average is clearly zero.

Another basis of much importance to MR is the complex representation of vectors in the transverse plane (cf. Sec. 2.3.5). Recall that in this basis the real part is the x-component and the imaginary part is the y-component. In terms of a given amplitude B_1, left-handed and right-handed rf fields can be written, respectively, as

$$B_1^{left} \equiv B_1^L \tag{3.44}$$

$$B_1^{right} \equiv B_1^R \tag{3.45}$$

where the clockwise (left-handed or 'negative') component is

$$B_1^L = B_1 e^{-i\omega t} \tag{3.46}$$

and the counterclockwise (right-handed or 'positive') component is

$$B_1^R = B_1 e^{i\omega t} \tag{3.47}$$

Only the former component (3.46) is effective, on-resonance, in tipping spins.

The linear (along x) rf field (3.15) can be rewritten as

$$B_1^{lin} = B_1^L + B_1^R = 2B_1 \cos\omega t \tag{3.48}$$

provided the identification is made that

$$B_1 = \frac{1}{2}b_1^{lin} \tag{3.49}$$

It is verified that only half of the original amplitude is present in the left-handed component in (3.48). A linear field must have a peak amplitude of $2B_1$ in order to have a weighting of B_1 in its left-handed component.

3.3.4 Laboratory Angle of Precession

A return to the general picture in the rotating reference frame, on- or off-resonance, can be made through the effective field (3.14). (Recall that ω is the rf frequency and $\omega_0 = \gamma B_0$ and they are not necessarily equal in this discussion.) For the combined static and rf fields,

$$\vec{B}_{eff} = (B_0 - \frac{\omega}{\gamma})\hat{z} + B_1\hat{x}' \tag{3.50}$$

rewriting (3.28). If the angle between $\vec{B}_{eff}$ and $\vec{B}_0$ is defined to be θ (Fig. 3.4),

$$\cos\theta = \frac{B_0 - \omega/\gamma}{B_{eff}} = \frac{\omega_0 - \omega}{\omega_{eff}} \tag{3.51}$$

$$\sin\theta = \frac{\omega_1}{\omega_{eff}} \tag{3.52}$$

where

$$\omega_{eff} = \gamma B_{eff} = \gamma\sqrt{(B_0 - \omega/\gamma)^2 + B_1^2} = \sqrt{(\omega_0 - \omega)^2 + \omega_1^2} \tag{3.53}$$

The equation of motion (3.26) dictates that, for constant ω_0 and ω_1, the magnetic moment precesses around $\vec{B}_{eff}$ in the rotating reference frame with frequency ω_{eff}, as exemplified in Fig. 3.4 (see also Fig. 3.3). This precession incorporates the primary lessons of both the present and previous chapters.

The angle α between the spin magnetic moment $\vec{\mu}$ and the static field direction $\hat{z}$ shown in Fig. 3.4 is the subject of the next problem. There the request is to show that

$$\cos\alpha(t) = \cos^2\theta + \cos\omega_{eff}t\,\sin^2\theta = 1 - 2\sin^2\theta\,\sin^2\frac{\omega_{eff}t}{2} \tag{3.54}$$

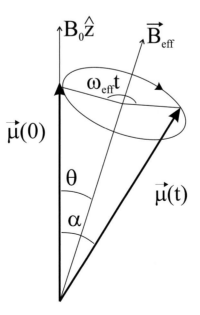

Fig. 3.4: The precession of a magnetic moment around the effective magnetic field in the rotating reference frame.

The expression (3.54) yields the behavior of the z-component of the magnetic moment as a function of time.

Problem 3.6

Let $\alpha(t)$ be the angle between $\vec{\mu}(0)$ and $\vec{\mu}(t)$ as shown in Fig. 3.4. Assume $\vec{\mu}(0)$ is parallel to the $\hat{z}$-direction. Show that $\cos\alpha(t)$, measuring the amount of magnetic moment, or spin, left along $\hat{z}$, is given in terms of θ and ω_{eff} by (3.54). Hint: Decompose $\vec{\mu}(t)$ into components parallel and perpendicular to $\vec{B}_{eff}$. Then project these components onto the z-axis.

Suggested Reading

A review of the relevant general concepts of rotation and precession in classical mechanics and NMR can be found in the following two texts:

- H. Goldstein. *Classical Mechanics: Pearson New International Edition.* Pearson, 3rd ed., London, 2014.

- C. P. Slichter. *Principles of Magnetic Resonance.* Springer Verlag, 3rd ed., New York, 2010.

The next article presents an outstanding discussion of NMR in rotating reference frames:

- I. I. Rabi, N. F. Ramsey and J. Schwinger. Rotating coordinates in magnetic resonance problems. *Rev. Modern Phys.*, 26: 167, 1954.

Chapter 4

Magnetization, Relaxation, and the Bloch Equation

Chapter Contents

Summary: The interactions of spins with their surroundings are modeled in the presence of external field effects by the phenomenological Bloch equation. The relaxation decay times T_1, T_2, T_2', and T_2^* are introduced. Solutions of the Bloch equation are given for constant and harmonic fields.

Introduction

Thus far, the response of an isolated proton's spin in an external magnetic field has been modeled by the classical equations of motion of a single magnetic moment. The interactions of the proton spin with its neighboring atoms lead to important modifications to this behavior. The local fields change the spin precession frequency, and the proton can exchange spin energy with the surroundings. In this chapter, we model these effects, as guided by experiment, after introducing the average magnetic dipole moment density ('magnetization').

4.1 Magnetization Vector

For images of a macroscopic body, we focus on protons, introducing their local magnetic moment per unit volume, or magnetization, as $\vec{M}(\vec{r}, t)$. Consider a volume element ('voxel') with volume V small enough that external fields are to a good approximation constant over V,[1] but big enough to contain a large number of protons. The magnetization as defined is the sum of the individual magnetic moments divided by the total volume

$$\vec{M} = \frac{1}{V} \sum_{i = \text{protons in V}} \vec{\mu}_i \qquad (4.1)$$

The set of spins in V is called a spin 'isochromat,' which can be defined to be an ensemble or domain of spins with the same phase. With the neglect of the proton interactions with their environment, a sum over the equations of motion for the individual spins (2.24) yields

$$\frac{1}{V} \sum_i \frac{d\vec{\mu}_i}{dt} = \frac{\gamma}{V} \sum_i \vec{\mu}_i \times \vec{B}_{ext} \qquad (4.2)$$

or

$$\frac{d\vec{M}}{dt} = \gamma \vec{M} \times \vec{B}_{ext} \qquad \text{(non-interacting protons)} \qquad (4.3)$$

It is most advantageous to analyze the magnetization, and its differential equation, in terms of parallel and perpendicular components defined relative to the static main magnetic field, $\vec{B}_{ext} = B_0 \hat{z}$. The parallel, or 'longitudinal' component of the magnetization is

$$M_\parallel = M_z \qquad (4.4)$$

The transverse components are

$$\vec{M}_\perp = M_x \hat{x} + M_y \hat{y} \qquad (4.5)$$

The corresponding components of the cross product in (4.3) lead to decoupled equations

$$\frac{dM_z}{dt} = 0 \qquad \text{(non-interacting protons)} \qquad (4.6)$$

and

$$\frac{d\vec{M}_\perp}{dt} = \gamma \vec{M}_\perp \times \vec{B}_{ext} \qquad \text{(non-interacting protons)} \qquad (4.7)$$

The modeling of the proton interactions with its neighborhood leads to additional terms in (4.6) and (4.7) which depend on decay parameters, and these parameters are different in the two equations. This difference is related to the fact that, in contrast to a given magnetic moment, the magnitude of the macroscopic magnetization is not fixed, since it is the vector sum of (many) proton spins. The components of $\vec{M}$ parallel and perpendicular to the external field 'relax' differently in the approach to their equilibrium values.

4.2 Spin-Lattice Interaction and Regrowth Solution

Equation (4.6) is certainly wrong for interacting protons, insomuch as their moments try to align with the external field through the exchange of energy with the surroundings. To understand the origin of the missing term, an energy argument is helpful.

---

[1]The external fields are assumed to vary spatially only over scales much larger than $V^{\frac{1}{3}}$.

The classical formula for the potential energy associated with a magnetic moment immersed in a magnetic field is (Appendix A)

$$U = -\vec{\mu} \cdot \vec{B} \tag{4.8}$$

This implies that the moment will tend to line up parallel to the field in order to reach its minimum energy state, if energy can be transferred away. Since the protons are considered to be in thermal contact with the lattice of nearby atoms, the thermal motion present in the lattice can account for any change in a given proton spin energy (4.8). In the quantum language developed in the next chapter, a spin can exchange a quantum of energy with the lattice.

The magnetization version of (4.8) is the potential energy density

$$U_M = -\vec{M} \cdot \vec{B} = -M_{\parallel} B_0 \tag{4.9}$$

involving only the longitudinal component of the magnetization. Although the transverse components can be ignored in discussing the energy, it follows that, as the longitudinal magnetization returns to its equilibrium value M_0, the transverse magnetization must vanish. (In fact, the transverse magnetization can vanish more quickly due to 'dephasing,' see the next section.) The equilibrium value relevant to room temperatures obeys Curie's law in its dependence on the absolute temperature T and the external field,

$$M_0 = C\frac{B_0}{T} \tag{4.10}$$

The constant C is derived in Ch. 6 for protons as well as for other particles with different spins.

It is helpful to preview some of the discussion in Ch. 6 with respect to (4.10). In the applications to MRI, (4.10) is very small compared to the maximum possible magnetization (which would be the product of the spin density times the individual spin magnetic moment). Since the proton spin energy (4.8) is tiny compared with the thermal energy scale kT (k is the Boltzmann's constant and T is in kelvin) at room temperature, there is only a minuscule energy advantage for a spin moment to be aligned with the magnetic field. In consequence, only a very small fraction (about five in one million for a field strength of 1.5 T) of parallel spins exceed anti-parallel spins for field strengths of interest. Fortunately, Avogadro's number is so large, that, for example, on the order of 10^{18} excess proton spins are aligned along a 0.5 T field in one mole of water (see Ch. 6). Hence the magnetization M_0 is still big enough to be measured.

Suppose the equilibrium magnetization of a body is disturbed (by, say, the temporary application of an rf pulse) from its equilibrium value. As a result of the continued presence of the static field, the magnetization returns to its equilibrium magnetization vector $M_0\hat{z}$. In the remainder of this section, the relaxation of the longitudinal component to M_0 is discussed, and, in the next section, the relaxation of the transverse components to zero is described.

Introduction of T_1

A constant interaction growth rate from the proton interactions with the lattice (see Ch. 6) implies that the rate of change of the longitudinal magnetization, $dM_z(t)/dt$, is proportional to the difference $M_0 - M_z$. The proportionality constant is empirically determined, and represents the inverse of the time scale of the growth rate. Equation (4.6) is replaced by[2]

$$\frac{dM_z}{dt} = \frac{1}{T_1}(M_0 - M_z) \qquad (\vec{B}_{ext} \parallel \hat{z}) \qquad (4.11)$$

where T_1 is the experimental 'spin-lattice relaxation time.' The relaxation parameter T_1 ranges from tens to thousands of milliseconds for protons in human tissue over the B_0 field strengths of interest (0.01 T and higher). Typical values for various tissues are shown in Table 4.1.

The solution of (4.11) can be found, for example, by the procedures outlined in Prob. 4.1. After the application of an rf pulse, the longitudinal magnetization displays an exponential form showing the evolution from the initial value, $M_z(0)$, to the equilibrium value, M_0:

$$M_z(t) = M_z(0)e^{-t/T_1} + M_0(1 - e^{-t/T_1}) \qquad (\vec{B}_{ext} \parallel \hat{z}) \qquad (4.12)$$

Tissue	T_1 (ms)	T_2 (ms)
gray matter (GM)	950	100
white matter (WM)	600	80
muscle	900	50
cerebrospinal fluid (CSF)	4500	2200
fat	250	60
blood[3]	1200	100–200[4]

Table 4.1: Representative values of relaxation parameters T_1 (see Sec. 4.2) and T_2 (see Sec. 4.3), in milliseconds, for hydrogen components of different human body tissues at $B_0 = 1.5$ T and 37 °C (human body temperature). These are only approximate values; see Ch. 22.

Problem 4.1

Derive (4.12) by solving the first-order differential equation (4.11). Hint: One method is to use an integrating factor. Another is simply to put the magnetization and time variables on the opposite sides of the equation and integrate.

We reiterate that this solution corresponds to the situation where $\vec{B} = B_0\hat{z}$ and M_0 is the equilibrium value.[5] The solution for an arbitrary starting point will be of value in multiple rf pulse experiments:

$$M_z(t) = M_z(t_0)e^{-(t-t_0)/T_1} + M_0(1 - e^{-(t-t_0)/T_1}) \qquad (\vec{B}_{ext} \parallel \hat{z}) \qquad (4.13)$$

---

[2]The absence of an explicit field dependence in the solution should not be misunderstood. It is only because of the external field that the longitudinal magnetization evolves to M_0.

[3]See Sec. 25.6.1.

[4]The higher value pertains to arterial blood and the lower value to venous blood.

[5]If the external field were not uniform, the solution would only refer to a given point in space. The dependence on $\vec{r}$ has been suppressed.

Problem 4.2

The key equation (4.12) can be used to investigate general questions. If unmagnetized material is placed in a region with a finite static field at $t = 0$ ($M_z(0) = 0$):

a) Find the time it takes, in units of T_1, for the longitudinal magnetization to reach 90% of M_0.

b) Find an approximate formula for $M_z(t)$ of this material in the limit that $t \ll T_1$. Use this formula to find the initial ($t = 0$) slope of $M_z(t)$, and compare the answer to the general formula indicated in Fig. 4.1, when $M_z(0) = 0$.

Equation (4.12) is the key to understanding the regrowth, after an initial disturbance, *of longitudinal magnetization.* Throughout the discussion in later chapters of this book, it is often necessary to determine how much longitudinal magnetization is available to be rotated back into the transverse plane by a given sequence of rf pulses. An illustration of the exponential regrowth for a given initial value is presented in Fig. 4.1a. The time scale for regrowth is seen to be determined by T_1.

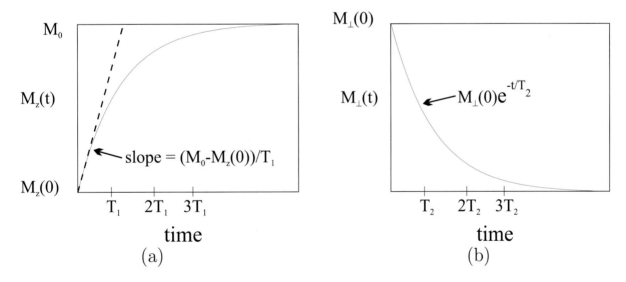

Fig. 4.1: (a) The regrowth of the longitudinal component of magnetization from the initial value $M_z(0)$ to the equilibrium value M_0. (b) The decay of the magnitude of the transverse magnetization from an initial value.

4.3 Spin-Spin Interaction and Transverse Decay

An important mechanism for the decay of the transverse magnetization is as follows. Spins experience local fields which are combinations of the applied field and the fields of their neighbors. Since variations in the local fields lead to different local precessional frequencies, the individual spins tend to fan out in time, as shown in Fig. 4.2, reducing the net magnetization vector. The 'fanning out' is usually referred to as 'dephasing.' The total transverse magnetization is the vector (or complex) sum of all the individual transverse components.

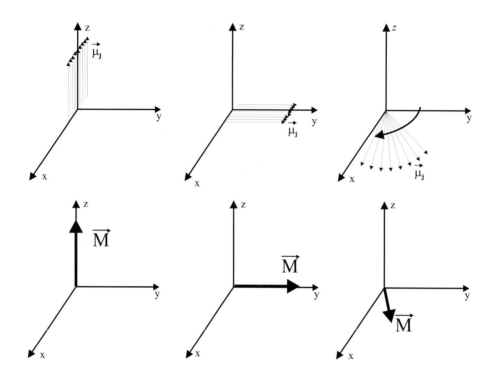

Fig. 4.2: The upper sequence shows a 90° tip of a set of spins (isochromats) into the transverse plane such that they all lie along the y-axis (laboratory frame) at some instant in time, as shown in the middle figure. Precession of the individual spins in the x-y plane immediately follows (the recovery of longitudinal magnetization is ignored since the focus is on transverse magnetization dephasing effects). The lower sequence shows the same process in terms of the net transverse magnetization which decreases in magnitude during the precession because of the fanning out of the spins.

Introduction of T_2

The characterization of the overall rate of reduction in transverse magnetization brings forth another experimental parameter, the 'spin-spin' relaxation time T_2. The differential equation (4.7) is changed by the addition of a decay rate term

$$\frac{d\vec{M}_\perp}{dt} = \gamma \vec{M}_\perp \times \vec{B}_{ext} - \frac{1}{T_2}\vec{M}_\perp \tag{4.14}$$

The additional term leads to exponential decay of any initial value for $\vec{M}_\perp$. This is most easily seen in the rotating reference frame, where the differential equation has a standard decay-rate form[6]

$$\left(\frac{d\vec{M}_\perp}{dt}\right)' = -\frac{1}{T_2}\vec{M}_\perp \qquad \text{(rotating frame)} \qquad (4.15)$$

with the solution

$$\vec{M}_\perp(t) = \vec{M}_\perp(0)e^{-t/T_2} \qquad \text{(rotating frame)} \qquad (4.16)$$

Equation (4.16) describes the exponential decay of the magnitude $M_\perp \equiv |\vec{M}_\perp|$ of the transverse magnetization in either the laboratory or the rotating reference frame. A sample curve for the decay is displayed in Fig. 4.1b.

Owing to the fact that the 'spin-spin' interactions include the collective dephasing effect, where no energy is lost, as well as the same spin-lattice couplings giving rise to T_1 effects, (4.14) corresponds to a higher relaxation rate than (4.11). Define the relaxation rates by

$$R_1 \equiv 1/T_1 \qquad \text{and} \qquad R_2 \equiv 1/T_2 \qquad (4.17)$$

Then

$$R_2 > R_1 \qquad \text{or} \qquad T_2 < T_1 \qquad (4.18)$$

The relaxation parameter T_2 is on the order of tens of milliseconds for protons in most human tissue (see Table 4.1 for a variety of T_2 tissue values). It is approximately constant over the B_0 range of interest for a given tissue. The values of T_2 are much shorter for solids (on the order of microseconds) and much longer for liquids (on the order of seconds).

Introduction of T_2^* and T_2'

In practice, there is an additional dephasing of the magnetization introduced by external field inhomogeneities. This reduction in an initial value of $\vec{M}_\perp$ can sometimes be characterized by a separate decay time T_2'.[7] The total relaxation rate, defined as R_2^*, is the sum of the internal and external relaxation rates ($R_2' \equiv 1/T_2'$)

$$R_2^* = R_2 + R_2' \qquad (4.19)$$

In terms of an overall relaxation time $T_2^* \equiv 1/R_2^*$,

$$\frac{1}{T_2^*} = \frac{1}{T_2} + \frac{1}{T_2'} \qquad (4.20)$$

As we shall see later, the loss of transverse magnetization due to T_2' is 'recoverable.' To the extent that T_2' effects dominate the 'fan out' shown in Fig. 4.2, an additional pulse can be designed so as to lead to a rephasing of the spins, a reversal of the dephasing caused by the external field inhomogeneities. It is possible to recover their initial phase relationship corresponding to the initial value of $\vec{M}_\perp$. Referred to as 'creating an echo,' this process will be described in detail in Ch. 8. The intrinsic T_2 losses are not recoverable; they are related to local, random, time-dependent field variations.

---

[6]Recall from Ch. 3 that there is no need to distinguish between $\vec{M}$ and $\vec{M}'$.

[7]There is no guarantee that local field inhomogeneities lead to an exponential signal decay, but they are assumed to do so in this discussion.

4.4   Bloch Equation and Static-Field Solutions

The differential equations (4.11) and (4.14) for magnetization in the presence of a magnetic field and with relaxation terms can be combined into one vector equation,

$$\frac{d\vec{M}}{dt} = \gamma \vec{M} \times \vec{B}_{ext} + \frac{1}{T_1}(M_0 - M_z)\hat{z} - \frac{1}{T_2}\vec{M}_\perp \qquad (4.21)$$

This empirical vector equation is referred to as the Bloch equation. The relaxation terms describe the return to equilibrium, but only for a field pointing along the z-axis. The quantum mechanical underpinnings of the Bloch equation are described in Chs. 5 and 6.

Let us solve the Bloch equation for the constant field case, $\vec{B}_{ext} = B_0\hat{z}$. A calculation of the components of the cross product in (4.21) produces the three component equations

$$\frac{dM_z}{dt} = \frac{M_0 - M_z}{T_1} \qquad (4.22)$$

$$\frac{dM_x}{dt} = \omega_0 M_y - \frac{M_x}{T_2} \qquad (4.23)$$

$$\frac{dM_y}{dt} = -\omega_0 M_x - \frac{M_y}{T_2} \qquad (4.24)$$

where $\omega_0 \equiv \gamma B_0$. The first equation is the same as (4.11) whose solution is (4.12). For the last two equations, the relaxation terms can be easily eliminated by the change of variables, $M_x = m_x e^{-t/T_2}$ and $M_y = m_y e^{-t/T_2}$ (i.e., by the introduction of integrating factors). The resulting differential equations for m_x and m_y have exactly the form of the equations found, and solved, for μ_x and μ_y in Ch. 2.[8] In terms of the original variables, the complete set of solutions is therefore

$$M_x(t) = e^{-t/T_2}\left(M_x(0)\cos\omega_0 t + M_y(0)\sin\omega_0 t\right) \qquad (4.25)$$

$$M_y(t) = e^{-t/T_2}\left(M_y(0)\cos\omega_0 t - M_x(0)\sin\omega_0 t\right) \qquad (4.26)$$

$$M_z(t) = M_z(0)e^{-t/T_1} + M_0(1 - e^{-t/T_1}) \qquad (4.27)$$

The equilibrium or steady-state solution can be found from the asymptotic limit $t \to \infty$ of (4.25)–(4.27). In that limit, all the exponentials vanish implying the steady-state solution

$$M_x(\infty) = M_y(\infty) = 0, \quad M_z(\infty) = M_0 \qquad (4.28)$$

The general time-dependent solution for the transverse components, (4.25) and (4.26), is seen to have sinusoidal terms modified by a decay factor. The sinusoidal terms correspond to the precessional motion discussed in Ch. 2, and the damping factor comes from the transverse relaxation effect. The magnitude $|\vec{M}|$ is not fixed: The longitudinal component relaxes from its initial value to the equilibrium value M_0; the transverse component rotates clockwise and it decreases in magnitude. Recall that the transverse decay time T_2 is in general different from (smaller than) the longitudinal decay time T_1. An example of the resulting left-handed 'corkscrew' trajectory for an initial magnetization lying in the transverse plane is illustrated in Fig. 4.3.

---

[8]See, in particular, Prob. 2.6.

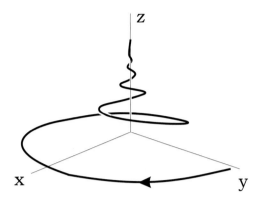

Fig. 4.3: The trajectory of the tip of the magnetization vector showing the combined regrowth of the longitudinal magnetization and decay of the transverse components. The initial value was along the y-axis and the reference frame is the laboratory.

Problem 4.3

A direct derivation of the steady-state solution, when it exists, of a system of differential equations can often be found by the following procedure. Assuming that the system evolves to constant values for large times, all time derivatives can be set to zero. The problem reduces to a system that can often be solved analytically. Use this procedure to find the steady-state solution directly from (4.22), (4.23), and (4.24), verifying (4.28).

Phase Description

The general solutions could also be simplified[9] in their description by employing the complex representation of Sec. 2.3.5

$$M_+(t) \equiv M_x(t) + iM_y(t) \tag{4.29}$$

With the details left to the next problem, the solution for a static field in this representation is

$$M_+(t) = e^{-i\omega_0 t - t/T_2} M_+(0) \tag{4.30}$$

As a follow-up on the remarks of Sec. 2.3.5 about the phase of a single moment, *the phase of the complex representation of the magnetization in solutions like (4.30) plays a key role in characterizing imaging signals.* The generalization of (2.41) is

$$M_+(t) = |M_+(t)|e^{i\phi(t)} = M_\perp(t)e^{i\phi(t)} \tag{4.31}$$

noting that the magnitude of the complex magnetization (4.29) is the same as the magnitude $M_\perp$ of the transverse vector (4.5). For the static-field solution,

$$M_\perp(t) = e^{-t/T_2} M_\perp(0) \tag{4.32}$$

---

[9]The solutions may also be described in terms of the rotation matrices introduced in Ch. 2.

and

$$\phi(t) = -\omega_0 t + \phi(0) \tag{4.33}$$

In addition, the phase is often given with reference to rotating frames where, for the static-field case in the Larmor rotating frame, it becomes a constant, $\phi = \phi(0)$.

Problem 4.4

---

a) Find the differential equation for $M_+(t)$ analogous to (2.40) and show that its solution is (4.30).

b) Show that (4.30) is equivalent to (4.25) and (4.26).

c) Repeat (a) for

$$M_- \equiv M_x - iM_y = -i(M_y + iM_x) \tag{4.34}$$

4.5   The Combination of Static and RF Fields

An rf field needs to be added to the static field in order to tip $\vec{M}$ from its equilibrium direction. The precession of the resulting transverse component of magnetization produces its own (rotating) field, which can be detected with a nearby coil (see Ch. 7). The analysis of the resulting motion is done expeditiously, as we have shown in Ch. 3, in rotating reference frames.

4.5.1   Bloch Equation for $\vec{B}_{ext} = B_0\hat{z} + B_1\hat{x}'$

Following Sec. 3.3.3, we add a left-circularly polarized rf field $\vec{B}_1$ which is at rest in the rotating frame and parallel to $\hat{x}'$ (see Ch. 3). The total external field is

$$\vec{B}_{ext} = B_0\hat{z} + B_1\hat{x}' \tag{4.35}$$

The effective field in that frame is

$$\vec{B}_{eff} = (B_0 - \frac{\omega}{\gamma})\hat{z} + B_1\hat{x}' \tag{4.36}$$

For the addition of an rf field $\vec{B}_1$ to the Bloch equation,[10] it is supposed that there still exists a z-component equilibrium value M_0, and decay constants T_1 and T_2. The reader is asked to show that the corresponding rectangular vector components of the Bloch equation *in the primed coordinates* are

$$\left(\frac{dM_z}{dt}\right)' = -\omega_1 M_{y'} + \frac{M_0 - M_z}{T_1} \tag{4.37}$$

---

[10]For many imaging applications, the magnitude of the rf field is much smaller than B_0 and, moreover, the rf field is turned off for a large fraction of the time.

$$\left(\frac{dM_{x'}}{dt}\right)' = \Delta\omega\, M_{y'} - \frac{M_{x'}}{T_2} \tag{4.38}$$

$$\left(\frac{dM_{y'}}{dt}\right)' = -\Delta\omega\, M_{x'} + \omega_1 M_z - \frac{M_{y'}}{T_2} \tag{4.39}$$

with

$$\Delta\omega \equiv \omega_0 - \omega \tag{4.40}$$

We are reminded that ω_0 is the Larmor frequency, ω_1 is the spin frequency due to the rf field, and ω is the rf laboratory frequency of oscillation. The $\Delta\omega$ terms in the above equations are 'off-resonance' contributions. They may represent deviations from ideal conditions due to static field impurities or variations in the applied rf frequency.

Problem 4.5

Taking note of (3.26), demonstrate that in the primed basis (4.21) reduces to (4.37)–(4.39).

The above differential equations contain frequency terms, which combine to produce an instantaneous rotation about an effective field, and decay constant terms. On-resonance $(\omega = \omega_0)$ precession (with frequency $\omega_1 = \gamma B_1$) around $\vec{B}_1$ of the components transverse to $\hat{x}'$ is evidently superimposed on the relaxation decay in (4.37) and (4.39). In the original unprimed frame, this is a nutation superimposed on the decay.

4.5.2   Short-Lived RF Pulses

The rf pulses in most MR measurements are designed to have a very short time duration, τ_{rf}, and, consistent with the correspondingly large bandwidth, the typical values for ω_1 are much greater than the decay rates $1/T_1$ and $1/T_2$. Therefore the differential equations (4.37)–(4.39) can be simplified both when the rf pulse is turned on and when it is turned off.

When the rf pulse is turned on for short times, the relaxation terms can be ignored relative to the frequency terms. Upon the replacement $\vec{M} \to \vec{\mu}$, the resulting equations are identical to (3.26) for which the solutions have already been found.

When the rf pulse is considered to be turned off, $(\omega_1 = 0)$, the Bloch equations are just what was solved in the previous section, aside from a transformation to the rf rotating reference frame. Upon the replacement $\omega_0 \to \Delta\omega$ in (4.25)–(4.27), the motion in the rotating frame is described by

$$M_{x'}(t) = e^{-t/T_2}\left(M_{x'}(0)\cos\Delta\omega t + M_{y'}(0)\sin\Delta\omega t\right) \tag{4.41}$$

$$M_{y'}(t) = e^{-t/T_2}\left(M_{y'}(0)\cos\Delta\omega t - M_{x'}(0)\sin\Delta\omega t\right) \tag{4.42}$$

$$M_z(t) = M_z(0)e^{-t/T_1} + M_0(1 - e^{-t/T_1}) \tag{4.43}$$

4.5.3   Long-Lived RF Pulses

The rf field is kept on for a relatively long time in some applications. The sample is then said to be 'saturated' and the long-term behavior of the magnetization can be described by steady-state solutions.

Steady State

To find the steady-state solutions, all time derivatives are set equal to zero in (4.37)–(4.39). We shall first derive them in the limit, $\omega_1 = 0$. In this limit, the steady-state solution is easily seen to be

$$M_z^{ss} = M_0, \quad M_{x'}^{ss} = M_{y'}^{ss} = 0 \tag{4.44}$$

The above zeroth-order (in ω_1) solution implies that as $\omega_1 \to 0$ the transverse magnetization components must vanish. Hence, for small but nonzero ω_1, $M_{x'}$ and $M_{y'}$ must be $\mathcal{O}(\omega_1)$ (i.e., at most first-order in ω_1).[11] Therefore, from (4.37) we find $M_0 - M_z = \mathcal{O}(\omega_1^2)$. Then, correct in first-order ω_1, the steady-state solution must satisfy

$$M_z^{ss} = M_0 \tag{4.45}$$

$$M_{y'}^{ss}\Delta\omega - \frac{1}{T_2}M_{x'}^{ss} = 0 \tag{4.46}$$

$$M_{x'}^{ss}\Delta\omega + \frac{1}{T_2}M_{y'}^{ss} = M_0\omega_1 \tag{4.47}$$

The solutions of (4.46) and (4.47) are

$$M_{x'}^{ss} = M_0\frac{\Delta\omega\, T_2}{1 + (\Delta\omega\, T_2)^2}\omega_1 T_2 \tag{4.48}$$

$$M_{y'}^{ss} = M_0\frac{1}{1 + (\Delta\omega\, T_2)^2}\omega_1 T_2 \tag{4.49}$$

correct to $\mathcal{O}(\omega_1^2)$. The general-order solutions are treated in a problem.

Problem 4.6

Return to the Bloch equations (4.37)–(4.39) and solve them in the steady state for arbitrary B_1, obtaining

$$M_{x'}^{ss} = M_0\frac{\Delta\omega\, T_2}{D}\omega_1 T_2 \tag{4.50}$$

$$M_{y'}^{ss} = M_0\frac{1}{D}\omega_1 T_2 \tag{4.51}$$

$$M_z^{ss} = M_0\frac{1 + (\Delta\omega\, T_2)^2}{D} \tag{4.52}$$

---

[11] $\mathcal{O}(x^n)$ means that the terms vanish at least as fast as x^n as $x \to 0$. In the Taylor series for a function $f(x)$, $f(x) = f(0) + xf'(0) + x^2 f''(0)/2 + \ldots$, the first term is $\mathcal{O}(1)$, the second is $\mathcal{O}(x)$, the third is $\mathcal{O}(x^2)$, and so forth.

with

$$D = 1 + (\Delta\omega\, T_2)^2 + \omega_1^2 T_1 T_2 \qquad (4.53)$$

Notice that these reduce to (4.48), (4.49), and (4.45), respectively, for small ω_1. In particular, show that $M_{x'}^{ss}$ and $M_{y'}^{ss}$ are $\mathcal{O}(\omega_1)$ and that $M_0 - M_z^{ss} = \mathcal{O}(\omega_1^2)$, consistent with the previous discussion. Also, show that the steady-state magnetization develops a phase shift in the x'-y' plane

$$\Delta\phi = \cot^{-1}(\Delta\omega T_2) \qquad (\text{mod } \pi) \qquad (4.54)$$

Suggested Reading

The basic concepts of NMR appear in the following early papers:

- F. A. Bloch. Nuclear induction. *Phys. Rev.*, 70: 460, 1946.

- F. A. Bloch, W. W. Hansen and M. Packard. Nuclear induction. *Phys. Rev.*, 69: 127, 1946.

- F. A. Bloch, W. W. Hansen and M. Packard. The nuclear induction experiment. *Phys. Rev.*, 70: 474, 1946.

- E. M. Purcell, H. C. Torrey and R. V. Pound. Resonance absorption by nuclear magnetic moments in a solid. *Phys. Rev.*, 69: 37, 1946.

Chapter 5

The Quantum Mechanical Basis of Precession and Excitation

Chapter Contents

Summary: The history of the quantization of spin is briefly reviewed. A derivation of precession in a constant field is presented in the context of quantum mechanics. A quantum mechanical derivation of the action of an rf field is also derived. This chapter and the following one (Ch. 6) could be omitted in a first MRI study.

Introduction

In quantum mechanics, the wave nature of matter associated with probability amplitudes leads to discrete values for energy, momentum, and angular momentum, just as the waves on violin strings lead to discrete values of frequency, or harmonics. The primary implication for the spin vector of a proton is that only two discrete (quantized) values are found for any measurement of a given spin component. The objective in the present chapter is to show that this is consistent with the classical picture of spins precessing about a magnetic field.

We begin with a little of the history of the measurements of quantum spin interactions with magnetic fields. The quantum mechanical framework for calculations of these interactions, in which the Schrödinger equation plays the central role, is introduced. The use of the classical precession picture for static fields, and of the rf induced rotation of magnetic moments in the rotating reference frame, is justified by specific quantum analysis. In each case, we choose to make an explicit matrix element derivation of the corresponding

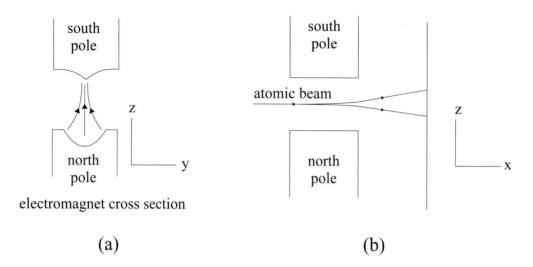

(a)   (b)

Fig. 5.1: The historical Stern-Gerlach experiment: Using a vertical (z-axis) magnetic field gradient from an electromagnet to split a beam of silver atoms in the direction of the gradient. Two views of the experiment are shown. In (a), the direction of the beam is out of the page. In (b), a side view of the beam is shown.

MRI phenomenon, rather than one based on quantum operator techniques. The latter[1] are important, especially in NMR studies, but perhaps what is presented here is more quickly assimilated for the issues directly at hand. The quantum basis for the thermal interactions of spins and the spin relaxation phenomena is the subject of Ch. 6.

5.1   Discrete Angular Momentum and Energy

Discreteness of the energy levels of the proton's magnetic moment interaction with a magnetic field is related to the discreteness of the proton's intrinsic angular momentum, or spin. In fact, this is the historical path along which scientists came to the conclusion that spin was quantized. In the early 1920's, Stern and Gerlach experimented with a beam of neutral silver atoms passing through a perpendicular (vertical) magnetic field gradient (see Fig. 5.1). Even with zero electric charge, a magnetic force is exerted on any atom that possesses a nonzero magnetic moment, as is the case for a silver atom, in a spatially varying magnetic field.

To see this, an expression for the force can be found from the gradient of the magnetic potential energy U in (4.8). For a field $\vec{B}$,

$$\vec{F} = -\vec{\nabla}U = \vec{\nabla}(\vec{\mu} \cdot \vec{B}) \qquad (5.1)$$

The field produced by the magnet in the figure has y- and z-components, and both are spatially varying. But, averaged over time, the y-component of the magnetic moment (and its spatial gradient) in the central region is zero. This follows from the expected classical precession[2] about the z-axis. Therefore, $\vec{\mu} \cdot \vec{B}$ may be replaced by $\mu_z B_z$ in (5.1) and, since

---

[1] Operator techniques are described in the references.

[2] The quantum mechanical justification of the precession picture is the subject of Secs. 5.3 and 5.4.

$\vec{\mu}$ is independent of position, the z-component of (5.1) becomes

$$F_z = \mu_z \frac{\partial B_z}{\partial z} \equiv \mu_z G_z \qquad (5.2)$$

The notation G_z for the z-derivative of the vertical component of the field will be useful in later imaging discussions about 'field gradients.'

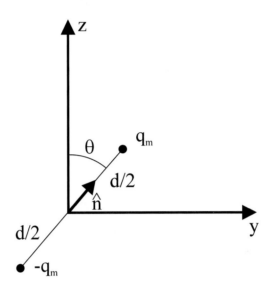

Fig. 5.2: Illustration for Prob. 5.1. Two magnetic monopoles, of equal and opposite charge, lie a distance d apart in the y-z plane with their center at the origin. The unit vector $\hat{n}$ is directed from the negative charge toward the positive charge.

Problem 5.1

For this problem, we refer back to the concept of a magnetic charge, and the corresponding magnetic moment and force equations, (2.11) and (2.12), respectively, in Ch. 2. Two oppositely charged magnetic monopoles, as shown in Fig. 5.2, have a magnetic moment given by $\vec{\mu} = q_m d\hat{n}$, and the force on a magnetic charge q_m due to a magnetic field $\vec{B}$ is given by $\vec{F} = q_m \vec{B}$. We are consistent with Maxwell's equations in assuming the z-component of the magnetic field depends only on z in the y-z plane, so that its Taylor series is

$$B_z(z) = B_z(0) + z\frac{dB_z(0)}{dz} + \ldots \qquad (5.3)$$

In the limit of small separation d (point dipole limit), show that the z-component of the force on the two monopoles is $q_m d \cos\theta \frac{dB_z(0)}{dz}$ and compare this answer to (5.2).

The experiment of Stern and Gerlach had the two necessary ingredients entering into (5.2), gradients and moments. They used electromagnets with vertical pole faces where the z-component of the field increases as the upper pole is approached (Fig. 5.1a). The angular momentum of an unpaired electron in a silver atom gives rise to an atomic magnetic moment[3] whose component parallel to the field gradient would lead to a deflection according to (5.2). The relation analogous to (2.16) is

$$\vec{\mu}_e = \gamma_e \vec{J}_e \tag{5.4}$$

in terms of the spin angular momentum $\vec{J}_e$ associated with the electron.

The classical conclusion from (5.2) and (5.4) is that the beam should be deflected through a spread of angles, due to a continuous spread of magnetic moment values, or more fundamentally, a continuous spread of angular momentum values. Working at the time when many profound quantum discoveries were being made, Stern and Gerlach had the specific goal of searching for quantization effects, and they found them. Instead of a smear of deflection angles, *their measurements showed that the beam split vertically into two beams, corresponding to two discrete values for the z-component of the angular momentum of the electron.* Although it was not known at that time, we now understand the angular momentum of the unpaired silver electron to be entirely due to its spin; there is no orbital angular momentum for this electron state. The spin component in (5.2) must be quantized.

With the motivation given above, let us describe, as an experimental fact, the quantization of angular momentum for the general case. (It is to be kept in mind, however, that the theoretical underpinnings discussed in the next section can be used to derive these results.) A measurement of, say, the z-component of any atomic or nuclear angular momentum $\vec{J}$ leads to integer (or half-integer) multiples of $\hbar$, which is Planck's constant divided by 2π,

$$\hbar \equiv \frac{h}{2\pi} \tag{5.5}$$

The measured values are

$$J_z = m_j \hbar \tag{5.6}$$

where the $2j+1$ values of m_j are

$$m_j = -j, -j+1, ..., j-1, j \tag{5.7}$$

and j is an integer or half-integer whose relation to the total angular momentum is discussed below. The m_j are sometimes called magnetic quantum numbers because of their role in magnetic field experiments like that of Stern and Gerlach.

The quantum number j is associated with the magnitude of the total angular momentum $\vec{J}$ according to

$$J^2 = j(j+1)\hbar^2 \tag{5.8}$$

where

$$j = 0, 1, 2, ... \quad \text{or} \quad \frac{1}{2}, \frac{3}{2}, \frac{5}{2}, ... \tag{5.9}$$

---

[3]In this case, the nuclear magnetic moment is negligible; the reader is referred to the discussion in Ch. 2.

Problem 5.2

A theoretical argument can be made to derive (5.8) from (5.7). Consider making many measurements of J_z^2 for some isolated system (or over a large ensemble of identical systems) which has a fixed magnitude J. With no outside interaction, each m_j value is equally probable. Furthermore, the average values of all components-squared must come out the same for this isotropic situation. (Separate measurements of the components are contemplated, since sharp, simultaneous measurements of more than one component cannot be made. See Secs. 5.2 and 5.3 for a further discussion of these quantum effects.) It is thus assumed that

$$< J_x^2 >=< J_y^2 >=< J_z^2 > \tag{5.10}$$

Starting with the relation between the magnitude and the components, $J^2 = J_x^2 + J_y^2 + J_z^2$, find (5.8) from an average value of J_z^2. Hint:

$$\sum_{-j}^{j} m_j^2 = \frac{j(2j+1)(j+1)}{3} \tag{5.11}$$

The total angular momentum for atomic and nuclear systems has a contribution $\vec{L}$ from orbital motion and a contribution $\vec{S}$ from the intrinsic spin,

$$\vec{J} = \vec{L} + \vec{S} \tag{5.12}$$

Each of these vectors has analogous quantum numbers. For the orbital angular momentum $\vec{L}$, the number corresponding to j is called l and is an integer only. Its magnitude satisfies

$$L^2 = l(l+1)\hbar^2 \qquad \text{where } l = 0, 1, 2, ... \tag{5.13}$$

There are $2l + 1$ observed values of m_l such that $L_z = m_l\hbar$ for any experiment set up to measure the z-component of orbital momentum. The spin angular momentum vector $\vec{S}$ has a quantum number s that can take on either integer or half-integer values. The same form holds for its magnitude that

$$S^2 = s(s+1)\hbar^2 \qquad \text{where } s = 0, 1, 2, ... \quad \text{or} \quad \frac{1}{2}, \frac{3}{2}, \frac{5}{2}, ... \tag{5.14}$$

with $2s+1$ values of m_s pertaining to the z-component $S_z = m_s\hbar$ of the spin vector. Finally, the range of j values for a given set of l and s is found from

$$j = |l - s|, |l - s| + 1, ..., l + s - 1, l + s \tag{5.15}$$

The two deflection angles observed in the Stern-Gerlach experiment determine the spin quantum number s for the electron. From the above discussion, and for no orbital angular momentum, it must be that $s = \frac{1}{2}$ and $m_s = \pm\frac{1}{2}$. The electron has 'spin one-half.' At the time of the experiment, by the way, it was not known whether an electron had any spin at all. We see that the existence of spin itself is inferred from such measurements.

Return now to the proton. Experiments in the years following the work of Stern and Gerlach showed the proton to have spin one-half as well. Thus the magnetic moment (2.16) is discretized and (4.8) leads to discrete energy values.

$$E = -\vec{\mu} \cdot \vec{B} = -\mu_z B_z = -\gamma m_s \hbar B_z \tag{5.16}$$

with[4]

$$m_s = \pm\frac{1}{2} \Rightarrow \begin{matrix} \text{spin parallel to field} \\ \text{spin anti-parallel to field} \end{matrix} \tag{5.17}$$

The two proton energy levels predicted by (5.16) are exhibited in Fig. 5.3. *This is an example of the general Zeeman effect where atomic or nuclear magnetic moments in the presence of an external magnetic field lead to splittings in the atomic or nuclear energy levels.*

Problem 5.3

In atomic physics, the magnetic moment associated with an intrinsic spin angular momentum $\vec{S}$ is written in terms of the Landé g-factor,

$$\vec{\mu} = \gamma \vec{S} \tag{5.18}$$

where the gyromagnetic ratio is given by

$$\gamma = g\mu_M \tag{5.19}$$

with the 'magneton' factor

$$\mu_M = \frac{e}{2M} \tag{5.20}$$

In (5.20), e is the magnitude of the particle charge (1.60×10^{-19} coulomb for electrons and protons) and M is the particle mass (9.11×10^{-31} kg for the electron and 1.67×10^{-27} kg for the proton, leading to the Bohr magneton and the nuclear magneton factor, respectively; see Ch. 2). Calculate the gyromagnetic γ factors (5.19) for the electron and proton, respectively, given the experimental g-factors, $g_e = 2.00$ and $g_p = 5.59$. Compare your answers with those in Sec. 2.2.

5.2   Quantum Operators and the Schrödinger Equation

The challenge that arises in view of the quantum nature of the proton spin degree of freedom is to justify the use of classical precession for the proton spin motion. In this section, the tools needed for a quantum analysis are introduced after a simple, but important, connection between precession and quantum energy differences is made. The precession justification is presented in Sec. 5.3.

---

[4]The two m_s values are also referred to as 'spin-up' and 'spin-down,' respectively, stemming from a reference to the z-axis.

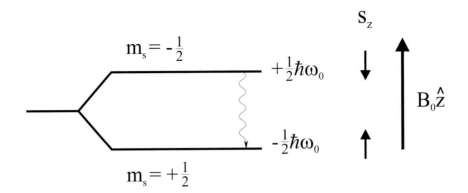

Fig. 5.3: The Zeeman energy levels for a spin one-half system and a positive gyromagnetic ratio. The spin is parallel to the external field $B_0\hat{z}$ in the lower energy state. The wavy vertical line represents a transition from the higher to the lower state by photon emission.

The magnitude of the energy absorbed or released by the proton spin system, upon a transition (up or down) between the higher and the lower energy states, is found from (5.16) to be

$$\Delta E = E\left(m_s = -\frac{1}{2}\right) - E\left(m_s = +\frac{1}{2}\right) = \frac{1}{2}\gamma\hbar B_0 - \left(-\frac{1}{2}\gamma\hbar B_0\right) = \hbar\omega_0 \qquad (5.21)$$

for a constant field $\vec{B} = B_0\hat{z}$. *The frequency in (5.21) associated with the emission or absorption of the quantum of energy (the photon) is nothing other than the Larmor precession frequency*

$$\omega_0 = \gamma B_0 \qquad (5.22)$$

It is observed that the frequency of the rf photon that is emitted during such transitions (Fig. 5.3), or that can be used to stimulate such transitions, is the same as the classical precession frequency of the proton magnetic moment. In Larmor precession, however, the magnetic potential energy is constant.

5.2.1 Wave Functions

To uncover the full quantum description of precession, and to understand better the identity between the frequency associated with the transition from one state to the next and the Larmor frequency, let us develop predictions for the measurement of the magnetic moment. Quantum mechanics is the description of physical states and transitions between those states by wave functions (or wave amplitudes). These wave functions are complex numbers, now a necessity and not merely a convenience, and the square of their modulus (absolute value) is a probability density. For example, a particle wave function $\Psi(\vec{r}, t)$ implies

$$\int_{\Delta V} |\Psi(\vec{r}, t)|^2 dV = \text{probability of finding the particle in volume } \Delta V \text{ at time t} \qquad (5.23)$$

ignoring spin for the moment.

It is the wave nature of Ψ that leads to discrete energy levels. In defining the framework of quantum mechanics, the wave functions are assumed to satisfy the *Schrödinger differential wave equation*

$$H\Psi = i\hbar \frac{\partial \Psi}{\partial t} \tag{5.24}$$

subject to boundary and initial conditions. The 'operator' H (the energy or Hamiltonian operator) is typically a combination of functions and derivatives; it operates on Ψ. The method of separation of variables, $\Psi = \psi(\vec{r})f(t)$, can be used to solve (5.24) if H has no explicit time dependence. In that case, a solution is

$$\Psi = \psi(\vec{r})e^{-\frac{i}{\hbar}Et} \tag{5.25}$$

provided the time-independent Schrödinger equation is satisfied,

$$H\psi = E\psi \tag{5.26}$$

According to (5.26), the Hamiltonian operates on ψ to give the energy E of 'stationary states,' i.e., those states described by the single term (5.25). For single-particle systems with interactions describable by force potentials[5]

$$H = \frac{\vec{p}^2}{2m} + U = \frac{-\hbar^2}{2m}\nabla^2 + U \tag{5.27}$$

where $\vec{p}$ is the particle momentum and m its mass. The operator $\nabla^2 = \partial^2/\partial x^2 + \partial^2/\partial y^2 + \partial^2/\partial z^2$ arises from the kinetic energy term and U is the potential energy term.

5.2.2   Momentum and Angular Momentum Operators

The operator representation of the kinetic energy in the second step of (5.27) follows from the momentum operator[6]

$$\vec{p} = -i\hbar\vec{\nabla} \tag{5.28}$$

Components of (5.28), such as $p_x = -i\hbar\frac{\partial}{\partial x}$, satisfy the commutation relations[7]

$$[p_x, x] = [p_y, y] = [p_z, z] = -i\hbar$$
$$[p_x, y] = [p_x, z] = [p_y, x] = [p_y, z] = [p_z, x] = [p_z, y] = 0 \tag{5.29}$$

with

$$[A, B] \equiv AB - BA \tag{5.30}$$

---

[5]These are 'non-relativistic' particles, meaning the speeds are much less than the speed of light. The deeply bound electrons in heavy elements have important relativistic corrections to the Hamiltonian.

[6]For example, the action of this operator on the 'plane-wave' state $e^{i\vec{k}\cdot\vec{r}}$ yields the momentum 'eigenvalue' $\vec{p} = \hbar\vec{k}$. A particle parameter has thereby been connected with a wave parameter (the wave vector $\vec{k}$) consistent with the de Broglie relation $p = h/\lambda$ where $k = 2\pi/\lambda$ with wavelength λ.

[7]To verify these, distribute the action of the derivative in, for example, the quantity $[p_x, x]f(x)$ for an arbitrary function $f(x)$.

Commutation relations for spin operators are of special interest. The quantum algebra for angular momentum components, in general, is the set

$$[J_x, J_y] = i\hbar J_z, \ [J_y, J_z] = i\hbar J_x, \ [J_z, J_x] = i\hbar J_y \tag{5.31}$$

which also holds for the components of the orbital angular momentum $\vec{L}$ and intrinsic spin $\vec{S}$, separately. In fact, it is straightforward, though tedious, to use (5.29) to check that the components of the operator representation

$$\vec{L} = \vec{r} \times \vec{p} = -i\hbar \vec{r} \times \vec{\nabla} \tag{5.32}$$

satisfy (5.31) with J_x, J_y, J_z replaced by L_x, L_y, L_z, respectively.

We shall represent spin angular momenta with finite matrices, instead of derivatives. (Because of the difference in the commutation relations, matrix representations of linear momenta and position need to be infinite-dimensional.) In particular, the matrix representation for the spin one-half vector is

$$\vec{S} = \frac{\hbar}{2}\vec{\sigma} \tag{5.33}$$

where the three linearly independent 'Pauli spin matrices' are

$$\sigma_x = \begin{pmatrix} 0 & 1 \\ 1 & 0 \end{pmatrix}, \ \sigma_y = \begin{pmatrix} 0 & -i \\ i & 0 \end{pmatrix}, \ \sigma_z = \begin{pmatrix} 1 & 0 \\ 0 & -1 \end{pmatrix} \tag{5.34}$$

It is left for Prob. 5.4 to show that this spin vector has the correct magnitude and that its components satisfy the correct algebra. The two spin states of a spin-1/2 system can be represented by two-component column vectors. The two-by-two matrices of (5.34) correspond to operators on the spin states.

Problem 5.4

Consider the spin one-half vector given by (5.33) in terms of (5.34).

a) Show that its square satisfies (5.14) for $s = \frac{1}{2}$. Note that the right-hand side of (5.14), in this case, is a matrix proportional to the 2×2 identity matrix $I = \begin{pmatrix} 1 & 0 \\ 0 & 1 \end{pmatrix}$.

b) Show that the components satisfy the same algebra as in (5.31), but with $\vec{J}$ replaced by $\vec{S}$. Explain why the algebra itself is a restriction on the magnitude.

For the record, it is noted that the well-known Heisenberg uncertainty principle corresponds to the fact that certain operators do not commute. The non-commutativity of p_x, x, for example, is intimately related to the impossibility of measuring them at the same time. Similarly, the commutation relations (5.31) imply that no two (or more) components of angular momentum can be simultaneously measured. In the limit $\hbar \to 0$, all commutators are zero and the classical determinism is recovered. The reader is referred to standard textbooks on quantum mechanics for elaboration of these remarks.

5.2.3   Spin Solutions for Constant Fields

Consider the magnetic-moment interaction (only) of a particle, with a gyromagnetic ratio γ, in a constant external (non-operator) magnetic field $\vec{B} = B_0 \hat{z}$. The general solution will be described first, and its derivation for an example is detailed afterward. The potential energy is

$$U = -\vec{\mu} \cdot \vec{B} = -\gamma J_z B_0 \tag{5.35}$$

in terms of the operator J_z. The use of a (square) matrix representation for J_z implies that the wave function ψ in (5.26) on which it operates is a column matrix. For states with fixed angular momentum j, the column entries ψ_{j,m_j} refer to different values m_j of the angular momentum component J_z as previewed in (5.7). A general solution of the linear Schrödinger differential equation for a given j, but possibly different energies, is the superposition of terms of the form (5.25). If only the m_j dependence of the energies is shown, the superposition is

$$\Psi(\vec{r}, t) = \sum_{m_j=-j}^{+j} C_{m_j} \psi_{j,m_j}(\vec{r}) e^{-\frac{i}{\hbar} E_{m_j} t} \tag{5.36}$$

The coefficients C_{m_j} are complex numbers to be determined by initial conditions. With the neglect of the kinetic energy contribution, the energies are the eigenvalues of (5.35)

$$E_{m_j} = -\gamma m_j \hbar B_0 \tag{5.37}$$

to be compared to (5.16). A concrete example of (5.36) is derived below for the spin one-half case.

Consider the specific case of a proton at rest and immersed in the constant external field. Let us show how the solution of the Schrödinger equation for zero kinetic energy leads to the quantum numbers and matrix elements introduced above, for a spin one-half particle with no orbital motion. Using the potential energy (5.35), the equality $\vec{J} = \vec{S}$, and the representation (5.33), the Hamiltonian in (5.27) becomes

$$H = -\gamma B_0 S_z = \begin{pmatrix} -\frac{1}{2}\hbar\omega_0 & 0 \\ 0 & +\frac{1}{2}\hbar\omega_0 \end{pmatrix} \tag{5.38}$$

The Pauli representation for σ_z has led to a Hamiltonian that is already diagonalized. The two solutions[8] to (5.26) are thus easily found by inspection to be

$$\psi_+ \; \equiv \; \psi_{+1/2} = \begin{pmatrix} 1 \\ 0 \end{pmatrix} \qquad\qquad \text{spin parallel ('spin up')} \tag{5.39}$$

$$\psi_- \; \equiv \; \psi_{-1/2} = \begin{pmatrix} 0 \\ 1 \end{pmatrix} \qquad\qquad \text{spin anti-parallel ('spin down')} \tag{5.40}$$

such that $H\psi_\pm = E_\pm \psi_\pm$ where

$$E_\pm = \mp\frac{1}{2}\hbar\omega_0 \tag{5.41}$$

---

[8]There are two linearly independent column matrices.

The solutions ψ_+ and ψ_- are indeed 'eigenfunctions' of S_z as well as of H

$$S_z \psi_\pm = \pm \frac{1}{2} \hbar \psi_\pm \qquad (5.42)$$

with the expected 'eigenvalues' $m_s \hbar = \pm \frac{1}{2} \hbar$.

We have found that the simplest matrix representation satisfying the spin commutator algebra leads to Schrödinger solutions with the eigenvalues for the energy and the z-component of the angular momentum expected for a spin one-half particle. In simplified subscript form, the version of (5.36) for the proton is

$$\Psi(t) = \sum_{m=\pm\frac{1}{2}} C_m \psi_m e^{-\frac{i}{\hbar} E_m t} \qquad (5.43)$$

It is noticed that the absence of any $\vec{r}$ dependence originates from the neglect of the proton's orbital and translational motion.

5.3 Quantum Derivation of Precession

What does quantum mechanics predict for a measurement of the magnetic moment as a function of time, $\vec{\mu}(t)$, for a proton at rest in a constant field? In the quantum framework, this is defined by an average value[9] (or 'expectation value') for the general state described by (5.43),

$$
\begin{aligned}
< \Psi | \vec{\mu} | \Psi > &\equiv \int \Psi^\dagger \vec{\mu} \Psi \, dV = \Psi^\dagger \vec{\mu} \Psi V \\
&= \gamma V \sum_m \sum_{m'} C_{m'}^* C_m \psi_{m'}^\dagger \vec{S} \psi_m e^{\frac{i}{\hbar}(E_{m'} - E_m)t}
\end{aligned}
\qquad (5.44)
$$

where, as before, the subscripts on the magnetic quantum numbers are dropped (e.g., $m_s \equiv m = \pm \frac{1}{2} \equiv \pm$). The Hermitian adjoint of a matrix (such as $\Psi^\dagger$) is a combined transpose and complex conjugate operation. The positioning of $\vec{\mu} = \gamma \vec{S}$ between $\Psi^\dagger$ (a row matrix) and Ψ (a column matrix) reflects the operator nature of the spin angular momentum vector (and hence of the magnetic moment). The factor V arises from the trivial integration over the volume containing the proton; we recall Ψ is independent of $\vec{r}$.

The normalization condition on the total probability implies a condition on the complex coefficients in (5.43). The proton must be somewhere in V, i.e.,

$$< \Psi | \Psi > \equiv \int \Psi^\dagger \Psi \, dV = \Psi^\dagger \Psi V = V \sum_m \sum_{m'} C_{m'}^* C_m \psi_{m'}^\dagger \psi_m e^{\frac{i}{\hbar}(E_{m'} - E_m)t} = 1 \qquad (5.45)$$

This leads to (see Prob. 5.5)

$$V \sum_m |C_m|^2 = 1 \qquad (5.46)$$

---

[9]For a simple, classical probability density distribution $\rho(\theta)$, the average value of a quantity is found by evaluating the integral $< \theta > = \int dV \theta \rho(\theta)$. This is generalized in quantum mechanics, as shown, to a density matrix involving the wave functions.

Problem 5.5

We want to provide the derivation of (5.46). From the explicit solutions (5.39) and (5.40), show that

$$\psi_{m'}^{\dagger}\psi_m = \delta_{m'm} \tag{5.47}$$

where the Kronecker delta

$$\delta_{m'm} = \begin{cases} 1 & m = m' \\ 0 & m \neq m' \end{cases} \tag{5.48}$$

Thus show that (5.45) leads to (5.46).

The key ingredient in the reduction of (5.44) is $\psi_{m'}^{\dagger}\vec{S}\psi_m$. For example, (5.39), (5.40), and (5.34) can be used to show that $\psi_{m'}^{\dagger}\sigma_y\psi_m$ is zero if $m = m'$, $-i$ if $m' = 1/2$ and $m = -1/2$, or $+i$ if $m' = -1/2$ and $m = 1/2$. We can summarize all results as a vector equation

$$\psi_{m'}^{\dagger}\vec{\sigma}\psi_m = \hat{x}\delta_{m',-m} + 2mi\hat{y}\delta_{m',-m} + 2m\hat{z}\delta_{m'm} \tag{5.49}$$

Problem 5.6

Complete the derivation of (5.49).

With (5.41) and (5.49), the y-component of (5.44), for example, reduces to the real part of a complex number

$$
\begin{aligned}
< \mu_y > \equiv\ < \Psi|\mu_y(t)|\Psi > &= \frac{1}{2}\hbar\gamma V \left(-iC_+^*C_-e^{-i\omega_0 t} + iC_-^*C_+e^{+i\omega_0 t}\right) \\
&= \gamma\hbar V \operatorname{Re}\left(iC_-^*C_+e^{+i\omega_0 t}\right)
\end{aligned} \tag{5.50}
$$

in which $C_+ \equiv C_{+1/2}$, $C_- \equiv C_{-1/2}$. If a polar coordinate representation is used,

$$C_+ = a_+e^{i\alpha_+},\, C_- = a_-e^{i\alpha_-} \tag{5.51}$$

then (5.46) requires $V(a_+^2 + a_-^2) = 1$. This is satisfied by $a_+ \equiv \frac{1}{\sqrt{V}}\cos\Theta$, $a_- \equiv \frac{1}{\sqrt{V}}\sin\Theta$. Hence (5.50) becomes $< \mu_y > = \gamma\hbar\sin\Theta\cos\Theta\sin(\alpha_- - \alpha_+ - \omega_0 t)$. The calculation of the other two components (see Prob. 5.7) with $\Theta \equiv \theta/2$, $\alpha_- - \alpha_+ \equiv \phi_0$ leads to[10]

$$< \mu_x > = \frac{\gamma\hbar}{2}\sin\theta\cos(\phi_0 - \omega_0 t) \tag{5.52}$$

$$< \mu_y > = \frac{\gamma\hbar}{2}\sin\theta\sin(\phi_0 - \omega_0 t) \tag{5.53}$$

$$< \mu_z > = \frac{\gamma\hbar}{2}\cos\theta \tag{5.54}$$

---

[10]The reader may be interested in verifying that it is somewhat faster to use the matrix methods of the next section to derive the various results of this section.

The set of expectation values for the magnetic moment components represents a vector of magnitude $\gamma\hbar/2$ precessing clockwise about the z-axis at a fixed polar angle θ. The initial azimuthal angle is ϕ_0. The motion is illustrated in Fig. 5.4.

Problem 5.7

---

a) Derive the other two components (5.52) and (5.54).

b) What is the expectation value of $\mu_+ = \mu_x + i\mu_y$?

We observe that the quantum mechanical state consisting of an arbitrary superposition of a parallel spin state and an anti-parallel spin state leads to an expectation value which is precisely the clockwise precession predicted classically for a proton.[11] The relative weighting (a_+/a_-) determines the polar angle and the relative phase $(\alpha_- - \alpha_+)$ fixes the initial azimuthal angle.

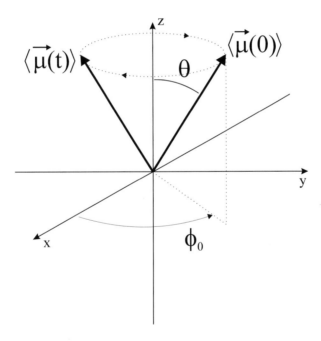

Fig. 5.4: The precession of the quantum expectation value of the magnetic moment operator in the presence of a constant external field pointed in the z-direction.

---

[11]Quantum mechanics shows itself only through the $\hbar$ factor coming from the spin dependence of the moment magnitude $\gamma\hbar/2$. The proton spin is fundamentally a quantum property.

5.4   Quantum Derivation of RF Spin Tipping

Attention is now turned to a magnetic moment immersed in the combined static and left-circularly polarized rf field (3.41)

$$\vec{B}(t) = B_0\hat{z} + B_1(\hat{x}\cos\omega t - \hat{y}\sin\omega t) \qquad (5.55)$$

We should like to justify the classical picture where, in the rotating reference frame defined by the rf field, and on-resonance, the motion is simply a rotation of the magnetic moment about the x'-axis (the rf field direction). The calculations proceed in a manner similar to those in the preceding section.

   The Hamiltonian for a proton at rest in the field (5.55) is

$$H(t) = -\vec{\mu}\cdot\vec{B}(t) = -\frac{\gamma\hbar}{2}\left(\sigma_z B_0 + (\sigma_x\cos\omega t - \sigma_y\sin\omega t)B_1\right) \qquad (5.56)$$

recalling the Pauli spin vector definition of (5.33). The time dependence of the Hamiltonian will have to be considered, but it is still possible to use the method of separation of variables in the solution of the Schrödinger equation for the present case.

   It is useful to write (5.24) in terms of the matrix elements of $H(t)$. From (5.34), the static-field term is

$$-\frac{\gamma\hbar}{2}\sigma_z B_0 = -\frac{\hbar\omega_0}{2}\begin{pmatrix} 1 & 0 \\ 0 & -1 \end{pmatrix} \qquad (5.57)$$

and the component of $\vec{\sigma}$ along $\hat{x}'$ is

$$\sigma_{x'} = \sigma_x\cos\omega t - \sigma_y\sin\omega t = \begin{pmatrix} 0 & e^{i\omega t} \\ e^{-i\omega t} & 0 \end{pmatrix} \qquad (5.58)$$

The Schrödinger equation becomes

$$i\hbar\frac{\partial\Psi}{\partial t} = -\frac{\hbar}{2}\begin{pmatrix} \omega_0 & \omega_1 e^{i\omega t} \\ \omega_1 e^{-i\omega t} & -\omega_0 \end{pmatrix}\Psi \qquad (5.59)$$

with the usual identifications for the frequencies, $\omega_0 \equiv \gamma B_0$ and $\omega_1 \equiv \gamma B_1$. Note that, as in the previous section, the $\hbar$ factor can be canceled out, a first indication that classical behavior will be recovered.

   A simple set of differential equations can be found by a change of variables. Consider the following (completely general) form for the wave function

$$\Psi = \psi_1'(t)\psi_+ e^{i\omega_0 t/2} + \psi_2'(t)\psi_- e^{-i\omega_0 t/2} = \begin{pmatrix} \psi_1'(t)e^{i\omega_0 t/2} \\ \psi_2'(t)e^{-i\omega_0 t/2} \end{pmatrix} \qquad (5.60)$$

The superposition of the 'complete set' of column matrices, ψ_+ and ψ_-, leads to differential equations, with no ω_0 terms, for the new wave variables, $\psi_1'(t)$ and $\psi_2'(t)$.[12] After a cancelation of those terms by the time derivatives of the $e^{\pm i\omega_0 t/2}$ factors and the assumption that the rf

---

[12]In fact, the change of variables (5.60), as the primes suggest, is the wave function transformation from the laboratory to the Larmor rotating frame.

field is on-resonance (i.e., $\omega = \omega_0$), the result is the coupled system for the column-matrix components

$$\frac{d\psi_1'}{dt} = \frac{i}{2}\omega_1\psi_2' \tag{5.61}$$

$$\frac{d\psi_2'}{dt} = \frac{i}{2}\omega_1\psi_1' \tag{5.62}$$

Because of the on-resonance condition, the coupled equations have no explicit time dependence in their coefficient. Taking a second time-derivative of (5.61) and (5.62), a technique that was used to decouple a similar set of differential equations in Sec. 2.3.3 (Prob. 2.6), we find

$$\frac{d^2\psi_{1,2}'}{dt^2} = -\frac{1}{4}\omega_1^2\psi_{1,2}' \tag{5.63}$$

Equations (5.63) have the general solutions

$$\psi_1'(t) = c_1\cos\frac{\omega_1 t}{2} + c_2\sin\frac{\omega_1 t}{2} \tag{5.64}$$

$$\psi_2'(t) = c_3\cos\frac{\omega_1 t}{2} + c_4\sin\frac{\omega_1 t}{2} \tag{5.65}$$

where the c_i are, in general, complex constants. Also, from (5.61) and (5.62),

$$c_3 = -ic_2 \tag{5.66}$$

$$c_4 = ic_1 \tag{5.67}$$

With the wave function known, the expectation values of the different components of the magnetic moment vector can be computed. The expectation values of interest are $\langle\mu_z\rangle$, and the rotating transverse components, $\langle\mu_{x'}\rangle$ and $\langle\mu_{y'}\rangle$, since the classical behavior predicts precession about the x'-axis. From (5.44), the first calculation yields

$$\langle\mu_z\rangle \equiv \langle\Psi|\mu_z|\Psi\rangle = \frac{1}{2}\hbar\gamma V\left(|\psi_1'|^2 - |\psi_2'|^2\right) \tag{5.68}$$

To determine $\langle\mu_{x'}\rangle$ and $\langle\mu_{y'}\rangle$, the combinations of Pauli spin matrices that arise are $\sigma_{x'}$ given in (5.58), and

$$\sigma_{y'} = \sigma_x\sin\omega t + \sigma_y\cos\omega t = i\begin{pmatrix} 0 & -e^{i\omega t} \\ e^{-i\omega t} & 0 \end{pmatrix} \tag{5.69}$$

The remaining 2×2 matrix elements can be reduced to

$$\langle\mu_{x'}\rangle = \gamma\hbar V\mathrm{Re}\left(\psi_1'^*\psi_2'\right) \tag{5.70}$$

$$\langle\mu_{y'}\rangle = \gamma\hbar V\mathrm{Im}\left(\psi_1'^*\psi_2'\right) \tag{5.71}$$

Problem 5.8

Provide the details for the calculations leading from (5.64) and (5.65) to (5.68), (5.70), and (5.71).

The next step is to write the magnetic moment expectation values in terms of the explicit solutions, (5.64) and (5.65). Two computations provide the necessary ingredients

$$|\psi_1'|^2 - |\psi_2'|^2 = (|c_1|^2 - |c_2|^2)\cos\omega_1 t + 2\mathrm{Re}\,(c_1^* c_2)\sin\omega_1 t \tag{5.72}$$

$$(\psi_1')^* \psi_2' = i\frac{1}{2}(|c_1|^2 - |c_2|^2)\sin\omega_1 t - i\mathrm{Re}\,(c_1^* c_2)\cos\omega_1 t + \mathrm{Im}\,(c_1^* c_2) \tag{5.73}$$

The condition (5.45) on the wave function normalization is now

$$\langle \Psi \mid \Psi \rangle = V\left(|\psi_1'|^2 + |\psi_2'|^2\right) = V\left(|c_1|^2 + |c_2|^2\right) = 1 \tag{5.74}$$

The general solution of the constraint (5.74) is $c_1 \equiv \frac{1}{\sqrt{V}}\cos\frac{\Theta}{2}e^{-i\phi_1}$ and $c_2 \equiv \frac{1}{\sqrt{V}}\sin\frac{\Theta}{2}e^{-i\phi_2}$.

The combination (5.72), (5.73), and the constraint solutions transforms (5.68), (5.70), and (5.71) into

$$\langle \mu_{x'}(t) \rangle = \frac{\gamma\hbar}{2}\sin\Theta\cos\Phi \tag{5.75}$$

$$\langle \mu_{y'}(t) \rangle = \frac{\gamma\hbar}{2}\left[\cos\Theta\sin\omega_1 t + \sin\Theta\cos\omega_1 t\sin\Phi\right] \tag{5.76}$$

$$\langle \mu_z(t) \rangle = \frac{\gamma\hbar}{2}\left[\cos\Theta\cos\omega_1 t - \sin\Theta\sin\omega_1 t\sin\Phi\right] \tag{5.77}$$

with $\Phi \equiv \phi_1 - \phi_2 - \pi/2$. The initial values of the expectation components are

$$\langle \mu_{x'}(0) \rangle = \frac{\gamma\hbar}{2}\sin\Theta\cos\Phi \tag{5.78}$$

$$\langle \mu_{y'}(0) \rangle = \frac{\gamma\hbar}{2}\sin\Theta\sin\Phi \tag{5.79}$$

$$\langle \mu_z(0) \rangle = \frac{\gamma\hbar}{2}\cos\Theta \tag{5.80}$$

where it is noted that $\langle \mu_{x'}(t) \rangle$ is independent of time. Equations (5.78)–(5.80) describe an arbitrary initial orientation for a vector of magnitude $\frac{\gamma\hbar}{2}$. In spherical coordinates, the initial direction is seen to have a polar angle of Θ and an azimuthal angle of Φ.

The expectation-value components (5.75)–(5.77) can be rewritten in terms of the initial components (5.78)–(5.80),

$$\langle \mu_{x'}(t) \rangle = \langle \mu_{x'}(0) \rangle \tag{5.81}$$
$$\langle \mu_{y'}(t) \rangle = \langle \mu_{y'}(0) \rangle \cos\omega_1 t + \langle \mu_z(0) \rangle \sin\omega_1 t \tag{5.82}$$
$$\langle \mu_z(t) \rangle = -\langle \mu_{y'}(0) \rangle \sin\omega_1 t + \langle \mu_z(0) \rangle \cos\omega_1 t \tag{5.83}$$

Equations (5.82) and (5.83) represent a vector, of fixed magnitude, which is precessing clockwise about the x'-axis, in the rotating reference frame, with a precession frequency ω_1 as predicted by classical theory. Arbitrary initial conditions are obviously accommodated.

Suggested Reading

Excellent reviews of the basic quantum aspects required to understand the NMR signal appear in the following three references:

- A. Abragam. *The Principles of Nuclear Magnetism.* Clarendon Press, New York, 1961.

- I. I. Rabi, N. F. Ramsey and J. Schwinger. Rotating coordinates in magnetic resonance problems. *Rev. Modern Phys.*, 26: 167, 1954.

- C. P. Slichter. *Principles of Magnetic Resonance.* Springer-Verlag, 3rd ed., New York, 2010.

Chapter 6

The Quantum Mechanical Basis of Thermal Equilibrium and Longitudinal Relaxation

Chapter Contents

Summary: The equilibrium magnetization M_0 is derived for a system of particles with spin at temperature T in the presence of a static external field. The thermal quantum basis of the Bloch equations for combined static and rf fields is briefly discussed.

Introduction

In the quantum description of precession in both the laboratory and rotating reference frames, given in Ch. 5, the relaxation mechanisms were ignored. We turn here to the quantum description of the interactions that lead to both spin-lattice and spin-spin relaxation. The thermal equilibrium value of the magnetization is determined, in the presence of relaxation, for a constant external magnetic field. This can be referred to as the Boltzmann equilibrium value; it applies when the time between experiments is long compared to the relaxation time scale. The relaxation terms used in the previous chapters can themselves be derived in a quantum framework. The quantum basis for these terms and the driving terms used to model an rf magnetic field is very briefly touched upon. Transient and steady-state solutions of simple versions of the Bloch equations are studied.

6.1   Boltzmann Equilibrium Values

The equilibrium value M_0 was required in the solution (4.12) of the Bloch equation for the longitudinal magnetization, $M_z(t)$. This value, arising in the relaxation limit $M_z(\infty) = M_0$, represents the trade-off between the tendency of a spin system to align itself with the external field (the lowest energy state), and its ability to gain energy from thermal contact. Interactions beyond those with the external fields are at the heart of these exchanges.

To set the stage for a discussion of the exchange interactions, consider two systems in external magnetic fields, with gravity ignored. First, the classical motion of a point particle with charge q and velocity $\vec{v}$ is governed by the Lorentz magnetic force law (see Appendix A)

$$\vec{F} = q\vec{v} \times \vec{B} \tag{6.1}$$

in the presence of an external magnetic field $\vec{B}$. The particle traces out helical paths along the field lines as time goes on. Although the Lorentz force is observed to be perpendicular to the motion, so that no work is performed on the particle, radiation and other dissipative interactions will eventually leave the particle at rest. The second system is a compass needle initially swinging back and forth in response to torque from an external field (see Ch. 2). It will slow down due to friction, with smaller and smaller oscillations around the position of zero torque. The point particle stops, and the bar magnet ultimately settles down along the field direction, because energy is given off to the surroundings.

On the other hand, if the particle and the bar magnet were in thermal contact with other material, and at (absolute) temperature T, they would retain kinetic energy on the order of kT, where k is Boltzmann's constant. The exchange interactions will leave these systems (as well as a system of spins) in equilibrium somewhere above the (ground) state of lowest energy, depending on how large kT is. The probability of finding a system with energy ϵ, while in contact with a much larger system (the 'reservoir' depicted in Fig. 6.1) at temperature T, is equal to the normalized Boltzmann factor,[1]

$$P(\epsilon) = \frac{e^{-\epsilon/kT}}{Z} \tag{6.2}$$

The normalization divisor is the partition function, the sum over all weighting factors,

$$Z = \sum_{\epsilon} e^{-\epsilon/kT} \tag{6.3}$$

A system of interest is a spin in thermal contact with the rest of a set of N spins and with the background lattice all at temperature T. The number N is taken to be very large along with the size of the lattice. To find the thermal equilibrium value of M_z, consider the calculation of the z-component of the average total magnetic moment for N spins distributed over all possible magnetic spin states, neglecting translational motion. This brings together the thermal interactions and the quantum basis of the magnetization. The quantization axis is chosen along the external field direction (the z-axis, as usual) and the case of a general

---

[1]See any introductory thermal physics text for a discussion of the Boltzmann factor.

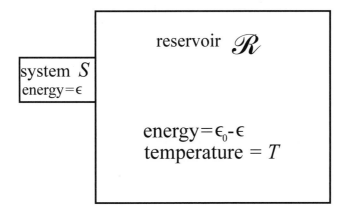

Fig. 6.1: A small system in thermal equilibrium with a reservoir at temperature T. The total energy ϵ_0 is conserved between the two systems.

spin s, with magnetic number $m_s \equiv m$, is analyzed. The thermal average of the z component of the magnetization is

$$M_0 = \rho_0 \sum_{m=-s}^{s} P(\epsilon(m))\mu_z(m) \tag{6.4}$$

where $\rho_0 = N/V$ is the density of spins per unit volume in the homogeneous isochromat of volume V.[2] From (5.16),

$$\epsilon = -m\hbar\omega_0 \tag{6.5}$$

$$\mu_z = m\gamma\hbar \tag{6.6}$$

The explicit expression for the equilibrium magnetization is

$$M_0 = \frac{N\gamma\hbar}{V} \frac{\displaystyle\sum_{m=-s}^{s} m e^{mu}}{\displaystyle\sum_{m=-s}^{s} e^{mu}} \tag{6.7}$$

with

$$u \equiv \frac{\hbar\omega_0}{kT} \tag{6.8}$$

The expression (6.7) can be simplified in MR, because the nuclear magnetic energies are so much smaller than room-temperature thermal energies. Having referred, in Ch. 4, to the extremely small 'excess spin' in the direction of the magnetic field, we can now explain that it comes from the Boltzmann factor. For human body temperature (310 K), and protons, the basic exponent unit in (6.7)–(6.8) has the numerical value $u \simeq 6.6 \times 10^{-6} B_0$ for B_0 in

---

[2]In this chapter, ρ_0 describes the true density of spins per unit volume. However, in later chapters, other factors will be absorbed into ρ_0, and it will be used to describe the sensitivity of the MRI experiment to a group of spins. The term 'spin density' is still employed in these instances, but the reader is cautioned that it is not always a measure of the number of spins per unit volume.

tesla. Hence the basic exponential is unity to within ten parts per million for field strengths in that range,

$$\exp\left(\frac{\hbar\omega_0}{kT}\right) = 1 + \frac{\hbar\omega_0}{kT} + \mathcal{O}\left(\left(\frac{\hbar\omega_0}{kT}\right)^2\right) + \dots$$

$$\simeq 1 + 6.6 \times 10^{-6} B_0 \tag{6.9}$$

For the finite m values of interest, e^{mu} is also very close to unity, leading to a simplified limit for (6.7). For arbitrary spins, it is to be shown in Prob. 6.2 that

$$M_0 \simeq \rho_0 \frac{s(s+1)\gamma^2\hbar^2}{3kT} B_0 \qquad (\hbar\omega_0 \ll kT) \tag{6.10}$$

This form of M_0 will be used in Ch. 7 for defining the relative signal strengths of different elements in an MR experiment.

Problem 6.1

Find the value of (6.7) in the limits

a) $T \to \infty$. Your limit should be consistent with the expectation of the spins being equally distributed over all $2s+1$ states.

b) $T \to 0$. Your limit should be consistent with the spins all dropping to the bottom (ground) state. Hint: The maximum magnetization is

$$M_0^{max} = \rho_0\gamma\hbar s \tag{6.11}$$

corresponding to $m = m_{max} = s$ for every spin. There is no longer any thermal interaction.

Problem 6.2

Derive (6.10) as the leading term in a $1/T$ expansion of (6.7) using $e^{mu} \simeq 1 + mu$. Hint: Since $\sum_{-s}^{s} m = 0$, the first-order term, such as that in (6.9), must be kept. Now see Prob. 5.2.

The limit (6.10) constitutes a quantum derivation of the experimental Curie's law for magnetization, which states that the magnetization should be proportional to $1/T$, but with the bonus of determining the coefficient. Its vanishing in the limit of $T \to \infty$ should agree with the reader's result for part (a) in Prob. 6.1. For a proton ($s = 1/2$), (6.10) becomes

$$M_0 \simeq \frac{1}{4}\rho_0 \frac{\gamma^2\hbar^2}{kT} B_0 \qquad (\text{proton}, \hbar\omega_0 \ll kT) \tag{6.12}$$

Finally, let us revisit these results in terms of the proton spin excess, defined by the difference between the number of spins parallel $(N(\uparrow))$ and anti-parallel $(N(\downarrow))$ to the external field

$$
\begin{aligned}
\Delta N &\equiv N(\uparrow) - N(\downarrow) \\
&= N(P_+ - P_-) \\
&\simeq \frac{Nu}{2}
\end{aligned}
\tag{6.13}
$$

where the Boltzmann probability (6.2) for the two spin-$\frac{1}{2}$ states ($m = \pm\frac{1}{2}$ or $\epsilon = \mp\frac{1}{2}\hbar\omega_0$) is

$$
P_\pm = \frac{e^{\pm u/2}}{e^{u/2} + e^{-u/2}}
\tag{6.14}
$$

Problem 6.3

A homogeneous sample of protons with gyromagnetic ratio γ is immersed in a uniform static field B_0 and at arbitrary absolute temperature T. Find an expression in terms of the hyperbolic tangent for the average value (thermal equilibrium) of the z-component of the magnetic moment vector for one of these protons. Show that this gives the expected $T \to 0$ and $T \to \infty$ results.

Problem 6.4

---

a) Derive the approximation in (6.13).

b) Show that (6.13) implies an excess of 5 out of every 10^6 spins at 1.5 T.

6.2 Quantum Basis of Longitudinal Relaxation

The next task is to understand, by an example, how the Bloch relaxation terms themselves can be derived within the quantum approach. The local interactions leading to relaxation are treated as perturbations of the spin-system external magnetic-field quantum states. The example to be considered is the z-component of the Bloch equations for a constant external field.

Suppose there are N protons at rest and subjected to the constant magnetic field $B_0\hat{z}$, with no other external fields. (We return later to the description of the rf field interactions in this framework.) Each can be in either of the two spin states, $m = \pm 1/2$. The lower energy state pertains to $m = +1/2$ where the magnetic moment and the field are parallel. None of the protons could make a change of state without additional forces, reminiscent of the earlier remarks about point charges and compass needles.

Turning on the interactions with the neighborhood atomic and nuclear lattice allows state transitions. These small disturbances can be analyzed in 'time-dependent perturbation theory.'[3] The lowest-order transition probability rate to go from state i to state f (or a set of final states $\{f\}$) due to a small perturbation potential V, as it occurs in the Schrödinger equation, is

$$W_{fi} = \frac{2\pi}{\hbar} | < f|V|i > |^2 \rho(E_f) \tag{6.15}$$

The importance of this formula in quantum calculations has led to it being called the 'golden rule number two.' The occurrence of the square of the modulus of the first-order transition amplitude in (6.15) is the familiar connection between wave amplitude and probability. The notation for the off-diagonal transition matrix element $< f|V|i >$ follows that in Ch. 5. The density $\rho(E_f)$ of final states per unit energy reduces for one final state to a Dirac delta function (see Ch. 10 for the definition of this function) expressing the conservation of energy

$$\rho(E_f) = \delta(E_f - E_i) \tag{6.16}$$

The derivation of (6.15) can be found in the references.

Labels are needed for the transition probabilities and the number of states. Any transition down in energy from $m = -1/2$ to $m = +1/2$ for one proton must be accompanied by a transition upwards in energy from some lower lattice state l to a higher lattice state h $(l- \rightarrow h+)$. The energy jumps, up and down, must be equal, by the law of conservation of energy. The lattice states must include other nucleon spin states. For the transition up in energy for a proton, the picture is reversed $(h+ \rightarrow l-)$. See Fig. 6.2. We denote the respective probability rates (6.15) for these two processes by $W_{h+,l-}$ and $W_{l-,h+}$. (Strictly speaking, these are the rates per proton per lattice site.) Finally, if $N_\pm$ is the initial number of spins with $m = \pm 1/2$, respectively, and if n_h (n_l) is the number of initial lattice states with the higher (lower) energy, the rate of change of the $+1/2$ spin-state number is

$$\frac{dN_+}{dt} = W_{h+,l-}N_- n_l - W_{l-,h+}N_+ n_h \tag{6.17}$$

The (large) numbers of lattice states, n_h and n_l, are independent of changes in N_+, and are related to each other by the Boltzmann factor ratio,

$$\frac{n_h}{n_l} = e^{-\gamma\hbar B_0/kT} \tag{6.18}$$

which is just the ratio of the average values for n_h and n_l.

The probabilities in (6.17) are equal in lowest-order perturbation theory,

$$W_{h+,l-} = W_{l-,h+} \equiv W \tag{6.19}$$

This follows from the 'detailed balance' relation $W_{fi} = W_{if}$ which holds for any Hermitian[4] potential V. In that case, $< f|V|i > = < i|V|f >^*$ in the formula (6.15), using (6.16) for a single state f. Also, in terms of the spin excess pointing along the field,

$$\Delta N \equiv N_+ - N_- \tag{6.20}$$

---

[3]For a detailed discussion of time-dependent perturbation theory, see any introductory quantum mechanics text.

[4]Recall from Sec. 5.3 that Hermiticity of a matrix M implies that $M^\dagger \equiv M^{*T} = M$.

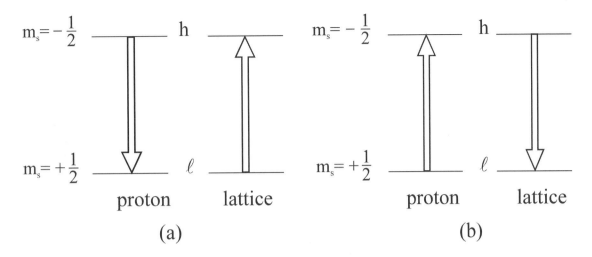

Fig. 6.2: The response of the lattice to transitions between the two proton spin states. The labeling is explained in the text.

and the (fixed) total number of spin states

$$N = N_+ + N_- \tag{6.21}$$

the spin-state numbers can be rewritten

$$N_\pm = \frac{N \pm \Delta N}{2} \tag{6.22}$$

From (6.17), (6.19) and (6.22),

$$\frac{d(\Delta N)}{dt} = WN(n_l - n_h) - W\Delta N(n_l + n_h) \tag{6.23}$$

In the relaxed or equilibrium steady state, $d(\Delta N)/dt = 0$, leading to

$$(\Delta N)_0 = \frac{(n_l - n_h)}{(n_l + n_h)} N \qquad \text{(equilibrium)} \tag{6.24}$$

The zero subscript refers to the equilibrium value, achieved in the long-time limit.

With the coefficient of ΔN on the right-hand side of (6.23) identified as the spin-relaxation decay rate,

$$\frac{1}{T_1} \equiv W(n_l + n_h) \tag{6.25}$$

then

$$\frac{d(\Delta N)}{dt} = \frac{(\Delta N)_0 - \Delta N}{T_1} \tag{6.26}$$

Finally, multiply (6.26) by the z-component of the magnetic moment, $\frac{1}{2}\gamma\hbar$, and average over the volume, as in (4.1), to get M_z for a proton. The result is

$$\frac{dM_z}{dt} = \frac{M_0 - M_z}{T_1} \tag{6.27}$$

This is the same form as that in (4.11).

Problem 6.5

Show that (6.24) and (6.18) yield

    a) the common ratio for the equilibrium values

$$\left(\frac{N_-}{N_+}\right)_0 = \frac{n_h}{n_l} = e^{-\gamma \hbar B_0/kT} \tag{6.28}$$

    b) a high temperature limit consistent with (6.12).

6.3   The RF Field

The external field cross products in the Bloch differential equations, which drive the solutions, are the remaining terms to be justified. For the constant external field, the quantum derivation of the expression $\gamma \vec{M} \times \vec{B}_0$ follows from a volume average of the magnetic moment equations of motion found by the methods of Ch. 4. The time-dependent rf field cannot be found quite so straightforwardly. However, we can analyze effects of rf fields with amplitudes that are small compared to the constant field, using the same perturbation theory used in the discussion of relaxation.

Consider N protons at rest and immersed in the constant magnetic field $B_0 \hat{z}$, but with no lattice interactions. Turning on the rf field can cause transitions between the two spin states for each proton. The fact that the rf field is perpendicular to the z-axis produces complications in the quantum calculations. The amplitude in the transition rate (6.15) involves a perturbation potential $-\vec{\mu} \cdot \vec{B}_1$, where spin-vector components transverse to the quantization axis arise. Spin operators σ_x and σ_y, which were discussed in Ch. 5, lead to off-diagonal matrix elements, and hence to cross terms in the square of the probability amplitudes. The different magnetization components become mixed together in the Bloch equations, as a result of these complications.

If the vector nature of both the rf field and the magnetization is ignored, the origin of an external field driving term is easy to understand. For the remainder of this argument, we shall make that simplification. For such rf fields, define the probability rate for a proton to drop to $m = +1/2$ from $m = -1/2$ as w_{+-}. The probability rate for the proton to go up to $m = -1/2$ from $m = +1/2$ is w_{-+}. It is important to note that energy exchange takes place through the interaction with the external field; no lattice neighborhood interaction is needed for the exchange, so that interaction is also ignored. The 'detailed balance' relation is

$$w_{+-} = w_{-+} \equiv w \tag{6.29}$$

so

$$\frac{dN_+}{dt} = N_- w_{+-} - N_+ w_{-+} = (N_- - N_+)w \tag{6.30}$$

Here, Boltzmann factors and lattice population numbers have not entered into the analysis. Using (6.22) for $N_\pm$, we obtain

$$\frac{d(\Delta N)}{dt} = -2w\Delta N \tag{6.31}$$

for constant N.

Problem 6.6

Solve the differential equation (6.31) in terms of the initial condition $\Delta N(0)$. Conclude from the solution that any initial spin excess disappears for constant w.

Within the approximations of the model, the driving term, due to the external rf field, can be joined to the relaxation rate (6.26)

$$\frac{d(\Delta N)}{dt} = \frac{(\Delta N)_0 - \Delta N}{T_1} - 2w\Delta N \tag{6.32}$$

Equation (6.32) is an uncoupled version of the z-component Bloch equation (4.21). To derive the correctly coupled form of the equations (4.22)–(4.24), a more detailed examination of the quantum transition amplitudes is required. It can be shown, however, that the general relaxation-plus-driving-term structure arises in much the same way as in the above. And the solutions of the diagonal version (6.32) are also instructive. For example, the steady-state, or equilibrium, solution is

$$\Delta N_{eq} = \frac{(\Delta N)_0}{1 + 2wT_1} \tag{6.33}$$

Suggested Reading

The fundamental concepts of the quantum processes are given in the following four references:

- N. Bloembergen, E. M. Purcell and R. V. Pound. Relaxation effects in nuclear magnetic resonance experiments. *Phys. Rev.*, 73: 679, 1948.

- E. M. Purcell, H. C. Torrey and R. V. Pound. Resonance absorption by nuclear magnetic moments in a solid. *Phys. Rev.*, 69: 37, 1946.

- I. I. Rabi, N. F. Ramsey and J. Schwinger. Rotating coordinates in magnetic resonance problems. *Rev. Modern Phys.*, 26: 167, 1954.

- C. P. Slichter. *Principles of Magnetic Resonance.* Springer Verlag, 3rd ed., New York, 2010.

Chapter 7

Signal Detection Concepts

Chapter Contents

Summary: The physical principles of MR signal detection are derived from Faraday's law of electromagnetic induction. The principle of reciprocity is used to obtain an expression for the MR signal in terms of the sample magnetization and the field of the detector coils. Both real valued and complex valued demodulated signal formulas are presented. The strength of the MR signal as a function of the static and rf fields, the gyromagnetic ratio, the natural abundance, and other parameters is discussed.

Introduction

In the previous chapters, the central theme has been to detail the changes in the magnetization of a sample that are produced by external magnetic fields. One such case included rotating the magnetization away from its alignment along a static field by the application of a perturbing, transient rf field perpendicular to the static field direction. The rotation is actually a spiraling-downward motion due to the continuing precession about the static field direction. Once the magnetization has a transverse component, the detection of its precession about B_0 can be considered. It is the spin's own magnetic field lines that are swept along with the precession which forms the key to observing the magnetization. An electromotive force (emf) would be created in any coil through which the spin's magnetic flux sweeps, a consequence of Faraday's law. The time-dependent form of this current carries the information that is eventually transformed into an image of the sample.

Let us look more closely at the signal generated by the precessing magnetization. Consider a single magnetic moment as a bar magnet precessing about an axis perpendicular to its length. The magnetic flux of a rotating bar magnet is rotated as well, and an *emf* may be induced in nearby coil elements. We refer the reader to Fig. 7.1. On a macroscopic scale, this system is recognized as an electrical generator. The electrical power in use today is generally produced by forcibly spinning giant electromagnets near conducting coils. The MR signal is detected using the same principles: an rf coil is placed near a body which contains a large number of tiny rotating nuclear magnetic moments. Both the transmit and receive coils are designed for optimal performance at the same Larmor frequency so they may efficiently tip the magnetization and detect the resulting signal, respectively. Indeed, a single coil can be used for both purposes.

A great deal of interesting engineering goes into the detection of the MR signal. In this chapter, the basic physical principles involved will be discussed, and the engineering issues will be considered in later chapters dealing with coil design. Below, the relationship between the strength of the MR signal and the magnetization of the sample is quantified, starting with coil *emf* considerations. The different variables upon which the signal depends are exhibited, and the signal processing issues, such as demodulation, are explored. In the next chapter, simple but important signal detection experiments are introduced.

7.1   Faraday Induction

The *emf* induced in a coil by a change in its magnetic flux environment can be calculated by Faraday's law of induction (see Appendix A):

$$emf = -\frac{d\Phi}{dt} \tag{7.1}$$

where Φ is the flux through the coil,[1]

$$\Phi = \int_{\text{coil area}} \vec{B} \cdot d\vec{S} \tag{7.2}$$

The flux can be thought of as proportional to the number of field lines penetrating the effective area presented by the loops making up the coil. The number of flux lines is a convenient picture, and is arbitrarily normalized. Equation (7.2) is, by contrast, well-defined. The currents induced in a conducting loop by a changing flux produce a field which opposes the changes induced by the external field.[2]

In the application of (7.1) to MRI, a study of elementary examples with wire loops is helpful. The first example is a fixed coil in a time-dependent, fixed-axis magnetic field. Consider a harmonic (i.e., sinusoidal in time) magnetic field with angular frequency ω making an angle θ to the normal of the plane of the square coil shown in Fig. 7.2a. The magnetic field is given by

$$\vec{B}(t) = B(\sin\theta\hat{y} + \cos\theta\hat{z})\sin\omega t \tag{7.3}$$

---

[1]The vector $d\vec{S}$ has magnitude dS and is normal to the differential area in the direction chosen for the definition of positive flux.

[2]The result that induced currents produce fields that oppose externally induced flux changes is referred to as Lenz's law.

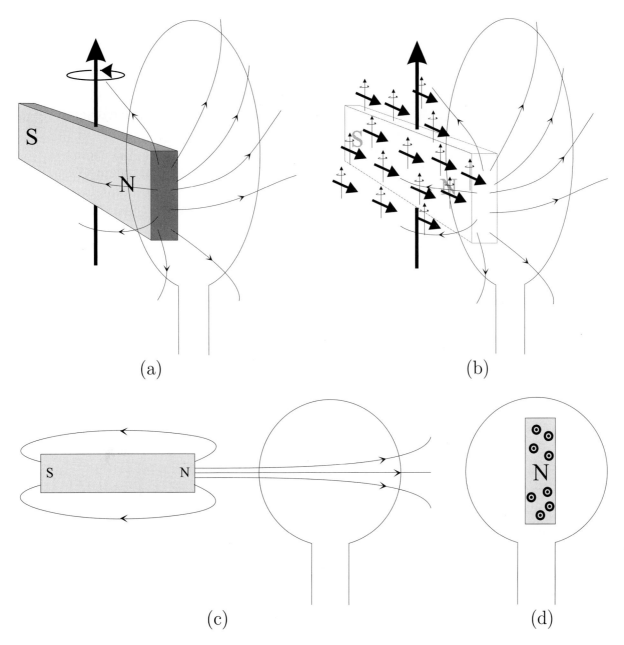

Fig. 7.1: This figure illustrates the flux coupling of a magnet with a loop of wire. A single rotating macroscopic bar magnet is shown in (a). Part (b) of the figure models the magnet as the combined effect of many individual spins (small dark arrows). The depiction of individual spins in (b) is only symbolic since an average sample contains trillions of trillions of nuclei. According to the discussion in Sec. 7.1, the flux through the coil is minimized when the bar length is in the plane of the coil (c) and maximized when it is perpendicular to that plane (d). In order for the *emf* to be nonzero, the flux must change in time and some coil element must have a component of its direction that is perpendicular to the applied flux.

for constant $B > 0$. The field (7.3) is taken to be uniform over the space of the coil, at any instant in time.[3] The coil is chosen to lie in the x-y plane so that $d\vec{S} = dx\,dy\,\hat{z}$. From (7.1) and (7.2), the *emf* generated in the coil by the time-varying magnetic field is

$$emf \;=\; -\frac{d}{dt}\int_{-L/2}^{L/2} dx \int_{-L/2}^{L/2} dy\,\hat{z}\cdot\vec{B}(t)$$

$$=\; -L^2 B\omega\cos\theta\cos\omega t \tag{7.4}$$

At $t = 0$, for example, the *emf* is negative, producing a clockwise (negative $\hat{\phi}$-direction) current in the loop. This can be verified by using the right-hand rule to see in which direction the current would have to flow to produce a field which opposes the change in the applied field $\vec{B}(t)$. The appearance of the ω factor in (7.4), which results from the time derivative, is an example of the significant fact that the *emf* increases with higher frequency.

The next example is a rotating coil in a constant field, which is the subject of Prob. 7.1. This case has an induced *emf* identical to that which would arise if, instead, the coil were stationary and the field rotated, a situation more closely related to the MRI experiment. In a standard MRI experiment, the field associated with a precessing magnetization sweeps past fixed receiving coils. Problem 7.2 addresses a simple situation of this kind.

Problem 7.1

---

a) A vertical circular loop of wire with radius a rotates about the z-axis at constant angular frequency, as shown in Fig. 7.2b, in a uniform magnetic field. If the loop lies initially in the y-z plane, the normal to the plane of the loop changes with time according to $\hat{n}(t) = \hat{x}\cos\omega t + \hat{y}\sin\omega t$. The magnetic field is given by $\vec{B} = B\hat{x}$. Find the *emf* induced in this coil.

b) Consider another orientation of the loop, assuming that $\vec{B}$ remains the same, i.e., $\vec{B} = B\hat{x}$. What *emf* will be induced in the loop if it initially lies in the x-y plane, and is rotated about the x-axis? In this case, $\hat{n}(t) = \hat{y}\sin\omega t + \hat{z}\cos\omega t$.

Problem 7.2

Consider the situation in Fig. 7.2c where the coil lies in the x-y plane and a spatially independent field rotates about the x-axis:

$$\vec{B}(t) = -B\sin\omega t\,\hat{z} + B\cos\omega t\,\hat{y}$$

Show that the *emf* induced in the coil is $L^2 B\omega\cos\omega t$. (Note that such fields can be produced by, for example, 'birdcage' coils, provided the rf wavelengths are not too small. See Ch. 27.)

---

[3]A magnetic field that varies in time must also vary in space, according to Maxwell's equations (see Appendix A). However, such spatial variations may be ignored for distances small compared to the wavelength, $\lambda = 2\pi c/\omega$. At 1.0 T the free-space wavelength for electromagnetic radiation is about 7 m.

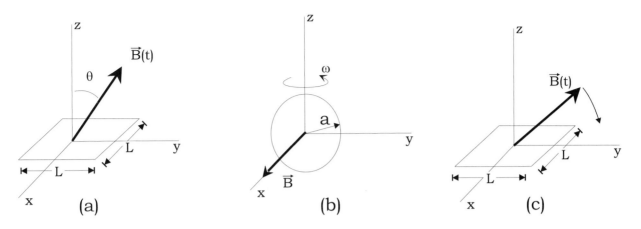

Fig. 7.2: Three related examples of loops of wires experiencing changing flux as a function of time: (a) A square coil is stationary, and the applied field oscillates along a fixed axis. (b) A circular coil rotates in a static field. (c) A stationary coil is immersed in a rotating, fixed-magnitude field (an example of special relevance to MR measurements).

7.2   The MRI Signal and the Principle of Reciprocity

Equation (7.2) can be converted into a form which is more useful for MRI, where the roles of the magnetization source and the detection coil are reversed. Switching their roles in an equation for the signal is an example of the principle of reciprocity which will be described later on in this section.

There is a magnetic field associated with the magnetization of a sample arising from the effective current density

$$\vec{J}_M(\vec{r}, t) = \vec{\nabla} \times \vec{M}(\vec{r}, t) \tag{7.5}$$

A current density $\vec{J}$ implies $|\vec{J}|$ charge per unit time per unit area in the direction of $\hat{J}$. The curl operation in (7.5) computes the net 'circulation' of the magnetization. To get a feel for this, magnetization can be approximated as a density distribution of many small current loops. The net currents associated with these loops correspond to the effective current density (7.5). Some background for the magnetization current and the vector calculus to follow is found in Appendix A.

The vector potential at position $\vec{r}$ stemming from a source current, such as (7.5), is

$$\vec{A}(\vec{r}) = \frac{\mu_0}{4\pi} \int d^3r' \frac{\vec{J}(\vec{r}')}{|\vec{r} - \vec{r}'|} \tag{7.6}$$

where the time dependence has been suppressed and the 'gauge choice' is left understood. The effects due to the time delay between the source and the measurement of the field are ignored. The magnetic field is calculated from

$$\vec{B} = \vec{\nabla} \times \vec{A} \tag{7.7}$$

Using (7.7) and Stokes' theorem,[4] it is possible to write the flux (7.2) through a coil in terms

---

[4]Stokes' theorem states that the surface integral of the scalar product between the curl of an arbitrary

of the vector potential

$$\Phi = \int_{area} \vec{B} \cdot d\vec{S} = \int_{area} (\vec{\nabla} \times \vec{A}) \cdot d\vec{S} = \oint d\vec{l} \cdot \vec{A} \tag{7.8}$$

A detailed derivation demonstrating that the flux Φ_M through a coil due to a magnetization source can be related to a flux due to the coil that goes through the magnetization is given next. The use of (7.5), (7.6) and (7.8), an integration by parts (where a surface term can be ignored for finite sources), and the vector identity, $\vec{A} \cdot (\vec{B} \times \vec{C}) = -(\vec{A} \times \vec{C}) \cdot \vec{B}$, respectively, give

$$\begin{aligned} \Phi_M &= \oint d\vec{l} \cdot \left[\frac{\mu_0}{4\pi} \int d^3 r' \frac{\vec{\nabla}' \times \vec{M}(\vec{r}')}{|\vec{r} - \vec{r}'|} \right] \\ &= \frac{\mu_0}{4\pi} \int d^3 r' \oint d\vec{l} \cdot \left[\left(-\vec{\nabla}' \frac{1}{|\vec{r} - \vec{r}'|} \right) \times \vec{M}(\vec{r}') \right] \\ &= \frac{\mu_0}{4\pi} \int d^3 r' \vec{M}(\vec{r}') \cdot \left[\vec{\nabla}' \times \left(\oint \frac{d\vec{l}}{|\vec{r} - \vec{r}'|} \right) \right] \end{aligned} \tag{7.9}$$

The version of (7.6) for current loops, now evaluated at position $\vec{r}'$,

$$\vec{A}(\vec{r}') = \frac{\mu_0}{4\pi} \oint \frac{I d\vec{l}}{|\vec{r} - \vec{r}'|} \tag{7.10}$$

shows that the curl of the line integral over the current path in (7.9) is actually $\vec{\mathcal{B}}^{receive}$, the magnetic field per unit current that would be produced by the coil at the point $\vec{r}'$,

$$\vec{\mathcal{B}}^{receive}(\vec{r}') = \vec{B}(\vec{r}')/I = \vec{\nabla}' \times \left(\frac{\mu_0}{4\pi} \oint \frac{d\vec{l}}{|\vec{r} - \vec{r}'|} \right) \tag{7.11}$$

Finally, the flux can be written as

$$\Phi_M(t) = \int_{sample} d^3 r \vec{\mathcal{B}}^{receive}(\vec{r}) \cdot \vec{M}(\vec{r}, t) \tag{7.12}$$

where the time dependence of the magnetization is now made explicit. The fact that the flux in (7.12) depends upon $\vec{\mathcal{B}}^{receive}$, the 'receive' field[5] produced by the detection coil at all points where the magnetization is nonzero, is an example of the principle of reciprocity. The original expression as a surface integration over the detection coil area has been replaced by a volume integration over the region of nonzero magnetization. That is, the flux through the detection coil due to the magnetization can be found instead by calculating the flux that would emanate from the detection coil, per unit current, through the (rotating) magnetization.

---

vector function $\vec{a}$ and the normal to the surface is equal to the line integral of $\vec{a}$ around the closed path bounding the surface: $\int d\vec{S} \cdot (\vec{\nabla} \times \vec{a}) = \oint d\vec{l} \cdot \vec{a}$

[5]Recall that the term 'magnetic field per unit current' refers to magnetic field divided by a constant current, $\vec{B}$. In later discussions, the notation $\vec{\mathcal{B}}$ will be used to describe this quantity.

The *emf* induced in the coil is expressed as

$$emf = -\frac{d}{dt}\Phi_M(t)$$

$$= -\frac{d}{dt}\int_{sample} d^3r\, \vec{M}(\vec{r},t) \cdot \vec{\mathcal{B}}^{receive}(\vec{r}) \tag{7.13}$$

Equation (7.13) is a key formula for understanding the factors which affect signal amplitude. The dependence of the *emf* on the excitation or transmit field $B_1^{transmit}$ is implicit in the dependence of (7.13) on the magnetization $\vec{M}$.

Problem 7.3

Consider two fixed loops of wire, each carrying the same current $I(t)$. Show that the *emf* induced in coil 1 by coil 2 is identical to the *emf* induced in coil 2 by coil 1, an example of a reciprocity relation. Hint: Consider (7.8) and the vector potential for current loops (7.10).

7.3 Signal from Precessing Magnetization

The fundamental signal in an MR experiment comes from the detection of the *emf* predicted by (7.13) for precessing magnetization. In this section, the prediction is analyzed further, in terms of variables involving the static and rf fields, and the properties of the sample of spins. The experiment described below from a given sample is generally referred to as a 'free induction decay.' This experiment is discussed in more detail in the next chapter.

7.3.1 General Expression

It is assumed that the sample is immersed in a static, uniform field $B_0\hat{z}$ and has been 'excited' by some rf pulse so that there exists, at time t, transverse components, M_x, M_y of magnetization, in addition to a longitudinal component, M_z. The signal measured by some system of electronics is proportional[6] to (7.13), which can be written out in terms of the individual components as

$$\text{signal} \propto -\frac{d}{dt}\int d^3r \left[\mathcal{B}_x^{receive}(\vec{r})M_x(\vec{r},t) + \mathcal{B}_y^{receive}(\vec{r})M_y(\vec{r},t) + \mathcal{B}_z^{receive}(\vec{r})M_z(\vec{r},t) \right] \tag{7.14}$$

When the known solutions for $\vec{M}(\vec{r},t)$ are inserted into the integrand, the evaluation of the time-derivative, discussed below, shows that the longitudinal magnetization can be neglected, even when there is a nonzero z-component for the receive-coil field.

The static-field solutions (4.25)–(4.27) hold for each $\vec{r}$. The longitudinal generalization is

$$M_z(\vec{r},t) = e^{-t/T_1(\vec{r})}M_z(\vec{r},0) + (1 - e^{-t/T_1(\vec{r})})M_0 \tag{7.15}$$

---

[6]The proportionality factor depends on amplifier gain and other factors, as determined by the detection scheme.

It is especially useful to employ the complex representation for the transverse components, not just in taking the time derivative, but for a variety of phase discussions to follow in subsequent chapters. Noting (4.31) through (4.33),

$$
\begin{aligned}
M_+(\vec{r},t) &= e^{-t/T_2(\vec{r})}e^{-i\omega_0 t}M_+(\vec{r},0) \\
&= e^{-t/T_2(\vec{r})}e^{-i\omega_0 t+i\phi_0(\vec{r})}M_\perp(\vec{r},0)
\end{aligned}
\tag{7.16}
$$

The phase ϕ_0 and magnitude $M_\perp(\vec{r},0)$ are determined by the initial rf pulse conditions. The rectangular components are found through the real and imaginary parts,

$$
M_x = \mathrm{Re}M_+ , \quad M_y = \mathrm{Im}M_+
\tag{7.17}
$$

The time derivative in (7.14) can be taken inside the integrand (and inside the Re and Im operations when (7.16) and (7.17) are substituted into (7.14)) to operate directly on (7.15) and (7.16). For static fields at the tesla level and protons, the Larmor frequency ω_0 is at least four orders-of-magnitude larger than typical values of $1/T_1$ and $1/T_2$. Hence the derivative of the e^{-t/T_1} and e^{-t/T_2} factors most certainly can be neglected,[7] compared with the derivative of the $e^{-i\omega_0 t}$ factor. With that approximation understood,

$$
\begin{aligned}
\text{signal} &\propto \omega_0\int d^3 r e^{-t/T_2(\vec{r})}\left[\mathcal{B}_x^{receive}(\vec{r})\,\mathrm{Re}\left(iM_+(\vec{r},0)e^{-i\omega_0 t}\right)+\mathcal{B}_y^{receive}(\vec{r})\,\mathrm{Im}\left(iM_+(\vec{r},0)e^{-i\omega_0 t}\right)\right] \\
&\propto \omega_0\int d^3 r e^{-t/T_2(\vec{r})}M_\perp(\vec{r},0)[\mathcal{B}_x^{receive}(\vec{r})\sin\left(\omega_0 t-\phi_0(\vec{r})\right) \\
&\qquad\qquad\qquad\qquad\qquad\qquad +\mathcal{B}_y^{receive}(\vec{r})\cos\left(\omega_0 t-\phi_0(\vec{r})\right)]
\end{aligned}
\tag{7.18}
$$

The leading term in the time-derivative calculation indicates that *the rapid Larmor oscillations of the transverse magnetization induce the dominant signal in the receive coil.* It also explains why the transverse magnetization M_+, or its magnitude $M_\perp = \sqrt{M_x^2 + M_y^2}$, is referenced, heuristically, as the 'signal.'[8]

The expression for the signal can be further simplified. The receive field laboratory components may be written quite generally in terms of the magnitude $\mathcal{B}_\perp$ and angle $\theta_\mathcal{B}$ in the parametrization

$$
\mathcal{B}_x^{receive} \equiv \mathcal{B}_\perp\cos\theta_\mathcal{B}, \quad \mathcal{B}_y^{receive} \equiv \mathcal{B}_\perp\sin\theta_\mathcal{B}
\tag{7.19}
$$

With the possible position dependence made explicit and the trigonometric identity $\sin(a+b) = \sin a\cos b + \cos a\sin b$,

$$
\text{signal} \propto \omega_0\int d^3 r e^{-t/T_2(\vec{r})}M_\perp(\vec{r},0)\mathcal{B}_\perp(\vec{r})\sin\left(\omega_0 t+\theta_\mathcal{B}(\vec{r})-\phi_0(\vec{r})\right)
\tag{7.20}
$$

The expression (7.20) for the signal is easily modified for the more general situation. The replacement $T_2 \to T_2^*$ must be made in the presence of external field inhomogeneities, although this distinction is ignored in the current chapter. A time-independent (or time-averaged) variation in the z-component of the local magnetic field, other than those already

---

[7]There are certain cases, such as in solids, where T_2 is on the order of a microsecond or less, and such approximations may no longer be valid.

[8]The complete Larmor-frequency dependence of the signal, including implicit ω_0 dependence in M_+, is discussed in the next section.

taken into account through T_2', may arise, for example, from the gradient fields used in imaging as detailed in later chapters. These field variations change the precession frequency according to

$$\omega(\vec{r}) = \omega_0 + \Delta\omega(\vec{r}) \tag{7.21}$$

The correction $\Delta\omega(\vec{r})$ has been ignored in the outside factor ω_0 in (7.18), but *it cannot be omitted in the phase of the sinusoid.*[9] Finally, in the case where additional fields have time dependence (e.g., when they are turned on and off), the phase $-i\omega(\vec{r})t$ is replaced by $-i\int_0^t dt'\,\omega(\vec{r},t')$; see (3.37).

7.3.2 Spatial Independence

The limit where all spatial dependence can be neglected, applies, for example, to studies of small homogeneous samples. Consider all quantities inside the integral (7.20) to be independent of $\vec{r}$. If the sample volume is V_s, then

$$\text{signal} \propto \omega_0 V_s e^{-t/T_2} M_\perp \mathcal{B}_\perp \sin\left(\omega_0 t + \theta_{\mathcal{B}} - \phi_0\right) \quad \text{(space-independent limit)} \tag{7.22}$$

For the precession frequency to be constant everywhere, the static field B_0 must also be uniform throughout space.

The constant phases in (7.22) are especially important in the comparison of signals from different sources where, for example, it is necessary to see whether cancelations occur. Practice in their computation is the subject of Prob. 7.4.

Problem 7.4

Consider a $\pi/2$-pulse produced by a left-circular $B_1^{transmit}$ field lying along $\hat{x}'$ in the rotating frame. It results in the rotation of the equilibrium magnetization of a sample into the $+\hat{y}'$ direction at $t = 0$ (at which time $\hat{y} = \hat{y}'$). (The magnetization would subsequently precess such that it remains pointed along the $+\hat{y}'$ direction in the rotating frame.)

a) Find the phase angle ϕ_0 in (7.22) corresponding to this initial condition.

b) Find ϕ_0 for the imaging scenario where the $\pi/2$-pulse is produced by $B_1^{transmit}$ along $-\hat{y}'$ (so that the magnetization is rotated into $+\hat{x}$ at $t = 0$ and remains pointed along the $+\hat{x}'$ direction in the rotating frame thereafter).

c) Repeat (b) for $B_1^{transmit}$ along $+\hat{y}'$.

d) Repeat (b) for $B_1^{transmit}$ along $-\hat{x}'$.

---

[9]A simple, but relevant example is $\cos(10^6 + \theta)$. Variations of θ in the interval $(0, 2\pi)$, though minuscule with respect to one million, can change the cosine value over the full range $(-1, 1)$.

7.3.3 Signal Demodulation

The rapid oscillations at the frequency ω_0 in the above signal expressions are removed, in practice, by an electronic step of 'demodulation,' which is tantamount to viewing the signal from a rotating reference frame. *Demodulation corresponds to the multiplication of the signal by a sinusoid or cosinusoid with a frequency at or near ω_0.* Strictly speaking, the transmit or 'irradiation' rf frequency ω_{rf} is this frequency, but in most experiments ω_{rf} is chosen equal to ω_0.

The space-independent formula (7.22) is used below to illustrate a demodulated signal. We take the reference signal, which is separately generated for the demodulation, to have frequency $\Omega = \omega_0 + \delta\omega$ where $\delta\omega$ is referred to as the 'offset' frequency from the Larmor frequency ω_0. Both sine and cosine multiplication are considered, corresponding, respectively, to data storage in two 'channels,' a 'real' array of numbers and an 'imaginary' array of numbers. The origin of the terminology is made evident in the following.

Real Channel

Consider first the multiplication of (7.22) by $\sin{(\omega_0 + \delta\omega)}t$.[10] With the suppression of the remaining factors, another trigonometric identity $\sin a \sin b = \frac{1}{2}(\cos{(a-b)} - \cos{(a+b)})$ leads to

$$
\begin{aligned}
\text{demodulated signal} \;&\propto\; \text{reference signal} \cdot \text{induced } emf \\
&\propto\; \sin{(\omega_0 + \delta\omega)}t \cdot \sin{(\omega_0 t + \zeta)} \\
&\propto\; \frac{1}{2}\left(\cos{(\delta\omega \cdot t - \zeta)} - \cos{((2\omega_0 + \delta\omega)t + \zeta)}\right)
\end{aligned}
\tag{7.23}
$$

with $\zeta \equiv \theta_{\mathcal{B}} - \phi_0$. A split into two frequencies is exhibited.

Low pass filtering[11] applied to the demodulated signal (Fig. 7.3) eliminates the high frequency component in (7.23),

$$
\text{demodulated and filtered signal} \propto \frac{1}{2}\cos{(\delta\omega \cdot t - \zeta)} = \frac{1}{2}\mathrm{Re}(e^{i\delta\omega\cdot t - i\zeta})
$$
$$
\text{(real channel)} \tag{7.24}
$$

Together with the T_2 envelope factor, this yields the time dependence of the so-called 'real' channel of the signal.

Imaginary Channel

The imaginary channel may be defined by multiplying the signal by the demodulation factor $-\cos{(\omega_0 + \delta\omega)}t$ (the negative rather than positive cosinusoid has been chosen as a convention) and carrying out steps analogous to the above analysis. The result is

---

[10]An analog-multiplier electronic circuit is used to combine the signal with the reference sinusoid.

[11]In the past, this has been done with analog filters such as the Butterworth filter which have slow falloff away from zero frequency. Today, however, digital filters which have much improved step-like edges are used to perform low pass filtering.

$$\text{demodulated and filtered signal} \propto \frac{1}{2}\sin\left(\delta\omega \cdot t - \zeta\right) = \frac{1}{2}\text{Im}(e^{i\delta\omega\cdot t - i\zeta})$$

$$\text{(imaginary channel)} \qquad (7.25)$$

Problem 7.5

Derive the time-dependence (7.25) for the imaginary channel of the demodulated and filtered signal.

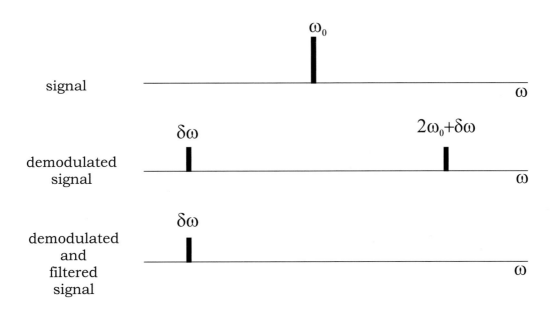

Fig. 7.3: The shifts in frequency for signals from a uniform sample due to demodulation and filtering, with small offset $\delta\omega$. The thick bars represent the signal at the indicated frequencies.

Laboratory Versus Demodulated Signals

The frequencies of the original and demodulated signals are compared in Fig. 7.3. The figure is applicable for either the real or imaginary channel, showing how the original signal at the Larmor frequency is demodulated into two components, one close to zero frequency and the other nearly twice the Larmor frequency, for small offset $\delta\omega$. See (7.23), for example. The filtered signal, (7.24) or (7.25), is left with only the small frequency component.

In summary, the signal, as measured in the laboratory, oscillates rapidly near the Larmor frequency. The demodulated[12] signal, essentially the signal measured in the rotating frame

---

[12]From now on, demodulation will usually refer to the combined demodulation and filtering operation.

defined by the reference frequency $\Omega = \omega_0 + \delta\omega$, is free of the rapid Larmor oscillation. It oscillates at the offset frequency $\delta\omega$.

Problem 7.6

Consider the signal resulting from two spin isochromats with identical spin densities but different frequencies of precession $\omega_a = \omega_0 + \Delta\omega$ and $\omega_b = \omega_0 - \Delta\omega$. The total signal for this experiment is just the linear addition of the signal from each isochromat. Find the demodulated signal (with zero offset, $\delta\omega = 0$) from the two-spin system and compare it to the demodulated signal (with offset) represented by (7.24) or (7.25).

Note: It will be evident in the solution that the signal from two spin isochromats with slightly different frequencies (a difference represented by a small $\Delta\omega$) exhibits beats. See the discussion on beating in Ch. 8.

Complex Signal

The real and imaginary forms of the two channel signals, (7.24) or (7.25), suggest the definition of a complex quantity that is quite useful. Consider the complex demodulated signal, $s(t)$, defined as

$$s(t) \equiv s_{re}(t) + i s_{im}(t) \tag{7.26}$$

where s_{re} and s_{im} refer to the real and imaginary channel demodulated signals. In place of (7.22), we have

$$s(t) \propto \omega_0 V_s e^{-t/T_2} M_\perp \mathcal{B}_\perp e^{i[(\Omega-\omega_0)t+\phi_0-\theta_\mathcal{B}]} \qquad \text{(space-independent limit)} \tag{7.27}$$

in terms of the reference signal frequency Ω. The real (imaginary) part of this expression yields the real (imaginary) channels.

More generally, (7.20) is replaced by

$$s(t) \propto \omega_0 \int d^3r \, e^{-t/T_2(\vec{r})} M_\perp(\vec{r},0) \mathcal{B}_\perp(\vec{r}) e^{i((\Omega-\omega_0)t+\phi_0(\vec{r})-\theta_\mathcal{B}(\vec{r}))} \tag{7.28}$$

Alternate forms with a change in the overall sign on the phase are possible. The integrand can also be written in complex notation. From (7.16) and the related definition based upon (7.19)

$$\mathcal{B}_+ \equiv \mathcal{B}_x^{receive} + i\mathcal{B}_y^{receive} = \mathcal{B}_\perp e^{i\theta_\mathcal{B}} \tag{7.29}$$

we obtain with $\Omega = \omega_0$,

$$s(t) \propto \omega_0 \int d^3r \, M_+(\vec{r},t) \mathcal{B}_+^*(\vec{r}) \tag{7.30}$$

This expression can itself be generalized for the more detailed experiments involving additional rf pulses and gradient fields.

7.3.4 Dependent Channels and Independent Coils

The above derivation of the real and imaginary channel demodulated signals was performed for arbitrary receive coil field directions. Whether $\vec{\mathcal{B}}^{receive}$ pointed in the laboratory x-direction ($\theta_\mathcal{B} = 0$) or along the y-direction ($\theta_\mathcal{B} = \pi/2$), or any other (spatially independent) direction in the x-y plane, the complex signal remained proportional to $e^{i\delta\omega t}$. Only the phase $\theta_\mathcal{B}$ changes in (7.27). In this sense, one coil is as good as another, and two (or more) coils do not yield any more information. The signal from two uncoupled coils (coils that have small flux 'linkage') can be used, however, to obtain an improvement in the ratio of signal to noise. The noise in one of these uncoupled coils is independent of the noise in the other whereas, for a single coil, the noise in one channel is the same as that in the other (i.e., the noise is correlated between the channels). These issues are discussed in more detail in Ch. 15.

A single quadrature, or circularly polarized (CP), receive coil can also be used to increase the signal.[13] This corresponds to demodulation with a sinusoid in the x-direction, say, and a cosinusoid in the y-direction. The resulting signal is the same for both: (7.24), with $\theta_\mathcal{B} = 0$, is the same as (7.25), with $\theta_\mathcal{B} = \pi/2$. To the extent that the 'cross-channel' noise is uncorrelated, the CP coil will also increase the signal-to-noise ratio.

7.4 Dependence on System Parameters

Let us investigate what (7.22) tells us about the variables on which the signal depends. Despite its lack of spatial information, this simple approximation is quite useful in understanding various imaging issues.

7.4.1 Homogeneous Limit

Suppose that the equilibrium magnetization $M_0\hat{z}$ is independent of position (i.e., the sample is homogeneous), and it is uniformly rotated (i.e., the rf field is homogeneous) into the transverse plane with an on-resonance $\pi/2$-pulse. Further, suppose that relaxation effects may be neglected, and that the static field is also perfectly homogeneous. The proportionality (7.27) can be turned into an equation for the signal amplitude, if the electronic amplification factors are ignored,[14]

$$|s| = \omega_0 M_0 \mathcal{B}_\perp V_s \tag{7.31}$$

Recall that M_0 is proportional to B_0 from (6.12). Therefore, in the small sample limit, (7.31) predicts a growth of B_0^2 (or, equivalently, ω_0^2 from $\omega_0 = \gamma B_0$) in the signal as a function of field. A general analysis, including space dependence and differences in the sampled nuclei, is complicated, and electronic and sample noise must also be considered. For example, at high fields, noise also increases linearly with B_0 so that, by the above estimate, the more pertinent quantity, the signal-to-noise ratio, is proportional to B_0.[15] *It is the increase of signal-to-noise ratio with frequency that accounts for the interest in higher-field imaging in*

---

[13]Such coils are discussed further in Ch. 27.

[14]Even in the presence of T_2 decay and without demodulation, the expression (7.31) still represents the peak signal obtained at $t = 0$ for a homogeneous sample.

[15]More general expressions for signal-to-noise in MR experiments are discussed in Ch. 15.

MRI. Indeed, fields in excess of 10 T are already in use for NMR microscopy experiments. Higher fields have additional attraction for spectroscopists since the chemical shift dispersion increases linearly with field strength.

Problem 7.7

The following problem will be of recurring interest when signal-to-noise issues are discussed. Consider a cubical volume of a uniform water sample, 10 cm on a side, in a constant magnetic field of 1 T, and at a temperature of 300 K. Assume the approximation given by (7.31).

a) Estimate the maximum *emf* that could be induced in a coil which, by reciprocity, can produce a constant magnetic field per unit current of 1 gauss/A over the sample. Assume a proton NMR experiment was performed.

b) What is the percentage increase or decrease in the signal from this sample if the length of the cubical side is increased to 20 cm?

c) For the new cubical dimension of 20 cm, how much must you change either B_0 or the temperature to keep the signal the same as in part (a)?

There are a number of technical difficulties associated with higher field imaging, however, and whether there is an optimal field strength for MRI remains to be seen. (See Ch. 15 for some additional insight into this question.) Optimal field strength is also likely to depend upon the application. The signal dependence on V_s is crucial to very high resolution imaging, since the signal in each voxel is limited by its volume and the available magnetization for the given field and temperature conditions. In general, as resolution is increased, the available signal decreases. This is easy to understand by considering the volume integral over the entire sample as a summation over smaller volumes (voxels, say) within the sample. The smaller the individual volume, the less signal it will produce. In order to obtain enough signal from the tiny volumes ($\approx 1000\,\mu m^3$ for μm = one micron) sought after by microscopists, fields of approximately 7 T and higher are usually employed.

7.4.2   Relative Signal Strength

What we call the relative signal strength $\mathcal{R}$ of an MR experiment for a particular nuclear species can also be analyzed through (7.31).[16] The first step is to find the dependence of the equilibrium-magnetization formula (6.10) on the gyromagnetic ratio γ_i and spin s_i of a specific nucleus i:

$$M_{0_i} \propto a_i s_i (s_i + 1)\gamma_i^2 \tag{7.32}$$

---

[16]The more common definition for the sensitivity of an MR experiment is based on the signal-to-noise ratio of a given chemical species relative to a fixed standard species, usually ^{1}H, which is normalized to have a sensitivity of unity.

where a_i is the natural abundance (the fractional occurrence of a given stable isotope relative to all stable isotopes). The relative signal strength $\mathcal{R}_i$ of a given nuclear species i can be defined from the species-dependent factors in (7.31) combined with (7.32). Noting $\omega_0 \propto \gamma$, we find

$$\mathcal{R}_i \equiv |\gamma_i|^3 r_i a_i s_i (s_i + 1) \tag{7.33}$$

The weighting r_i is the relative abundance in the human body of the given element referenced to some nucleus. In this text, signal strength is quoted relative to ^{1}H in gray matter.

Using γ instead of ω_0 means that only for the same static field can a comparison of two different elements be made through (7.33). The parameters for several other elements relative to ^{1}H are presented in Table 7.1. Its sizable gyromagnetic ratio and large fractional presence explain why ^{1}H is the subject of choice for imaging of humans by nuclear magnetic resonance.

Problem 7.8

Using (7.33) and the data from Table 7.1, verify the calculated values given in that table for the relative signal strengths $\mathcal{R}_i/\mathcal{R}(^1\text{H})$ of the following nuclear species: (i) ^{23}Na   (ii) ^{17}O   (iii) ^{31}P.

Nucleus i	γ_i (MHz/T)	r_i	a_i	s_i	$\mathcal{R}_i/\mathcal{R}(^1\text{H})$ at $1\,T$
^{1}H, gray matter	42.58	1.0	1.0	$\frac{1}{2}$	1.0
^{23}Na, average tissue	11.27	9.1×10^{-4}	1.0	$\frac{3}{2}$	8.4×10^{-5}
^{31}P, average tissue	17.25	8.5×10^{-4}	1.0	$\frac{1}{2}$	5.7×10^{-5}
^{17}O, gray matter	-5.77	0.5	3.8×10^{-4}	$\frac{5}{2}$	5.5×10^{-6}
^{19}F, average tissue	40.08	4.5×10^{-8}	1.0	$\frac{1}{2}$	3.8×10^{-8}

Table 7.1: Table of γ, natural abundance a, fraction of all isotopes r relative to ^{1}H in gray matter, spin s in units of $\hbar$ (see Ch. 5), and calculated relative sensitivity of other elements of interest. The values presented refer to a fixed field strength. Note that a negative value of γ means that precession occurs in the counterclockwise direction. The product of $a_i r_i$ and the molarity 88 M for ^{1}H in gray matter yields the relative body abundances of Table 2.1.

7.4.3   Radiofrequency Field Effects

Up to now, we have assumed that the transmit and receive rf coils produce uniform fields over the imaging volume. If this is not the case, the image intensity will vary as a function of position, even for a uniform sample. The image will appear to be brighter or darker in regions where either one or both of the rf fields, referred to by $B_1^{transmit}$ (tips spins) or $\mathcal{B}^{receive}$ (measures signal), vary. The changes in image intensity as a function of field depend on flip angle and which field is being discussed. Assuming a uniform rotation by the transmit coil, the image will be darker in regions where $\mathcal{B}^{receive}$ is smaller, and brighter where $\mathcal{B}^{receive}$ is larger.

The effect of the transmit field is more complex. Consider the case of a $\pi/2$ flip angle. Any field which is greater or less than ideal (i.e., than that strength resulting in exactly a 90° rotation) results in reduced transverse magnetization and, therefore, a decrease in available signal. This statement is valid for a single pulse experiment only. However, if a flip angle of less than $\pi/2$ is desired, the picture is more complicated, and will be discussed in Ch. 8.

Specific imaging conditions can lead to a quadratic dependence on B_1 if the same coil is used for tipping the spins and detecting the signal, or if similar field profiles exist in $B_1^{transmit}$ and $\mathcal{B}^{receive}$. Transmit and receive coils are carefully chosen in each imaging situation to maximize image quality, but it is still necessary to be aware of coil effects when viewing an image. More of these considerations will be discussed in later chapters where specific applications and design issues are addressed.

Problem 7.9

Investigate the effect of using different combinations of rf systems to tip the spins and measure the resulting signal.

a) Assume two identical spins are excited by a uniform field, such that they both receive a perfect $\pi/2$-rotation into the transverse plane. What will be the relative difference in the signal between the two spins if $\mathcal{B}^{receive}(spin\ 1) = C$, a constant, and $\mathcal{B}^{receive}(spin\ 2) = 1/2\ C$?

b) Assume now that the two spins from (a) are excited by different transmit fields. The first spin experiences $B_1^{transmit}(spin\ 1) = C'$, another constant, and receives a $\pi/2$ flip. The second spin only experiences a field of $B_1^{transmit}(spin\ 2) = 1/2\ C'$, and therefore is not rotated by the same angle. If $\mathcal{B}^{receive}$ is identical for the two spins, what is the relative difference in their measured signal?

c) It appears from the preceding problems that if only one of the transmit and receive fields is inhomogeneous, but not both, then it might be best to transmit with an inhomogeneous rf field, and receive with a homogeneous field. However, this is not how experiments are normally performed. Explain why this might be the case. Hint: Recall that the received signal depends upon $\mathcal{B} = B/I$ and preview Ch. 15.

Suggested Reading

A good introduction to basic NMR signal detection is given in:

- W. S. Hinshaw and A. H. Lent. An introduction to NMR imaging: From the Bloch equation to the imaging equation. *Proc. IEEE*, 71: 338, 1983.

The basic interaction between the nuclear magnetic moment and the rf coil as well as the reciprocity concept are introduced in this widely quoted paper:

- D. I. Hoult and R. E. Richards. The signal-to-noise ratio of the nuclear magnetic resonance experiment. *J. Magn. Reson.*, 24: 71, 1976.

A complete description of magnetic moments appears in the following text:

- J. D. Jackson. *Classical Electrodynamics.* John Wiley and Sons, 3rd ed., Hoboken, 1999.

A list of other NMR active elements (i.e., those with nonzero spin) can be found in:

- P. T. Beall, S. R. Amtey and S. R. Kasturi. *NMR Data Handbook for Biomedical Applications.* Pergamon Press, New York, 1984.

Chapter 8

Introductory Signal Acquisition Methods: Free Induction Decay, Spin Echoes, Inversion Recovery, and Spectroscopy

Chapter Contents

Summary: Basic MR experiments are described, including the detection of a global signal from all the excited spins in a sample, the measurement of field inhomogeneities through T_2^* decay, the reduction of such field effects through the spin echo method, and variations on that method. The signals for commonly repeated sequences, such as the free induction decay and spin echo, are analyzed. A discussion of chemical shifts is based on differences in the Larmor frequency for the same nucleus in different chemical structures.

Introduction

The signal received by the rf detector coil is determined not just by the properties of the body but also by a rich set of magnetic field possibilities. In this chapter, we begin the study of the signal by considering simple, though important, rf field choices. The first is a single rf excitation pulse applied uniformly to the sample, producing a signal associated with the collective Larmor precession of all excited spins. The second is a pair of rf pulses;

the excitation pulse followed by another pulse whose purpose is to help recover, via an 'echo,' some of the signal lost to T_2' relaxation. The third is one of repeating, in various combinations, a given set of rf pulses. The fourth corresponds to an important method called 'inversion recovery,' where the spins are inverted prior to creating the transverse magnetization. Inversion recovery is useful in highlighting differences in T_1 behavior, and in 'nulling' the signal from tissues. Four sections are devoted to these choices and a first-pass approach for measuring T_2 and T_1 is also presented. A more in-depth study of these parameters using modern imaging sequences appears in Ch. 22.

The 'sequence diagram' is also introduced, which represents all rf pulses and other relevant quantities (field gradients will be included in Ch. 9) that are applied during the entire experiment in an easy-to-understand format. As more complex sequence diagrams are introduced in future chapters, it will be seen that a single experiment may involve changing certain parameters and repeating the modified rf structure or, in the case of 'multiple data acquisitions,' simply repeating a fixed rf structure.

Spectroscopy is briefly introduced in the last section. The signal from components with different Larmor frequencies is collected to obtain information about the constituents of the sample.

8.1   Free Induction Decay and T_2^*

The simplest MRI experiment involves detecting a global signal from a sample. Consider a $\pi/2$-pulse applied uniformly to proton spins in a static magnetic field associated, say, with any hydrogen atoms present (a macroscopic set). The pulse rotates the longitudinal magnetization (the excess spins) into the transverse plane after which the tipped spins freely and collectively precess. As discussed in Ch. 7, the total time-varying coherent magnetic field derived from the sum over all precessing proton spin fields would induce a small *emf* in any rf coil properly oriented to detect the corresponding flux changes. This experiment is called a free induction decay (FID). The signal expressions from the previous chapter can be applied directly to its analysis.

An FID is performed routinely on MRI machines to tune rf coils and optimize system response. It can be used to locate the resonance peak for water and determine the rf amplitude and duration necessary to produce a maximum signal.

8.1.1   FID Signal

The groundwork for the theoretical expression for the FID signal has been laid in Ch. 7. From (7.28), the complex form for a demodulated signal due to an rf spin flip at $t = 0$ is

$$s(t) \propto \omega_0 \int d^3r\, e^{-t/T_2(\vec{r})} \mathcal{B}_\perp(\vec{r}) M_\perp(\vec{r}, 0) e^{i((\Omega - \omega(\vec{r}))t + \phi_0(\vec{r}) - \theta_\mathcal{B}(\vec{r}))} \qquad (8.1)$$

with demodulation reference frequency Ω and field angle $\theta_\mathcal{B}$. Over the whole sample, there is, in general, spatial dependence in T_2 and the initial magnetization (even with a perfect $\pi/2$-pulse, the equilibrium value M_0 depends on the local spin density). The possibility that the precession frequency can change with position has also been included, $\omega = \omega(\vec{r})$.

Consider the following simple FID experiment. Assume that, in fact, the precession frequency is constant ($\omega = \omega_0$) over all space, and that the initial magnetization phase, the direction of the receive field, and the decay constant are also space-independent. The associated factors can be taken outside of the integral in (8.1)

$$s(t) \quad \propto \quad \omega_0 e^{-t/T_2} e^{i((\Omega-\omega_0)t+\phi_0-\theta_\mathcal{B})} \int d^3r \mathcal{B}_\perp(\vec{r}) M_\perp(\vec{r},0) \tag{8.2}$$

Nonuniformities in the receive coil, and especially in the sample, are still taken into account. The complex exponential gives way to a cosine or a sine depending on whether the real or the imaginary channel signal is detected.

The expression (8.2) can be used to understand several examples of signal time dependence. In the laboratory frame, where no demodulation is applied ($\Omega = 0$), rapid oscillations at frequency ω are damped by the relaxation factor, as shown in Fig. 8.1a. Demodulation on-resonance ($\Omega = \omega_0$) eliminates the sinusoid, with only the T_2 envelope remaining (Fig. 8.1b). A demodulation slightly off-resonance ($\Omega - \omega = \delta\omega$) leaves a low frequency component in Fig. 8.1c. Lastly, the superposition of demodulated signals (at some central value for Ω) from several spin populations, each with a different Larmor frequency, leads to a sum of terms (8.2), yielding a signal that decays faster than a single demodulated signal which only has T_2 damping (Fig. 8.1d). The dephasing among the populations causes the reduced signal, resembling a T_2' effect.

The transmit rf field pulses shown in Fig. 8.1 show rapid oscillations in the laboratory and none in the rotating frame. Indeed, the left-circular B_1 field, given by (3.24), is sinusoidal in the x, y coordinates, and it is constant in the x', y' coordinates. The remaining figures of this chapter show the Larmor-frame rf pulses. It is important to note that narrow 'boxcar' pulses (or 'hard pulses') correspond to larger frequency spreads than what is generally desired. In fact, time profiles such as 'sinc' functions (Ch. 9) are required in imaging applications, where rf pulses with sufficiently limited frequency spread are utilized.[1] The more relevant rf pulse time graphs are discussed and illustrated in Ch. 10.

8.1.2 Phase Behavior and Phase Conventions

It is recalled that the contribution to the phase of (8.1) due to the magnetization (or spin isochromat) at $\vec{r}$ is

$$\phi(\vec{r},t) = -\omega(\vec{r})t + \phi_0(\vec{r}) = -\gamma B_z(\vec{r})t + \phi_0(\vec{r}) \tag{8.3}$$

Starting at the initial value ϕ_0 at $t = 0$, the phase ϕ is seen to accumulate an additional amount, at time t, due to the precession about the z-component of the field. From the discussion in Sec. 7.3.1, where it was assumed that the transverse magnetization is created by an initial rf pulse, the angle ϕ_0, the phase of the initial magnetization $M_+(\vec{r},0)$, is determined by the direction of the rf pulse. See Prob. 7.4.

Initial phases, such as those in (8.3), often can (and will) be redefined or ignored in subsequent equations. It is possible to choose the origin along any axis of convenience. Although polar coordinates in the x-y plane are usually defined such that $\phi = 0$ along

---

[1]Nevertheless, narrow boxcar pulses, or hard pulses, will be the staple for the remainder of this and the following chapters.

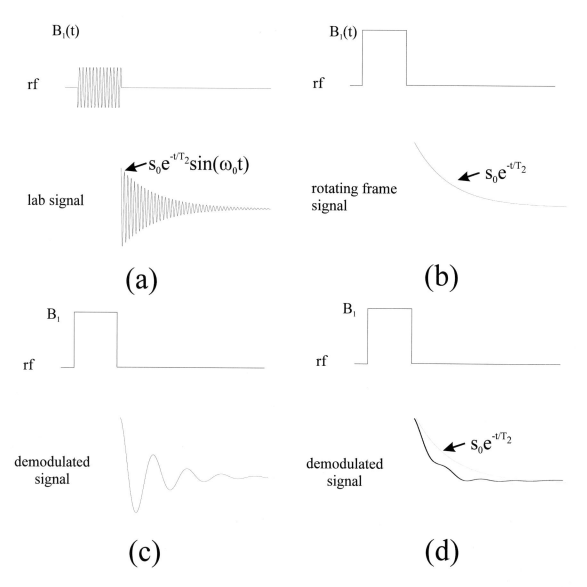

Fig. 8.1: (a) The FID signal in the laboratory frame for all spins precessing at the same Larmor frequency. The laboratory rf transmit field oscillates at that frequency. (b) The same experiment but as measured in the Larmor rotating frame (i.e., demodulated). The rotating frame rf field is at 'rest.' (c) The demodulated FID signal when the demodulation is not exactly at the Larmor frequency. (d) The total demodulated FID signal from several isochromats, each with slightly different Larmor frequencies, exhibiting a decay, with slow oscillations, that is faster than T_2 decay alone, due to dephasing. The demodulation in (d) is determined by the average (fast) frequency. Note that the laboratory signal in (a) is only suggestive since the oscillations seen in practice are too rapid to display. The T_2' effects have not been included in any of the curves; note that the differences in case (d) could be considered, alternatively, to be due to field inhomogeneities.

the positive x-axis, it is frequently useful to choose the zero point to be along the initial magnetization. For example, the choice for the zero angle would be along the y-axis for a $\pi/2$-pulse (field) direction along $\hat{x}$. At $t = 0$, $\hat{x}$ and $\hat{y}$ coincide with their respective primed, rotating counterparts, $\hat{x}'$ and $\hat{y}'$. However, the counterclockwise rotation for the definition of increasing ϕ will be maintained.

8.1.3 T_2^* Decay

It has been discussed previously that the dephasing of the magnetization caused by field inhomogeneities produces additional suppression of the signal in (8.1). The damping of the magnitude of the transverse magnetization was described in Ch. 4 by the replacement of T_2 by T_2^*

$$M_\perp(\vec{r}, t) = M_\perp(\vec{r}, 0)e^{-t/T_2^*} \tag{8.4}$$

Although qualitatively the same shape as shown in Fig. 8.1b, the new envelope factor typically decays much faster in time. The decay time T_2^* represents a combination of external field induced (T_2') and thermodynamic (T_2) effects,

$$\frac{1}{T_2^*} = \frac{1}{T_2} + \frac{1}{T_2'} \tag{8.5}$$

The quantity T_2' is both machine and sample dependent.[2] The characteristic which most distinguishes it from T_2, besides the fact that it can be much smaller, is that the T_2' signal loss is recoverable (reversible). The details behind the reversibility are presented in Sec. 8.2.

The T_2' dependence is used in FID measurements to determine whether the homogeneity of the main magnet is adequate. A uniform sample is placed in the magnet, and the FID is then observed. If the decay is too rapid (Fig. 8.1d), poor magnet homogeneity is indicated, and corrections to the main field are made in an attempt to recover the pristine signal. The reader is referred to Ch. 27, where static-field coil construction issues are discussed. Although T_2^* can be obtained by fitting the data to the exponential form in (8.4), separating T_2 and T_2' is more difficult. A method for measuring T_2 is presented in this chapter after an introduction of the spin echo.

T_2' Estimates

The origin of the T_2' part of the decay is the collective effect of the dephasing of the isochromats of spins. This can be described by a dephasing limit (i.e., $t \to \infty$)

$$\sum_{\text{sample}} e^{i\phi(\vec{r}, t)} \xrightarrow[\text{dephasing}]{} 0 \tag{8.6}$$

A demonstration of the vanishing of the sum in (8.6) for randomly distributed phases is contained in Sec. 21.1, while a related integral version is found in Sec. 10.2. The sum corresponds to a discrete version of the demodulated signal (8.1) where the remaining field and

---

[2]In particular, T_2' is a local quantity, and images are frequently found to be of poorer quality away from the main-coil center. The static field variations across a unit voxel are smaller near the center where the field uniformity is usually best.

magnetization factors have been suppressed. It has been noted in Ch. 4, that only under certain circumstances would the sum be proportional to the exponential form $e^{-t/T_2'}$ (and consistent with the T_2' dependence in (8.4)).

A simple phase argument can be applied to estimate the size of the decay time T_2'. This argument carries the additional benefit of introducing a way to connect other field variations, such as external linear fields and internal susceptibility effects (Ch. 25), to phase changes. Consider the phase (8.3) for a spin isochromat at position $\vec{r}$ where there is a time-independent spatial variation $\Delta B(\vec{r})$ in the z-component of the total magnetic field. With the neglect of the initial phase, the laboratory accumulated phase is

$$\phi(\vec{r}, t) = -\gamma \left(B_0 + \Delta B(\vec{r}) \right) t \tag{8.7}$$

The reader is asked to carry out a numerical estimate of T_2', using (8.7), in Prob. 8.1.

Problem 8.1

It is not necessary to consider how the sum of phases in (8.6) leads to an exponential decay, in order to find an estimate of the value of T_2' and to understand how it is affected by field strength and homogeneity. The following modest calculation will suffice.

Suppose two proton spins are positioned at $\vec{r}_1$ and $\vec{r}_2$, respectively, where $\Delta B(\vec{r}_1) = +\delta$ ppm (parts per million) $\equiv (\delta/10^6) \cdot B_0$, and $\Delta B(\vec{r}_2) = -\delta$ ppm, with respect to an arbitrary B_0. Find a formula for the time it takes the two spins to become π radians out of phase with each other, so that the net magnetization of the pair is zero. Discuss the dependence of this time on δ and B_0 and thus find a numerical estimate of T_2', as the time of the first zero crossing of the signal for $\delta = 1.0$ and $B_0 = 1.5$ T.

This problem is also representative of two spins with symmetrically chemically shifted frequencies relative to some base-line frequency. The concept of chemical shift is introduced later in this chapter.

Although simple phase arguments are most useful in understanding various effects, care must be taken not to double count. For example, external field inhomogeneities are already accounted for when the exponential factor $e^{-t/T_2'}$ is included, as in the formula for the magnitude of the magnetization, (8.4). The phase ϕ of the complex magnetization M_+ is redefined, when that factor is present, so as not to include the effects of those inhomogeneities. A similar situation occurs for the intrinsic T_2 damping; local field effects are already included, at least in part, by the factor e^{-t/T_2}. An experimental method for removing the dephasing represented by the $e^{-t/T_2'}$ factor is described in the next section. The following problem is also on phase dispersion, where an approximate value of a field gradient is to be calculated.

Problem 8.2

The parameter T_2' is associated with the (relatively smooth) variation in the z-component of the external field. An estimate of the average gradient in this component can be found from a given phase variation. If the z-component changes from $B_0 + \Delta B(\vec{r}_1)$ to $B_0 + \Delta B(\vec{r}_2)$, then the average gradient of that component between the two points $\vec{r}_1$ and $\vec{r}_2$ can be defined as

$$\overline{G} \equiv \frac{|\Delta B(\vec{r}_2) - \Delta B(\vec{r}_1)|}{|\vec{r}_2 - \vec{r}_1|} \tag{8.8}$$

Suppose two protons are situated at these points. If $|\vec{r}_2 - \vec{r}_1|$ is 2 mm, and if there is no initial phase difference between their spins, find the value of $\overline{G}$ leading to a 2π difference in phase, after a time 5 ms, for the two proton spins.

The average gradient found in this problem is not dissimilar to that present in the body, at the interface between tissue and air, as caused by magnetic susceptibility differences, for static fields at the tesla level. That is, even for a perfectly homogeneous static field, there are inhomogeneities due to differences in local field shielding (see Ch. 20).

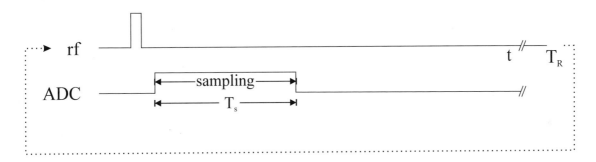

Fig. 8.2: Sequence diagram for a repeated FID experiment. Repetition of the rf pulse and sampling, with repeat time T_R, is indicated by the dotted line and arrow in this figure, but the fact that the process, or 'cycle,' is usually repeated is left understood in most diagrams. The ADC line represents the activity of the analog-to-digital converter, which is the device used to sample the signal over time T_s.

8.1.4   The FID Sequence Diagram and Sampling

Figure 8.2 is a sequence diagram representing one cycle of a simple FID experiment in which the repetition is indicated explicitly by a dotted line. This chapter notwithstanding, the dotted line and the repeat time T_R are customarily left out of the sequence diagrams, and the repetition is implied by other features, such as broken lines or 'gradient tables' (see Ch. 10).

The continuous emf signal is measured by the analog-to-digital converter (ADC) as shown in Fig. 8.2. The measurement is carried out at a finite set of discrete steps in time. If N points are collected at uniform Δt intervals, the total sampling time is

$$T_s = (N - 1)\Delta t \qquad (8.9)$$

Such sampling represents an approximation of the signal. The number and frequency of such steps needed for an accurate representation is discussed in Ch. 12.

8.2   The Spin Echo and T_2 Measurements

In the circumstance where the external field is not particularly uniform, the time constant T_2' can often be sufficiently small that $1/T_2'$ dominates $1/T_2$, and a severe extrinsic signal loss may result. Fortunately, this effect can be reversed by a well-known rf pulse sequence called the 'spin echo method.'

8.2.1   The Spin Echo Method

The spin echo sequence is based on the application of two rf pulses: a $\pi/2$-pulse followed by a π-pulse (or 'refocusing' pulse). The plot showing the recovery of T_2' signal loss resulting from this sequence is shown in Fig. 8.3. To understand the signal plot, we shall analyze three steps.

In the first step, it is sufficiently general to assume that the magnetization of a sample is tipped by the first pulse immediately into the transverse plane. Suppose this happens instantaneously at $t = 0$ such that, initially, the (excess) spins point along the $\hat{y}'$ axis. (Recall that (the field of) such a pulse lies along $\hat{x}'$, where the pulse is assumed to be applied in the rotating frame.) The spins at different positions $\vec{r}$ begin to dephase, relative to each other, as they experience different field strengths, each of which, in general, is not exactly equal to B_0. The accumulated phase of a spin at $\vec{r}$ in the rotating frame is found by subtracting the Larmor term in (8.7). The phase ϕ in this frame relative to the y'-axis is

$$\phi(\vec{r}, t) = -\gamma \Delta B(\vec{r})\, t \qquad \text{for } 0 < t < \tau \qquad (8.10)$$

where $\phi_0 = 0$ in (8.3).

The entire second step, for present purposes, is considered to be instantaneous. Another rf pulse with twice the amplitude, but otherwise identical to the first, is then applied. The second pulse is along $\hat{y}'$, rotating the spins about the y'-axis through the angle π, at time τ. The spins which had previously accumulated extra positive phase now have, at the instant after the π-pulse,[3] the negative of that phase, and vice versa,[4]

$$\begin{aligned}
\phi(\vec{r}, \tau^+) &= -\phi(\vec{r}, \tau^-) \\
&= \gamma \Delta B(\vec{r})\, \tau \qquad (8.11)
\end{aligned}$$

---

[3]We shall use the notation $f(t^{\pm})$ to refer to the limits $\lim\limits_{\epsilon \to 0} f(t \pm |\epsilon|)$.

[4]The action of the π-pulse, $\phi \to -\phi$, would be changed to $\phi \to \pi - \phi$, for example, if the $\phi = 0$ line were redefined to lie along the x'-axis.

In the third step, the spins continue, after time τ, to accumulate phase according to (8.10)

$$\begin{aligned}
\phi(\vec{r}, t) &= \phi(\vec{r}, \tau^+) - \gamma \Delta B(\vec{r})(t - \tau) \\
&= -\gamma \Delta B(\vec{r})(t - 2\tau) \\
&= -\gamma \Delta B(\vec{r})(t - T_E), \qquad t > \tau
\end{aligned} \qquad (8.12)$$

with the echo time defined by

$$T_E \equiv 2\tau \qquad (8.13)$$

Since the rate at which phase is accumulated by each spin is unchanged, all of the spins will return to $\phi = 0$ at the same time, the echo time. *Equation (8.12) shows that the accumulated phase of all spins experiencing a time-independent field variation will return to*

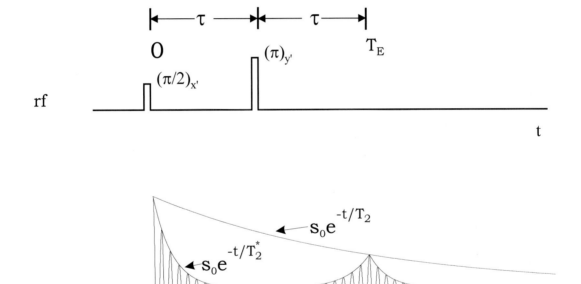

Fig. 8.3: A $\pi/2$-pulse is applied along the positive x'-axis at $t = 0$, and a π-pulse is applied along the positive y'-axis at $t = \tau$ to invert the phase that the spins have accumulated. The spins then 'rephase,' producing what is called an 'echo.' Notice that the signal strength is still limited by the T_2 envelope at the echo time $T_E = 2\tau$, as measured from the center of the rf pulse. The corresponding exponentials for the decay envelopes are found in (8.18). Here, and in later figures, the π-pulse is drawn at twice the height, for the same width, as the $\pi/2$-pulse, corresponding to the need for twice the B_1 amplitude to get twice the angle of spin rotation. The echo shows a positive local maximum, instead of a negative local minimum, since the magnetization is rephased along $+\hat{y}'$. The subscripts on the rf pulse brackets denote the axis along which the rf field is applied.

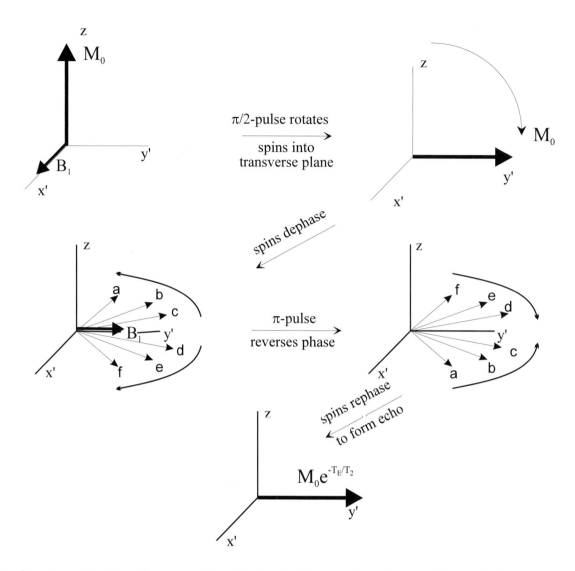

Fig. 8.4: A simulation of an ensemble of spins in the rotating reference frame during a spin echo experiment. A $\pi/2$-pulse rotates the spins, around the x'-axis, into the transverse plane where they begin to precess. The spins accumulate extra phase, until this accumulation is inverted by the π-pulse. The spins continue to collect extra phase at the same rate and, at a later time, all spins return to the positive y'-axis together, forming an echo. The echo amplitude is still reduced, however, by the intrinsic T_2 decay.

zero at $t = T_E$, *regardless of the value of* ΔB *and the position* $\vec{r}$. *Therefore, it is obvious that all of the spins will be realigned at the same time, and the realignment of the spins is called a spin echo.*[5] This particular rf pulse combination produces a positive echo along $\hat{y}'$ (i.e., the echo refocuses all spins along the positive y' direction). Figure 8.4 presents a simplified picture of the behavior of the individual spins during the experiment.

---

[5]This type of echo is also called a Hahn or rf echo.

Problem 8.3

It is also possible to generate a spin echo with the same rotational axis for the $\pi/2$ and π-pulses. Consider, for example, the case where the $\pi/2$ and π-pulses are both applied along the x'-axis (so the spins are always rotated clockwise about the x'-axis). Write the equations for the phase during the experiment in analogy with (8.11)–(8.12), using the convention that the phase is zero when $\vec{M}$ is parallel to $\hat{y}'$. Show that an echo is produced along the direction opposite to that which the magnetization had immediately after the $\pi/2$ excitation (i.e., a negative-echo along $\hat{y}'$). Signal plots would therefore display a 'negative' peak at the echo.

8.2.2   Spin Echo Envelopes

The next question is about the explicit form of the decay-and-growth echo exponentials. The envelope of $M_\perp(\vec{r}, t)$ for the spin echo experiment can be found by addressing the time dependence in the relaxation rate R_2^{SE} for the spin echo experiment. This is determined by the time rate of change in the rotating reference frame (see Ch. 4)

$$\left(\frac{dM_\perp}{dt}\right)'_{relaxation} = -R_2^{SE} M_\perp \tag{8.14}$$

where the primed derivative is defined in (3.10). All other terms in the Bloch equation for the transverse magnetization are neglected. It has been noted in an earlier discussion that the microscopic justification for the rate equation (8.14), which is based on an analysis of the dephasing cancelations, is found in Ch. 20.

Before the π-pulse and after the echo, R_2^{SE} is the usual sum of extrinsic and intrinsic terms. Between the π-pulse and the echo, the extrinsic rate is negative, because the phase differences due to field inhomogeneities are being refocused. This corresponds to the change in sign implied by (8.12) for $d\phi/dt$.[6] We have

$$R_2^{SE}(t) = \begin{cases} R_2' + R_2 & 0 < t < \tau \\ -R_2' + R_2 & \tau < t < 2\tau = T_E \\ R_2' + R_2 & t > 2\tau = T_E \end{cases} \tag{8.15}$$

to be compared with the simple FID rate

$$R_2^* = R_2' + R_2 \tag{8.16}$$

Within each interval, R_2^{SE} is constant, and the solution to (8.14) has the usual exponential form

$$M_\perp(t) = M_\perp(t_0)e^{-(t-t_0)R_2^{SE}} \qquad \text{(each interval)} \tag{8.17}$$

---

[6]If there is exponential decay during dephasing then there is exponential growth during rephasing.

Although any t_0 within the given interval can be taken as an initial time, the intention is to use (8.17) to evolve the magnetization from the beginning of each interval ($t_0 = 0, \tau, T_E$, respectively).

Matching the exponential solutions of the separate differential equations at the two boundaries of the three intervals leads to the spin echo envelope (magnitude) for the whole experiment. Leaving the details to a problem, we find

$$M_\perp(t) = M_\perp(0) \begin{cases} e^{-t/T_2^*} & 0 < t < \tau \\ e^{-t/T_2}e^{-(T_E-t)/T_2'} & \tau < t < 2\tau = T_E \\ e^{-t/T_2}e^{-(t-T_E)/T_2'} = e^{-t/T_2^*}e^{T_E/T_2'} & t > 2\tau = T_E \end{cases} \quad (8.18)$$

in terms of the decay times[7] and the initial magnetization $M_\perp(0)$ at $t = 0$. The spatial dependence has been suppressed everywhere. The envelope shown in Fig. 8.3 corresponds to (8.18).

Problem 8.4

Derive (8.18) from the solutions to the differential equations in each of the three intervals. The corresponding changes in the relaxation rate are given by (8.15). The initial value is $M_\perp(0)$ at $t = 0$, and $M_\perp(t)$ is continuous over time.

8.2.3   Limitations of the Spin Echo

The signal peaks at the echo, as seen in Fig. 8.3, but it recovers only to the level dictated by the T_2 envelope. *The spin echo does not reduce the effect of T_2 decay on the signal.* The reason lies in the rapid time fluctuations in the intrinsic local fields. The inhomogeneities in these internal fields do not stay fixed in time after the π-pulse, the rates at which phase is accumulated change with time, and, in general, no refocusing is possible. Fortunately, the irreversibility of the intrinsic T_2 loss is not a severe limitation for liquids (T_2 is often three orders of magnitude shorter for solids). The time interval over which data are collected often can be made short compared with T_2.

Examples of other time-dependent spin effects include motion (macroscopic or microscopic) where the spins move from place to place during the experiment, such that they experience different fields at different locations. The spin echo will not refocus these types of inhomogeneities.[8]

Although the spin echo presents a way of reversing the effect of T_2', the recovery is complete only when $\phi(t)$ backtracks to zero for all of the spins. If the spins are not at this point, then the data will be tainted by T_2' decay, despite the effort to refocus the spins. For instance, in Fig. 8.3, only the data point collected at $t = T_E$ is completely refocused. The problem is acute when B_0 is rather inhomogeneous, since a very short T_2' implies a rapid drop-off in either direction away from the echo.

---

[7]Recall from Ch. 4 that $R_2 \equiv 1/T_2$, $R_2^* \equiv 1/T_2^*$, and $R_2' \equiv 1/T_2'$.

[8]The effects that coherent motion can have on MRI will be discussed in the chapter on flow (Ch. 24). Inferior rf pulses and coils can also affect the phase of the signal.

8.2.4   Spin Echo Sampling

The measurement of the signal raises the question of how the data are to be collected. We have noted that data will be sampled at multiple time points (i.e., a time series). The acquisition of single data points[9] at two different echo times can be used to determine the spin-spin decay constant, if its spatial dependence is ignored. From the combination of (8.18) and (8.2), the demodulated signal at the spin echo, $t = T_E$, is

$$s(T_E) \propto \omega_0 e^{-T_E/T_2} \int d^3 r \mathcal{B}_\perp(\vec{r}) M_\perp(\vec{r}, 0)$$ (8.19)

where the initial phases have been ignored. Varying the time of the π-pulse in a second experiment leads to a different echo time ($T_E' > T_E$, say) where

$$s(T_E') \propto \omega_0 e^{-T_E'/T_2} \int d^3 r \mathcal{B}_\perp(\vec{r}) M_\perp(\vec{r}, 0)$$ (8.20)

From these two data points, an estimate for T_2 can be obtained from the ratio of the two signals, (8.19) and (8.20). The explicit and implicit proportionality constants can be taken to be the same, and the ratio can be solved to find

$$T_2 = \frac{T_E' - T_E}{\ln\left(s(T_E)/s(T_E')\right)}$$ (8.21)

Multiple points can be sampled near a single echo for more information. A sufficiently large time series may be used to spectrally resolve the signal, a subject of importance in 'chemical shift' imaging. See Sec. 8.5 and Ch. 10.

8.2.5   Multiple Spin Echo Experiments

Rather than repeating an experiment with a different echo time to measure T_2, it is common to collect data for more than one echo of the original rf excitation. This is accomplished by applying multiple π-pulses after a single $\pi/2$-pulse (see Fig. 8.5). For definiteness, it may be assumed that these are all along the $\hat{y}'$ axis, so that the repeated refocusing is always along that same axis; this is not a general rule. For uniform spacing, the nth π-pulse is at the time $(2n - 1)\tau$. The signal at each echo can be measured and plotted, as a function of time or n, on a semi-log scale where the echoes occur at $t_n = 2n\tau = nT_E$. A fit to a straight line will reveal the relaxation rate.

The spin echo experiments to measure T_2 are conceptually simple but turn out to be fraught with difficulties. In an introductory discussion such as given here, the π-pulses are assumed to be perfect: The flip angle rotations are taken to be instantaneous and exactly $\pi/2$ or π over the whole sample. Also, the spatial diffusion of the spins is ignored. Diffusion is a problem because field inhomogeneities lead to changes in the Larmor frequency when spins meander into different spatial regions. These and other factors lead to accumulated errors in the determination of relaxation parameters. We shall return to such issues in Chs. 16, 21, and 22, where realistic rf pulses and methods to overcome a variety of difficulties are discussed.

---

[9]The need for a small frequency spread or 'bandwidth,' provided by a low pass filter with a narrow window to suppress high frequency noise, is investigated in Ch. 12.

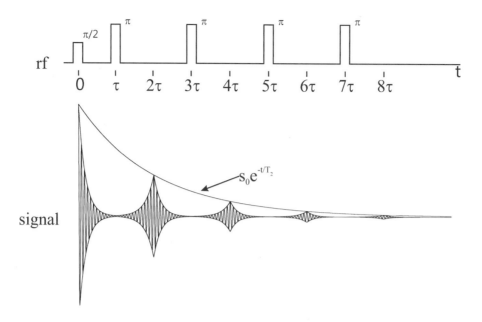

Fig. 8.5: A signal arising from multiple spin echoes generated by regularly repeated π pulses.

8.3   Repeated RF Pulse Structures

A major issue in imaging, and indeed in NMR experiments in general, is the requirement of an adequate signal, relative to the noise present. It may be necessary to repeat the experiment a number of times, averaging the measurements for a final result. This yields a general improvement in the ratio of signal to noise, in terms of the number of repetitions, as will be discussed in Ch. 15. For an experiment with repeated sequences, however, the available transverse magnetization (and hence the signal) will depend upon the repetition time T_R, which determines the amount of regrowth of longitudinal magnetization $M_z(t)$.[10] Recall that the transverse magnetization is established initially by the tipping of the longitudinal magnetization into the transverse plane. Fig. 8.6 illustrates the magnetization history of a repeated FID example.

An important issue, consequently, is the choice of T_R. Repeating the rf pulse structure (as it is defined in the sequence diagram) after too short an interval will not leave time for $M_z(t)$ to relax to the maximum longitudinal equilibrium magnetization, M_0. (For very short T_R, the signal becomes so small, it is referred to as being 'saturated.' See Ch. 6.) Waiting a longer time to repeat the data acquisition step is inefficient. A compromise must be reached.

In this section, formulas for the longitudinal and transverse magnetization will be derived for experiments in which FID and spin echo sequences are repeated. It is kept in mind that the signal is directly related to an integration over the transverse magnetization in expressions such as (8.2). The integrals and spatial dependence will be left understood in what follows, phases are neglected, and the $\vec{r}$ dependence will be suppressed in the equations. *Since the signal is directly proportional to the transverse magnetization, the magnitude $M_\perp$ will be studied as a function of time.* The important variables are the repeat time T_R and, where

---

[10]See Ch. 18 for a more detailed discussion of signal behavior for arbitrary T_R and flip angle.

applicable, the π-pulse time τ. We also introduce the nomenclature of repeated rf pulse structures and cycles within a loop structure of sequence diagrams.

The detailed question of finding the optimal value of T_R is considered in Ch. 15. There it will be seen that the choice depends upon the desired 'contrast' in the image.

8.3.1   The FID Signal from Repeated RF Pulse Structures

In the canonical FID experiment, a single $\pi/2$-pulse is applied and the signal can be measured immediately. In this section, an expression for the FID signal as a function of time for regularly repeated $\pi/2$-pulses (i.e., constant T_R) will be found. The simplifying assumption, $T_R \gg T_2^*$, is used, implying that the transverse magnetization has decayed completely by the end of any given repetition (prior to the next $\pi/2$-pulse).

Assume that the longitudinal magnetization available for the first sequence is M_0. Since the interest here is to perform an efficient experiment, the repeat time will not be too large: $T_R \lesssim T_1$. In this case, only the first rf pulse may see the maximum longitudinal magnetization M_0. From the second sequence onwards, the longitudinal magnetization will recover only as far as T_R allows. As we will see, the signal behavior after the first cycle will be similar

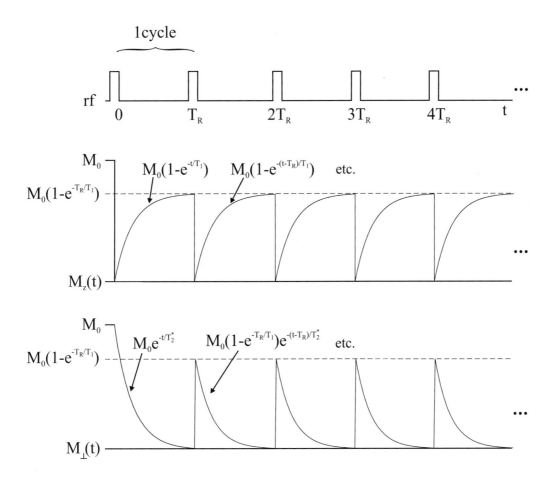

Fig. 8.6: The behavior of the transverse and longitudinal magnetization for a regularly repeated FID experiment, with fixed repeat time T_R.

from one repetition of the rf pulse structure to the next, so a straightforward averaging will improve the signal-to-noise ratio.[11] The signal from the first cycle is usually not used, since the initial magnetization may be different from the equilibrium value.

Define $t = 0$ at the center of the first $\pi/2$-pulse. The pulse is assumed to be sufficiently narrow that its action is instantaneously to tip the magnetization from the z-axis into the transverse plane

$$
\begin{aligned}
M_z(0^+) &= 0 \tag{8.22}\\
M_\perp(0^+) &= M_z(0^-) = M_0 \tag{8.23}
\end{aligned}
$$

Following the pulse, the time-evolution of the transverse and longitudinal magnetization are described by the Bloch solutions (Ch. 4) in terms of the initial values (8.22) and (8.23)

$$
\begin{aligned}
M_z(t) &= M_z(0^+)e^{-t/T_1} + M_0(1 - e^{-t/T_1}) = M_0(1 - e^{-t/T_1}) \tag{8.24}\\
M_\perp(t) &= M_\perp(0^+)e^{-t/T_2^*} = M_0 e^{-t/T_2^*} \tag{8.25}
\end{aligned}
$$

for $0 < t < T_R$.

After the first cycle, (8.22) and (8.23) are replaced by the action of the second pulse at $t = T_R$

$$
\begin{aligned}
M_z(T_R^+) &= 0 \tag{8.26}\\
M_\perp(T_R^+) &= M_z(T_R) = M_0(1 - e^{-T_R/T_1}) \tag{8.27}
\end{aligned}
$$

in which (8.24) was used to evaluate $M_z(T_R^-)$. (Remember it is assumed that there is no transverse magnetization left at $t = T_R^-$ to get tipped into the z-direction.) The Bloch solutions for the second interval are combined with (8.26) and (8.27) to give

$$
\begin{aligned}
M_z(t) &= M_z(T_R^+)e^{-(t-T_R)/T_1} + M_0\left(1 - e^{-(t-T_R)/T_1}\right) = M_0\left(1 - e^{-(t-T_R)/T_1}\right) \tag{8.28}\\
M_\perp(t) &= M_\perp(T_R^+)e^{-(t-T_R)/T_2^*} = M_0\left(1 - e^{-T_R/T_1}\right)e^{-(t-T_R)/T_2^*} \tag{8.29}
\end{aligned}
$$

for $T_R < t < 2T_R$.

The pattern is now clear. For the nth cycle, the longitudinal magnetization is zero at the beginning and evolves to a common value at the end

$$
M_z(t = nT_R^-) = M_0(1 - e^{-T_R/T_1}) \tag{8.30}
$$

independent of n. Therefore, the same longitudinal value, for $n \geq 2$, is tipped into the transverse plane at the start of each cycle, to initialize the evolution of the transverse magnetization. The 'signal' as a function of time in the nth cycle is universally[12]

$$
M_\perp(t_n) = M_0(1 - e^{-T_R/T_1})e^{-t_n/T_2^*} \qquad (n \geq 2) \tag{8.31}
$$

---

[11]This is only true when $\pi/2$-pulses are employed. For the more general case of variable flip angles, see Ch. 18.

[12]We might very well use t', in place of t_n, to describe the cycle time in view of the lack of dependence on n.

for $0 < t_n < T_R$ where the time during the cycle t_n is defined in terms of the total experimental time t by

$$t \equiv t_n + (n-1)T_R \tag{8.32}$$

The signal for the repeated FID experiment[13] is thus reduced by the factor $1 - e^{-T_R/T_1}$ at each instant in time, relative to that for a single FID run. It is essentially this factor that is plotted in Fig. 8.7, which shows the maximum value of the signal, in each interval, for the repeated FID measurement. This corresponds to (8.31) at $t_n = 0$ as a function of T_R.

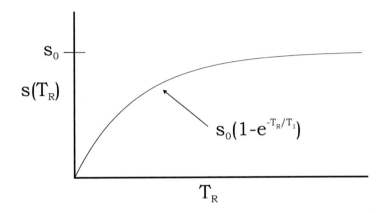

Fig. 8.7: The demodulated signal, for a repeated FID experiment, as a function of T_R. The signal is assumed to be measured immediately following the $\pi/2$-pulse, in a given cycle.

Problem 8.5

Experiments with $\pi/2$-pulses and short T_R can be expected to have reduced signal. That is, in the limit that T_R becomes much less than T_1 (but still much larger than T_2^*), show that $M_z(nT_R^-)$ is proportional to T_R/T_1.

8.3.2 The Spin Echo Signal from Repeated RF Pulse Structures

Consider a spin echo experiment with regularly repeated rf pulse structures under the same simplifying assumption that $T_R \gg T_2^*$. The sequence is diagramed in Fig. 8.8. Again, the effect of the $\pi/2$-pulse for the first cycle is given by

$$M_z(0^+) = 0 \tag{8.33}$$
$$M_\perp(0^+) = M_z(0^-) = M_0 \tag{8.34}$$

The Bloch solution (4.12) for the longitudinal magnetization can be applied to the two intervals before and after the π-pulse at $t = \tau$. Noting (8.34),

$$M_z(t) = \begin{cases} M_z(0^+)e^{-t/T_1} + M_0(1 - e^{-t/T_1}) = M_0(1 - e^{-t/T_1}) & 0 < t < \tau \\ M_z(\tau^+)e^{-(t-\tau)/T_1} + M_0(1 - e^{-(t-\tau)/T_1}) & \tau < t < T_R \end{cases} \tag{8.35}$$

---

[13] For short T_R, this is sometimes called a 'partial saturation' experiment.

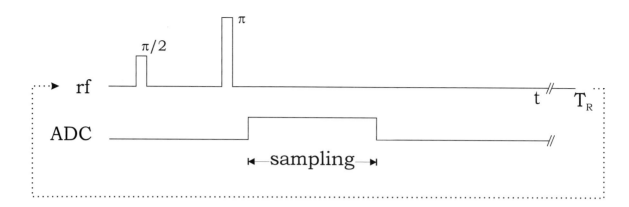

Fig. 8.8: The sequence diagram for a repeated spin echo experiment. A long sampling time is not required when only one data point is measured.

From the action of the π-pulse and the first solution in (8.35), M_z changes sign so that

$$M_z(\tau^+) = -M_z(\tau^-) = -M_0(1 - e^{-\tau/T_1}) \tag{8.36}$$

The second solution in (8.35) thus becomes

$$M_z(t) = M_0(1 - 2e^{-(t-\tau)/T_1} + e^{-t/T_1}) \qquad \tau < t < T_R \tag{8.37}$$

The transverse magnetization is given by (8.18) with $M_\perp(0^+) = M_0$. At the echo, with all T_2' effects rephased, it is

$$M_\perp(T_E) = M_0 e^{-T_E/T_2} \tag{8.38}$$

The longitudinal magnetization at the end of the first cycle, with the value $M_z(T_R^-)$, gets tipped into the transverse plane by the next $\pi/2$-pulse. The transverse magnetization evolves with this initial value to its magnitude at the echo in the second cycle

$$M_\perp(T_R + T_E) = M_z(T_R^-)e^{-T_E/T_2} \tag{8.39}$$

where, from (8.37),

$$M_z(T_R^-) = M_0(1 - 2e^{-(T_R-\tau)/T_1} + e^{-T_R/T_1}) \tag{8.40}$$

In practice, for $\tau \ll T_R$, (8.40) is well approximated by[14]

$$M_z(T_R^-) \simeq M_0(1 - e^{-T_R/T_1}) \qquad \tau \ll T_R \tag{8.41}$$

The longitudinal magnetization at the end of the second cycle has an expression identical to (8.37), because its initial value was again zero. (As in the FID case, the limit $T_R \gg T_2^*$ implies that $M_\perp(T_R) = 0$ so that the excitation pulse will not tip any longitudinal magnetization back along the z-axis, i.e., $M_z(0_n^+) = 0$.)

---

[14]This answer could have been written down immediately. In the limit that $\tau \to 0$, (8.37) reduces to the corresponding FID expression (8.30).

For each ensuing cycle, the answers repeat. The longitudinal magnetization evolves to the approximate answer

$$M_z(nT_R^-) \simeq M_0(1 - e^{-T_R/T_1}) \qquad n \geq 1 \tag{8.42}$$

The transverse magnetization at an arbitrary echo is

$$M_\perp(2\tau + nT_R) \simeq M_0(1 - e^{-T_R/T_1})e^{-2\tau/T_2} \qquad n \geq 1 \tag{8.43}$$

recalling $T_E = 2\tau$. For other times in each cycle, formulas for the signal can be adapted from (8.18).

In conclusion, the measured signal at any echo has the same T_R/T_1 dependence, for $\tau \ll T_R$, as the repeated FID experiment, but without the severe T_2^* suppression. As expected, the π-pulse continues to serve to refocus static field inhomogeneities, so that the magnetization at the center of the echo is only a function of T_2. The variability of the signal as a function of sequence timing (through the parameters T_R or τ) is quite evident in (8.43). This variability is of great utility to MRI in defining image contrast, as will be seen throughout the remainder of the text.

Multiple Spin Echo Sequence Diagram

Consider a pulse structure in which a single $\pi/2$-pulse is followed by multiple π-pulses. After each π-pulse, a new echo can be measured. The signal and sequence diagram are exemplified by Figs. 8.5 and 8.9, corresponding to four and three π-pulses, respectively. A related problem for two π-pulses appears next.

Problem 8.6

A repeated 'double spin echo' sequence is a pulse structure with a single $\pi/2$-pulse followed by two π-pulses. The first π-pulse follows the $\pi/2$-pulse by a time interval τ and the two π-pulses are separated from each other by 2τ. Assume $\tau \ll T_1$.

  a) Draw the sequence diagram for this experiment.

  b) Derive the signal expression at the two echoes.

8.4 Inversion Recovery and T_1 Measurements

The FID and spin echo experiments are useful for determining the T_2 properties of a sample. As single experiments, however, they are not sensitive to T_1. As repeated experiments, on the other hand, their signals do depend on T_1, and the spin-lattice parameters could, in principle, be determined by performing a number of repeated sequences with different values of T_R. Such experiments, however, take a relatively long time.

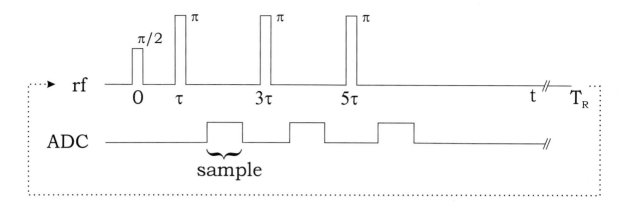

Fig. 8.9: Sequence diagram for a three-echo example of the multi-echo spin echo experiment.

There is another experiment, called 'inversion recovery,' that is sensitive to T_1. Although this method can be employed to get an accurate value of T_1, the determination likewise cannot be made from a single experiment. Inversion recovery is similar to an FID experiment, but with an additional π-pulse employed to invert the magnetization and defined to occur at a time interval T_I before the $\pi/2$-pulse. The sequence diagram is found in Fig. 8.10a. The regrowth of the longitudinal component of the magnetization between these pulses leads to a strong signal dependence on T_I.

8.4.1 T_1 Measurement

In the measurement of T_1 through inversion recovery, it is necessary to keep track of the longitudinal component of the magnetization during the period between the π- and $\pi/2$-pulses. The longitudinal magnetization right after the initial π-pulse is the negative of the equilibrium value

$$M_z(0^+) \;=\; -M_0 \tag{8.44}$$

The time $t = T_I$ has been defined as the time of the $\pi/2$-pulse. The magnetization grows toward its equilibrium value in the interval between the pulses according to (4.12)

$$M_z(t) = -M_0 e^{-t/T_1} + M_0(1 - e^{-t/T_1}) = M_0(1 - 2e^{-t/T_1}), \quad 0 < t < T_I \tag{8.45}$$

After the longitudinal magnetization is tipped into the transverse plane to provide the initial signal, the magnitude of the transverse magnetization evolves as

$$M_\perp(t) = \left| M_0(1 - 2e^{-T_I/T_1}) \right| e^{-(t-T_I)/T_2^*}, \quad t > T_I \tag{8.46}$$

As advertised, the magnitude of the measured signal is modulated by the T_1-dependent factor $\left|1 - 2e^{-T_I/T_1}\right|$. This can be compared with the factor $\left|1 - e^{-T_R/T_1}\right|$ from (8.43) for the repeated spin echo experiment. The factor of 2 occurring in (8.46) makes it possible to find a finite value of T_I where the signal is zero. Therefore, an accurate way to determine T_1 is to use the fact that the signal vanishes when

$$T_{I,null} = T_1 \ln 2 \tag{8.47}$$

This implies that the signal is a sensitive function of T_I, and, hence, of T_1, as illustrated in Fig. 8.11. To find T_1, T_I is varied until a zero in the signal is located. Signal zeros can be accurately determined, so that T_1, at least for a uniform sample, can be precisely measured using this method.

There is additional utility associated with the zero in the signal. If a sample is being studied which contains two substances or tissues with different values of T_1, then an experiment can be performed with T_I chosen such that the signal from one of the tissues is zero. That component is said to be 'nulled.' In this way, different components of a sample may be studied selectively.

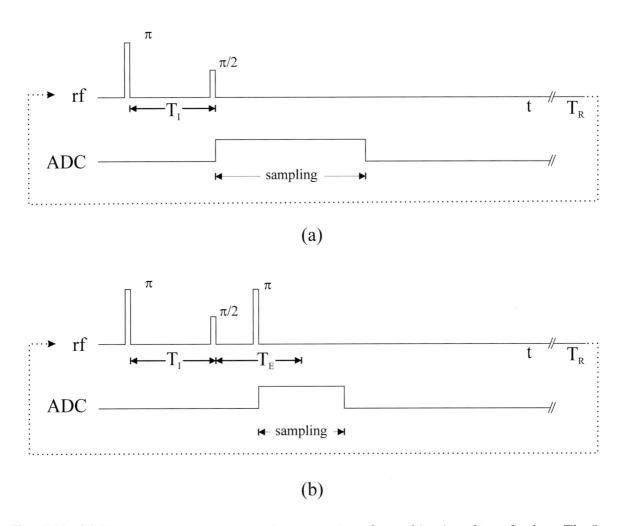

(a)

(b)

Fig. 8.10: (a) The inversion recovery experiment consists of a combination of two rf pulses. The first pulse inverts the longitudinal magnetization. The second pulse tips the longitudinal magnetization into the transverse plane so an FID signal may be measured. (b) The spin echo inversion recovery experiment consists of three rf pulses. The first pulse inverts the longitudinal magnetization, the second pulse tips the longitudinal magnetization into the transverse plane, and the third pulse inverts both the longitudinal and transverse magnetization leading to an echo. This experiment and a repeated version are the subjects of Prob. 8.7 and Prob. 8.10, respectively.

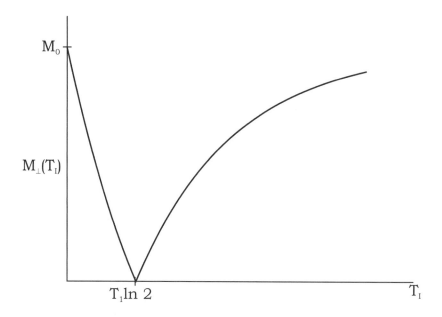

Fig. 8.11: The magnitude of the signal for an inversion recovery as a function of T_I, the time between rf pulses. Notice that the signal vanishes at $T_I = T_1 \ln 2$ which corresponds to the point where the longitudinal magnetization has regrown from $-M_0$ to zero.

Problem 8.7

For a single repetition of the cycle of the spin echo inversion recovery sequence in Fig. 8.10b, show that $M_\perp(T_E + T_I)$ is given by

$$M_\perp(T_E + T_I) = M_0 \left| 1 - 2e^{-T_I/T_1} \right| e^{-T_E/T_2} \qquad (8.48)$$

8.4.2   Repeated Inversion Recovery

Following Sec. 8.3, a natural extension is to consider a repeated sequence of the inversion recovery rf structure. The repeated inversion recovery experiment is diagramed in Fig. 8.12. The effect of the first π-pulse is to invert the equilibrium magnetization, but no transverse magnetization is created, i.e.,

$$M_z(0^+) = -M_z(0^-) = -M_0 \qquad \text{(first cycle)} \qquad (8.49)$$
$$M_\perp(0^+) = 0 \qquad (8.50)$$

An increasingly familiar calculation leads to the magnetization (the longitudinal component and the magnitude of the transverse component) during the period between the π-pulse and the $\pi/2$-pulse as given by

$$M_z(t) = -M_z(0^-)e^{-t/T_1} + M_0(1 - e^{-t/T_1}) = M_0(1 - 2e^{-t/T_1})$$
$$M_\perp(t) = 0$$
$$0 < t < T_I \qquad (8.51)$$

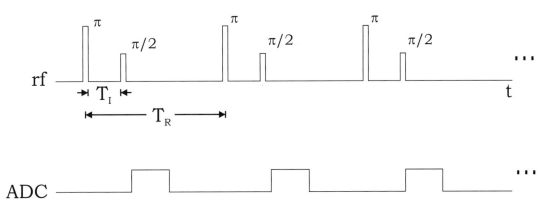

Fig. 8.12: A repeated inversion recovery experiment.

The $\pi/2$-pulse converts the longitudinal magnetization into transverse magnetization whose precession can be detected as the MR signal

$$M_z(T_I^+) = 0 \tag{8.52}$$

$$M_\perp(T_I^+) = \left| -M_z(0^-)e^{-T_I/T_1} + M_0(1 - e^{-T_I/T_1}) \right| = \left| M_0(1 - 2e^{-T_I/T_1}) \right| \tag{8.53}$$

The longitudinal magnetization and the magnitude of the transverse magnetization for the time interval between the $\pi/2$-pulse and the next π-pulse are found in the usual way to be

$$M_z(t) = M_0 \left(1 - e^{-(t-T_I)/T_1} \right) \tag{8.54}$$

$$M_\perp(t) = \left| -M_z(0^-)e^{-T_I/T_1} + M_0(1 - e^{-T_I/T_1}) \right| e^{-(t-T_I)/T_2^*}$$

$$= \left| M_0(1 - 2e^{-T_I/T_1}) \right| e^{-(t-T_I)/T_2^*}$$

$$T_I < t < T_R \tag{8.55}$$

The longitudinal magnetization at $t = T_R^-$,

$$M_z(T_R^-) = M_0 \left(1 - e^{-(T_R - T_I)/T_1} \right) \tag{8.56}$$

corresponds to the regrowth from $t = T_I$, the time the $\pi/2$-pulse tipped all of the magnetization into the transverse plane, to the end of the repetition. Since $M_z(T_I^+) = 0$ for all repetitions of the sequence, $M_z(T_R)$ will also be the same in every cycle.

The signal during the nth cycle of the repeated experiment is simple to find, if it is assumed that $T_R \gg T_2^*$. This condition implies $M_\perp(t_n = T_R^-) = 0$ at the end of each cycle. Substituting the expression (8.56) for $M_z(0^-)$ generalizes (8.55) to

$$M_\perp(t_n) = \left| -M_0(1 - e^{-(T_R - T_I)/T_1})e^{-T_I/T_1} + M_0(1 - e^{-T_I/T_1}) \right| e^{-(t_n - T_I)/T_2^*}$$

$$= M_0 \left| 1 + e^{-T_R/T_1} - 2e^{-T_I/T_1} \right| e^{-(t_n - T_I)/T_2^*}$$

$$T_I < t_n < T_R \tag{8.57}$$

in each cycle.

Problem 8.8

Design a double inversion recovery sequence to null both CSF and gray matter so that abnormalities in gray matter can be better seen. Often the CSF in the sulci causes a major partial volume effect (see Sec. 15.6) with gray matter and it is best removed for a good T_1-weighted image. However, there are times such as in imaging multiple sclerosis when suppressing the gray matter itself in an otherwise T_2-weighted sequence can be useful in revealing abnormalities or increases in water content in the gray matter. Derive the equations associated with your sequence and simulate what would happen at 1.5 T if the edematous signal in the gray matter had a T_1 and T_2 of 1500 ms and 200 ms, respectively, compared to the actual values of gray matter listed in Table 4.1.

Problem 8.9

As a generalization of (8.47), show that the value of T_I for which the signal from a repeated inversion recovery experiment is zero is

$$T_I = T_1 \ln \left(\frac{2}{1 + e^{-T_R/T_1}} \right) \tag{8.58}$$

Problem 8.10

Derive the following formula, for the magnitude of the transverse magnetization, for any repetition of a $\pi/2$ spin echo inversion recovery experiment, Fig. 8.10b,

$$M_\perp(T_E + T_I) = M_0 \left| 1 + 2e^{-(T_R - T_E/2)/T_1} - e^{-T_R/T_1} - 2e^{-T_I/T_1} \right| e^{-T_E/T_2} \tag{8.59}$$

Assume $T_R \gg T_2$ and all transverse magnetization $M_\perp \to 0$ at T_R has vanished at $t = T_R$.

8.5   Spectroscopy and Chemical Shift

The FID experiment can be used to determine the presence of a particular nuclear species. Consider a sample immersed in a perfectly homogeneous static field long enough to reach equilibrium magnetization. The Larmor frequency for the sample depends on the species

$$\omega_{0_i} = \gamma_i B_0 \tag{8.60}$$

where i denotes the nucleus of interest. A narrow-band rf pulse can be applied at the Larmor frequency of a particular nuclear species, such that other species with different frequencies are left unexcited. The abundance of a given species may be found by calibrating the signal intensity against samples with known properties. The frequencies which give rise to an FID signal help to determine the composition of a sample based upon knowledge of γ_i for various nuclei. In this experiment, only the presence of the desired element is determined, not its spatial distribution.

A more practical approach involves applying a broad-band transmit rf pulse, containing a wide spectrum of frequencies, and obtaining a more complicated FID signal. This signal contains information about the set of all nuclear species in the sample whose frequencies lie within the pulse spectrum. The bandwidth of the analog receive filter must also be wide enough to accommodate the range of excited frequencies. A decomposition of the signal using Fourier analysis can lead to a resolution of which species are present, and of their relative population.

Such experiments are sensitive to the molecular environment in which the nucleus finds itself. There are small, but measurable, differences in the degree of magnetic shielding due to the local environment, implying slightly different Larmor frequencies. These frequency changes can be described in terms of 'chemical shifts.' The shielding constant σ is an assumed linear response of the electronic structure to the external field, and it is defined by

$$B_{\text{shifted}}(j) = (1 - \sigma_j)B_0 \qquad (8.61)$$

where j refers to the chemical compound. A positive (negative) chemical shift $f_\sigma = -\sigma\gamma B_0$ implies shielding (anti-shielding). The chemical shift usually refers to a frequency shift. However, in order to quote the chemical shift with a dimensionless quantity, a reference frequency is chosen and the ppm difference between the shifted frequency and the reference frequency is calculated. Thus in (8.61), if the Larmor frequency is chosen as the reference, the shielding constant σ becomes the dimensionless chemical shift. Therefore, in the rest of this book, the symbol σ is also referred to as the chemical shift. Details about the role of chemical shifts in imaging are presented in Ch. 17 and other chapters dealing with sequence design.

As an example, hydrogen nuclei in water are not the only source of signal for ^{1}H MR. They can also be found in many organic compounds, where there are differences in their frequencies. Body fat (lipids) have a mean chemical shift of roughly 3.35 ppm. This corresponds, for instance, to a Larmor frequency shift f_σ of 214 Hz at 1.5 T relative to water.

In general, an MR experiment designed to determine the abundance, but not the spatial distribution, of different molecules or nuclei in a sample is referred to as an MR spectroscopic experiment. Hybrid experiments that provide information about the spatial distribution and abundance of different chemical species are referred to as chemical shift imaging experiments (see Chs. 10 and 17). The primary focus of this text, however, is the spatial imaging of a single chemical species or MRI, and not MR spectroscopy (MRS).

Sampling and Spectroscopy Experiments

Consider a population of different nuclear species. Let the jth species contain $\mathcal{N}_j$ hydrogen nuclei with shielding constant σ_j. The phase of each nucleus as a function of time is

$$\phi_j(t) = -\gamma B_0(1 - \sigma_j)t \qquad (8.62)$$

assuming a homogeneous field B_0. If all other spatial dependence is ignored as well,[15] the demodulated signal from this set of spins is given by

$$s(t) \propto \sum_j \mathcal{N}_j e^{i\gamma\sigma_j B_0 t} \qquad (8.63)$$

Relaxation damping has also been neglected. The spatial integral (8.1) is replaced by a sum over the individual spins, and $\mathcal{N}_j$ is related to $M_\perp$ according to the discussion in Ch. 4. A spectral analysis is made of the signal in order to extract estimates of the relative spin densities corresponding to each $\mathcal{N}_j$.

The data can be collected using the FID structure shown in Fig. 8.1 or the spin echo structure of Fig. 8.3. In both cases, multiple data points are needed to resolve the contributions from the different species, as discussed in Sec. 8.2.4.

For a continuous set of $\mathcal{N}_j$, the sum is replaced by an integral over a continuous distribution in σ, and the signal becomes

$$s(t) \propto \int d\sigma\, \mathcal{N}(\sigma) e^{i\gamma\sigma B_0 t} \qquad (8.64)$$

where, as a portent of things to come, we observe that the signal (8.64) is a Fourier transform. It is through inverse transforms (or inverse Fourier series) that the signal can be processed in order to determine the original species profile, and the next chapter presents the transform connection as a central theme.

---

[15]Such assumptions are quite reasonable for the small samples used in NMR spectroscopy.

Suggested Reading

The fundamental concept of an echo is introduced in:

- E. L. Hahn. Spin echoes. *Phys. Rev.*, 80: 580, 1950.

Basic Fourier transform concepts as applied to NMR are presented in:

- T. C. Farrar and E. D. Becker. *Pulse and Fourier Transform NMR: Introduction to Theory and Methods.* Academic Press, New York, 1971.

The concepts of nulling two tissues are presented in:

- T. W. Redpath and F. W. Smith. Imaging gray brain matter with a double-inversion pulse sequence to suppress CSF and white matter signals. *MAGMA*, 2: 451, 1994.

- K. Turetschek, P. Wunderbaldinger, A. A. Bankier, T. Zontsich, O. Graf, R. Mallek and K. Hittmair. Double inversion recovery imaging of the brain: Initial experience and comparison with fluid attenuated inversion recovery imaging. *Magn. Reson. Imag.*, 16: 127, 1998.

Chapter 9

One-Dimensional Fourier Imaging, k-Space, and Gradient Echoes

Chapter Contents

Summary: The basic tenets are established for imaging with linear gradient fields. The MR signal is connected to the Fourier transform of the spin density, and the image reconstruction is described in terms of the inverse Fourier transform. The role of the gradient structure is studied with respect to phase refocusing, k-space coverage, and alternative gradient directions. Sequence diagrams are generalized to include gradient field information.

Introduction

In the previous chapter, a discussion of the global magnetic resonance signal from a sample was presented. The goal of MR imaging, however, is not only to establish the presence of different nuclei, but also to determine the spatial distribution of a given species within the sample. Since identical nuclei precess at different rates in locations where the magnetic field has changed, the local spatial distribution of the spins can be determined from the frequency content of the resulting MR signal, provided a well-defined spatial field variation is superimposed on the homogeneous static field.

To impose spatial dependence, the uniform static field can be augmented by a smaller, linearly varying magnetic field. In this chapter, an analysis of the signals resulting from a 'linear gradient field' is given. For clarity, we can restrict ourselves to one dimension in learning the basic concepts and the principal role of the gradient fields. The fact that the signal is effectively a Fourier transform of the spin density is already evident in this case. A simple two-spin model and other examples serve to highlight some signal processing mathematics, such as that involving the Dirac delta function. The 2D and 3D imaging problems are considered in the next chapter.

The coverage of k-space is pivotal to reconstructing an image of the sample by inverse-Fourier-transform techniques. The relationship between the choice of gradient fields and the way in which k-space is covered is introduced. The standard sequence diagram is expanded to include the gradient structures. The implications of arbitrary gradient directions and more general gradient behavior are discussed at the end of the chapter.

9.1   Signal and Effective Spin Density

The imaging of a body commonly refers to the determination of the amplitude (magnitude) of the spin distribution, or spin density, rather than the magnetization. Groundwork on the relationship between the signal and the spin density is laid in this section. The definition of what is meant by a spin density, in three dimensions as well as in one dimension, is addressed. While it is convenient to ignore relaxation effects in an introductory discussion of imaging, the results are not entirely academic. They are valid for data sampling taking place over times small compared to T_2^*.

9.1.1   Complex Demodulated Signal

Let us define $s(t)$ as the complex demodulated signal given by an adaptation of (7.28). To turn the proportionality into an equation, Λ is introduced as a constant which includes the gain factors from the electronic detection system. The transmitting and receiving rf coils are considered to be sufficiently uniform, so that the initial magnetization phase ϕ_0, the receive field directional phase $\theta_{\mathcal{B}}$, and the receive field amplitude $\mathcal{B}_\perp$ are all independent of position. In view of the focus on position dependence, all constant phases can be set equal to zero or absorbed into Λ. The signal[1] is generalized to include a space- and time-dependent precession frequency $\omega(\vec{r}, t)$. With the neglect of relaxation effects

$$s(t) = \omega_0 \Lambda \mathcal{B}_\perp \int d^3 r \, M_\perp(\vec{r}, 0) e^{i(\Omega t + \phi(\vec{r}, t))} \tag{9.1}$$

where Ω is the reference (demodulation) frequency (with no offset, $\Omega = \omega_0$). The angle ϕ is the accumulated phase (3.37) with the counterclockwise positive sign convention

$$\phi(\vec{r}, t) = -\int_0^t dt' \omega(\vec{r}, t') \tag{9.2}$$

where $\omega = \omega_0$ only if there is a uniform static field. In the discussions of this chapter, the addition of a gradient field is assumed to be the primary reason that the precession frequency ω is a function of both position and time. When the gradient field is not present, the static field is assumed to be strictly homogeneous (and ω_0 strictly constant).

---

[1]Hereafter, the fact that the signal is demodulated and complex is left understood.

9.1.2 Magnetization and Effective Spin Density

With the neglect of relaxation effects, and the assumption of, say, a perfect $\pi/2$-pulse applied uniformly over the sample, the initial transverse magnetization is simply the equilibrium magnetization M_0. From (6.12), the equilibrium magnetization can be expressed in terms of the proton spin density. The resulting expression involving the temperature T and static field B_0 (the gradient field is not yet turned on) is

$$M_\perp(\vec{r}, 0) = M_0(\vec{r}) = \frac{1}{4}\rho_0(\vec{r})\frac{\gamma^2\hbar^2}{kT}B_0 \tag{9.3}$$

No restriction to one dimension has yet been made; the quantity $\rho_0(\vec{r})$ is the number of proton spins per unit volume in three dimensions.

From the combination of (9.1) and (9.3),

$$s(t) = \int d^3r\rho(\vec{r})e^{i(\Omega t + \phi(\vec{r},t))} \tag{9.4}$$

where the effective spin density[2] $\rho(\vec{r})$ has been introduced

$$\rho(\vec{r}) \equiv \omega_0\Lambda\mathcal{B}_\perp M_0(\vec{r}) = \frac{1}{4}\omega_0\Lambda\mathcal{B}_\perp\rho_0(\vec{r})\frac{\gamma^2\hbar^2}{kT}B_0 \tag{9.5}$$

If the receive field magnitude $\mathcal{B}_\perp$, for example, is not homogeneous, its spatial dependence can be included in (9.5). The relaxation factors may also be incorporated in the definition.

The present interest is the case where the phase factor in (9.4) depends only on one dimension, which can be defined as the z coordinate. The signal can then be written as

$$s(t) = \int dz\rho(z)e^{i(\Omega t + \phi(z,t))} \tag{9.6}$$

in terms of the effective 1D spin density[3]

$$\rho(z) \equiv \int\int dx\,dy\,\rho(\vec{r}) \tag{9.7}$$

All integration limits are determined by the region of nonzero spin density. The 'linear density' $\rho(z)$ is thus obtained by projection of the other two dimensions onto the z-axis. The integration over the other two coordinates leaves a one-dimensional problem.

A caveat is that the same symbol ρ is used for both the three-dimensional and one-dimensional effective densities. Also, it is observed that they are not equal to, but rather, only proportional to, the actual number of proton spins per unit volume or length, respectively, with a proportionality coefficient including temperature, frequency, electronics, field, and other factors. Nevertheless, we shall, for convenience, call them 'spin densities.'

Neglecting relaxation effects causes little error in a 'single-acquisition' experiment, as alluded to earlier, if the total sampling time T_s is much less than T_2^*. (In (9.6), $0 \leq t \leq T_s$.)

---

[2]When the constant phases ϕ_0 and $\theta_\mathcal{B}$ are retained, the effective spin density is complex.

[3]Differences in the precession frequencies of the various nuclear species excited by the given rf pulse are ignored.

For multiple acquisitions, the examples in Ch. 8 have shown that there are both T_1 and T_2 dependencies in spin echo experiments. Equation (9.6) remains valid for such repeated experiments, provided the repetition time is large enough, i.e., $T_R \gg T_1$, and the echo time is small enough, i.e., $T_E \ll T_2$. Under these conditions, e^{-T_R/T_1} is negligible, and e^{-T_E/T_2} is close to unity. When relaxation effects cannot be ignored, $\rho(z)$ should be replaced by $\rho(z, T_1, T_2)$, and in the general case, $\rho(\vec{r})$ by $\rho(\vec{r}, T_1, T_2)$.

9.2   Frequency Encoding and the Fourier Transform

The object of imaging is to determine the spin density $\rho(z)$ of a sample from the measurement of the signal as a function of time. The first step is to connect the spin precession to its position, and the second is to recognize that this connection implies that the signal is a well-known linear integral transform of the spin density.

9.2.1   Frequency Encoding of the Spin Position

The Larmor frequency of a spin will be linearly proportional to its position z if the static field is augmented with a linearly varying field.[4] The maximum of the linearly changing field at any point in the system is usually considerably smaller in magnitude than the static field.[5] The magnetization is considered to have been tipped, initially, into the transverse plane, so that it is already precessing freely with angular frequency ω_0, before the gradient field is brought into play. (Throughout the discussion of this chapter, it is assumed that the rf pulses and the gradient fields are not applied at the same time. In the next chapter, important techniques arising from their simultaneous application are considered.)

If a (spatially) linearly varying field is added to the static field, then the z-component of the field is

$$B_z(z,t) = B_0 + zG(t) \tag{9.8}$$

The quantity G is the (spatially) constant gradient in the z-direction,

$$G_z \equiv \partial B_z/\partial z \tag{9.9}$$

and for now G is set equal to G_z. The time dependence of $G(t)$ reminds us that the gradient may undergo quite general modifications during the course of an experiment. Define the variation in the angular frequency of the spins by

$$\omega(z,t) \equiv \omega_0 + \omega_G(z,t) \tag{9.10}$$

---

[4]The 'linear field gradient' must have other components in order to satisfy the basic Maxwell's equations, $\vec{\nabla} \cdot \vec{B} = 0$ and $\vec{\nabla} \times \vec{B} = 0$. If these components are very small compared to B_0 they may, in general, be ignored (see Ch. 27), although their effects in certain 'phase sensitive' methods are not always negligible.

[5]In MRI experiments, G is on the order of tens of mT/m while the spatial extent is on the order of a few tens of cm. As a result, the gradient creates frequencies on the order of a few dozen to a few hundred kHz at most. The signal frequency components induced in the receiving coil have differences in the audiofrequency range forming the envelope for the extremely fast oscillations at the Larmor frequency (on the order of MHz) in the radiofrequency range. This situation is analogous to the waves transmitted by FM radio stations, with the Larmor frequency playing the role of the carrier frequency.

For (9.8), the deviation from the Larmor frequency is linear in both z and G

$$\omega_G(z,t) = \gamma z G(t) \tag{9.11}$$

The use of a gradient to establish a relation, such as (9.11), between the position of spins along some direction and their precessional rates is referred to as frequency encoding along that direction.[6] The object of the standard MR imaging of humans is to extract information about the hydrogen distribution of the sample, in this case by looking at the signal due to frequency encoded proton spins.

The accumulated phase, up to time t, due to the applied gradient is

$$\phi_G(z,t) \;=\; -\int_0^t dt'\,\omega_G(z,t') \tag{9.12}$$

$$\;=\; -\gamma z \int_0^t dt'\,G(t') \tag{9.13}$$

where it is recalled that the gradient is assumed to be applied only after the initial rf excitation at $t = 0$.

Problem 9.1

Assume a typical clinical static field of $B_0 = 1.5\,\text{T}$ and a linear gradient field with $G \equiv \partial B_z/\partial z = 10\,\text{mT/m}$. The volume of the sample to be imaged (the 'imaging volume') is $50\,\text{cm}$ DSV ('diameter spherical volume').

a) Compare the maximum change in the field introduced by the gradient with that introduced by field inhomogeneities of $10\,\text{ppm}$.

b) Compare the maximum change in frequency induced by the gradient with the Larmor frequency produced by the main field.

c) Explain (qualitatively) how field inhomogeneities might affect the image.

9.2.2 The 1D Imaging Equation and the Fourier Transform

The signal (9.6), with demodulating frequency $\Omega = \omega_0$ and precession frequency (9.10), is given by

$$s(t) = \int dz\, \rho(z)\, e^{i\phi_G(z,t)} \tag{9.14}$$

where the phase, after demodulation, is determined by the gradient field. Equation (9.14) is applicable to measurements with gradient fields that have arbitrary z dependence; it is often referred to as the *1D imaging equation*. It can be generalized by replacing ϕ_G by the angle

---

[6]It is this simple but critical realization that is the cornerstone of MR imaging and led to the seminal paper by Lauterbur (see the list of references at the end of this chapter).

ϕ due to all gradient and rf field variations. Remember that any initial (spatially constant) phase is ignored.

The explicit z-dependence in the phase (9.12) for the linear field leads to

$$s(k) = \int dz \rho(z) e^{-i2\pi kz} \tag{9.15}$$

where the time dependence resides implicitly in the *spatial frequency* $k = k(t)$ with

$$k(t) = \gamma \int_0^t dt' G(t') \tag{9.16}$$

This expression shows that, when linear gradients are implemented, *the signal $s(k)$ is the Fourier transform of the spin density* of the sample. The spin density is said to be *Fourier encoded* along z by the linear gradient.

The fact that the signal and the density are related by such a well-studied linear transform is a boon to MRI. A detailed treatment of the Fourier transform and some of its properties is found in Ch. 11. The foremost property of the Fourier transform is its well-defined inverse. Given $s(k)$ for all k, *the spin density of the sample can be found by taking the inverse Fourier transform of the signal*

$$\rho(z) = \int dk \, s(k) e^{+i2\pi kz} \tag{9.17}$$

The signal $s(k)$ and the image $\rho(z)$ are a 'Fourier transform pair.' It is important to understand that any direction could have been chosen for this one-dimensional example. In future chapters, the 'frequency encoding' or 'read direction' is chosen as the x-direction, rather than the z-direction.

9.2.3   The Coverage of k-Space

It is most useful to formulate imaging arguments in terms of image (z) space and data (k) space, in view of the Fourier transform connection. The inverse transform implies that the spin density can be reconstructed from the signal, if the latter is collected over a sufficiently large set of k values. The integration in (9.17) requires 'good coverage' of k-space.

The dependence on time and the applied gradient amplitude is the key to covering a large enough range in k. In the case where the applied gradient is constant over the whole time interval $(0, t)$, (9.16) reduces to

$$k = \gamma G t \tag{9.18}$$

Therefore, to collect a uniform distribution of points in k-space, it is only necessary to sample the signal at a constant rate in the presence of a constant gradient. Sampling both negative and positive values for k can be achieved by changing the sign of the gradient. Specific procedures for such coverage are detailed in Sec. 9.4.

If the signal could be measured continuously over a very long time and an accurate integration carried out in (9.17), then a faithful picture of the spin density would be found. However, several factors prevent collection of continuous data over all k-space. First, the signal must be sampled in a finite amount of time and second, relaxation effects wipe out the signal within a finite period. In actuality, the data collected will be a truncated and discretized version of $s(k)$, and it is necessary to carefully study the discrete Fourier transform to understand the impact these two modifications have upon the resulting image (see Chs. 11 and 12) relative to the continuous analytic form given in (9.17).

9.2.4 Rect and Sinc Functions

There are two important functions in upcoming discussions of signal analysis, the 'boxcar' or rect function

$$\text{rect}(z) \equiv \begin{cases} 0 & z < -1/2 \\ 1 & -1/2 \leq z \leq 1/2 \\ 0 & z > 1/2 \end{cases} \tag{9.19}$$

and the sinc function

$$\text{sinc}(z) = \frac{\sin z}{z} \tag{9.20}$$

The functions $\text{rect}(z)$ and $\text{sinc}(k)$ are a Fourier transform pair, a fact highlighted in the first problem to follow.

Following the previous chapter, time profiles of the rf pulses continue to be shown as rect functions (recall that narrow rect functions have been referred to as hard pulses). It was also noted there that, in general, rect functions are more appropriately used for the frequency profiles, rather than the time profiles, of the rf fields. It is now seen that this means realistic rf time profiles should be modeled by sinc functions. Such profiles are implemented in Ch. 10.

Problem 9.2

Consider a boxcar spin-density distribution with width z_0, centered at $z = 0$, and given by $\rho(z) = \rho_0 \text{rect}(z/z_0)$. Find the signal $s(k)$ for this spin density from (9.15). The answer will involve the sinc function, $\text{sinc}(\pi k z_0)$. Then check, using integral tables for example, that the answer gives back the correct spin density through the inverse transform (9.17). (See also Prob. 9.3.)

9.3 Simple Two-Spin Example

Consider a pair of classical spins[7] (a 'dumbbell' of two point spins) lying along the z-axis, at $z = \pm z_0$. Although individual classical spins are not experimentally relevant, the simplicity of the model is useful in demonstrating the 1D imaging method. Suppose the spins have reached equilibrium alignment along the static field (Fig. 9.1a). If an rf pulse is applied to tip the spins into the transverse plane, a single-frequency signal results in the absence of a gradient. If the signal shown in Fig. 9.1b were demodulated at the Larmor frequency, it would be constant.

---

[7]It is perhaps more appropriate to think of these as two spin isochromats. In any case, we wish to consider continuous changes in the spin direction; we avoid referring to (quantum mechanical) proton spins for this reason.

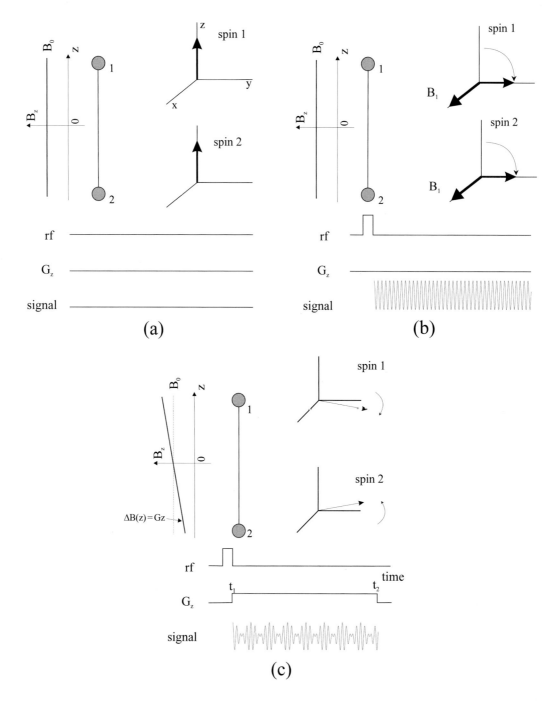

Fig. 9.1: Example of a 1D MRI experiment. The positions of two point spins (depicted as circles on a 'spin dumbbell' with no MRI signal from the connecting rod) are to be determined by imaging. The z-component of the laboratory magnetic field is plotted to the left of the dumbbells. The rotating frame orientation of the spin in each dumbbell is displayed at the right of the diagram. The sequence diagrams underneath represent the rotating frame input rf (assumed to be along $\hat{x}'$ and producing a $\pi/2$ rotation), the applied gradient, and the laboratory received signal (with T_2 decay neglected), before demodulation, as a function of time. Steps (a), (b), and (c) are described in the text. Note that G_z has the constant value G in part (c) between the times t_1 and t_2.

If the experiment is run again in the presence of the field gradient (Fig. 9.1c), during the time interval (t_1, t_2), the precessional rates of the two spins will differ slightly from the Larmor frequency. For $G > 0$ and gyromagnetic ratio γ, the spin at z_0 rotates clockwise and the spin at $-z_0$ rotates counterclockwise at the same rate, in the rotating reference frame. Therefore, while the constant gradient G is applied, with $t_1 < t < t_2$, the spin at z_0 has rotated through an angle, $\phi(z_0, t) = -\gamma G z_0 (t - t_1)$, and the spin at $-z_0$ through an angle, $\phi(-z_0, t) = \gamma G z_0 (t - t_1)$.

The signal in this case can be directly calculated since the integrals over the spin density reduce to the sum of the contributions from each spin. Recall the analogous sum in (8.63) and let $t_1 = 0$ for convenience. The net signal is

$$
\begin{aligned}
s(t) &= s_0 e^{-i\gamma G z_0 t} + s_0 e^{i\gamma G z_0 t} \\
&= 2s_0 \cos(\gamma G t z_0) \qquad 0 < t < t_2
\end{aligned}
\tag{9.21}
$$

or

$$
s(k) = 2s_0 \cos(2\pi k z_0) \qquad 0 < k < k_2 \equiv \gamma G t_2
\tag{9.22}
$$

with k from (9.18) and s_0 the (common) magnitude of the signal associated with each spin. Equation (9.21) exhibits the expected beat envelope from two identical sources at different frequencies. (The superposition of the envelope on the fast carrier frequency corresponds to the laboratory signal shown in Fig. 9.1c.) Given this signal, and knowledge of the applied gradient, the distribution of the spins follows. In this case, the beat frequency $\gamma G z_0$ implies the distance between the spins is $2z_0$. Albeit a very simple example, this demonstrates how the frequencies imposed by gradients yield information about the spatial distribution of the spins in a sample.

It is useful to verify that the signal leads directly to $\rho(z)$ through the inverse Fourier transform. By changing the sign on G, (9.22) may be considered to be valid for all k; a later discussion is directed to techniques for acquiring data at both positive and negative k values. From (9.17)

$$
\begin{aligned}
\rho(z) &= \int_{-\infty}^{\infty} dk \, 2s_0 \cos(2\pi k z_0) e^{i2\pi k z} \\
&= s_0 \int_{-\infty}^{\infty} dk \left(e^{i2\pi k(z+z_0)} + e^{i2\pi k(z-z_0)} \right) \\
&= s_0 [\delta(z + z_0) + \delta(z - z_0)]
\end{aligned}
\tag{9.23}
$$

In the last step, it is recognized that the integrals over the exponentials are Dirac delta functions. For now, it need only be noted that the delta function $\delta(z - z_0)$ is, qualitatively, a spike at $z = z_0$ with, in the limit, an infinite height, zero width, and unit area. In the next section, the Dirac delta function is discussed in more detail. Also, in view of its importance in signal processing, the representation

$$
\delta(z) = \int_{-\infty}^{\infty} dk \, e^{i2\pi k z}
\tag{9.24}
$$

is derived in the same section. Thus, the spin density (9.23) is exactly what is expected, for two point spins at $\pm z_0$.

9.3.1   Dirac Delta Function

The Dirac delta function[8] is the zero width limit of a sharply peaked distribution with fixed unit area

$$\delta(z - a) = 0 \quad \text{if } z \neq a \tag{9.25}$$

and

$$\int_{z_1}^{z_2} dz\, \delta(z - a) = \begin{cases} 1 & a \in (z_1, z_2) \\ 0 & a \notin (z_1, z_2) \end{cases} \tag{9.26}$$

The delta function is a filter or sifting function since it has the property of being able to select a particular value of a function according to

$$\int_{-\infty}^{\infty} dz\, \delta(z - a) f(z) = f(a) \tag{9.27}$$

Let us derive, as a limit, the representation of the delta function in (9.24). Define

$$\begin{aligned} I(z, K) &\equiv \int_{-K}^{K} dk\, e^{i2\pi k z} \\ &= \frac{\sin(2\pi K z)}{\pi z} \\ &= 2K \operatorname{sinc}(2\pi K z) \end{aligned} \tag{9.28}$$

The integrated result has been written in terms of the sinc function (9.20). Next, the large K limits of (9.28) and its integral need to be investigated. Note that, for $z = 0$, $\lim_{K \to \infty} I(0, K) = \infty$, since, as a limit, $\operatorname{sinc}(0) = 1$. For $z \neq 0$, $I(z, K)$ oscillates increasingly rapidly as K grows. As K approaches infinity, the function oscillates so rapidly that any function $f(z)$ it multiplies will be averaged to zero everywhere except near $z = 0$, where it will sift out the value $f(0)$. Finally, an integration over any interval including the origin gives unity for $K \to \infty$. The remaining details of the arguments showing that

$$\lim_{K \to \infty} I(z, K) = \delta(z) \tag{9.29}$$

are the subject of Prob. 9.3.

Problem 9.3

---

a) In order to obtain a qualitative understanding of how the function $I(z, K) = 2K \operatorname{sinc}(2\pi K z)$ approaches a delta function, plot it as a function of z around the origin for the following values of K

i) $K = 1/\pi$ ii) $K = 10/\pi$ iii) $K = 100/\pi$

It will be noticed that, as K grows larger, the first zero crossing occurs closer and closer to zero, the function oscillates faster, and its 'energy' is more and more concentrated at the origin.

---

[8]The Dirac delta function is an example of a generalized function which, despite its singular properties, can be manipulated according to the usual rules of calculus.

b) Show that for any positive pair, $a > 0, b > 0$

$$\lim_{K \to \infty} \int_{-a}^{b} 2K \operatorname{sinc}(2\pi K z)\, dz = 1 \qquad (9.30)$$

given the integral value

$$\int_{-\infty}^{\infty} dw\, \frac{\sin w}{w} = \pi \qquad (9.31)$$

9.3.2 Imaging Sequence Diagrams Revisited

Sequence diagrams have been introduced in the previous chapter. In Fig. 9.1, the sequence diagrams have been generalized to include gradient structure. More examples appear in subsequent figures of this chapter, and gradients for additional dimensions are added to the diagrams of the next chapter in the discussion of multi-dimensional imaging. The diagrams remain easy to understand. Recall that time is displayed on the horizontal axis. The vertical axis indicates whether the given quantity is active or not, and the activation refers, for example, to the B_1 magnetic field on the rf axis or $G_z = dB_z/dz$ on the gradient axis.

9.4 Gradient Echo and k-Space Diagrams

Suppose the two spins in the dumbbell example are replaced by a 'cylinder' of an arbitrary z-distribution of spins (Fig. 9.2). The positions of the spins are frequency encoded by an applied gradient, and Fourier techniques are available, as discussed, to image the spin distribution. Figure 9.2 carries us through an MR experiment where the equilibrium magnetization M_0 is attained (see Fig. 9.2a) and acted upon by a 90° rf pulse along $\hat{x}'$ to create a transverse magnetization also of amplitude M_0 over the whole sample. The decaying signal in Fig. 9.2b represents the FID in the laboratory frame. Applying a gradient along $\hat{z}$ causes a more rapid decay exhibiting beat frequencies (Fig. 9.2c). The transverse components of spins at different z-locations are shown projected onto the x-y plane to illustrate the dephasing of the signal. By reversing the gradient polarity, an echo can be formed at $t' = 0$ (Fig. 9.2d), according to the following explanation.

Signal measurements over a sufficient range of k are needed to reasonably reconstruct the spin density. The principal technique for obtaining negative, as well as positive, k values is the 'gradient echo' method. A single, constant gradient (such as in Fig. 9.2c) is restricted in the k interval it generates, while a combination of gradients (such as in Fig. 9.2d) can be used to expand the k range from negative to positive k values. The time at which the data corresponding to the $k = 0$ point (the echo) is measured can be moved, for example, to the center of a particular gradient 'lobe.'

In particular, combinations of gradient lobes permit the recovery of a signal loss due to the presence of the gradients themselves. The net signal from a set of spins will begin to disappear, after a gradient field is applied, for the same reason as that underlying T_2'

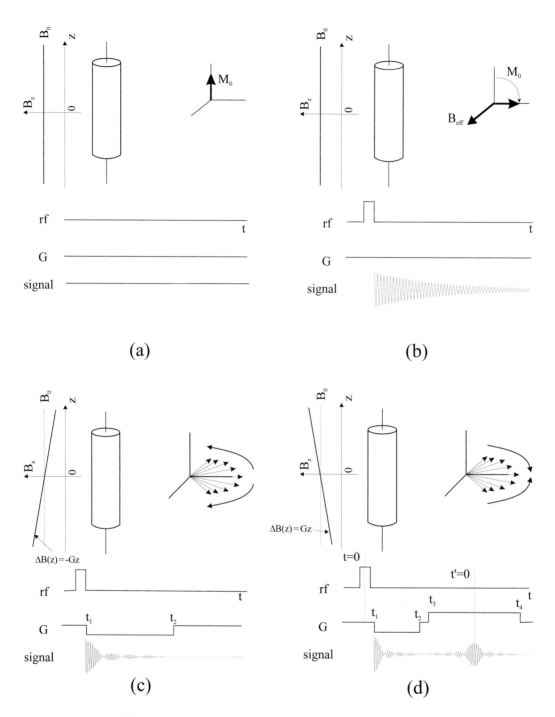

Fig. 9.2: A consecutive set of time events in a 1D MRI experiment. This illustration follows
the description of Fig. 9.1, except the two point spins are replaced by a 'cylinder' containing an
arbitrary distribution of spins. Parts (a) and (b) are the same as in the previous figure, and (c)
and (d) are described in the text. The magnetic field plotted at the left of the cylinder in (c) refers
to the field in the time interval (t_1, t_2), and, in (d), to the interval (t_3, t_4). For comparison, the spin
isochromats are pictured lying in a single plane, despite their different z coordinates. Note that
$G_z = -G$ in part (c) and has both a negative and a positive lobe of strength G in part (d).

decay.[9] Since the applied gradient is a field inhomogeneity, the spins dephase, as illustrated by the 'fan out' around $\phi = 0$ in Fig. 9.2c for constant gradients. (For a given sign on the gradient, both positive and negative phases are found for any distribution of spins straddling the origin, $z = 0$.) A series of gradient pulses can be used to form an echo similar to the spin, or rf, echo described in Ch. 8. A simple example of a gradient echo is developed below.

It should be noted that the loss of signal due to the presence of the gradient is expected from the property of the Fourier transform. Roughly speaking, the Fourier transform is a (continuous) sum of different phases which interfere with each other. The longer the cylinder of spins, the faster the Fourier transform drops off with k (i.e., with time in the imaging experiment). It is observed in Fig. 9.2c that the signal is (half of) a sinc function with a falloff expected from the dephasing arguments. (Rephasing can be achieved, as discussed below, such that the full sinc function signal is produced (Fig. 9.2d).) *In essence, the details of the dephasing determine the Fourier transform, and this dephasing represents the encoded information content.*

The associated coverage of k values can be described by a *k-space diagram*. The k-space diagram for the simple boxcar gradient in Fig. 9.1c is shown in Fig. 9.3. For a constant gradient, the k value is proportional to the imaging time according to (9.18). In this case, only half of k-space is covered for a gradient with a given sign. Other examples are exhibited below for gradient echo experiments. The effect on the signal due to the gradient manipulation is studied through the expression for the signal strength, (9.14). Recall that the relation between the phase and an arbitrary linear gradient in the z-direction is given by (9.13).

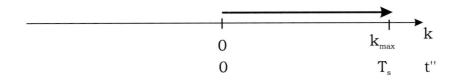

Fig. 9.3: The k-space coverage for an FID imaging experiment. The time $t'' = (t - t_1)$ is defined from the beginning of the gradient. The total sampling time is T_s. Notice that only half of k-space is covered by this experiment. There is no progression through k-space until time t_1 in Fig. 9.1c which is equivalent to $t'' = 0$.

9.4.1 The Gradient Echo

The gradient dephasing of spins in an object can be understood using phase arguments similar to those employed in Ch. 8 for the rf echo. Let us analyze the specific gradient sequence included in Fig. 9.2d.

A constant negative gradient ($G_z = -G$ for $G > 0$) is present in the time interval (t_1, t_2). From (9.13), the phase accumulation due to the gradients for a spin at z, and at a time t, during the application of the first gradient lobe is

$$\phi_G(z, t) = +\gamma G z(t - t_1) \qquad t_1 < t < t_2 \qquad (9.32)$$

---

[9]The total signal decay in the presence of an applied gradient is sometimes characterized by the relaxation time, T_2^{**}, analogous to T_2^* for static-field inhomogeneities.

The sign is consistent with the counterclockwise precession expected for a negative gradient and positive z-coordinate.

The second gradient lobe is positive ($G_z = G$ in terms of the same parameter G) during the time interval (t_3, t_4). The phase behavior relative to the y'-axis at any time in this interval is

$$\phi_G(z,t) = +\gamma Gz(t_2 - t_1) - \gamma Gz(t - t_3) \qquad t_3 < t < t_4 \tag{9.33}$$

Notice that there is no phase change during the period when the applied gradient is zero.

The gradient echo is now evident. The phase (9.33) returns to zero (Fig. 9.2d) at

$$t = t_3 + t_2 - t_1 \equiv T_E \tag{9.34}$$

for all z. The echo corresponds to that time during the second gradient lobe where the evolved area under the second lobe just cancels the area of the first lobe. *The cancelation suggests the general condition for a gradient echo,*

$$\int G(t)dt = 0 \tag{9.35}$$

i.e., the zeroth moment of $G(t)$ vanishes. The gradient echo analysis in imaging revolves around this criterion.

Returning to the example, the second gradient time interval can be chosen, as in Fig. 9.2d, such that the echo occurs at its center; that is, when $(t_4 - t_3)/2 = t_2 - t_1$. It is useful to define a new time coordinate with its origin at the echo

$$t' \equiv t - t_3 - (t_2 - t_1) = t - T_E \tag{9.36}$$

Thus, (9.33) can be rewritten

$$\phi_G(z,t) = -\gamma Gzt' \qquad -(t_4 - t_3)/2 < t' < (t_4 - t_3)/2 \tag{9.37}$$

with an obvious zero at $t' = 0$. It is during the time interval indicated in (9.37) that the data are usually sampled.

The signal (9.14) can be written as a function of t' over the region in which $G_z = G$. During the time the second gradient is turned on, the signal is

$$\begin{aligned} s(t') &= \int dz\rho(z)e^{-i\gamma Gzt'} \\ &= \int dz\rho(z)e^{-i2\pi k(t')z} \qquad -(t_4 - t_3)/2 < t' < (t_4 - t_3)/2 \end{aligned} \tag{9.38}$$

where $k = \gamma Gt'$ from (9.16). With the time-shift to t', the signal (9.38) is expressed in a form convenient to analyze the data as referenced from the center of the second lobe. (The second lobe is called the 'rephasing gradient lobe' of the read gradient, while the first lobe is referred to as the 'dephasing lobe' for that gradient.) Such time-shifts are regularly used in MR analysis.

The above experiment thus leads to a range of negative and positive k-space points for measurements made symmetrically about the echo. The negative gradient lobe has been utilized to create an echo in the middle of the positive rephasing gradient where $k = 0$.

A k-space diagram for the gradient echo experiment is shown in Fig. 9.4a. The signal in k-space is a simple transcription of (9.38),

$$s(k) = \int dz\rho(z)e^{-i2\pi kz} \qquad -k_{max} < k < k_{max} \tag{9.39}$$

where $k_{max} = \gamma G(t_4 - t_3)/2$.

Image reconstruction is also possible with just positive k-space values (see Ch. 13 for a further discussion of FID imaging with partial Fourier reconstruction). In this case, the imaging experiment is performed with a single, positive, read gradient lobe. A k-space diagram for the FID imaging experiment has already appeared in Fig. 9.3. The limits on k-space sampling are $0 < k < k_{max}$, where $k_{max} = \gamma G T_s$, for a constant gradient $G > 0$ and sampling time T_s.

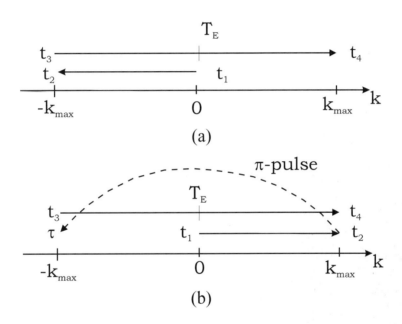

Fig. 9.4: The k-space coverage for the basic gradient echo experiment and the two variants of the spin echo experiment presented in the text. Diagram (a) applies to the basic gradient echo experiment and to the spin echo variant where all frequency encoding occurs after the π-pulse (see Fig. 9.6). Diagram (b) shows the spin echo variant where both gradient lobes are positive (see Fig. 9.5). In all cases, $k_{max} = \gamma G(t_4 - t_3)/2$. The dashed line represents the action of the π-pulse which changes k to $-k$.

Problem 9.4

Spins with gyromagnetic ratio γ are uniformly distributed with uniform spin density ρ_0 along the z-axis from $-z_0$ to z_0 in a 1D imaging experiment. Suppose they are excited at $t = 0$ by an rf pulse such that the signal at that instant would be given by

$$s(t=0) = \int_{-z_0}^{z_0} dz\, \rho_0 = 2z_0\rho_0 \qquad (9.40)$$

A negative constant gradient field $-G$ is immediately applied at $t = 0^+$ and flipped to the positive constant gradient field $+G$ at time $t = T$. Find an expression for the signal for $t > T$ and show that it exhibits a gradient echo at time $t = 2T$.

9.4.2   General Spin Echo Imaging

In Ch. 8, the spin echo experiment was introduced as a method to refocus the phase accumulation due to static-field inhomogeneities. While the gradient echo refocuses the phase induced by the application of gradients, it does not refocus the dephasing due to static-field inhomogeneities. In many cases, T_2^* decay can cause a significant reduction in signal before the gradient echo is performed. Under these circumstances, it may be beneficial to perform a spin echo in concert with the gradient echo, to refocus the static field inhomogeneities and, thereby, increase the signal at the gradient echo.

In general, the use of both a gradient echo and a spin echo during an imaging experiment is referred to simply as a spin echo experiment. It is necessary, however, to distinguish an imaging spin echo experiment from the global spin echo method described in Ch. 8.[10] If imaging is being discussed, then the spin echo sequence is a combination of multiple rf pulses and a set of applied gradients,[11] but, in a global signal detection experiment, it may only refer to the rf pulses.

Two Variants of the 1D Spin Echo Imaging Experiment

There are two primary methods in which the spin echo may be incorporated with imaging. The first is to apply a π-pulse in between two gradient pulses, where both gradient pulses have the same polarity. See Fig. 9.5 for the timing and gradient parameters. In the presence of magnetic field inhomogeneities, the phase behavior for a spin isochromat at the position z during the first gradient pulse is

$$\phi(z,t) = -\gamma \Delta B(z)t - \gamma G z(t - t_1) \qquad t_1 < t < t_2 \qquad (9.41)$$

for the initial $\pi/2$-pulse (field) applied along $\hat{x}'$ and ϕ defined with respect to the y'-axis so that $\phi(z,0) = 0$ (see Sec. 8.2). In (9.41), the z-component of the static field is $B_0 + \Delta B(z)$, and the constant gradient G is taken to be positive. For the π-pulse applied along $\hat{y}'$ at $t = \tau$, all of the phase, including that due to the gradients, is inverted, $\phi \to -\phi$.[12] During

---

[10]An alternate description is to refer to spin echoes induced by rf pulses as rf echoes or Hahn echoes. Both rf echoes and gradient echoes are, after all, spin rephasing, or spin echoes.

[11]The time variations of gradients will be referred to as 'gradient pulses.'

[12]The conclusions in these discussions do not depend on the choices of the rf pulse field directions and the $\phi = 0$ axis. For other choices, constant phases may arise that are nonzero, but that are the same for all isochromats.

the application of the second gradient lobe, the phase evolves according to

$$\phi(z,t) = \gamma \Delta B(z)\tau + \gamma G z(t_2 - t_1) - \gamma \Delta B(z)(t - \tau) - \gamma G z(t - t_3) \quad t_3 < t < t_4 \quad (9.42)$$

If, as indicated in the figure, the time of the spin echo, $t = 2\tau$, coincides with the time of the gradient echo, $T_E \equiv t_3 + (t_2 - t_1)$, then the expression (9.42) for the phase vanishes at that common point. With this constraint on τ, the total phase induced by the applied-gradient and static-field inhomogeneities has been refocused.

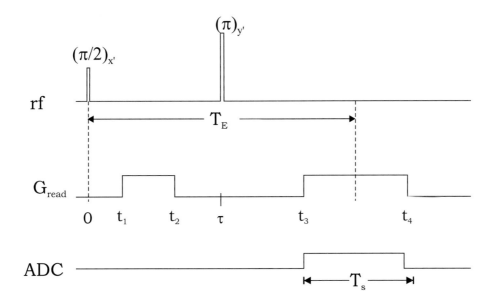

Fig. 9.5: Sequence diagram for a spin echo 1D imaging experiment with a π-pulse between two gradient lobes of the same polarity. The directions along which the rf fields point are indicated by the subscripts and correspond to the choices in the text, but the echo is independent of these choices.

The key to the arrangement is that the π-pulse effectively changes the sign on the first gradient, so that the two gradient lobes can produce the same cancelation seen in (9.33). The associated k-space coverage is displayed in Fig. 9.4b.

A second, essentially equivalent method of collecting spin echo data in conjunction with a gradient echo uses a 'bipolar' gradient structure. Two gradient lobes of opposite polarity follow the π-pulse (Fig. 9.6). The evolution of the phase is worked out in the following problem, with the result that the phase expression pertaining to the time interval of the second gradient lobe shows the same zero as in (9.42). With the times t_i redefined by Fig. 9.6, it is clear that $\phi(z, T_E) = 0$, if $2\tau = t_3 + (t_2 - t_1)$. The rf echo and gradient echo mechanisms work independently in the second method and, as before, they combine to give maximal signal at T_E. Therefore, the k-space diagram is the same as that for the regular gradient echo sequence, which was shown in Fig. 9.4a and similar forms of (9.37) to (9.39) are valid for the spin echo as well. *This exercise demonstrates that several different data acquisition schemes can lead to the same k-space coverage.*

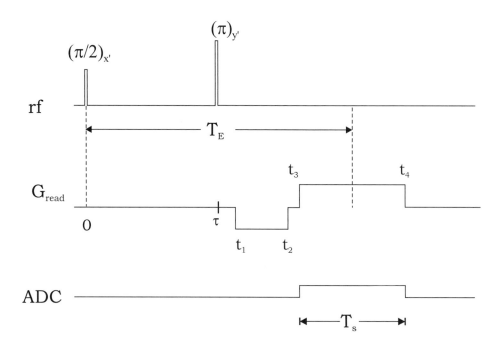

Fig. 9.6: Sequence diagram for a spin echo 1D imaging experiment with a π-pulse preceding two gradient lobes of opposite polarity. The subscripts on the rf flip angles again denote the direction of the applied magnetic field $\vec{B}_1$.

Problem 9.5

---

a) In terms of the timing and gradient parameters shown in Fig. 9.6, show that the phase during the first (negative) gradient lobe is

$$\phi(z,t) \;=\; \gamma G z(t-t_1) - \gamma \Delta B(z)(t-2\tau) \qquad t_1 < t < t_2 \quad (9.43)$$

b) Show that the phase during the second (positive) gradient lobe is

$$\phi(z,t) = \gamma G z(t_2 - t_1) - \gamma \Delta B(z)(t-2\tau) - \gamma G z(t-t_3) \qquad t_3 < t < t_4$$
$$(9.44)$$

which is identical to (9.42).

In both sequences, the common denominator is the occurrence of the gradient echo and spin echo at the same time. Although more advanced imaging discussions are necessary to fully understand differences between these two sequences, it is possible to give one reason for favoring the second method. The position encoding in the second example takes place at a time closer to the sampling of the data and, as may be anticipated, motion effects will be minimized (see Ch. 23).

9.4.3   Image Profiles

MR images, in general, are shown in a grayscale format where brightness (whiteness) indicates higher spin density. Most images are displayed such that only the highest spin density in an object appears white and areas with lower values of $\hat{\rho}$ appear in correspondingly darker shades of gray. Zero spin density appears black.

Figure 9.7 demonstrates how a 1D projection of an object is related to both an effective spin density and an image. In Fig. 9.7a, a pencil is shown where the spin density in the eraser end is constant and only half of that of the constant spin density found in the remainder of the pencil. The pencil also tapers linearly to zero at the nib. Figure 9.7b is a plot of the 1D (projected) physical spin density in the pencil as a function of z. The linear gradient field shown in Fig. 9.7c could be used to obtain the k-space data necessary to reconstruct a 1D image. In order to view the reconstructed 1D 'line' image, the density $\hat{\rho}(z)$ is shown as a row of pixels with finite width in Fig. 9.7d. Notice that in this 1D imaging discussion, where all spins at a given frequency have been projected onto the same z-position, relaxation effects have been neglected.

The image profile of the pencil in Fig. 9.7b is an example of a conventional graph of effective spin density along the imaging axis. In general, this may be generated along an arbitrary line in higher dimensions, and it is useful for the determination of specific properties of the reconstructed 3D spin density which are difficult to otherwise discern. For instance, consider the linear decrease in signal at the end of the pencil. This feature is immediately evident in the profile, but the linearity may not be readily apparent in the 1D image (Fig. 9.7d).

Problem 9.6

In this problem, we study the effects of relaxation on the signal for the pencil described above and in Fig. 9.7. Assume that $\rho_0 = 1$ and that relaxation effects during data sampling can be neglected, i.e., $T_s \ll T_2^*$. A simple gradient echo experiment (Fig. 9.2d) with a $\pi/2$-pulse is considered.

   a) Assume that all data are collected in one excitation so that the longitudinal relaxation of the sample is not a factor. For $T_{2,eraser}^* = 20\,\text{ms}$, $T_{2,pencil}^* = 50\,\text{ms}$, and $T_E = 30\,\text{ms}$, plot the reconstructed image profile (where only the relaxation effects are taken into account).

   b) Instead, assume that the experiment must be repeated many times to acquire an adequate amount of data. Assume that $T_E \simeq 0$, $T_{1,eraser} = 400\,\text{ms}$, $T_{1,pencil} = 3000\,\text{ms}$, and $T_R = 500\,\text{ms}$. Plot the reconstructed image profile in this case to see the effect of T_1 on the image. See Sec. 8.3.

This problem is an introductory example of how imaging parameters can affect the resulting reconstructed profile. Contrast mechanisms based on differences in relaxation times are developed further in Ch. 15.

A practical illustration of the concepts of the previous discussion is found by performing a gradient echo experiment. A spatially uniform cuboidal gel (a 'phantom') is imaged along its longest dimension. The other two dimensions are much smaller in comparison. The resultant 1D image is shown in Fig. 9.8b, where the oscillations at the edge in the object profile are an example of Gibbs ringing (see Ch. 12). The concave dip in the image profile is presumably due to an rf nonuniformity caused by the gel electrical conductivity (see Ch. 27).

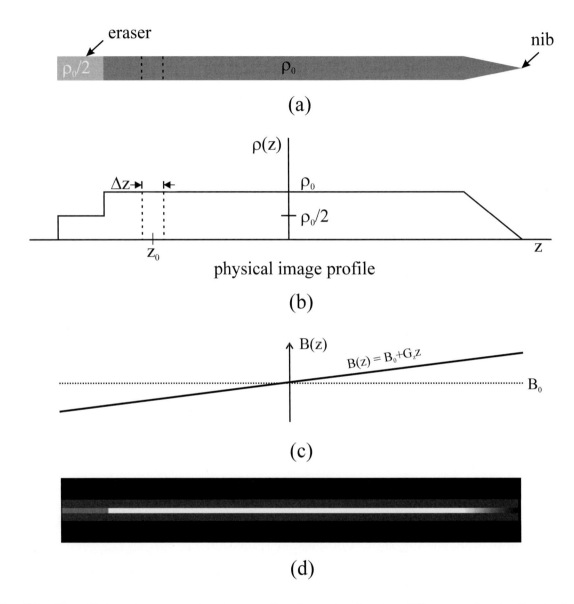

Fig. 9.7: The 1D imaging example of a pencil (where the density differences due to the lead and lead tip are ignored). The physical object being imaged is shown in (a), and the physical 1D projected spin density, or image profile, is plotted in (b). A 1D MRI of the pencil can be carried out using the magnetic field with the linear gradient plotted in (c). In (d), the resulting image is shown as a line of pixels Δz, where the thick black border is added for visual contrast. The projection onto 1D at z_0, for example, is carried out by three integrations: Two integrations are over the transverse dimensions of the pencil, and the third integration is over Δz.

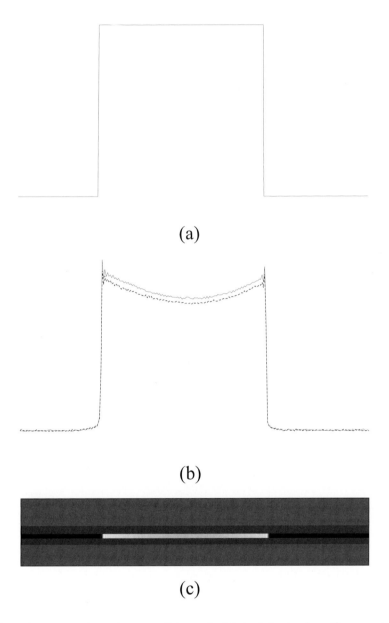

(a)

(b)

(c)

Fig. 9.8: A 1D imaging experiment on a thin cuboidal object of uniform spin density using a gradient echo sequence. (a) Expected physical 1D profile. (b) Measured profile at two different T_E values (the solid line is obtained at $T_E = 6\,\text{ms}$ and the dashed line is obtained at $T_E = 20\,\text{ms}$). As expected, there is a drop in signal at the longer T_E value. (c) A 1D image where the line of pixels is constructed as in Fig. 9.7d. The thickness of the line is exaggerated for visualization purposes. Due to the choice of relationship between image brightness and signal strength, the profile variations seen in (b) are not visible in the image.

9.5   Gradient Directionality and Nonlinearity

9.5.1   Frequency Encoding in an Arbitrary Direction

Although the z-direction was chosen for the 1D spatial encoding of spins, there is no restriction on the direction along which the gradient can be applied. A constant gradient vector $\vec{G}$ may be used to define an arbitrary coordinate direction, with respect to which the z-component of the associated applied magnetic field $\vec{B}^g$ is linearly changing.[13] The superscript g is used to remind the reader that an applied gradient is being considered. The gradient vector is defined by[14]

$$
\begin{aligned}
\vec{G}(t) &\equiv \vec{\nabla} B_z^g(\vec{r}) \\
&= \hat{x}\frac{\partial}{\partial x}B_z^g + \hat{y}\frac{\partial}{\partial y}B_z^g + \hat{z}\frac{\partial}{\partial z}B_z^g \\
&\equiv G_x(t)\hat{x} + G_y(t)\hat{y} + G_z(t)\hat{z}
\end{aligned}
\tag{9.45}
$$

The general linear gradient is a superposition of three linear gradients, G_x, G_y, G_z along the three orthogonal directions. *Each gradient corresponds to a magnetic field whose z-component varies linearly along the given direction* and this same z-component augments the static field. The x-gradient, y-gradient, and z-gradient z-components of the magnetic field vary linearly in x, y, and z, respectively.

A gradient $\vec{G}$ with a fixed direction[15] corresponds to one coordinate along one direction. The z-component of the total (static plus linear) magnetic field can be written as

$$
B_z(\xi, t) = B_0 + \vec{G}(t) \cdot \vec{r} = B_0 + G(t)\xi
\tag{9.46}
$$

where the magnitude of the gradient vector is G, and the variable ξ is defined as the position along the direction of $\vec{G}$,

$$
\xi \equiv \hat{G} \cdot \vec{r}
\tag{9.47}
$$

The application of the field (9.46) leads to a formula for the (spatially varying) precessional frequency,

$$
\omega(\xi, t) = \omega_0 + \gamma\vec{G}(t) \cdot \vec{r} = \omega_0 + \gamma G(t)\xi
\tag{9.48}
$$

as a generalization of (9.10). The associated phase accumulation is

$$
\phi_G(\xi, t) = -\gamma\vec{r} \cdot \int_0^t dt' \vec{G}(t') = -\gamma\xi \int_0^t dt' G(t')
\tag{9.49}
$$

Equation (9.16) is now extended to

$$
\vec{k}(t) = \gamma \int_0^t \vec{G}(t') dt'
\tag{9.50}
$$

---

[13]The fact that $\vec{G}$ is constant in space means that B_z grows linearly in that direction.

[14]We remind the reader that the unprimed coordinates are assigned to the laboratory, rather than the rotating, reference frame.

[15]This implies that the individual components of $\vec{G}$ have exactly the same time dependence. Their ratios are (any) constants.

The combination of these results gives the more general 1D imaging equation

$$s(t) = \int d^3r \rho(\vec{r}) e^{-i2\pi \vec{k}(t)\cdot\vec{r}} = \int d\xi \rho(\xi) e^{-i2\pi k(t)\xi} \qquad (9.51)$$

A fuller reference to the k-space directions is obtained by rewriting (9.51) as

$$s(\vec{k}) = \int d^3r \rho(\vec{r}) e^{-i2\pi \vec{k}\cdot\vec{r}} \qquad (9.52)$$

The 1D spin density along ξ is

$$\rho(\xi) \equiv \int \int d\eta d\chi \rho(\vec{r}) \qquad (9.53)$$

The variables η and χ are coordinates for a plane perpendicular to the gradient $\vec{G}$ direction.

The resultant signal (9.51) remains a Fourier integral and one-dimensional imaging can thus be conducted in the direction of $\vec{G}$. The image along the direction of $\vec{G}$, as before, can be reconstructed using an inverse Fourier transform. *The directionality of the gradient field and, hence, of the image can be varied by changing the relative amplitudes of the three components* G_x, G_y, *and* G_z; more details concerning the relationship of the components to the net direction are found in Sec. 10.1. (This is also a topic of discussion in Ch. 14 where radial k-space coverage is considered.) In fact, now the reader begins to see some of the flexibility inherent in MRI, that, without physically rotating the sample, *the viewing angle or imaging direction can be modified by manipulation of the imaging gradients.*

9.5.2 Nonlinear Gradients

It is possible to alter the uniform static field with something other than a linear gradient field. As long as there are no points where B_z has the same value, i.e., as long as it is single-valued, the Fourier transform of the signal can be constructed. The Fourier transform, and knowledge of the magnetic field, can then be combined to relate the frequency and position information, and to create a faithful image.

It is actually impossible to generate a perfectly linear gradient in free space and, in some imaging circumstances, it is necessary to account for the distortion associated with the gradients after the Fourier transform is performed. Still, gradient coil designers strive for linearity over a limited imaging volume, and consider linearity, speed, and image quality in their specifications. In most whole-body MRI machines, the maximum gradient deviation remains within 5% of the desired value (see Ch. 20 for specific image distortion discussions). If an application presented itself where extremely fast data acquisition were required, and unlimited computing power were available, poorer gradients might be a practical alternative.

Suggested Reading

The following two references discuss basic k-space concepts:

- S. Ljunggren. A simple graphical representation of Fourier-based imaging methods. *J. Magn. Reson.*, 54: 338, 1983.

- D. B. Twieg. The k-trajectory formulation of the NMR imaging process with applications in analysis and synthesis of imaging methods. *Med. Phys.*, 10: 610, 1983.

Elementary aspects of sampling and Nyquist limits are presented in:

- O. E. Brigham. *The Fast Fourier Transform.* Prentice-Hall, Englewood Cliffs, New Jersey, 1974.

The basic pioneering concepts of magnetic resonance imaging are introduced in:

- P. C. Lauterbur. Image formation by induced local interactions. Examples employing magnetic resonance. *Nature*, 243: 190, 1973.

- P. Mansfield and P. K. Grannell. NMR 'diffraction' in solids? *J. Phys. C: Solid State Phys.*, 6: L422, 1973.

Chapter 10

Multi-Dimensional Fourier Imaging and Slice Excitation

Chapter Contents

Summary: Imaging in more than one dimension is introduced. The notion of k-space is extended to multiple dimensions. Generic 2D and 3D imaging sequences are introduced. Excitation of a specific slice is described as a technique for the creation of 2D images. The signals contributed by different chemical species during the same experiment are studied as imaging in an additional dimension.

Introduction

The previous chapter focused on the 1D version of an MR imaging experiment. It was discovered there that the signal from the excited spins with a transverse component precessing in a linearly changing magnetic field is a Fourier transform of the effective spin density along the linear gradient direction (ξ, say). The transform variable of the data is the spatial frequency k_ξ, which may be varied by virtue of its dependence on time and the gradient strength. The signal can be inverse Fourier transformed in the ξ direction to profile the effective spin density.

In the first section of this chapter, the generalization of 1D Fourier encoding to two and three dimensions is introduced. A component of the spatial frequency vector $\vec{k}$ is associated with each direction, and with a gradient-vector component for that direction. The resulting

165

expression for the signal is a two- or three-dimensional Fourier transform of the effective spin density. The technique of covering k-space by varying gradient amplitudes and the notion of 'phase encoding' are introduced. Rather than collecting data over the entire third dimension, a 'slice select' technique is introduced in Sec. 10.2 whereby the signal is limited by an rf excitation with a sufficiently narrow bandwidth to that from a thin slice perpendicular to the third direction. The two 'in-plane' dimensions of the slice are those referred to in '2D Fourier imaging' in Sec. 10.3. Two common techniques for working in three dimensions, multi-slice 2D imaging and 3D imaging, are introduced in the fourth section. The multi-slices are obtained by a series of rf pulses with different center frequencies. The 3D imaging is the partitioning of a single slab by the use of a phase encoding gradient. A central consideration is the time taken to collect data. The last section examines the difference in signals from protons in different molecular environments due to chemical shifts. The chemical shift is an additional degree of freedom and the distribution of the signal in this variable can be couched as a dependence on an additional imaging dimension.

10.1   Imaging in More Dimensions

Imaging in 1D was predicated on separating out the unique information associated with each spatial position by frequency encoding the data. A new construct, k-space, could be used to express the data in terms of the Fourier transform of the spin density. Different points in k-space can then be collected by sampling the data during the ADC on-time, T_s, as shown in Fig. 10.1. This would produce a k-space representation of $s(k_x)$ as a set of points sampled along the continuous line in Fig. 10.1b. Similarly, enough information must be collected in the y and z directions to make it possible to extract $\rho(\vec{r})$ in three dimensions. In the following discussion, we first assert that the same Fourier transform representation of the data can be found in 3D and that the gradients in y and z can be used to extend k-space to 3D as well. Afterward, we shall demonstrate how to physically accomplish this, despite the loss of signal due to relaxation.

10.1.1   The Imaging Equation

The 3D Representation

Consider the extension of the one-dimensional imaging equation (9.15) to all three spatial dimensions.[1] The signal from a single rf excitation of the whole sample in the presence of a set of three orthogonal gradients may be written as the 3D Fourier transform[2]

$$s(\vec{k}) \;=\; \int d^3 r \rho(\vec{r}) e^{-i2\pi \vec{k}\cdot\vec{r}} \tag{10.1}$$

or

$$s(k_x, k_y, k_z) \;=\; \int\int\int dx\, dy\, dz\, \rho(x,y,z) e^{-i2\pi(k_x x + k_y y + k_z z)}$$
$$=\; \mathcal{F}[\rho(x,y,z)] \tag{10.2}$$

---

[1]For the moment, we defer the question concerning the way the image is to be viewed or presented.

[2]Although they are important, relaxation factors continue to be omitted in the introductory imaging equations.

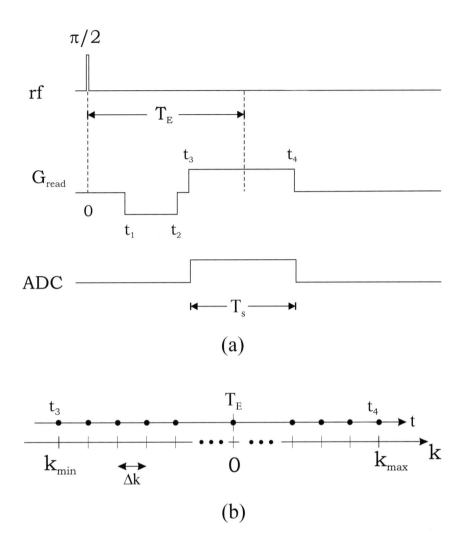

Fig. 10.1: (a) A 1D imaging protocol for a gradient echo sequence structure with sampling restricted to the ADC period T_s between t_3 and t_4. (b) The associated sampled k-space coverage running from k_{min} to k_{max}. Although $|k_{min}| \simeq k_{max}$, the fact that they need not be the same is illustrated in this diagram and is a subject of interest in later chapters.

This is called the *3D imaging equation*. The three implicitly time-dependent components of $\vec{k}$ are related to the respective gradient-component integrals (cf. 9.16)

$$k_x(t) = \gamma \!\!\!\!\!\!\!\!\!\!- \int^t G_x(t')dt', \quad k_y(t) = \gamma \!\!\!\!\!\!\!\!\!\!- \int^t G_y(t')dt', \quad k_z(t) = \gamma \!\!\!\!\!\!\!\!\!\!- \int^t G_z(t')dt' \qquad (10.3)$$

where the integrations run from the onset of the gradient to time t. The challenge is to manipulate the application of the gradients in such a way that *3D k-space* can be sampled sufficiently. This is required in order that the reconstructed image $\hat{\rho}(\vec{r})$, which is the inverse Fourier transform of the measured data, $s_m(\vec{k})$ (a density distribution derived from a set of discrete data, see Ch. 12),

$$\hat{\rho}(\vec{r}) \;=\; \int d^3k \, s_m(\vec{k}) e^{i2\pi \vec{k}\cdot\vec{r}} \qquad (10.4)$$

be an accurate estimate of the physical density $\rho(\vec{r})$. In the discussions to follow, this will be accomplished by independently varying G_x, G_y, and G_z to sweep over the 3D k-space.

The 2D Representation

For a planar object, or for a thin slice through a 3D object, where 2D information alone is required, only k_x and k_y need to be sampled. The sequence diagram in Fig. 10.2 employs just one rf pulse to cover 2D k-space with a set of discretely sampled parallel lines as shown in Fig. 10.3. Each set of points along a given k_y line represents the acquisition of 'phase encoded' 1D data, since the phase of each point along y is encoded as $\gamma G_y \tau_y y$. *This y-dependent phase contribution is unchanged during data sampling along the k_x-axis.*[3] We return to a detailed discussion of Figs. 10.2 and 10.3 in Sec. 10.1.2.

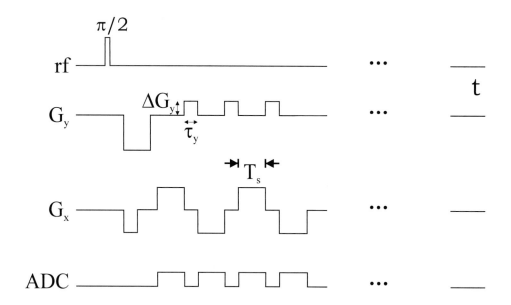

Fig. 10.2: Sequence diagram for coverage of 2D k-space with a single rf excitation. To continue echoing the data, the read gradient is reversed after each application of ΔG_y. The 'phase encoding' steps ΔG_y are applied when the read gradient is off.

Consider the imaging of a planar portion of a three-dimensional object with physical density $\rho(\vec{r})$. As an example of the phase encoding described above, all information along y at a given x is projected onto x for the line $k_y = 0$, i.e.,

$$s(k_x, 0) = \int d^3r\, \rho(\vec{r}) e^{-i2\pi k_x x} \tag{10.5}$$

An inverse Fourier transformation of this line of data leads to the 1D projection reconstructed image according to the following calculation

$$\hat{\rho}_{1D}(x) = \int dk_x\, s(k_x, 0) e^{i2\pi k_x x} = \int d^3r'\, \rho(\vec{r'}) \int dk_x\, e^{-i2\pi k_x (x - x')}$$

---

[3]The use of the phrase 'phase encoding' can be misleading, since all gradients or field inhomogeneities add phase to the magnetization, but it is universally used when the encoding gradient is varied in stepwise fashion.

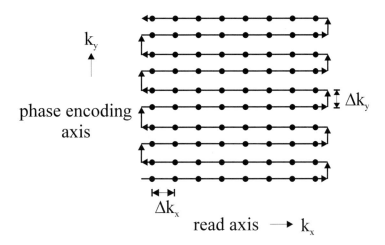

Fig. 10.3: The k-space coverage for a 2D example. Each dot represents a sampled point. Lines of connected dots are shown to be along the read direction, referring to data collected during the same read period. The arrows indicate the chronological order of data acquisition.

$$= \int \int \int dx'dy'dz' \, \rho(x',y',z') \, \delta(x - x') = \int \int dy \, dz \, \rho(x,y,z) \qquad (10.6)$$

The generalization of the encoding to arbitrary k_y is

$$s(k_x, k_y) = \int \int \int dx \, dy \, dz \, \rho(x,y,z) e^{-i2\pi(k_x x + k_y y)} \qquad (10.7)$$

After a calculation similar to (10.6), the result of inverse Fourier transformation with respect to both k_x and k_y is the 2D image projected along $\hat{z}$

$$\hat{\rho}(x,y) = \int dk_x s(k_x, k_y) e^{i2\pi(k_x x + k_y y)} = \int dz \, \rho(x,y,z) \qquad (10.8)$$

10.1.2 Single Excitation Traversal of k-Space

1D Coverage

In the 1D example of the gradient echo sequence, the path through k-space was seen to start at zero and then move to the left as the negative gradient was applied from t_1 to t_2 (Fig. 10.1). Just after it is turned off, a large negative k value has been reached. When the gradient is switched on again, this time to a positive value, *the direction of coverage in k-space is reversed*, and the data are sampled between t_3 and t_4. The 'dephasing gradient' is seen to be a gradient which determines the starting point of the sampling in k-space, but data usually are not taken over this lobe.

2D Coverage

A standard coverage of 2D k-space corresponds to the series of parallel lines in a plane. The first two gradients along $\hat{x}$ and $\hat{y}$ in Fig. 10.2 move the position in k-space from the origin to the bottom left corner in Fig. 10.3. This traversal of 2D k-space is obtained by alternately turning on the G_x gradient and then the G_y gradient as illustrated in Fig. 10.2. The bottom line in k-space is obtained by the usual read gradient structure during sampling of the data. Applying a positive ΔG_y with just enough amplitude to carry k_y up one line moves the position in k-space to the right-side of the second line from the bottom. To bring it back across k_x requires applying a negative lobe of the same time duration as the positive rephasing gradient applied for the bottom line. Repeating the same steps, and each time reversing the polarity of the x-gradient, will carry the position up through the (k_x, k_y) plane. The vertical spacing of the set of horizontal read gradient lines is determined by the step size in k_y which is in turn determined by ΔG_y (see below). The data are not collected during the short vertical steps drawn in Fig. 10.3. We return to a detailed analysis of the signal in 2D imaging in Sec. 10.3.

3D Coverage and Data Collection

The above coverage of 2D k-space can be generalized to 3D by considering a series of planes leading to a three-dimensional set of parallel lines. The set can be obtained in 3D k-space by discrete sampling, or phase encoding, in both of the directions k_y and k_z.[4] The imaging of three dimensions by the use of two phase encoding directions perpendicular to the read direction is called '3D imaging,' to contrast it with 'multi-slice 2D imaging.' The difference between the two approaches has to do with how the rf excitation is carried out. In the latter, a series of rf pulses defines the series of slices filling out the third dimension. In the former, an rf pulse may be used to excite a 'thicker' slice which is then phase encoded (or, as it is often called, 'partition encoded') in the slice select gradient direction; a series of such rf pulses is needed to run through all the partition encoding and phase encoding gradient values. (See Sec. 10.4 for further details about both approaches.)

How do we change the gradients to achieve the discretized coverage in 3D imaging? Let the x-gradient define the read direction of the set of lines. The read sampling along the line may be carried out, as before, with measurements at finite time steps Δt during the continuous application of a gradient G_x. The associated step in the k_x direction is

$$\Delta k_x = \gamma\!\!\!\!/ \, G_x \Delta t \qquad (10.9)$$

The orthogonal gradients, G_y and G_z, are turned off during the read sampling, in order to keep each line parallel to the x-axis. Before the read data are taken, the (k_y, k_z) position of each line is determined by applying the orthogonal gradients for, say, times τ_y and τ_z. After a given line has been sampled, an adjacent parallel line is approached by turning the orthogonal gradients back on, for the same times τ_y or τ_z with the same amplitudes, either ΔG_y or ΔG_z. The corresponding shifts in k-space are

$$\begin{aligned}\Delta k_y &= \gamma\!\!\!\!/ \, \Delta G_y \tau_y \\ \Delta k_z &= \gamma\!\!\!\!/ \, \Delta G_z \tau_z\end{aligned} \qquad (10.10)$$

Once again, to continue echoing, the $k_x = 0$ point is traversed alternately either left-to-right or right-to-left while the read gradient oscillates from a positive to a negative value from one

---

[4]The relationships of both the spacings and the limitations on the number of steps to the degradation of the image quality are detailed in Chs. 12 and 13.

line to the next. The phases associated with the orthogonal, or phase encoding, gradients, G_y and G_z, are indeed fixed along each line during the taking of data.

10.1.3   Time Constraints and Collecting Data over Multiple Cycles

It is rare to collect all k-space points following a single rf excitation. Only a small number of lines of k-space can be collected after each rf excitation before the signal is lost due to T_2 or T_2^* decay. In conventional imaging, often only one line of k-space data is collected following an rf excitation (the process is illustrated in Fig. 10.4). After a new rf pulse, the

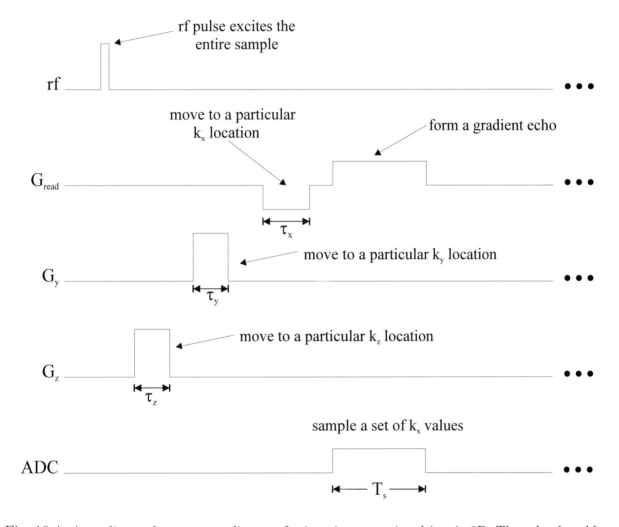

Fig. 10.4: A gradient echo sequence diagram for imaging an entire object in 3D. The role played by each gradient in the experiment is described in the figure. The location of a sampled point in each direction of k-space is proportional to the area under the corresponding applied gradients between the rf excitation pulse and the sampled point (see Sec. 10.3). The ellipses denote the systematic repetition of the cycle of rf and variable gradient pulse amplitudes shown above required to cover k-space. In later chapters, we discuss the manner in which the transverse magnetization is suppressed or 'spoiled' just before the start of each new cycle.

phase encoding gradients are incrementally increased/decreased with step sizes ΔG_y and ΔG_z appearing in (10.10), followed by the acquisition of another line of k-space data. This process is repeated every T_R until all of the necessary k-space data are acquired. In terms of a sequence diagram, the set of phase encoding gradient values corresponding to their incrementation as carried out over the multiple T_R intervals is represented as a 'table' (such as shown in Fig. 10.5c), with an arrow pointing in the direction of incrementation, which also indicates the direction of k-space traversal in the phase encoding direction. In this case, as suggested in Figs. 10.4 and 10.5, all k_x lines are collected from left-to-right in contrast to the example in Fig. 10.3.

The possible loss of signal due to transverse relaxation effects is best discussed in terms of the 'total acquisition time' for an MR experiment. Consider first a 3D k-space data collection and let N_y and N_z denote the phase encoding steps for the two directions perpendicular to the read axis. It takes $N_y N_z$ different repetitions (different lines) of the experiment for each unique pair of phase encoding gradient values (each line). The total time for a 3D imaging method is given by

$$T_{acq} = N_y N_z T_R \qquad (10.11)$$

For a 2D imaging experiment, the total acquisition time is simply

$$T_{acq} = N_y T_R \qquad (10.12)$$

See Prob. 10.1 for an example calculation of the total acquisition time for a 3D experiment. Given the large amount of data which needs to be calculated, it is understood why k-space coverage, at least for simpler MR systems, is often limited to one line at a time.[5] For both 3D and 2D experiments, when data is collected N_{acq} times to improve signal-to-noise, the total MR imaging time is increased by a factor N_{acq}.

Problem 10.1

Consider a uniform cubical sample of water.

a) If the entire sample is excited, how long would it take to collect 64×64 lines (64 phase encoding points along each of the transverse axes, i.e., those axes perpendicular to the original 'read' line of data), if $T_R = 20\,\mathrm{ms}$? This is the procedure described as 3D volume imaging in Sec. 10.5.

b) Based on part (a) and the values of T_2 in Table 4.1, explain why k-space data is often collected only one line at a time (but see Ch. 19).

---

[5]When signal-to-noise and gradient capabilities are sufficient, either multiple gradient echo or short-T_R sequences can be used to shorten acquisition times. These concepts are discussed in detail in Chs. 18 and 19.

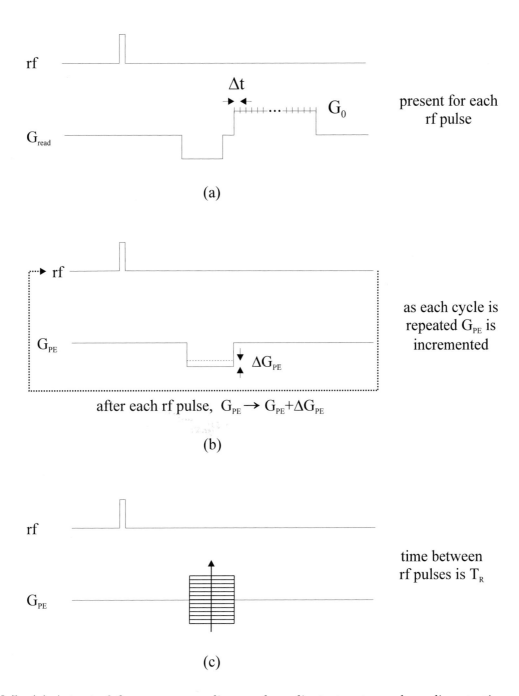

present for each
rf pulse

as each cycle is
repeated G_{PE} is
incremented

time between
rf pulses is T_R

Fig. 10.5: (a) A typical frequency encoding read gradient structure where discrete time samples lead to discrete 1D k-space coverage along a read direction. (b) The coverage along a given phase encoding direction is carried out with one k-space step for each rf pulse. Different k-space samples are obtained by varying the amplitude of the gradient for each pulse repetition. The dotted line (with the arrowhead at the end pointing to rf) indicates that this 'cycle' of the sequence structure is repeated. (c) A simpler representation of the entire sequence structure indicated in (b). The series of gradient amplitudes, and the direction of changing amplitude, are now represented by the stepped column or 'phase encoding table' and its arrow. It is noted that either frequency encoding or phase encoding could be used for coverage of any k-space line, see Sec. 10.1.4.

10.1.4   Variations in k-Space Coverage

Recall that phase encoding is the process of stepping to a specific location in k-space in a plane defined by two orthogonal dimensions before a line of data is acquired along the read direction perpendicular to that plane. Whatever the scheme, *the basic requirement of sampling the data is to visit each lattice point of the k-space volume-of-interest.* The plane or set of lines in 2D or 3D imaging could be replaced, in principle, by an arbitrary trajectory through the k-space region-of-interest as long as the same points are sampled. A rich variety of rf and gradient combinations can be used to effect the same coverage of k-space, as will be discovered throughout the text.

In fact, there are alternatives for the coverage of a single line itself. Instead of the series of time steps Δt made during the application of a constant gradient G_0 (Fig. 10.5a), the gradient strength may be stepped by an amount ΔG_x to generate the same Δk_x (Fig. 10.5b). The time the variable gradient is applied may be fixed at τ_x and a gradient table used to step through k_x-space. This is exactly how the phase encoding shifts (10.10) are generated, and it would have been possible to introduce phase encoding by first showing this as an alternative to frequency encoding of the line (see Prob. 10.2). A new rf excitation is required for each new gradient strength, however, and the time taken is increased thereby.[6]

Problem 10.2

We have introduced the concept of phase encoding as a separate means to image the spatial distribution of $\rho(\vec{r})$ orthogonal to the read gradient. However, it can also be used to replace the read gradient. To accomplish this, assume that the 1D experiment is repeated N_x times with a repeat time T_R. Use only the dephasing lobe of the read gradient, of length τ. The readout portion is not used. Further, assume that the amplitude of the gradient is changed from rf pulse to rf pulse by an amount ΔG_x. Sampling takes place at the same point in time after the new x-direction phase encoding gradient is applied from one rf pulse to the next (i.e., only a single point would be sampled in each T_R in this scenario).

a) Describe how the amplitude of the dephasing lobe must be varied from one rf pulse to the next to get the equivalent coverage of k-space to that in Fig. 10.5a where

$$\Delta k_x \;=\; \gamma G_x \Delta t \qquad\qquad (10.13)$$

Specifically show that

$$\Delta G_x \tau \;=\; G_x \Delta t \qquad\qquad (10.14)$$

if the sampling in k-space is identical for each approach.

b) What are the disadvantages and advantages of this method?

---

[6]A third alternative is to increase the time τ_x with G_x fixed. The acquisition time is increased even more.

10.2 Slice Selection with Boxcar Excitations

In general, magnetic resonance images are produced by exciting a single thin slice of the body by using a combination of gradient fields and 'spatially selective' rf pulses. The slices are thinner for the 2D imaging methods. Radiofrequency pulses are spatially selective by having a finite region of support in the frequency content of the transmitted pulse, i.e., by having a finite bandwidth. The presence beforehand of a linear gradient means that only the slice corresponding to the region of support in the Larmor frequency domain is excited. The one-to-one correspondence of a given distance along the gradient direction to a particular Larmor frequency leads to the possibility of tuning the rf pulse frequency to excite a slice at a desired spatial location.

10.2.1 Slice Selection

Let us define the 'slice select axis' as the direction perpendicular to the plane of the desired slice. Accordingly, the gradient along this axis is defined as the slice select gradient. Choosing the *z-axis* as the slice select axis leads to a *transverse* slice of the body. If the *y-axis* is chosen, the slice is referred to as *coronal*. Finally, if the *x-axis* is chosen, the slice is said to be *sagittal*. The nomenclature is exhibited in Fig. 10.6, and summarized in Table 10.1.

The presence of a slice select gradient causes the frequency of precession to be a linear function of position along the corresponding slice select axis. The usual convention is to choose the *z*-direction as this axis (corresponding to transverse slices). The frequency at

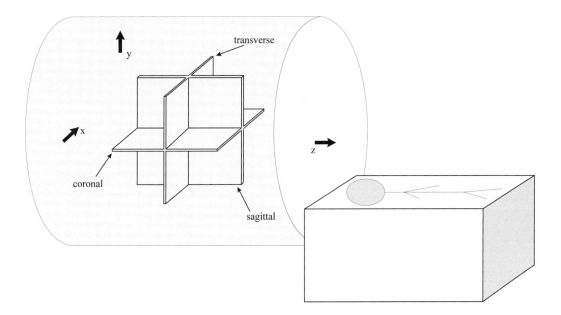

Fig. 10.6: The orientation of the orthogonal slice planes correlated with the standard axes of a whole-body MRI magnet system. The subject is usually placed head first into the magnet and carried in by a sliding gantry on the patient table. The feet point along the $+\hat{z}$, left shoulder along $+\hat{x}$, and nose along $+\hat{y}$ when the person is supine (lying on his/her back).

Applied slice select gradient	Name	Slice plane orientation
G_x	sagittal	parallel to y-z plane
G_y	coronal	parallel to x-z plane
G_z	transverse	parallel to x-y plane

Table 10.1: The relationship between the slice select gradient used and the orientation of the slice plane produced by it. The names have an anatomical basis. It is common in MRI to define these planes in terms of the magnet axes.

position z (in cycles per second) is

$$f(z) = f_0 + \gamma G_z z \tag{10.15}$$

where $f_0 = \gamma B_0$ is the Larmor precession frequency at $z = 0$. This linear relation between $f(z)$ and z is illustrated in Fig. 10.7.

The specific goal is to excite uniformly a slice such that all spins in the slice have identical phase and flip angle after slice selection. To excite an infinitesimal slice through z_0, the rf pulse must be tuned to the frequency $f(z_0)$ given by (10.15). Since the frequency spread of a realistic rf pulse is bounded (i.e., bandlimited), a region of finite thickness along the z direction within the object would have its spins tipped, while spins outside this region would ideally remain aligned with B_0.

To excite a slice of finite thickness extending from $z_0 - \Delta z/2$ to $z_0 + \Delta z/2$, the rf pulse should have a frequency profile, in the rotating frame, which is unity over the range Δf of frequencies from $(\gamma G_z z_0 - \gamma G_z \Delta z/2)$ to $(\gamma G_z z_0 + \gamma G_z \Delta z/2)$ and zero outside (Fig. 10.8). The bandwidth BW_{rf} of the rf pulse, i.e., the width Δf of its region-of-support in the frequency domain, is given by

$$\begin{aligned} BW_{rf} &\equiv \Delta f \tag{10.16}\\ &= (\gamma G_z z_0 + \gamma G_z \Delta z/2) - (\gamma G_z z_0 - \gamma G_z \Delta z/2) \tag{10.17}\\ &= \gamma G_z \Delta z \tag{10.18} \end{aligned}$$

In summary, thanks to the presence of the gradient G_z, there is a range of frequencies which can be excited to create transverse magnetization in a slice with thickness Δz orthogonal to the z-axis. This range of frequencies of bandwidth BW_{rf} is effected by the electronics driving the transmit coil.

It is convenient to introduce a notation for the slice thickness[7]

$$\Delta z \equiv TH \tag{10.19}$$

As a result, the slice thickness TH is a function of the bandwidth BW_{rf} of the rf pulse and the applied gradient

$$TH = \frac{BW_{rf}}{\gamma G_z} \tag{10.20}$$

---

[7]In the case of 2D imaging, the thickness of the imaging slice Δz and the excited slice TH are equivalent. However, in the case of 3D imaging, the thickness of the entire excited region TH is divided up into a series of effective 2D images of thickness Δz. See Secs. 10.1 and 10.4.

Note that the various quantities defined in the above discussion are illustrated in Figs. 10.7 and 10.8.

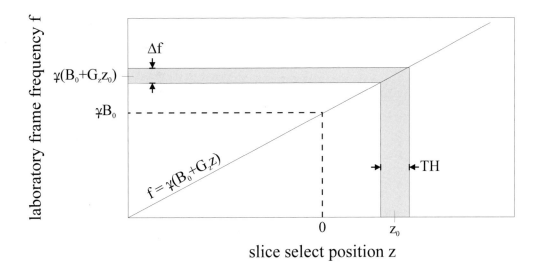

Fig. 10.7: The precession frequency (f) in the laboratory frame as a function of position along the slice select axis when a gradient G_z is applied along the z-direction. The frequency bandwidth $\Delta f \equiv BW_{rf}$ (the shaded horizontal strip) is such that the slice region of thickness Δz (the shaded vertical strip) is symmetrically excited. Since the slice is offset from the origin in the z direction by z_0, the center frequency of the rf pulse is offset from the static Larmor frequency γB_0 by $\gamma G_z z_0$ as indicated.

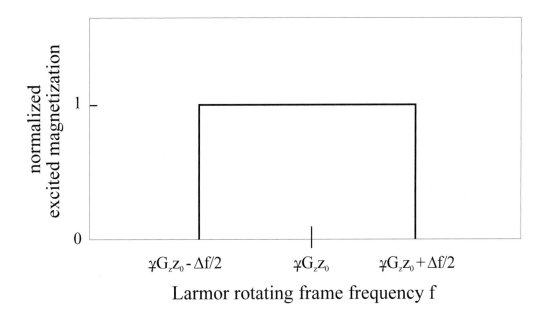

Fig. 10.8: Excited magnetization (normalized) boxcar frequency profile in the Larmor rotating frame. Its temporal profile is that of an ideal (infinitely long) sinc pulse.

In order to get a uniform flip angle across the slice, the analytic form of the rf excitation profile, as a function of frequency, must be proportional to a boxcar function, rect$(f/\Delta f)$ of bandwidth Δf. This implies that the temporal envelope of the rf pulse $B_1(t)$, which is the inverse Fourier transform of the frequency profile (see Ch. 16), is a sinc function. Using the results of Prob. 9.2 in the time-frequency domain

$$B_1(t) \propto \text{sinc}(\pi \Delta f\, t) \tag{10.21}$$

The sinc envelope corresponds to the amplitude modulation of the rf oscillations in the laboratory frame.[8] The center frequency of the excited bandwidth is $\gamma G_z z_0$ in the Larmor rotating frame (Fig. 10.8) and $f_0 + \gamma G_z z_0$ in the laboratory frame (Fig. 10.7). The former is in the audiofrequency (kHz) range while the latter frequency is in the radiofrequency (MHz) range in MRI applications. (Compare this comment to footnote 5 in Sec. 9.2.)

It is observed that the first zero crossing of the expression (10.21) occurs at a time $t_1 = 1/\Delta f$. (The zeros of $\text{sinc}(x) \equiv \sin x/x$ are $x = n\pi$ for all nonzero integers n.) While the sinc function is ultimately damped to zero only at infinity, a realistic rf pulse is necessarily a time-truncated version of the sinc function, being on only for time τ_{rf}, say. The number n_{zc} of sinc zero crossings in this time is an important quantity in the design of an rf pulse. The total number of crossings is given by[9]

$$n_{zc} = [\tau_{rf}/t_1] = [\Delta f\, \tau_{rf}] \tag{10.22}$$

where the square brackets $\lfloor\ \rfloor$ are used to specify the operation 'largest integer less than or equal to.' The larger the number of zero crossings, the closer the excitation profile approaches the ideal boxcar. More discussion on the design of rf pulses is found in Ch. 16.

Problem 10.3

Suppose a slice select gradient $G_z = 20\,\text{mT/m}$ is used to excite a slice which is 10 mm thick.

a) What is the required rf bandwidth?

b) If G_z is reduced to $5\,\text{mT/m}$, but τ_{rf} is unchanged, by what factor is the total number of zero crossings increased or decreased?

10.2.2 Gradient Rephasing After Slice Selection

Any attempt to uniformly excite a slice faces the same signal-loss mechanism discussed in Sec. 9.4 concerning the gradient echo method. The slice select gradient induces dephasing in the slice select direction across the finite slice thickness. Moreover, the defocusing begins

---

[8]The temporal envelopes in the sequence diagrams are shown henceforth as sinc functions; they are sometimes called 'soft pulses,' in contrast to the 'hard pulses' described in earlier chapters.

[9]To guarantee an even number of zero crossings, set $n_{zc} = 2[\tau_{rf}/2t_1]$.

to occur during the excitation, since the slice select gradient is assumed to be turned on already by the time the rf pulse is initiated. (In comparison, all sequences treated in Ch. 9 had gradients that were not applied during the rf pulse.) *As in the gradient echo 1D imaging case, when an echo is sought, the signal can be recovered by adding a rephasing gradient.*

To set the stage for a good first approximation of the structure needed for the follow-up gradient, consider the slice to be excited instantaneously at $t = 0$ (see Fig. 10.9) in the midst of a constant gradient strength, $G_z = G_{ss}$. The transverse magnetization at position z along the excited slice gains phase $\phi(z,t)$ at the time t in the Larmor rotating frame, given by (9.13)

$$\phi(z,t) = -\gamma G_{ss} z t \qquad (10.23)$$

Since the rf pulse excites magnetization only across the slice of thickness Δz, the signal at time t follows the form (9.14) involving the (effectively) one-dimensional spin density $\rho(z)$ defined earlier in (9.7). The spin density can, in addition, be taken as constant over thin slices (but not the phase ϕ which is a function of z) yielding

$$s(t) \simeq \rho(z_0) \int_{z_0 - \frac{\Delta z}{2}}^{z_0 + \frac{\Delta z}{2}} e^{i\phi(z,t)} dz \qquad (10.24)$$

As time progresses, spins at different z positions accumulate different amounts of phase. The resulting decrease in the signal stems from the vanishing of the integral

$$\int_{z_0 - \frac{\Delta z}{2}}^{z_0 + \frac{\Delta z}{2}} e^{i\phi(z,t)} dz \xrightarrow[\text{dephasing}]{} 0 \qquad (10.25)$$

which is an example of the general dephasing result (8.6). The dephasing occurs along the gradient direction (i.e., perpendicular to the slice) and the signal, in general, decreases with an increase in the slice thickness and/or gradient strength.

The procedure to correct for this phase accumulation is to have the gradient reversed after the rf pulse is turned off, such that the spins realign in the transverse plane at the end of the reversed gradient lobe (see Fig. 10.9). (The simple relationship between these two gradient lobes is discussed below.) *As a result, the excited spins in the slice are all at zero phase after the application of this rephasing lobe.* The slice is now ready to be imaged.

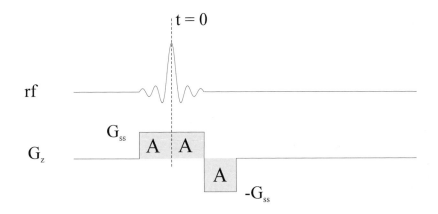

Fig. 10.9: A slice select gradient to excite a slice parallel to the x-y plane.

In the aforementioned approximation, where it is assumed that the spins are tipped instantaneously into the transverse plane at the center of the rf pulse (at $t = 0$), the dephasing takes place only during the second half of the slice select gradient applied during the rf pulse. The requirement on the rephasing-gradient structure is easy to find. Recall from (9.35) that the total area under the gradients, from the time $t = 0$, will evolve to zero at the instant of refocusing. For a symmetric slice select gradient with $|G_z| = |G_{\text{rephase}}|$

$$\left| \frac{\int dt G_{\text{rephase}}}{\int dt G_{ss}} \right| = \left| \frac{\text{total area under } G_{\text{rephase}}}{\text{total area under } G_{ss}} \right| = 50\% \tag{10.26}$$

including the possibility of arbitrary time dependence for each gradient lobe. The signs of G_{ss} and $G_{rephase}$ are assumed to be fixed and opposite to each other. If, for example, they are both boxcar pulses, and are related by $G_{rephase} = -2G_{ss}$, then the rephase gradient would have to be applied for only one quarter of the total length of time as the slice select gradient. See the forthcoming problem and figures for more examples.

We shall return later in this book to the fact that the 50% result of (10.26) is only valid for small flip angles. In a more accurate calculation, the constraint on the rephasing gradient depends upon the details of the rf pulse. For the example of a slice selective $\pi/2$-pulse with a sinc envelope, the ideal rephasing gradient should have an area which is about 50.6% of the area of the original slice select gradient. This is discussed further in Ch. 16. In practice, the amplitude of the rephasing gradient is varied until the maximum signal is obtained.

Problem 10.4

Consider the excitation of a slice of thickness $\Delta z = 4\,\text{mm}$, by a bandlimited rf pulse on for a time duration $\tau_{rf} = 4\,\text{ms}$. Assume that the flip angles of the spins are dominated by the exact (time) center of the rf pulse. If the applied gradient strength is given as $10\,\text{mT/m}$:

a) Find the difference in accumulated phase between two spins on opposite sides of the slice (i.e., at $z = z_0 \pm \Delta z/2$) at the end of the rf pulse.

b) Show that, in general, $\phi = 0$ for all spins at the end of the rephase gradient lobe, under the constraint (10.26).

c) How long must the rephasing gradient be applied, for complete refocusing, if $G_{rephase} = -G_{ss}$ and the two gradients are boxcar pulses? What is the duration of the total slice select process, including the time that both G_{ss} and $G_{rephase}$ are applied?

10.2.3   Arbitrary Slice Orientation

An advantage of MRI is that an arbitrary slice direction can be selected without using moving parts or repositioning the body. The expression for the precessional frequency of spins in the presence of an arbitrary gradient vector was obtained in (9.51). Slice excitation, as shown in Fig. 10.7, is a frequency encoding process. When an arbitrary gradient vector is used in combination with a sinc pulse in the time domain, a slice perpendicular to that gradient vector is selected (see Fig. 10.10).

The creation of an arbitrary gradient vector requires all three Cartesian gradients to be used simultaneously, and has been discussed already in Sec. 9.5.1. Their time dependence must be the same, to within an overall positive or negative proportionality constant. A sequence diagram corresponding to excitation of an arbitrary slice is presented in Fig. 10.11.

The different weightings of the Cartesian gradients can be transcribed into spherical angles. If $\vec{G} = (G_{0x}, G_{0y}, G_{0z})$, the slice select axis defined by $\vec{G}$ is at the angle Θ relative to the z-axis given by

$$\Theta = \tan^{-1} \frac{\sqrt{G_{0x}^2 + G_{0y}^2}}{G_{0z}} \tag{10.27}$$

Its projection into the x-y plane makes an angle Φ relative to the x-axis where

$$\Phi = \tan^{-1} \frac{G_{0y}}{G_{0x}} \tag{10.28}$$

The angles are shown in Fig. 10.10.

It must also be remembered that the read and phase encoding directions are required to be orthogonal to the slice select direction. The Cartesian components for the associated gradients must therefore satisfy the orthogonality conditions $\vec{G}_R \cdot \vec{G}_{ss} = \vec{G}_{PE} \cdot \vec{G}_{ss} = 0$.

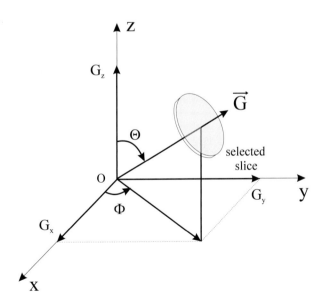

Fig. 10.10: Slice selection at an arbitrary direction by a gradient vector perpendicular to the slice selection axis. Here the arbitrary gradient vector requires all three gradients G_x, G_y, and G_z to be used. The spherical angles of the gradient vector are the polar angle Θ and the azimuthal angle Φ.

The slice excited along an arbitrary direction is thus described by the same number of angles as that used for a rigid body (for example, the Euler angles). If the slice requires only one angle to fix its orientation (say, one rotation from a standard z-slice configuration), it is called an 'oblique slice.' If two are required, it is called 'double oblique.' Images for conventional slice orientations and an oblique-slice orientation are shown in Fig. 10.12.

Problem 10.5

Assume that the slice select gradient amplitudes are changed from those shown in Fig. 10.11 to be $G_{0x} = -G_{0y} = 2G_{0z}$. What are the angles Φ and Θ of the resulting slice? Draw the excited plane (use Fig. 10.10 as a guide).

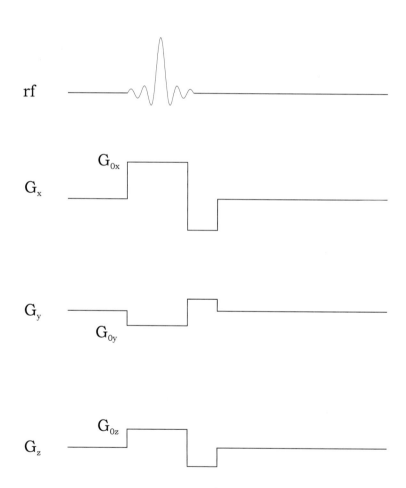

Fig. 10.11: Sequence diagram showing gradient waveforms (with rephasing lobes) required to excite an arbitrary slice. The ratios of the different components are fixed during the time the three gradients are applied.

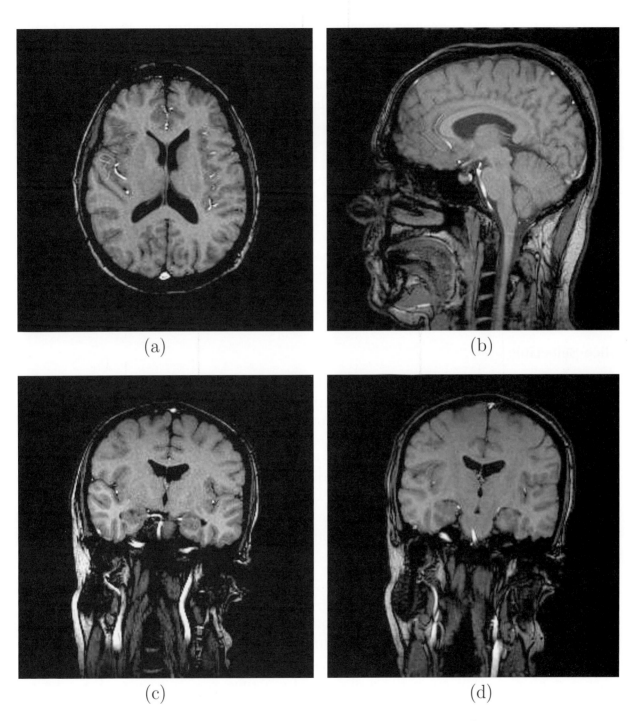

(a)

(b)

(c)

(d)

Fig. 10.12: Images of the human brain, obtained with a 2D gradient echo imaging sequence, in the three standard orientations along with an image for an oblique orientation. (a) Transverse image, (b) sagittal image, (c) coronal image, and (d) an oblique plane obtained by tilting slightly (by 9°) the slice select plane for a coronal image toward the transverse plane (by applying a small G_z component in addition to G_y for the slice select gradient).

10.3   2D Imaging and k-Space

Two classes of typical 2D imaging sequences are described. The first involves the $\pi/2$-pulse gradient echo sequence, which is one of the simplest to analyze. Second, attention is turned to spin echo experiments. Coverage of k-space for both cases is given. In these examples, the convention will be to take the two imaging dimensions in the x-y plane, implying that the slice select gradient is along the z-axis. The phase encoding and read gradients are along the y-axis and x-axis, respectively.

10.3.1   Gradient Echo Example

Figure 10.13 depicts a conventional 2D gradient echo experiment. A constant z-gradient is applied during the rf pulse for a total time τ_{rf}, and then reversed immediately following the pulse. To rephase the spins in the slice, the requirement from (10.26) is that, if the amplitude $G_{rephase}$ of the follow-up lobe equals $-G_{ss}$, it must be on for a time $\tau_{rf}/2$. As required, the area under the rephase lobe then counterbalances half of the area under the slice select lobe[10] (these areas are denoted by $-B/2$ and B, respectively, in the notation of the figure).

Slice Selecting

At the end of the rephase lobe of the slice select gradient, all the transverse magnetization components within the slice are in phase, with a common accumulated phase value $\phi = 0$. The signal from the whole slice, as defined by a demodulated version of (9.4), is the zero phase slice integration

$$s(\tau_{rf}) = \int\int dx\,dy \left[\int_{z_0-\frac{\Delta z}{2}}^{z_0+\frac{\Delta z}{2}} \rho(x,y,z)dz\right] \tag{10.29}$$

For the given slice in z, the purpose of the next steps is to probe the two-dimensional dependence of the effective 3D spin density $\rho(x,y,z)$ via gradients applied along the x- and y-directions.

Phase Encoding the Data

After the slice select gradient is turned off, it is followed by a phase encoding gradient (the second gradient labeled $G_{y,PE}$ in Fig. 10.13). Assume for the moment that no other gradient is applied during this period. The magnetization accumulates a y-dependent phase when a gradient is kept on in the y direction for a time $\tau_{PE} = \tau_y$, say. For a boxcar gradient G_y ($\equiv G_{y,PE}$), a simple y-dependent adaptation of the phase (10.23) leads to a signal immediately following the phase encoding (see Fig. 10.13) given by

$$s(\tau_{rf}+\tau_y) = \int \left[\int\left[\int_{z_0-\frac{\Delta z}{2}}^{z_0+\frac{\Delta z}{2}} \rho(x,y,z)\,dz\right] e^{-i2\pi\bar\gamma G_y\tau_y y}\,dy\right]dx$$
$$\text{(only } G_y \text{ is applied during } \tau_y) \tag{10.30}$$

---

[10]Hereafter, the total gradient structure including the rephasing lobe is referred to as the slice select gradient. In this case, it is $G_z(t)$ for all t.

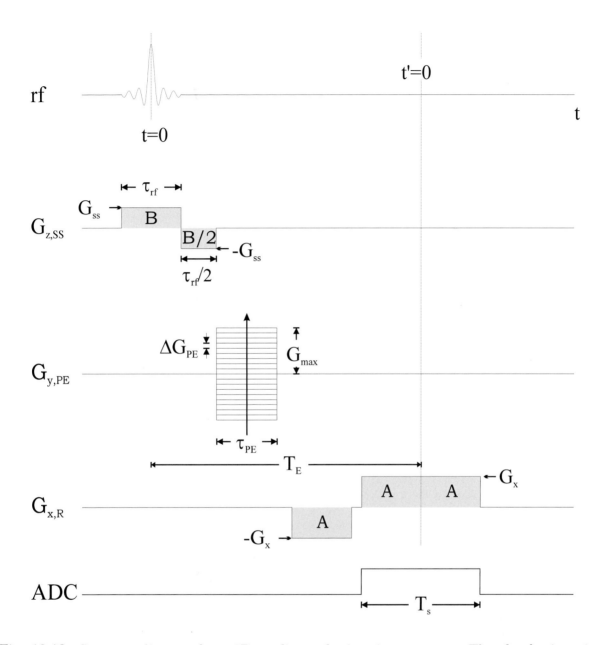

Fig. 10.13: Sequence diagram for a 2D gradient echo imaging sequence. The rf pulse is a sinc function in time, corresponding to a boxcar frequency spectrum. The design of the rephasing lobe of the slice select z-gradient is described in Sec. 10.2.2. The phase encoding y-gradient is pictured as a series of horizontal lines to denote that it is being stepped regularly through increasing values during different repetition periods. The x-gradient has the read gradient echo structure explained in Sec. 9.4. The symbols A, B, and $B/2$ refer to areas under the gradient lobes, and important timings and gradient strengths are also marked. Note that in this 2D sequence structure no gradients overlap each other in time, in contradistinction to the structure shown in Fig. 10.14.

The encoded phase[11] can be written in terms of the k-space spatial frequency associated with the y direction

$$k_y(G_y) = \gamma G_y \tau_y \tag{10.31}$$

The independent variable G_y will be varied in steplike fashion (step sizes ΔG_{PE}), ultimately to gather information about the y dependence of the spin density. This will be a repeated experiment (see Figs. 10.5b and 10.5c) where τ_y stays the same in every cycle. We return later to the manner in which G_y and, hence, k_y are stepped in value.

To establish a k_y value before the data are collected, the phase encoding gradient waveform should appear before the read lobe (i.e., the gradient lobe(s) applied during data sampling) of the third, or read, gradient G_x. It can, however, be superimposed on the dephasing lobe of the read gradient and/or on the rephasing lobe of the slice select gradient; see the later discussion on the gradient superposition principle.

Reading the Data

The third linear magnetic field to be applied corresponds to the read gradient echo structure already detailed in the previous chapter. The gradient G_x has a negative dephasing lobe followed by the read (or rephasing) lobe (a previous example is found in Fig. 9.6 for the 'constant gradient' or boxcar case), during which time the signal is measured. The position along the x-axis is encoded according to the 1D Fourier discussion in Ch. 9; that axis determines the so-called 'frequency encoding' direction. In terms of the time-shifted variable $t' \equiv t - T_E$, the phase in (9.49) can be augmented by the x-axis version of (10.30), to give an expression for the signal. (The magnetic fields, and hence the phases, can be superposed: see the discussion below.) For the boxcar gradient and timing parameters defined in Fig. 10.13,

$$s(t', G_y) = \int \left[\int \left[\int_{z_0 - \frac{\Delta z}{2}}^{z_0 + \frac{\Delta z}{2}} \rho(x, y, z)\, dz \right] e^{-i2\pi\gamma G_y \tau_y y}\, dy \right] e^{-i2\pi\gamma G_x t' x}\, dx$$

$$-T_s/2 < t' < T_s/2 \tag{10.32}$$

where z_0 refers to the center of the excited slice. The spatial frequency[12] associated with the x-direction is

$$k_x(t') = \gamma G_x t' \tag{10.33}$$

A change of independent variables in (10.32) leads to[13]

$$s(k_x, k_y) = \int \int \left[\int_{z_0 - \frac{\Delta z}{2}}^{z_0 + \frac{\Delta z}{2}} \rho(x, y, z) dz \right] e^{-i2\pi(k_x x + k_y y)} dx\, dy \tag{10.34}$$

---

[11]Following earlier notation, the gradient G_y and the k-space variable k_y used to describe the phase encoding direction are more generally referred to as G_{PE} and k_{PE}, respectively.

[12]Also following earlier notation, the read gradient G_x and its k-space variable k_x are more generally referred to as G_R and k_R, respectively.

[13]As before, the symbol s for signal is used in both cases for convenience. This use reminds us once again about the notational trap that (10.34) is not obtained from (10.32) by a strict substitution, for example, of k_x for t.

The integrated z-dependence is often suppressed, giving for a slice centered at z_0

$$s(k_x, k_y) = \int \int \rho(x, y, z_0) e^{-i2\pi(k_x x + k_y y)} dx \, dy \qquad (10.35)$$

Of course, the integral over z in (10.34) reminds us that the 2D image contains a sum or projection over all information in the slice.

It is evident in (10.32) that *the signal obtained by measuring the received emf over a period of time T_s, in the presence of a gradient echo structure in the read direction after it is phase encoded by a fixed value of G_y, gives a line in the k-space set of 2D Fourier transform values of the effective 2D spin density for the selected slice.* The phase encoding line in k-space is itself sampled at discrete points during the time interval T_s. Thus, stepped changes in G_y produce a series of sampled lines (see Fig. 10.15a), in a coverage of the 2D k-space pertaining to the 2D Fourier transform.

The z-, y-, and x-axes of Fig. 10.6 are the conventional choices for the slice select, phase encoding, and read directions, respectively, for 2D imaging. Experiments may be performed with different axes for the different gradients. It is important to identify the gradient axes in the interpretation of the images produced, because artifacts[14] are often formed in the image which are unique to each axis. For example, several artifacts associated with physiological motion are more pronounced along the phase encoding axis.

The appearance and location of these artifacts can be altered by using a different choice of encoding axes (see Ch. 23).

Problem 10.6

---

a) In both the slice select and read directions, it is often desirable to keep the gradients used prior to sampling the data as short as possible to reduce the effects of motion. Neglecting the phase encoding time, how can this be accomplished while satisfying the conditions on the area of the slice select rephasing and the read dephasing gradients if G_{ss}, G_R, τ_{rf}, and T_s are fixed for other reasons? Remember that you are constrained by a maximum possible gradient strength in each direction.

b) Draw a sequence diagram showing the shortest possible echo time, assuming that the slice select and read gradients used are $0.1G_{max}$, where G_{max} is the maximum available gradient strength for either gradient. Label the magnitudes and duration of all gradients used in terms of τ_{rf}, T_s, and G_{max}. Assume $t_{ramp} = 0$.

Superposition of Phase Effects

It was noted earlier that the phase encoding gradient and the dephasing lobe of the read gradient in the 2D gradient echo sequence shown in Fig. 10.13 can be applied simultaneously.

---

[14] An artifact is defined as a false feature in the image. It is created by some imperfect process in the data collection or in the inverse Fourier transform. See Chs. 11 and 12.

The rephasing lobe of the slice select gradient can also be applied at the same time. In examples of sequences to follow this discussion, all these three lobes are generally shown to coincide in time with each other (see, for example, Fig. 10.14 where these three lobes are all turned on simultaneously). How is it that we can have these gradients on simultaneously before the data are read out, given that they act as a single effective gradient vector if applied during slice selection or during data sampling?

The answer is that the phase accumulation for any superposition of contributions to the z-component of the magnetic field, referring back to the general precession solutions of Chs. 2 and 3, is just the sum of the phases for each contribution. Any additional field just adds a term to the exponent in solutions such as those in (2.41) including the generalizations to time dependent fields and the associated phase integrals in (3.37). This superposition principle for the phase has already been used, in effect, in the discussions for the construction of arbitrary gradient directions in Secs. 9.5 and 10.2.3. The point now is that the gradient components must have different time dependence as well.

In the typical 2D sequence, such as in Fig. 10.14, the phase along each direction serves a different purpose. The terms along $\hat{x}$ and $\hat{y}$ encode the data to extract information in the excited plane, while the gradient lobe in the $\hat{z}$ direction serves the purpose of completing the slice selection process. The processes just described are independent of the occurrences in the other directions. The only exceptions to this rule of independence of action are during the time periods of slice selection and the data measurement (where there is rf excitation or signal detection). In these two cases, the presence of additional gradients would lead to a rotation of the encoded spatial axis (just as the slice select gradient axis is changed by adding other gradient components).

k-Space Coverage

A sufficiently large set of k_x and k_y values is required in order to invert the 2D Fourier transform (10.32) and accurately reconstruct the image of the spin density. A measure of how large this set must be is the subject of Ch. 12. Presently, the discussion is focused on the procedure for covering a given set of k-space data.

The k-space coverages associated with the sequences shown in Figs. 10.13 and 10.14 are pictured in Fig. 10.15. The initial phase, before the application of the phase encoding and read gradients, corresponds to the 2D origin, $k_x = k_y = 0$ for every repeat cycle. (Any initial phase from the slice select gradient is rephased to zero by its rephasing lobe.) The combination of the first (dephasing) lobe of the read gradient and a particular step of the phase encoding gradient lobe is applied to locate the point $(k_{R,min}, k_y(G_y))$ in k-space, where $k_y(G_y)$ is given in (10.31) and

$$k_{R,min} = -\gamma G_x T_s/2 \qquad (10.36)$$

This is represented by the long dark arrows which are right-angled in Fig. 10.15a where the read gradient dephasing lobe follows the phase encoding lobe and which are diagonal in Fig. 10.15b when these lobes overlap. The second, positive part of the read gradient lobe moves the signal through a set of (N_x, say) steps while data are collected (the series of short sequential horizontal arrows in Fig. 10.15). Multiple lines in the phase encoding gradient indicate the stepped changes (N_y in all, say) for each repetition of the experiment. Each time this gradient is altered, a new value of k_y is chosen (the long-dashed dark arrows), and

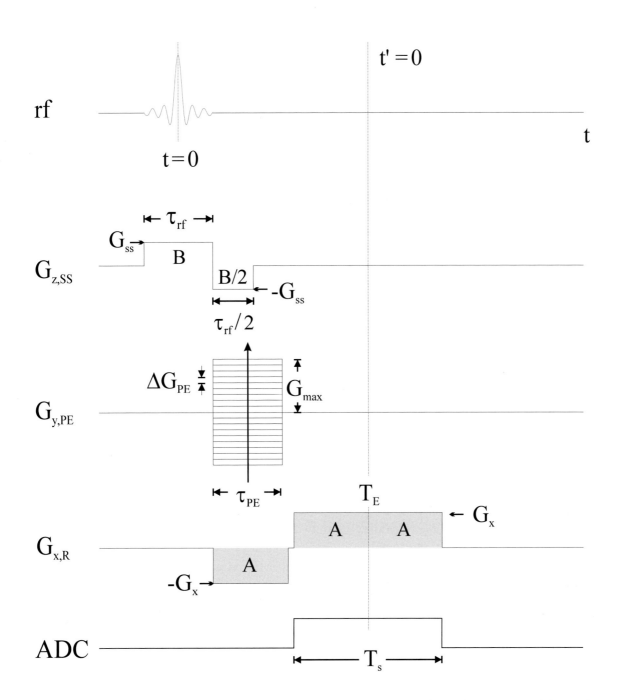

Fig. 10.14: A 2D gradient echo sequence that is more typical than that of Fig. 10.13. The rephase lobe of the slice select gradient, the dephase lobe of the read gradient, and the phase encoding gradient table are all switched on at the same time. This shortens the echo time, a desirable feature in most applications.

a new set of data is sampled along k_x. The complete path that a sequence takes through k-space is often referred to as its *k-space trajectory*. The sizes of the vertical and horizontal steps taken in k-space are considered next.

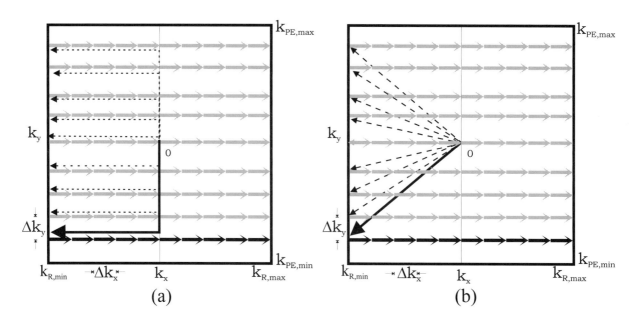

Fig. 10.15: Traversal of k-space for typical gradient echo experiments   The signal may be considered to be initialized at $k_x = k_y = 0$ with any accumulated phase due to the slice select gradient reset to zero by its rephasing lobe. (a) For the sequence in Fig. 10.13, the phase encoding gradient and the dephasing lobe of the read gradient are applied at different times. After each new rf pulse, the k-space trajectory would first move vertically along the k_y direction (dark solid arrow and dark small dashed arrows) to the current phase encoded spatial frequency over the period of time the phase encoding gradient lobe is applied. This is then followed by a horizontal traversal to $k_{R,min}$ while the read dephasing lobe is on (lightened arrows). (b) For the sequence shown in Fig. 10.14, the combined effect of the phase encoding lobe, at a given (stepped) G_y value, and the dephasing read gradient lobe is to move the signal to a chosen k-space value moving along a diagonal trajectory where both k_x and k_y change simultaneously as a function of time (long bold arrow). The read gradient is then reversed to bring the spins back through a complete set of k_x values (short bold arrows) leaving k_y unaltered during data sampling. The experiment is repeated by returning to a new starting k_y value (long-dashed dark arrows) to obtain a complete set of data (lightened arrows). The effects of the slice select rephasing gradient (the third dimension) are not included in the 2D k-space description.

Phase Encoding Order

The k-space coverage for the 2D imaging sequences has been found in the above discussion to be represented by N_y horizontal lines of 2D k-space each with N_x sampled points. Practically, a desire to have N_y an even number in 'fast Fourier transform' analysis has been noted (i.e., $N_y \equiv 2n_y$), so that the lines are typically indexed in a minimally asymmetric manner from $m = -n_y$ to $m = (n_y - 1)$ (see Chs. 11 and 12). The value of G_y is incremented by a fixed amount ΔG_y at each step, such that $G_{y,min} = -n_y\Delta G_y$ and $G_{y,max} = (n_y - 1)\Delta G_y$.[15] At the step corresponding to index m, the y-gradient is $G_y(m) = m\Delta G_y$. This particular stepping order is referred to as a sequential acquisition or 'sequential ordering' of the phase encoding steps. Recall that the arrow on the sequence representation, or gradient table, of the phase encoding, such as in Fig. 10.13, indicates the direction of the steps taken in the phase encoding k-space direction. An arrow pointing upward represents k-space coverage from $k_{y,min} = \gamma G_{y,min}\tau_y \equiv k_{PE,min}$ to $k_{y,max} = \gamma G_{y,max}\tau_y \equiv k_{PE,max}$ while a downward-pointing arrow would have indicated the opposite coverage.

Although sequential ordering is the most commonly used ordering of phase encoding steps, there are two other ordering schemes that are used occasionally (see Chs. 18 and 19 for discussions of the circumstances under which they are advantageous). The first is called a 'centric reordering' scheme where the $k_{PE} = 0$ line is collected first, then followed by $k_{PE} = -\Delta k_y$, $k_{PE} = \Delta k_y$, $k_{PE} = -2\Delta k_y$, $k_{PE} = 2\Delta k_y$, and so on outward. An expression for Δk_y is found below. The other scheme is a reordering such that the lines in k-space are collected starting from the outermost lines, alternating between positive and negative values, and moving inward until the $k_{PE} = 0$ line is collected last. This is referred to as 'reverse centric' coverage and leads to what can be thought of as a high pass filter since it enhances the larger spatial frequencies. These three phase encoding ordering schemes are illustrated in Fig. 10.16.

k_x-k_y Coverage and Time

In the archetypal sequential acquisition schemes shown in Fig. 10.14, the neighboring lines of data,[16] each of which are at a constant k_{PE}, are separated by

$$\Delta k_y \equiv \Delta k_{PE} = \gamma \Delta G_y \tau_y \equiv \gamma \Delta G_{PE} \tau_{PE} \tag{10.37}$$

The position of the k-space samples in the read direction, on the other hand, is determined by the sampling rate rather than a change in gradient strength. If the data are sampled in time steps Δt, then the associated k-space sampling interval in the read direction is

$$\Delta k_x \equiv \Delta k_R = \gamma G_x \Delta t \equiv \gamma G_R \Delta t \tag{10.38}$$

The signal is measured over $N_x \equiv N_R$ steps for a given value of m in the gradient table.

Each new rf excitation is performed a time T_R after the previous excitation, until k-space has been adequately sampled along both directions. How sparse this sampling can be (that is, how large Δt and ΔG_{PE} can be) is dictated by the Nyquist criterion, which is discussed in detail in Ch. 12. How far out k-space is sampled is defined by $k_{R,min}$, $k_{R,max}$, $k_{PE,min}$, and $k_{PE,max}$, and these boundaries determine the spatial resolution (see Chs. 12 and 13). Although a vertical pair of neighboring sampled points may be separated by an identical distance in k-space as for a neighboring horizontal pair ($\Delta k_x = \Delta k_y$), they may be very much separated in their times of acquisition. In the present case, nearest neighbors on the x-axis are separated by Δt, but adjacent points along the y-axis will be separated by a time interval of T_R per acquisition.

---

[15]Thus, for large n_y, k-space coverage is approximately symmetric about $G_y = 0$.

[16]We refer to different phase encoding 'lines' as the data collected for a given k_y value. These are also referred to as phase encoding 'views.'

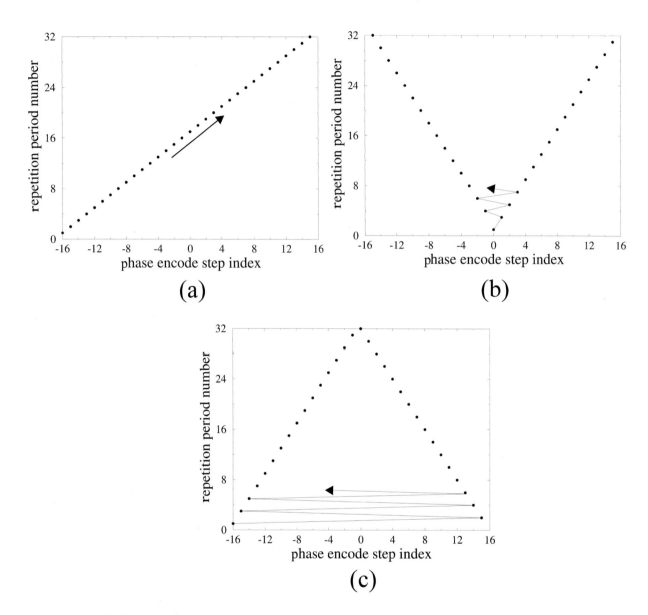

Fig. 10.16: Different ordering schemes for the phase encoding gradient table. (a) A sequential ordering scheme showing the acquisition of a linearly increasing phase encoding line number as a function of rf pulse number. (b) A centric reordering scheme where the first gradient amplitude is zero, the second ΔG, the third $-\Delta G$, the fourth $2\Delta G$, and so on. (c) A reverse-centric reordering scheme where the gradient settings begin at the maximum magnitudes and work inward. The arrows shown indicate the time direction of the collection of the phase encoding steps.

Alternate Phase Encoding Scheme

In the sequential phase encoding scheme discussed above, the phase encoding gradient is increased through a table of values starting from a negative maximum to a positive maximum by steps of ΔG_y. It has been assumed that a pulsed gradient waveform with a variable amplitude G_y is switched on for a time τ_y, so that $k_y(G_y) = \gamma G_y \tau_y$. The same phase encoding could have been done by using a constant gradient value G_y^0 (say) while varying the time t_y for each given phase encoding step. Then $k_y(t_y) = \gamma G_y^0 t_y$. While of historical interest,[17] this scheme leads to longer and longer echo times and hence an increase in the minimum-achievable T_R value. However, for systems which do not have variable gradient strengths, this is an alternative method for phase encoding, and offers the same k-space coverage.

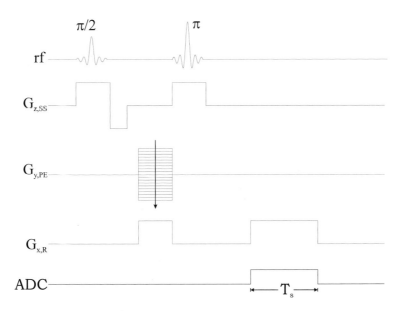

Fig. 10.17: Sequence diagram for a 2D spin echo imaging sequence. The arrow pointing downwards in the gradient table, indicating that the phase encoding gradient is stepped sequentially from its most positive value to its most negative value, has the same effect as an upward arrow in a sequence without a π-pulse. There is no rephasing gradient required for the π-pulse as a symmetric slice select gradient is self refocusing.

10.3.2 Spin Echo Example

The sequence diagram for a conventional 2D spin echo imaging experiment is shown in Fig. 10.17. As discussed in Sec. 9.4.2, there are two options for doing the 1D spin echo imaging experiment based on the placement of the readout gradient dephasing lobe. There are also two options for the phase encoding gradient in the 2D spin echo imaging sequence, corresponding to placing it either before or after the π-pulse. The phase encoding gradient

---

[17]See the reference to Kumar, Welti, and Ernst in the Suggested Reading.

is placed before the π-pulse in the example in the figure. While it can be shown that the full 2D k-space is covered in both cases, there is a difference in how this space is covered. This is the subject of Prob. 10.7. The practical implications of these two phase encoding choices are discussed in Chs. 23 and 26.

Problem 10.7

Assume that the phase ϕ is defined such that a π-pulse reverses the accumulated phase of all spins: $\phi \rightarrow -\phi$. In terms of k-space, the π-pulse is equivalent to a reflection through the origin: $\vec{k} \rightarrow -\vec{k}$.

  a) Show that the k-space diagram for the spin echo experiment shown in Fig. 10.17 is identical to that in Fig. 10.15b which corresponds to the gradient echo sequence shown in Fig. 10.14.

  b) Find the k-space diagram for the spin echo experiment shown in Fig. 10.17 if the phase encoding gradient table is applied after the π-pulse, but before the read gradient. (The dephasing read gradient lobe is unchanged.)

10.4   3D Volume Imaging

More often than not, information is required over a three-dimensional volume for imaging. In Sec. 10.1, we have introduced the two approaches to be described here. One involves 3D methods with short T_R values (see Ch. 18 for a discussion of fast imaging). The other is the multi-slice 2D method where the 2D imaging techniques of the previous section are generalized to a series of slices for the coverage of a 3D volume.

10.4.1   Short-T_R 3D Gradient Echo Imaging

The conventional 3D imaging sequence is created from a 2D imaging sequence by adding a gradient table in order to phase encode along the slice select direction as well. An example is shown for a gradient echo sequence in Fig. 10.18. As mentioned, the process of phase encoding the slice select direction is often called partition encoding. The excited slice is usually called a *slab* (with thickness TH) and the reconstructed multiple slices (with thickness $\Delta z = TH/N_z$ according to the Nyquist discussions in Chs. 12 and 13) are known as *partitions*. Each new rf pulse excites the same slab, but is followed by a different phase encoding gradient setting.

What are the possible advantages to collecting data with a 3D volume method, in comparison with multi-slice imaging? First, the ability to change the number of the N_z phase encoding steps over the slab means that there is control over the smallness of the partition thickness $\Delta z = TH/N_z$ without any limitation on the rf amplitude or duration. Second, consecutive slices can be adjacent, in contrast to 2D imaging where the rf pulse leaks into the neighboring slices and there is always a slice gap in practice. Third, larger rf bandwidths can be used for thicker slabs in 3D imaging, and the rf pulse time τ_{rf} can be shortened, making it possible to reduce T_E. Fourth, both short T_E and the high spatial resolution achievable in the partition encoding direction help reduce signal loss due to T_2^* dephasing (see Ch. 20 for a detailed discussion). Fifth, the signal-to-noise ratio can be enhanced even for thin slices because of the parameters available in 3D imaging (see Ch. 15 for the dependence of SNR on T_R and N_z), but achieving this may come at the expense of increased imaging time.

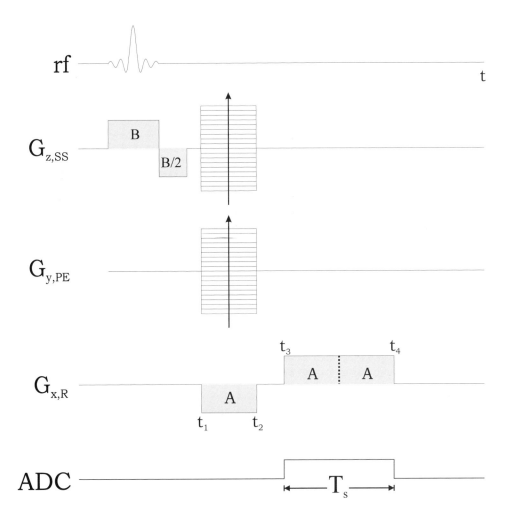

Fig. 10.18: A 3D gradient echo imaging sequence where the two directions orthogonal to the read direction are phase encoded.

10.4.2 Multi-Slice 2D Imaging

The multi-slice 2D approach for the coverage of a 3D volume-of-interest (VOI) is accomplished by the application of a number of rf pulses within a single repeat time. Each rf pulse is centered at a different frequency and excites a different slice. In an original single rf pulse short-T_E, intermediate-T_R sequence, the additional rf pulses can be applied during the idle time between the end of data sampling and the rest of the cycle time T_R to excite other slices in the VOI.

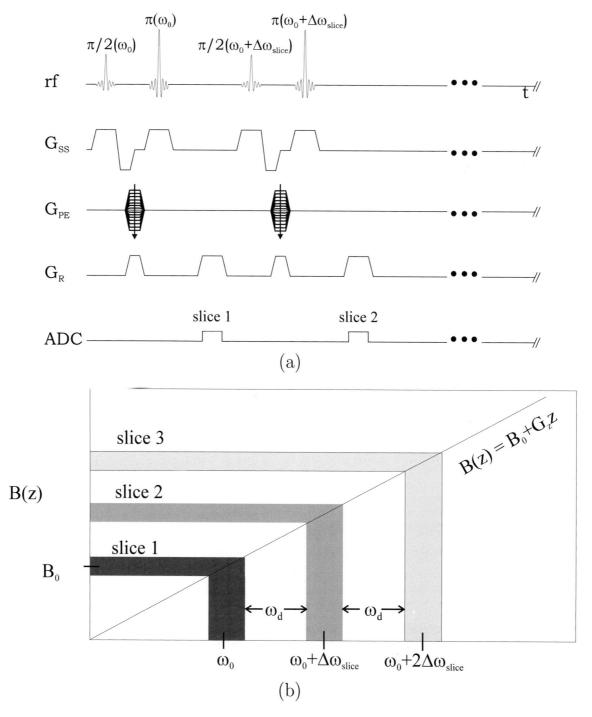

(a)

(b)

Fig. 10.19: (a) A multi-slice imaging experiment where a number of slices are collected during each T_R by stepping through a series rf pulse frequencies. (b) The field-frequency plot where the center frequency of the rf pulse is varied from one slice to the next in the presence of the slice select gradient. To insert a gap between two adjacent slices, the quantity $\omega_d = \Delta\omega_{\text{slice}} - 2\pi BW$ must be positive, in order to avoid 'interslice crosstalk.' The frequency bandwidth is BW for all rf pulses.

Because of imperfect rf profiles, however, the immediate neighborhood of an excited slice is also partly excited. Hence, this region cannot be included in the following slice, if the spins do not have time to recover toward equilibrium. In multi-slice methods, it is common either to leave a gap between slices so that contiguous coverage is not obtained, or to excite all the odd-numbered slices first and then all the even-numbered slices afterward (the slices are said to be 'interleaved' in the odd-even procedure), in order to avoid the 'slice crosstalk' effect (the alteration of signal in one slice caused by overlapping rf pulses from an adjacent slice). Figure 10.19 exhibits the sequence diagram and frequency encoding graph for leaving gaps between slices. In this figure, ω_d represents the frequency associated with a slice gap (d) such that $\omega_d < \Delta\omega_{\text{slice}}$. Specifically,

$$d = \omega_d / \gamma G_z = \frac{\Delta\omega_{\text{slice}} - 2\pi BW}{\gamma G_z} \qquad (10.39)$$

Although the multi-slice 2D method appears to be rather time consuming (inefficient) for large T_R, scans with longer repeat times can be made more efficient through the usage of multiple gradient echoes and spin echoes (see Ch. 19). Very long values of T_R with a reduced number of repetitions and reduced scan time are possible; see the discussion of segmented k-space coverage in Ch. 19.

For comparison, a set of images obtained with a 2D spin echo sequence and a set of images with a 3D short-T_R gradient echo sequence are shown in Fig. 10.20. Although comparable volume coverage was obtained (with the 2D method) for one image orientation in about one-third the time of the 3D imaging experiment, the total acquisition time for obtaining 2D images in all three orientations would be about the same as the 3D imaging time. While all three slice orientations can be reconstructed from a single 3D data set, the resulting image quality may suffer if the resolution in each direction is not the same. The image quality is reduced by the interpolation required to view the 3D data from different orientations.

10.5 Chemical Shift Imaging

In previous discussions in this chapter, the chemical shift effect has been ignored. The MRI signal for living tissue is largely made up of ^{1}H in water, and the effects on the image from other hydrogen nuclei are typically small. An important exception to this assumption, however, is fat (CH_2 based tissue elements), which is chemically shifted from H_2O and can have a significant signal associated with it. The encoding of measurable contributions from different species such as water, fat, choline, creatine, n-acctyl aspartate (NAA), and lactate, leads to an additional dimension for imaging.[18]

---

[18]Studies in the biomedical sciences are addressed to other chemical species contributing to the ^{1}H spectrum in humans. For example, one of the species seen in a hydrogen spectrum is a lactate spectral peak; an elevated lactate content in some location in the human body points to an inefficient and typically anomalous anaerobic glucose metabolism for energy production as opposed to the more efficient and typically normal aerobic glucose metabolism.

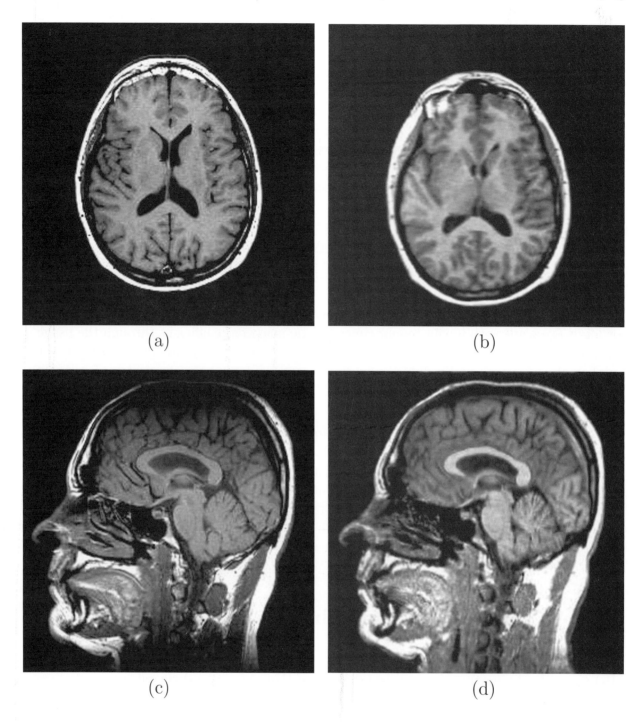

(a)   (b)

(c)   (d)

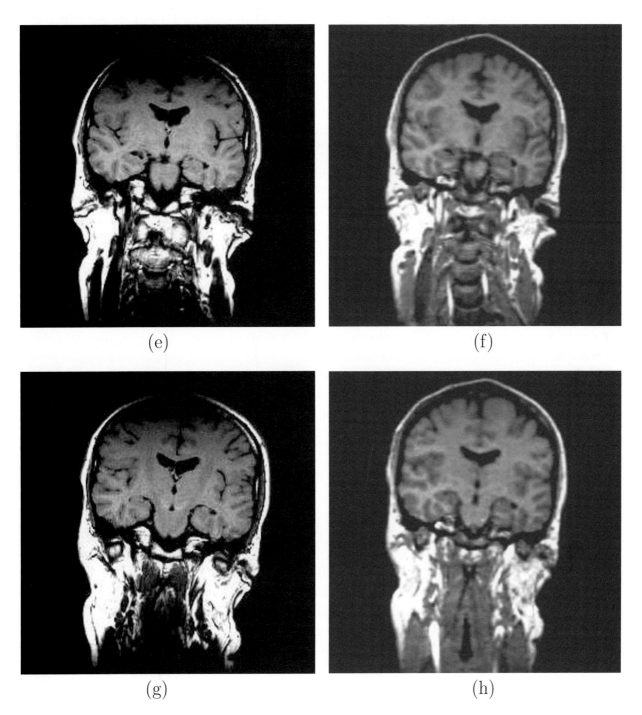

Fig. 10.20: Images acquired using a 2D spin echo sequence in (a) the transverse plane, (c) the sagittal plane, (e) the coronal plane, and (g) a plane obtained such that the selected slice is slightly rotated from the coronal plane into the transverse plane (see Fig. 10.12). Images of the same slices (b), (d), (f), and (h) reconstructed from a 3D whole-head imaging experiment with a short-T_R, 3D gradient echo sequence. Image (b) is slightly offset from (a) due to subject motion. Note the reasonably similar tissue differentiation in both sets of images. The signal from the top of the head is reduced in the spin echo case relative to the gradient echo because of a drop-off in rf excitation sensitivity. This effect is discussed later in Ch. 18.

Chemical shift imaging refers to the process of selectively imaging (or obtaining the spatial distribution of) identical nuclei that experience different levels of magnetic shielding due to their chemical environments. These shielding effects cause chemical shifts which were briefly introduced in Sec. 8.5. There are a number of methodologies for performing a spectrally selective MRI sequence, including 'selective excitation,' 'selective saturation,' and using the chemical shift to generate additional frequency or phase encoding of the spins. The last method is detailed below in terms of an added imaging dimension. Other methods for chemical shift imaging are discussed in Ch. 17.

We noted in Sec. 8.5 that differences in magnetic shielding cause nuclei in various chemical compounds to precess at slightly different rates. It is possible to use this frequency variation in a manner similar to that employed by frequency encoding gradients. From (8.61), the shift in the frequency due to the shielding factor σ is

$$\Delta\omega(\sigma) = -\sigma\gamma B_0 = -\sigma\omega_0 \tag{10.40}$$

Hence, a chemical shift frequency encoding 'axis' can be defined in terms of $\sigma = -\Delta\omega/\omega_0$, which is typically quoted in ppm. This creates another effective imaging axis, leading to, for example, a 4D space (or 3D) made up of three spatial dimensions x, y, z, (or two spatial dimensions x, y) and a spectral dimension σ.

In the corresponding expression for the signal, the chemical shift phase effects are to be added to those due to a general set of applied gradients leading altogether to a 4D Fourier transform for 3D spatial volume imaging, for example. Assuming a perfectly uniform B_0, the generalization of (9.15) is

$$s(\vec{k}, t) = \int d^3r\, d\sigma\, \rho(\vec{r}, \sigma)e^{-i2\pi(\vec{k}\cdot\vec{r}-\sigma f_0 t)} \tag{10.41}$$

in terms of the Larmor frequency f_0. The signal is now expressed in terms of an additional Fourier transform over the population of chemically shifted species evaluated at the point in the dimensionless space given by $f_0 t$.

In order to image along the 'chemical shift' dimension, some modifications are made in the previous sequences. In typical chemical shift imaging, data are read along the time axis which means that the transverse magnetization is allowed to evolve over time under the influence of the chemical shifts while data is measured. That is, each spatial axis is treated as a phase encoding axis with gradients used to locate a position in 2D or 3D k-space before data are taken. A line of chemical shift data is collected at a specific point in k-space during each repetition of the experiment. A sequence that could be utilized for the phase encoding of a 2D k-space in the chemical shift data collection is shown in Fig. 10.21. Note that no imaging gradients are applied during the time data would be measured around the echo.

10.5.1   A 2D-Spatial 1D-Spectral Method

Consider how a set of 2D images of different chemical species might be found from the 2D chemical shift imaging (2D CSI) experiment of Fig. 10.21. A simple illustration of the associated 2D k-space data from such an experiment is given in Fig. 10.22, while the corresponding 2D-spatial, 1D-spectral representation might look like that in Fig. 10.23. The set

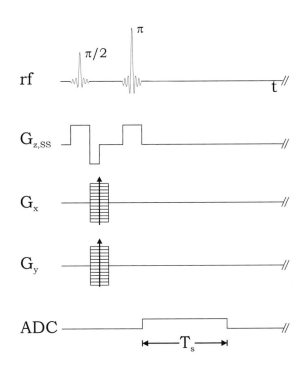

Fig. 10.21: A 2D spin echo chemical shift imaging sequence for the acquisition of a chemical shift spectrum.

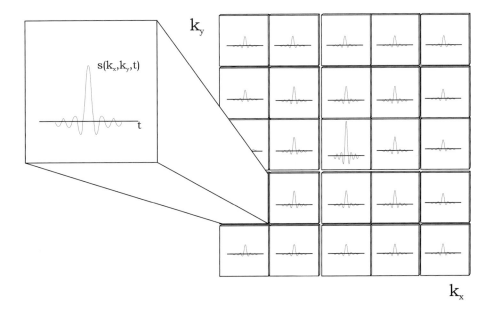

Fig. 10.22: The real part of the signal centered around the spin echo shown as a function of time for each sampled k-space point for a boxcar chemical shift distribution (i.e., a sample where the different spectral components are present in equal amounts). The frequency content of the signal at each point contains chemical shift information, as well as the spatial information encoded by the gradients. The latter is represented by the variation (reduction) in the spin echo signal observed with an increase in distance from the origin of k-space.

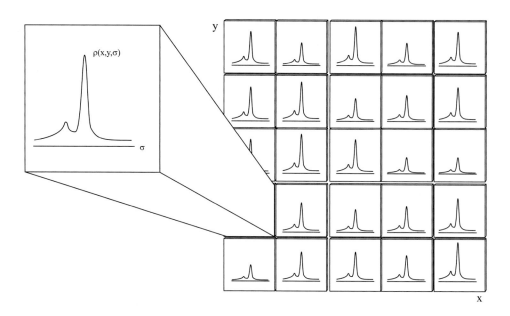

Fig. 10.23: A simple illustration of an example of a chemical shift spectrum collected at every point in 2D x-space. Note that the spatially varying spectral distribution is illustrated by the varying shape and strength of peaks in the spectra shown for each voxel.

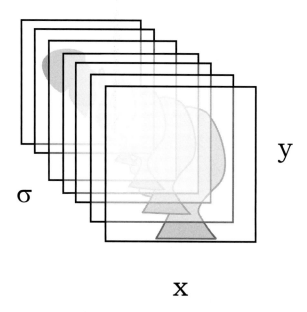

Fig. 10.24: The layers of images obtained with the chemical shift techniques described in Sec. 10.5.1. The image is sliced along the chemical shift axis to provide images of the different chemically shifted nuclei in the sample. For example, one can think of creating a water image, a lactate image, an NAA (n-acetyl aspartate) image, and a fat image.

of images for the different chemical species generated is suggested by the stack of cartoons in Fig. 10.24.

In more detail and following the previous discussions, a thin slice of the body is chosen with a combination of rf pulses and gradients, leading to an effective 2D spin density. For this chemical shift experiment, each point in 2D k-space is encoded with two phase encoding tables, one in x and one in y. After spatial phase encoding, the data are sampled at n points each separated in time by Δt to obtain information along the chemical shift axis. A 3D Fourier inverse transform of the collected data leads to an image whose third axis contains information about different chemical species. By 'slicing' the created 3D image set, it is possible to produce a set of images, each corresponding to a particular value of σ (Fig. 10.24).

In this manner, it is possible to obtain separate images of water, fat, lactate, and so forth, showing their respective spatial distributions in the body. The presence of field inhomogeneities complicates the process, and methods to deal with this in the simplified two-species case of extracting water and fat images are discussed in Ch. 17. Generalizations to the multi-species case are also considered in that chapter.

As in the previous formula development, the 2D CSI signal can be conveniently written as a function of t', the time defined about the echo. It is given by

$$s(k_x, k_y, t') = \int d\sigma \int dx\, dy\, \rho(x, y, \sigma) e^{-i2\pi(k_x x + k_y y - \sigma f_0 t')} \tag{10.42}$$

A 3D inverse Fourier transformation of the signal thus yields an image $\hat{\rho}(x, y, \sigma)$ over a slice defined by slice selection in the z-direction. The similarity between this experiment and the standard spatial 3D imaging is reflected by the formula for the total 2D CSI acquisition time which is the same as (10.11) with N_z replaced by N_x

$$T_{acq} = N_x N_y T_R \tag{10.43}$$

Problem 10.8

---

   a) Show that the information collected at each time point prior to Fourier transformation of the signal along t' in (10.42) already provides a useful 2D image at $t' = 0$.

   b) What changes in the image as t' increases?

The 2D CSI experiment could also be performed using an FID rather than a spin echo to collect the data. Such an idea is attractive at first sight since it is possible to begin collecting data immediately after the phase encoding gradients, leading to shortened T_R values and reduced imaging time. As mentioned in Ch. 8, an FID signal contains an adequate amount of information to obtain spectral information. There are a number of technical problems, however, which are primarily associated with the difficulty in collecting data about the $t = 0$ point. The absence of this data can lead to baseline or low frequency signal loss errors in the reconstructed images. These associated problems are eliminated in the spin echo case, where the chemical species come together in phase at the echo, defining the total integrated (over all chemical species) spin density information correctly for each voxel.

Problem 10.9

Given the following imaging parameters, determine T_{acq} in each case.

a) Find T_{acq} for a 2D spatial imaging experiment with $N_y = 256$ and $T_R = 1000\,\text{ms}$.

b) Find T_{acq} for a 2D spatial 1D spectral CSI experiment with $N_x = N_y = 256$ and $T_R = 1000\,\text{ms}$.

c) Find T_{acq} for a 3D spatial imaging experiment with $N_x = N_y = 256$, $N_z = 128$, and $T_R = 1000\,\text{ms}$.

d) Find T_{acq} for a 4D imaging experiment with $N_x = N_y = N_z = 16$ and $T_R = 1000\,\text{ms}$.

e) Discuss the implications of your results to the imaging of humans. Assume it is difficult for an average patient to stay in the imaging environment (lying still inside the bore of a magnet) for more than 30 minutes without becoming uncomfortable. Usually 10 minutes is assumed to be an upper limit for a single MRI scan. Assume also that you are imaging the entire human head which requires about 19.2 cm (left-to-right) × 25.6 cm (head-to-foot with oversampling) × 22.4 cm (front-to-back) of total spatial coverage. Given that the spatial resolution, as defined later in Ch. 13, is the ratio of FOV (the area over which the image is acquired) to number of encoded points, discuss the trade-off in spatial resolution versus imaging time in going from part (c) to part (d).

10.5.2   A 3D-Spatial, 1D-Spectral Method

It is apparent that 4D imaging is also possible, but with a significantly longer imaging time. All three spatial directions can be phase encoded before data are read along the σ-direction. The 3D CSI signal for data acquisition about the center of a spin echo in terms of t' for each read period is

$$s(k_x, k_y, k_z, t') = \int d\sigma \int d^3r\, \rho(x, y, z, \sigma) e^{-i2\pi(k_x x + k_y y + k_z z - \sigma f_0 t')} \qquad (10.44)$$

The total acquisition time when all three axes are phase encoded is given by

$$T_{acq} = N_x N_y N_z T_R \qquad (10.45)$$

The extra factor of N_z in comparison with (10.43) makes 4D imaging impractical for human imaging in most situations. It is, nevertheless, a powerful method for imaging and spectroscopy of inanimate samples and sedated animals at high fields where times on the order of hours are taken to perform the experiments to obtain high SNR. On humans, it would be necessary to sacrifice spatial resolution or spatial coverage for reduced imaging time and reasonable SNR, when all four dimensions need to be encoded.

Suggested Reading

The current approach to phase encoding appears in:

- J. M. Hutchison, R. J. Sutherland and J. R. Mallard. NMR imaging: image recovery under magnetic fields with large nonuniformities. *J. Phys. E.: Scient. Instrum.*, 11: 217, 1978.

The 'alternate phase encoding scheme' for Fourier imaging was introduced in the following paper:

- A. Kumar, D. Welti and R. R. Ernst. NMR Fourier Zeugmatography. *J. Magn. Reson.*, 18: 69, 1975.

The concepts of k-space are introduced in:

- S. Ljunggren. A simple graphical representation of Fourier-based imaging methods. *J. Magn. Reson.*, 54: 338, 1983.

- D. B. Twieg. The k-trajectory formulation of the NMR imaging process with applications in analysis and synthesis of imaging methods. *Med. Phys.*, 10: 610, 1983.

An introduction to chemical shift imaging can be found in:

- T. R. Brown, B. M. Kincaid and K. Ugurbil. NMR chemical shift imaging in three dimensions. *Proc. Natl. Acad. Sci. U.S.A.*, 79: 3523, 1982.

- R. E. Sepponen, J. T. Sipponen and J. I. Tanttu. A method for chemical shift imaging: demonstration of bone marrow involvement with proton chemical shift imaging. *J. Comput. Assist. Tomogr.*, 8: 858, 1984.

Chapter 11

The Continuous and Discrete Fourier Transforms

Chapter Contents

Summary: Continuous and discrete Fourier transforms pertinent to MRI are detailed. A set of tables describing various Fourier transform pairs and general properties is given. Features of imaging that are directly related to the properties are described and analyzed. Phase imaging is introduced. Although the discussions in this chapter are addressed to 1D transforms, the results are easily generalized to higher dimensions.

Introduction

An important connection between the MR signal and the continuous Fourier transform has been demonstrated in the previous two chapters. In the absence of relaxation effects, the signal $s(\vec{k})$ was shown to be the Fourier transform of the spin density $\rho(\vec{r})$, so an inverse Fourier transform performed on the data leads to a reconstructed spatial image $\hat{\rho}(\vec{r})$. The caret sign over the ρ indicates that this represents an estimate of the effective spin density. To better understand this transformation and its numerical approximations, basic properties of the continuous and discrete Fourier transforms are studied in the present chapter. Descriptions of certain experimental imaging results in terms of the transform properties and theorems are included, particularly with respect to artifacts in the data. Certain artifacts are connected with the fact that $\hat{\rho}$ may be complex, and its phase leads to the concept of 'phase imaging.'

The definitions and properties of the continuous transform are contained in the first and second sections, respectively. Properties refer to theorems, symmetries, and convolution, and the experimental relevance of some of these properties is also a subject of the second section. Among the Fourier transform pairs (functions and their transforms) of importance to MRI, and discussed in the third section, is the sampling function and its transform, both of which are 'comb' functions. The definitions and properties of the discrete transform round out the chapter in the last two sections.

11.1   The Continuous Fourier Transform

The primary function of the Fourier transform is to map from position space to its 'conjugate' space, and vice versa through the inverse transform. The ability to represent a function in the two domains is important in many applications. In the case of MRI, the one-dimensional imaging problem leads to the Fourier integral

$$s(k) = \int_{-\infty}^{\infty} dx\, \rho(x) e^{-i2\pi kx} \tag{11.1}$$

as shown in (9.15). The spin density in x-space (position space) is transformed into its associated k-space (spatial-frequency space) counterpart, which is directly related to the signal.

In the following, several basic Fourier transform concepts and properties are presented, with only a little attention paid to general theory. The emphasis will be on useful formulas for the evaluation of (11.1). Although only one-dimensional transforms are considered in what follows, 2D and 3D transforms are straightforward generalizations.

In a more general notation,[1] the 1D transform can be written[2]

$$H(k) \equiv \mathcal{F}(h(x)) = \int_{-\infty}^{\infty} dx\, h(x) e^{-i2\pi kx} \tag{11.2}$$

along with its inverse

$$h(x) \equiv \mathcal{F}^{-1}(H(k)) = \int_{-\infty}^{\infty} dk\, H(k) e^{+i2\pi kx} \tag{11.3}$$

The consistency of the pair of equations (11.2) and (11.3) can be shown using the Dirac delta function (or impulse function) introduced in Ch. 9. The delta functions in either space (x-space and k-space) have the following representations (cf.(9.24))

$$\delta(k - k_0) = \int_{-\infty}^{\infty} dx\, e^{-i2\pi(k-k_0)x} \tag{11.4}$$

$$\delta(x - x_0) = \int_{-\infty}^{\infty} dk\, e^{+i2\pi k(x-x_0)} \tag{11.5}$$

---

[1] The inclusion of the 2π factors in the exponentials, a convention already employed in the imaging equations, eliminates the need for $1/2\pi$ (or $1/\sqrt{2\pi}$) normalization coefficients outside of one or the other (or both) Fourier integrals.

[2] A lower-case letter is generally used to denote a function in one domain, and its transform is denoted by the corresponding upper-case letter. This convention has not been followed in the connection between $\rho(x)$ and $s(k)$.

Insertion of (11.2) into (11.3) yields[3]

$$
\begin{aligned}
h(x) &= \int_{-\infty}^{\infty} dx'\, h(x') \int_{-\infty}^{\infty} dk\, e^{-i2\pi k(x'-x)} \\
&= \int_{-\infty}^{\infty} dx'\, h(x')\delta(x-x') \\
&= h(x)
\end{aligned}
\tag{11.6}
$$

The inverse Fourier transform can now be put to work. If the signal $s(k)$ were known for all k, (11.1) could be inverted to give

$$
\rho(x) = \int_{-\infty}^{\infty} dk\, s(k)e^{i2\pi kx}
\tag{11.7}
$$

In fact, as has been emphasized in various portions of the past three chapters, the signal can only be finitely sampled, corresponding to the so-called measured signal distribution $s_m(k)$.[4] The (continuous) inverse Fourier transform of s_m yields the reconstructed image

$$
\hat{\rho}(x) = \int_{-\infty}^{\infty} dk\, s_m(k)e^{i2\pi kx}
\tag{11.8}
$$

The differences between $\hat{\rho}(x)$ and $\rho(x)$ comprise an important topic recurring throughout this book and especially in Chs. 12–15.

Problem 11.1

---

a) Write the Cartesian 2D forms of (11.2) and (11.3).

b) If $s(k_x, k_y) = \rho_0 AB\, \mathrm{sinc}(\pi k_x A)\, \mathrm{sinc}(\pi k_y B)$, describe the object $\rho(x, y)$ that produced this signal. (See Ch. 9 or Table 11.3.) An illustration of this 2D Fourier pair is in Figs. 11.1a and 11.1b.

11.2 Continuous Transform Properties and Phase Imaging

It is necessary to study the general properties of the continuous Fourier transform in order to understand the differences between the reconstructed MR image $\hat{\rho}(x)$ and the physical spin density $\rho(x)$. Besides the discrete nature of the sampling, differences between $\rho(x)$ and $\hat{\rho}(x)$ can be the result of errors in data acquisition and signal processing. *The term artifact introduced in Ch. 10 is generally used to describe any of the differences between $\hat{\rho}(x)$ and*

---

[3]It is assumed throughout that for the physical applications considered the mathematical steps employed, e.g., changing order of integration, are valid. In particular, the steps taken are justified even for generalized functions, such as the Dirac delta function, which are neither continuous, differentiable, nor square integrable.

[4]While we often refer to this as simply the 'measured signal,' it is seen in Ch. 12 that this is in fact a sum of delta functions.

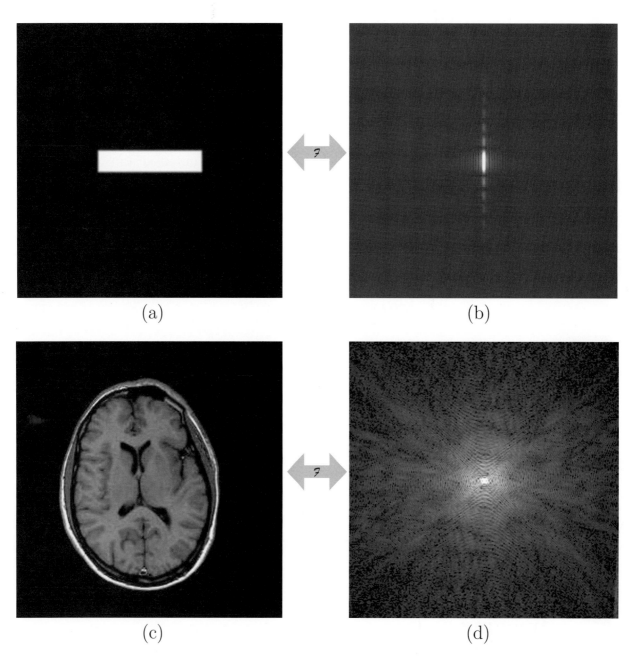

Fig. 11.1: Examples of the relationship between the magnitude of the signal $s(k)$ and the magnitude of the reconstructed spin density $\hat{\rho}(x)$. An image (a) of a rectangular object is shown alongside its k-space representation (b). The k-space data are more spread out along the direction parallel to the shorter side of the rectangle, reflecting the increase in higher spatial frequency components expected for smaller objects; see Prob. 11.1. The image and the data shown in (c) and (d), respectively, are for a transverse slice through a human head. The fact that the k-space data has the shape of a ball is a result of the roundness of the head and the shape is not very different from circular-phantom data (see Ch. 14).

$\rho(x)$. Specific differences can often be directly related to a particular feature of the Fourier transform. For instance, $\hat{\rho}(x)$ often appears complex because of experimental conditions (see below). Some Fourier transform properties of particular interest to MRI are discussed in the remainder of this section. A summary of general Fourier transform properties can be found in the tables.

11.2.1 Complexity of the Reconstructed Image

Although $\rho(x)$ is strictly a real quantity, $\hat{\rho}(x)$ need not be real. The simplest example that demonstrates this is the presence of a global (constant) phase shift ϕ_0 leading to a modified signal

$$\tilde{s}(k) = e^{i\phi_0} s(k) \tag{11.9}$$

where the 'true' $s(k)$ is defined as the Fourier transform of $\rho(x)$. This can arise from the real and imaginary channels being switched or from incorrect demodulation and leads to

$$\hat{\rho}(x) = e^{i\phi_0} \rho(x) \tag{11.10}$$

The real part of $\hat{\rho}(x)$ will not give the physical image, unless the presence of ϕ_0 is understood and a correction made. One solution is to take the magnitude of $\hat{\rho}(x)$ to get $\rho(x)$ independent of ϕ_0, a common practice owing to the many sources of global phase errors creeping into the data. This 'magnitude' image is the image most commonly used. The local phase error is the subject of the next subsection.

11.2.2 The Shift Theorem

The 'time shifting' relation (or Fourier transform shift theorem) found in Table 11.1 tells of the consequences of shifts in the echo relative to its expected location or of incorrectly referenced signal demodulation (i.e., demodulation at the wrong frequency). This will now be seen to lead to a complex reconstructed image $\hat{\rho}(x)$.

Consider a signal which is shifted in k-space by k_0 so that $s_m(k) \rightarrow s_m(k - k_0)$. In particular, the center, or echo, of the signal is moved to $k = k_0$ (the shift of the signal to the left in Fig. 11.2 corresponds to $k_0 < 0$). The effect of this shift on a reconstructed image $\hat{\rho}(x)$ is found by taking the inverse Fourier transform of $s_m(k - k_0)$

$$
\begin{aligned}
\hat{\rho}(x) &= \mathcal{F}^{-1}\left(s_m(k - k_0)\right) \\
&= \int_{-\infty}^{\infty} dk\, s_m(k - k_0) e^{i2\pi k x} \\
&= e^{i2\pi k_0 x} \int_{-\infty}^{\infty} dk'\, s_m(k') e^{i2\pi k' x} \\
&= e^{i2\pi k_0 x} \hat{\rho}_{expected}(x)
\end{aligned}
\tag{11.11}
$$

Equation (11.11) implies that *a shift of the origin in k-space creates an additional phase (which is linear in that shift) in the reconstructed image $\hat{\rho}(x)$*. Since the magnitude is not altered, $\rho(x)$ is faithfully reconstructed by a magnitude operation (i.e., $|\hat{\rho}| = \rho$ in this case). Local phase errors are removed in the same manner as global ones.

The other case to be considered is the introduction of a linear phase shift in the k-space data. The following problem demonstrates that a linear phase shift of the signal, $s_m(k) \rightarrow s_m(k)e^{-i2\pi kx_0}$, leads to a spatial shift of x_0 in the position of the reconstructed image.

Problem 11.2

Show that $h(x - x_0) = \mathcal{F}^{-1}(H(k)e^{-i2\pi kx_0})$. Explain how this result leads to a spatial shift in the reconstructed image when the signal is incorrectly demodulated, so that $s_m(t) \rightarrow s_m(t)e^{-i\Delta\omega t}$. To what demodulation frequency does this correspond?

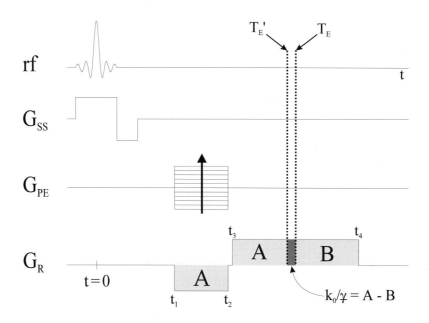

Fig. 11.2: Example of a read gradient structure leading to a shift of the echo in the sampling window. The area under the gradient between t_1 and t_2 is A and the area under the read gradient itself is $2B$. The echo is shifted from T_E to $T'_E < T_E$ if A is chosen to be less than B. This results in a shift of $k_0 < 0$ in the read direction k-space variable.

11.2.3   Phase Imaging and Phase Aliasing

This is an appropriate place to introduce 'phase imaging,' following the establishment of both image reconstruction and the shift theorem. While it is a magnitude image that is typically presented in the 2D plots viewed, additional information remains in the phase of the complex reconstructed image $\hat{\rho}$. It is useful to plot 2D phase images where each pixel intensity is proportional to the calculated phase value for the complex local signal (or 'voxel signal'). We shall see that the phase artifact due to an uncentered gradient echo is best visualized in such a phase image.

The phase image $\phi(x, y)$ is obtained from

$$\phi(x, y) \equiv \mathrm{Arg}\, \hat{\rho}(x, y) = \tan^{-1}\left(\frac{\mathrm{Im}\, \hat{\rho}(x, y)}{\mathrm{Re}\, \hat{\rho}(x, y)}\right) \qquad (11.12)$$

The inverse-tangent function shown is calculated to find the 2D intensity plots. Since the inverse-tangent is periodic with period 2π, the phase image can only be mapped into the interval $[-\pi, \pi)$, although the true phase value might take on any real value. The end result of this is a form of phase aliasing[5] where spins with phase values differing by multiples of 2π would have the same intensity.[6] If this occurs predominately in one of the two dimensions, it shows up as bands, or 'zebra stripe' artifacts, in (x, y) intensity plots, and it is illustrated in Figs. 11.3c and 11.3d.

One cause of the zebra stripes is an 'asymmetry' in the echo position. The gradient-induced echo corresponds to the point $k = 0$ ($k \equiv k_x \equiv k_R$) where the readout gradient phase is zero for all spins. The assumption is made that the echo occurs at the center of the sampling window. However, when the gradient echo is not centered in this window, either by design or by an error, the measured signal ($s_a(k)$, say) with $k = 0$ still defined at the center is not the true $s(k)$. It is instead $s_a(k) = s(k - k_0)$, in terms of the shift k_0 in the k-space origin along the read direction. According to the shift theorem, this changes the phase in the reconstructed x-space image by the amount

$$\Delta\phi(x) = 2\pi k_0\, x \qquad (11.13)$$

In a plot over a given range of x-values, the phase shift (11.13) will lead to a phase image with more and more aliasing bands, the larger the value of k_0. Measurements, such as the widths of the horizontal bands in Fig. 11.3 (where the x-axis is vertical), can be used to find the spatial frequency k_0 associated with the zebra stripe artifact. With this analysis, adjustments can be made to recenter the echo.

Problem 11.3

Explain how you could use the result (11.13) of the Fourier shift theorem analysis to find the time of the center of the echo given a zebra stripe (a region where phase changes from $-\pi$ to π) of width A and a readout gradient strength G.

In general, the time point where the echo occurs may have spatial dependence on y as well as x. Local field inhomogeneities lead to such dependence for local phases in $\hat{\rho}(x, y)$ and can cause serious artifacts, but by studying the phase variations, field inhomogeneities can be probed. The deviations from strictly parallel bands seen in Figs. 11.3c and 11.3d are due to the presence of local field errors.

---

[5]This is also referred to as phase 'wrapping,' 'foldover,' or 'wraparound.'

[6]The usefulness of knowing the true phase value such as in MR velocity quantification (Ch. 24) and in computing the actual echo shift in the case considered next, prompts the need for 'phase unwrapping' algorithms.

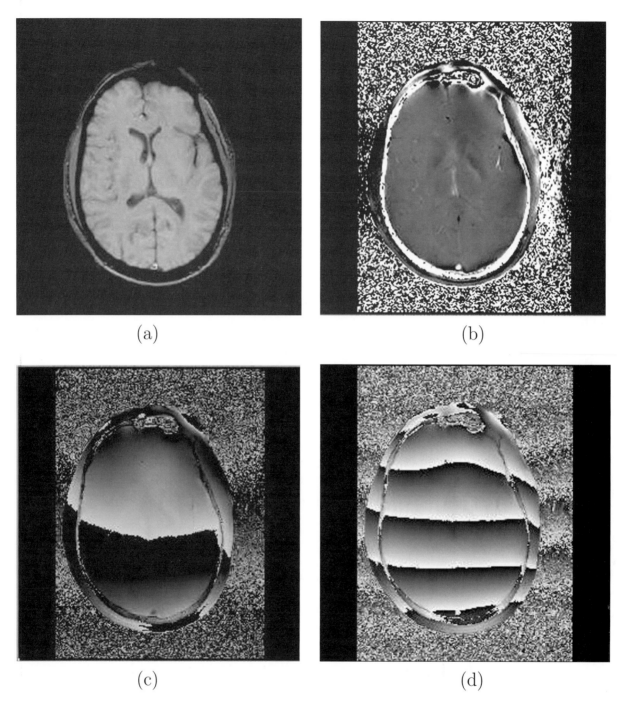

(a)   (b)

(c)   (d)

Fig. 11.3: (a) A 2D gradient echo magnitude image of the head. (b) The corresponding phase image of the head when the echo is centered in the read data acquisition window. (c) A phase image taken from the same data that produced (b) except that the echo is shifted 'one sample point' away from the center of the sampling window. (d) A phase image where the echo is shifted five points away from the center of the sampling window. The restricted variation of the phase from $-\pi$ to π creates the banding referred to as the 'zebra stripe' artifact. The phase shift occurs along the read (vertical) direction, and the bands are perpendicular to this direction. This is an example of how knowledge of the theory behind an artifact gives information about the sequence acquisition.

11.2.4 Duality

The shift theorem is also evident in the transform of a shifted delta function, $\delta(x) \rightarrow \delta(x-x_0)$. With $H(k)$ found from (11.2), the transform pair exhibit the expected phase shift

$$
\begin{aligned}
h(x) &= \delta(x - x_0) \\
H(k) &= e^{-i2\pi k\, x_0}
\end{aligned}
\tag{11.14}
$$

Alternatively, the shifted delta function is seen to give rise to a periodic transform with period $1/x_0$ (i.e., invariance under $k \rightarrow k + 1/x_0$). This is relevant to sampling, as will be seen in Ch. 12.

Another Fourier pair is given by

$$
\begin{aligned}
H(-x) &= e^{i2\pi k_0 x} \\
h(k) &= \delta(k - k_0)
\end{aligned}
\tag{11.15}
$$

which is a simple illustration of the general duality property of the Fourier transform. This is the property that the replacement of $x \rightarrow k$ and $k \rightarrow -x$ in a transform pair $h(x) \overset{\mathcal{F}}{\Leftrightarrow} H(k)$, yields a new transform pair $H(-x) \overset{\mathcal{F}}{\Leftrightarrow} h(k)$. Knowledge of one Fourier transform pair leads to another pair without additional calculations.

11.2.5 Convolution Theorem

Many signal modifications leading to variations in $\hat{\rho}(x)$ can be described in terms of functions or 'filters' that multiply the unperturbed signal (see Chs. 12 and 13). As an example, consider T_2^* decay during data acquisition. The measured signal can be modeled as the product of $s(k)$ in the absence of relaxation and an exponential decaying function. The (inverse) Fourier transform of products of such functions is needed for the reconstructed spin density.

The convolution theorem provides a method for understanding the Fourier transform of the product of two or more functions in terms of their individual transforms. *The Fourier transform of the product of two functions is the convolution of the Fourier transforms of each function*

$$
\mathcal{F}\left(g(x) \cdot h(x)\right) = G(k) * H(k)
\tag{11.16}
$$

where the convolution operator $*$ is defined by

$$
G(k) * H(k) \equiv \int_{-\infty}^{+\infty} dk'\, G(k') H(k - k')
\tag{11.17}
$$

The proof of the convolution theorem is left to Prob. 11.4.

The integral in (11.17) shows that finding the convolution of two functions at the position x involves reflecting one function through the origin, displacing it by x, and finding the area of the product of the two functions. A graphical representation is useful for a qualitative, and sometimes quantitative, understanding of convolution.

As an example, consider the convolution of a right-triangular (ramp) function with itself. The ramp function is defined by

$$
h(x) = \begin{cases} x & 0 < x < 1 \\ 0 & \text{otherwise} \end{cases}
\tag{11.18}
$$

The convolution is described graphically in Fig. 11.4. The value of the convolution is displayed at the right for five different x values. Consistent with the five cases shown, a direct integration leads to

$$h(x) * h(x) = \begin{cases} \frac{1}{6}x^3 & 0 < x < 1 \\ \frac{1}{6}(2-x)(x^2 + 2x - 2) & 1 \le x < 2 \\ 0 & 0 \text{ otherwise} \end{cases} \qquad (11.19)$$

The details are the subject of Prob. 11.5, after which appears a similar, but simpler, example.

Problem 11.4

a) Prove the convolution theorem given in (11.16) and Table 11.1,

$$\mathcal{F}(g(x)h(x)) = G(k) * H(k) \equiv \int_{-\infty}^{\infty} dk'\, G(k')H(k - k')$$

Hint: Replace $g(x)$ and $h(x)$ by their Fourier transform representations inside the transform of the product.

b) Show that Parseval's theorem of Table 11.1 follows directly from the convolution theorem upon the replacement of $h(x)$ by $g^*(x)$.

Problem 11.5

Derive (11.19) by direct integration.

Problem 11.6

a) Show that the (isosceles) triangle function $\Lambda(x)$ defined as

$$\Lambda(x) = \begin{cases} 1 - |x| & -1 \le x \le 1 \\ 0 & \text{elsewhere} \end{cases} \qquad (11.20)$$

can be obtained as the convolution of two rect functions with both unit width and unit height

$$\Lambda(x) = \text{rect}(x) * \text{rect}(x) \qquad (11.21)$$

as shown in Fig. 11.5. Do this either graphically or by direct integration.

b) Derive the Fourier transform of $\Lambda(x)$ by direct integration of (11.20).

c) Rederive the same Fourier transform using the convolution theorem.

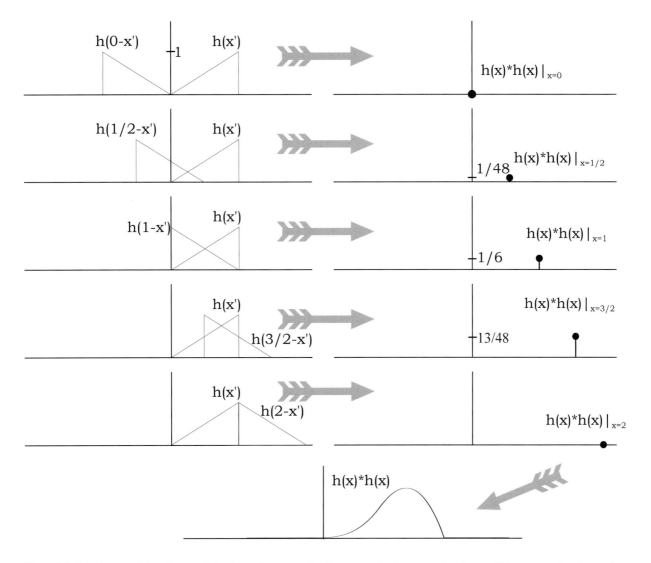

Fig. 11.4: A combined graphical and numerical example in convolution. The convolution of a ramp function with itself involves an integration over the product (which is not shown) of the mirror-reflected ramp functions $h(x')$ and $h(x - x')$ both of which are plotted for five different x values. See (11.18), (11.19), and Prob. 11.5.

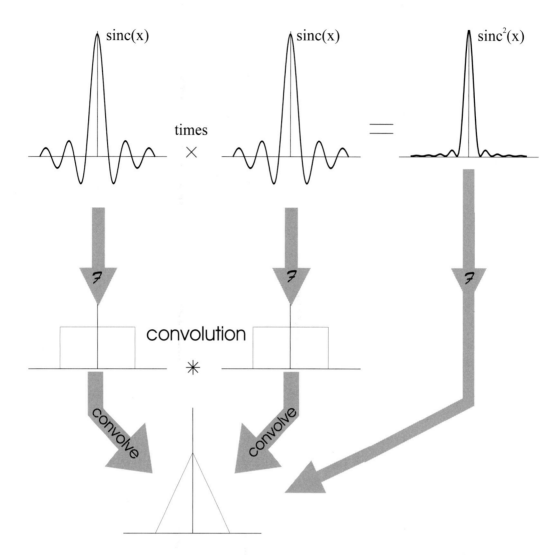

Fig. 11.5: A shortcut to the Fourier transform of the product of two sinc functions through the convolution of two boxcars.

11.2.6   Convolution Associativity

The convolution of three functions arises in the analysis of the effect of finite sampling of k-space data on the reconstructed image in Ch. 12. In that analysis, the first convolution includes the sampling effect, while a second convolution is required to include the finite length of data collection. It does not matter in which order the convolutions are done, since the convolution operation is associative.

Problem 11.7

Prove the associativity: $a(x) * (b(x) * c(x)) = (a(x) * b(x)) * c(x)$.

11.2.7 Derivative Theorem

It is possible to derive important information about the boundaries in an object by analyzing the derivative of the image. The derivative theorem states that if $f(x)$ and $F(k)$ are Fourier transform pairs, then

$$\mathcal{F}\left(f'(x)\right) = i2\pi k F(k) \tag{11.22}$$

(See the following problem.) As a result, a 'derivative image' $\hat{\rho}'(x)$ can be found directly by taking the inverse Fourier transform of the product of $s(k)$ with $i2\pi k$. An example is shown in Fig. 11.6 which also illustrates the fact that derivative images magnify the effects of noise $\eta(k)$. Upon multiplication by k, the measured signal, $s_m(k) + \eta_m(k)$, is enhanced at large k values, where noise is relatively more important.

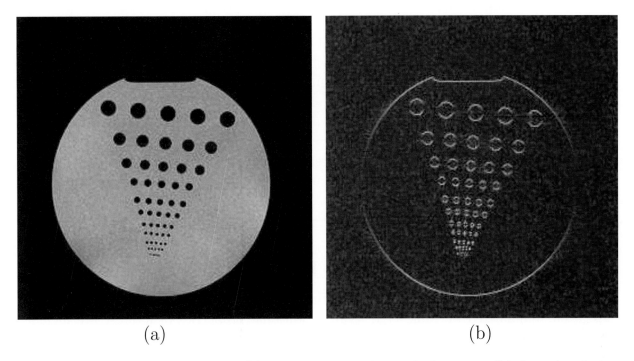

(a)   (b)

Fig. 11.6: A 2D magnitude image (a) and an image of the 1D-derivative (b) for a 'resolution phantom.' The 1D derivative is taken in the vertical direction, so that the derivative image shows enhanced upper and lower edges (those edges with components perpendicular to the vertical direction). Notice that noise is also enhanced in the derivative image.

Problem 11.8

Derive the Fourier derivative theorem (see Table 11.1).

11.2.8   Fourier Transform Symmetries

Odd and even symmetries play a significant role in the Fourier transform description of imaging and in certain image reconstruction methods. As an example, consider a real function $h(x) = h^*(x)$, of particular interest since the spin density is just such a function. The real and imaginary parts of its transform are even (symmetric) and odd (anti-symmetric), respectively, under $k \rightarrow -k$, $\mathrm{Re}[H(k)] = \mathrm{Re}[H(-k)]$ and $\mathrm{Im}[H(k)] = -\mathrm{Im}[H(-k)]$ (see Table 11.2). In order to see this, the transform (11.2) can be rewritten in terms of cosine and sine transforms

$$H(k) = \int_{-\infty}^{\infty} dx\, h(x)[\cos(2\pi kx) - i\sin(2\pi kx)] \tag{11.23}$$

With $h(x)$ real, the real (imaginary) part of $H(k)$ is given by the cosinusoid (sinusoid) term in (11.23), which is even (odd) in k.

The above example implies that the Fourier transform of a purely real function possesses complex conjugate symmetry: $H(k) = H^*(-k)$. When $\rho(x)$ is real, the signal $s(k)$ has this symmetry, a fact which is exploited in 'partial Fourier imaging' (see Ch. 13). The procedure is to cover only half of k-space, with the other half is generated by assuming conjugate symmetry. The following problem requires similar analysis for a purely imaginary $h(x)$.

Problem 11.9

Find the even/odd symmetries for the real and imaginary parts of the transform of a purely imaginary function $h(x)$. Compare your answers with those given in Table 11.2.

11.2.9   Summary of Continuous Fourier Transform Properties

The properties of the Fourier transform and their relevance to MRI discussed in this section have been summarized in Table 11.1. Some additional properties of interest are included in that table. The compilation should prove useful in certain Fourier applications in the remainder of the text, and the reader may wish to make note of its location.

Another table noted in the previous problem catalogs the odd/even, real/imaginary, and continuous/discrete properties of Fourier transform pairs. Table 11.2 is of particular value in MRI where knowledge of the sample can be used to predict properties of the measured signal. In particular, the fact that the object is real is exploited in half Fourier or partial Fourier imaging, as mentioned earlier in this section. A detailed discussion of partial Fourier imaging appears in Ch. 13.

11.3   Fourier Transform Pairs

There are several Fourier transform pairs which are ubiquitous in discussions of MRI. The derivations of some of the more involved Fourier transforms are presented below. Table 11.3 contains five transform pairs of importance and appears at the end of the section.

Property	Mathematical expression
linearity	$\mathcal{F}(h_1(x) + h_2(x)) = \mathcal{F}(h_1(x)) + \mathcal{F}(h_2(x))$ $\mathcal{F}(\beta h(x)) = \beta \mathcal{F}(h(x))$
duality	if $h(x) \overset{\mathcal{F}}{\Leftrightarrow} H(k)$ then $H(-x) \overset{\mathcal{F}}{\Leftrightarrow} h(k)$
space scaling	$\mathcal{F}(h(\alpha x)) = \frac{1}{|\alpha|} H\left(\frac{k}{\alpha}\right)$
space shifting	$\mathcal{F}(h(x - x_0)) = H(k)e^{-i2\pi k x_0}$
alternate form	$h^*(x) = \int_{-\infty}^{\infty} dk\, H^*(k)e^{-i2\pi kx}$ $\quad = \mathcal{F}^{-1}(H^*(-k))$
even $h(x)$	$H(k) = \int_0^{\infty} dx\, h(x)e^{-i2\pi kx} + \int_{-\infty}^{0} dx\, h(x)e^{-i2\pi kx}$ $\quad = \int_0^{\infty} dx\, h(x)\left(e^{-i2\pi kx} + e^{i2\pi kx}\right)$ $\quad = 2\int_0^{\infty} dx\, h(x)\cos 2\pi kx$
odd $h(x)$	$H(k) = \int_0^{\infty} dx\, h(x)\left(e^{-i2\pi kx} - e^{i2\pi kx}\right)$ $\quad = -2i\int_0^{\infty} dx\, h(x)\sin 2\pi kx$
convolution	$\mathcal{F}(g(x)h(x)) = G(k) * H(k)$ $\qquad\qquad = \int_{-\infty}^{\infty} dk'\, G(k')H(k - k')$
derivative	$\mathcal{F}\left(\frac{dh}{dx}\right) = i2\pi k H(k)$
Parseval	$\int_{-\infty}^{\infty} dx\, |h(x)|^2 = \int_{-\infty}^{\infty} dk\, |H(k)|^2$

Table 11.1: Summary of the mathematical properties of the continuous Fourier transform.

$h(x)$	$H(k)$	
	Real part	Imaginary part
real	even	odd
imaginary	odd	even

Table 11.2: Symmetry properties of the continuous Fourier transform important for imaging applications.

11.3.1   Heaviside Function

As an example of a Fourier transform important to MRI, consider the Heaviside function $\Theta(k)$,

$$\Theta(k) = \begin{cases} 1 & k > 0 \\ 1/2 & k = 0 \\ 0 & k < 0 \end{cases} \tag{11.24}$$

The inverse Fourier transform of $\Theta(k)$ is given in terms of a Dirac delta function. To derive this distribution, insert an exponential $e^{-2\pi\epsilon|k|}$ where the limit $\epsilon \to 0^+$ is to be taken after the other operations are completed. The transform now becomes

$$
\begin{aligned}
h_\Theta(x) = \mathcal{F}^{-1}(\Theta(k)) &= \lim_{\epsilon \to 0^+} \int_{-\infty}^{\infty} dk\, \Theta(k) e^{i2\pi kx} e^{-2\pi\epsilon|k|} = \lim_{\epsilon \to 0^+} \int_0^{\infty} dk\, e^{-2\pi k(\epsilon - ix)} \\
&= \frac{1}{2\pi} \lim_{\epsilon \to 0^+} \frac{1}{\epsilon - ix} = \frac{1}{2\pi} \lim_{\epsilon \to 0^+} \left(\frac{\epsilon}{\epsilon^2 + x^2} + i \frac{x}{\epsilon^2 + x^2} \right) \\
&= \frac{1}{2}\delta(x) + \frac{i}{2\pi} P\left(\frac{1}{x}\right)
\end{aligned}
\tag{11.25}
$$

where $h_\Theta(x)$ has been used to denote the Fourier transform of $\Theta(k)$ to avoid conflict with the use of θ as an angle. The identification of the δ-function and the principal value operation[7] P is based on the identities

$$\delta(x) = \lim_{\epsilon \to 0^+} \frac{1}{\pi} \frac{\epsilon}{\epsilon^2 + x^2} \tag{11.26}$$

$$P\left(\frac{1}{x}\right) = \lim_{\epsilon \to 0^+} \frac{x}{\epsilon^2 + x^2} \tag{11.27}$$

11.3.2   Lorentzian Form

The Fourier transform of exponentials representing signal decay around echoes yields a 'Lorentzian' function, an example of which is described in the following problem.

Problem 11.10

Spectroscopists study 'metabolites' by consideration of the area under the frequency or spectral response of the MR signal. Assume that the effective signal decay in the time domain is of the form $h(t) = e^{-|t|/T_2}$. Note that f and t are the Fourier conjugate variables in this problem, instead of x and k.

a) Derive $H(f)$ and compare your answer to that in Table 11.3.

b) Using the form found in part (a), find the total area under the curve $H(f)$. How does it depend upon T_2?

c) Alternatively, can you find the area under $H(f)$ from $h(t)$?

d) In practice, the true $t = 0$ point is not sampled. Why does this imply that the area must be found in the frequency domain?

---

[7]The principal value instruction requires that the region $(-\epsilon, \epsilon)$ be excluded in the integration over the $x = 0$ singularity of the function $1/x$.

11.3.3   The Sampling Function

The modeling of uniform sampling is discussed in the next chapter. Discrete sampling is represented by the product of the continuous signal with a sampling function, and the convolution theorem can be used to find the Fourier transform of the product. However, before convolution can be applied, the Fourier transform of the sampling function must be known.

The sampling function, defined as $u(k)$, is a sum of delta functions such that its product with the continuous signal is zero except at the points where the data were sampled, as desired. It is

$$u(k) = \Delta k \sum_{p=-\infty}^{\infty} \delta(k - p\Delta k) \tag{11.28}$$

By substituting (11.28) into (11.3), an intermediate step in finding $U(x)$, the inverse Fourier transform of $u(k)$, is given by

$$U(x) = \mathcal{F}(u(k)) = \Delta k \sum_{p=-\infty}^{\infty} \int_{-\infty}^{\infty} dk\, \delta(k - p\Delta k) e^{i2\pi kx} = \Delta k \sum_{p=-\infty}^{\infty} e^{i2\pi p\Delta k\, x} \tag{11.29}$$

Using the Fourier series identity (see the following problem)

$$\sum_{n=-\infty}^{\infty} e^{i2\pi na} = \sum_{m=-\infty}^{\infty} \delta(a - m) \tag{11.30}$$

gives[8]

$$U(x) = \sum_{q=-\infty}^{\infty} \delta(x - q/\Delta k) \tag{11.31}$$

Therefore, the Fourier transform $U(x)$ is also a sampling function. This property plays an important role in establishing the periodicity of the reconstructed spin density image $\hat{\rho}(x)$.

Problem 11.11

---

a) Prove the identity given in (11.30). Hint: Consider integrations over small intervals that either include or exclude the region where the argument of one of the δ-functions vanishes.

b) Show that the Fourier transform of $U(x)$ collapses back to (11.28).

11.4   The Discrete Fourier Transform

The discrete Fourier transform (DFT) can be introduced independently as a mathematical tool which maps a function defined at a finite set of uniformly spaced points into a like number of uniformly sampled points in conjugate space. A discrete inverse Fourier transform

---

[8]Note the delta function identity $\delta(ax) = \delta(x)/|a|$.

rect function	$\mathrm{rect}\left(\frac{x}{W}\right)$	$\overset{\mathcal{F}}{\Longleftrightarrow}$	$W\,\mathrm{sinc}(\pi W k)$
Gaussian	e^{-ax^2}	$\overset{\mathcal{F}}{\Longleftrightarrow}$	$\sqrt{\frac{\pi}{a}}e^{-\frac{\pi^2 k^2}{2}}$
sampling (or 'comb') function	$\sum\limits_{n=-\infty}^{\infty}\delta(x-n/\Delta k)$	$\overset{\mathcal{F}}{\Longleftrightarrow}$	$\Delta k\sum\limits_{p=-\infty}^{\infty}\delta(k-p\Delta k)$
Lorentzian form	$\frac{2\pi}{1+4\pi^2 x^2}$	$\overset{\mathcal{F}}{\Longleftrightarrow}$	$\pi e^{-|k|}$
Heaviside step function	$\Theta(x)$	$\overset{\mathcal{F}}{\Longleftrightarrow}$	$\frac{1}{2}\delta(k)-\frac{i}{2\pi}P(\frac{1}{k})$

Table 11.3: Fourier transform pairs which are relevant to a large number of MRI discussions found throughout the text. Note that the P in the expression of the Heaviside function refers to the principal value of the integral.

(DIFT) can also be defined, leading to a discrete Fourier transform pair. The discrete Fourier transform represents an exact transform, and it can be viewed as a special case of the continuous Fourier transform.[9]

As used in MRI, the discrete Fourier transform is an approximation of the continuous Fourier transform. Although the signal in MRI is continuous over all k-space, uniform sampling over a finite amount of time leads to a measured signal that is best described as a finite set of uniformly spaced measurements approximating the continuous signal. The measured signal describes a function which may be transformed using the discrete Fourier transform. Chapters 12 and 13 contain a detailed analysis of the effects of approximating the continuous signal. The discrete Fourier transform as a special case of the continuous Fourier transform is developed in anticipation of these discussions in Ch. 12.

It is also useful to present discrete Fourier transform properties similar to those laid out in Sec. 11.1 for the continuous Fourier transform. Multi-dimensional generalizations are not difficult to make for the various properties discussed.

A notation is used where h and H are replaced by g and G, respectively, to highlight the difference between the continuous pairs and the discrete pairs. With a length scale L, the discrete Fourier transform is defined by

$$G\left(\frac{p}{L}\right) \equiv \mathcal{D}(g) = \sum_{q=-n}^{n-1} g\left(\frac{qL}{2n}\right)e^{-i2\pi pq/2n}$$

$$p = -n, -n+1, ..., 0, ..., n-2, n-1 \qquad (11.32)$$

which can be written in terms of more familiar x-space and k-space notation if $\Delta k = 1/L$

---

[9]It may also be viewed as a truncated version of an infinite Fourier series, the latter the periodic limit of a Fourier transform.

and $L = 2n\Delta x$

$$G(p\Delta k) = \sum_{q=-n}^{n-1} g(q\Delta x)e^{-i2\pi pq\Delta x\Delta k} \tag{11.33}$$

This notation will be further developed, and explained in Ch. 12. The corresponding definition for the discrete inverse Fourier transform is

$$g\left(\frac{qL}{2n}\right) \equiv \mathcal{D}^{-1}(G) = \frac{1}{2n}\sum_{p=-n}^{n-1} G\left(\frac{p}{L}\right)e^{i2\pi pq/2n}$$

$$q = -n, -n+1, ..., 0, ..., n-2, n-1 \tag{11.34}$$

The coefficient $1/2n$ is the normalization factor that could be inserted into one or the other of the summations. Again, (11.34) can be written in terms of k-space and x-space,

$$g(q\Delta x) = \frac{1}{2n}\sum_{p=-n}^{n-1} G(p\Delta k)\,e^{i2\pi pq/2n} \tag{11.35}$$

The demonstration that (11.32) and (11.34) constitute a discrete Fourier pair rests on the identity

$$\sum_{k=-n}^{n-1} e^{i2\pi pk/N}e^{-i2\pi rk/N} = N\delta_{pr} \tag{11.36}$$

with

$$N = 2n \tag{11.37}$$

The Kronecker delta function δ_{pr} was defined in Ch. 5 as

$$\delta_{pr} = \begin{cases} 1 & \text{for } p = r \\ 0 & \text{otherwise} \end{cases} \tag{11.38}$$

Using (11.34), the object is recovered perfectly by using the discrete inverse Fourier transform only if it is actually a set of points of amplitude $g\left(\frac{qL}{2n}\right)$.

Problem 11.12

---

a) Prove the identity (11.36).

b) Substitute (11.32) into (11.34) to show that the discrete Fourier transform in fact gives rise to a transform pair.

11.5 Discrete Transform Properties

Mirroring those of the continuous transform, some discrete transform properties are shown in Table 11.4, where $g(q)$ and $G(p)$ are shorthand, in the remainder of this section, for the respective quantities (11.34) and (11.32). Since many properties of the two transforms are similar, and have already been outlined for the continuous transform, fewer are presented here. The proofs of several properties are left to a problem. This section serves more as an illustration of how to manipulate the finite sums than a further demonstration of transform properties. The development of these properties parallels the steps required for the derivation of the properties in Table 11.1.

11.5.1   The Discrete Convolution Theorem

The convolution theorem states that

$$g_1(q) \cdot g_2(q) \overset{\mathcal{D}}{\Leftrightarrow} G_1(p) * G_2(p) \tag{11.39}$$

where discrete convolution is defined by[10]

$$G_1(p) * G_2(p) = \frac{1}{2n} \sum_{r=-n}^{n-1} G_1(r) G_2(p-r) \tag{11.40}$$

To prove the theorem, substitute the discrete Fourier transform definitions of G_1 and G_2 on the right-hand side of (11.40) and use (11.36) to show

$$
\begin{aligned}
G_1(p) * G_2(p) &= \frac{1}{2n} \sum_{r=-n}^{n-1} \sum_{q=-n}^{n-1} g_1(q) e^{-i2\pi r q/2n} \sum_{q'=-n}^{n-1} g_2(q') e^{-i2\pi (p-r) q'/2n} \\
&= \frac{1}{2n} \sum_{q=-n}^{n-1} \sum_{q'=-n}^{n-1} g_1(q) g_2(q') 2n \delta_{q\,q'} e^{-i2\pi p q'/2n} \\
&= \sum_{q=-n}^{n-1} g_1(q) g_2(q) e^{-i2\pi p q/2n} \\
&= \mathcal{D}\left(g_1(q) \cdot g_2(q)\right) \tag{11.41}
\end{aligned}
$$

Problem 11.13

Assuming periodicity of $g(q)$

    a) Prove the space shifting property of Table 11.4.

    b) Prove Parseval's theorem as shown in Table 11.4.

Problem 11.14

Find the even/odd symmetries for the real and imaginary parts of the transform $G(p)$ of a purely real function $g(q)$. Compare your result with the entry in Table 11.2.

---

[10]Arguments that lie outside the range $(-n, n-1)$ must be mapped back into the range by the 'mod $2n$' operation.

11.5.2 Summary of Discrete Fourier Transform Properties

As was the case with the continuous Fourier transform, only a selection of transform properties have been discussed in detail. Table 11.4 includes additional properties of the discrete Fourier transform.

Description of property	Mathematical expression
convolution	$\mathcal{D}(g_1(q) \cdot g_2(q)) = G_1(p) * G_2(p) = \frac{1}{2n} \sum\limits_{r=-n}^{n-1} G_1(r) G_2(p-r)$
linearity	$\mathcal{D}(g_1(q) + g_2(q)) = \mathcal{D}(g_1(q)) + \mathcal{D}(g_2(q))$
symmetry	$g(q) \to G(p)$ $\frac{1}{N} G(p) \to g(-q)$
space shifting	$\mathcal{D}(g(q-j)) = G(p) e^{-i2\pi p j / 2n}$
alternate form	$g(q) = \left(\frac{1}{2n} \sum\limits_{p=-n}^{n-1} G^*(p) e^{-i2\pi p q / 2n} \right)^*$
Parseval's Theorem	$\sum\limits_{q=-n}^{n-1} |g(q)|^2 = \frac{1}{2n} \sum\limits_{p=-n}^{n-1} |G(p)|^2$

Table 11.4: Properties of $\mathcal{D}$, the discrete Fourier transform.

Suggested Reading

Some notation and several conventions have been borrowed for this chapter from:

- O. E. Brigham. *The Fast Fourier Transform.* Prentice-Hall, Englewood Cliffs, New Jersey, 1974.

Another excellent text from which to study the Fourier transform is:

- R. N. Bracewell. *The Fourier Transform and Its Applications.* McGraw Hill, New York, 1986.

Chapter 12

Sampling and Aliasing in Image Reconstruction

Chapter Contents

Summary: Signal sampling and the Nyquist sampling criterion are presented. Image reconstruction and the role of the discrete Fourier transform are discussed, along with a first introduction to resolution. Descriptions of aliasing artifacts, analog filtering, nonuniform sampling and other practical imaging considerations are made.

Introduction

This chapter addresses some of the effects that data collection methods have on the image. It is recalled that the signal is proportional to the emf induced in the receive coil by the rotating magnetization. This emf gives rise to a continuous or analog signal which is detected, sampled, and stored as finite, digitized data. Measurements of the MRI signal necessarily involve truncations and discrete sampling of k-space.

It is critical to acquire data in such a way as to generate a faithful representation of the spin density after a Fourier transform is performed on the signal. In the first section, discretization of infinite data is shown to lead to the Nyquist sampling rule for minimizing certain aliasing image errors (reconstruction artifacts). Truncation of the data is discussed in the second section, along with the truncated and discretized reconstructed image. The conditions under which the sampled signal and the sampled image are connected by the discrete version of the Fourier transform are also described. The relationship of aliasing to rf coil properties, noise, and analog filters is considered in Sec. 12.3. Several consequences of inadequate or incorrect sampling, especially with respect to nonuniformities in k-space, are covered in the last section.

12.1   Infinite Sampling, Aliasing, and the Nyquist Criterion

We consider in this section the mathematical modeling of infinite sampling, using the sampling function introduced in Ch. 11.

12.1.1   Infinite Sampling

Consider the discretization of the measurement, but without any limitation on the (infinite) number of discrete steps. Although it is not possible to collect an infinite set of data, it is instructive to understand first the consequences of such 'infinite samplings.' A subsequent step will be to consider a finite sample size.

The MR signal is generally collected over a set of uniformly spaced points in k-space. For a constant read gradient G_R, such sampling is achieved along the read direction by taking data at uniform intervals Δt in time, with the by now familiar relationship between the k-space step $\Delta k_R \equiv \Delta k$ and Δt

$$\Delta k = \gamma G_R \Delta t \tag{12.1}$$

The measured signal is $s(p\Delta k)$ at the step denoted by the integer p. The set of all (positive and negative) integers corresponds to the infinite sampling limit.

Consider the multiplication of the continuous signal by a 'comb' or 'sampling' function. Recall that the sampling function is the infinite sum of evenly spaced Dirac delta functions introduced in Ch. 11

$$\text{comb function}(k) \equiv \text{sampling function}(k) \equiv u(k) = \Delta k \sum_{p=-\infty}^{\infty} \delta(k - p\Delta k) \tag{12.2}$$

with a generic constant spacing Δk. The multiplication yields the signal distribution[1] corresponding to infinite sampling

$$\begin{aligned} s_\infty(k) &\equiv s(k) \cdot u(k) \\ &= \Delta k \sum_{p=-\infty}^{\infty} s(p\Delta k)\delta(k - p\Delta k) \end{aligned} \tag{12.3}$$

The coefficients of the delta functions are the aforementioned sampled signals $s(p\Delta k)$. The sampling function, a signal example, their respective Fourier transforms, and the signal distribution are all shown in Fig. 12.1.

The inverse transform of $s_\infty(k)$ leads to an approximation, or reconstructed image, of the physical density $\rho(x)$. With a portion of the notation already introduced in (11.8), the

---

[1]This distribution is an infinite sum of delta functions, but it has the same units as a signal. It is a 'signal density' multiplied by Δk.

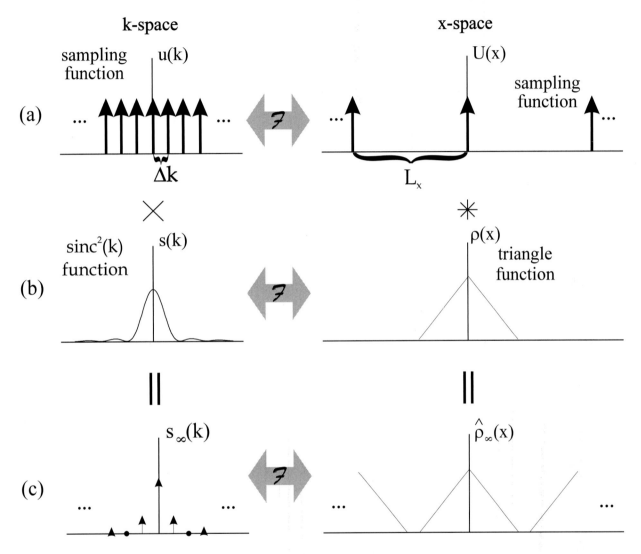

Fig. 12.1: The Fourier transform pairs for a signal example and the sampling function are illustrated in (a) and (b). The functions $\text{sinc}^2(k)$ and $u(k)$, and their respective (inverse) transforms, are the subjects of problems in Ch. 11. The product of the sampling function in (a) with the signal in (b) yields the sampled signal, and its inverse transform, in (c). The Fourier transform of the sampled signal, which may also be computed by the indicated convolution of the individual inverse transforms, is the first topic in the present chapter. Aliasing, the second topic, is avoided in this figure by the choice of a sufficiently small k-space step Δk and, hence, a sufficiently large 'field-of-view' $L_x \equiv 1/\Delta k$.

reconstructed image for infinite sampling is found to be

$$
\begin{aligned}
\hat{\rho}_\infty(x) &= \int_{-\infty}^{\infty} dk\, s_\infty(k) e^{i2\pi k x} \\[2mm]
&= \int_{-\infty}^{\infty} dk \left[\Delta k \sum_{p=-\infty}^{\infty} s(p\Delta k)\delta(k - p\Delta k) \right] e^{i2\pi k x} \\[2mm]
&= \Delta k \sum_{p=-\infty}^{\infty} s(p\Delta k) e^{i2\pi p \Delta k\, x}
\end{aligned}
\tag{12.4}
$$

This expression is an infinite Fourier series and represents a histogram approximation of the continuous inverse transform (11.7), i.e., of $\rho(x)$. In the event that $\rho(x)$ vanishes outside of a finite interval, the periodic Fourier series yields an infinite set of exact copies of the physical spin density, provided that the period associated with the copies is larger than the interval. A period that is too small gives rise to an 'aliasing' problem discussed in the next subsection. Before addressing the important question of the relation of the period to Δk, we show how convolution of delta functions is a simple way to examine the multiple copies.

The product of $s(k)$ and $u(k)$ in the definition of the sampled signal (12.3) implies that $\hat{\rho}_\infty(x)$ can be described equivalently by the convolution of $\rho(x)$ and $U(x)$ (the latter is the inverse Fourier transform of $u(k)$ discussed in Ch. 11)

$$
\hat{\rho}_\infty(x) = \rho(x) * U(x)
\tag{12.5}
$$

The function $U(x)$ is again a comb, as shown in Sec. 11.3.3,

$$
U(x) = \sum_{q=-\infty}^{\infty} \delta(x - q/\Delta k)
\tag{12.6}
$$

The convolution of any function $f(x)$ with a delta function $\delta(x - x_0)$ is easily seen to be

$$
f(x) * \delta(x - x_0) = \int dx'\, f(x')\delta(x - x' - x_0) = f(x - x_0)
\tag{12.7}
$$

Thus the convolution of the infinite sum (12.6) with any function gives an infinite series, each term of which is a copy of the function displaced from the next by the interval $1/\Delta k$. That is, (12.5) becomes

$$
\hat{\rho}_\infty(x) = \sum_{q=-\infty}^{\infty} \rho(x - q/\Delta k)
\tag{12.8}
$$

An infinite series of copies of the triangle function is illustrated in Fig. 12.2, which focuses on the convolution indicated in Fig. 12.1.

12.1.2   Nyquist Sampling Criterion

From the above discussion and the figures, spatial periodicity is a prominent feature of $\hat{\rho}_\infty(x)$. It is observed from the expression (12.4) that the periodicity corresponds to the fact that $e^{i2\pi p \Delta k\, x}$ is unchanged, for any p, if $x \to x + 1/\Delta k$. This replication concept is evident from (12.8) and demonstrates that $\hat{\rho}_\infty(x)$ is translationally invariant. That is,

$$
\hat{\rho}_\infty(x) = \hat{\rho}_\infty(x + 1/\Delta k)
\tag{12.9}
$$

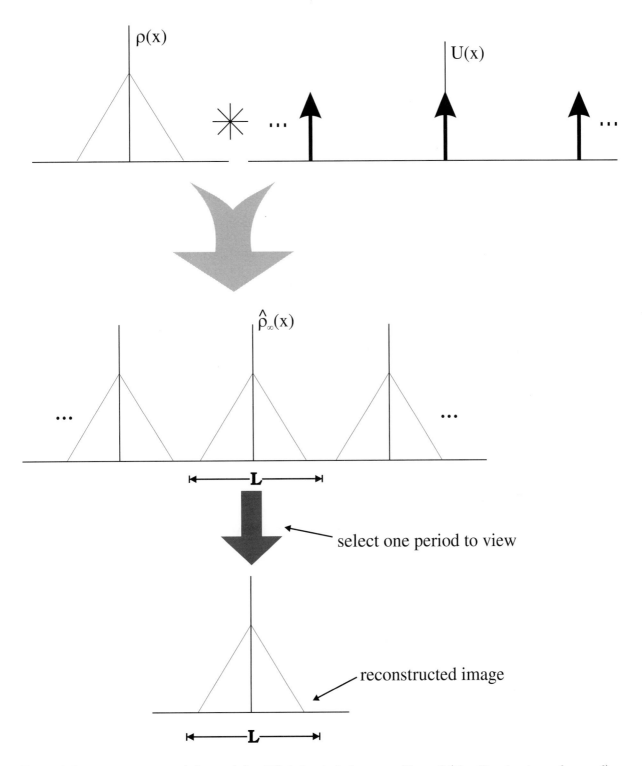

Fig. 12.2: The image $\hat{\rho}_\infty(x) = \rho(x) * U(x)$ for infinite sampling of (the Fourier transform of) a triangle function (see Fig. 12.1). Notice that the physical spin density is now repeated over all space, with periodicity $\hat{\rho}_\infty(x) = \hat{\rho}_\infty(x + L)$, where $L = 1/\Delta k$ (Sec. 12.1.2). The spacing Δk is small enough that L exceeds the object (triangle) size and aliasing is avoided.

Thus the periodicity of $\hat{\rho}_\infty(x)$ is given by the reciprocal of the spacing of the delta functions in the Fourier transform of the sampling function,

$$1/\Delta k \equiv L \equiv \text{FOV} \tag{12.10}$$

The uniform spacing between data points Δk is $1/L$ where L is the spatial interval over which the reconstructed image repeats itself. The interval L is called the field-of-view (FOV).

To construct an image, one of these copies is chosen. Although the copies of $\rho(x)$ are adequately separated in Fig. 12.2, this need not be the case. If the images overlap, then there will be significant differences between $\rho(x)$ and what is displayed as an image. This type of artifact is generally referred to as 'aliasing.'[2] It is possible to find a general requirement, or criterion, for the sampling rate to eliminate this artifact.

The criterion can be introduced by considering what happens if L is too small. The example at the top of Fig. 12.3 depicts a case where the spatial period L of the images in x-space is greater than the length (call it A) of the object being imaged. However, if $L < A$, then those parts of the image corresponding to the pixels near the edges of the object, which have to be assigned somewhere in the image, will be mapped back inside of L. The object is 'aliased' due to the overlap of the repeated images, with the left edge mapped into the right-side of the interval L, and vice versa for the right edge. See the example at the bottom of Fig. 12.3. An image illustration of such aliasing appears in Fig. 12.4. To avoid this type of image error, data must be sampled such that the inverse of the sampling step in k-space is larger than the size A of the object to be imaged. In one dimension, this means that the FOV must be larger than the object size

$$L > A \ \ \text{or} \ \ \Delta k < \frac{1}{A} \tag{12.11}$$

Equation (12.11) is referred to as the Nyquist sampling criterion.

The above discussion carries the hidden assumption that the signals from all spins in the object are detected. The ability to suppress aliasing by reducing the region to which the receive coil is sensitive is considered in Sec. 12.3.

Problem 12.1

a) Redraw Fig. 12.3 for a boxcar spin density function.

b) Redraw Fig. 12.3 for the triangular spin density function of Figs. 12.1 and 12.2.

c) In imaging the human torso, including the shoulders and arms, it is typical to acquire a 2D coronal image. Discuss what aliasing might look like for an FOV along the shoulder-to-shoulder axis that only covers the width of the chest but not the arms.

---

[2]Besides the names of phase wrapping, foldover, and wraparound indicated in Sec. 12.4.1, aliasing is also called 'ghosting.'

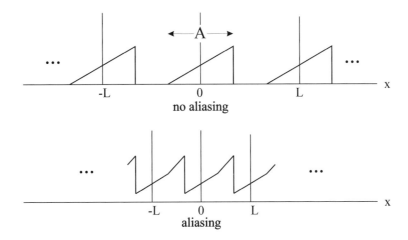

Fig. 12.3: The infinite sampling image $\hat{\rho}_\infty(x)$ is reconstructed for a ramp-like spin density. The Nyquist relation is satisfied in the top figure where the sample size is less than the FOV ($A < L$) while it is not satisfied in the bottom figure where $A > L$. Aliasing occurs for the latter, where copies of the object overlap and image distortion results, assuming the receive coil detects the signal from the entire object. The left (right) piece of the ramp is mapped inside the right (left) border of the L interval.

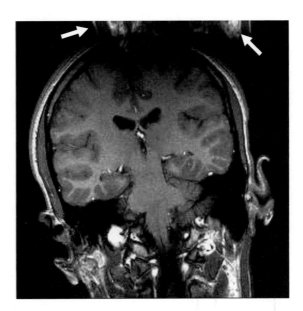

Fig. 12.4: An aliased image of the head and neck. Notice that the base of the neck is seen to appear at the top of the head (see arrows). In this example, the FOV parallel to the head-foot (cranial-caudal) axis was chosen to be too short, resulting in the aliasing. That is, the rf coil picked up signal from a region larger than the FOV.

Nyquist in the Read Direction

In the case where sampled data are separated by a time interval Δt and a gradient $G_R(t)$ is applied along the read direction, (12.11) can be rewritten as

$$\Delta k_R \equiv \gamma \int_t^{t+\Delta t} dt' \, G_R(t') = \frac{1}{L_R} < \frac{1}{A_R} \tag{12.12}$$

where the dimension of the sample in the read direction is A_R. For the special case of a boxcar gradient, the left-hand side of (12.12) is

$$\Delta k_R = \gamma G_R \Delta t \quad \text{(rectangular gradient lobe)} \tag{12.13}$$

The combination of (12.12) and (12.13) is often taken as an equality

$$\gamma G_R \Delta t L_R = 1 \tag{12.14}$$

which can be used to find one parameter when the others are fixed. Although it is easier to consider the Nyquist relation in terms of x- and k-space, for practical reasons it is necessary to understand the rate at which data must be sampled in time. The definition of the associated Nyquist sampling frequency during the application of a constant read gradient G_R leads to

$$f_R \equiv BW_{read} \equiv \frac{1}{\Delta t} = \gamma G_R L_R > \gamma G_R A_R \tag{12.15}$$

Problem 12.2

Determine the Nyquist frequency and the maximum allowable value Δk_{max}, before aliasing occurs, of a 1D water sample of 0.5 m in length. Assume that the applied gradient strength is either a) $G_R = 10\,\text{mT/m}$, b) $G_R = 25\,\text{mT/m}$, or c) $G_R = 50\,\text{mT/m}$.

Nyquist in the Phase Encoding Direction

The Nyquist relation applies to all three orthogonal directions. In the phase encoding direction (or partition encoding direction in 3D imaging) the Nyquist criterion specifies that

$$\Delta k_{PE} \equiv \gamma \int_t^{t+\tau_{PE}} dt' \, \Delta G_{PE}(t') = \frac{1}{L_{PE}} < \frac{1}{A_{PE}} \tag{12.16}$$

Once again, for the special case of a boxcar gradient, the left-hand side of (12.16) is

$$\Delta k_{PE} = \gamma \Delta G_{PE} \tau_{PE} \quad \text{(rectangular gradient lobe)} \tag{12.17}$$

where τ_{PE} is the duration of the phase encoding gradient pulse. The dimension of the sample along the direction under consideration is A_{PE}. In this case, the strength of the phase encoding gradient is being varied, but the duration of the gradient is fixed.

12.2 Finite Sampling, Image Reconstruction, and the Discrete Fourier Transform

The treatment of the MRI signal is not complete until the limits are imposed on the time during which measurements are taken. It is the reconstructed image derived from the corresponding truncated data set that is defined by the function $\hat{\rho}(x)$. For infinite sampling, this has the previous function $\hat{\rho}_\infty(x)$ as its limit.

12.2.1 Finite Sampling

The data truncation, or 'windowing,' is modeled mathematically by multiplying the sampled data by the rect function introduced in Ch. 9. The boundaries of the rect function must be defined carefully, so that the product of the sampling and the window functions reduces to the standard MRI sampling convention previewed in Sec. 10.3, and reintroduced in the last chapter through the discrete Fourier transform. The details are left to Prob. 12.3 and the result is

$$u(k) \cdot \text{rect}\left(\frac{k + \frac{1}{2}\Delta k}{W}\right) \;=\; \Delta k \sum_{p=-n}^{n-1} \delta(k - p\Delta k) \tag{12.18}$$

where the total number of points is $N = 2n$ and

$$W \equiv 2n\Delta k = N\Delta k \tag{12.19}$$

An integration over (12.18) yields Δk for each sampled point, which may be interpreted as $\Delta k/2$ on each side of the point. Thus $2n\Delta k$, and not $(2n-1)\Delta k$, is the total interval covered in k-space, encompassing $2n$ total points.

Problem 12.3

Derive (12.18). That is, show that the summation limits on the right-hand side follow from (12.2) and the argument in the rect function given on the left-hand side.

The final expression for the signal distribution corresponding to finite sampling, or 'measured' signal distribution, $s_m(k)$, is the product of three functions (signal, sampling, and window) given by

$$\begin{aligned} s_m(k) \;&=\; s(k) \cdot u(k) \cdot \text{rect}\left(\frac{k + \frac{1}{2}\Delta k}{W}\right) \\ &=\; \Delta k \sum_{p=-n}^{n-1} s(p\Delta k)\delta(k - p\Delta k) \end{aligned} \tag{12.20}$$

The result is the expected discrete and finite sum of delta function terms whose coefficients are again the sampled signals $s(p\Delta k)$. We consider the inverse Fourier transform of this signal in the next subsection.

Standard MRI Sampling

It has been noted that the distribution of points in (12.20) follows the standard convention where k-space is sampled slightly asymmetrically with an even number of points $N = 2n$ spread uniformly over the region $[-n\Delta k, (n-1)\Delta k]$. If $n \gg 1$, then the sampling is symmetric, to good numerical approximation. The reason for this convention is that an even number of points (usually 2^p points, for some p) is sampled in the implementation of a 'fast Fourier transform.' The FFT is an efficient computer algorithm for calculating the discrete Fourier transform of an object.

Consider what happens to the window function in (12.18) if it instead had been defined symmetrically with respect to the origin. With all points sampled at intervals of Δk, $2n+1$ points would then have fallen inside the sampling window (just barely: two would lie on its edges). By contrast, the shift of $(1/2)\Delta k$ to the left in the rect argument leads to only $2n$ sampled points, each separated by Δk and covering the range of integers $[-n, n-1]$. See the examples in Fig. 12.5.

The Nyquist theorem ensures adequate sampling of the data, but does not directly address what happens when the data are not sampled at the assumed points. For example, shifts in the sampled points are common in MRI, either due to experimental design or physical errors. The subject of Prob. 12.4 is to show that a uniform k-space shift in the data leads to a phase shift in the image that varies linearly as a function of position. The phase shift is anticipated from the continuous Fourier transform analysis in Sec. 11.2.2, but there are other errors present in the truncated and sampled data owing to the k-space shift, which can be analyzed with the discrete Fourier transform. An important signal loss arises if the shift is great enough to leave the signal peak at $k = 0$ close to the edge or even out of the sampling window (see Prob. 20.8). Nevertheless, the phase shift artifact is the principal difficulty, leading to artifacts in Re $\hat{\rho}(x)$. The procedure described in Ch. 11 involving the magnitude $|\hat{\rho}(x)|$ is *a fortiori* a method of choice in displaying images.

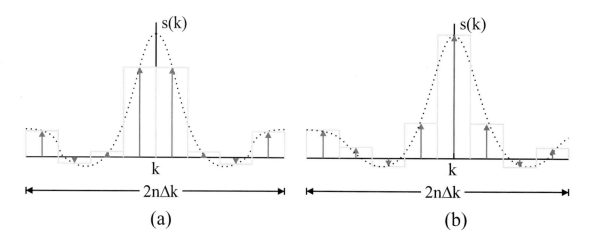

Fig. 12.5: Simple examples of (a) 'truly' symmetric sampling of k-space and (b) standard sampling as defined in MRI, both with an even number of points. In (a), both the sampling function $u(k)$ and the window function have been displaced from their standard MRI sampling definitions by the amount $\Delta k/2$ to the right. In (b), both are in standard position.

12.2.2 Reconstructed Spin Density

The reconstructed spin density for finite sampling is called $\hat{\rho}(x)$ and it is defined by the inverse Fourier transform of (12.20)

$$
\begin{aligned}
\hat{\rho}(x) &\equiv \int_{-\infty}^{\infty} dk\, s_m(k) e^{i2\pi kx} \\
&= \Delta k \int_{-\infty}^{\infty} dk \sum_{p=-n}^{n-1} s(p\Delta k)\delta(k - p\Delta k) e^{i2\pi kx} \\
&= \Delta k \sum_{p=-n}^{n-1} s(p\Delta k) e^{i2\pi p\Delta kx}
\end{aligned}
\tag{12.21}
$$

It is apparent that the periodicity (12.9) survives in (12.21)

$$
\hat{\rho}(x) = \hat{\rho}(x + 1/\Delta k)
\tag{12.22}
$$

so the Nyquist criterion applies to the truncated data as well.

Problem 12.4

Consider a shift K in the k-space data that can be acceptably approximated by $K = r\Delta k$ for some integer r. Assume that the entire echo signal remains within the sampling window. Justify the use of the discrete Fourier transform shift theorem in Table 11.4 for this situation and show that the theorem leads to a spatially varying linear phase in the reconstructed image (12.21). As a special case, explain how the results for truly symmetric sampling (for example, Fig. 12.5a) can be used to derive the results expected for 'MRI-symmetric' sampling (for example, Fig. 12.5b). Discuss the complications that arise for a shift that is not an integer multiple of Δk.

The fact that $\hat{\rho}(x)$ is not expected to represent exactly the physical spin density $\rho(x)$, in view of the limited data set, is made evident in (12.21). The finite sampling has led to a reconstructed spin density that is an approximation of the result (12.4) for infinite sampling, which, in turn, is a Fourier series representation of the physical spin density. Recall that the latter leads to exact copies of a localized $\rho(x)$ for sufficiently small values of Δk. The fact that the former is a discrete Fourier transform that may give an accurate representation of the physical spin density for a given 'resolution' is the subject we shall develop in the discussion to follow. The relationship between n and resolution will be part of that discussion.

It is recalled that differences between $\hat{\rho}(x)$ and $\rho(x)$ are defined as artifacts (Ch. 11). An artifact arising from the truncation is 'blurring' and it, along with other features, can be illustrated as follows. Since s_m is the product shown in (12.20), the Fourier transform in (12.21) may be reconsidered as a convolution of the three functions

$$
\hat{\rho}(x) = \rho(x) * U(x) * \left(W \operatorname{sinc}(\pi W x)\, e^{-i\pi x \Delta k} \right)
\tag{12.23}
$$

where the Fourier transform of the rect function in (12.23) is found by using the shift theorem on the transform of rect(k/W) (see Ch. 11). The result of the convolution of the first two functions, obtained in (12.4) and shown in the top portion of Fig. 12.6, is itself to be convolved with the sinc function (the next portion of the figure), the inverse Fourier transform of the rect function.[3] The reconstructed image $\hat{\rho}(x)$ obtained after the modifications of sampling and truncation is shown at the bottom of the figure. Notice that the convolution of the infinitely sampled signal with the sinc function slightly blurs the bandlimited images into each other since the sinc function is not bandlimited. All images include this effect, but only objects that occupy less than a few pixels show noticeable blurring effect. The blurring effect is generally negligible for a wide rect function (long boxcar) in the k-space, except when sharp boundaries are present in $\hat{\rho}(x)$ (see Ch. 13). A long boxcar gives rise to a narrowly peaked sinc function, approaching a delta function in the limit of infinite boxcar sampling. In this regard, and for a connection to resolution, see Prob. 12.5.

12.2.3 Discrete and Truncated Sampling of $\hat{\rho}(x)$: Resolution

The measurement of x-space is itself discretized and truncated. The spatial range, or spatial period, over which the spin density is imaged has already been defined as L. The truncation is for the obvious reason that there is no new information to be gained from the repetitions of the image. The discretization is over spatial steps (with uniform step size Δx) since there is a lower limit to the spatial information, or 'resolution,' available in the reconstructed spin density (see Prob. 12.5). A fundamental reason for the lower limit is the fact that truncation of k-space data leads to the x-space blurring described previously.

Problem 12.5

For convenience, consider a symmetric window, rect(k/W), in this problem. Show that the product of W with the first zero crossing of the Fourier transform of this window is constant, and find that constant. Compare this result to (12.30), noting that the first zero crossing distance represents the accuracy of measuring distances in x-space, the 'spatial resolution' discussed in Sec. 12.2.3 and in Ch. 13. This result is reminiscent of the Heisenberg uncertainty principle in quantum mechanics (Ch. 5). Given that W controls how small a window in k-space is examined, what does this 'uncertainty' result imply about blurring in MRI?

As in the k-space discussion, finite sampling can be modeled as the product of $\hat{\rho}(x)$, a sampling function, and a rect function. The sampling function in the image domain resembles (12.6), but with steps Δx; it is given by [4]

$$\tilde{U}(x) = \Delta x \sum_{q=-\infty}^{\infty} \delta(x - q\Delta x) \tag{12.24}$$

---

[3]It is remembered from Ch. 11 that the convolution operation is associative so that the order does not matter here.

[4]Note that this is not the same function as $U(x)$ in (12.6) and, apart from the extra factor of Δx, the key difference is the step size which is now Δx instead of L.

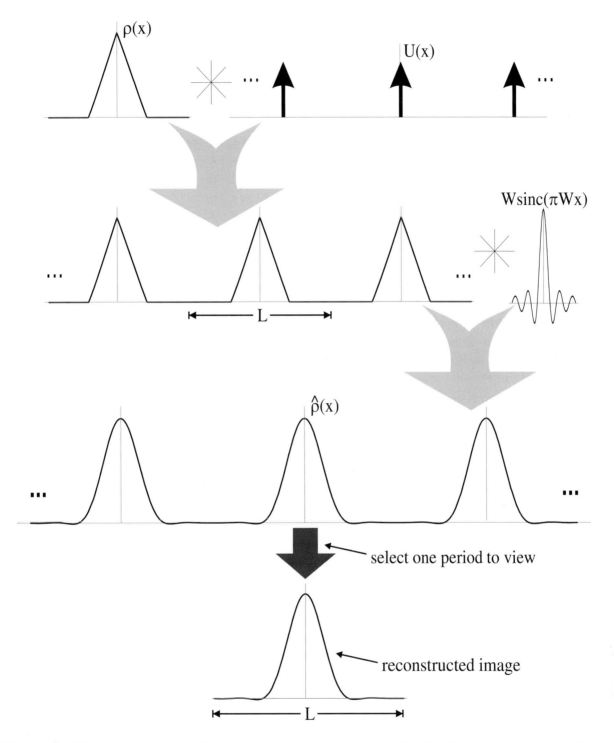

Fig. 12.6: The convolution of the unperturbed spin density with the Fourier transforms of the sampling and rect functions. The blurring and creation of multiple images shown here exist in all MRI images, even with L chosen to be larger than the object size. A single image is chosen from the set and the blurring is minimized if a wide rect function is employed (so that the sinc function is approximately a delta function). In order to show the blurring effect, the width of the object (triangle) is taken to be $4/W$ and the field-of-view to be $10/W$. Also, the phase accompanying asymmetric sampling has been ignored.

For the moment, we consider the number of sampling points to be equal to $2n'$ rather than $2n$ and we perform a calculation like that in (12.20). The complete expression of the 'measured' reconstructed spin density distribution for $2n'$ sampled points becomes

$$\hat{\rho}_m(x) \;=\; \hat{\rho}(x) \cdot \tilde{U}(x) \cdot \text{rect}\left(\frac{x + \frac{1}{2}\Delta x}{L}\right)$$

$$=\; \Delta x \sum_{q=-n'}^{n'-1} \hat{\rho}(q\Delta x)\delta(x - q\Delta x) \qquad (12.25)$$

with the relation

$$L = 2n'\Delta x \qquad (12.26)$$

analogous to that for W in (12.19). The resolution $\Delta x = L/(2n')$ is thus fixed by n' and L, and is commonly referred to as the image voxel (or pixel) size.

We observe that the coefficients of the delta functions (and Δx) are the sampled reconstructed densities $\hat{\rho}(q\Delta x)$ in parallel with the way that the sampled signals $s(p\Delta k)$ appeared in (12.20). Recall that the inverse Fourier transform of the signal distribution $s_m(k)$ gave the reconstructed spin density function $\hat{\rho}(x)$. Similarly, the Fourier transform of the measured reconstructed spin density distribution $\hat{\rho}_m(x)$ is a signal function, which we shall call $\hat{s}(k)$, given by

$$\hat{s}(k) \;=\; \int dx\, \hat{\rho}_m(x)e^{-i2\pi kx}$$

$$=\; \Delta x \sum_{q=-n'}^{n'-1} \hat{\rho}(q\Delta x)e^{-i2\pi kq\Delta x} \qquad (12.27)$$

It is seen that, for large n' and small Δx, (12.27) approaches the continuous Fourier transform of $\hat{\rho}(x)$, and $\hat{\rho}(x)$ approaches the continuous inverse transform of $\hat{s}(k)$.

But for large n and small Δk, we have already seen in (12.21) that $\hat{\rho}(x)$ approaches the continuous inverse transform of $s(k)$. The question addressed in the next subsection is about the conditions under which $\hat{s}(k)$ may be identified with $s(k)$. This will lead to the result that the discrete set of signals $s(p\Delta k)$ may be mapped into the discrete set of reconstructed spin densities $\hat{\rho}(q\Delta x)$ by the discrete inverse Fourier transform.

12.2.4   Discrete Fourier Transform

The condition that the two sets $s(p\Delta k)$ and $\hat{\rho}(q\Delta x)$ form a discrete Fourier transform pair is simply that the number of steps in both domains (k-space and x-space) must be equal

$$n = n' \qquad (12.28)$$

It is reasonable that the same size of data sets is needed to transform back and forth between domains.

To reach this result, we begin by showing that $\hat{s}(r\Delta k)$ reduces to $s(r\Delta k)$ under (12.28) for integer r. Replace $\hat{\rho}(q\Delta x)$ in (12.27) by the sum (12.21) of terms $s(p\Delta k)$

$$\hat{s}(r\Delta k) \;=\; \Delta x \Delta k \sum_{p=-n}^{n-1} \sum_{q=-n'}^{n'-1} s(p\Delta k)e^{i2\pi p\Delta k\, q\Delta x}e^{-i2\pi r\Delta k\, q\Delta x}$$

$$= \Delta x \Delta k \sum_{p=-n}^{n-1} \sum_{q=-n'}^{n'-1} s(p\Delta k)e^{i2\pi(p-r)\Delta k\, q\Delta x} \quad (12.29)$$

The combination of (12.10) and (12.26) leads to

$$\Delta k \Delta x = \frac{1}{L} \cdot \frac{L}{2n'} = \frac{1}{2n'} \quad (12.30)$$

and (12.29) reduces to

$$\hat{s}(r/L) = \frac{1}{2n'} \sum_{p=-n}^{n-1} \sum_{q=-n'}^{n'-1} s(p/L)e^{i\pi q(p-r)/n'} \quad (12.31)$$

Using the identity (11.36),

$$\sum_{q=-n'}^{n'-1} e^{i\pi q(p-r)/n'} = 2n'\delta_{pr} \quad (12.32)$$

it is found that $\hat{s}(r/L)$ is point by point equal to the signal where it is originally sampled

$$\hat{s}(r/L) = \sum_{p=-n}^{n-1} s(p/L)\delta_{pr} = s(r/L) \quad (12.33)$$

It follows that the two discrete and truncated (or bandlimited) functions, the sampled signal and the sampled reconstructed spin density, are related by

$$s(p\Delta k) = \Delta x \sum_{q=-n'}^{n'-1} \hat{\rho}(q\Delta x)e^{-i\pi pq/n'}$$

$$\hat{\rho}(q\Delta x) = \Delta k \sum_{p=-n}^{n-1} s(p\Delta k)e^{i\pi pq/n'} \quad (12.34)$$

Consider

$$\hat{\rho}(r\Delta x) = \Delta k \sum_{p=-n}^{n-1} s(p\Delta k)e^{i\pi pr/n'}$$

$$= \Delta k \Delta x \sum_{q=-n'}^{n'-1} \hat{\rho}(q\Delta x) \sum_{p=-n}^{n-1} e^{i\pi p(r-q)n/(n'n)}$$

$$= \frac{n}{n'} \sum_{q=-n'}^{n'-1} \hat{\rho}(q\Delta x)\delta_{rn/n',\, qn/n'} \quad (12.35)$$

The condition to recover any arbitrary $\hat{\rho}(r\Delta x)$ in (12.35) is possible only if $n = n'$.

Defining

$$\hat{\rho}_{MRI}(qL/2n) = \hat{\rho}(qL/2n)\Delta x \quad (12.36)$$

then

$$s(p/L) = \sum_{q=-n}^{n-1} \hat{\rho}_{MRI}(qL/2n)e^{-i\pi pq/n}$$

$$\hat{\rho}_{MRI}(qL/2n) = \frac{1}{2n} \sum_{p=-n}^{n-1} s(p/L)e^{i\pi pq/n} \quad (12.37)$$

This is precisely the discrete Fourier transform pair discussed in Ch. 11. It is also easy to show that the Nyquist symmetry continues to hold for this pair. Further, it demonstrates that $\hat{\rho}_{MRI}(x)$, *the discrete Fourier transform of* $s(p/L)$, *which is what is displayed in an MRI image, is proportional to the physical spin density times the volume of the voxel.* However, for the sake of brevity, and where no ambiguity occurs, we continue to use $\hat{\rho}(\vec{r})$, the effective spin density, to discuss the MR image.

Problem 12.6

Nyquist symmetry: Show that the expression for $\hat{\rho}(q\Delta x)$ in (12.34) is invariant under $x \rightarrow x + L$, i.e., under $q \rightarrow q + L/\Delta x$.

12.2.5 Practical Parameters

The following problem provides a summary for sampling parameters. The role of the Nyquist criterion is highlighted in the calculations for both 2D and 3D imaging.

Problem 12.7

Assume the following 2D imaging parameters: $L_x = L_y = 256\,\text{mm}$; $N_x = N_y = 256$; $TH = 5\,\text{mm}$; $T_R = 600\,\text{ms}$. Assume that $\hat{x}$, $\hat{y}$, and $\hat{z}$ are the read, phase encoding, and slice select directions, respectively. Also suppose that $T_s = 5.12\,\text{ms}$ and $\tau_{PE} = 2.56\,\text{ms}$ and that the rf excitation bandwidth BW_{rf} is 2 kHz. See Ch. 10 for the sequence diagrams.

a) Find the readout bandwidth, BW_{read}, the Nyquist sampling interval Δt in the read direction, the Nyquist sampling interval Δk_x in the k_x direction, and the strength of the read gradient (G_x) used.

b) What is the Nyquist sampling interval Δk_y in the k_y direction? What is the gradient step size ΔG_y in the phase encoding table? What is the strength of the maximum value $G_{y,max} = N_y \Delta G_y/2$ of the phase encoding gradient?

c) What is the slice select gradient G_{ss} used?

d) What is the total imaging time T_{acq}?

e) What happens to G_x, $G_{y,max}$, and G_{ss} when N_x and N_y are doubled at the same time that TH is halved while all other quantities are unchanged?

f) How does G_x change when L_x is halved while all other parameters are held fixed? How does it change if, instead, T_s is changed to 2.56 ms while L_x is unchanged from 256 mm and N_x is fixed at 256?

g) Suppose the imaging is performed as a 3D imaging experiment with $L_z \equiv TH = 32\,\text{mm}$ and $N_z = 16$, with all other parameters the same as in the original problem statement (the partition encoding and phase encoding gradient times are the same: $\tau_z = \tau_{PE} = 2.56\,\text{ms}$).

i) What is G_{ss}? (The z-axis is now the 'slab' selection axis and the partition encoding gradient is referred to as G_z.)

ii) What is ΔG_z and what is $G_{z,max}$?

iii) What is the total imaging time if (i) T_R were 600 ms (ii) T_R were 60 ms? How does T_{acq} in either case compare with the imaging time in the 2D imaging experiment?

iv) How does G_{ss} compare between the 2D and 3D imaging experiments?

12.3   RF Coils, Noise, and Filtering

The choice of FOV rests on a number of additional factors in imaging, besides the size of the object. We consider in this section the effects of variations in the spatial regions that are excited by the rf transmission coils, or that are receive-coil-sensitive, or that are directly filtered by electronic means. An illustration of these considerations may be made involving the rf receive coil. If that coil is sensitive to MR signals or noise outside of the frequency range determined by G_R and L_R in the read direction ($BW_{read} = \gamma G_R L_R$), then there will be aliasing in the reconstructed image according to the Nyquist relation. The effective size of the spin system may be larger than the body size A_R.

12.3.1   RF Field-of-View Considerations

In order to avoid aliasing and still image efficiently, $L_R \equiv L$ must be chosen carefully. A simple set of 1D imaging situations is presented in Fig. 12.7 to illustrate different factors that determine a proper choice of L. In Fig. 12.7a, L is determined by the actual physical extent A of $\rho(x)$ since the entire object is excited by the rf pulse. The region of receive coil sensitivity matches the excitation range. In Fig. 12.7b, L has been chosen to be less than the physical extent of $\rho(x)$ because the region of rf excitation is less than the length of the sample. Since there will be no signal from regions where the spins have not been tipped into the transverse plane there is no reason for L to be larger than the rf excited region. (See later for complications due to noise stemming from those regions.) In Fig. 12.7c, the receive coil is only sensitive to a region smaller than A. There will be no signal detected outside of the receive coil sensitivity, and therefore L does not need to extend beyond this range.

12.3.2   Analog Filtering

The subject of noise in the MR signal is an important one and Ch. 15 is devoted to its detailed discussion. As a preliminary topic, we describe here some aspects of the filtering of noise, as they relate to the FOV. The total measured signal can be modeled by the sum of a signal $s(k)$ and a noise function $\epsilon(k)$. In view of the results of the previous section, the total signal is considered to be the finite and discretized set of measurements related to the finite and discretized set of reconstructed spin density data through the discrete Fourier transform. Since the transform is linear, the reconstructed image is also the summation of the MR image and a noise image

$$s(k) + \epsilon(k) \overset{\mathcal{D}}{\Leftrightarrow} \hat{\rho}(x) + \hat{\eta}(x) \tag{12.38}$$

where $\hat{\eta}(x) \equiv \mathcal{D}^{-1}\left(\epsilon(k)\right)$.

The noise in MR is usually assumed to be white in nature, i.e., power is uniformly distributed as a function of frequency. This means that a reconstructed image will have

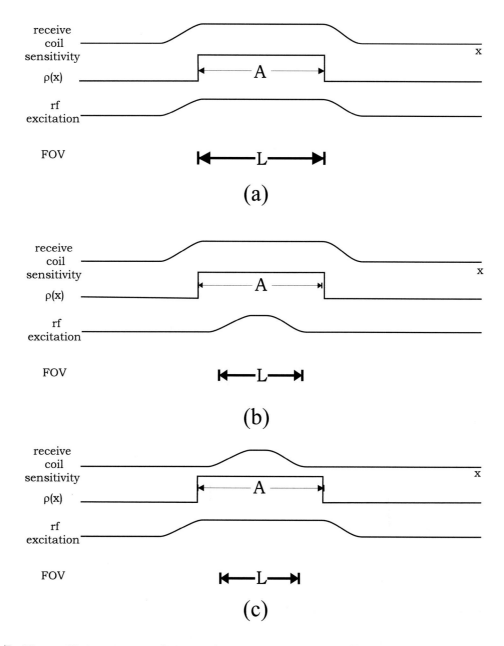

Fig. 12.7: Three 1D imaging conditions where the parameters affecting the choice of L have been varied. As described in the text, the FOV is chosen in each case such that no aliasing appears in the reconstructed image.

noise aliased into the image from frequencies outside of the region-of-interest (ROI). In the read direction, however, it is possible to limit the frequency content of the measured signal to a narrow frequency band by filtering the data. *In general, modifications of the signal in MRI are referred to as filters.* In Ch. 13, filters corresponding to multiplication of the k-space data will be discussed at length. The specific electronics of frequency filters relevant to the present topic is beyond the scope of this text, but the filter effects on the reconstructed image can be examined.

Since the data received in the read direction by the electronics are continuously acquired, they can be analog filtered before sampling. Analog filtering is equivalent to multiplying the signal as a function of frequency by a filter function $H(f)$ as shown in Fig. 12.8. The linear relationship between frequency and position in an MRI experiment implies the filter can also be thought of as modifying the x-space image. Phase encoding, however, is performed before data are read, so analog filtering cannot be carried out along the phase encoding direction.

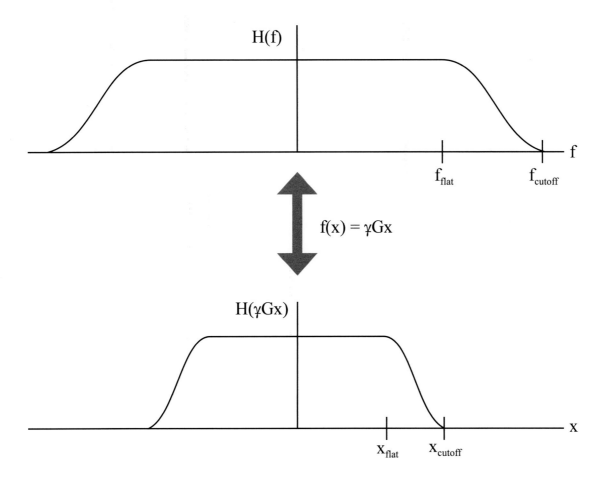

Fig. 12.8: Example of a low pass frequency response (top figure) for an electronics analog filter. Frequency encoding along the read direction leads directly to its corresponding spatial response (bottom figure). The negative frequencies are a result of the demodulation of the Larmor frequency in the signal. The transition frequencies, f_{flat} and f_{cutoff}, are described in the text, and correspond to the spatial positions, x_{flat} and x_{cutoff}, respectively.

There are two primary reasons to perform analog filtering of the MRI data. The first, as mentioned, is to limit the effects of noise from outside of the desired bandwidth. The second includes cases where the body excited in the read direction is larger than the ROI of the imaging experiment. For example, measurements for a transverse image of the human chest for the study of the heart (the ROI) may include the signal from the body over the whole arm-to-arm range (the read direction). A filter can be used to limit the frequency content of the signal in order to get an image of the heart alone.

In the ideal case, the analog filter behaves like a rect function allowing all frequencies within its bandwidth and rejecting all frequencies outside its bandwidth. However, filters with such sharp frequency transitions are unrealistic. The typical filter has a smooth roll-off from 'pass-band' to 'reject-band' (e.g., Fig. 12.8), the roll-off rate being determined by the type of the filter. In this case, it is possible to identify a flat pass-band, or low pass, region $|f| < f_{flat}$, in terms of a maximum flat frequency f_{flat}. The reject-band region may be defined by $|f| > f_{cutoff}$, introducing an outer edge cutoff frequency f_{cutoff}. The transition roll-off region lies between the flat and cutoff frequencies.

In Fig. 12.9, three possible implementations of analog filtering are illustrated. Figure 12.9a shows the case where the filtered frequency band closely matches the size of the object being imaged ($2x_{flat} \approx A_R$).[5] In this case, the FOV in the read direction L_R can be chosen equal to $2x_{cutoff}$, so that there is no noise outside of the imaging region that leaks back inside. Therefore, the filtered reconstructed image, defined by $\hat{\rho}_f$, is given by

$$\hat{\rho}_f(x) = H(x)\left(\hat{\rho}(x) + \hat{\eta}(x)\right) \tag{12.39}$$

It is necessary to be careful in matching the filter with the object size since, if $A_R > 2x_{flat}$, the image will lose intensity near the edges of the object being imaged.

Figure 12.9b shows the case where the filter extends beyond the physical body and includes some frequencies that are not of interest. Since L_R is less than $2x_{cutoff}$, any data obtained outside of this region will alias back into the image. The noise between the filter cutoffs and the boundaries of the FOV on the left (right) will be mapped in reverse order inside and to the right (left) of the FOV interval. If the filter range is not so large (i.e., $x_{cutoff} < L_R$) that multiple aliasing has to be considered, a formula for the filtered reconstructed spin density may be given by

$$\hat{\rho}_f(x) = \begin{cases} H(x)\left(\hat{\rho}(x) + \hat{\eta}(x)\right) + \underbrace{H(x - L_R)\hat{\eta}(x - L_R)}_{\text{aliased noise}} & 0 \leq x \leq L_R/2 \\[2em] H(x)\left(\hat{\rho}(x) + \hat{\eta}(x)\right) + \underbrace{H(x + L_R)\hat{\eta}(x + L_R)}_{\text{aliased noise}} & -L_R/2 < x < 0 \end{cases} \tag{12.40}$$

The fact that $\rho(x) = 0$ for $|x| \geq L_R/2$ (i.e., $A_R < L_R$) means there is aliasing only of noise and not of the MR spin signal. The noise profile does not have uniform variance, due to the aliasing effect, and is a function of the width of the filter. As an example, if L is only slightly less than $2x_{cutoff}$, the noise will appear slightly larger at the outer edges of the image than in the center.

---

[5]The encoded positions x_{flat} and x_{cutoff} are illustrated in Fig. 12.8.

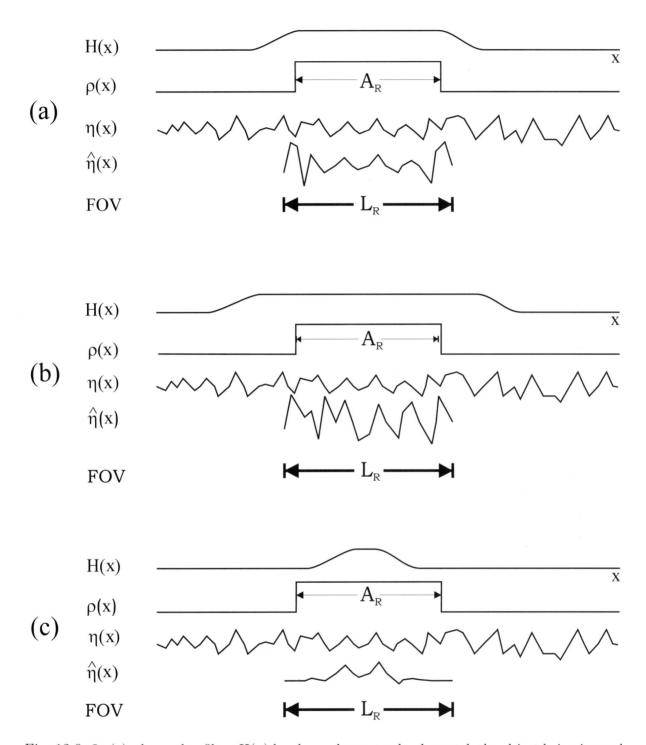

Fig. 12.9: In (a), the analog filter $H(x)$ has been chosen to closely match the object being imaged, minimizing the effect of noise $\eta(x)$ outside of the body. In (b), the applied analog filter extends beyond the boundaries of the desired object, and thereby includes additional noise contributions that will be aliased back into a reconstructed image. In (c), the analog filter is used to isolate a region within the body by filtering out the contribution from those areas not being imaged.

Finally, in Fig. 12.9c the case is shown where $2x_{cutoff} < A_R$. In this case, part of the object will be truncated by the filter, and the subinterval in x that is reconstructed may be found from (12.39). This method can be used to select a small volume or avoid aliasing of a large object.

In the above cases, the range of the filter was varied for a fixed FOV and body size. In fact, noise and signal aliasing both can be eliminated for the read direction if L_R is made larger than either the filter range or A_R (keeping sampling time fixed). This will not alter the resolution Δx, nor change the SNR of the experiment (see Ch. 15). The only cost is in the increased storage and processing time needed for the additional data. *Sampling extra data outside of the ROI in order to ensure that aliasing is avoided is generally referred to as oversampling.*

12.3.3   Avoiding Aliasing in 3D Imaging

In 3D imaging, L_z is often chosen to be equal to TH. However, this choice implies that the signal contributions of spins that are excited outside the slice or slab profile (Fig. 12.10a) due to rf leakage will be aliased into the imaging region as shown in Fig. 12.10b. Images with and without this aliasing are displayed in Fig. 12.11. It is clear that the artifact seriously degrades the quality of the resulting images. Aliasing can be avoided in this situation by choosing L_z to be greater than TH (Fig. 12.10c). Unfortunately, since $\Delta z = L_z/(2n_z)$, an increase in L_z forces the partition number n_z to be larger for the same resolution, Δz, and, accordingly, data acquisition time also increases.

12.4   Nonuniform Sampling

Along any line of k-space data there exist factors such as eddy currents, analog-to-digital conversion errors, and timing errors that may lead to nonuniform spacing of the data points. These types of error may occur along read lines, or along phase/partition encoding lines perpendicular to a given read position. The nonuniform sampling is shown to lead to aliasing in the images.

In the situation where k-space sampling of a line is not uniform, it is generally possible to model the data as being made up of several uniformly sampled data sets that are shifted in k-space from each other. To investigate the presence of aliasing, Fourier transforms are taken along the read lines or the phase encoding lines. In the following subsection, a prototypical 1D situation where two uniformly spaced data sets are combined to generate an image is studied. Afterward, a brief introduction to analog-to-digital errors is made in Sec. 12.4.2.

12.4.1   Aliasing from Interleaved Sampling

Suppose the reciprocal of the minimum required FOV for a given 1D object is $\Delta k = 1/L$, and the data sets containing the odd points,[6] $s_o(k)$, and even points, $s_e(k)$, are collected

---

[6]More generally, we might refer to odd lines and even lines in 2D imaging as those lines in k-space with odd index or even index where the line running through the origin is even. These are the perpendicular phase encoding lines referred to just previously.

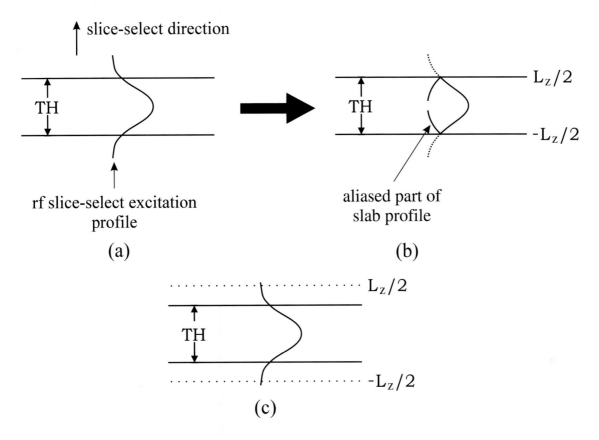

Fig. 12.10: The rf excitation profile of a typical slice select pulse in a 3D imaging experiment is shown in (a) along with the assumed slab thickness TH. If L_z is chosen to be equal to TH, then a significant amount of aliasing from the tail of the excitation will be aliased into the slab as shown in (b). Recall that the upper tail in (a) aliases into the lower portion in (b), as indicated by the long arrow, and vice versa. If L_z is chosen larger, as shown in (c), then there will be no aliasing, but the number of partitions will have to be increased to maintain the same resolution Δz. Also, the imaging amplitude drops to zero outside the slab.

along a line such that the separation between two adjacent points in either data set is $2\Delta k$. A complete set obtained by interleaving the odd and even points symmetrically would have the uniform k-space step size (Δk) required to avoid aliasing.

Correctly Interleaved Data

The sampling function $u(k)$ can be written as the sum of two functions $u_e(k)$ and $u_o(k)$

$$u(k) = u_e(k) + u_o(k) \tag{12.41}$$

which are defined as

$$u_e(k) = \Delta k \sum_{m=-\infty}^{\infty} \delta(k - 2m\Delta k) \tag{12.42}$$

$$u_o(k) = \Delta k \sum_{m=-\infty}^{\infty} \delta(k - (2m+1)\Delta k) \tag{12.43}$$

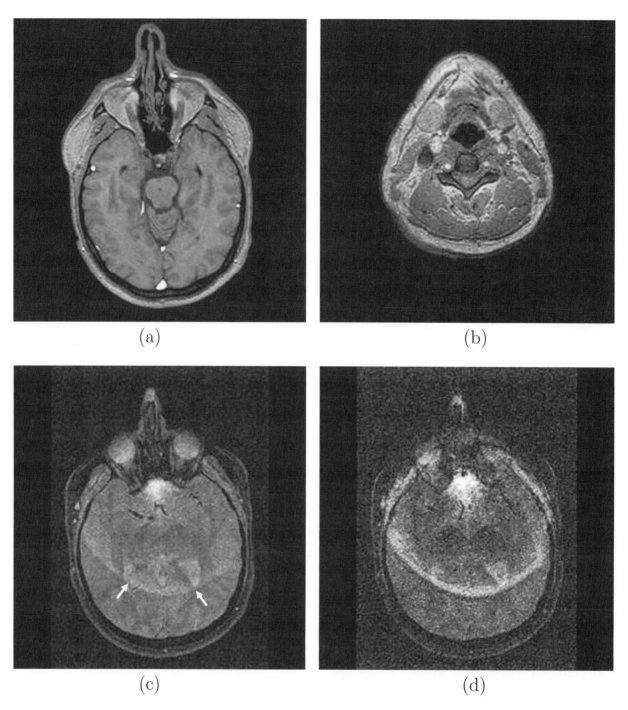

Fig. 12.11: Four partitions from a single 3D experiment where images (a) and (b) show two una-liased images and (c) and (d) exhibit aliasing. The head image (a) and neck image (b) correspond to partitions closer to the middle of the total slab, while the head image in (c) is from the top of the slab and shows aliasing of the neck into the brain (white arrows). The neck image in (d) shows significant aliasing from the brain. The fact that the aliased information from the brain is as bright as the neck tissue in (d) is due to the inhomogeneity of the rf coil used for both receive and transmit (see Ch. 16) resulting in a reduced flip angle in the neck region.

That is, $u_e(k)$ samples the even index k-space points whereas $u_o(k)$ samples the odd points. Multiplication in k-space by these comb functions leads to measured data sets $s_e(2m\Delta k)$ and $s_o((2m+1)\Delta k)$, respectively.[7]

The reconstructed image for infinite sampling is a convolution of the physical spin density and $U(x)$, the inverse transform of the sampling function. The latter is found to be

$$U(x) = U_e(x) + U_o(x) \tag{12.44}$$

where the identity (11.30) can be employed to obtain

$$
\begin{aligned}
U_e(x) &= \mathcal{F}^{-1}\{u_e(k)\} = \Delta k \sum_{q=-\infty}^{\infty} \delta\left(2\Delta k\, x - q\right) \\
&= \frac{1}{2} \sum_{q=-\infty}^{\infty} \delta\left(x - q\frac{L}{2}\right)
\end{aligned}
\tag{12.45}
$$

and, with further assistance from the shift theorem (11.11),

$$
\begin{aligned}
U_o(x) &\equiv \mathcal{F}^{-1}\{u_o(k)\} = \mathcal{F}^{-1}\{u_e(k - \Delta k)\} \\
&= \frac{1}{2} e^{i2\pi\Delta k x} \sum_{q=-\infty}^{\infty} \delta\left(x - q\frac{L}{2}\right) \\
&= \frac{1}{2} \sum_{q=-\infty}^{\infty} \delta\left(x - q\frac{L}{2}\right) e^{iq\pi}
\end{aligned}
\tag{12.46}
$$

The simple result (12.7) for any convolution involving a delta function leads to the respective series for the convolution of $\rho(x)$ with $U_e(x)$ and $U_o(x)$

$$\hat{\rho}_e(x) \equiv \rho(x) * U_e(x) = \frac{1}{2} \sum_{q=-\infty}^{\infty} \rho\left(x - q\frac{L}{2}\right) \tag{12.47}$$

and

$$\hat{\rho}_o(x) \equiv \rho(x) * U_o(x) = \frac{1}{2} \sum_{q=-\infty}^{\infty} \rho\left(x - q\frac{L}{2}\right) e^{iq\pi} \tag{12.48}$$

The expressions (12.47) and (12.48) are the ingredients for the following image formula

$$
\begin{aligned}
\hat{\rho}_\infty(x) &= \mathcal{F}^{-1}\{s_\infty(k)\} = \mathcal{F}^{-1}\{s_e(k)\} + \mathcal{F}^{-1}\{s_o(k)\} \\
&= \hat{\rho}_e(x) + \hat{\rho}_o(x)
\end{aligned}
\tag{12.49}
$$

Since the odd terms cancel between the two series, the standard result for infinite sampling is recovered,

$$\hat{\rho}_\infty(x) = \sum_{r=-\infty}^{\infty} \rho(x - rL) \tag{12.50}$$

---

[7]Infinite sampling is considered for simplicity but without losing too much generality. As shown earlier, the finite data collection window leads to another convolution in the image domain and blurring occurs. Effects on the image reconstruction of discrete sampling can be considered independent of these windowing effects since the convolution operator is associative as shown in Ch. 11.

which exhibits an infinite number of Nyquist copies.

In the interval $x = -L/2$ to $x = L/2$, the series (12.50) reduces to one term, $\hat{\rho}_\infty(x) = \rho(x)$ under the assumption that the spin density vanishes outside that interval, and there is no aliasing. There is aliasing, however, in the individual odd and even series where the range of nonzero values for $\rho(x)$ implies that three terms $q = -1$, 0, and $+1$ contribute to the series (12.47) and (12.48). Also, these contributions can be better circumscribed by splitting the physical spin density into its left-side and right-side values defined by

$$\rho(x) = \rho_l(x) + \rho_r(x) \tag{12.51}$$

where

$$\rho_l(x) \equiv \begin{cases} \rho(x) & -L/2 < x \le 0 \\ 0 & \text{otherwise} \end{cases} \tag{12.52}$$

and

$$\rho_r(x) \equiv \begin{cases} \rho(x) & 0 < x < L/2 \\ 0 & \text{otherwise} \end{cases} \tag{12.53}$$

The left/right decomposition is particularly useful for describing aliasing features inside the FOV and leads to

$$
\begin{aligned}
\hat{\rho}_e(x) &= \frac{1}{2}\left[\rho\left(x + \frac{L}{2}\right) + \rho(x) + \rho\left(x - \frac{L}{2}\right)\right] \\
&= \frac{1}{2}\rho(x) + \frac{1}{2}\left[\rho_r\left(x + \frac{L}{2}\right) + \rho_l\left(x - \frac{L}{2}\right)\right] \quad -L/2 < x < L/2 \quad (12.54)
\end{aligned}
$$

$$
\begin{aligned}
\hat{\rho}_o(x) &= \frac{1}{2}\left[-\rho\left(x + \frac{L}{2}\right) + \rho(x) - \rho\left(x - \frac{L}{2}\right)\right] \\
&= \frac{1}{2}\rho(x) - \frac{1}{2}\left[\rho_r\left(x + \frac{L}{2}\right) + \rho_l\left(x - \frac{L}{2}\right)\right] \quad -L/2 < x < L/2 \quad (12.55)
\end{aligned}
$$

The extra terms in each equation are left-side and right-side functions representing aliasing that cancels if the even and odd sets are combined according to (12.49).

The aliasing effect in images reconstructed with just the even or odd points alone can be investigated from (12.54) and (12.55). Consider the simple boxcar spin density illustrated in Fig. 12.12. The reader is asked to verify the plots shown for $\hat{\rho}_e(x)$ and $\hat{\rho}_o(x)$ in the figure, which exhibit aliasing features adjacent to the object (the object is only one-third of the FOV). Their sum, however, is correctly interleaved and gives the expected result $\hat{\rho}_\infty(x)$.

Problem 12.8

Employ (12.54) and (12.55) to derive the plots showing aliased features for $\hat{\rho}_e(x)$ and $\hat{\rho}_o(x)$ for the boxcar object in Fig. 12.12.

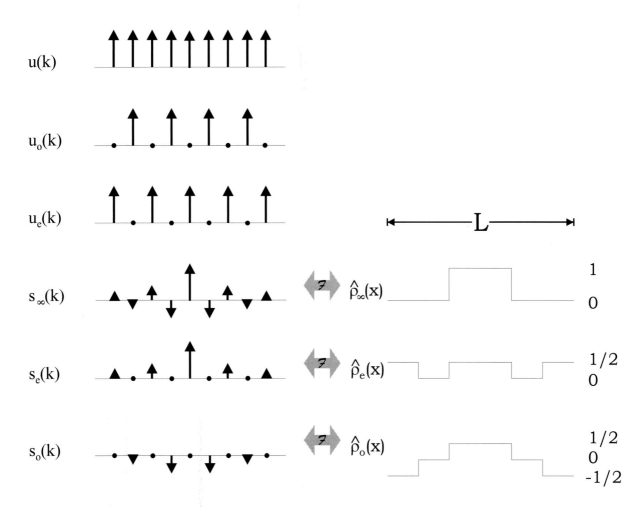

Fig. 12.12: Reconstructed images for infinite sampling of a unit boxcar object centered in the FOV with width equal to $L/3$. Aliasing in the uniform 1D k-space sampling case occurs whenever the odd points or even points are missing along a line in k-space. There is no aliasing for the given FOV, however, provided that the point separation is as shown for $u(k)$, and, indeed, interleaving the even and odd series leads to $\hat{\rho}_\infty(x) = \rho(x)$. The vertical arrows represent the relative strengths of the delta functions and there is an infinite number of sampling points in each row of vertical arrows.

Incorrectly Interleaved Data

In the incorrectly interleaved case, the separation between the interleaved points is not equal to Δk. Consider the case where $u_e(k)$ is still given by (12.42), but the odd sampling function is shifted slightly in k-space and is modeled by

$$u_{o,i}(k) = \Delta k \sum_{m=-\infty}^{\infty} \delta(k - (2m + 1 - \alpha)\Delta k) \qquad (12.56)$$

where $-1 < \alpha < 1$ ($\alpha = 0$ represents perfect sampling for the odd points). The subscript i is present to remind the reader that this is the 'incorrectly interleaved case' for the odd-point sampling function. From the shift theorem for the Fourier transform of (12.56), the x-space sampling function is found to be

$$U_{o,i}(x) = \frac{1}{2} \sum_{q=-\infty}^{\infty} \delta\left(x - q\frac{L}{2}\right) e^{i\pi q(1-\alpha)} \tag{12.57}$$

Steps taken in the previous, correctly interleaved, case can be repeated such that $\hat{\rho}_{o,i}(x)$ is found to be

$$
\begin{aligned}
\hat{\rho}_{o,i}(x) &= \frac{1}{2}\left[\rho\left(x + \frac{L}{2}\right)e^{-i\pi(1-\alpha)} + \rho(x) + \rho\left(x - \frac{L}{2}\right)e^{i\pi(1-\alpha)}\right] \\
&= \frac{1}{2}\rho(x) + \frac{1}{2}\left[\rho_r\left(x + \frac{L}{2}\right)e^{-i\pi(1-\alpha)} + \rho_l\left(x - \frac{L}{2}\right)e^{i\pi(1-\alpha)}\right]
\end{aligned}
$$

$$-L/2 < x < L/2 \tag{12.58}$$

The aliasing terms exhibit additional phase shifts beyond those found previously, and now would not cancel their counterparts in (12.54).

Let $\hat{\rho}_i(x)$ represent the incorrectly interleaved reconstructed image. The combination of (12.54) and (12.58) gives

$$\hat{\rho}_i(x) = \rho(x) + \frac{1 + e^{-i\pi(1-\alpha)}}{2}\rho_r\left(x + \frac{L}{2}\right) + \frac{1 + e^{i\pi(1-\alpha)}}{2}\rho_l\left(x - \frac{L}{2}\right)$$

$$-L/2 < x < L/2 \tag{12.59}$$

It is observed that, for $\alpha \neq 0$, the aliased information is not canceled by the addition of the two data sets. Furthermore, neither adding the magnitudes of the separate series nor taking the magnitude of the sum (12.59) eliminates aliasing.

Problem 12.9

Redo Fig. 12.12 for both the real and imaginary parts of all three images, $\hat{\rho}_i(x)$, $\hat{\rho}_e(x)$, and $\hat{\rho}_{o,i}(x)$ utilizing (12.54), (12.58), (12.59), and $\alpha = 0.5$. Comment on the amplitude of the ghosts relative to the original object. The object is the same boxcar distribution as in Fig. 12.12.

Another advantage of describing these images in terms of their right-side and left-side values is that the final image can be written in terms of matrix equations for the left- and right-sides of $\hat{\rho}_e$ and $\hat{\rho}_{o,i}$. This treatment gives a more manageable analytical approach to an arbitrary number of interleaves, and it also lends itself more readily to numerical computer work.

Consider a matrix representation for (12.59). As right-side values can be produced by $\rho_l(x - L/2)$, the right-side of the reconstructed image, in particular, can be written as

$$\hat{\rho}_r(x) = \hat{\rho}_{r_e}(x) + \hat{\rho}_{r_{o,i}}(x) \tag{12.60}$$

The even and odd components of the right-side of the reconstructed image can be written in matrix notation as

$$\begin{pmatrix} \hat{\rho}_{r_e}(x) \\ \hat{\rho}_{r_{o,i}}(x) \end{pmatrix} = \frac{1}{2} \begin{pmatrix} 1 & 1 \\ 1 & e^{i\pi(1-\alpha)} \end{pmatrix} \begin{pmatrix} \rho_r(x) \\ \rho_l\left(x - \frac{L}{2}\right) \end{pmatrix} \qquad 0 < x < \frac{L}{2} \qquad (12.61)$$

The right-side and left-side parts of $\rho(x)$ may now be found by inverting the matrix transformation in (12.61), yielding

$$\begin{pmatrix} \rho_r(x) \\ \rho_l\left(x - \frac{L}{2}\right) \end{pmatrix} = \frac{2}{(e^{i\pi(1-\alpha)} - 1)} \begin{pmatrix} e^{i\pi(1-\alpha)} & -1 \\ -1 & 1 \end{pmatrix} \begin{pmatrix} \hat{\rho}_{r_e}(x) \\ \hat{\rho}_{r_{o,i}}(x) \end{pmatrix} \qquad 0 < x < \frac{L}{2} \quad (12.62)$$

By translating $\rho_l(x - L/2)$ to $\rho_l(x)$, the original physical spin density is recovered.

When α is known, two images, $\hat{\rho}_e(x)$ and $\hat{\rho}_{o,i}(x)$, are reconstructed. This is accomplished by taking the full data set $s(k)$ and replacing all $s_{o,i}(k)$ points with zero to get the $s_e(k)$ data set and replacing all $s_e(k)$ points with zero to obtain the $s_{o,i}(k)$ data set, respectively. The resulting two images, both of them aliased in this case, are then processed using (12.62) to extract an unaliased image.

Problem 12.10

Using (12.62) and $\alpha = 0$, show that $\rho_r(x)$ and $\rho_l(x - L/2)$ turn out to give the correct right and left sides of $\rho(x)$, respectively. Hint: See (12.54) and (12.55).

Aliasing in the incorrectly interleaved case occurs simply because there are two different k-space step sizes. If this is extended to many different step sizes, the above methods can be generalized to multiple k-space interleaves. In certain sequences, the most efficiently implemented versions cover k-space in such a way that nonuniform samples in k-space are obtained, and this nonuniformity, together with any resulting aliasing, can be analyzed using multiple interleave formalisms. Problem 12.11 deals with such a generalization of the interleaved k-space sampling problem.

Problem 12.11

---

a) Consider a four-point interleaved problem (i.e., the case where every fourth point is collected in one experiment, and the entire k-space coverage is obtained after four experiments) where the four sampling functions are defined as

$$u_j(k) = \Delta k \sum_{m=-\infty}^{\infty} \delta(k - (4m + j)\Delta k) \qquad (12.63)$$

and $j = 0, 1, 2, 3$. Generalize the analysis carried out in the previous discussion to this case. Note that, in this case, the FOV must be divided into quarters for a similar analysis to be performed. Verify the following matrix equation in this case

$$\begin{pmatrix} \hat{\rho}_0(x) \\ \hat{\rho}_1(x) \\ \hat{\rho}_2(x) \\ \hat{\rho}_3(x) \end{pmatrix} = \frac{1}{4} \begin{pmatrix} 1 & 1 & 1 & 1 \\ 1 & i & -1 & -i \\ 1 & -1 & 1 & -1 \\ 1 & -i & -1 & i \end{pmatrix} \begin{pmatrix} \rho(x) \\ \rho(x - L/4) \\ \rho(x - L/2) \\ \rho(x - 3L/4) \end{pmatrix} \qquad \frac{L}{4} < x < \frac{L}{2}$$

$$(12.64)$$

b) Rewrite the 4×4 matrix in (a) for the case where sampling functions $1, 2, 3$ are shifted in k-space by $\alpha_1 \Delta k$, $\alpha_2 \Delta k$, and $\alpha_3 \Delta k$, respectively.

c) Qualitatively describe the effect on the image when α_1, α_2, and α_3 are all nonzero in terms of the aliasing and the noise present in the reconstructed image.

12.4.2　Aliasing from Digital-to-Analog Error in the Gradient Specification

The gradient step $\Delta G_y \equiv \Delta G$ for phase encoding required to give a large field-of-view can be sufficiently small that round-off errors result. Consider an example where $\Delta G = 12.5 \, \Delta G_{DAC,min}$ where $\Delta G_{DAC,min}$ is the smallest possible step size that the MR gradient amplifier can produce. The phase encoding table would lead to the series 12.5, 25, 37.5, 50, ... (in units of $\Delta G_{DAC,min}$), but, since only integer units are possible in the digital-to-analog conversion (DAC), the series 13, 25, 38, 50, ... is realized instead. In terms of gradient steps, the series would be characterized as $\Delta G'$, $2\Delta G$, $2\Delta G+\Delta G'$, $4\Delta G$, etc., where $\Delta G' = 13 \, \Delta G_{DAC,min}$. This is an example of the even and odd interleaving problem where, ignoring the change in units, the series corresponds to $\Delta k = 12.5 \, \Delta k_{DAC,min}$ and $\alpha \Delta k = -0.5 \, \Delta k_{DAC,min}$ in the earlier notation. Aliasing would arise from the indicated shift for nonzero α values.

Problem 12.12

Assume that the round-off error for a system is such that

$$\left(\frac{\Delta G_y}{\Delta G_{DAC,min}} \right) = \frac{15}{4} \qquad (12.65)$$

Answer the following questions.

a) What is α for the point where $G_y = \Delta G_y$?

b) One in how many points will be sampled at the correct location in k-space given the above error? The nonuniform sampling that occurs in this case varies periodically throughout k-space.

c) If there is no round-off error, then only one object will appear in the image (there will be no ghosting or aliasing). Based upon the sampling variations, how many repeated objects do you expect to see in the image? Hint: Review Prob. 12.11.

Suggested Reading

Sampling principles are addressed in detail in:

- R. N. Bracewell. *The Fourier Transform and its Applications.* McGraw Hill, New York, 1986.

- O. E. Brigham. *The Fast Fourier Transform.* Prentice-Hall, Englewood Cliffs, New Jersey, 1974.

- A. V. Oppenheim and R. W. Schafer. *Discrete-time Signal Processing.* Prentice-Hall, Englewood Cliffs, New Jersey, 1989.

- A. Papoulis. *The Fourier Integral and its Applications.* McGraw-Hill, New York, 1987.

Chapter 13

Filtering and Resolution in Fourier Transform Image Reconstruction

Chapter Contents

Summary: The point spread function introduced by reconstruction from limited Fourier data is established. The Gibbs ringing associated with truncated data is considered along with its reduction by image filtering. The spatial resolution of an image reconstruction method is formally defined and discussed. Partial Fourier data collection and image reconstruction of asymmetric k-space data are presented. Digital data truncation effects and methods to overcome them are also reviewed.

Introduction

Studying discrete Fourier transforms is only the initial step in developing an accurate MR image reconstruction. The effects of Fourier inversion from sampled and limited data ('filtered' data) are quantitatively modeled in terms of the 'point spread' or 'blur' function (Sec. 13.2).

The point spread function arises from the convolution of the Fourier transforms of the signal and the filters. One of the artifacts that arises from the presence of an oscillatory point spread function is Gibbs ringing which occurs at all step-like discontinuities in the object (Sec. 13.3). Spatial filtering is used to reduce Gibbs ringing at the expense of blurring the reconstructed image.

Spatial resolution of a given reconstruction method is also formally defined (Sec. 13.4). From this definition, it is shown that, when transverse relaxation effects during sampling can be neglected, the spatial resolution is described by the pixel size. When spatial filtering is used to reduce Gibbs ringing, the effective spatial resolution is degraded. Similarly, transverse decay (T_2^* related signal loss) during data sampling can reduce the spatial resolution. This signal loss acts as a low pass filter when the sampling points after the echo are used for partial Fourier image reconstruction (Sec. 13.5). When points before the echo are used, it acts as a high pass filter in k-space.

Zero filling is often used in partial Fourier image reconstruction (Sec. 13.6). A zero filled image can also be reconstructed from the original image with sub-voxel shifts, which can recover signal loss due to a point-like object in the image. Some criteria, approaches, and limitations of partial Fourier image reconstruction are discussed in Sec. 13.7. An object that has only a real part can be correctly reconstructed from the partial k-space data when at least half of k-space is acquired. For a complex object, an iterative procedure is presented to better reconstruct an estimate of the true object. Finally, the digital truncation of the k-space signal through an analog-to-digital converter (ADC) is introduced (Sec. 13.8). The dynamic range of the ADC has to be wide enough such that the information of small structures can be differentiated above the noise level in an image.

13.1   Review of Fourier Transform Image Reconstruction

In Ch. 12, the MR imaging experiment has been introduced as one where the data are discretely collected over a finite region of k-space, and an image is subsequently obtained by a discrete inverse Fourier transform of that data. Chapter 12 contained, in particular, an explanation of the necessary density of k-space sampling so that the image can be reconstructed without aliasing. All these discussions describe the simplest data collection strategies for a given object. In this section, the progress made so far on the image reconstruction problem is reviewed and summarized.

13.1.1   Fourier Encoding and Fourier Inversion

In Chs. 9 and 10, it was shown that the measured MR data are equivalent to a k-space representation of the excited magnetization of the sample. That is, 3D spatial encoding through magnetic field gradients leads to a signal which is a Fourier integral of the effective spin density

$$s(k_x, k_y, k_z) = \int \int \int dx\, dy\, dz\, \rho(x, y, z) e^{-i2\pi(k_x x + k_y y + k_z z)} \tag{13.1}$$

Such developments are referred to as *Fourier encoding* methods. The reconstruction method for finding $\rho(x, y, z)$ through the inverse Fourier integral

$$\rho(x, y, z) = \int \int \int dk_x \, dk_y \, dk_z \, s(k_x, k_y, k_z) e^{i2\pi(k_x x + k_y y + k_z z)} \tag{13.2}$$

is referred to as *Fourier inversion*.

13.1.2 Infinite Sampling and Fourier Series

Data measurement, as described in Ch. 12, is done by sampling the Fourier encoded data rather than by continuous monitoring, leading to discrete k-space coverage. When infinite k-space sampling is carried out, an inverse Fourier series replaces the continuous inverse Fourier transform. The 1D series[1] has been defined previously as $\hat{\rho}_\infty(x)$ and given by (12.4)

$$\hat{\rho}_\infty(x) = \Delta k \sum_{p=-\infty}^{\infty} s(p\Delta k) e^{i2\pi p \Delta k x} \tag{13.3}$$

For example, the reconstructed $\hat{\rho}_\infty(x)$ converges, in the absence of aliasing, to $\rho(x)$ in the mean squared sense when the object $\rho(x)$ has no step discontinuities, and to $(\rho(x_0^+) + \rho(x_0^-))/2$ when a step discontinuity occurs at $x = x_0$.

13.1.3 Limited-Fourier Imaging and Aliasing

Time limitations restrict the number of data samples collected per readout (N_x), as well as the number of phase encoding (N_y) and partition encoding (N_z) steps. With only partial coverage of k-space, the inversion problem is called a *limited-Fourier inversion* problem. The 1D reconstructed image, defined as $\hat{\rho}(x)$ in (12.21), is the truncated version of (13.3)

$$\hat{\rho}(x) = \Delta k \sum_{p=-n}^{n-1} s(p\Delta k) e^{i2\pi p \Delta k x} \tag{13.4}$$

Now it is the theory of discrete Fourier transforms that is relevant. The transform is over $N = 2n$ data points in k-space, with individual widths Δk for each of the N points. The total width W of k-space coverage is

$$W = N\Delta k = 2n\Delta k = k_{max} - k_{min} + \Delta k \tag{13.5}$$

We recall that (13.4) follows (13.3) in exhibiting the periodicity when $x \to x + 1/\Delta k$. Therefore, to avoid aliasing, the intervals Δk must satisfy the Nyquist criterion

$$\Delta k \equiv \frac{1}{L} \leq \frac{1}{A} \tag{13.6}$$

That is, the FOV, L, must be greater than the physical size A of the object (more generally, the region to which the experiment is sensitive).

---

[1]As in previous chapters, often we restrict ourselves to one dimension. Thanks to the separability of the discrete Fourier transform, the image reconstruction in the other two dimensions can be assumed to be carried out independently and in a similar fashion.

13.1.4   Signal Series and Spatial Resolution

The other member of the discrete transform pair (12.34) is the finite series for the signal
over truncated and discretized spatial positions

$$s(k) = \Delta x \sum_{q=-n}^{n-1} \hat{\rho}(q\Delta x)e^{-i2\pi k q \Delta x} \tag{13.7}$$

The evaluations of $\hat{\rho}(x)$ are in terms of the spatial step size Δx,

$$\Delta x = \frac{L}{N} = \frac{1}{N\Delta k} = \frac{1}{W} \tag{13.8}$$

Equation (13.8) provides a starting point in the discussion of 'spatial resolution,' or the
size of the smallest feature that can be measured for a given object. A familiar aspect of
Fourier analysis is the need for large values of k in order to describe smaller and smaller
spatial features; this is reflected in the combination of (13.5) and (13.8). Given the linear
dependence of k on the applied gradient, it follows that an increase in gradient strength
implies a smaller value for Δx. The effects of the size of W on image quality are considered
in Sec. 13.4.

There are other important factors in the determination of the best possible spatial resolution, such as the signal-to-noise ratio, which is the subject of Ch. 15. The filtering of data
is fundamentally connected to spatial resolution and is introduced in Sec. 13.2. These issues
notwithstanding, a naive lower limit on Δx is instructive, especially in comparison with the
more realistic estimates addressed later in the chapter. This is considered in the following
problem.

Problem 13.1

What is the best resolution Δx that can be expected from proton imaging for
a read gradient of 20 mT/m, without regard to signal-to-noise? Assume that
the sampling time is limited by the intrinsic spin-spin relaxation time, taking a
representative value for T_2 of 50 ms. Investigate the change in your answer for
the largest read gradient strength in commercial use.

13.2   Filters and Point Spread Functions

In this section, a framework for quantitatively understanding the effects of sampling and
truncation in terms of 'filters' and their associated Fourier transforms is developed. *A k-
space filter[2] is any function $H(k)$ that multiplies the k-space MRI data. The inverse Fourier
transform of a k-space filter is defined to be the associated point spread function $h(x)$. The*

---

[2]For consistent notation, an x-space filter, such as that already introduced in Sec. 12.3, is referred to
as $H(x)$. The caveat again arises that $H(k)$ and $H(x)$ are generic labels and there is no implied relation
between them.

reconstructed image $\hat{\rho}(x)$ may then be found by convolution of $h(x)$ with $\rho(x)$. The convolution operation is a convenient procedure for the investigation of any 'blurring' that occurs due to the filter, as noted in the last chapter. The imaging artifacts created by different filters, such as truncation and sampling, are considered below.

An easy way to understand the effect of a filter is to look at the simple example of $\rho(x) = \delta(x)$. In this case, $\hat{\rho}(x)$ will be equal to the Fourier transform of the filter (hence the name, 'point spread function'), since convolution of a function with $\delta(x)$ returns the function.[3] The reconstructed image will now have finite values at locations other than the origin; it has been smeared or 'blurred' by the effect of the filter and the reconstructed image is not equivalent to the physical spin density. This example gives insight into how a filter will affect an arbitrary image, since any object spin density can be described as a sum of individual spins or delta functions. As an image of a delta function produced by the filter, the point spread function is also called the 'impulse response function.'

13.2.1 Point Spread Due to Truncation

Truncation of data is equivalent to saying that $s(k)$ has been filtered by the rect function. Suppose that the k-space data are collected continuously, but only from $-n\Delta k$ to $(n-1)\Delta k$, the limits in (13.4). Then the collected data are said to be truncated, or *windowed*, by the filter $H_w(k)$ given by the rect function in (12.18)

$$H_w(k) \equiv \text{rect}\left(\frac{k + \frac{1}{2}\Delta k}{W}\right) \tag{13.9}$$

The collected data are computed by

$$s_w(k) = s(k)H_w(k) \tag{13.10}$$

where $s(k)$ is the untruncated continuous Fourier transform of $\rho(x)$. The reconstructed image from this data is

$$\begin{aligned} \hat{\rho}_w(x) &= \mathcal{F}^{-1}\left(s(k)H_w(k)\right) \\ &= \rho(x) * h_w(x) \end{aligned} \tag{13.11}$$

where $h_w(x)$ is defined to be the inverse Fourier transform, or the point spread function, of $H_w(k)$. As used in (12.23),

$$h_w(x) = W\text{sinc}(\pi W x)e^{-i\pi\Delta k\,x} \tag{13.12}$$

The blurring due to the convolution of the spin density with (13.12) has been described earlier in Sec. 12.2. In the present language, the function $h_w(x)$ spreads the information from each point in the image and maps spin information from a range of physical locations into each position x. That is, the reconstructed image $\hat{\rho}_w(x)$ is corrupted by information from its neighbors. Attention is now directed to include the effects of discrete sampling.

---

[3]From Sec. 12.1.1, we recall that the convolution of $f(x)$ with $\delta(x - x_0)$ is equal to $f(x - x_0)$.

13.2.2   Point Spread for Truncated and Sampled Data

The modeling of both windowing and discrete sampling is through the product (12.18) of a rect function with the sampling function,

$$H_{ws}(k) \equiv \Delta k \, \text{rect}\left(\frac{k + \frac{1}{2}\Delta k}{W}\right) \sum_{p=-\infty}^{\infty} \delta(k - p\Delta k) = \Delta k \sum_{p=-n}^{n-1} \delta(k - p\Delta k) \qquad (13.13)$$

The measured data are the finite set of $s(p\Delta k)$ arising as coefficients in the distribution $s_m(k)$ given in (12.20)

$$s_m(k) \equiv s_{ws}(k) = s(k)H_{ws}(k) = \Delta k \sum_{p=-n}^{n-1} s(p\Delta k)\delta(k - p\Delta k) \qquad (13.14)$$

From (13.13) and (13.14), the Fourier inversion yields the image (12.21)

$$\hat{\rho}(x) \equiv \hat{\rho}_{ws}(x) = \int_{-\infty}^{\infty} dk \, s_m(k)e^{i2\pi kx} = \Delta k \sum_{p=-n}^{n-1} s(p\Delta k)e^{i2\pi p\Delta kx} \qquad (13.15)$$

The original notation had no subscript for the finitely sampled reconstructed spin density. Alternatively, $\hat{\rho}(x)$ can be expressed as the convolution

$$\hat{\rho}(x) = \rho(x) * h_{ws}(x) \qquad (13.16)$$

The inverse Fourier transform $h_{ws}(x)$, or the point spread function in the finite Fourier inversion case, is found simply by replacing $s(k)$ by unity in (13.15). The result is

$$h_{ws}(x) = \Delta k \sum_{p=-n}^{n-1} e^{i2\pi p\Delta kx} \qquad (13.17)$$

The explicit summation of (13.17) is given in Prob. 13.2, and the following simplified expression is obtained

$$h_{ws}(x) = W \frac{\text{sinc}(\pi W x)}{\text{sinc}(\pi \Delta kx)}e^{-i\pi \Delta k\,x} \qquad (13.18)$$

Problem 13.2

---

a) Derive the identity

$$\sum_{p=-n}^{n-1} x^p = x^{-n}\frac{1 - x^{2n}}{1 - x} \qquad (13.19)$$

b) Derive (13.18) from (13.17).

c) Show that the phase factor $e^{-i\pi x\Delta k}$ is eliminated by symmetrizing the sum from $-n$ to n, rather than from $-n$ to $n-1$.

As in the continuous case, the point spread function $h_{ws}(x)$ creates a blurred version of $\rho(x)$ to yield $\hat{\rho}(x)$. The primary difference between $h_w(x)$ and $h_{ws}(x)$ is that the latter also leads to aliasing, or overlapping, of the images corresponding to the blurring of the spatially repeated images into one another. However, while $h_w(x)$ only includes the effect of truncation, it accounts for most of the blur in an image.

13.2.3 Point Spread for Additional Filters

Other factors that modify the MRI signal may also be modeled as filters. They include the relaxation exponentials, involving T_2 or T_2^*, which change the magnitude of the signal. Furthermore, it is sometimes useful to modify the data after collection (i.e., 'post-process' the data) in order to modify the 'blurring' caused by $h_{ws}(k)$, minimize other artifacts, or enhance certain image features. This is often done by applying another filter to the data.

The filters in this text will be denoted by $H_{filter}(k)$ where the generic subscript *filter* will be the name of the specific filter under discussion. The same subscript will be added to the reconstruction spin density or image, so that, for several filters, we would write $\hat{\rho}_{filter\,1,filter\,2,\cdots}$. The standard windowing and sampling filters will be left understood, consistent with the previous usage in representing the signal (13.14) and the reconstructed image (13.15). The signal obtained by the addition of one filter to the standard windowing and sampling can be written in a variety of ways

$$
\begin{aligned}
\hat{s}_{m,filter}(k) &= s_m(k) \cdot H_{filter}(k) = s(k) \cdot H_{ws}(k) \cdot H_{filter}(k) \\
&\equiv s(k) \cdot H_{ws,filter}(k)
\end{aligned}
\tag{13.20}
$$

where $H_{ws,filter}(k)$ is shorthand for all three filters applied to the data. As a result, the reconstructed image can be written in terms of various convolutions

$$
\begin{aligned}
\tilde{\rho}_{filter}(x) &= \hat{\rho}(x) * h_{filter}(x) = \rho(x) * h_{ws}(x) * h_{filter}(x) \\
&\equiv \rho(x) * h_{ws,filter}(x)
\end{aligned}
\tag{13.21}
$$

Throughout the remainder of this text, filters will be considered in terms of their own point spread functions $h_{filter}(x)$, or of the combined point spread function $h_{ws,filter}(x)$ for all filters. Examples of such k-space filters are treated throughout the remainder of this chapter.

13.3 Gibbs Ringing

It is well-known that *Gibbs ringing* accompanies Fourier series representations of functions with step discontinuities. The presence of any bright objects or sharp transitions from one tissue to another can lead to the Gibbs effect as an artifact in MRI. This is particularly serious if it mimics certain disease states. In the present section, Gibbs ringing is introduced, illustrations are provided, and the reduction of the Gibbs effect by filtering is discussed.

13.3.1 Gibbs Overshoot and Undershoot

In the numerical evaluation of a Fourier series, and especially in the finite series defined in the discrete Fourier transform, Gibbs ringing arises as an oscillating overshoot and undershoot in the immediate neighborhood of a step discontinuity. The overshoot (above the top of the step) and undershoot (below the bottom of the step) have the property that, as the total number N of terms in the series tends to infinity, both the peak overshoot and the peak undershoot approach a limiting value of approximately 9% of the step height. Using the reconstructed spin density as an example, and assuming that a step discontinuity occurs at $x = x_0$,

$$\lim_{N \to \infty} \left| \hat{\rho}(x_0^{\pm}) - \rho(x_0^{\pm}) \right| \simeq 0.09 \left| \rho(x_0^{+}) - \rho(x_0^{-}) \right| \tag{13.22}$$

where $x_0^{\pm} \equiv \lim_{\epsilon \to 0^+} (x_0 \pm \epsilon)$. A derivation of the '9%' result employing the convolution (13.16) is presented next. This derivation also is useful for showing how other properties of Gibbs ringing may be analyzed with the convolution representation. An alternative demonstration using Fourier series is presented in Prob. 13.3.

Suppose we have a function $f(x)$ which is continuous at all points except at $x = 0$, where it has a step discontinuity. With a step amplitude of $|f(0^+) - f(0^-)|$ at that discontinuity, $f(x)$ can be represented by

$$f(x) = f_c(x) + (f(0^+) - f(0^-))\Theta(x) \tag{13.23}$$

where $f_c(x)$ is a continuous function and $\Theta(x)$ is the by-now familiar Heaviside step-function. Since the Gibbs effect originates from windowing the data, a window filter is assumed to be applied to the k-space representation of $f(x)$. For convenience, consider a symmetric window with width W

$$H_w^{sym}(k) = \mathrm{rect}(k/W) \tag{13.24}$$

which implies that the reconstructed image is given by the convolution

$$\hat{f}(x) = f(x) * h_w^{sym}(x) \tag{13.25}$$

where the symmetric point spread function is (13.12) without the phase factor

$$h_w^{sym}(x) = W\mathrm{sinc}(\pi W x) \tag{13.26}$$

The next step is to compare the values of the reconstructed function at the two different positions, $x = 0$ and $x = \Delta x$, in the limit $\Delta x \to 0$ or $W = 1/\Delta x \to \infty$. The identity (9.29) gives

$$\lim_{W \to \infty} h_w^{sym}(x) = \delta(x) \tag{13.27}$$

Equations (13.23), (13.25), (13.27), and (12.7) combine to give

$$\lim_{W \to \infty} \hat{f}(x) = f_c(x) + (f(0^+) - f(0^-)) \lim_{W \to \infty} \int_0^{\infty} h_w^{sym}(x - x')dx' \tag{13.28}$$

Before taking the limit, the integral in (13.28) can be reduced to

$$\begin{aligned}
\int_0^{\infty} h_w^{sym}(x - x')dx' &= \int_{-\infty}^{x} h_w^{sym}(X)dX \qquad \text{where } X \equiv x - x' \\
&= \frac{1}{\pi} \int_{-\infty}^{\pi W x} \frac{\sin y}{y}dy \\
&= \frac{1}{2} + \frac{1}{\pi}Si(\pi W x) \tag{13.29}
\end{aligned}$$

where $Si(x)$ is the 'Sine integral' defined as

$$Si(x) \equiv \int_0^{x} \frac{\sin y}{y}dy \tag{13.30}$$

and $Si(-\infty) = -\pi/2.$[4] With $Si(0) = 0$ and $Si(\pi) \simeq 1.8519$,

$$
\begin{aligned}
\lim_{W \to \infty} \hat{f}(0) &= f(0^-) + \frac{1}{2}(f(0^+) - f(0^-)) \\
&= \frac{1}{2}(f(0^-) + f(0^+))
\end{aligned}
\tag{13.31}
$$

To estimate the Gibbs ringing effect, we take the limit of $W \to \infty$ (recall $W = 1/\Delta x$)

$$
\begin{aligned}
\lim_{W \to \infty} \hat{f}(\Delta x) &\simeq f_c(\Delta x) + (f(0^+) - f(0^-))\left(\frac{1}{2} + \frac{1.8519}{\pi}\right) \\
&\simeq f(\Delta x) + 0.09(f(0^+) - f(0^-))
\end{aligned}
\tag{13.32}
$$

noting $f(\Delta x) = f_c(\Delta x) + (f(0^+) - f(0^-))$. In a similar fashion, it can be shown that $\lim_{W \to \infty} \hat{f}(-\Delta x) = f(-\Delta x) - 0.09(f(0^+) - f(0^-))$.

Problem 13.3

This problem provides an alternate demonstration of the Gibbs ringing artifact. Consider a periodic function $f(x) = \text{rect}(x/A)$ with its two discontinuities at $x = \pm A/2$ and with a period of $L = 2A$.

   a) Decompose $f(x)$ into a cosine Fourier series and investigate the Gibbs ringing at one of the discontinuities, say $A/2 + \Delta x$, by numerical evaluation of the first N terms with $A = N\Delta x/2$ and $N > 128$. The sum of the Fourier series from the first N terms leads to the 9% overshoot and undershoot peaks, and the distance of these peaks from the discontinuity is proportional to $1/N$ for large N. The latter fact indicates the invariance property for Gibbs ringing as discussed in the text.

   b) Also comment on the possible increase in the effective amplitude of the Gibbs ringing when these two edges are at some separation which leads to a coherent addition of the ringing. Hint: Look ahead at discussions on page 276 and Fig. 13.3b in particular.

13.3.2   Gibbs Oscillation Frequency

The above demonstration makes it clear that, if N is large and $N \to 2N$, the peak-to-peak difference in the ringing is invariant. However, the peaks of the overshoot and undershoot move half the distance closer to the discontinuity than before. For an infinite Fourier series, the oscillations are thereby squeezed into an infinitesimal physical region. For a finite Fourier series (such as in the discrete Fourier transform), the oscillations have a finite width. In particular, an invariance property of Gibbs ringing can be seen from the expression (13.18)

---

[4]See also (9.31).

for $h_{ws}(x)$. For a fixed FOV and $N \to 2N$, we have $W \to 2W$ and $\Delta x = 1/W \to \Delta x/2$. More generally, the product $Wx = Wq\Delta x = q$ depends only on the pixel number q. Thus the oscillations in the $\text{sinc}(\pi Wx)$ factor in the numerator[5] of (13.18), which are responsible for the Gibbs effect, scale with the pixel size. The filter is effectively invariant in that it is a function of pixel number only in $\hat{\rho}(x)$ from (13.16).

This property of invariance for Gibbs ringing is also illustrated in Prob. 13.3. Both properties are shown in Fig. 13.1.

Problem 13.4

Gibbs ringing can occur from a discontinuity in magnitude or phase. Investigate the effects of finite sampling for $f(x) = \text{rect}(x/L)e^{i\phi(x)}$ where a phase $\phi(x) = 0$ for $x \leq 0$ and $\phi(x) = \pi/2$ for $x > 0$. Find the Fourier transform of $f(x)/L$ and then use a discrete inverse Fourier transform to reconstruct the image. Assume $k = q\Delta k$ where $L\Delta k = 1$ and q is from -128 to $+127$.

13.3.3   Reducing Gibbs Ringing by Filtering

Gibbs ringing can seriously degrade an image and its interpretation. Increasing N for a fixed FOV alleviates the problem in view of the fact that the spatial distance over which the ringing propagates is reduced. Hence, running a scan twice with two different values of N can help determine whether or not an object is a Gibbs artifact (see Fig. 13.1).

There may be insufficient time, however, to double the number of scans whenever artifacts appear. A different remedy is the use of an additional filter to smooth out the image, retrospectively evaluate, or post-process the data. If the data set is multiplied by a function which vanishes, along with its first derivative, at $k = \pm k_{max}$, it is said to have been apodized. Again, for convenience, k-space is filtered symmetrically, with $W = 2k_{max}$. For example, if $s(k)$ is multiplied by

$$H_{Hanning}(k) = \frac{1 + \cos\left(\frac{2\pi k}{W}\right)}{2} = \cos^2\left(\frac{\pi k}{W}\right) \tag{13.33}$$

it has been apodized with a *Hanning filter*. If $k \to \pm k_{max}$, then $2\pi k/W \to \pm\pi$, and it is verified that $H_{Hanning}(k) \to 0$ and $H'_{Hanning}(k) \to 0$. The inverse Fourier transform of $H_{Hanning}(k)$ easily follows from its decomposition into exponentials,

$$h_{Hanning}(x) = \frac{1}{2}\delta(x) + \frac{1}{4}(\delta(x - \Delta x) + \delta(x + \Delta x)) \tag{13.34}$$

The corresponding filtered reconstructed spin density is also simple to determine

$$\begin{aligned} \hat{\rho}_{Hanning}(x) &= h_{Hanning}(x) * \hat{\rho}(x) \\ &= \frac{1}{4}\hat{\rho}(x - \Delta x) + \frac{1}{2}\hat{\rho}(x) + \frac{1}{4}\hat{\rho}(x + \Delta x) \end{aligned} \tag{13.35}$$

It is seen that this k-space filter corresponds to an 'averaging' in the image domain.

---

[5]The argument, or spatial frequency, of the sinc function in the denominator is reduced by a factor of N, in comparison with that of the numerator.

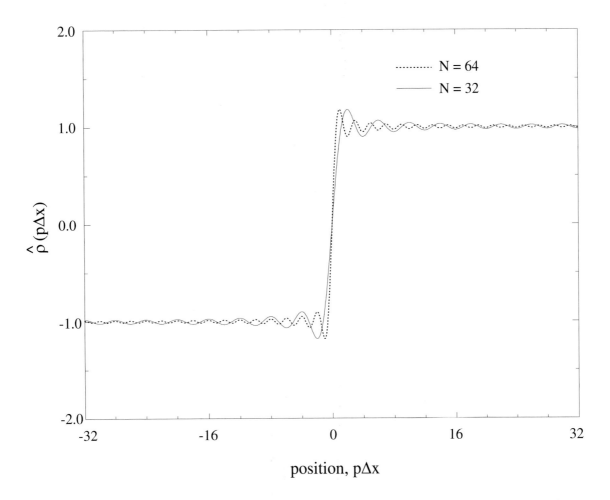

Fig. 13.1: Gibbs oscillations resulting from the convolution of a step discontinuity with the point spread function associated with finite and discrete sampling in k-space. The curves are displayed on a fixed field-of-view with the $N = 32$ case interpolated to $N = 64$. For large N, the amplitude of the truncation artifact remains invariant as a function of pixel number. The oscillations, however, increase in spatial frequency, with a scale set by the resolution.

Convolution Masks

Since images are generally presented as pixel maps, the images and the point spread function of filters may be specified discretely and indexed by integers. In this representation, a 2D image, for example, is a 2D matrix of numbers. A 1D filter such as $h(x)$ is represented by a 1D vector that is usually referred to as a *convolution mask*. The physical dimensions are added separately as scales.

The Hanning filter result (13.35) may be rewritten as

$$
\begin{aligned}
\hat{\rho}_{Hanning}(q\Delta x) &= \sum_r m_{Hanning,r}(q)\hat{\rho}(r\Delta x) \\
&= \frac{1}{4}\hat{\rho}\left((q-1)\Delta x\right) + \frac{1}{2}\hat{\rho}(q\Delta x) + \frac{1}{4}\hat{\rho}\left((q+1)\Delta x\right) \qquad (13.36)
\end{aligned}
$$

where the Hanning three-point mask has been defined by

$$
m_{Hanning,r}(q) = \begin{cases} 1/4 & r = q - 1 \\ 1/2 & r = q \\ 1/4 & r = q + 1 \\ 0 & \text{otherwise} \end{cases} \tag{13.37}
$$

The Hanning mask acts only on the pixel q under consideration and its two immediate neighbors. Since masks are specified by a vector of length equaling the number of affected neighborhood pixels, $h_{Hanning}(x)$ is said to be represented by a vector of length 3.

The number 3 for the Hanning mask vector length is related to the requirement that the function and its first derivative vanish at the maximum k values. It leads to smoothing of oscillations due to sharp features in the data. In the convolution picture, Gibbs ringing is understood by the oscillations from one pixel to the next produced, in symmetric windowing, by the function

$$
h_w^{sym}(x) = W \text{sinc}(\pi W x) \tag{13.38}
$$

The averaging over three neighboring pixels implied by (13.36) reduces much of the ringing, as illustrated in Fig. 13.2.

13.4   Spatial Resolution in MRI

The spatial resolution of an imaging method refers to the smallest resolvable distance between two different objects, or two different features of the same object. The definition for this distance is subject, however, to the choice of object, the limitations on measurements, psychological matters, and more. It is recalled that the point spread function can be used to quantify the spread or blur due to the reconstruction method. Indeed, the point spread function for a perfect experiment with infinite data could be described by a delta function. The convolution with a delta function yields a perfect reconstruction[6] with vanishing voxel size. In a real experiment, a nonzero spatial resolution may be defined in terms of a point spread function.

A first definition of spatial resolution may be chosen to be the area under $h_{filter}(x)$, for an arbitrary imaging method with a point spread function $h_{filter}(x)$, divided by the value of the filter at the origin:

$$
\text{spatial resolution of filter} \equiv \Delta x_{filter} \equiv \text{`blur' of filter} = \frac{1}{h_{filter}(0)} \int_{-\infty}^{\infty} dx\, h_{filter}(x)
$$
$$
= \frac{H_{filter}(0)}{h_{filter}(0)} \tag{13.39}
$$

This gives an effective measure of the spread or width of the point spread function.[7] For a boxcar function, for example, whose height is $h_{filter}(0)$, Δx_{filter} is its width. In general, it

---

[6]The reader is warned about ambiguities in the language used to describe resolution. Better or improved or 'higher' resolution means smaller or lower or decreased resolvable distances. Worse or 'lower' resolution means larger or increased distances.

[7]As indicated in the equation, the spatial resolution Δx_{filter} is also called the 'blur' of the given set of filters.

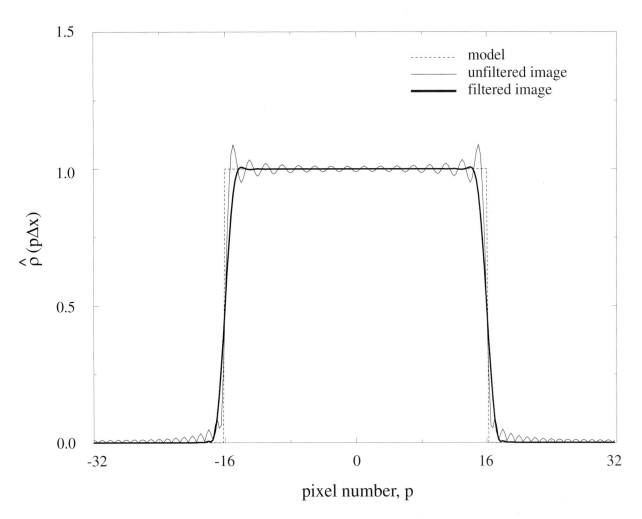

Fig. 13.2: The model object is a rect function. The reconstructed unfiltered image is obtained by windowing and sampling (DFT image reconstruction). The filtered image is found by apodization with the Hanning filter. The Gibbs ringing is dramatically reduced after filtering but at the expense of a loss of resolution.

may be assumed that the filter has a global maximum at the origin, $H(k) \le H(0)$. In those cases where distributions, such as delta functions, are used, the spatial resolution may need to be defined as a limit.

Problem 13.5

Find the spatial resolution $\Delta x_{Gaussian}$ associated with a Gaussian filter

$$h_{filter}(x) = e^{-ax^2}$$

for a real constant $a > 0$.

In the discrete Fourier transform reconstruction case, $h_{ws}(x)$ is periodic with period L and the definition (13.39) would lead to an infinite width. Consider, instead, the spatial resolution of the windowed and sampled MR image to be defined in terms of the area within the FOV

$$\Delta x_{MRI,filter} \equiv \text{MR spatial resolution with filter} = \frac{1}{h_{ws,filter}(0)} \int_{-L/2}^{L/2} dx \, h_{ws,filter}(x)$$
(13.40)

This definition is used to estimate the smallest separation between two objects that can be determined with a standard MRI reconstruction with additional filters.

The integration in (13.40) is readily carried out, in the absence of an additional filter, utilizing the representation (13.17) and giving

$$
\begin{aligned}
\Delta x_{MRI} &\equiv \text{window and sampling resolution with no additional filtering} \\
&= \frac{\sum_{p=-n}^{n-1} \int_{-L/2}^{L/2} dx \, e^{i2\pi p \Delta k x}}{\sum_{p'=-n}^{n-1} 1} \\
&= \frac{1}{2n} \sum_{p=-n}^{n-1} L \delta_{p0} \\
&= \frac{1}{2n\Delta k} = \frac{1}{W} = \Delta x = \text{the Fourier pixel size}
\end{aligned}
$$
(13.41)

According to the definition (13.40), the smallest distance that can be resolved with a discrete Fourier transform reconstruction is exactly the same as the 'Fourier pixel size' Δx already introduced in Ch. 12 and in Sec. 13.1.4.

Spatial Resolution and k-Space Coverage

The broader the coverage in k-space, the better the MR spatial resolution. This well-known statement follows from (13.41) and brings up the relationship of k-space coverage to the reconstruction of objects with structures over different scales. Consider 2D images with sampling windows of variable sizes $N_x \times N_y$ and fixed FOV. Increases in N_x and N_y lead to decreases in Δx and Δy, respectively. The reduced voxel size (in this case, a pixel size) should lead to improved or higher resolution.

An example is presented in Fig. 13.3 involving a 'resolution phantom,' where a hierarchy of different sized 'holes' (regions with no signal in the MR images) are studied under changes in the voxel size.[8] The results of reconstructing images from windows of size 64 × 64, 128 × 128, 256 × 256, and 512 × 512 with a fixed FOV of 256 mm are shown. The coverage of a larger window in k-space improves the definition of the small holes or 'resolution elements.' In particular, the Gibbs ringing pattern becomes less noticeable as the voxel size decreases. An additional effect to be discussed in Ch. 15 is that a halving of voxel size in each direction by doubling the sampling points leads to a $\sqrt{2}$ loss in signal-to-noise ratio. An interesting

---

[8]This resolution phantom has a series of parallel plastic cylinders embedded in water. Any resulting MR image of this phantom when taken in a plane perpendicular to the long axis of these cylinders leads to regions with no signal, i.e., the 'holes' referred to in this discussion.

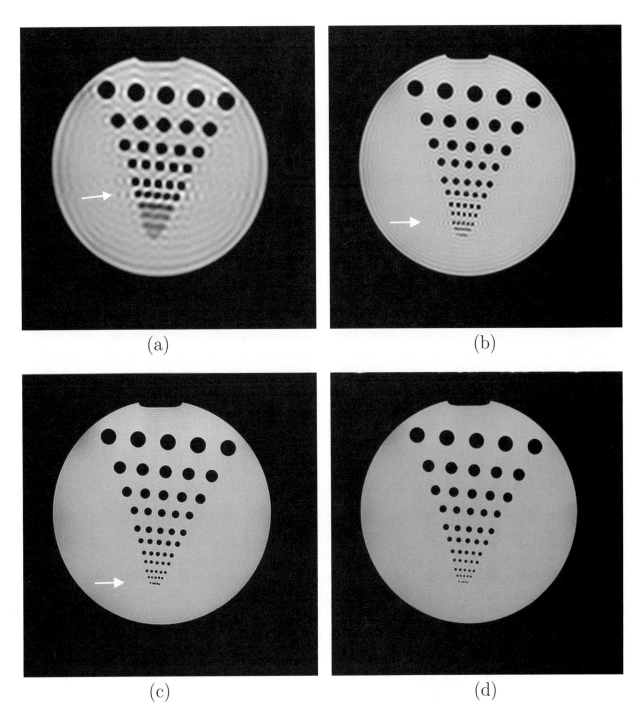

Fig. 13.3: Resolution phantom images reconstructed from filtering a 512×512 matrix size acquisition in a fixed FOV of 256 mm. The reconstructions are from the reduction of the full window down to a (a) 64×64 window, (b) 128×128 window, (c) 256×256 window, and also the full (d) 512×512 window. The improved resolution and reduction in Gibbs ringing effects are evident for each increase in the window size, which implies a decrease in the pixel size $\Delta x \Delta y$.

enhancement of the Gibbs artifact occurs when two or more edges from a series of objects in a row come close enough together that the ringing from each edge coherently combines with that from other edges. In this instance, the ringing extends significantly past the edge of the outermost object (see arrows in Figs. 13.3a through 13.3c). The row where this occurs shifts as a function of resolution.

Information Content in k-Space

The improvement in spatial resolution brought about by the inclusion of larger k-space values brings up a more general point. Pictures in k-space show the spatial frequency components necessary for the Fourier representation of the physical spin density function. Low spatial frequency (k-space) components are needed for spatially slowly changing parts of the object, while the high spatial frequency (k-space) components should be included to better depict small structures whose size is on the order of the voxel size. Small features of particular interest in MRI are tissue boundaries.

The relationship of regions in k-space to different scales may be better understood by considering two extreme limits: a 1D object filling the entire FOV and a 1D object whose size equals Δx. For a constant profile, the first object maps to an 'impulse' at $k = 0$; see Prob. 13.6. More generally, data points in the neighborhood containing the $k = 0$ point are needed to represent such slowly varying structures in the object. An example of the information content in the 'low frequency components' was demonstrated in Fig. 13.3a, where the 512-point data set was truncated down to 64 points (effectively, a low pass filter was applied in each direction). Evidently, almost all information about the large structures is already contained in the central $1/64^{th}$ fraction of the 512×512 data set.

Problem 13.6

In this problem, some very familiar calculations are revisited in the context of the information content of k-space. It is helpful to recall that sampling and filtering in k-space correspond to processing the analog signal obtained from the continuous Fourier transform of the spin density. To reconstruct the image from the sampled signal data, a discrete Fourier transform is analyzed.

a) Find the analog signal for a constant spin density filling the FOV, where $\rho(x) = \rho_0 \operatorname{rect}(x/L)$. Show that sampling this signal at intervals of $p\Delta k$ (Δk is determined by the Nyquist criterion) for any integer p gives zero except at $p = 0$.

b) Find the sinc function that represents the analog signal for a constant spin density occupying only one voxel, $\rho(x) = \rho_0 \operatorname{rect}(x/\Delta x)$. Discuss the implications of the first zero crossing of the sinc function. How many pixels wide would the object have to be so that the first zero crossing of the sinc function is at the edge of k-space?

The small resolution elements, on the other hand, are indistinguishable in Fig. 13.3a because of severe blurring, in contrast to the high resolution image of Fig. 13.3d. An object with constant profile whose size equals Δx has a sinc function for its k-space representation, whose first zero crossing occurs only at $\pm 2k_{max}$; this is also expanded upon in Prob. 13.6. While this means that all collected k-space points contain some information about such small objects, the high spatial frequency components are especially necessary. The image in Fig. 13.4b has been obtained by setting the central part of k-space to zero (the high pass filtering depicted in Fig. 13.4a), the complement to data used for reconstructing the image shown in Fig. 13.3a. The edges of the hierarchy of small holes and of the disk itself are the only features remaining in the image.

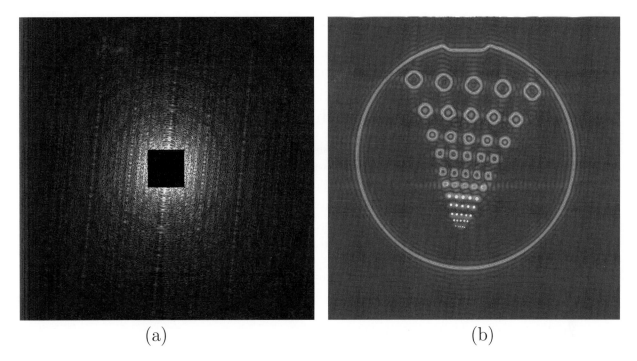

(a)   (b)

Fig. 13.4: A result of high pass filtering, in k-space, of the same imaging object as in Fig. 13.3. (a) The removal of a central portion of k-space signal data (a center square that is $1/64^{th}$ of the 512×512 window has been replaced by zeros). (b) The corresponding reconstructed image is left with only the edges (i.e., the rapid spatial variations) and the small resolution elements highlighted. Although the image is similar to the 1D derivative image in Fig. 11.6, it is more akin to a 2D derivative image since a 2D k-space filter was used.

13.4.1   Resolution after Additional Filtering of the Data

The addition of another filter to the windowing and sampling of data implies the multiplication of the signal by both $H_{ws}(k)$ and $H_{filter}(k)$ in k-space. From (13.13), it is easy to see that the corresponding point spread function $h_{ws,filter}(x)$ may be expressed by

$$h_{ws,filter}(x) = \Delta k \sum_{p=-n}^{n-1} H_{filter}(p\Delta k)e^{i2\pi p\Delta kx} \qquad (13.42)$$

Starting with (13.40) and (13.42), it is also simple to follow the steps in (13.41) to obtain

$$
\begin{aligned}
\Delta x_{MRI,filter} &\equiv \text{MR spatial resolution with filter} \\
&= \frac{H_{filter}(0)}{\Delta k \sum\limits_{p'=-n}^{n-1} H_{filter}(p'\Delta k)}
\end{aligned}
\tag{13.43}
$$

It may be assumed that the global maximum of the k-space filters occurs at $k = 0$, i.e., $H_{filter}(0) \geq H_{filter}(k)$ for all k since these filters generally are required to be low pass filters. The result (13.43) then leads to

$$
\Delta x_{MRI,filter} \geq \frac{1}{2n\Delta k} \equiv \frac{1}{W} = \Delta x
\tag{13.44}
$$

In consequence, the resolution with additional filtering is worse than the resolution from direct discrete inverse Fourier transform reconstruction alone.

13.4.2   Other Measures of Resolution

There is a separate approach to defining $\Delta x_{filter\,1,filter\,2,\cdots}$ that does not require a calculation such as that in (13.40). Instead, it is based on the intrinsic blurring of a point isochromat created by the filter. Imagine two point objects affected by a filter $H_{filter}(k)$ with a point spread function $h_{filter}(x)$. Consider the signal due to the two objects, A (with magnitude a) at $x = 0$ and B (with magnitude b) at $x = x_B$, as shown in Fig. 13.5. Since the image at x_B will be affected by A because of the filter blur, the contribution at the point x_B due to A is

$$
\begin{aligned}
\hat{\rho}_{filter}^{due\,to\,A}(x_B) &= a\delta(x) * h_{filter}(x)|_{x=x_B} \\
&= a \cdot h_{filter}(x_B)
\end{aligned}
\tag{13.45}
$$

The contribution at x_B due to object B itself is

$$
\begin{aligned}
\hat{\rho}_{filter}^{due\,to\,B}(x_B) &= b\delta(x - x_B) * h_{filter}(x)|_{x=x_B} \\
&= b \cdot h_{filter}(0)
\end{aligned}
\tag{13.46}
$$

Thus, the final reconstructed image at x_B is given by

$$
\hat{\rho}_{filter}^{two\,spins}(x_B) = b \cdot h_{filter}(0) + a \cdot h_{filter}(x_B)
\tag{13.47}
$$

In addition, at any position x,

$$
\hat{\rho}_{filter}^{two\,spins}(x) = a \cdot h_{filter}(x) + b \cdot h_{filter}(x - x_B)
\tag{13.48}
$$

Equation (13.48) demonstrates the obscuring of the point object at x_B due to the blur from A. For illustration purposes, consider the filter to be a window function. It is assumed that object B can be resolved in the presence of A when the distance between the two objects is greater than or equal to the distance of the first zero crossing of the filter. With this definition, the first zero crossing of (13.12), or (13.18), gives a resolution of $1/W$, which is equivalent to the earlier result for Δx_{MRI} in (13.41).

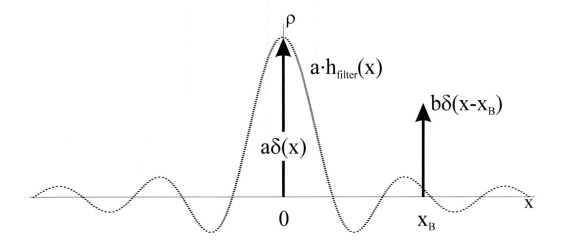

Fig. 13.5: The spin density for two point objects A and B is given by $\rho(x) = a\delta(x) + b\delta(x - x_B)$. The reconstructed spin density for object A is also shown (dashed line), corresponding to a truncation k-space filter, and given by the point spread function times the magnitude a. In contrast to Fig. 13.6, spatial resolution can be defined in terms of the zero crossings of the point spread function.

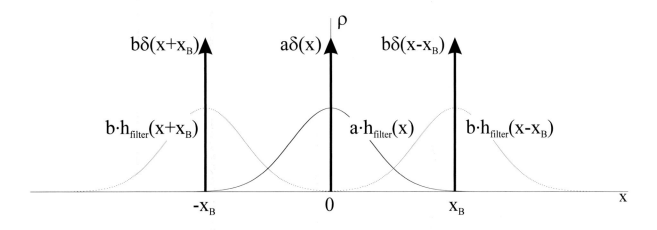

Fig. 13.6: Example of several impulse objects, and their convolution with a positive definite point spread function. The spatial resolution may be defined in terms of the 'width' of the point spread function.

Full Width at Half Maximum (FWHM) and Full Width at Tenth Maximum (FWTM) Approximations

The definition of spatial resolution in terms of zero crossings is not appropriate for a positive definite, or negative definite, point spread function, such as that shown in Fig. 13.6. An alternate criterion based on the filter profile is often used.[9] The Δx_{filter} may be defined as

---

[9]In general, a statistical analysis is necessary to determine the probability that two objects may be distinguished given any resulting overlap. Nevertheless, the expressions given in the text for $\Delta x_{MRI, filter}$ work well for the filters commonly applied in MRI.

the 'width' of the filter, for a symmetric filter with a maximum at its center. The 'width' may, in turn, be defined as twice the distance from the center to the point where the filter has fallen to a fraction κ of its maximum. Therefore, Δx_{filter} is found by solving the equation given by

$$h_{filter}(\Delta x_{filter}/2) = \kappa\, h_{filter}(0) \tag{13.49}$$

The ambiguity in determining whether two objects can be resolved is reflected in the choice of κ. A well-known convention is to employ the full width at half maximum for the width,

$$\Delta x_{filter} \equiv \text{FWHM}_{filter} \tag{13.50}$$

corresponding to $\kappa = 1/2$. A more demanding criterion follows from the use of the full width at tenth maximum,

$$\Delta x_{filter} \equiv \text{FWTM}_{filter} \tag{13.51}$$

for which $\kappa = 1/10$.

Problem 13.7

a) Find the $\Delta x_{Gaussian}$ using both the FWHM and the FWTM definitions for the Gaussian filter of Prob. 13.5, and compare your answers to the result for that problem.

b) Repeat the two determinations in (a) but for the window filter whose point spread function is $h_{filter}(x) = W \text{sinc}(\pi W x)$. Only consider the solution when $|x| < 1/W$. Compare your answer to the definition based on the first zero crossing result.

A question arises about how to find the total resolution for two or more filters applied to the same data. If two filters of the same shape are multiplied in the k-space domain, it is common to add their individual resolution, or blur, together via

$$\Delta x_{filter\,1, filter\,2} \approx \Delta x_{filter\,1} + \Delta x_{filter\,2} \tag{13.52}$$

This is an identity if the FWHM rule is used to define Δx_{filter} and both filters have exponential form in the k-space domain (see Prob. 13.8). If one or another does not have exponential form, the total blur may have to be calculated for the combined filtering, including the effects of finite sampling. While it is tempting to write $\Delta x_{MRI,filter} \approx \Delta x_{MRI} + \Delta x_{filter}$, the MRI window and sampling filter are not exponential in form and, in general, this approximation is not valid. One example is given in Sec. 13.5.

Problem 13.8

Prove that (13.52) is an identity for exponential forms, by adding the FWHM for the inverse Fourier transforms of $e^{-a|k|}$ and $e^{-b|k|}$ and comparing the result to the FWHM for the inverse Fourier transform of $e^{-(a+b)|k|}$. These forms are pertinent to imaging.

13.5   Hanning Filter and T_2^* Decay Effects

Sampling and windowing are a natural part of the data processing used in MR imaging. Signal variations as a function of time due to T_2^* decay during data sampling in the read direction can be determined from the exponential expressions found earlier for transverse relaxation. In particular, such innate filtering imposes limits on the best spatial resolution which can be achieved in an experiment. Even if infinite time were available for sampling, and continuous data could be acquired, the signal would still be filtered by the transverse decay envelope leading to a limited resolution.

13.5.1   Resolution Due to the Hanning Filter

To get a flavor for the effect on resolution of filtering the data, consider the Hanning filter (13.33) that represents a simple model of symmetric windowing. Using (13.43) and the identify given in (13.19), the spatial resolution with the presence of the Hanning filter can be easily calculated as

$$\Delta x_{Hanning} = 2\Delta x \tag{13.53}$$

This means that when a Hanning filter is applied to k-space data, the image resolution is reduced by a factor of 2.

Problem 13.9

Derive (13.53).

13.5.2   Partial Fourier T_2^* Reconstruction Effects

The result of (13.44), for which the Fourier pixel size was the lower limit on the spatial resolution, depended on the implicit assumption that the sampling time T_s is short compared to T_2^*. When T_s is comparable to T_2^*, the exponential decay of the signal during sampling can lead to a significant filtering action on $s(k)$. In order to demonstrate this effect, let us consider an image reconstructed from sampling points that are acquired at and after the echo. This partial Fourier reconstruction was introduced in Sec. 11.2.8 and more will be discussed under Sec. 13.7. From the discussions in Ch. 8, T_2^* decay occurs in both spin echo and gradient echo acquisitions. The filter is modeled by $e^{-|t'|/T_2^*}$ where $t' = 0$ is the time of echo. Since $k = \gamma G t'$, the k-space filter in addition to the usual windowing and sampling is

$$H_{filter}(k) = e^{-|k|/(\gamma|G|T_2^*)} \tag{13.54}$$

The T_2^* Filter Effect on Resolution

The MR spatial resolution with filter due to the T_2^* effect can be calculated using (13.54) and (13.43). The resolution is

$$\Delta x_{T_2^* \, filter} = \frac{e^{\Delta k/(\gamma|G|T_2^*)} - 1}{\Delta k \left(1 + e^{\Delta k/(\gamma|G|T_2^*)}\right)\left(1 - e^{-T_s/(2T_2^*)}\right)} \tag{13.55}$$

where

$$T_s = \frac{2n\Delta k}{\gamma|G|} = \frac{1}{\gamma|G|\Delta x} \tag{13.56}$$

Since $\Delta k \equiv \gamma|G|\Delta t \ll \gamma|G|T_2^*$ in most MRI cases, (13.55) can be well approximated by

$$\Delta x_{T_2^* \, filter} = \Delta x \frac{\alpha}{1 - e^{-\alpha}} \tag{13.57}$$

where $\alpha \equiv T_s/(2T_2^*)$. As α is always positive, it can be shown that $\Delta x_{T_2^* \, filter}$ always has a worse resolution than the Fourier pixel size Δx. It is also clear that when the sampling time T_s is much shorter than T_2^*, the image resolution approaches the lower limit, Δx.

Problem 13.10

---

a) Prove that $\Delta x_{T_2^* \, filter} \geq \Delta x$ from (13.57). Hint: Prove that $\alpha + e^{-\alpha} - 1 \geq 0$, for $\alpha \geq 0$. The equality holds only when $\alpha = 0$.

b) If $T_2^* = 20 \, \text{ms}$, $N = 256$, $G = 5 \, \text{mT/m}$, and $L = 256 \, \text{mm}$, find T_s and $\Delta x_{T_2^* \, filter}$ for the gradient echo experiment shown in Fig. 10.14.

If an image is reconstructed from sampling points acquired prior to the echo time, (13.43) is no longer suitable for the calculation of resolution. This is because (13.43) is valid only when $H_{filter}(0)$ is the largest value in k-space. In fact, the filter due to T_2^* (or T_2) decay will act as a high pass filter. As the signals at large $|\vec{k}|$ values (i.e., the initial sampling points) are enhanced by the T_2^* effects, the edges of objects in the image will be sharpened. This is similar to the case of multiplying the k-space signal by $|\vec{k}|$, described by the Fourier derivative theorem under Sec. 11.2.7. Using only the negative k-space data (i.e., replacing $-|k|$ with $|k|$ in (13.54)) will still yield a real only filter effect on the images.

The FWHM Approximation

Inverse Fourier transformation of (13.54) leads to the point spread function $h_{filter}(x)$ whose full width at half maximum gives an estimate of the spatial extent of the blur caused by the filter. The FWHM may be a reasonable first-order guess of the spatial resolution when (13.43) is difficult to evaluate.

From the derivation used in Prob. 13.8, the FWHM of the point spread function is

$$\text{FWHM}_{T_2^*} = \frac{\Delta x}{\pi} \left(\frac{T_s}{T_2^*} \right) \tag{13.58}$$

This FWHM represents an additional blur over and above that caused by the usual finite sampling window. As discussed under Sec. 13.4, the addition of Δx to (13.58) is clearly not equal to the exact total resolution (13.57).

Quantitative Values of Filtering Due to Transverse Relaxation for the Spin Echo

From the discussions in Ch. 8 and Fig. 8.3, it can be seen that a spin echo acquisition contains the asymmetric T_2 decay and the symmetric T_2' decay envelope centered about the echo (and, hence, around the k-space origin). The symmetric effect of the T_2' envelope fits the above discussion on partial Fourier reconstruction and T_2' can replace T_2^* in (13.55), (13.57), and even (13.58).

In order to avoid significant loss of spatial resolution due to transverse relaxation, it is always good to keep T_s as short as possible. Since blurring due to T_2' decay always exists after the echo in the spin echo images, it is especially important to maintain $T_s \ll T_2'$, which is related to the magnetic susceptibility via the relation found later in (20.86). This means that field inhomogeneities of the system can dictate upper limits on T_s through T_2'. The lower limit of T_s is typically constrained by the available maximum gradient strength for a given Δx. Further, it will be shown in Ch. 15 that the SNR per pixel in the reconstructed image is proportional to $\sqrt{T_s}$, so SNR is yet another criterion that limits T_s. Nevertheless, one might want to increase T_s, at the expense of a loss in resolution, in order to increase SNR.

13.6 Zero Filled Interpolation, Sub-Voxel Fourier Transform Shift Concepts, and Point Spread Function Effects

One method of interpolating incomplete k-space data is to fill out the data with additional zeros such that the pixel size after image reconstruction meets the desired interpolation. In this section, the equivalence of zero padded interpolation and sub-voxel shift using the shift theorem is shown. A discussion on the effects of the point spread function on the interpolated images shows that up to a 36% signal loss can be obtained if a point-like object is not centered within a reconstructed voxel. Sub-voxel shifts performed by using the shift theorem can be used to recover this signal loss.

After the zero filling, despite the apparent high resolution in terms of image voxel size in the image display, the spatial resolution does not change; it is still determined by the Fourier pixel size since the point spread function does not change its form.

13.6.1 Zero Padding and the Fast Fourier Transform

In the conventional N-sample case, the discrete inverse Fourier transform reconstruction gives

$$\hat{\rho}(q\Delta x) = \Delta k \sum_{p=-N/2}^{N/2-1} s(p\Delta k)e^{i2\pi pq/N} \tag{13.59}$$

When N is a power of 2, a very efficient version of the discrete Fourier transform called the fast Fourier transform (FFT) can be used for image reconstruction. When N is not a power of 2, the k-space data are often 'zero padded' (or zero filled) to the nearest power of 2, say $N_{\text{image}} > N$, and an N_{image}-point image is reconstructed using the FFT.

In the FFT reconstruction, the *pixel size* Δx_{pixel} is given by

$$\Delta x_{pixel} = \frac{L}{N_{\text{image}}} = \frac{1}{N_{\text{image}}\Delta k} < \frac{1}{N\Delta k} = \Delta x \qquad (13.60)$$

When $N_{\text{image}} = N$,

$$\Delta x_{pixel} = \frac{1}{N\Delta k} = \Delta x = \frac{1}{W} \qquad (13.61)$$

When Δx_{pixel} equals $1/W$, the reciprocal of the extent of k-space coverage, the pixel size is the Fourier pixel size, Δx. When the k-space data are zero padded to some other size, the image is reconstructed at a pixel size smaller than the Fourier pixel size. Zero padding adds no new information at the level of Δx_{pixel} but it does provide an interpolated image (i.e., Δx is interpolated to Δx_{pixel}).

13.6.2   Equivalence of Zero Filled Image and the Sub-Voxel Shifted Image

Assume that N k-space data points are zero filled to $2N$ points. Reconstructing the image at $2N$ points allows the image to have a voxel size of $\Delta x' = \Delta x/2$ while the spatial resolution of the image still remains Δx. Suppose $s_{m,zero}(k)$ represents the zero filled data set. Then

$$s_{m,zero}(p\Delta k) = \begin{cases} s(p\Delta k) & -\frac{N}{2} \leq p \leq \frac{N}{2} - 1 \\ 0 & -N \leq p \leq -\frac{N}{2} - 1 \text{ and } \frac{N}{2} \leq p \leq N - 1 \end{cases} \qquad (13.62)$$

If $\mathcal{D}_{2N}^{-1}$ represents the $2N$-point discrete inverse Fourier transform operator, then $\hat{\rho}_{zero}(q\Delta x') = \hat{\rho}_{zero}(q\Delta x/2) = \mathcal{D}_{2N}^{-1}\{s_{m,zero}(p\Delta k)\}$ and $\hat{\rho}(q\Delta x) = \mathcal{D}_N^{-1}\{s_m(k)\}$

$$\begin{aligned} \hat{\rho}_{zero}(q\Delta x/2) &= \Delta k \sum_{p=-N}^{N-1} s_{m,zero}(p\Delta k)e^{i2\pi qp/(2N)} \\ &= \Delta k \sum_{p=-N/2}^{N/2-1} s(p\Delta k)e^{i\pi qp/N} \end{aligned} \qquad (13.63)$$

where $-N \leq q \leq N - 1$.

Two separate images can also be constructed from the zero filled data set by constructing images at the even and odd data points separately. Consider only the even data points $q = 2r$ where $-N/2 \leq r \leq N/2 - 1$. The image reconstructed from these points is

$$\hat{\rho}_{zero,even}(2r\Delta x') = \Delta k \sum_{p=-N/2}^{N/2-1} s(p\Delta k)e^{i2\pi pr/N} = \hat{\rho}(r\Delta x) \qquad (13.64)$$

$$= \text{ spin density from the even-indexed voxels of the zero filled image}$$

The result of (13.64) indicates that the spin density from the even-indexed voxel is identical to the spin density from the voxel of the original image. However, a definition such as (12.36) implies that the signal from the even-indexed voxel is half of the signal from the voxel of the original image.

The spin density from the odd-indexed zero filled image voxels is

$$
\begin{aligned}
\hat{\rho}_{zero,odd}((2r+1)\Delta x') &= \Delta k \sum_{p=-N/2}^{N/2-1} s(p\Delta k)e^{i\pi(2r+1)p/N} \\
&= \Delta k \sum_{p=-N/2}^{N/2-1} \left[s(p\Delta k)e^{i\pi p/N} \right] e^{i2\pi rp/N}
\end{aligned}
\tag{13.65}
$$

If the half-voxel shifted image obtained using the shift theorem is $\hat{\rho}_{\text{shift}}(q\Delta x)$ whose N-point discrete Fourier transform is equal to

$$
s_{\text{shift}}(p\Delta k) = e^{i\pi p/N} s(p\Delta k)
\tag{13.66}
$$

then $\hat{\rho}_{\text{shift}}(q\Delta x)$ is given by

$$
\hat{\rho}_{\text{shift}}(q\Delta x) = \Delta k \sum_{p=-N/2}^{N/2-1} s(p\Delta k)e^{i\pi p/N}e^{i2\pi qp/N}
\tag{13.67}
$$

Comparing (13.65) and (13.67), along with the result of (13.64), it can be seen that the zero filled image can be obtained from the original image by applying the sub-voxel shift using the shift theorem.

13.6.3 Point Spread Effects on the Image Based on the Object Position Relative to the Reconstructed Voxels

From Sec. 13.2.2, (13.16) shows that the reconstructed image is the convolution of the original object with the point spread function $h_{ws}(x)$. From (13.67), it is clear that $\hat{\rho}_{\text{shift}}(q\Delta x) = \hat{\rho}((q+1/2)\Delta x)$, which can be quickly evaluated from the convolution of $\rho(x)$ with $h_{ws}(x)$. For example, consider a boxcar object of a unit signal and an infinitesimal width $w \ll \Delta x$ centered about $x = x_s$ with $|x_s| \le \Delta x/2$. The reconstructed image is given by

$$
\hat{\rho}_{bc}(q\Delta x) = \int dx'\, \rho(x')h_{ws}(q\Delta x - x')
\tag{13.68}
$$

where the subscript 'bc' indicates 'boxcar object.' The signal obtained at $q = 0$, the voxel nearest to the center of the object, is

$$
\begin{aligned}
\hat{\rho}_{bc}(0) &= \int_{x_s-w/2}^{x_s+w/2} dx'\, h_{ws}(-x') \\
&\simeq w h_{ws}(-x_s)
\end{aligned}
\tag{13.69}
$$

The approximation in (13.69) is valid since w is an infinitesimal width, and $h_{ws}(x)$ is a smoothly varying function about $x = x_s$. If the image is reconstructed on a grid that is shifted by half a pixel by using the shift theorem, the reconstructed signal would have been

$$
\hat{\rho}_{bc}^s(0) \simeq w h_{ws}(\Delta x/2 - x_s)
\tag{13.70}
$$

where the superscript s is used to indicate the shifted reconstruction. Comparing the reconstructed signals in (13.69) and (13.70), the signal is changed in the unshifted case by the ratio

$$R = |\hat{\rho}_{bc}(0)|/|\hat{\rho}_{bc}^s(0)| \tag{13.71}$$

which, for $x_s = \Delta x/2$, gives

$$R = |h_{wo}(-\Delta x/2)|/|h_{ws}(0)| \tag{13.72}$$

Since $\Delta k \Delta x = 1/N \ll 1$, (13.18) indicates that $|h_{ws}(-\Delta x/2)|$ can be approximated by $W \mathrm{sinc}(\pi/2) = 2W/\pi = 0.64W$. This leads to $R \simeq 0.64$; a 36% reduced signal is obtained when the object is centered half a voxel away from the voxel center. The shift theorem allows us to overcome this worst-case 36% underestimation of the signal by centering the object within a reconstructed voxel. However, recovering the 'missing' 36% from a shifted object does not imply that the image is resolved any more accurately. Resolution is still limited to Δx.

This property of the Fourier transform shift theorem, used to recover the reconstructed signal loss, can be taken advantage of in a number of practical situations. For example, zero filled interpolation has been in use for a long time in NMR spectroscopy for improved spectral peak estimation. The improved peak estimation leads to improved estimates of the spectral position. Extending the same ideas to imaging, it has been increasingly used for improved object signal estimation by overcoming the partial volume averaging[10] effect due to sharing of the object by two neighboring voxels. This is particularly helpful for MR angiographic applications (Ch. 24) and another reason why the shift theorem plays an important role in visualizing vessels.

13.7   Partial Fourier Imaging and Reconstruction

In certain cases, the number of data points on one side of the k-space origin is much more than the number of points on the other side (i.e., the data are highly asymmetric). In some applications where minimizing imaging time is of the essence, k-space is covered highly asymmetrically in the phase encoding direction. For example, the number of phase encoding lines required by the Nyquist condition is collected only in one half of k-space, while the other half (often the negative half of k-space) is covered only partially. Since phase encoding lines are usually separated in time by T_R, collecting fewer phase encoding lines implies a shortening of the total imaging time. The amount of time saved is determined by the 'degree of asymmetry.' In other applications such as MR angiography where shorter field echoes provide less sensitivity to rapid flow (Ch. 24), very short echo times can be achieved. One of the most popular means to achieve this is to obtain asymmetric echoes in the readout direction. These methods of asymmetric k-space coverage are generically classified as *partial Fourier imaging methods*.

Any Fourier imaging performed such that k-space is covered over the region $[-n_-\Delta k, (n_+ - 1)\Delta k]$, where practically $n_- \leq n_+$, is classified as a partial Fourier imaging scheme. The

---

[10]Partial volume averaging is defined and discussed in Ch. 15.

degree of asymmetry 'asym' is defined as

$$asym = \frac{n_+ - n_-}{n_- + n_+} \tag{13.73}$$

In the partial Fourier imaging scheme, n_- can be in the range $[0, n_+]$. As a result, the value of *asym* can be between 1 (completely asymmetric case, i.e., when only the non-negative half of k-space is covered) and 0 (completely symmetric case, i.e., symmetric k-space coverage). For example, consider the read gradient in Fig. 13.7. It has n_- points before the echo and $n_+ - 1$ points after. The total read sampling time is $N\Delta t$ where N is defined to be

$$N = n_- + n_+ \tag{13.74}$$

The field echo time F_E in Fig. 13.7 is referred to as the time from the beginning of the application of gradients in the read direction until the echo occurs in the sampling window. The minimum field echo time is given by

$$F_E = 2.5\tau_{rt} + 2n_-\Delta t \tag{13.75}$$

This is the first and only gradient field echo along the read direction in this sequence.[11] The echo time is then

$$T_E = 0.5\tau_{rf} + 2.5\tau_{rt} + 2n_-\Delta t \tag{13.76}$$

Clearly, as n_- approaches zero, T_E can be reduced to its minimum value.

Problem 13.11

Derive (13.75).

Ideally, the image is reconstructed from the asymmetric echo data by finding $s(-k)$ via the complex conjugate symmetry relation

$$s(-k) = s^*(k) \tag{13.77}$$

when $\rho(x)$ is a real function. Now, recreating a new data set with $2n_+$ points symmetrically distributed about the echo is straightforward. If n_+ is not a multiple of 2, the data can be zero filled to accommodate the FFT algorithm.

Another way to view totally asymmetric data (i.e., $n_- = 0$) is to look at the case when the data $s(k)$ is multiplied by a filter equivalent to the Heaviside step function $\Theta(k)$.

$$\begin{aligned} h_\Theta(x) &= \mathcal{F}^{-1}(\Theta(k)) \\ &= \frac{1}{2}\delta(x) + \frac{i}{2\pi}P\left(\frac{1}{x}\right) \end{aligned} \tag{13.78}$$

---

[11]The reader is reminded that field echoes, gradient echoes, or gradient field echoes all refer to times, after the initiation of the first read lobe, when the net area under the read gradient goes to zero. The phase, due to the read gradients *only*, is zero for all stationary spins at these times. These echoes should not be confused with spin echoes which are rf echoes that occur when the phase due to static field inhomogeneities for stationary spins is everywhere returned to zero.

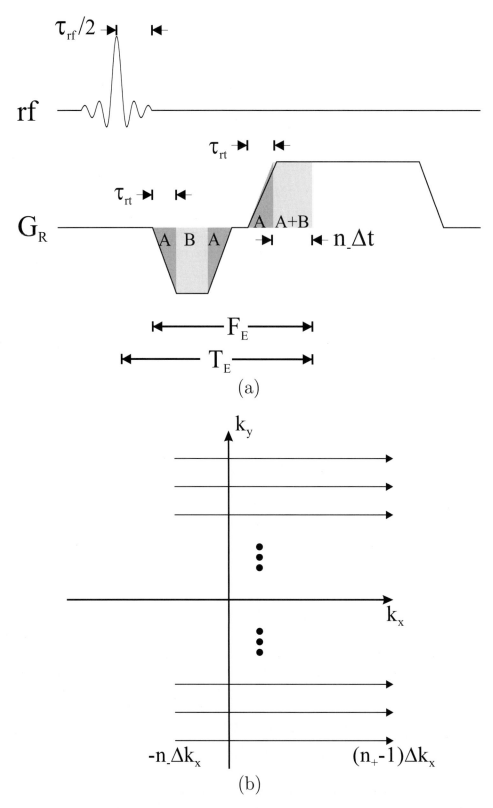

Fig. 13.7: (a) Readout gradient waveform and timings for the asymmetric sampling scheme, and (b) the corresponding k-space coverage. The shaded regions A and B have been shown explicitly to clarify the location of the gradient echo.

The details of this Fourier transform are shown in (11.25). Application of this filter leads to the following reconstructed spin density

$$
\begin{aligned}
\hat{\rho}_H(x) &= \rho(x) * h_\Theta(x) \\
&= \frac{1}{2}\rho(x) + \frac{1}{2}\rho(x) * \frac{i}{\pi}P\left(\frac{1}{x}\right)
\end{aligned}
\tag{13.79}
$$

This shows that when $\rho(x)$ is real, it can be found by taking $2\mathrm{Re}\,\hat{\rho}_H(x)$ after this filter is applied. In practice, because of field inhomogeneities and flow, $\rho(x)$ is effectively complex, $\rho(x) = \rho_{re}(x) + i\rho_{im}(x)$. This means that $2\mathrm{Re}\,\hat{\rho}_H(x)$ will no longer represent $\rho(x)$ since (13.77) is not valid and the complex terms in $\rho(x)$ and $\mathcal{F}^{-1}(\Theta(k))$ will mix components. More complicated schemes need to be designed to deal with this problem in that case.

The above discussion of the Heaviside function did not take into account sampling or truncation, which will also alter the reconstructed spin density. If partial Fourier reconstruction is considered from a discrete perspective, the filter $H_{filter}(k)$ (equivalent to the Heaviside unit step function $\Theta(k)$ in the continuous case) becomes

$$
H_{\Theta_+}(k) = \begin{cases} 0 & k < 0 \\ \frac{1}{2} & k = 0 \\ 1 & k > 0 \end{cases}
\tag{13.80}
$$

The factor of 1/2 at the origin can be understood by assuming that symmetric sampling should be recovered by the addition of two Heaviside functions. This is the case, if $H_{\Theta_-}(k)$ is defined to be

$$
H_{\Theta_-}(k) = \begin{cases} 1 & k < 0 \\ \frac{1}{2} & k = 0 \\ 0 & k > 0 \end{cases}
\tag{13.81}
$$

Problem 13.12

In Ch. 19, a short discussion on k-space sampling during gradient ramp-up will be presented. This technique finds practical use in short-T_E asymmetric echo imaging. For each sequence, some minimum number of points must be collected before the echo for a stable partial Fourier reconstruction to be performed. In certain ultrashort imaging applications, even the time required to collect as few as 32 points before the echo is considered to be too long. In such applications, sampling during gradient ramp-up provides the required shortening of T_E. Partial Fourier image reconstruction is then applied on these data to obtain improved image information. How many extra k-space points would be obtained if the ramp-up time of the read gradient lobe is 1 ms and Δt is a) 20 μs or b) 4 μs? With this particular design, the number of points recovered from the ramp-up to a constant read gradient can replace part of the usual uniform sampling before the echo. Those points sampled during the ramp-up will need to be nonuniform in time to create uniformly sampled points in k-space.

13.7.1   Forcing Conjugate Symmetry on Complex Objects

One approach to reconstructing a real image from asymmetric data is to force the data to obey complex conjugate symmetry. However, for a complex object

$$\rho(x) = \rho_{re}(x) + i\rho_{im}(x) \tag{13.82}$$

where $\rho_{re}(x)$ and $\rho_{im}(x)$ are real functions, this will result in an image that does not represent the actual object. Due to the linearity of the Fourier transform, it is possible to view this object as giving rise to two separate signals

$$\begin{aligned} s_{re}(k) &\equiv \mathcal{F}\left(\rho_{re}(x)\right) \\ s_{im}(k) &\equiv \mathcal{F}\left(i\rho_{im}(x)\right) \end{aligned} \tag{13.83}$$

Suppose the k-space data $s(k)$ are acquired only for $k \geq 0$. Then, complex conjugate symmetry is forced to create the uncollected data

$$\begin{aligned} s_c(k) &= \begin{cases} s(k) & k \geq 0 \\ s^*(-k) & k < 0 \end{cases} \\ &= \begin{cases} s_{re}(k) + s_{im}(k) & k \geq 0 \\ s_{re}^*(-k) + s_{im}^*(-k) & k < 0 \end{cases} \end{aligned} \tag{13.84}$$

Note that the actual signal for $k < 0$ should be $s_{re}^*(-k) - s_{im}^*(-k)$, as the signal from $i\rho_{im}(x)$ obeys the relation

$$s_{im}(k) = -s_{im}^*(-k) \tag{13.85}$$

Taking the inverse Fourier transform of this merged data set ($s_c(k)$) gives

$$\begin{aligned} \rho_c(x) &= 2\mathrm{Re}\left(\int_0^\infty dk (s_{re}(k) + s_{im}(k))e^{i2\pi kx}\right) \\ &= 2\mathrm{Re}\left(\mathcal{F}^{-1}((s_{re}(k) + s_{im}(k))\Theta(k))\right) \\ &= 2\mathrm{Re}\left(\rho_{re}(x) * h_\Theta(x)\right) + 2\mathrm{Re}\left(i\rho_{im}(x) * h_\Theta(x)\right) \\ &= \rho_{re}(x) - \rho_{im}(x) * \frac{1}{\pi}P\left(\frac{1}{x}\right) \end{aligned} \tag{13.86}$$

which is clearly not equal to $\rho(x)$ unless $\rho_{im}(x)$ is zero. Therefore, if an object is complex and a partial Fourier reconstruction method assuming a real object is applied, the resulting image will not be an accurate representation of $\rho(x)$.

13.7.2   Iterative Reconstruction

Collecting only part of the negative half of k-space allows for an iterative, constrained image reconstruction scheme. Two powerful constraints that can be used in the reconstruction are: (i) the k-space data that were collected represent the best knowledge about the object; new k-space data will therefore be created only for the $n_+ - n_-$ uncollected points, and (ii) the low spatial frequency phase image that can be reconstructed with the first $2n_-$ points covering $-n_- \leq k \leq n_- - 1$ represents our first estimate about the phase of the complex spatial domain data. The new $2n_+$-point image will then have its phase constrained to that of the $2n_-$ original low k-space data zero filled to $2n_+$ points. It is also assumed that the $n-1$ dimensions of an n-dimensional k-space data set have already been reconstructed by inverse Fourier transformation.

The iterative reconstruction algorithm is detailed in a stepwise fashion next.

Step 1: Create a truncated and zero padded (to $2n_+$ points) data set $\tilde{s}_\phi(p\Delta k)$ from the measured data set $s_m(p\Delta k)$ as follows

$$\tilde{s}_\phi(p\Delta k) = \begin{cases} 0 & n_- \leq p \leq n_+ - 1 \\ s_m(p\Delta k) & -n_- \leq p \leq n_- - 1 \\ 0 & -n_+ \leq p \leq -n_- - 1 \end{cases} \tag{13.87}$$

Step 2: This data set is used to obtain a low frequency phase estimate $\hat{\phi}(q\Delta x)$

$$\hat{\phi}(q\Delta x) \equiv \arg\left[\mathcal{F}^{-1}\left(\tilde{s}_\phi(p\Delta k) \right) \right] \tag{13.88}$$

Step 3: Initialize an iteration counter j to zero. An initial $2n_+$-point image is obtained from a zero padded version of the measured data set, say, $s_0(p\Delta k)$

$$s_0(p\Delta k) = \begin{cases} s_m(p\Delta k) & -n_- \leq p \leq n_+ - 1 \\ 0 & -n_+ \leq p \leq -n_- - 1 \end{cases} \tag{13.89}$$

The reconstructed image, $\mathcal{F}^{-1}\left(s_0(p\Delta k)\right)$, is denoted by $\hat{\rho}_0(q\Delta x)$.

The actual iterative part of the algorithm starts from the next step.

Step 4: An intermediate $(j+1)^{st}$ iterated complex image is obtained from

$$\tilde{\rho}_{j+1}(q\Delta x) = |\hat{\rho}_j(q\Delta x)| \, e^{i\hat{\phi}(q\Delta x)} \tag{13.90}$$

Step 5: This intermediate complex image is then Fourier transformed to create an intermediate k-space data set $\tilde{s}_{j+1}(p\Delta k)$ given by

$$\tilde{s}_{j+1}(p\Delta k) \equiv \mathcal{F}\left(\tilde{\rho}_{j+1}(q\Delta x)\right) \tag{13.91}$$

Step 6: Unlike the measured data $s_m(p\Delta k)$, $\tilde{s}_{j+1}(p\Delta k)$ has nonzero data for $-n_+ \leq p \leq n_+ - 1$. The complex data $\tilde{s}_{j+1}(p\Delta k)$ in the range from $-n_-\Delta k$ to $(n_+ - 1)\Delta k$ are substituted by the measured k-space data

$$s_{j+1}(p\Delta k) = \begin{cases} s_m(p\Delta k) & -n_- \leq p \leq n_+ - 1 \\ \tilde{s}_{j+1}(p\Delta k) & -n_+ \leq p \leq -n_- - 1 \end{cases} \tag{13.92}$$

Step 7: This is inverse Fourier transformed to create the $(j+1)^{st}$ complex image

$$\hat{\rho}_{j+1}(q\Delta x) = \mathcal{F}^{-1}\left(s_{j+1}(p\Delta k)\right) \tag{13.93}$$

Step 8: If $|\hat{\rho}_{j+1}(q\Delta x) - \hat{\rho}_j(q\Delta x)|$ is 'sufficiently small' (as determined by a predesigned convergence criterion), then go to step 9; otherwise, go to step 10.

Step 9: Output $\hat{\rho}_{j+1}(q\Delta x)$ as the final reconstructed image and end the algorithm.

Step 10: Increment iteration counter j by 1 and return to step 4.

In the above algorithm, it is important that the replacement data $\tilde{s}_{j+1}(p\Delta k)$ for each iteration are smoothed with the collected data $s_m(p\Delta k)$ around the merging point. Otherwise truncation artifacts due to the k-space discontinuity can be found in the reconstructed image. It is therefore useful to merge the two data sets with a u-point Hanning filter using an averaging procedure during the last iteration to avoid these artifacts. That is, the last k-space iterate is given by

$$
s_{j+1}(p\Delta k) = \begin{cases} s_m(p\Delta k) & -n_- + u \leq p \leq n_+ - 1 \\ \frac{1}{2}\left\{ s_m(p\Delta k)\left[1 - \cos\frac{\pi(p+n_-)}{u}\right] + \right. & \\ \left. \tilde{s}_{j+1}(p\Delta k)\left[1 + \cos\frac{\pi(p+n_-)}{u}\right]\right\} & -n_- \leq p \leq -n_- + u - 1 \\ \tilde{s}_{j+1}(p\Delta k) & -n_+ \leq p \leq -n_- - 1 \end{cases}
\tag{13.94}
$$

13.7.3   Some Implementation Issues

The previous discussion of the algorithm was built on a 1D basis. Consider the general asymmetrically collected 3D k-space data $s(k_x, k_y, k_z)$. What kind of complex conjugate symmetry does this data set possess when $\rho(x, y, z)$ is real? To answer this question, write out the expression for the complex conjugate of $s(k_x, k_y, k_z)$ in terms of a Fourier transform

$$
\begin{aligned}
s^*(k_x, k_y, k_z) &= \left(\int\int\int dx\, dy\, dz\, \rho(x,y,z)e^{-i2\pi(k_x x + k_y y + k_z z)} \right)^* \\
&= \int\int\int dx\, dy\, dz\, \rho^*(x,y,z)e^{i2\pi(k_x x + k_y y + k_z z)} \\
&= s(-k_x, -k_y, -k_z)
\end{aligned}
\tag{13.95}
$$

In short, for multi-dimensional k-space data, complex conjugate symmetry holds for points that are reflections of each other about the k-space origin. How does this important property manifest itself from a practical point of view? For example, in the 2D case, it is tempting to ask whether collecting data from only a single quadrant of k-space would be enough to reconstruct the image using complex conjugate symmetrization. The answer is simply no. Suppose that points were collected such that they covered only the first quadrant of k-space. The conjugate symmetry property (13.95) implies that only k-space samples which lie in the third quadrant can be obtained; the second and fourth quadrants are not filled at all.

When Is the Complex Conjugate Step Performed for Multi-Dimensional Data

Data can only be collected asymmetrically in one dimension such as the read direction to reduce T_E, or one of the phase encoding directions to reduce the total acquisition time. The property (13.95) also has another implication from an efficient algorithmic point of view.

There are two ways in which asymmetrically collected multi-dimensional k-space data can be reconstructed: one is to store the complete multi-dimensional k-space data into an array and complex conjugate symmetrize the data using (13.95). The second method is first to inverse Fourier transform all other directions in which data were collected symmetrically, and then apply a 1D complex conjugate symmetrization to the remaining 1D k-space data. Suppose data were collected symmetrically along k_y and asymmetrically along k_x to obtain a k-space data set $s(k_x, k_y)$. Fourier inverting along y yields a function with a single spatial dimension and a single k-space dimension, say $\hat{\rho}_y(k_x, y)$

$$
\begin{aligned}
\hat{\rho}_y(k_x, y) &= \int dk_y \, s(k_x, k_y) e^{i2\pi k_y y} \\
&= \int dx \, \rho(x, y) e^{-i2\pi k_x x}
\end{aligned}
\tag{13.96}
$$

Now, $\hat{\rho}_y(k_x, y)$ satisfies (13.77), i.e.,

$$
\hat{\rho}_y(-k_x, y) = \hat{\rho}_y^*(k_x, y)
\tag{13.97}
$$

Using (13.97) the uncollected data points can be filled for Fourier inversion. Obviously, the second method is more efficiently implemented from a memory size requirement point of view since all operations are separable in the different directions.

Faster Convergence of the Iterative Method

In practice, the imaged object may have significant imaginary parts because of rapidly varying background field inhomogeneities. As seen from (13.86), it is then possible to have significant reduction in the image amplitude by forcing complex conjugate symmetry on the data. This is the reason why $|\hat{\rho}_0(q\Delta x)|$ was used as a starting constraint in the iterative reconstruction method. However, this image still suffers from the complex blurring, introduced by the multiplication by the Heaviside step function in k-space, which can often be significant, and can lead to a rather slow convergence of the iterative process. For small phase errors, $|\hat{\rho}_0(q\Delta x)|$ in step 4 can be replaced by the absolute value of the image created after forcing complex conjugate symmetry on the original data.

13.8   Digital Truncation

When the data are sampled, they are converted from an analog (or continuous) signal into a digital signal (i.e., a combination of bits) via an ADC (analog-to-digital converter). Today, a 16-bit ADC is often used. How does an ADC operate? An ADC has a peak input voltage dynamic range specification (from say $-V$ to $+V$ volts) over which it works. A 16-bit ADC, for example, would take any input voltage V_{in} and allocate it to a certain 16-bit output stream. This bit stream contains 2^{16} voltage levels of V_{in}. Since the voltage range between $-V$ and $+V$ has to be allocated to a total of 2^{16} voltage levels, the voltage difference separating two levels is $2V/10^{16} = 2^{-15}V$. For a commercially available ADC, V is on the order of a few tens of volts. In order to distinguish small structures as discussed below, the detected and demodulated emf corresponding to the MR signal (which can vary from $10\,\mathrm{nV}$

to $1\,\mu V$) has to be amplified prior to its input to the ADC. Suppose the amplification is fixed based on the signal from a homogeneous object of spin density ρ_0 which fills the entire field-of-view of interest using the entire dynamic range of the ADC. The k-space signal for such an object is

$$s(k_x, k_y) = \begin{cases} \rho_0 L_x L_y & k_x = k_y = 0 \\ 0 & \text{elsewhere} \end{cases} \tag{13.98}$$

In terms of the reconstructed voxel size and number of collected k-space samples,

$$\begin{aligned} s(k_x, k_y) &= \begin{cases} N_x N_y \rho_0 \Delta x \Delta y & k_x = k_y = 0 \\ 0 & \text{elsewhere} \end{cases} \\ &= \begin{cases} N^2 \rho_0 \Delta^2 & k_x = k_y = 0 \\ 0 & \text{elsewhere} \end{cases} \end{aligned} \tag{13.99}$$

if $N_x = N_y = N$ and $\Delta x = \Delta y = \Delta$. Suppose now that the amplification is such that $\rho_0 \Delta^2$, the signal per voxel, corresponds to the voltage difference between two adjacent voltage levels. Then, for $N = 256 = 2^8$, the range of the 16-bit ADC will have been fully used. For an image of an object twice the size of the first object, i.e., for $N = 512$, $N^2 = 2^{18}$ and the last two bits of the 18-bit data will be lost when the data are acquired by the 16-bit ADC. For the homogeneous object, this loss does not matter since there is only one nonzero k-space sample. However, assume that another object occupying exactly one voxel with spin density ρ_0 is superimposed exactly at the center of the homogeneous object. The signal from this object, say $\Delta s(k_x, k_y)$, is

$$\Delta s(k_x, k_y) = \rho_0 \Delta^2 \tag{13.100}$$

This adds a constant voltage level corresponding to the unit voltage level that is usually represented only by the last bit with the value 1. Unfortunately, since the last 2 bits are lost, i.e., all signal values below 4 units will be suppressed to level 0, this single-voxel object will not be seen at all!

This problem of visibility loss of small objects is especially exacerbated in 3D imaging, as number of voxels becomes $N_x N_y N_z$. Consider that N_z slices, each with unit thickness, are reconstructed (N_z can be 64 or 128 in practice). If the same amplifier gain is used, any object whose signal is less than $N_z \rho_0 \Delta^2 \Delta z$ may be suppressed in the digitized k-space signal. Most information about these objects will be lost, and they will appear as noise in the image. This noise is usually referred to as 'digitization or discretization noise.'

One possible solution to avoid this problem is to collect the data twice, once with central k-space and once with the remaining part of k-space (see Fig. 13.8) so that neither has peak amplitudes which exceed 2^{16}. An alternate method would be to apply an automatic gain control (AGC) to the data to enhance signal at the edge of k-space so that the overall dynamic range is reduced. Then the data could be rescaled digitally to the values that would have been measured had an AGC filter not been applied.

Recall that Fourier transform is a linear operation. After proper zero filling, different portions of the k-space data can be independently reconstructed into different images, which can be combined into the original image. The central portion of the k-space data represented by the finite window W_1 (see Fig. 13.8) leads to a lower resolution and somewhat flat image. After the discrete inverse Fourier transform, the data from the high k-space region $W_2 - W_1$ will be rescaled appropriately and added to improve the resolution of the image.

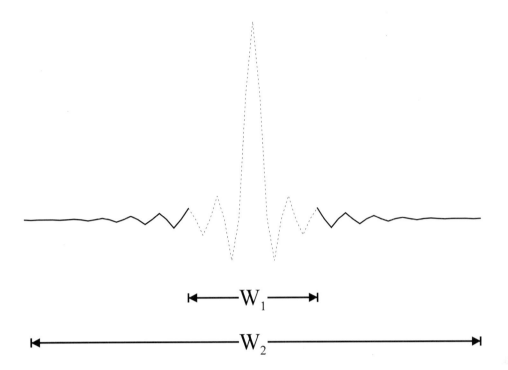

Fig. 13.8: Scheme for overcoming the data truncation artifact by acquiring the central k-space first and acquiring the higher k-space a second time so that both scans are automatically gain-controlled.

Problem 13.13

Consider a 3D object that fills the FOV and has either unit or zero spin density for each voxel. When a 3D data set is collected with $N_x = N_y = 128$ and $N_z = 32$, the maximum signal at $k_x = k_y = k_z = 0$ will be 2^{19} units in voltage. Generally, the ADC is only 16 bits (i.e., it will recognize 2^{16} individual voltage levels).

a) If the system rounds off signal to zero for any voltage less than unity, explain how an insufficient ADC range can act as a filter on the data.

b) What effect does this have on resolution in this problem and in general? Assume that the underlying object fills the FOV.

Imagine a narrow object, of volume $\Delta x \Delta y \Delta z / 4$ and amplitude ρ_1, superimposed on the original object that now has a unit spin density for each voxel. The signal $s(k)$ from this little object will be spread out over all k-space with a constant amplitude.

c) Show for $\rho_1 < 32$ that the signal from the entire object outside $\vec{k} = 0$ will be rounded off to either 0 or 1 when the peak signal is normalized to 2^{16}.

Suggested Reading

The following articles present methods for constrained partial Fourier image reconstruction:

- E. M. Haacke, E. D. Lindskog and W. Lin. A fast, iterative partial Fourier technique capable of local phase recovery. *J. Magn. Reson.*, 92: 126, 1991.

- Z.-P. Liang, F. E. Boada, R. T. Constable, E. M. Haacke, P. C. Lauterbur and M. R. Smith. Constrained reconstruction methods in MR imaging. *Rev. Magn. Reson. Med.*, 4: 67, 1992.

- P. Margosian, F. Schmitt and D. E. Purdy. Faster MR imaging: Imaging with half the data. *Health Care Instr.*, 1: 195, 1986.

The following articles present the filtering effects of T_2 and T_2^* decay during data sampling:

- E. M. Haacke. The effects of finite sampling in spin echo or field-echo magnetic resonance imaging. *Magn. Reson. Med.*, 4: 407, 1987.

- J. P. Mugler III and J. R. Brookeman. The optimum data sampling period for maximum signal-to-noise ratio in MR imaging. *Rev. Magn. Reson. Med.*, 3: 761, 1993.

The next text is an excellent reference on how to design and implement digital filters:

- R. W. Hamming. *Digital Filters.* III edition. Prentice-Hall, Englewood Cliffs, New Jersey, 1989.

General integral formulas and the concept of principal value can be found in the next two references, respectively:

- M. Abramowitz and I. A. Stegun, eds. *Handbook of Mathematical Functions with Formulas, Graphs, and Mathematical Tables.* National Bureau of Standards, Applied Mathematics Series 55, U.S. Govt. Printing Office, Washington, D.C., 1964.

- R. V. Churchill and J. W. Brown. *Complex Variables and Applications.* McGraw Hill, New York, 1990.

Chapter 14

Projection Reconstruction of Images

Chapter Contents

Summary: Radial methods of k-space coverage are detailed as alternatives to Cartesian Fourier k-space coverage. Reconstruction methods for such data are also discussed. The relationship between different reconstruction approaches is addressed. Certain advantages and disadvantages of the radial k-space coverage method are presented.

Introduction

The traversal of k-space can be carried out in a variety of ways, most of which have real physical analogs in terms of sequence design. In this chapter, radial coverage of k-space is considered, a method of historical consequence and of contemporary interest for specialized applications. The method is commonly known as projection reconstruction.[1] There is a broad experience that exists in this approach to image reconstruction in the world of x-ray tomography where there are entire books devoted to the subject. The advantages and difficulties in projection reconstruction are the present subject, but it is to be kept in mind that a variety of other ways to cover k-space are addressed in later chapters.

---

[1]It might be argued that this term should be reserved for the process of creating the image from the radially collected data. However, in keeping with the spirit of the common usage of the term in the MR literature, we reserve the usage of projection reconstruction to mean both the radial k-space coverage method and the reconstruction method.

The choice of reconstruction method is critical, in general, and is especially true in image reconstruction from radially collected data because of the many available methods for their reconstruction. *Artifacts associated with one method may be eliminated by resorting to other methods.* Although new artifacts necessarily replace the old when this change is made, the new artifacts may be more acceptable. It is such practical issues which ultimately decide which reconstruction method and what type of k-space coverage are used in a given application.

Projection reconstruction techniques are used on data collected with the aforementioned radial k-space coverage, whereas Fourier reconstruction methods are used to transform data obtained using rectangular k-space coverage. The theory behind various reconstruction methods for radially acquired data and some discussion on the implementation issues are presented in this chapter. The chapter begins with a rewriting of the measured signal in terms of polar coordinates which are better suited for the description of radially covered k-space data. This is followed by a discussion on how the gradients have to be varied so that radial k-space coverage can be obtained. Image reconstruction in polar coordinates is then briefly described to set the stage for later discussions.

14.1   Radial k-Space Coverage

To set the stage for a different approach to taking k-space data, the standard coverage described in Ch. 10 should be reviewed. The archetypical 2D imaging method encodes in the k_x and k_y directions by reading out a line of data with both read gradient G_x and phase encoding gradient G_y fixed. The latter is changed in amplitude at each subsequent rf pulse structure. The corresponding signal at time t is

$$s(t, \tau_y, G_x, G_y) = \int_{\Delta z} dz \int \int dx\, dy\, \rho(x, y, z) e^{-i2\pi \gamma (G_x x t + G_y y \tau_y)} \tag{14.1}$$

for a slice of thickness Δz perpendicular to the z-axis. The phase encoding has taken place during time τ_y. The relaxation effects and overall constants are absorbed into the spin density. With the z integration over the slice thickness included in a further redefinition of the spin density, a more compact formula for the signal can be written as

$$s(t, \tau_y, G_x, G_y) = \int \int dx\, dy\, \rho(x, y) e^{-i2\pi \gamma (G_x x t + G_y y \tau_y)} \tag{14.2}$$

The measurements implied by (14.2) are a horizontal line-by-line accumulation of the points in the (k_x, k_y) plane where, for pulsed gradients, the coordinates $k_x(t)$ and $k_y(\tau_y)$ are determined by

$$k_x = \gamma G_x t \text{ and } k_y = \gamma G_y \tau_y \tag{14.3}$$

leading to the more conventional form

$$s(k_x, k_y) = \int \int dx\, dy\, \rho(x, y) e^{-i2\pi \vec{k} \cdot \vec{r}} \tag{14.4}$$

where $\vec{k} = (k_x, k_y)$ and $\vec{r} = (x, y)$.

14.1.1 Coverage of *k*-Space at Different Angles

Rather than varying just the phase encoding gradient, suppose that the two gradients G_x and G_y are turned on at the same time. Then the net gradient vector points (and the data are frequency encoded) along an arbitrary angle θ with respect to the x-axis (the reader is referred back to Ch. 9 to the discussion about readout in an arbitrary direction).[2] The overall gradient strength G and angle θ are given by

$$G = \sqrt{G_x^2 + G_y^2} \quad \text{and} \quad \theta = \tan^{-1}\left(\frac{G_y}{G_x}\right) \tag{14.5}$$

such that

$$G_x = G\cos\theta \text{ and } G_y = G\sin\theta \tag{14.6}$$

Under these circumstances, the signal can be written[3]

$$s(t, G, \theta) = \int\int dx\, dy\, \rho(x, y) e^{-i2\pi\gamma G(x\cos\theta + y\sin\theta)t} \tag{14.7}$$

Following Ch. 9, the connection to $\vec{k}$-space is made through the definition of the k-space vector along the frequency encoding direction as

$$\vec{k} \equiv \gamma \vec{G} t \tag{14.8}$$

where $\vec{G} = (G_x, G_y)$. So equations analogous to (14.5) and (14.6) hold in terms of k and the same angle θ, where

$$k = \sqrt{k_x^2 + k_y^2} \quad \text{and} \quad \theta = \tan^{-1}\left(\frac{k_y}{k_x}\right) \tag{14.9}$$

such that

$$k_x = k\cos\theta \quad \text{and} \quad k_y = k\sin\theta \tag{14.10}$$

Substituting $\vec{k} = (k_x, k_y)$ from (14.10) and $\vec{r} = (x, y)$ into (14.4),

$$s(k, \theta) = \int\int dx\, dy\, \rho(x, y) e^{-i2\pi k(x\cos\theta + y\sin\theta)} \tag{14.11}$$

Finally, the polar variables k, θ spur a corresponding change from rectangular to polar coordinates in (x, y). Letting

$$x = r\cos\phi \text{ and } y = r\sin\phi \tag{14.12}$$

the signal becomes

$$s(k, \theta) = \int\int r\, dr\, d\phi\, \rho(r, \phi) e^{-i2\pi kr\cos(\phi - \theta)} \tag{14.13}$$

The angles θ and ϕ are displayed in Fig. 14.1.

---

[2]Recall that a given gradient direction means that the z-component of the magnetic field changes linearly along that direction.

[3]Throughout this chapter, and elsewhere in the book, it will be most convenient if the same symbol can be used for a function, even though the variables have been changed. For example, we may refer to $f(x, y)$ or $f(r, \phi)$ depending on whether Cartesian or polar coordinates are used. We may also use the same symbol for more variables, i.e., $f(x, y, z)$.

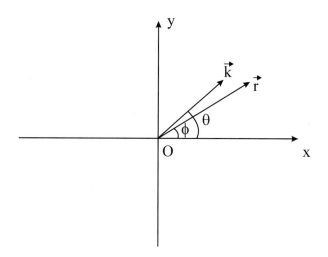

Fig. 14.1: The familiar polar and Cartesian relationships are shown for (r, ϕ) and (k, θ).

14.1.2   Two Radial Fourier Transform Examples

Consider two examples of spin densities independent of the polar angle ϕ. First, a spin density representing an infinitesimally thin ring at $r = r_0$ is

$$\rho(r) = N_0 \delta(r - r_0) \tag{14.14}$$

where N_0 is the number of spins at any given angle. The double integration (14.13) is reduced to a form independent of θ, as expected, owing to the periodicity in the ϕ integration[4]

$$
\begin{aligned}
s_{ring}(k) &= N_0 r_0 \int_0^{2\pi} d\phi \, e^{-i2\pi k r_0 \cos(\phi - \theta)} \\
&= 2\pi N_0 r_0 J_0(2\pi k r_0)
\end{aligned}
\tag{14.15}
$$

The transform has been related to the zeroth order Bessel function J_0. The general expression for the nth-order Bessel function is

$$J_n(u) \equiv \frac{i^n}{2\pi} \int_0^{2\pi} d\phi \, e^{-iu \cos\phi + in\phi} \tag{14.16}$$

These functions serve as a set of radial basis functions analogous to the trigonometric Fourier series.

The second example is that of a disk of spins,

$$\rho(r) = \rho_0 \Theta(r_0 - r) \tag{14.17}$$

in which the Heaviside or Θ step function is utilized

$$\Theta(u) \equiv \left\{ \begin{array}{l} 1, \text{ if } u > 0 \\ 0, \text{ if } u < 0 \end{array} \right. \tag{14.18}$$

---

[4]A shift in the integration variable may be used to show that integrals such as $\int_0^{2\pi} d\phi \, f(\cos(\phi - \theta))$ are independent of θ for any function f.

With the identity $uJ_0(u) = \frac{d}{du}(uJ_1(u))$, the Fourier transform (14.13) for the disk is found to be

$$s_{disk}(k) = 2\pi\rho_0 \int_0^{r_0} dr\, rJ_0(2\pi kr) \tag{14.19}$$

$$= \rho_0 r_0 J_1(2\pi kr_0)/k \tag{14.20}$$

In Fig. 14.2, a plot of (14.20) is compared with the product of sinc functions found in the 2D Cartesian transform of a box-shaped spin density. The shapes in k-space are similar.

Problem 14.1

Compare the Taylor series expansions up to and including fourth-order in k for $\text{sinc}(k\pi A)$ and $J_1(\pi kd)/(\pi kd/2)$ where A is the width of the rect function and d is the diameter of the disk. Using these series, or some other computation, compare the two functions through a plot on the same graph for $A = d$.

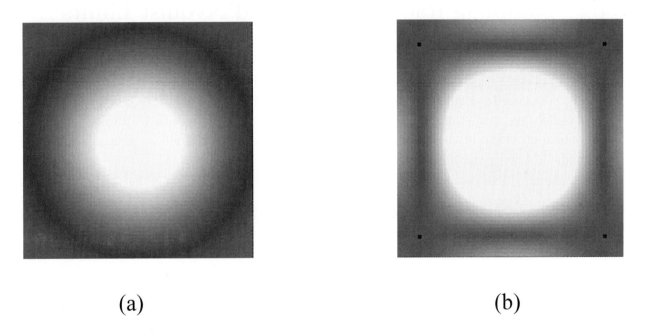

(a)   (b)

Fig. 14.2: Comparison between (a), the Fourier transform of a disk of diameter d of uniform spin density, and (b), the Fourier transform of a square of side d with uniform spin density.

14.1.3   Inversion for Image Reconstruction

Sufficient k-space data will allow a determination of the image through the inverse Fourier transform of (14.4) or (14.13). In Cartesian coordinates the image is found from

$$\rho(x, y) = \int\int dk_x\, dk_y\, s(k_x, k_y) e^{i2\pi(k_x x + k_y y)} \tag{14.21}$$

and in polar coordinates from

$$\rho(r, \phi) = \int \int k\, dk\, d\theta\, s(k, \theta) e^{i2\pi kr \cos(\theta - \phi)} \tag{14.22}$$

The degree to which the image is faithfully reconstructed depends on the completeness of k-space coverage.

The next question is the manner in which the array of vector values of $\vec{k}$ needed for the above inverse transforms is measured. Different points along a line in k-space collinear with a given $\vec{G}$ can be sampled over time, or by changing the magnitude of the gradient. To sample lines at different angles, and sweep out a 2D area in k-space, the gradient vector direction can be changed systematically. After a discussion of the number of data points required, various formulas for analyzing data gathered in radial sweeps of k-space are detailed in the rest of the chapter. Data can also be sampled in k-space and then interpolated to a Cartesian coverage to allow the use of (14.21). Similarly, $\rho(r, \phi)$ is usually interpolated to a Cartesian grid to display the image.

14.2   Sampling Radial k-Space and Nyquist Limits

Radial Coverage with an Echo

Assume for a given readout that it is possible by gradient reversal or by the appropriate spin echo sequence to cover both positive and negative halves of each line covered in k-space for a fixed θ (see, for example, Fig. 14.3a). Then the θ interval can be limited to 180°. To maintain coverage of the complete k_x-k_y plane, k can be redefined as plus or minus the magnitude of $\vec{k}$ with the limits,

$$-k_{max} \le k \le k_{max} \tag{14.23}$$

where $k_{max} = \gamma G T_s / 2$. The angular coverage is also limited to collect a finite number of angles. For N uniformly spaced readouts (N different gradient directions, Fig. 14.3b),

$$N\Delta\theta = \pi \tag{14.24}$$

Problem 14.2

For the convention using both positive and negative values of k, show that the polar variable relations (14.10) are replaced by

a) $k = \text{sgn}(k_y)\sqrt{k_x^2 + k_y^2}$

b) $\theta = \tan^{-1}(\frac{k_y}{k_x}) \bmod \pi$

Radial Coverage with FIDs

Although there is an inherent advantage to using an echo to collect a frequency encoded symmetric data set, the original benefit gained in radial coverage (i.e., not having to wait for the phase encoding before readout) is lost. Most of the current applications of radial k-space coverage involve imaging of short T_2 or T_2^* tissues. Sampling of the $k = 0$ point as quickly as possible is achieved only in the limit of sampling an FID. In this case, each readout covers the range $0 \leq k \leq k_{max}$, and the gradient angle θ must now be varied over the range $0 \leq \theta < 2\pi$ to cover a circular region of radius k_{max} in k-space. The sequence diagram for such an acquisition method is shown in Fig. 14.3c.

In any FID sampling scheme, the true $k = 0$ point, i.e., the time point where all isochromats are in phase, is not adequately sampled because of the finite width of the rf pulse. In those cases, the measured k-space function is actually a shifted version of $s(k, \theta)$, $(s(k+\Delta, \theta)$, say). This k-space shift manifests itself as a spatially linearly varying phase when the measured data are inverse Fourier transformed and image reconstruction then creates artifacts due to phase cancelation. An estimate of this linearly varying phase is therefore required before image reconstruction can be successfully performed on a newly created data set corrected for this shift. Even if the phase shift is successfully used to estimate the k-space shift Δ, it is still difficult to extrapolate the collected data to estimate $s(0, \theta)$ especially in an imaging experiment performed over a large sample because of the presence of B_0 inhomogeneities. However, as seen later (in Sec. 14.4.4), the signal at the $k = 0$ sample is not required for image reconstruction as it is forced to be zero in the reconstruction method anyway (see the description of 'filtered back projection' and the 'M-filter' in Sec. 14.4.4). Another major disadvantage with FID sampling is that if there are any remnant eddy currents (discussed in Ch. 27) immediately after the ramp-up of the read gradients, these might cause missampling of k-space, making the prediction of the $s(0, \theta)$ point difficult in practice.

As a result of the difficulties with the FID method, the sampling scheme is often a compromise between the ease of reconstruction of the symmetric radial coverage and the short intervals of the first readout sample of the FID radial coverage method (see Fig. 14.3c). This compromise is achieved by using highly asymmetric spin echoes or gradient echoes. The collection of a few negative k-space points in an asymmetric data collection scheme also allows image reconstruction with $0 \leq \theta \leq \pi$ and the use of partial Fourier image reconstruction (see Ch. 13).

Nyquist Limits in Radial Sampling

The Nyquist limitations on the step sizes in k-space need to be adapted to the polar coordinates. The differences compared to Cartesian step sizes change the nature of aliasing in important ways. The step sizes in the radial direction and in the θ direction, respectively, Δk_r and Δk_θ, are illustrated in Fig. 14.4. The key is that the latter depends on the distance from the origin

$$\Delta k_\theta = k\Delta\theta \leq k_{max}\Delta\theta \qquad (14.25)$$

To prevent aliasing, the largest angular step for fixed $\Delta\theta$ must follow the Nyquist criterion (Ch. 12)

$$k_{max}\Delta\theta \equiv 1/L \qquad (14.26)$$

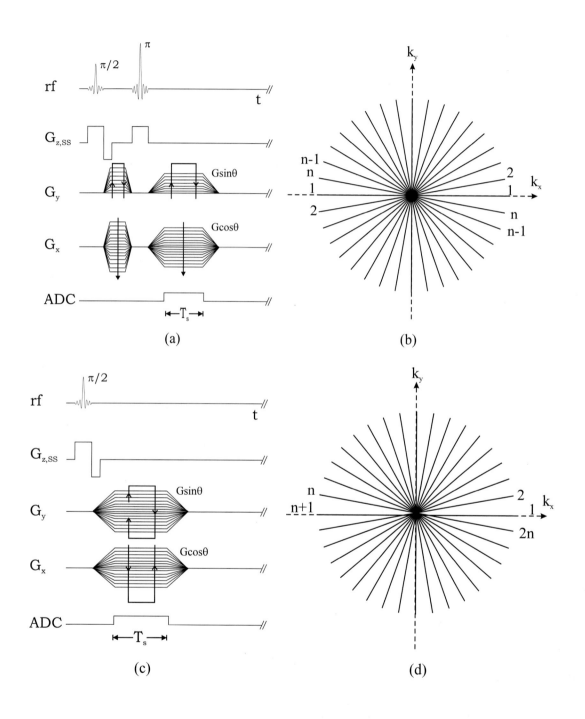

(a)

(b)

(c)

(d)

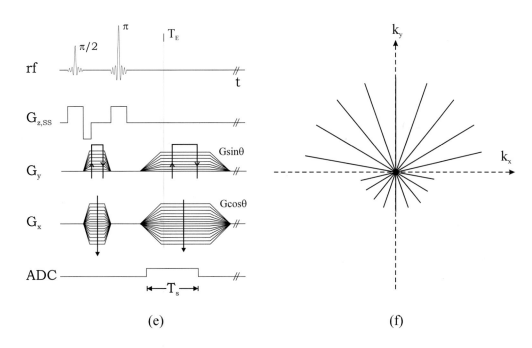

$$(e) \qquad\qquad\qquad (f)$$

Fig. 14.3: Sequence diagrams and associated k-space coverage for radial coverage. Spin echo sampling is illustrated in (a) and (b). The frequency encoding gradients, one of which steps through a cosinusoidal table, and the other which steps through a sinusoidal table, are varied such that θ lies in the range $0 \leq \theta \leq \pi$. FID sampling is illustrated in (c) and (d), where the frequency encoding gradients vary such that θ lies in the range $0 \leq \theta \leq 2\pi$. This variant has found increasing usage in imaging short T_2 or short T_2^* tissues. A partial Fourier method necessitates the use of asymmetric radial sampling as shown in (e) and (f).

for the field-of-view L. Hence the minimum number of angular views required to avoid aliasing is

$$n_\theta = \pi/\Delta\theta \geq \pi k_{max} L \qquad (14.27)$$

The radial step must similarly satisfy

$$\Delta k_r = 1/L \qquad (14.28)$$

From (14.8), the time steps along the gradient direction are thereby limited to

$$\Delta t = \Delta k_r/(\gamma G) \leq 1/(\gamma G L) \qquad (14.29)$$

The minimum total number of samples required in radial sampling is

$$n_r = 2k_{max}/\Delta k_r \geq 2k_{max} L \qquad (14.30)$$

This is the same condition as that for the read direction in the Cartesian k-space coverage method. Therefore the total number of points required to obtain an unaliased image with equal spatial resolution in both directions, i.e., with equal radial and angular spatial resolution when an echo is collected, is

$$n_r n_\theta \geq 2\pi(k_{max} L)^2 \qquad (14.31)$$

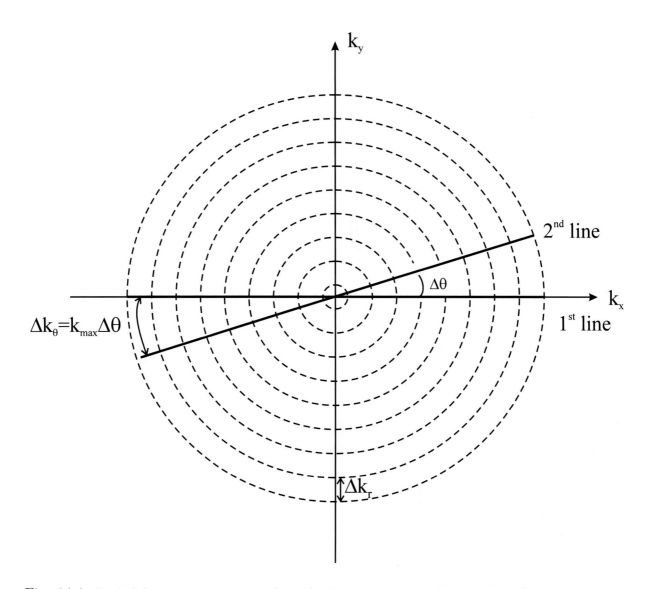

Fig. 14.4: Radial k-space coverage involves obtaining samples in k-space that fall on concentric circles. The separation between any two adjacent circles defines the separation Δk_r in the radial sampling direction, whereas, the angular separation between any two successive angular lines in k-space (such as between the two example lines shown in the figure) defines $\Delta\theta$. The two quantities Δk_r and $\Delta\theta$ are constrained by the Nyquist sampling criterion.

Comparison of Projection Reconstruction and 2D k-Space

The number (14.31) can be compared to the number of points required in Cartesian coverage. The number in either the x or y directions is the same as (14.30), so the total for the standard two-dimensional imaging method is[5]

$$n_x n_y \geq 4(k_{max} L)^2 \qquad (14.32)$$

The simple fact that $2\pi > 4$ means there are more sampling points in the circle of diameter L (pertinent to the radial coverage) than there are in the (larger) square of side L (pertinent to Cartesian coverage). In order to get adequate sampling at large k, there is oversampling (i.e., sampling more densely than Nyquist requires) of the smaller k values where Δk_θ is reduced proportionate to the k value. The total acquisition time for the projection reconstruction method is thus $\pi/2$ times longer, and the extra points collected result from the increased scan time. Looking ahead to Ch. 15, it is noted that this translates into better signal to noise for the 'radial readout,' but the price paid is the longer time taken for the measurement. Furthermore, this potential increase in SNR is realized only for a subregion of sampled points.

The illustration that the density of coverage in k-space varies inversely as the distance from the origin in k-space is presented in Fig. 14.4. We are reminded that the density of coverage in Cartesian methods is uniform. This varying density of coverage (leading to nonuniform coverage) usually has implications that relate to aliasing artifacts (as discussed briefly in Ch. 12). On the other hand, because the denser sampling of small k-space values implies relatively more information about the large structures of the image, the corresponding image reconstruction creates an image with a higher signal to noise ratio at the large distance scales in contrast with images reconstructed from Cartesian data. The high density in the center of k-space can lead to coherent or colored (in comparison with incoherent or white) noise in the object which can create a streaking of noise across pixels (see Ch. 15).

Problem 14.3

---

a) For a circular field-of-view of diameter $L = 256\,\text{mm}$ and $k_{max} = 1\,\text{mm}^{-1}$, find the minimum number of angular views (n_θ) that would be required to avoid aliasing in (i) an FID radial sampling scheme, and (ii) a spin echo sampling scheme.

b) Similarly, find the minimum number of views (n_r) required along the radial k-space variable direction.

c) If $T_R = 600\,\text{ms}$, what is the minimum total imaging time for (i) the FID radial sampling scheme, and (ii) the spin echo sampling scheme?

It is interesting to note that the spatial resolution in the x or y direction is limited in the 2D approach, since each gradient has an upper limit, which in turn restricts k-space coverage. But for $\Delta\theta$, the resolution in the θ direction, no such limit exists. Therefore, by an increase in angular acquisition, an object, such as a wheel with many spokes, can be resolved to the degree of accuracy desired.

---

[5]We consider the same maximum for k in both coverages in order to have the same spatial resolution in the radial direction, $\Delta r = 1/(2k_{max})$, as in either x or y direction.

14.3   Projections and the Radon Transform

A rotated coordinate system can be exploited for the case of a fixed gradient direction. It is observed that the phase in (14.11) depends only on the combination

$$x' = x\cos\theta + y\sin\theta \tag{14.33}$$

This is expected since the rotation through an angle θ to a new coordinate system leads to a frequency encoding axis x' parallel to the gradient direction ($\vec{G}\cdot\vec{r} = Gx'$) (see Ch. 9). It is natural to go to an integration over the primed coordinates since all spins along a given line perpendicular to the x' axis have constant phase.

A change of integration variables in (14.11) from (x, y) to (x', y'), for example, yields[6]

$$s(k,\theta) = \int\int_{\hat{x}'\|\vec{k}} dx'dy'\rho(x',y')e^{-i2\pi kx'} \tag{14.34}$$

where $\rho(x', y')$ can be written

$$\rho(x', y') \equiv \int\int dx\,dy\,\rho(x,y)\delta(x' - x\cos\theta - y\sin\theta)\delta(y' + x\sin\theta - y\cos\theta) \tag{14.35}$$

The integration restrictions indicated imply that the Cartesian coordinates x', y' must be chosen such that the x'-axis is at an angle θ with respect to the original x-axis. That is, x' is given by (14.33) and y' by

$$y' = -x\sin\theta + y\cos\theta \tag{14.36}$$

The (x', y') axes are a (counterclockwise) rotated version of the (x, y) axes.

The fact that the phase in (14.34) is independent of y' focuses attention onto the integral

$$P(x',\theta) = \int_{x',\theta} dy'\rho(x',y') \tag{14.37}$$

In the above notation, the projection $P(x',\theta)$ represents an integration along a line, at an angle of $\pi/2 + \theta$ with respect to the x-axis, passing through the point x'. This line integral follows the Cartesian ray perpendicular to the gradient direction, and is sometimes referred to as a 'ray sum,' a nomenclature growing out of the x-ray analog discussed below. The ray for $x' = x_0'$ and a given θ is shown in Fig. 14.5.

The reference to a 'ray sum' is appropriate in view of the discrete steps taken in measurements and in numerical integration over that discrete data set. The (discrete) set of all ray sums at a given θ is the full 'projection' for a specified gradient direction. The continuous set of projections at all possible angles of an object $\rho(x, y)$ comprise the set of Radon transforms $\check{\rho}$. The Radon transform is defined as

$$\check{\rho}(x',\theta) \equiv \mathcal{R}\rho \equiv \int_{-\infty}^{\infty}\int_{-\infty}^{\infty} dx\,dy\,\rho(x,y)\delta(x' - x\cos\theta - y\sin\theta) \quad 0 \le \theta \le \pi \tag{14.38}$$

which is nothing more than what is shown pictorially in Fig. 14.6. Hence, a set of 'projections' as defined above and collected at some finite set of angles, is a discrete approximation to the Radon transform of $\rho(x, y)$.

---

[6]The Jacobian for the transformation represented by (14.33) and (14.36) is unity. More simply, $dx\,dy = dx'dy'$ for the same reason a rotated pixel is unchanged in area or shape.

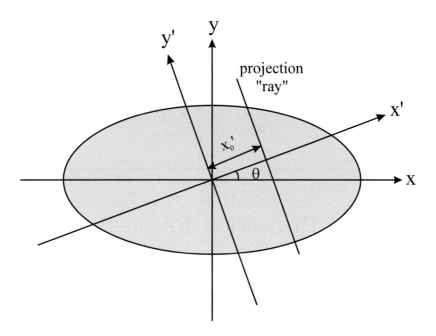

Fig. 14.5: Notation and framework for defining the projection of an object (shown here as a shaded surface) for rays (such as the one shown at a normal distance of x_0') making some arbitrary angle θ with respect to the x-axis.

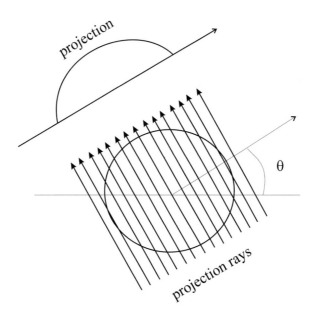

Fig. 14.6: A complete sampled set of sums for a set of parallel rays defined by the gradient direction. A continuous version of this so-called 'parallel ray projection' for a given object measured over all possible angles is the Radon transform of the object.

Problem 14.4

Compute the Radon transform of the following circular disk of uniform spin density

$$\rho(x,y) = \begin{cases} \rho_0 & x^2 + y^2 \leq r_0^2 \\ 0 & \text{elsewhere} \end{cases}$$

14.4   Methods of Projection Reconstruction with Radial Coverage

There are several ways of extracting an image from the data obtained by the projection approach. We consider three methods of projection reconstruction, the first a trivial and coarse approximation of the object, and the other two the most commonly used methods, after a brief connection to the reconstruction technique used in x-ray tomography is made.

14.4.1   X-Ray Analog

The gathering of data over rays projected through objects has its historical precedence in x-ray tomography. An x-ray beam is attenuated as it passes through the body to be imaged. With an initial rate I_0 of photons per unit time (at the same energy), the attenuation through a homogeneous thickness L is given by the familiar exponential formula,

$$I = I_0 e^{-\mu L} \tag{14.39}$$

where μ is an absorption constant that depends on the electron density of the material. For a heterogeneous body with a spatially varying attenuation constant $\mu(x,y)$ and a beam direction of $\pi/2 + \theta$ with respect to the x-axis, the primed coordinates in the previous projection discussion can also be employed in the more general attenuation formula, giving

$$I(x') = I_0(x')e^{-\int_L dy' \mu(x',y')} \tag{14.40}$$

The tomographic ray sum is defined by the exponent in (14.40)

$$P_{\text{x-ray}}(x',\theta) = \ln\left(I_0(x')/I(x')\right) = \int_{L,\theta} dy' \mu(x',y') \tag{14.41}$$

This measures the shading found in x-ray film and represents the total (i.e., integrated) absorption along the ray defined by the polar coordinate pair (x',θ). Comparison of (14.37) with (14.41) shows a close connection between x-ray imaging and the radial readout measurement in MRI.

14.4.2 Back-Projection Method

The line integral in (14.37) or (14.41), associated with a ray such as that shown in Fig. 14.5, constitutes a signal whose components come from somewhere along the line of pixels orthogonal to the x'-axis at some fixed x' value. A first approximation to image inversion from this data is to assume the signal has had equal contributions from each pixel in the line; a graphical representation of this assumption is to shade each pixel with its share of the total weight corresponding to the value of the original line integral. (Thus, in first approximation, the share is $1/n_r$ of the integral value.) Each daughter signal (the line integral) is apportioned back equally on each parent pixel (in the reconstructed image). The image obtained is the net shading achieved when all rays are added together. This process of image formation is called 'back-projection.'

In Fig. 14.7, a set of four rays is illustrated along with the corresponding signal shading. The example of back-projection shows only a rough similarity to the original object. Although a larger number of rays can improve the result, residual 'starring' remains at the edges, and corrections must be applied. A filtered version of the method is discussed after the next subsection. There is also some residual nonzero signal (bleeding out of the signal) in the reconstructed image where originally the spin density was zero.

This bleeding out (or smearing) artifact can be demonstrated easily with the simple example of an object with a point spin density. Suppose that the spin density model is such that it has unit spin density at the point $x = x_0$ (illustrated as point P in Fig. 14.8a). Then

$$\rho(x, y) = \delta(x - x_0)\delta(y) \tag{14.42}$$

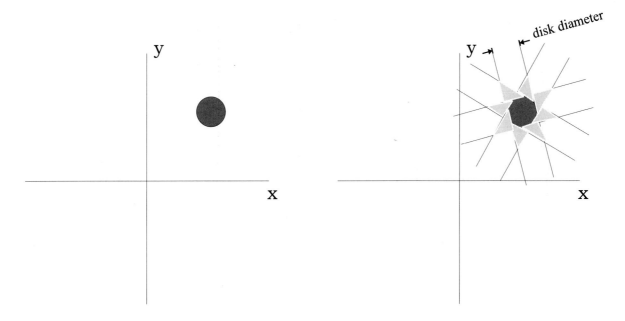

Fig. 14.7: The back-projection method is the simplest first approximation to the image in reconstruction from projections. Note the 'starring' artifact is obtained even for the simple case of a disk of uniform spin density.

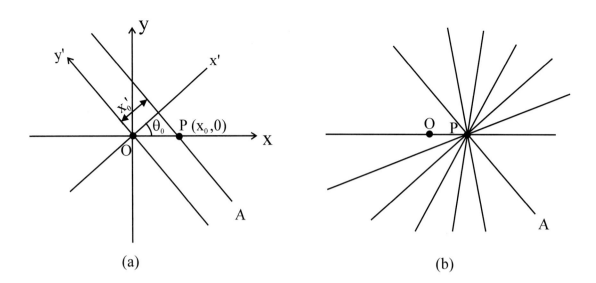

(a)   (b)

Fig. 14.8: (a) Pictorial representation for a particular projection computed such that the point P is mapped to the point where $x'_0 = x_0 \cos\theta_0$ on the projection. See Fig. 14.5 for details. (b) The reprojection of the collected projection data creates lines of unit intensity, all of which pass through P, but only one of which passes through any other point. The final back-projected image has a value n_θ at point P and a value of unity everywhere else.

and the Radon transform (or projection) of ρ evaluated at a distance x' away from the origin along a direction making an angle θ_0 is given as

$$\check{\rho}(x', \theta_0) = \delta(x' - x_0 \cos\theta_0) \tag{14.43}$$

Back-projection of some discrete set of projections representing samples of the continuous Radon transform of the object requires that each given projection be taken and reprojected into the image matrix and the intensities at a given pixel from all reprojected rays be summed to give the final image $R(x,y)$. Since each projection at angle θ has unit amplitude at $x' = x \cos\theta$, and is zero everywhere else (from (14.43)), each reprojection will create a line of unit intensity, each of which passes the point P in the reconstructed image, while one and only one reprojected nonzero ray passes through every other point (see Fig. 14.8b). In other words, the reconstructed image has unit intensity everywhere, and an intensity n_θ at P. The nonzero background intensity represents the starring or blurring effect, and the relative intensity of the artifact is reduced as the number of angular samples n_θ increases.

In summary, in the case where θ is covered continuously over 0 to π, the back-projected image $R(x,y)$, represented by $\mathbf{B}\rho$, is given by

$$R(x,y) \equiv \mathbf{B}\rho = \int_0^\pi d\theta P(x\cos\theta + y\sin\theta, \theta) \tag{14.44}$$

The formula for the back-projected image that allows for rays that are not necessarily distributed continuously, but covers 0 through π with the most general case of unequal angular intervals of $\Delta\theta_i$ is

$$R(x,y) = \sum_i P(x\cos\theta_i + y\sin\theta_i)\Delta\theta_i \tag{14.45}$$

Aside from units, $R(x, y)$ reflects the reconstructed spin density corresponding to the starred construction described earlier. For a given x, y, the expression (14.33) changes from angle to angle, and is generalized to give

$$x_i' = x \cos \theta_i + y \sin \theta_i \qquad (14.46)$$

The inherent difficulty in using the back-projection method to recover an acceptable approximation of the object spin density, even in the ideal case, has been made evident. It is usually discussed as a method of projection reconstruction, however, since it is a useful tool for laying the groundwork for other reconstruction methods to follow.

14.4.3 Projection Slice Theorem and the Fourier Reconstruction Method

In another approach to image reconstruction from projections, we return to the relation of the measured signal to the two-dimensional Fourier transform of the spin density in k-space.

Projection Slice Theorem

In terms of the line projection (14.37), (14.34) becomes

$$s(k, \theta) = \int dx' P(x', \theta) e^{-i2\pi k x'} \qquad (14.47)$$

The angle θ is fixed in this integration and, hence, it is seen that $s(k, \theta)$ is the Fourier transform, with respect to x', of the line projection P, with θ a fixed spectator parameter. This is the *projection slice or central slice theorem* which says that the two-dimensional Fourier transform $s(\vec{k})$ of the spin density is the one-dimensional Fourier transform of the line projection integral. The one-dimensional transform is with respect to the coordinate along the direction of $\vec{k}$. The interrelationship among ρ, $\check{\rho}$, and s, as represented by the projection slice theorem, is illustrated in Fig. 14.9.

Fourier Reconstruction

In review of the standard 2D Fourier MR imaging method, position (with respect to the two orthogonal directions within the slice) is encoded into the phase of the collected data at different instants of time. Recall that one direction involves 'phase encoding' and the other, 'frequency encoding.' Because the encodings are independent of each other, the Fourier inversion operator is separable in the two directions, and it can be implemented as two 1D inversions, one following the other. However, in the radial sampling method, both spatial variables are encoded at the same instant of time. Therefore, a true 2D inversion would be needed if the reconstruction were performed directly on the collected data, for which certain fast Fourier implementation algorithms do not apply.

Fortunately, we can make use of the projection slice theorem in a conversion from radial k-space data to an interpolated rectangular grid. The 2D Fourier inversion can then be employed and fast Fourier transform numerical techniques can be utilized in such a 'Fourier reconstruction method.' Problems occur near the edge of k-space in accurately doing this

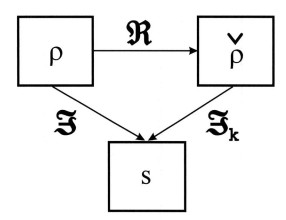

Fig. 14.9: Interrelationships among the original spin density ρ, its Radon transform $\check{\rho}$, and its 2D Fourier transform s. In the figure, $\mathcal{F}$ represents the 2D Fourier transform operator, and $\mathcal{F}_k$ represents the 1D radial Fourier transform operating on each projection.

(because of the reduced density of k-space samples there), leading to aliasing of edges (represented mainly by the high spatial frequency data) unless oversampling is done in the θ direction to improve interpolation.

14.4.4   Filtered Back-Projection Method

There is a way to find the two-dimensional Fourier transform of $\rho(x,y)$ directly from the back-projection formulas. Consider (14.44), which is the integral limit of (14.45),

$$R(x,y) = \int_0^\pi d\theta\, P(x',\theta) \tag{14.48}$$

remembering that there is additional θ dependence in x' through (14.33). The projection slice theorem (14.47) implies that the line projection $P(x',\theta)$ is given by a 1D inverse Fourier transform of $s(k,\theta)$ along the k direction. Substitution of $P(x',\theta)$ in (14.48) yields

$$R(x,y) = \int_0^\pi d\theta \int_{-\infty}^\infty dk\, s(k,\theta)e^{i2\pi kx'} \tag{14.49}$$

Note that the k-integration in (14.49) includes negative values. We can reduce the k range to the positive axis, returning to a magnitude definition for k by doubling the θ integration range,

$$R(x,y) = \int_0^{2\pi} d\theta \int_0^\infty dk\, s(k,\theta)e^{i2\pi \vec{k}\cdot\vec{r}} \tag{14.50}$$

where we have also backtracked to the original form of the exponent in (14.50) involving the two-dimensional vectors $\vec{k}$ and $\vec{r}$.

It is observed in (14.50) that, if the integrand is multiplied and divided by k, the full polar-variable measure of $k\,dk\,d\theta = d^2k$ appears. Thus $1/k$ times $s(k,\theta)$ must be the Fourier transform of R. We have the Fourier pair in 2D

$$R(x,y) = \int d^2k \frac{s(k,\theta)}{k}e^{i2\pi\vec{k}\cdot\vec{r}} = \mathcal{F}^{-1}(s/k) \tag{14.51}$$

$$\frac{s(k,\theta)}{k} = \int d^2r R(x,y) e^{-i2\pi \vec{k}\cdot\vec{r}} = \mathcal{F}(R) \tag{14.52}$$

The procedure can now be made clear. The Fourier transform $s(k,\theta)$ of an object is found by first determining the Fourier transform of $R(x,y)$ and then multiplying it by k (or $|k|$, if we go back to including negative values for k). In detail, rewriting the spin density as the inverse Fourier transform of $s(k,\theta)$ but integrated over the ranges suitable for projection variables and expressing the exponent $\vec{k}\cdot\vec{r} = kx'$ (from (14.22)) yields

$$\rho(x,y) = \int_0^\pi d\theta \int_{-\infty}^\infty |k|dk \; s(k,\theta) e^{i2\pi kx'} \tag{14.53}$$

The integrand now suggests the use of a 'filtered' projection that is the inverse Fourier transform of $|k|s(k,\theta)$ instead of $s(k,\theta)$, as it naturally arises in (14.53), by

$$P_{\text{filter}}(x',\theta) = \int_{-\infty}^\infty |k|dk \; s(k_x,k_y) e^{i2\pi kx'} \tag{14.54}$$

Finally, the image is obtained from the inverse Fourier transform of the filtered k-space data.

Multiplication by $|k|$ is both a cure and disease for this image reconstruction problem. Note that this 'M-filter' (so-called because of its 'M'-like shape in k-space; see Fig. 14.10) is a high pass filter since it enhances the high spatial frequencies while eliminating the zero spatial frequency. Remember the comment in the back-projection section that the simple reprojection of the collected projections creates blurring and the starring artifact. This high pass filter serves to remove the blurring, and an acceptable image is obtained using the filtered back-projection method (see Fig. 14.11 for a comparison between images reconstructed by back-projection and filtered back-projection). Although the object is now ideally reconstructed, the noise at the higher k-space samples gets exaggerated by the linear filter $|k|$. As a result, the reconstructed image has noise which becomes correlated even though the noise in the collected data is white and uncorrelated.

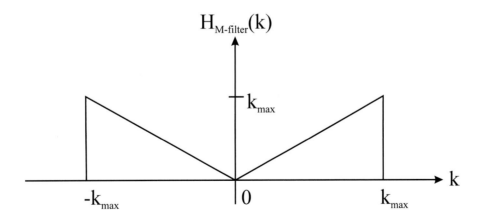

Fig. 14.10: The M-filter k-space response. In practice, it is common to smooth the M-filter transition to zero at $\pm k_{max}$ to avoid truncation artifacts (ringing) at tissue boundaries by applying a Hanning filter following the M-filter.

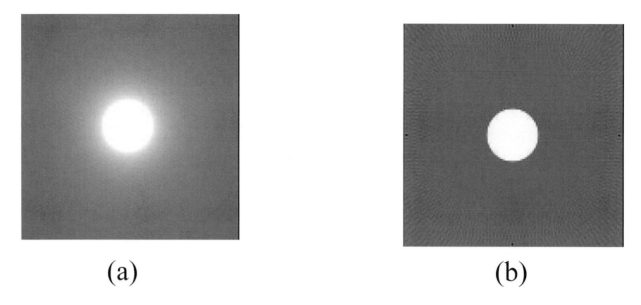

(a)   (b)

Fig. 14.11: Comparison between (a) back-projection and (b) filtered back-projection reconstruction from projections of a disk of uniform spin density. Note that the filtering has eliminated the star artifact seen in the back-projection.

14.4.5   Reconstruction of MR Images from Radial Data

Note that the data collected in the projection reconstruction scheme are the 1D Fourier transforms of projections of the spin density function along different directions. Therefore, methods such as filtered back-projection have the added advantage of needing less reconstruction time because the time required for the 1D Fourier transforms is saved. Therefore, the filtered back-projection method applicable to MR data is to apply the M-filter to $s(k,\theta)$ by multiplying it by $|k|$. Then take the inverse Fourier transform and back-project to create the image. In operator form, this translates into

$$\hat{\rho}(x,y) = \{[\mathbf{B}\mathcal{F}_k^{-1}]|k|s(k,\theta)\}(x,y) \tag{14.55}$$

Similarly, the Fourier regridding and reconstruction of MR images is made easier by the data already being in k-space. The only required operation on the collected data is to regrid the radially sampled data to Cartesian coordinates so that a 2D fast Fourier transformation would yield the final image.

One remark about a practical issue is worth mention here. If the projections obtained by inverse Fourier transforming each line of collected data at different angles have the origin mapped to different points, the reconstructed image will be badly blurred. One way to remedy this is to note that the center of mass of each projection is supposed to be spatially invariant. Using this fact, each projection can be centered correctly by estimating the center of mass of each projection and forcing them all to be at some arbitrary point.

Problem 14.5

In this problem, we will derive the form of another image reconstruction method which is equivalent to filtered back-projection, and is commonly known as the 'convolution back-projection' reconstruction method.

a) Starting with the final expression for the 'filtered projection' $P_{\text{filter}}(x', \theta)$ in (14.54) and the convolution theorem, show that

$$P_{\text{filter}}(x', \theta) = [\mathcal{F}^{-1}s(k, \theta)] * [\mathcal{F}^{-1}|k|] \qquad (14.56)$$

b) Show that the inverse 1D Fourier transform of $|k|$ evaluated at r is $-1/(2\pi^2 r^2)$. Hence, write an equivalent expression for the 'filtered projection' as a convolution integral.

c) Write the equivalent set of operations for convolution back-projection from radial MR data based on your result in part (b).

14.5 Three-Dimensional Radial k-Space Coverage

The signal measured from an experiment with an arbitrary frequency encoding gradient is the Fourier transform of the line integral or ray projection of the spin density distribution of the object along the gradient direction only when a slice selective pulse is used. When such a selective pulse is not applied, and instead a nonselective pulse is applied, the measured signal is now a planar projection or planar integration, the plane again being perpendicular to the gradient direction defined by the polar angle θ and azimuthal angle ϕ. Suppose we consider a gradient applied at an angle θ relative to the z-axis and angle ϕ relative to the x-axis. Then, for points P defined by the Cartesian coordinates (x, y, z) lying along some arbitrary plane perpendicular to some point R defining the projection plane and at a distance r away from the origin, defined by the spherical polar coordinates (r, θ, ϕ) (see Fig. 14.12), the vectors $\overrightarrow{OP}$ and $\overrightarrow{OR}$ are defined respectively, as:

$$\overrightarrow{OP} = x\hat{x} + y\hat{y} + z\hat{z} \qquad (14.57)$$

$$\overrightarrow{OR} = r\sin\theta\cos\phi\hat{x} + r\sin\theta\sin\phi\hat{y} + r\cos\theta\hat{z} \qquad (14.58)$$

Hence, the normal vector $\overrightarrow{PR}$ drawn from P to the line OR defining the frequency encoding axis is given by

$$\begin{aligned} \overrightarrow{RP} &= \overrightarrow{OP} - \overrightarrow{OR} \\ &= (x - r\sin\theta\cos\phi)\hat{x} + (y - r\sin\theta\sin\phi)\hat{y} + (z - r\cos\theta)\hat{z} \end{aligned} \qquad (14.59)$$

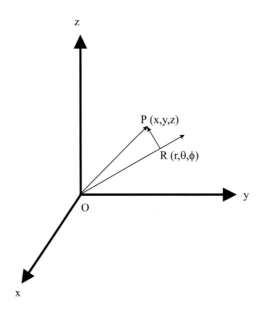

Fig. 14.12: Projection plane definition. Here the projection plane at $R(r, \theta, \phi)$ is defined to be perpendicular to the vector $\overrightarrow{OR}$. One such point on the projection plane is P, with $\overrightarrow{PR}$ being perpendicular to $\overrightarrow{OR}$.

Since $\overrightarrow{OR}$ and $\overrightarrow{RP}$ are perpendicular to each other, $\overrightarrow{OR} \cdot \overrightarrow{PR} = 0$, and that defines the equation of the projection plane, i.e.,

$$(x - r\sin\theta\cos\phi)(r\sin\theta\cos\phi) + (y - r\sin\theta\sin\phi)(r\sin\theta\sin\phi) + (z - r\cos\theta)(r\cos\theta) = 0 \tag{14.60}$$

which, on simplification yields the equation of the projection plane as:

$$r = x\sin\theta\cos\phi + y\sin\theta\sin\phi + z\cos\theta \quad \text{(projection plane equation)} \tag{14.61}$$

By collecting a set of these planar projections for different values of θ and ϕ covering a sphere for obtaining isotropic spatial resolution, the entire spherical volume can be reconstructed into voxels (or volume elements) that are represented by a uniform spin density estimate $\rho(x, y, z)$. This 3D spin density distribution can be written in terms of its 3D Fourier transform, $s(k_x, k_y, k_z)$ as:

$$\rho(x, y, z) = \int \int \int dk_x \, dk_y \, dk_z \, s(k_x, k_y, k_z) e^{i2\pi(k_x x + k_y y + k_z z)} \tag{14.62}$$

which is the same representation as the reconstructed image from the signal measured one line at a time in k-space by 'reading out' after the signal is phase encoded in the other two directions by constant phase encoding and partition encoding gradients. Repeating such an experiment with different values of the phase encoding and partition encoding gradients allows for the complete coverage of 3D k-space. This same k-space inversion method is valid for data encoded radially over a sphere such that one radial line is collected in k-space making angles θ and ϕ with respect to the z- and x-axes respectively, and parallel to the read gradient direction during a single readout. Repeated measurements with read gradients at different θ and ϕ values such that they cover the required extent in k-space within a spherical volume allow inversion by converting (14.62) into its polar form, giving

$$\rho(x, y, z) \equiv \rho(\vec{r}) = \int_0^{2\pi} d\phi \int_0^{\pi} d\theta \int_0^{\infty} dk\, k^2 \sin\theta s(k, \theta, \phi) e^{i2\pi\vec{k}\cdot\vec{r}} \qquad (14.63)$$

where $\vec{k}$ has spherical polar coordinates of (k, θ, ϕ).

Image reconstruction from 3D radial k-space data can be carried out similar to reconstruction from 2D data, using either the 3D version of the projection slice theorem or a new filtered back-projection method. To mathematically state the 3D projection slice theorem, we again define the planar projection along the (θ, ϕ) direction, $P_{\theta\phi}(r)$,[7] and its 1D radial Fourier transform, $\mathcal{F}_r\{P_{\theta\phi}(r)\}$ or $F_{\theta\phi}(k)$, say.

$$P_{\theta\phi}(r) = \int\int\int dx\, dy\, dz\, \rho(x, y, z)\delta(r - x\sin\theta\cos\phi - y\sin\theta\sin\phi - z\cos\theta) \qquad (14.64)$$

and

$$F_{\theta\phi}(k) \equiv \mathcal{F}_r\{P_{\theta\phi}(r)\}(k) \equiv \int_0^{\infty} dr\, P_{\theta\phi}(r) e^{-i2\pi kr} \qquad (14.65)$$

Given these notations, the projection slice theorem states that

$$s(k, \theta, \phi) = F_{\theta\phi}(k) \qquad (14.66)$$

In other words, each measured line $F_{\theta\phi}(k)$, the Fourier transform of the planar projection $P_{\theta\phi}(r)$, equals that line from the 3D k-space data $s(k, \theta, \phi)$ along the same orientation as the read gradient.

Therefore, either one of the two expressions (14.62) or (14.63) can be used for computing the required 3D spin density distribution $\rho(x, y, z)$. The main differences between using the radial representation and Cartesian representation is that there is no fast Fourier transform method to implement (14.63) as in the 2D case, whereas, once the Cartesian representation is obtained approximately by interpolating $s(k, \theta, \phi)$ into a Cartesian coordinate system, the 3D inversion can be achieved separably in the three directions using FFTs.

To derive the 3D filtered back-projection method, we first note that $P_{\theta\phi}(r)$ can be written in terms of $F_{\theta\phi}(k)$ as

$$\begin{aligned} P_{\theta\phi}(r) &= \int_0^{\infty} dk\, F_{\theta\phi}(k) e^{i2\pi kr} \\ &= \int_{-\infty}^{\infty} dk\, s(k, \theta, \phi) e^{i2\pi kr} \end{aligned} \qquad (14.67)$$

Using a previous notation (14.54), let us define a 'filtered projection:'

$$P_{\theta\phi}^{\text{filt}}(r) \equiv \int_0^{\infty} dk\, k^2 \sin\theta\, s(k, \theta, \phi) e^{i2\pi kr} \qquad (14.68)$$

---

[7]The set of all planar projections, defined over all possible (r, θ, ϕ), is the 3D Radon transform of the object.

Then, from (14.63) and (14.64)

$$\rho(\vec{r}) = \rho(x,y,z) = \int_0^{2\pi} \int_0^{\pi} d\theta\, d\phi\, P_{\theta\phi}^{\text{filt}}(x\sin\theta\cos\phi + y\sin\theta\sin\phi + z\cos\theta) \qquad (14.69)$$

If the 3D back-projection operator $\mathbf{B}^3$ acting on some set of planar projections $P_{\theta\phi}^{\text{filt}}(r)$ is defined as the operation

$$\mathbf{B}^3 P_{\theta\phi}^{\text{filt}}(r) \equiv R(x,y,z) \int_0^{\pi} \int_0^{2\pi} d\theta\, d\phi\, \sin\theta\, P_{\theta\phi}^{\text{filt}}(r)|_{r=x\sin\theta\cos\phi+y\sin\theta\sin\phi+z\cos\theta} \qquad (14.70)$$

then

$$\rho(x,y,z) = \left[\mathbf{B}^3 P_{\theta\phi}^{\text{filt}}(r)\right](x,y,z) \qquad (14.71)$$

i.e., the 3D spin density distribution is obtained as the 3D back-projection of the inverse Fourier transform of the collected k-space data $s(k,\theta,\phi)$ that is 'filtered' by the k-space function $k^2\sin\theta$.

Only the continuous case in k-space has been considered up to now. In reality, only samples are collected in k-space. Nyquist limits similar to the 2D case can be derived for the 3D case too. To determine how the gradient direction is stepped, the usual method is to assume that isotropic spatial resolution is required. This means that the solid angle[8] $\sin\theta\, d\theta d\phi$ formed by the elemental surface area strip on the unit sphere by some azimuthal angular increment $d\phi$ from some initial angle ϕ and by some polar angle increment $d\theta$ from some initial angle θ, is the same for all (θ,ϕ) pairs (see Fig. 14.13). Since the solid angle is $\sin\theta\, d\theta d\phi$, this means that if θ is incremented in uniform intervals of $\Delta\theta$, ϕ is incremented as $\frac{\Delta\phi}{\sin\theta}$. For isotropic resolution, $\Delta\theta = \Delta\phi$. Hence, the discrete filtered 3D back-projection is obtained as

$$\rho(x,y,z) = \Delta\theta^2 \sum_m \sum_n P_{\theta_m\phi_n}^{\text{filt}}(x\sin\theta_m\cos\phi_n + y\sin\theta_m\sin\phi_n + z\cos\theta_m) \qquad (14.72)$$

for such a k-space coverage.

14.6 Radial Coverage Versus Cartesian k-Space Coverage

In the Cartesian k-space sampling scheme, a finite amount of time is spent after the rf pulse for phase encoding to encode the directions other than the frequency encoding direction. In radial coverage, this finite time is saved, as the readout can be started as soon as the slice select rephase lobe is completed. This saving is very useful in imaging certain short T_2 tissues, and in microscopic imaging where susceptibility effects cause the T_2^* to be extremely short. Of course, with a nonselective rf pulse (rf pulse with a sharp boxcar rf envelope) with a frequency response broad enough to excite all spins in the object lying within the region of sensitivity of the transmit coil, even the finite time required for the rephase lobe of the slice select gradient is not required. Then, an FID sampling is approximately achieved.

---

[8]Remember, solid angles are defined as elemental surface areas on the unit sphere. For example, the solid angle subtended by the entire spherical surface is 4π steradians, since the total surface area of the unit sphere is in fact 4π.

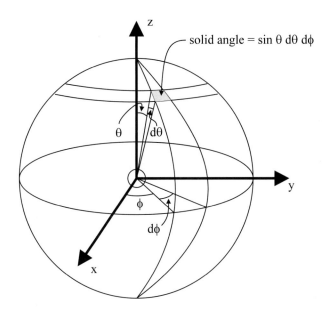

Fig. 14.13: Illustration of the solid angle defining the elemental area $\sin\theta\, d\theta\, d\phi$ on the unit circle. Note that for isotropic resolution in the final 3D reconstruction, this solid angle formed by elemental changes $d\theta$ and $d\phi$ in the azimuthal and polar angles remains constant for all θ and ϕ.

14.6.1 Image Distortion Due to Off-Resonance Effects: Cartesian Coverage Versus Radial Sampling

One difficulty with radial k-space coverage is the radial blurring of point objects that occurs in the presence of field inhomogeneities. On the other hand, in Fourier imaging, this resonance offset effect shifts the location of the affected spins along the read direction only. As a result, in both cases, the point spread function changes from point to point as a function of the field inhomogeneity relative to the read gradient strength.

Effects of B_0 Inhomogeneities in Cartesian Imaging

In this and the next subsection, the effects of field inhomogeneities on the imaging point spread function are considered (no discrete approximations are considered, and the data and image functions are (continuous) Fourier transform pairs; this implies that the point spread function in the absence of any inhomogeneity is a Dirac delta function in either case). To this effect, the image for data collected when the object is a point (i.e., an impulse at some arbitrary position) gives the point spread function. Let us consider the object to be a unit impulse at $\vec{r_0} = (x_0, y_0)$, i.e.,

$$\rho(x, y) = \delta(x - x_0)\delta(y - y_0) \tag{14.73}$$

Suppose that the field is inhomogeneous, and the inhomogeneity at (x_0, y_0) is $\Delta B(x_0, y_0)$. Therefore, the measured signal as a function of time is

$$s(t) = e^{-i2\pi\bar{\gamma}\Delta B(x_0,y_0)t} \cdot e^{-i2\pi(\bar{\gamma}G_R x_0(t-T_E)+k_y y_0)} \tag{14.74}$$

Since k_x equals $\gamma G_R t'$ where $t' = (t - T_E)$, $\gamma t'$ in the above expression can be replaced by k_x/G_R, and the signal can be written as a function of k_x as

$$s(k) = e^{-i2\pi k_x \frac{\Delta B(x_0,y_0)}{G_R}} \cdot e^{-i2\pi\gamma\Delta B(x_0,y_0)T_E} \cdot e^{-i2\pi(k_x x_0 + k_y y_0)} \tag{14.75}$$

Inverse Fourier transforming and neglecting the constant phase factor first term and recognizing that the third term is in fact the Fourier transform of $\rho(x, y)$ (from (11.5)) gives the generalized point spread function in the presence of an inhomogeneity at position (x, y) as

$$h_{\Delta B,c}(x, y) = \delta\left(x - x_0 - \frac{\Delta B(x_0, y_0)}{G_R}\right)\delta(y - y_0) \tag{14.76}$$

As before, this new point spread function only convolves with any other point spread function, whether it is due to signal decay during sampling or to the discrete Fourier transformation. Since this is a delta function, it obviously does not change the shape of imaging point spread function. The only effect is that the coordinate position in the read direction is translated by an amount $x_0 + \Delta B(x_0, y_0)/G_R$; in the presence of a continuously-varying field inhomogeneity function, this leads to a distortion of the object. This distortion effect is the subject of detailed discussion in Ch. 20.

Effects of B_0 Inhomogeneities in Radial Imaging

An analysis along lines similar to the one above is carried out for radial imaging here. The Radon transform of $\tilde{\rho}(x, y)$ (defined in (14.38)) yields the projection

$$P(x', \theta) = \int\int dx\, dy\, \delta(x - x_0)\delta(y - y_0)\delta(x' - x\cos\theta - y\sin\theta) \tag{14.77}$$

Similar to (14.47), the collected k-space data in the presence of $\Delta B(x_0, y_0)$ are then given by

$$s(k, \theta) = \int dx' e^{-i2\pi kx'}\left[\int\int dx\, dy\, \delta(x - x_0)\delta(y - y_0)\delta(x' - x\cos\theta - y\sin\theta)\right]e^{-i2\pi\gamma\Delta B(x_0,y_0)t} \tag{14.78}$$

In the above equation, the radial k-space variable k is given by $k \equiv \gamma G t'$, and $t \equiv (t' + T_E)$. Note that G is independent of θ, and is given by $G = \sqrt{G_x^2 + G_y^2}$ with G_x and G_y varying as $G\cos\theta$ and $G\sin\theta$ for a given projection angle θ. Upon simplification, (14.78) yields

$$s(k, \theta) = e^{-i2\pi k(x_0\cos\theta + y_0\sin\theta)} \cdot e^{-i2\pi k\Delta B(x_0,y_0)/G}e^{-i2\pi\gamma\Delta B(x_0,y_0)T_E} \tag{14.79}$$

Let us use the filtered back-projection method as a tool for illustration here. The reconstructed image evaluated at $\vec{r} = (x, y)$ (neglecting the constant phase term $e^{-i2\pi\gamma\Delta B(x_0,y_0)T_E}$) is given by

$$\hat{\rho}(x, y) = \int_0^{2\pi} d\theta \int_0^\infty dk\, k e^{i2\pi k(x\cos\theta + y\sin\theta)}\left(e^{-i2\pi k(x_0\cos\theta + y_0\sin\theta)}\right)\left(e^{-i2\pi k\Delta B(x_0,y_0)/G}\right) \tag{14.80}$$

To determine the relevant point spread function due to the presence of the field inhomogeneity, (14.80) is rewritten using the convolution theorem (see Ch. 11, for example) as

$$\hat{\rho}(x, y) = \mathcal{F}_{2D}^{-1}\left(e^{-i2\pi k(x_0\cos\theta + y_0\sin\theta)}\right) * \mathcal{F}_{2D}^{-1}\left(e^{-i2\pi k\Delta B(x_0,y_0)/G}\right) \tag{14.81}$$

From (11.5), the first term is a delta function positioned at $x = x_0, y = y_0$, the same as the object's spin density. The second term, the point spread function ($h^{\mathrm{radial}}_{\Delta B}(x,y)$), is clearly not a delta function, unless $\Delta B(x_0, y_0)$ is zero.

The 2D inverse Fourier transform needed to evaluate $h^{\mathrm{radial}}_{\Delta B}(x,y)$ can be performed in radial k-space, where each point is defined by the coordinates (k, θ). Let us define a r_0 as

$$r_0 \equiv \frac{\Delta B(x_0, y_0)}{G} \tag{14.82}$$

for convenience. Now, performing the integration over θ first gives the result

$$h^{\mathrm{radial}}_{\Delta B}(r, \phi) = 2\pi \int_0^\infty dk\, k e^{i2\pi r_0 k} J_0(2\pi k r) \tag{14.83}$$

which is independent of the polar angle ϕ in the spatial coordinate system used to describe the reconstruction point (x, y). This means that, instead of the local, spatial shifting of the point as occurs in Fourier imaging, the effect in radial k-space coverage is to create a radial smear. Frequency shifts due to chemical shifts also manifest themselves in a similar fashion.

14.6.2   Effects of Motion

One of the nice features of projection reconstruction on the other hand is the effect of object motion during data acquisition on the reconstructed image. In Fourier imaging, periodic motion causes periodic ghosts whose number within the FOV, and distance from each other, are determined by the period of the motion relative to T_R. In any case, the first ghost, which is closest to the object, is the most significant amongst these. In the worst-case scenario, this ghost might lie very close to the object of interest, leading sometimes to false diagnosis. On the other hand, periodic motion causes radial streaking in radial imaging. However, by nature, the streaks have very low intensity very close to the moving object, and the first significant streak occurs farther away from it. As a result, object visibility is not hindered by the presence of any significant nearby ghosts with projection reconstruction. However, there is still a smearing or blurring of the image due to the motion.

14.6.3   Cartesian Sampling of Radially Collected Data

It is not uncommon to resample radial data onto a Cartesian grid. This has the advantage of allowing a straightforward 2D Fourier transform reconstruction to be performed to create the image. The noise spatial frequency is white when a 2D DFT is used compared to a varied spatial frequency response for projection reconstruction. The latter has heavily filtered low spatial frequency noise. The effects of motion during data collection still cause a blur rather than ghosting despite the fact that a 2D DFT was performed. The regridding does lead to aliasing of the image due to insufficiently accurate data interpolation. This can be partially overcome by oversampling the radial data but requires increased data acquisition time.

Suggested Reading

Two excellent texts that cover the basic concepts and reconstruction of projection data are:

- S. R. Deans. *The Radon Transform and Some of its Applications.* John Wiley and Sons, New York, 1983.

- G. T. Herman. *Image Reconstruction from Projections: The Fundamentals of Computerized Tomography.* Academic Press, New York, 1980.

General sampling concepts for different k-space schemes are covered in:

- D. B. Twieg. The k-trajectory formulation of the NMR imaging process with applications in analysis and synthesis of imaging methods. *Med. Phys.*, 10: 610, 1983.

The point spread function resulting from polar sampling is given in the following two papers:

- M. L. Lauzon and B. K. Rutt. Effects of polar sampling in k-space. *Magn. Reson. Med.*, 36: 940, 1996.

- K. Scheffler and J. Hennig. Reduced circular field-of-view imaging. *Magn. Reson. Med.*, 40: 474, 1998.

Chapter 15

Signal, Contrast, and Noise

Chapter Contents

Summary: Quantitative methods for understanding the effects of noise in an image are introduced. The important imaging parameter, the signal-to-noise ratio (SNR), is studied in detail. The effects of imaging parameters such as spatial resolution, T_s, and the number of measured data samples N_x, N_y, and N_z on SNR are discussed. Contrast-to-noise ratio (CNR) and visibility concepts are developed as measures of useful information in an image. The issue of SNR as a function of field strength is briefly considered.

Introduction

All physical measurements include either random or systematic noise, which can seriously affect the accuracy or interpretation of a measurement. The degree to which noise affects a measurement is generally characterized by the signal-to-noise ratio (SNR). In MRI, the SNR is a key parameter for determining the effectiveness of any given imaging experiment. If the SNR is not high enough, it becomes impossible to differentiate tissues from one another or the background. Since the signal has already been discussed at some length in previous chapters, a study of the properties of the noise, and development of expressions for SNR which depend on the imaging parameters are made the major focus of this chapter.[1] SNR as a function of resolution, readout bandwidth (BW_{read}), and imaging time is developed. In MRI, every factor of $\sqrt{2}$ improvement in SNR allows a doubling of resolution in one direction and has an order of magnitude psychological effect on the quality of the image. It is, therefore, necessary to strive in all possible ways to optimize SNR for a fixed spatial resolution.

In Ch. 13, the issue of spatial resolution was studied, and it was determined that MRI can localize signals to very small regions. Localization of the signal is only half of the battle in an MRI experiment. If the signals from different tissues are all the same, a uniform image would be obtained giving no useful anatomic or diagnostic information. The real objective is to localize the signal and be able to differentiate diseased from healthy tissue and one tissue type from another. This implies that there must be a signal difference, referred to as contrast, between different tissues. Combining SNR with contrast leads to the quantity contrast-to-noise ratio (CNR) which is the real 'measure' of the usefulness of an experiment. The second half of this chapter deals with the study of CNR in MRI. It will be found that there are many variables which may be employed to generate contrast in the MRI experiment, and several specific forms of MRI contrast are discussed in depth.

15.1   Signal and Noise

The ability to ascertain whether some object is within a voxel or not depends critically on whether the signal for the object in that voxel can be distinguished from noise. It is the manifestation of the noise in the image, not the noise in the raw data, that is critical here. In this section, the translation from one domain to the other is considered.

15.1.1   The Voxel Signal

The general k-space signal encoding scheme leads to a signal expression (10.2)

$$s(\vec{k}) = \int_V d^3 r \rho(\vec{r}) e^{-i2\pi \vec{k} \cdot \vec{r}} \tag{15.1}$$

When the signal expression in (15.1) is written for the 3D Fourier imaging case, it becomes

$$s(k_x, k_y, k_z) = \int \int \int dx\, dy\, dz\, \rho(x, y, z) e^{-i2\pi(k_x x + k_y y + k_z z)} \tag{15.2}$$

As in earlier chapters, the data are assumed to be sampled at a set of points in 3D k-space. These points are separated by Δk_x, Δk_y, and Δk_z, respectively, in the three orthogonal k-space directions, and cover the range defined by the set of integers

$$p',\ q',\ \text{and } r' \in (-N_x, N_x - 1), (-N_y, N_y - 1), (-N_z, N_z - 1)$$

The image is reconstructed by applying a discrete inverse Fourier transform to the set of data represented by $s_m(p'\Delta k_x, q'\Delta k_y, r'\Delta k_z)$. Likewise, the image is represented by

---

[1]Imaging parameters are those variables which are free to be chosen in an experiment, such as T_R, T_E, readout bandwidth, etc., and not the physical constants associated with the sample such as ρ, T_1, or T_2.

$\hat{\rho}_m(p\Delta x, q\Delta y, r\Delta z)$ where p, q, and r typically cover the same range as p', q', and r'. The signal at a given point in the image is

$$\hat{\rho}_m(p\Delta x, q\Delta y, r\Delta z) = \frac{1}{N_x N_y N_z} \sum_{p',q',r'} s(p'\Delta k_x, q'\Delta k_y, r'\Delta k_z) e^{i2\pi\left(\frac{p\,p'}{N_x} + \frac{q\,q'}{N_y} + \frac{r\,r'}{N_z}\right)} \quad (15.3)$$

The effective spin-density $\hat{\rho}_m(p\Delta x, q\Delta y, r\Delta z)$ is also known as the 'voxel signal' $S(\vec{r})$ since it is the signal which will be represented in the volume element $\Delta x \Delta y \Delta z$ at position $(p\Delta x, q\Delta y, r\Delta z)$ in the reconstructed image.[2] Recall that $\hat{\rho}_m(p\Delta x, q\Delta y, r\Delta z)$ often not only represents the transverse magnetization within the voxel volume but also contains a handful of scaling factors and relaxation parameters.[3]

In Secs. 15.1–15.3, it is assumed that voxels are small volumes with uniform spin densities ($\rho(x) =$ a constant). Therefore, all arguments in these sections neglect the possibility of a voxel containing more than one tissue type. Section 15.4 introduces the subject of voxels which are not homogeneous. From Ch. 13, it must also be remembered that the presence of the finite-width point spread function of the discrete Fourier transform (13.17) and the finite blur due to T_2^* decay during sampling (13.57) cause the presence of a nonzero contribution from magnetization outside the voxel boundaries to overlap or contribute to the voxel of interest.

From the discussion on spatial resolution in Ch. 13, the voxel size also represents the area under the point spread function normalized to the zero value of the point spread function. As a result, whenever the spatial resolution is improved by reducing Δx, Δy, or Δz, the total contribution to the voxel signal is reduced proportionately (see, for example, (12.25)); for example, if Δx is halved, $\hat{\rho}_m(p\Delta x, q\Delta y, r\Delta z)$ is also halved. Therefore, in general

$$\hat{\rho}_m(p\Delta x, q\Delta y, r\Delta z) \propto \Delta x \Delta y \Delta z \equiv \text{voxel volume} \equiv V_{voxel} \quad (15.4)$$

The signal limit of (7.20) shows that the peak signal for a homogeneous sample (at $t = 0$ in an FID experiment, or at $t = T_E$ for a 90° gradient echo or spin echo imaging experiment) when transverse signal decay and amplification factors are neglected is given by (7.22)

$$\text{signal for homogeneous object} = \omega_0 M_0 \mathcal{B}_\perp V_{sample} \quad (15.5)$$

where $\mathcal{B}_\perp$ is the transverse field amplitude produced by the receive coil when a unit current is passed through it. Since the voxel is assumed to be a small homogeneous volume element in these discussions, (6.10) can be used to rewrite (15.5) for proton imaging as

$$
\begin{aligned}
S &\equiv \hat{\rho}_m(p\Delta x, q\Delta y, r\Delta z) \\
&\propto \omega_0 \cdot \frac{\frac{1}{2} \cdot \frac{3}{2} \cdot \gamma^2 \hbar^2}{3kT} \cdot B_0 \cdot \mathcal{B}_\perp(p\Delta x, q\Delta y, r\Delta z) \cdot \Delta x \Delta y \Delta z \\
&\propto \frac{\gamma^3 \hbar^2}{4kT} \cdot B_0^2 \cdot \mathcal{B}_\perp(p\Delta x, q\Delta y, r\Delta z) \cdot V_{voxel} \quad (15.6)
\end{aligned}
$$

---

[2]The reader may recall from Ch. 11 that the Fourier transform of a function represented by a lowercase letter is represented by an uppercase letter. Here lowercase s is used to represent k-space data, $s(\vec{k})$, and an uppercase S is used for the image $S(\vec{r})$, usually when the image voxel signal is being discussed.

[3]The use of effective spin density is no more appropriate than using transverse magnetization or number of spins in a voxel. It has been used in this way because all voxels in a conventional Fourier imaging approach have the same dimensions, and hence, the actual spin density times this volume has the same relative behavior from voxel to voxel as what we have called, for simplicity, effective spin density.

It is important to note the different dependencies in (15.6). Of interest is the direct dependence on the voxel volume, on $\vec{M} \cdot \vec{B}$ (which is proportional to $\rho_0 \mathcal{B}_\perp$) which is discussed in Secs. 7.3 and 7.4, and on B_0^2, the topic of discussion of a later section in this chapter, as well as the inverse dependence on the sample temperature (which is discussed in Ch. 6).

15.1.2   The Noise in MRI

One of the primary goals of a well-conducted MRI experiment is to obtain enough voxel signal relative to noise (as measured by the ratio of the voxel signal to the noise standard deviation, or signal-to-noise ratio SNR) to observe tissues of interest. Generally, the noise voltage derives from random fluctuations in the receive coil electronics and the sample. Even though there are other sources of signal fluctuations such as digitization noise and pseudo-random ghosting due to moving spins, these sources are minimized in an ideal experiment.

The variance[4] of the fluctuating noise voltage is presented here, without proof,[5] to be

$$\mathrm{var}(emf_{\mathrm{noise}}) \equiv \sigma_{thermal}^2 \propto \overline{(emf_{\mathrm{noise}} - \overline{emf_{\mathrm{noise}}})^2} = 4kT \cdot R \cdot BW \qquad (15.7)$$

where the horizontal bar over a value implies an average value, R is the effective resistance of the coil loaded by the body, and BW is the bandwidth of the noise-voltage detecting system (in NMR, both the signal and the noise are detected by the receive coil and the bandwidth of reception is determined by the cutoff frequency of the analog low pass filter, BW_{read}).

The proportionality to BW is the principal feature of (15.7), inasmuch as the temperature and resistance of the coils and bodies are not variable. The random thermal fluctuations in the measured signal (as represented in (15.7)) are called 'white' fluctuations because they are characterized by equal expected noise power components at all frequencies within the readout bandwidth.[6] The noise 'variance' of the body and coil together is the sum of variances since these statistical processes are independent, leading to

$$\sigma_{thermal}^2(\vec{k}) = \sigma_{body}^2(\vec{k}) + \sigma_{coil}^2(\vec{k}) + \sigma_{electronics}^2(\vec{k}) \qquad (15.8)$$

for all k-space values. For all further subsections, the shorthand notation σ_m^2 is typically used in place of $\sigma_{thermal}^2$ where the subscript 'm' connotes 'measured.' It is seen that an effective or total resistance can be inserted into (15.7) representing the sum of the individual components

$$R_{eff} = R_{body} + R_{coil} + R_{electronics} \qquad (15.9)$$

15.1.3   Dependence of the Noise on Imaging Parameters

Imaging parameters refer to those factors which can be chosen in an experiment and are not intrinsic properties of the sample. Imaging parameters include factors such as T_E, T_R,

---

[4]If the probability density function of a random variable x is $f(x)$ so that $\int dx\, f(x) = 1$, the mean of a function $g(x)$ denoted by $\overline{g(x)}$ is given by $\overline{g(x)} = \int dx\, g(x)f(x)$. The variance is defined to be $\mathrm{var}(g(x)) = \int dx f(x)(g(x) - \overline{g(x)})^2$.

[5]For a nice derivation of the Nyquist theorem, see, for example, Kittel in the Suggested Reading. This expression is generally valid up to the order of 10^{14} Hz for protons.

[6]Since white noise has zero mean, the standard deviation is also the square root of the mean of the noise emf squared, i.e., the root mean squared (or rms) value.

Δx, Δy, and Δz, etc., for example, which can be changed in the experiment. The number of spins in the sample, its temperature, and relaxation times are not usually considered imaging parameters. In this section, the effects of relaxation parameters on the experiment are neglected.

Just as the voxel signal depends on the voxel volume which is an imaging parameter, the variance of the voxel signal due to noise is also found to depend on the choice of imaging parameters through the discrete inverse Fourier transform. As before, the measured k-space signal can be thought of as the sum of the true k-space signal $s(k)$ with white noise $\epsilon(k)$ added to it to give the noisy measured signal $s_m(k)$:

$$s_m(k) = s(k) + \epsilon(k) \tag{15.10}$$

For this characterization, the noise autocorrelation function is defined as

$$R_\epsilon(\tau) \equiv \overline{\epsilon(k_p)\epsilon^*(k_q)}|_{\tau \equiv (k_p - k_q)} \tag{15.11}$$

and the Fourier transform of $R_\epsilon(\tau)$, $r_\eta(f)$, is known as the spectral density. $R_\epsilon(\tau)$ is given by an impulse of strength σ_m^2, i.e.,

$$R_\epsilon(\tau) = \sigma_m^2 \delta(\tau) \tag{15.12}$$

and the spectral density is seen to be white since

$$\begin{aligned} r_\eta(f) &\equiv \int d\tau\, R_\epsilon(\tau)e^{-i2\pi f\tau} \\ &= \sigma_m^2 \end{aligned} \tag{15.13}$$

The above expression is valid for continuous k-space data measurement. In the discrete case,

$$\overline{\epsilon(k_p)\epsilon^*(k_q)} = \sigma_m^2 \delta_{pq} \tag{15.14}$$

where now $k_p \equiv p\Delta k$ and $k_q = q\Delta k$ and the Dirac delta is replaced by a Kronecker delta. As before, this implies that any two white noise samples are uncorrelated and the expected noise power is σ_m^2.

White noise is also typically characterized as being Gaussian (or normal) distributed with zero mean and variance σ_m^2. This distribution is denoted by $\mathcal{N}(0, \sigma_m)$. Two Gaussian distributed random variables which are uncorrelated are also independent.

This information makes it possible to evaluate the statistical properties of the noise in the image domain. Using the definition of the discrete inverse Fourier transform acting on $\epsilon(k)$, the white noise transforms to

$$\eta(p\Delta x) = \frac{1}{N} \sum_{p'} \epsilon(p'\Delta k)e^{i2\pi p'\Delta k p\Delta x} \tag{15.15}$$

in the image domain. Recall that the k-space variable $\epsilon(p'\Delta k)$ is assumed to have a distribution of the form $\mathcal{N}(0, \sigma_m)$. Taking the expectation of both sides, we get

$$\begin{aligned} \overline{\eta(p\Delta x)} &= \frac{1}{N} \sum_{p'} \overline{\epsilon(p'\Delta k)}e^{i2\pi p'\Delta k p\Delta x} \\ &= 0 \end{aligned} \tag{15.16}$$

Taking the variance of both sides yields a result independent of p

$$\text{var}(\eta(p\Delta x)) \equiv \sigma_0^2(p\Delta x) = \frac{1}{N^2}\sum_{p'}\sum_{q'}\overline{\epsilon(p'\Delta k)\epsilon^*(q'\Delta k)}e^{i2\pi p\Delta x(p'\Delta k-q'\Delta k)}$$

$$= \frac{\sigma_m^2}{N^2}\sum_{p'}\sum_{q'}\delta_{p'q'}e^{i2\pi p\Delta x(p'\Delta k-q'\Delta k)}$$

$$= \frac{\sigma_m^2}{N} \tag{15.17}$$

where the independence of the random variables $\epsilon(p'\Delta k)$ and $\epsilon(q'\Delta k)$ as defined in (15.14) is used. Note that σ_m^2 is the measured variance of any point in k-space, while σ_0^2 will be used to indicate the noise variance in the image domain. *Hence, the variance measured in any voxel in image space is N times smaller than in the detected signal and is the same for all voxels.* It is also common to quote the noise as the standard deviation $\sigma_0(p\Delta x)$. *In conclusion, from (15.17), as N increases to aN ($a > 1$), $\sigma_0(p\Delta x)$ decreases by the factor $1/\sqrt{a}$.*

The image can now be rewritten, due to the linearity of the Fourier transform, as

$$\hat{\rho}_m(p\Delta x) = \hat{\rho}_{m,0}(p\Delta x) + \eta(p\Delta x) \tag{15.18}$$

where $\eta(p\Delta x)$ has mean 0 and variance $\sigma_0^2(p\Delta x)$ independent of p. In (15.18), $\hat{\rho}_{m,0}$ represents the pristine image without any noise. As a reminder, the generalization of the expression (15.17) to two dimensions gives

$$\sigma_0^2(p\Delta x)|_{2D} = \frac{\sigma_m^2}{N_x N_y} \tag{15.19}$$

and to three dimensions gives

$$\sigma_0^2(p\Delta x)|_{3D} = \frac{\sigma_m^2}{N_x N_y N_z} \tag{15.20}$$

Problem 15.1

Show that $\hat{\rho}(0)$ is nothing more than the average of all k-space data. Hence, rederive (15.17) for the voxel at $p = 0$.

Problem 15.2

In Ch. 13, the partial Fourier imaging problem was presented and the special form of its reconstruction was discussed in detail.

a) Suppose only half the number of k-space lines are collected in the phase encoding direction ($\hat{y}$) to save imaging time (i.e., only one half of k-space is covered). How does this affect the noise in the reconstructed image?

b) Generalize this to the case where n_- points are collected in the negative k_y direction and n_+ points are collected in the positive definite k_y direction (i.e., $k_y \leq 0$).

15.1.4 Improving SNR by Averaging over Multiple Acquisitions

Repeating an entire imaging experiment N_{acq} times[7] and averaging the signal over these N_{acq} measurements to improve the SNR is common practice. The MRI system typically adds the signals directly to one another, and does not store them separately, saving a great deal of data space. The averaged k-space sample $s_{m,av}(k)$ of $s_m(k)$ is:

$$s_{m,av}(k) = \frac{1}{N_{acq}} \sum_{i=1}^{N_{acq}} s_{m,i}(k) \tag{15.21}$$

This implies that

$$\overline{s_{m,av}(k)} = \frac{1}{N_{acq}} \sum_{i=1}^{N_{acq}} \overline{s_{m,i}(k)} = \frac{1}{N_{acq}}\left(N_{acq}s(k)\right) = s(k) \tag{15.22}$$

The noise from each of the N_{acq} acquisitions is assumed to be statistically independent from one acquisition to the next. As a result, the noise variance σ_m^2 from each measurement adds in quadrature to the total noise variance of the averaged signal $s_{m,av}(k)$, i.e.,

$$\sigma_{m,av}^2 \equiv \mathrm{var}(s_{m,av}(k)) = \frac{1}{N_{acq}^2} \sum_{i=1}^{N_{acq}} \mathrm{var}(s_{m,i}(k))$$

$$= \frac{\sigma_m^2(k)}{N_{acq}} \tag{15.23}$$

Therefore,

$$\sigma_{m,av}(k) = \frac{\sigma_m(k)}{\sqrt{N_{acq}}} \tag{15.24}$$

The SNR of the k-space signal becomes

$$\mathrm{SNR}(k) = \frac{\overline{s_{m,av}(k)}}{\sigma_{m,av}(k)} = \sqrt{N_{acq}}\frac{s(k)}{\sigma_m(k)} \tag{15.25}$$

i.e., *the SNR improves as the square root of the number of acquisitions if the noise is uncorrelated from one experiment to the next.* However, other sources of systematic noise from the MR experiment can lead to σ_m^2 being greater than $\sigma_{thermal}^2$ and these sources will not be reduced the same way by averaging (see Appendix B).

The noise for a given voxel has already been shown to be proportional to σ_m. Hence, the same $\sqrt{N_{acq}}$ dependence carries over into the expression for the SNR/voxel, i.e.,

$$\mathrm{SNR/voxel}(p\Delta x, q\Delta y, r\Delta z) \propto \frac{\sqrt{N_{acq}}}{\sigma_0} \tag{15.26}$$

as well.

---

[7]These repetitions are sometimes done in consecutive T_R intervals (with the phase encoding gradient(s) at the same value) for minimizing k-space data inconsistencies. In practice, the repetition rate for the acquisition loop is determined by the intended application of the sequence.

Phase Encoding Order When Multiple Acquisitions Are Averaged

Figure 15.1 shows one particular repetition structure for a sequence performing N_{acq} acquisitions before the phase encoding gradient amplitude is augmented. In other applications, this might not be the method of choice for averaging over multiple acquisitions. For example, it is typical in cardiac imaging to actually have the loop structure inside out from the case shown in the figure, i.e., a new acquisition is started after all phase encoding steps have been collected, and the images are averaged finally.

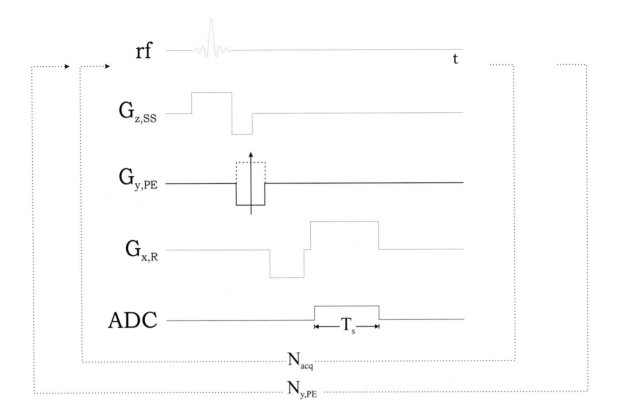

Fig. 15.1: Sequence diagram explicitly demonstrating multiple acquisitions for a 2D FT acquisition method. The phase encoding gradient table is shown in a different form from the usual to remind the reader that the phase encoding gradient is held at one constant value in the acquisition loop. The solid line is supposed to indicate this particular gradient value. The dashed line shows the limit to which the phase encoding gradient is increased at the end of the imaging experiment.

Averaging Unequal Voxel Signals from a Set of Multiple Coils

In MRI, it is becoming increasingly common to use multiple smaller coils to enhance the SNR. Smaller coils pick up less noise than larger coils since they magnetically couple to a smaller volume of the sample. The signal picked up by each coil is used to create individual images which are then combined in some way to create a final image. Unfortunately, these smaller coils, usually lying on the surface of the sample (surface coils), have progressively rapidly weakening B_1 receive fields as a function of distance away from the coil surface.

Therefore, the intensity of images reconstructed from these coils also varies spatially (see Sec. 7.4). In order to construct a final image with reasonable homogeneity of signal and optimal SNR, the images generated by the individual coils must be combined.

Problem 15.3

Suppose that a two-coil system is used such that the voxel signal picked up by coil 1 (S_1) at a point $\vec{x}_a$ equals a, and that picked up by coil 2 (S_2) at the same point equals αa with $\alpha \leq 1$. The standard deviation of the noise associated with either coil is assumed to be the same (say σ_0). Suppose that the two images are added together such that the voxel signal ($\hat{\rho}_m(\vec{x}_a)$) from coil 2 is multiplied by β where β is also ≤ 1.

   a) Write an expression for the SNR/voxel after addition of the two weighted voxel signals as a function of β given that the noise distributions in the two coils are statistically independent and are identically equal to each other.

   b) Maximize the SNR/voxel as a function of β and show that the SNR is maximized when β equals α.

   c) Maximize the SNR/voxel when $\sigma_2 = \beta' \sigma_1$, where β' is a real constant.

From Prob. 15.3, *the optimal linear combination of the two signals is not direct addition as a first guess might suggest. Instead, it is given by the sum-of-squares of the signals picked up by the two coils (the case where β equals α) normalized to the larger of the two signals.* What is the logic behind such a combination? If the two signals are equal, direct addition yields the optimal SNR. However, when one of the two signals is smaller than the other, weighting the smaller measurement by the square of the ratio of the smaller to larger signal produces the optimal SNR. For example, by the time the second signal is one-fifth of the first, there is no need to keep its signal since noise dominates in this case. In this squared sum scheme, the second signal contributes only 4% to the signal, preventing this domination by noise. Recall that the noise picked up by the coil manifests itself as noise with equal variance throughout the image so that, as $\mathcal{B}_\perp$ falls off, the voxel signal decreases while the noise does not.

15.1.5   Measurement of σ_0 and Estimation of SNR

As obtained in (15.19) and (15.20), the standard deviation of the signal in any voxel due to white noise added to the k-space data is independent of voxel number, i.e., the image white noise standard deviation is independent of position in the image. Henceforth, σ_0 and not $\sigma_0(p\Delta x)$ is used to denote the voxel signal standard deviation. In a homogeneous region of a tissue of interest in the image, the average voxel signal over that region is a good estimate of the tissue voxel signal S. In the absence of any systematic variations such as Gibbs ringing, when the SNR in that region is high enough, it is shown later in Sec. 15.7 that the standard deviation in this region is also a very good estimate of σ_0.

A better way to measure σ_0 is to measure the average value or standard deviation of a region-of-interest outside the object where there is no signal (see Fig. 15.2). As shown in Appendix B, the voxel signal here is 'Rayleigh distributed' in the magnitude image. The mean and standard deviation of this random variable are related to the standard deviation of the underlying Gaussian distributed white noise as $1.253\sigma_0$ and $0.665\sigma_0$, respectively. Obtaining σ_0 from either measurement in the background noise gives a more accurate estimate than trying to measure the standard deviation in the image itself (unless the image is perfectly uniform in the region being evaluated). The ratio of the average signal to the estimated value of σ_0 then gives an SNR estimate.

15.2   SNR Dependence on Imaging Parameters

In this section, several imaging parameter dependencies of the SNR on a voxel basis are summarized in different forms. The dependence of SNR/voxel on imaging parameters such as the number of acquisitions N_{acq}, the number of k-space samples N_x, N_y and N_z, the readout bandwidth dependence, and voxel dimensions $\Delta x, \Delta y$ and Δz (or TH in 2D) are discussed in detail. The dependence of SNR on spatial resolution is given utmost importance, and some compromises which have to be kept in mind while improving spatial resolution are presented.

15.2.1   Generalized Dependence of SNR in 3D Imaging on Imaging Parameters

The SNR dependence on imaging parameters is complicated by the noise behavior. Noise depends on many different imaging parameters. From (15.6), (15.7), and (15.19)

$$\text{SNR/voxel} \propto \frac{\Delta x \Delta y \Delta z \sqrt{N_{acq}}}{\sqrt{\frac{BW_{read}}{N_x N_y N_z}}} \tag{15.27}$$

Substituting $\Delta t = \frac{1}{BW_{read}}$ gives

$$\text{SNR/voxel} \propto \Delta x \Delta y \Delta z \sqrt{N_{acq} N_x N_y N_z \Delta t} \tag{15.28}$$

Since $T_s = N_x \Delta t$, substituting this into (15.28) yields

$$\text{SNR/voxel} \propto \Delta x \Delta y \Delta z \sqrt{N_{acq} N_y N_z T_s} \tag{15.29}$$

Equations (15.27)–(15.29) can be rewritten in a number of ways, depending on the parameters which are to be considered. It is necessary to keep in mind that although any parameter in (15.27)–(15.29) may be varied without altering the validity of the relations, the following relations hold

$$
\begin{array}{llll}
\text{(a)} & L_x = N_x \Delta x & \text{(b)} & L_y = N_y \Delta y \\
\text{(c)} & L_z = N_z \Delta z & \text{(d)} & T_s = N_x \Delta t \\
\text{(e)} & BW_{read} = \frac{1}{\Delta t} = \gamma G_x L_x & \text{(f)} & BW/\text{voxel} = BW_{read}/N_x
\end{array}
\tag{15.30}
$$

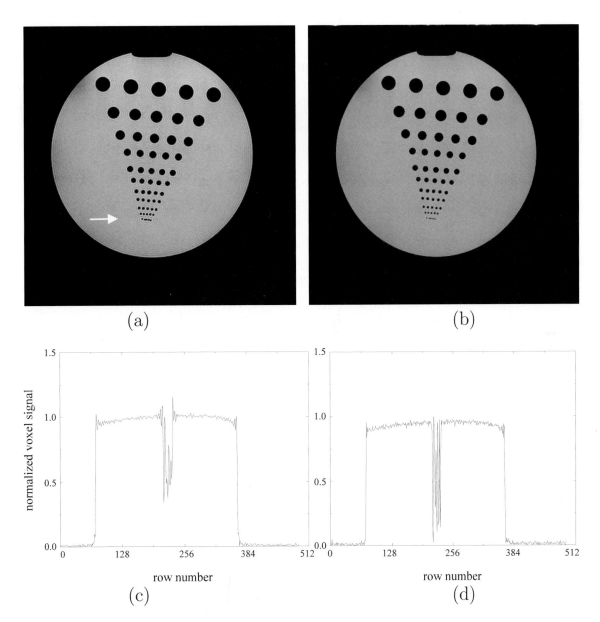

Fig. 15.2: Two images collected with identical T_R, T_E, and G_x. However, N_x, N_y, and T_s in (b) are two times the same values in (a), leading to an improvement in spatial resolution. This increase in resolution leads to a reduction of the SNR by a factor of 2. Noise standard deviation inside the object is estimated by taking $1/1.253 \simeq 0.8$ times the mean measured in a region outside the phantom where there is no signal (see Appendix B). This noise-only region has to lie reasonably away from the edge of the object, and there should be no artifacts nearby. The profiles in (c) and (d) illustrate the larger variation in noise for (a) versus (b), respectively. They also show the higher resolution associated with (d), where five distinct dips (each corresponding to one resolution element) are visible versus only three in (c). The profiles were taken through the row cutting through the last row of smallest resolution elements.

These interrelations exist implicitly in each of the above expressions for the SNR. Therefore, whenever a parameter in a given expression for SNR is varied, the resultant effects on the rest of the parameters must be checked. Also, it is obvious that through these relations a number of other expressions for the SNR may be developed to highlight the effects of varying a certain subset of these parameters. Often an expression for SNR will be accompanied by a condition that some quantity be kept constant which limits how certain parameters may be varied. Finally, there are other dependencies of the signal related to data acquisition and tissue properties, which will be dealt with in Sec. 15.4.

To calculate what happens in the case of a fixed variable, an implicit form can be substituted into (15.29). For example, since $\Delta x = L_x/N_x$, if Δx is fixed, L_x and N_x cannot vary arbitrarily and (15.28) or (15.29) are better written as

$$\text{SNR/voxel} \propto L_x \Delta y \Delta z \sqrt{\frac{N_y N_z \Delta t}{N_x}}\bigg|_{\Delta x = L_x/N_x = constant} \tag{15.31}$$

Other such specialized proportionalities can be derived.

An increase in the spatial resolution by a factor of 2 in both in-plane directions leads to a factor of 2 loss in SNR when the increased spatial resolution is achieved by maintaining the read gradient fixed while T_s is doubled (from (15.29)). Such an example is shown in Fig. 15.2, from which the mean and standard deviation estimates were obtained. Taking the ratio of the mean of the local background to the noise standard deviation in the two cases demonstrates the consistency of the measured SNR with that expected from (15.29). Doing this in a region where the profile is flat yields an SNR/voxel of 187.5 for Fig. 15.2a and 91.0 for Fig. 15.2b.

15.2.2 SNR Dependence on Read Direction Parameters

From (15.29), with all other parameters maintained constant, the SNR dependence on read direction parameters can be reduced to

$$\text{SNR/voxel}|_{read} \propto \Delta x \sqrt{T_s} \tag{15.32}$$

Although (15.32) depends only upon two parameters, dependencies on L_x, BW, etc. are implicit in this expression (see (15.29) and (15.30)). Due to the importance of understanding the effects of altering read direction parameters, several example situations are shown in Table 15.1. Case 1 is chosen as a reference and given an SNR of unity. Also, note that in order to simplify the treatment, all of the situations in Table 15.1 are restricted to doubling or halving the parameters involved. There are also practical aspects to these choices, which will be discussed below.

From (15.32), it appears that it might be possible to obtain very high resolution without reducing SNR by shrinking Δx while increasing T_s. Realistically, however, there is a limit to how long T_s can be before the signal is seriously degraded by T_2^* effects.

Oversampling to Avoid Aliasing

Although the topic of aliasing has been dealt with in Ch. 12, it is useful here to revisit it in terms of how changing the FOV affects the SNR in a given experiment. In Table 15.1, cases

Case	Δx	N_x	L_x	G_x	Δt	T_s	SNR

Reference case

Case	Δx	N_x	L_x	G_x	Δt	T_s	SNR
1	Δx_0	N_0	L_0	G_0	Δt_0	$T_{s,0}$	1

Data reduction and oversampling

Case	Δx	N_x	L_x	G_x	Δt	T_s	SNR
2	Δx_0	$N_0/2$	$L_0/2$	G_0	$2\Delta t_0$	$T_{s,0}$	1
3	Δx_0	$2N_0$	$2L_0$	G_0	$\Delta t_0/2$	$T_{s,0}$	1

Degrading spatial resolution

Case	Δx	N_x	L_x	G_x	Δt	T_s	SNR
4	$2\Delta x_0$	$N_0/2$	L_0	G_0	Δt_0	$T_{s,0}/2$	$\sqrt{2}$
5	$2\Delta x_0$	$N_0/2$	L_0	$G_0/2$	$2\Delta t_0$	$T_{s,0}$	2

Improving spatial resolution

Case	Δx	N_x	L_x	G_x	Δt	T_s	SNR
6	$\Delta x_0/2$	N_0	$L_0/2$	G_0	$2\Delta t_0$	$2T_{s,0}$	$1/\sqrt{2}$
7	$\Delta x_0/2$	N_0	$L_0/2$	$2G_0$	Δt_0	$T_{s,0}$	$1/2$
8	$\Delta x_0/2$	$2N_0$	L_0	$2G_0$	$\Delta t_0/2$	$T_{s,0}$	$1/2$
9	$\Delta x_0/2$	$2N_0$	L_0	G_0	Δt_0	$2T_{s,0}$	$1/\sqrt{2}$

Table 15.1: Table showing the SNR/voxel when the voxel size is changed in the read direction under different conditions. The SNR/voxel is given relative to that of case 1 and can be seen to correlate exactly with $\Delta x(T_s)^{1/2}$ or equivalently, $(\Delta x/G_x)^{1/2}$. Note that T_s and G_x vary similarly from baseline conditions in the different cases.

2 and 3 demonstrate that altering the FOV does not alter the SNR of an experiment as long as T_s and Δx are unchanged. There are two important implications of this result.

First, it is possible to avoid aliasing in a given experiment by doubling the FOV in the read direction. This is accomplished by collecting twice as many points without varying the read gradient G_x or T_s (referred to as oversampling (case 3)), which neither degrades nor improves the SNR of the experiment. Therefore, *in many practical imaging situations, oversampling is used to double the FOV in the read direction and reduce aliasing artifacts without sacrificing SNR or lengthening T_s or the acquisition time.* Consider acquiring a transverse image of the human chest, for example, where the left to right dimension of the experiment is very large and is most likely to be chosen as the read direction. Oversampling in the read direction is then used to guarantee that the FOV extends past the patient's arms without increasing imaging time, or degrading SNR.

Alternatively, for a small object, where aliasing is not a problem and data storage space is at a premium, choosing a smaller FOV and collecting fewer data points (case 2) does not reduce SNR.

Degrading Resolution to Increase SNR

In case 4, Δx is increased by a factor of 2, the number of data points collected is halved and T_s is also halved. As seen from Table 15.1, SNR is increased by $\sqrt{2}$. If lower resolution can be tolerated, this increase in SNR could lead to better tissue recognition, and the reduction in T_s could be beneficial in reducing the chemical shift artifact (discussed in detail in Ch. 17), in overcoming static field inhomogeneity effects (since $BW/$voxel is increased), and in reducing relaxation effects during sampling.

In case 5, resolution is reduced by a factor of 2, and SNR is doubled because this increase in resolution is achieved while T_s is held constant. A doubling of SNR is a significant SNR improvement. Note that this effect is achieved by reducing the read gradient by a factor of 2. In most cases, reducing the gradient is not a problem, but it must be kept in mind that if the applied gradient strength reduces to a level comparable to those produced by local field inhomogeneities, then severe image distortion will result (as detailed in Ch. 20). *This trick of using a fixed T_s with the read gradient halved to acquire low resolution images and obtain a factor of 2 improvement in SNR is commonly used in clinical applications.*

Improving Resolution in the Read Direction

In both cases 6 and 7, Δx is halved by reducing the FOV by a factor of 2 without changing the number of sampled points. This should be done only if the FOV in case 1 is greater than or equal to twice the width of the object in the read direction so that aliasing will be avoided. In case 6, T_s is doubled by doubling Δt. This method leads to a reduction of SNR of only $\sqrt{2}$ since $BW/$voxel is again halved. Realistically, T_s must be short enough in case 1 so that, when it is doubled, it is still much shorter than T_2^*. In case 7, L_x is halved by doubling the read gradient G_x. This approach requires that enough gradient power be available to double G_0. Unfortunately, SNR is reduced by a factor of 2, making this a very inefficient approach. In case 8, Δx is halved by doubling N_x and keeping L_x and T_s fixed, which requires doubling G_x and halving Δt_0. This also leads to a halving of the SNR. In case 9, Δx is halved by doubling N_x while keeping both L_x and G_x fixed. This requires doubling the total sampling time, but is accompanied by only a $\sqrt{2}$ reduction in SNR. This is probably the optimal way to double the resolution of the experiment as long as the increased T_s is not comparable to T_2^*, and storing the extra data is not a problem, although it is similar to case 6 which requires less storage space but a smaller object.

Problem 15.4

A better understanding and feel for the SNR variation in the read direction can be obtained by relating the SNR to a combination of Δx and the $BW/$voxel.

a) Show that SNR/voxel $\propto \Delta x/\sqrt{BW/\text{voxel}}$.

b) When Δx is halved with a corresponding doubling of G_x (as in cases 7 and 8 in Table 15.1), how does $BW/$voxel vary in these two cases? What happens to the voxel signal? What happens to the SNR/voxel? Does the FOV change?

c) When Δx is halved by increasing N_x without a corresponding doubling of G_x (as in case 9 in Table 15.1), how does $BW/$voxel vary? What happens to the voxel signal and the SNR/voxel?

d) Find two other ways to halve Δx of the experiment depicted in Table 15.1. Hint: See cases 6 through 9.

e) Given the following parameters, find Δx_0 and the proportional SNR/voxel as given in (15.32). FOV$_{read}$ = 256 mm, N_x = 256, G_x = 2.5 mT/m, G_{max} = 15 mT/m, with the T_2^* of the tissue of interest being 20 ms. Assume that you would like to reduce Δx_0 in this case to $\Delta x_0/2$. Discuss how you might best accomplish this in terms of getting optimal SNR/voxel. For deriving this result, assume that T_s has to be less than or equal to T_2^*.

Since T_s equals $1/(\gamma G_x \Delta x)$, the proportionality in (15.32) can be rewritten as

$$\text{SNR/voxel} \propto \sqrt{\frac{\Delta x}{G_x}}$$

$$\propto \Delta x \sqrt{T_s} \tag{15.33}$$

Either expression contains no hidden dependencies and requires none of the imaging parameters to be fixed, i.e., they can be applied to any situation for computing the relative SNR change. According to this expression, the SNR/voxel decreases only by a factor of $\sqrt{2}$ for every halving of Δx as long as the read gradient is fixed. SNR however reduces by a factor of 2 if this improvement in spatial resolution is accompanied by a doubling of G_x. Note consistency with these observations for cases 6 through 9 in Table 15.1. The only way to improve the SNR when Δx is made smaller is to increase T_s accordingly. Unfortunately, this is possible only up to a point, either before relaxation effects begin to reduce the k-space signal or before T_s starts to limit the minimum T_R value. The features in cases 6 through 9 are also summarized in Fig. 15.3.

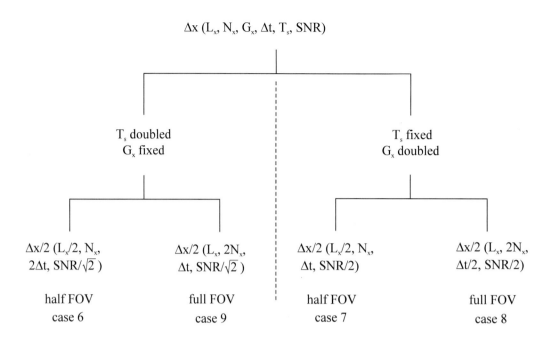

Fig. 15.3: Different ways of achieving improved spatial resolution in the read direction, and their effects on SNR. This figure summarizes cases 6 through 9 in Table 15.1, showing also what parameters were changed in comparison with case 1 to attain high resolution. For T_s fixed, either approach yields a loss of 2 in SNR while for T_s doubled, only a loss of square root of 2 in SNR occurs.

15.2.3   SNR Dependence on Phase Encoding Parameters

Pulling out just the SNR dependence on parameters which change only the image characteristics in the in-plane and through-plane phase encoding directions ($\hat{y}$ and $\hat{z}$, respectively) gives

$$\text{SNR/voxel} \propto \Delta y \Delta z \sqrt{N_y N_z} \qquad (15.34)$$

(recall $L_y = N_y \Delta y$ and $L_z = N_z \Delta z$). *There are only two alternate methods for improving spatial resolution in the phase encoding directions: first, decreasing Δy or Δz by increasing N_y or N_z while keeping L_y or L_z fixed (case 3 in Table 15.2), or second, decreasing Δy or Δz by decreasing L_y or L_z while keeping N_y or N_z fixed (case 2 in Table 15.2).*

Consider halving Δy using either of these methods. In the first method, the SNR decreases only by a factor of $\sqrt{2}$, whereas in the second method, the SNR decreases by a factor of 2. What are the advantages or disadvantages of either method? The first method, requiring doubling N_y, takes twice as long to complete compared to the second method. If the SNR is good enough and aliasing is avoided, the second method is twice as time-efficient as the first while having $\sqrt{2}$ worse SNR in comparison with the first. Of course, in the same imaging time as required by the first method, two acquisitions can be performed with the second method to reclaim the factor of $\sqrt{2}$ SNR loss, while maintaining the advantage of requiring less image storage space. These two cases are highlighted in Table 15.2.

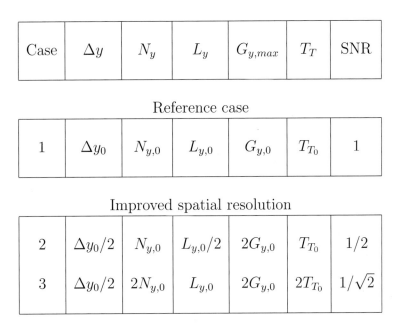

Case	Δy	N_y	L_y	$G_{y,max}$	T_T	SNR
Reference case						
1	Δy_0	$N_{y,0}$	$L_{y,0}$	$G_{y,0}$	T_{T_0}	1
Improved spatial resolution						
2	$\Delta y_0/2$	$N_{y,0}$	$L_{y,0}/2$	$2G_{y,0}$	T_{T_0}	$1/2$
3	$\Delta y_0/2$	$2N_{y,0}$	$L_{y,0}$	$2G_{y,0}$	$2T_{T_0}$	$1/\sqrt{2}$

Table 15.2: Two different ways to improve spatial resolution in the phase encoding direction, and their effects on the SNR and total imaging time.

15.2.4   SNR in 2D Imaging

The SNR expression in (15.29) can be rewritten for a 2D imaging experiment. The voxel now has dimensions of $\Delta x \times \Delta y \times TH$. Also, N_z is replaced by unity. Therefore

$$(\text{SNR/voxel})|_{2D} \propto \Delta x \Delta y TH \sqrt{N_y T_s} \qquad (15.35)$$

In other words, a 2D imaging experiment performed with exactly the same imaging parameters (including T_R, T_E, and flip angle) with $TH = \Delta z$ has $\sqrt{N_z}$ worse SNR in comparison with the 3D imaging experiment. However, the 2D imaging experiment requires an imaging time which is N_z times shorter than the 3D experiment. However, it is typically possible to collect the data for only one slice per T_R when the T_R value in the 2D imaging experiment equals the practically sensible choice of short T_R in the 3D imaging experiment. To obtain the same spatial coverage in the slice select direction requires N_z imaging experiments, increasing the total imaging time by N_z in the 2D imaging case. If the same imaging time is used for both the 2D and 3D imaging experiments, the same volume of coverage and the same contrast as the 3D can be achieved in 2D imaging albeit only with $\sqrt{N_z}$ less SNR. Or a single slice with the same SNR as the 3D experiment (obtained by imaging with $N_{acq2D} = N_z$) can be obtained. The most efficient means of collecting 2D data and covering the same region-of-interest as in the 3D imaging case is to use $T_{R_{2D}} = N_z T_{R_{3D}}$ and use a multi-slice acquisition[8] (although this guarantees neither that the 2D SNR is as good as the 3D SNR as discussed below nor that the contrast is comparable with the 3D imaging method).

---

[8]See Ch. 10 for more details.

15.2.5   Imaging Efficiency

In clinical applications, patient comfort and patient throughput are important day-to-day issues. The longer the imaging time per patient, the more patient discomfort and the less throughput. In Fourier imaging, the total imaging time for each imaging experiment is dependent directly on the number of sequence cycle repetitions. Consider the 3D imaging case, where the total imaging time is given by

$$T_T = N_{acq}N_yN_zT_R \tag{15.36}$$

The general wisdom is that, since

$$(\text{SNR/voxel})_{3D} \propto \Delta y \Delta z \sqrt{N_yN_z} \tag{15.37}$$

with L_y and L_z constant, if either N_y or N_z is halved and consequently Δy or Δz is doubled, respectively, not only is the SNR improved by a factor of $\sqrt{2}$, but the imaging time is also halved. As a consequence, if the same imaging time as that for the better resolution scan is used, the SNR can be improved further by an additional factor of $\sqrt{2}$ by averaging 2 acquisitions at lower resolution. Thereby, the SNR-per-unit-time is doubled in comparison with the high resolution image. *A time-normalized SNR is therefore considered a measure of imaging efficiency.* The normalization to time is done not on a per-unit-time basis, but on a per square root of time basis, since, for a fixed T_R, SNR is proportional to $\sqrt{T_T} = \sqrt{N_{acq}N_yN_zT_R}$. Therefore, for a fixed T_R, the imaging efficiency is defined as

$$\Upsilon \equiv \frac{(\text{SNR/voxel})_{3D}}{\sqrt{T_T}} \propto \frac{\Delta x \Delta y \Delta z \sqrt{N_{acq}N_yN_zT_s}}{\sqrt{N_{acq}N_yN_z}}$$
$$\propto \Delta x \Delta y \Delta z \sqrt{T_s} \tag{15.38}$$

In other words, an image with better spatial resolution, such as with Δy or Δz halved, is considered only half as SNR-efficient as an image acquired with voxel size Δy or Δz, respectively. Again, this measure does not include the role of voxel size relative to object size. The main conclusion is that high resolution can be achieved efficiently only in the read direction, and even that is limited by the need to keep T_s on the order of T_2^* or less.

15.3   Contrast, Contrast-to-Noise, and Visibility

Even the highest signal-to-noise ratio does not guarantee a useful image. An important aim of imaging for diagnostic purposes is to be able to distinguish between diseased and neighboring normal tissues. If the imaging method used does not have a signal-manipulating mechanism which produces different signals for the two tissues, distinguishing the two tissues is not possible. MRI is blessed with an abundance of signal-manipulating mechanisms, as the signal is dependent on a wide variety of tissue parameters. The problem of distinguishing a given (diseased) structure from surrounding (normal) tissue in the presence of added white noise falls under the broad category of the 'signal detection' problem, and requires an understanding of the importance of Contrast-to-Noise Ratio (CNR).

15.3.1 Contrast and Contrast-to-Noise Ratio

The common way to look at this problem is to examine the absolute difference in the signal between the two tissues of interest. If these tissues are labeled A and B, their signal difference[9] is defined as the 'contrast:'

$$C_{AB} \equiv S_A - S_B \tag{15.39}$$

where S_A and S_B are the voxel signals from tissues A and B, respectively. Although the inherent contrast may be large enough to detect a change, if the noise is too large, the signal difference would not be visible to the eye or to a simple signal difference threshold algorithm. The more appropriate measure is the ratio of the contrast to the noise standard deviation[10] known as the contrast-to-noise ratio, CNR:

$$\mathrm{CNR}_{AB} \equiv \frac{C_{AB}}{\sigma_0} = \frac{S_A - S_B}{\sigma_0} = \mathrm{SNR}_A - \mathrm{SNR}_B \tag{15.40}$$

The utility of this definition is best illustrated with a simple statistics discussion. For Gaussian distributed white noise, the probability that two tissues are different if CNR_{AB} equals $2\sqrt{2}$ is 95% and if CNR_{AB} equals $3\sqrt{2}$ is 99%. Ideally we would like to design the MR experiment to have sufficient spatial resolution to resolve the two tissues of interest (such as gray matter and white matter) and to have a high enough CNR that they can be distinguished from each other.

15.3.2 Object Visibility and the Rose Criterion

If multiple independent signal measurements N_{acq} are performed, an average of these signal measurements implies that the effective noise standard deviation becomes

$$\sigma_{eff} = \frac{\sigma_0}{\sqrt{N_{acq}}} \tag{15.41}$$

In an image where tissue A occupies n_{voxel} voxels, each of which has signal S_A with independent additive white noise with standard deviation σ_0, a similar voxel-averaging scenario can be incorporated into the detection criterion (with N_{acq} replaced by n_{voxel}) via a new measure referred to as the 'object visibility' or

$$\mathcal{V}_{AB} \equiv \frac{C_{AB}}{\sigma_{eff}} = \frac{C_{AB}}{\sigma_0}\sqrt{n_{voxel}} = \mathrm{CNR}_{AB}\sqrt{n_{voxel}} \tag{15.42}$$

Again, the noise in each voxel of the image, σ_0, is assumed to be the same for both tissues.

---

[9]It is also common to refer to contrast as C_{AB}/S_A or C_{AB}/S_B. We define these as relative contrast ratios.

[10]Since no physical subtraction is performed in the image, the standard deviation used is that common to both tissues A and B, i.e., σ_0. If a contrast image were created, then σ_0 would be replaced by $\sqrt{2}\sigma_0$.

The Rose Criterion

The visibility threshold can be determined empirically. Based on experiments with human observers detecting circular objects shone on a television screen, Rose found that random fluctuations in the photon flux forming the object confused the observer, and a minimum 'SNR' was required for confident object detection. Depending on the observer's expertise and what is being observed, a detection SNR threshold varying between 3 and 5 was found to be required for object recognition. This requirement is known as the 'Rose Criterion' in the diagnostic imaging literature.

A visibility threshold of about 4 can be reinterpreted for the tissue discrimination problem as follows: a Gaussian model for the additive white noise is found to be a rather good approximation for the thermal noise. With this assumption made, the image signal from tissues A and B can be modeled by two Gaussian distributions centered at S_A and S_B, respectively, with the same standard deviation σ_0. Now, if $(S_A - S_B) = 4\sigma_0$, as it would be for single-voxel tissues A and B, the two Gaussian distributions are separated by $4\sigma_0$ (see Fig. 15.4). Since a distance $2\sigma_0$ to one side of the mean covers about 97.5% of the area under a Gaussian distribution, it is reasonable to expect the human observer to choose a threshold which is $2\sigma_0$ away from either S_A or S_B. Then, the probability of the observer incorrectly classifying a voxel as belonging to one or the other tissue is 0.025, i.e., this is a 1-in-40 chance occurrence. That is, the probability of detection of the tissue is very high: for a multi-voxel object when $\mathcal{V}$ equals 4, only 1 in 40 voxels in the object will be classified incorrectly by the observer as a background voxel, and vice versa; for a single-voxel object, there is only a 1-in-40 chance of not detecting it.[11] This description is essentially a rule of thumb, as the perception of the object is likely to be much more complicated.

Problem 15.5

---

a) Show for cases 6 and 9 of Table 15.1 that $\mathcal{V}$ remains constant for a multi-voxel object.

b) It has been suggested that the Great Wall of China can be seen as the only man-made structure visible from outer space, yet it is only a few meters wide. Postulate why this might be possible based upon a visibility argument.

The effect of object size, σ_0, and contrast level on object visibility can be visually demonstrated to be determined by the quantity $\mathcal{V}$ as it was defined in (15.42) by observing the images in Fig. 15.5. The model image with no noise added is shown in Fig. 15.5a. The simulated objects are disk-like objects of linearly decreasing radius (one voxel radius to five voxel radius) going from top to bottom and linearly increasing signal values going from left to right (doubling from column 1 to column 5; actual values can be computed from SNR values quoted in the caption for Fig. 15.5) imaged in a zero signal background. The model image

---

[11]As for footnote 10, visibility has been defined relative to σ_0, not $\sqrt{2}\sigma_0$. If the latter were chosen, the above argument is still valid but the quoted visibility in the case being considered would be $2\sqrt{2}$ rather than 4.

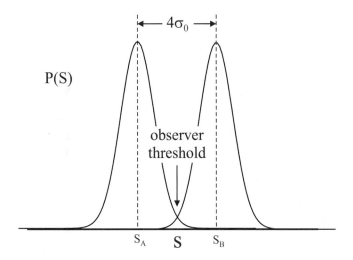

Fig. 15.4: Image signal distribution of two tissues A and B with added Gaussian distributed white noise. When $(S_A - S_B)$ equals $4\sigma_0$, the probability of an error in the detection of tissue A is about 0.025 when a threshold of $2\sigma_0$ is used. Likewise, the probability of mis-classifying a noise point as an object is also 0.025.

is assumed to be all real, whereas the noise is assumed to have uncorrelated and equal expected power in both the real and imaginary image channels. The noisy images were created by adding the real channel noise to the model and taking the magnitude of the two image channels after this addition. As described in the earlier discussion, the smaller disks become indistinguishable from noise at the lower SNR levels while the larger disks are detectable even at degraded SNR levels. Also, the higher the true contrast of the object, the higher the SNR degradation must be before such an object becomes undetectable. It is easy to note that at a given SNR level (images at different SNR levels are shown in Figs. 15.5b–15.5d), an imaginary diagonal line can be drawn separating the barely detectable objects from the undetectable objects and the clearly detectable objects. It is found that the objects along such a diagonal line have a constant value of the product of the signal with the square root of the number of voxels occupied by the object. This shows that the threshold of visibility is determined by the quantity $\mathcal{V}$ defined in (15.42).

15.4 Contrast Mechanisms in MRI and Contrast Maximization

As mentioned earlier, MRI has the flexibility to manipulate the tissue signal in many ways, leading to numerous contrast mechanisms. The flexibility arises from the MR signal dependence on many imaging parameters and tissue parameters. The most basic contrast generating mechanisms are based on spin density, and T_1 and T_2 differences between tissues. Others are flow, magnetic susceptibility differences, magnetization transfer contrast, tissue saturation methods, contrast enhancing agents and diffusion, all of which are discussed in one place or another in later chapters of this book. In this section, the focus is on three

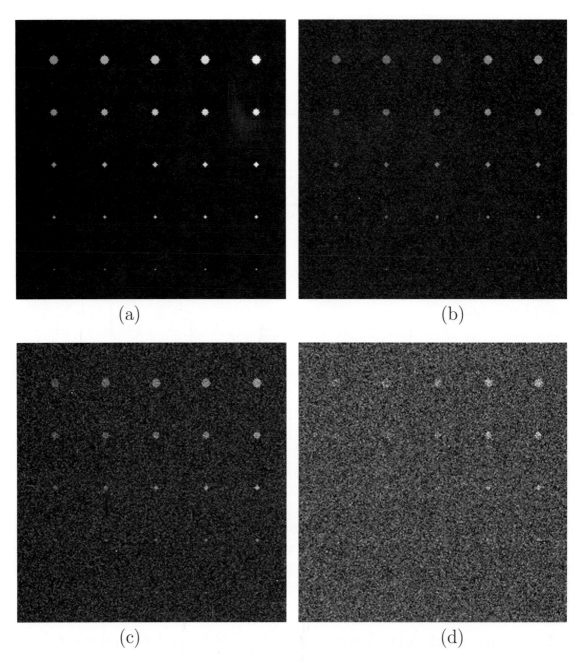

Fig. 15.5: Images designed to show how visibility of large and small objects changes as a function of CNR, and how their detection for a given CNR depends on the object size. For the cases shown, CNR is the same as SNR since each feature is being compared to the background noise. (a) Model of circles with no background noise (SNR $= \infty$); (b) SNR $= 4$; (c) SNR $= 2$; and (d) SNR $= 1$. (The SNR values quoted for these images are measured relative to the objects with lowest signal (column 1). As mentioned in the text, SNR doubles for the rightmost column in comparison with the leftmost column in each image.)

basic forms of contrast: spin-density weighted contrast, T_1-weighted contrast, and T_2- (or T_2^*-) weighted contrast.

A 90° gradient echo experiment is used as an example of how to obtain different forms of contrast. These results are identical to those that would be found for a 90° spin echo experiment under the assumption that $T_E \ll T_R$ and T_2 is replaced by T_2^*. Different expressions and relations must be derived for other imaging techniques.

15.4.1 Three Important Types of Contrast

Although each type of contrast is designed to enhance differences in one of the specified parameters (ρ_0, T_1, or T_2), the signal is a function of all three variables, and each must be kept in mind when determining overall image contrast. As an illustrative example, the contrast between tissues A and B for a 90° flip angle gradient echo experiment (see Fig. 15.6) is

$$C_{AB} = S_A(T_E) - S_B(T_E) = \rho_{0,A}(1 - e^{-T_R/T_{1,A}})e^{-T_E/T_{2,A}^*} - \rho_{0,B}(1 - e^{-T_R/T_{1,B}})e^{-T_E/T_{2,B}^*} \quad (15.43)$$

Note that the signal is assumed to be determined by the tissue signal solution from the Bloch equation at the echo time T_E. Remember, this time corresponds to the $k = 0$ sample in the read direction. C_{AB} can then be maximized with respect to either T_R or T_E.

15.4.2 Spin Density Weighting

In order to get contrast based primarily on ρ_0, the T_1 and T_2^* dependence of the gradient echo tissue signals must be minimized. When the argument of an exponential is small, an appropriate approximation to e^{-x} is $(1 - x)$ which is better written as $1 - \mathcal{O}(x)$. If the exponent is large and negative, e^{-x} can be approximated by zero. It is seen that in order to maintain adequate signal and get contrast based primarily upon spin density, appropriate choices of T_E and T_R would be

$$T_E \ll T_{2_{A,B}}^* \Rightarrow e^{-T_E/T_2^*} \to 1 \quad (15.44)$$

$$T_R \gg T_{1_{A,B}} \Rightarrow e^{-T_R/T_1} \to 0 \quad (15.45)$$

and expression (15.43) for the contrast between tissues becomes

$$
\begin{aligned}
C_{AB} &= (\rho_{0,A} - \rho_{0,B}) \\
&\quad - \rho_{0,A}\left(e^{-T_R/T_{1,A}} + \frac{T_E}{T_{2,A}^*}\right) + \rho_{0,B}\left(e^{-T_R/T_{1,B}} + \frac{T_E}{T_{2,B}^*}\right) \\
&\quad + \text{higher order and cross terms} \\
&\simeq \rho_{0,A} - \rho_{0,B} \quad (15.46)
\end{aligned}
$$

In this approximation, the contrast does not depend upon T_R or T_E, and need not be extremized relative to either T_R or T_E. This gives a general rule for spin density weighting: keep T_R much longer than the longest T_1 component; keep T_E much shorter than the shortest of $T_{2_{A,B}}^*$; the gradient echo image contrast is then primarily determined by spin density

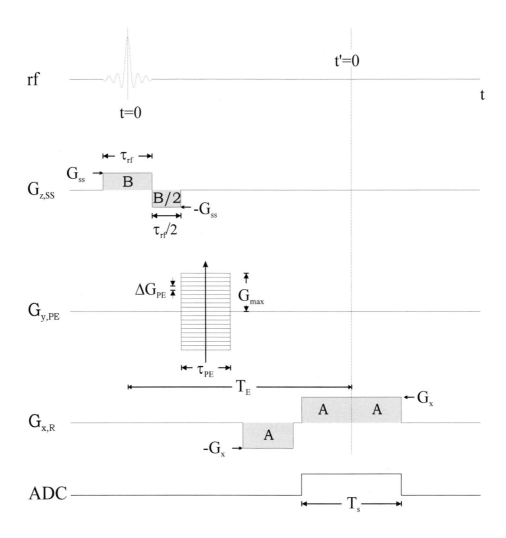

Fig. 15.6: A 2D gradient echo sequence diagram.

differences. Similar rules will be formed for T_1-weighting and T_2^*-weighting based on the practical limits imposed on T_E and T_R. These limits are summarized in Table 15.3. The actual error in this approximation of spin density weighting of the signal depends on the coefficients for T_E/T_2^* and T_R/T_1, the former vanishing only linearly in T_E/T_2^*. In practice, this means that most imaging experiments still have an error of a few percent even if T_E is as low as a few milliseconds since some typical T_2^* values are on the order of tens of milliseconds.

Problem 15.6

Estimating water content of one tissue relative to another from their contrast differences for a supposedly spin density weighted sequence may require including first-order effects of nonzero T_E and finite T_R. Consider a gradient echo experiment with $T_R = 5$ sec, $T_E = 5$ ms, and a $\pi/2$-pulse. Assume that ρ_0, T_1, and T_2^* for two adjacent tissues are 1.0, 2 sec, 40 ms and 0.8, 1 sec, 50 ms, respectively. The signal of the gradient echo dependence on T_E is found from

$$s = \rho_0(1 - e^{-T_R/T_1})e^{-T_E/T_2^*} \qquad (15.47)$$

a) What are the effects of nonzero T_E and finite T_R on the contrast in this supposedly spin density weighted sequence?

b) The signal of the spin echo dependence on T_E is more complicated since

$$s = \rho_0(1 - 2e^{-(T_R-\tau)/T_1} + e^{-T_R/T_1})e^{-T_E/T_2} \qquad (15.48)$$

Consider again $T_R = 5\,\text{sec}$ but $T_E = 20\,\text{ms}$ and a $\pi/2$-pulse, with T_2's of $40\,\text{ms}$ and $50\,\text{ms}$ respectively. How does the echo time affect contrast now?

Practically, the minimum T_E is limited by the available gradient strength. In fact, this limitation made the imaging of rigid solids impossible for many years because their T_2^* values are on the order of a few hundred microseconds to several milliseconds, and no hardware was available which could form an echo before the signal was gone. However, with modern hardware and modern imaging techniques, solids imaging is now viable. T_E is also limited by the highest acceptable readout bandwidth/voxel (or lowest possible T_s) for SNR and object visibility reasons. The maximum value of T_R, on the other hand, is constrained by imaging time and imaging efficiency reasons. Therefore, true spin density weighting using a 90° gradient echo sequence is practically achievable only for tissues with long enough T_2^*'s and short enough T_1's which allow T_E and T_R choices which satisfy the constraints imposed by the gradient strength limitation, the SNR and imaging time. Good spin density-weighted contrast is available for most purposes without requiring a zero T_E, or infinite T_R.

15.4.3 T_1-Weighting

Normal soft tissue T_1 values are quite different from one another. For this reason, T_1-weighted contrast offers a very powerful method for delineation of different tissues. To obtain spin density weighting, T_E and T_R were chosen to reduce the effect of T_1 and T_2. For T_1 and T_2 weighting, only the effects of T_2 and T_1 differences, respectively, can be minimized. The effects of spin density differences cannot be neglected.

For T_1 weighting, T_2^* effects have to be minimized. Using the gradient echo example as before, the choice of a very short T_E again reduces any T_2^* (or T_2) contrast, i.e., T_E is chosen such that

$$T_E \ll T_{2_{A,B}}^* \Rightarrow e^{-T_E/T_2^*} \to 1 \qquad (15.49)$$

and the expression for the contrast is now

$$
\begin{aligned}
C_{AB} &= S_A(T_E) - S_B(T_E) \\
&\simeq \rho_{0,A}(1 - e^{-T_R/T_{1,A}}) - \rho_{0,B}(1 - e^{-T_R/T_{1,B}}) \quad T_E \ll T_{2_{A,B}}^* \\
&= (\rho_{0,A} - \rho_{0,B}) - (\rho_{0,A}e^{-T_R/T_{1,A}} - \rho_{0,B}e^{-T_R/T_{1,B}})
\end{aligned} \qquad (15.50)
$$

Since there is no transverse relaxation dependence in the above expression, this expression is equally valid for a spin echo sequence as well. It is typical that T_1 and T_2 correlate with spin density, i.e., a tissue with higher spin density usually has longer T_1 and T_2 values, and tissues with lower spin density usually have shorter T_1 and T_2 values. As a result, while T_1 weighting depicts tissues with longer T_1 values with low signal and short-T_1 tissues with higher signal, the spin density contrast counteracts this effect. Hence, a unique choice of T_R which maximizes the T_1-weighted contrast should exist. To optimize the T_1-weighted contrast, (15.50) is extremized with respect to T_R. Differentiating C_{AB} with respect to T_R and setting it equal to zero leads to the relation

$$\frac{\rho_{0,A}e^{-T_R/T_{1,A}}}{T_{1,A}} = \frac{\rho_{0,B}e^{-T_R/T_{1,B}}}{T_{1,B}} \tag{15.51}$$

Solving for T_R from (15.51) gives the optimal T_R

$$T_{R_{opt}} = \frac{\ln\left(\frac{\rho_{0,B}}{T_{1,B}}\right) - \ln\left(\frac{\rho_{0,A}}{T_{1,A}}\right)}{\left(\frac{1}{T_{1,B}} - \frac{1}{T_{1,A}}\right)} \tag{15.52}$$

Some *a priori* knowledge of tissue properties is clearly very useful. When several tissues are present, it may be difficult to choose a single T_R which optimizes all contrast and two scans with two different T_R values would be required. In principle, T_1's of all tissues could then be found (see Ch. 22).

This optimal value of T_R can also be obtained graphically by plotting the expression for C_{AB} from (15.50) as a function of T_R. Consider one such plot shown in Fig. 15.7a. At long T_R values, all tissues will have relaxed completely, and only spin density contrast is obtained, i.e., the contrast curve approaches a constant value asymptotically. At low values of T_R such that $T_R \ll T_1$ (this defines the T_1-weighted contrast regime), where the signal is inversely proportional to T_1, the tissue with lower T_1 has a higher signal. In the case of gray matter and white matter, since white matter has the lower T_1, it has a higher signal at short T_R values. However, since white matter also has a smaller spin density than gray matter, once T_R becomes comparable to T_1, gray matter starts growing towards a higher value, crossing the white matter curve towards its higher spin density value. The crossover point represents a 'null point' between gray matter and white matter where there is no contrast. In between a T_R value of 0 where the contrast is zero and the null point, there must be a maximum, and this represents the T_R value which gives the optimal T_1-weighted gray matter/white matter contrast. Two other examples, GM/CSF (Fig. 15.7b) and GM/lesion[12] ($\rho_0 = 0.8$, $T_1 = 1.5\,\text{sec}$; Fig. 15.7c) are also shown for comparison. Again, the previous observations are obeyed in both cases, and the range of T_R choices for the spin density weighting or T_1 weighting regimes can be determined from these plots.

The presence of a null point in the contrast curves was already noted. Its determination for the particular case of GM/WM contrast is the subject of Prob. 15.7.

---

[12]A 'lesion' is used to indicate abnormal tissue which contains T_1 and T_2 values larger than those of normal gray matter.

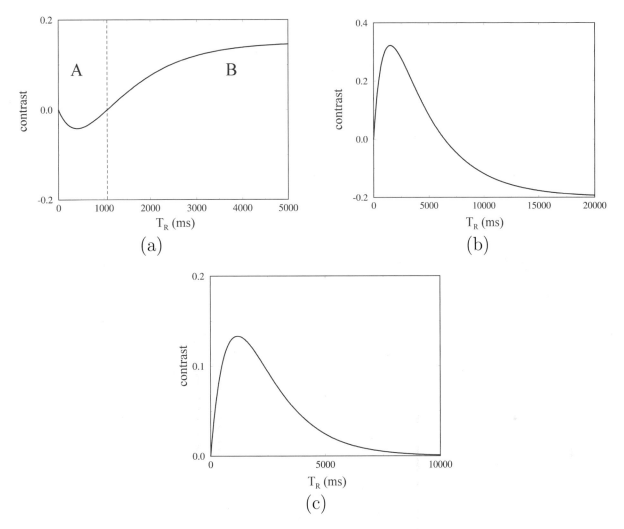

Fig. 15.7: C_{AB} as a function of T_R for (a) GM/WM (b) GM/CSF (c) GM/lesion in the case of a T_1-weighted 2D or 3D imaging experiment assuming ideal rf pulses. As demarcated in (a), two regions can be identified for each plot: one where the contrast is T_1 weighted (region A in (a) for example), and another where the contrast is spin density-weighted (region B in (a) for example). The figure shows that a unique T_R value which optimizes either contrast can be identified for each tissue pair of interest (which varies according to the intended application). The tissue parameters ρ_0 and T_1 used to simulate these figures came from Table 4.1 in Ch. 4. The lesion parameters were chosen to be $\rho_0 = 0.8$ and $T_1 = 1.5 \, \text{sec}$.

Problem 15.7

---

a) Show that for a 90° flip angle, short-T_E gradient echo sequence, there is a choice of T_R where gray matter (gray matter spin density relative to water $= 0.8$; $T_1 = 950\,\text{ms}$ at $1.5\,\text{T}$) and white matter (white matter spin density relative to water $= 0.65$; $T_1 = 600\,\text{ms}$ at $1.5\,\text{T}$) are iso-intense (i.e., they have the same signal). This represents a 'crossover point' on the contrast curve. What T_R does this crossover occur at?

b) Explain why there is such a crossover point (a plot of the two signals as a function of T_R would be helpful in making your argument).

c) From (15.52), find the T_R which optimizes the gray matter/white matter contrast.

The reader will find that these values are not perfect in real studies since the rf slice profile is not a boxcar function and all of the spins in the slice are not tipped by $\pi/2$. When this occurs, the tissues behave as if they have shorter than expected T_1.

Optimal T_R for Tissues with Similar Spin Densities and Fractionally Different T_1

The optimal value for T_R obtained in (15.52) represents the most general case of two tissues A and B which have different spin densities. In the early stages of the formation of certain diseased states, it is not uncommon to find the diseased tissue with a spin density which is very comparable to its normal neighbor, i.e.,

$$\rho_{0,A} \simeq \rho_{0,B} \equiv \rho_0 \tag{15.53}$$

and a T_1 which is fractionally different. That is,

$$T_{1,B} = T_{1,A}(1 + \delta) \quad \text{with} \quad \delta \to 0 \tag{15.54}$$

The expression for the contrast is

$$
\begin{aligned}
C_{AB} &= \rho_0 e^{-T_R/T_{1,A}} - e^{-T_R/((1+\delta)T_{1,A})} \\
&\simeq \rho_0 e^{-T_R/T_{1,A}} \left(e^{\delta T_R/T_{1,A}} - 1\right) \quad \text{since} \quad e^{-T_R/(1+\delta)T_{1,A}} \simeq e^{-(1-\delta)T_R/T_{1,A}} \\
&\simeq \rho_0 e^{-T_R/T_{1,A}} \left(\frac{T_R}{T_{1,A}}\right) \cdot \delta
\end{aligned}
\tag{15.55}
$$

which is again a function of T_R. Maximizing with respect to T_R then yields

$$T_{R_{opt}} = T_{1,A} \tag{15.56}$$

i.e., for two tissues with comparable spin density and slightly different T_1 values, the optimal T_R to choose is the T_1 value of the shorter T_1 tissue.

A similar approach can be taken for the arbitrary flip angle steady state incoherent method discussed in Sec. 18.1.5.

Problem 15.8

Derive an expression similar to (15.56) for a general value of δ. How does this value of $T_{R_{opt}}$ normalized to $T_{1,A}$ compare with the choice of a T_R of an average value of $T_{1,A}$ and $T_{1,B}$ normalized to $T_{1,A}$? What is the range of δ values up to which the average value serves as a reasonable approximation to the optimal T_R? The fact that the contrast is optimized by a T_R value comparable to the average of the T_1 values of the two tissues is used as a general rule of thumb for choosing T_R for tissues with comparable spin density values.

15.4.4 T_2^*-Weighting

The third basic contrast generating mechanism is based on differences in the transverse decay characteristics. Most disease states are characterized by an elevated T_2. Since the T_2 values are only on the order of tens of milliseconds whereas T_1 values are typically on the order of a second, a small increase in T_2 corresponds to a larger percentage increase than the same increase in T_1. As a result, T_2 is found to be a sensitive indicator of disease. T_2 weighting can be obtained by using spin echo sequences. T_2^* weighting also plays a useful role when local magnetic field susceptibility differences between tissues are present. If field changes occur sufficiently rapidly across a voxel, additional signal loss will occur when gradient echo sequences are used. For this reason, T_2^*-weighted images are used to study brain activity in brain functional imaging studies (as discussed in Ch. 25).

To avoid contributions from T_1 confounding the contrast, T_R is chosen such that[13]

$$T_R \gg T_{1_{A,B}} \Rightarrow e^{-T_R/T_1} \to 0 \tag{15.57}$$

in which case the gradient echo contrast is given by

$$C_{AB} = \rho_{0,A} e^{-T_E/T_{2,A}^*} - \rho_{0,B} e^{-T_E/T_{2,B}^*} \tag{15.58}$$

Figure 15.8b shows a plot of T_E versus contrast for (15.58) using gray matter ($\rho_0 = 0.8$ and $T_2 = 0.1\,\text{sec}$) and CSF ($\rho_0 = 1.0$ and $T_2 = 2\,\text{sec}$) as tissues A and B. Since GM has a T_2 value which is much shorter than that of CSF, the optimal T_E value is expected to be long compared to the T_2 value of gray matter and short compared to the T_2 value of CSF. On the other hand, when gray and white matter signals are considered as functions of T_E at long T_R values (Fig. 15.8a), WM ($\rho_0 = 0.65$ and $T_2 = 0.08\,\text{sec}$) always has a signal that is lower than that of GM. So, the optimal GM/WM contrast is produced by a very short T_E, in the spin density-weighted regime. A similar contrast curve can be generated for any two tissues

---

[13]It is also possible to obtain spin density or T_2^*-weighting with shorter T_R but then the rf pulse angle must be reduced to a value much less than $\pi/2$. A discussion of this class of experiments is reserved for the fast imaging discussion in Ch. 18.

of interest, whose relative spin density and T_2 values are known. For example, the case of GM/lesion contrast is considered in Fig. 15.8c. The lesion is assumed to have a ρ_0 of 0.8 and a T_2 of 350 ms. Since the contrast expression (15.58) contains only T_E dependence, optimal contrast is obtained by extremizing C_{AB} relative to T_E. The T_E at which the contrast is optimized is

$$T_{E_{opt}} = \frac{\ln\left(\frac{\rho_{0,B}}{T_{2,B}^*}\right) - \ln\left(\frac{\rho_{0,A}}{T_{2,A}^*}\right)}{\left(\frac{1}{T_{2,B}^*} - \frac{1}{T_{2,A}^*}\right)} \tag{15.59}$$

As previously discussed, a similar expression is obtained for a spin echo experiment in terms of T_E with T_2^* replaced by T_2. Expressions for the optimal T_E in the special case of only a fractional difference in T_2 also gives results identical in form to the T_R choice for optimal

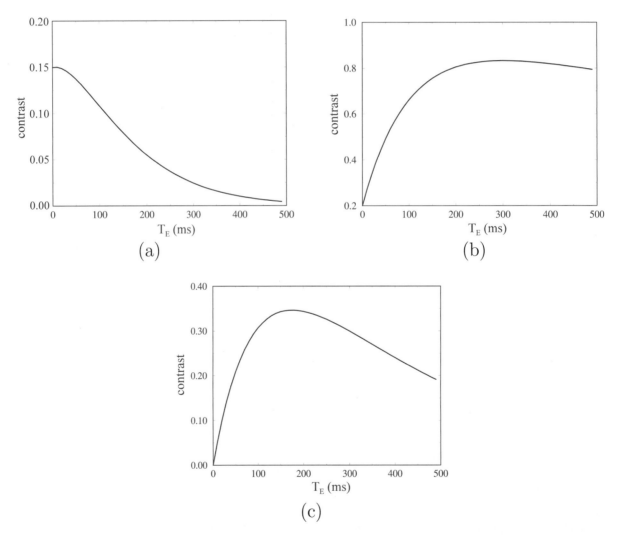

Fig. 15.8: C_{AB} as a function of T_E for (a) GM/WM (b) CSF/GM and (c) lesion/GM for a T_2-weighted scan. C_{AB} is given in units relative to a maximal value of unity. An optimal T_E value can also be obtained for each pair of tissues from such plots.

T_1-weighted contrast: that is, a T_E approximately equal to $T_{2,A}^*$ should be chosen.

Problem 15.9

a) Suppose that the relative spin density (ρ_0), T_1, and T_2 values of a certain tissue (gray matter, say) are 0.8, 1 s, and 100 ms, respectively. When disease sets in, suppose the local water content increases from 0 to 10% in each voxel. This two-compartment model implies that the fractional volume content of water in a voxel increases from 0 to 0.1 and that of the tissue decreases from 1.0 to 0.9. (This can happen when edema forms.) If the T_1 and T_2 of water are 4 s and 2 s, respectively, and the R_1 and R_2 values of healthy tissue and water average according to volume fraction of occupation of the voxel, what are the percentage increases in the effective T_1 and T_2 values in the diseased tissue?

b) Hence, which of the two mechanisms, T_1- or T_2-weighting, is more sensitive to small changes in local water content (compare the percentage change from values in normal tissues between T_1 and T_2)?

c) Find the optimal T_E for distinguishing this 'diseased tissue' from its normal neighbor, neglecting the change in spin density. Hence, show that the optimal T_E in the case of two tissues with comparable spin densities but different T_2 values such that $T_{2_B} = T_{2_A}(1 + \delta)$ is comparable to the average of the two T_2 values.

The conclusion from Prob. 15.9 is that T_2-weighting might be the intrinsic contrast mechanism of choice for distinguishing diseased states from normal tissue. In fact, it therefore comes as no surprise that T_2-weighted spin echo sequences are used for a variety of clinical applications.

15.4.5 Summary of Contrast Results

The general appearance of spin density, T_1- and T_2-weighted images of the brain is depicted in the images shown in Fig. 15.9. An optimal and yet practicable set of imaging parameters was used to obtain these images. Clearly, the T_1-weighted imaging method seems to be the most efficient in achieving the contrast required. An intermediate T_R value of about 600 ms gives optimal GM/WM contrast and shows good differentiation between these two structures and CSF and fat. Fat, with the lowest T_1 value amongst these four tissues, is shown as the brightest structure. On the other hand, CSF is shown with almost no noticeable signal because of its long T_1. White matter is the structure which is shown as the bright structure in the brain, while gray matter is shown with a lower gray level, all consistent with T_1 weighting. On the other hand, when it comes to spin density or T_2 weighting, it is impractical to design the sequence with a T_R which is on the order of a few T_1's of CSF. Therefore, it is typical to choose a T_R of about twice the T_1 of gray matter. At this T_R, CSF is almost iso-intense with white matter, and gray matter is found to have the highest signal. As described here, the spin density and T_2-weighted images shown in Figs. 15.9a and 15.9b were obtained using a T_R of 2.5 sec. On the T_2-weighted image, typically obtained using a longer T_E at the same T_R as the spin density-weighted image, CSF has the highest signal while white matter has the lowest signal. A set of general rules for choosing T_E and T_R for a $\pi/2$ gradient echo (or spin echo) experiment are outlined in Table 15.3.

Type of contrast	T_R	T_E
spin density	as long as possible	as short as possible
T_1-weighted	on the order of the T_1 values	as short as possible
T_2-weighted	as long as possible	on the order of the T_2 values

Table 15.3: General set of rules for generating tissue contrast.

Problem 15.10

Tissues A and B are found to have the following properties when imaged at a certain field strength

Quantity	A	B
T_1	600 ms	300 ms
intrinsic T_2^* ($\Delta B_0 = 0$)	80 ms	60 ms
normalized ρ_0	1.0	0.8

Assume that $\rho_{0,A}/\sigma_0$ is 40:1 and, in order for two tissues to be reliably differentiated, that the CNR must be greater than or equal to 4. Consider the gradient echo example presented earlier in this section.

a) If T_E is kept short (say $T_E = 20$ ms) to minimize T_2^* contrast, what is the minimum value of T_R that may be used to obtain a T_1-weighted image with adequate CNR such that A and B are reliably differentiated?

b) If T_R is 2000 ms, find the minimum and maximum values of T_E that could be used to obtain a T_2-weighted image with adequate CNR.

15.4.6   A Special Case: T_1-Weighting and Tissue Nulling with Inversion Recovery

Another commonly used mechanism for generating T_1 contrast is to use an inversion recovery (IR) sequence. Image contrast with the inversion recovery sequence can be adjusted with both T_R and T_I. There is interest in finding out the most time-efficient way to obtain T_1 weighting at some value (not necessarily the optimal value) of T_R or T_I. This is obtained by

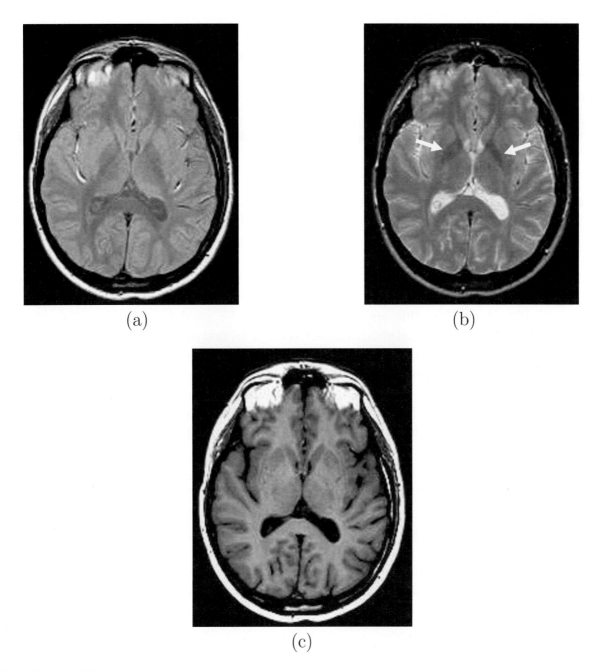

(a)

(b)

(c)

Fig. 15.9: Different forms of contrast generated by varying the imaging parameters with a spin echo sequence. (a) Spin density-weighted image. (b) T_2-weighted image. (c) T_1-weighted image. Although (a) is supposed to indicate spin density, it fails to do so for CSF since T_1 of CSF is too long (4.5 sec) relative to the T_R (2.5 sec). Gray/white matter contrast is good. In (b), the globus pallidus (arrow) appears quite dark (since the iron in it causes a diffusion weighted signal loss; see Ch. 21). As expected, CSF is bright because of its long T_2 (2 sec). Lastly, in (c), gray/white matter contrast is reversed and CSF is heavily suppressed. The dark CSF regions seem to visually enhance the overall contrast in the image.

looking at the differential change in signal relative to a differential increase in T_R or T_I. For the gradient echo sequence,

$$\frac{\partial C_{AB}}{\partial T_R} = \rho_{0,A}\frac{T_R}{T_{1,A}}e^{-T_R/T_{1,A}} - \rho_{0,B}\frac{T_R}{T_{1,B}}e^{-T_R/T_{1,B}} \tag{15.60}$$

whereas, for the inversion-recovery sequence (whose signal expression is given by (8.46))

$$\frac{\partial C_{AB}}{\partial T_I} = 2\left(\rho_{0,A}\frac{T_I}{T_{1,A}}e^{-T_I/T_{1,A}} - \rho_{0,B}\frac{T_I}{T_{1,B}}e^{-T_I/T_{1,B}}\right) \quad \text{for } T_R \gg T_1 \tag{15.61}$$

i.e., for the same increase in T_R or T_I, the inversion-recovery signal has twice the signal change as the spin echo signal change. If two tissues with only fractional T_1 differences are considered, this directly correlates to a doubling of the contrast in the inversion-recovery sequence. This was the reason for the early popularity of the inversion-recovery sequence for obtaining T_1 weighting.

The inversion process offers the ability to null a specific tissue by an appropriate choice of T_I. Some examples of this feature unique to the inversion recovery sequence are shown in Fig. 15.10. Here, four different choices of T_I can be used to null fat, white matter, gray matter, and cerebrospinal fluid, respectively. The first three are used in T_1-weighted IR imaging methods and the fourth in a T_2-weighted sequence to better differentiate small lesions otherwise obscured by CSF. The first is useful to image near the orbits where fat can obscure the optic nerve, for example. The third shows a more conventional T_1-weighted image. The fourth nulls CSF and any other water-like components but leaves good signal from pathological states with only slightly elevated water content relative to normal tissue.

Problem 15.11

Consider the implementation of an inversion-recovery sequence with T_I chosen to null the signal (implies $T_{I,null} = T_1 \ln 2$ in the limit that $T_R \gg T_1$) for either fat or water at 1.5 T. Find $T_{I,null}$ for water and fat whose T_1 values are $T_{1,w} = 4\,\text{s}$ and $T_{1,f} = 250\,\text{ms}$, respectively.

15.5 Contrast Enhancement with T_1-Shortening Agents

In fast imaging, where T_R is much less than T_1, the signal for a 90° flip angle is proportional to T_R/T_1 and, in this regime, tissues with shorter T_1 have a higher signal than tissues with longer T_1 and the contrast is predominantly T_1-weighted.

Certain external agents can be introduced into specific targeted tissues where these agents act to reduce the T_1 of that tissue. Figure 15.11 demonstrates the T_1-shortening effect of one of these agents. Suppose that the targeted tissue (in the case shown in Fig. 15.11, the targeted tissue is blood) has similar NMR properties as its neighboring tissue, causing an inability to differentiate the two using any of the three contrast mechanisms discussed in Sec. 15.4 but contains a different signal response to the contrast agent. By delivering the

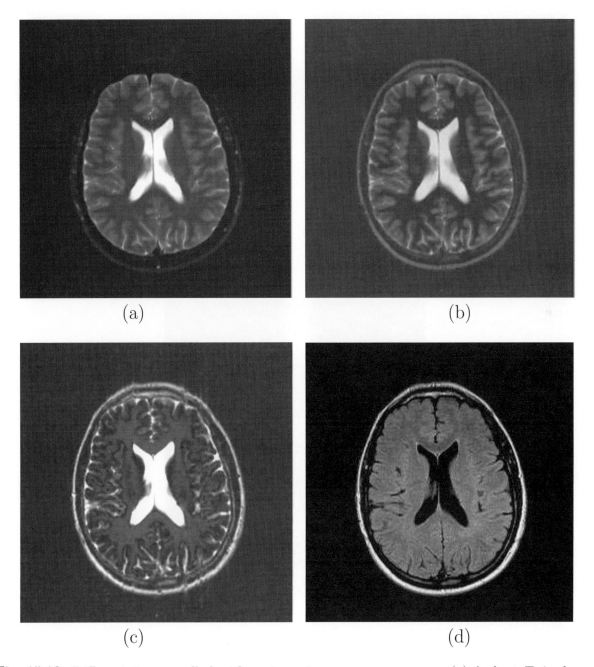

(a)

(b)

(c)

(d)

Fig. 15.10: Different tissues nulled with an inversion recovery sequence. (a) A short T_I is chosen to null fat. (b) An intermediate T_I is chosen to null WM. (c) A higher T_I nulls GM. (d) A very long T_I nulls CSF, which is typically used in a T_2-weighted sequence to null the otherwise very high signal producing CSF.

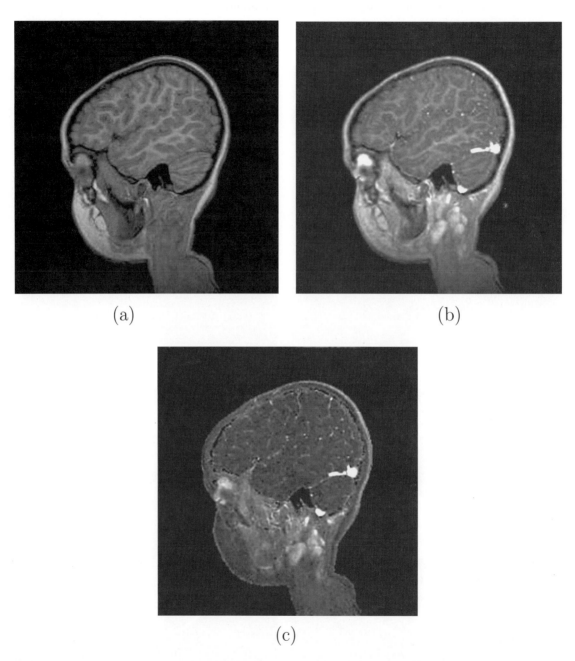

(a)   (b)

(c)

Fig. 15.11: T_1 reduction effects of a contrast agent. (a) A single slice from a 3D T_1-weighted data set before contrast agent was injected. (b) Image of the same slice after an intravenous injection of a T_1-shortening contrast agent. Since the T_1 of blood is shortened, the blood vessels light up, and are seen as bright spots in the image. Also, there is a loss of contrast between WM/GM because of the larger blood volume content of GM (hence, its signal increases more than that of WM, reducing contrast). (c) Subtraction of the first image from the second image depicts this signal increase predominantly in the blood vessels, but also from the blood-containing tissue itself. Only those voxels with a positive subtraction are shown; voxels with a negative subtraction are set to zero, leading to the isolated black dots in this image.

T_1-shortening agent to the tissue of interest, the targeted signal is increased while the signal from the background remains the same when a T_1-weighted sequence is used. This increases the contrast between the two tissues and, for this reason, such agents are commonly referred to as 'contrast agents.'

In general, the increase in relaxation rate after T_1 shortening is found to be directly proportional to the concentration C of the contrast agent delivered to the tissue. If $T_{1,0}$ is the intrinsic T_1 of the tissue and $T_1(C)$ is its shortened value, it is found that

$$R_1(C) \equiv \frac{1}{T_1(C)} = \frac{1}{T_{1,0}} + \alpha_1 C$$
$$\equiv R_{1,0} + \alpha_1 C \qquad (15.62)$$

where the constant of proportionality α_1 is called the longitudinal relaxivity (T_1 relaxivity) with units of $(mmol/l)^{-1}sec^{-1}$,[14] a property specific to the composition of the contrast agent. Figure 15.12a demonstrates the effect of a contrast agent *in vivo* on the T_1 of blood for which $T_{1,0} \simeq 1200\,ms$ at 1.5 T.

Problem 15.12

If a contrast agent at a dose of 0.1 mmol/kg is given to a 50 kg person with 5 liters of blood in his/her body, what is the expected T_1 of the blood when the contrast agent is well-mixed in the blood? Assume the T_1-relaxivity of the contrast agent is 5/mM/sec and T_1 of blood is 1200 ms. In practice, some of the agent is taken up by other organs in the body and this 'extravasation' can lead to the effective blood volume (or effective distributed volume of the contrast agent) being 10 liters for purposes of this calculation. How does this affect the above estimate for T_1?

In addition to shortening the T_1, these contrast agents also tend to shorten the T_2 of the tissue in a similar fashion to the T_1 shortening, i.e.,

$$R_2(C) \equiv \frac{1}{T_2(C)} = \frac{1}{T_{2,0}} + \alpha_2 C$$
$$= R_{2,0} + \alpha_2 C \qquad (15.63)$$

where α_2 is the transverse relaxivity of the contrast agent. Figure 15.12b shows the effect of contrast agent dosage on the T_2 of blood (which has an intrinsic T_2 ranging from 100 ms for venous blood to 200 ms for arterial blood). This concomitant decrease in T_2 tends to partly counterbalance the effects of shortened T_1. For many T_1-shortening contrast agents, the transverse and longitudinal relaxation rates are comparable in magnitude ($\alpha_1 \simeq \alpha_2$). Since $R_{2,0} > R_{1,0}$, a given increase in the concentration leads to a larger magnitude change in T_1 and, hence, in the signal due to this shortened T_1 effect than the effect caused by the T_2 reduction. It is only when $\alpha_2 C$ becomes comparable to $R_{2,0}$ that the signal loss due to the T_2 shortening becomes significant, and starts to overwhelm the enhanced T_1-weighted

---

[14]Recall that 1 mmol/l is also written as 1 mM (millimolar).

contrast. In fact, this crossover point between signal loss due to T_2 shortening and signal increase due to T_1 shortening defines an optimal contrast agent dosage.

A major clinical application of T_1 shortening contrast agents at present is intended for the improved detection of small lesions. Typically, these lesions have a fractionally increased water content leading to best depiction of these lesions in a T_2-weighted image before contrast agent is injected. Despite being the most sensitive contrast mechanism, it is not possible for the T_2-weighted image to depict very small lesions which are averaged with neighboring tissue of comparable NMR tissue properties. The use of an intravenous injection of a T_1

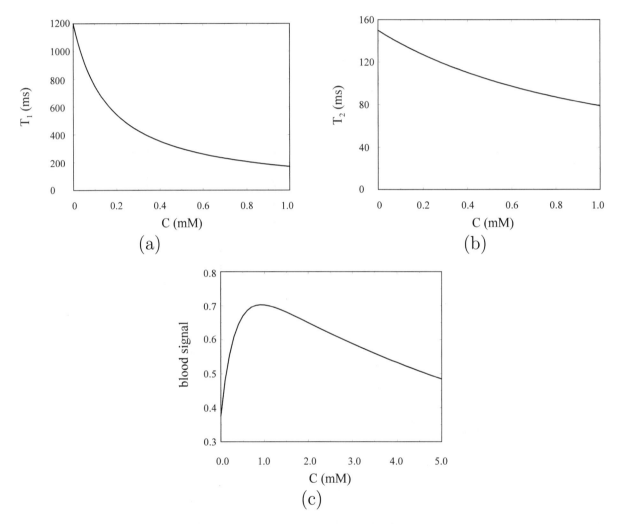

Fig. 15.12: T_1 and T_2 are plotted in (a) and (b), respectively, as functions of contrast agent concentration delivered to the tissue of interest. The contrast agent is supposed to have longitudinal and transverse relaxivities of 5/mM/sec and 6/mM/sec, respectively. Notice that the relative change in T_1 for a given concentration is much larger than that for T_2. (c) Blood signal in relative units as a function of contrast agent concentration plotted for a spin echo acquisition with 600 ms T_R and 20 ms T_E. (T_1 and T_2 of blood were taken to be 1200 ms and 150 ms, respectively.) Note that, as the concentration increases, the T_2 reduction effect takes over and causes a reduction of blood signal. In essence, an optimal concentration which maximizes the signal exists.

shortening agent is indicated for such patients. Most lesions are found to have a rich blood supply. Therefore, the lesions have contrast agent delivered locally, leading to lesion signal enhancement and improved lesion detection.

15.6 Partial Volume Effects, CNR, and Resolution

In the earlier discussion on object visibility, it was seen that $\mathcal{V}$ is invariant as a function of voxel size for multi-voxel objects under the assumption that the voxel signal came from a homogeneous chunk of tissue within the voxel. What then is the advantage of using a smaller voxel size if reducing the voxel size serves only to worsen the SNR while only maintaining object visibility? In this section, resolution effects on object visibility are discussed in detail, leading to a theoretical understanding of the effects of spatial resolution on the diagnostic value of an image.

If tissue A is smaller than a voxel, it shares the voxel with the background tissue, and tissue A is said to be 'partial volumed.' Such a partial volume model is shown in Fig. 15.13. If the point spread effects of the image reconstruction are neglected, a simple model for the combined signal from the voxel is the summed fractional signals of tissues A and B. Let S_A and S_B represent the signal for tissues A and B, respectively, when they occupy an entire voxel of size Δx (i.e., S_A is the signal from tissue A if α equals 1 in Fig. 15.13a). In the

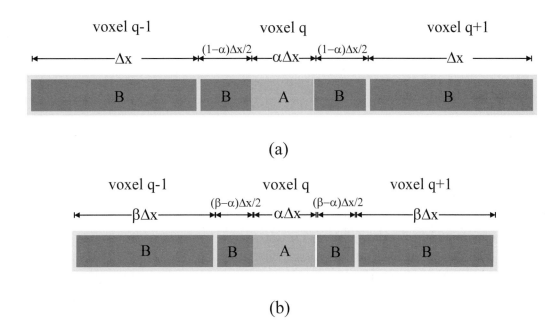

(a)

(b)

Fig. 15.13: Model of a 1D voxel q which is occupied by two different materials or tissues. Voxels $(q-1)$ and $(q+1)$ contain only background tissue with signal magnitude S_B in (a) where the voxel size is Δx, while the central voxel q contains a combination of tissues A and B, with tissue A of size $\alpha \Delta x$ ($\alpha < 1$) occupying a fraction α of the voxel. In (b), the voxel size is reduced to $\beta \Delta x$ ($\beta < 1$) and tissue A now occupies the fraction α/β of the central voxel while the signal from voxels $(q-1)$ and $(q+1)$ are also reduced to βS_B.

general case, if α is the fraction of voxel q occupied by tissue A, the signal for voxel q when $\beta = 1$ (Fig. 15.13a) is the sum of the voxel signal contributions $\hat{\rho}_{A,q}$ and $\hat{\rho}_{B,q}$ from A and B, respectively, i.e.,

$$\hat{\rho}_{voxel,q} = \hat{\rho}_{A,q} + \hat{\rho}_{B,q} \tag{15.64}$$

Now

$$\hat{\rho}_{A,q} \equiv \alpha S_A \quad \text{and} \tag{15.65}$$
$$\hat{\rho}_{B,q} \equiv (1 - \alpha)S_B \tag{15.66}$$

and hence from (15.64)

$$\hat{\rho}_{voxel,q} = \alpha S_A + (1 - \alpha)S_B \tag{15.67}$$

The image contrast is then

$$C_{q,q+1} = \underbrace{\hat{\rho}_{voxel,q}}_{\text{voxel with } A \text{ and } B} - \underbrace{\hat{\rho}_{voxel,q+1}}_{\text{homogeneous voxel with } B} = \alpha(S_A - S_B) \tag{15.68}$$

The conclusion is that if a certain tissue is partial volumed, its contrast is reduced according to the fraction of the voxel it is occupying.

In the case where the voxel size is reduced, i.e., $\beta < 1$, tissue A occupies the fraction $\frac{\alpha}{\beta}$ of the entire voxel volume and B occupies the remaining $1 - \frac{\alpha}{\beta}$ fraction of the voxel. Also, the signal from voxels $q - 1$ and $q + 1$ is now βS_B. In a similar fashion, the signal from A, when it occupies a complete voxel of size $\beta\Delta x$, is βS_A, leading to

$$\hat{\rho}_{q,A} \rightarrow \frac{\alpha}{\beta}(\beta S_A) \tag{15.69}$$

and

$$\hat{\rho}_{q,B} \rightarrow \frac{(\beta - \alpha)}{\beta}(\beta S_B) = (\beta - \alpha)S_B \tag{15.70}$$

Hence the contrast is

$$C_{q,q+1}|_{\beta<1} = \hat{\rho}_{voxel,q} - \hat{\rho}_{voxel,q\pm1} = (\alpha S_A + (\beta - \alpha)S_B) - \beta S_B = \alpha(S_A - S_B) \tag{15.71}$$

i.e., the contrast does not change.

Two cases can be considered for increasing the spatial resolution (say, making $\beta \rightarrow \beta/2$): case 1, doubling T_s or the number of phase encoding steps so that the SNR reduces by only $\sqrt{2}$ and case 2, halving the FOV keeping N fixed, leading to a loss of 2 in SNR. As the voxel size is decreased by a factor of 2, the CNR (and visibility) increases by $\sqrt{2}$ in case 1 and stays the same in case 2. If the SNR is good enough, this result indicates it is possible that a small partial volumed object will become visible as Δx is reduced.

In summary, the utility of high resolution lies in its ability to make partial volumed objects which are smaller than the voxel size visible, even though the SNR decreases as Δx is reduced. Although at first sight it seems like tissue A has been conveniently chosen to be at the center of the voxel in (a) for this improved visibility result, even in the more general case of an arbitrarily positioned A, it can always be moved into the center of the voxel by using the Fourier transform shift theorem (see Ch. 11 for details) for which case this improved visibility result holds.

Problem 15.13

Consider an object of size $\Delta x/4$ (say a small blood vessel) and centered in a 1D voxel of size Δx as shown in Fig. 15.14a. Suppose $(S_A - S_B)/\sigma_0$ is 2.0 when the voxel size is Δx. Now suppose the voxel size is halved (case 1) to $\Delta x/2$ (see Fig. 15.14b) and then halved again (case 2) to $\Delta x/4$ (see Fig. 15.14c).

a) If S_q/σ is 8.0 when the voxel size is Δx, what is the SNR at the two smaller voxel sizes shown in Figs. 15.14b and 15.14c? Assume that SNR_q is reduced by $\sqrt{2}$ each time the resolution is halved. The common misconception is that because the SNR is reduced, the diagnostic value of the image is lost. Evidently, object visibility, rather than SNR, is the more appropriate index of clinical utility.

b) What happens to $\mathcal{V}$ at the two smaller voxel sizes in (i) case 1, and (ii) case 2? Is the object visible at any of the three voxel sizes (i) in case 1, and (ii) case 2? Assume that the visibility threshold is 3. The important point is that if there is an object of interest which is invisible at a given voxel size because of partial volume effects, it may be possible to make it visible by reducing the voxel size. Other additional options include using a contrast agent to increase signal or averaging over multiple acquisitions to reduce the noise.

15.7 SNR in Magnitude and Phase Images

Phase offers some fascinating ways to enhance information about certain features in MR images. When the field is perfect and no motion is present, the expected phase is zero. White noise will also have a magnitude and phase. We consider here the contribution of noise to the magnitude and phase images ($|\hat{\rho}|$ and $\hat{\phi}$) in the case where the SNR is much greater than unity.

15.7.1 Magnitude Image SNR

The complex signal can be written as

$$\hat{\rho} = R + iI \tag{15.72}$$

or as

$$\hat{\rho} = \rho_m e^{i\phi} \tag{15.73}$$

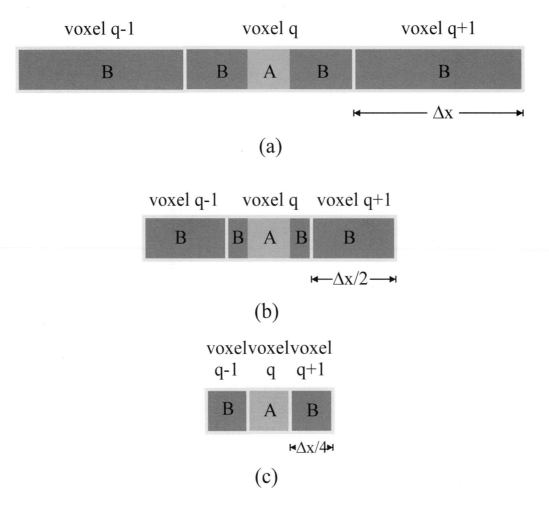

Fig. 15.14: (a) A 1D voxel of dimension Δx contains a square object $\Delta x/4$ in size. The voxel size is reduced to (b) $\Delta x/2$ and (c) $\Delta x/4$ to demonstrate the potential effects of partial voluming. For case 1, the actual CNR between tissues from (a) to (c) increases by a factor of 2 (as discussed in Sec. 15.6). This can also be understood by considering the change in voxel signal for A when B is zero. For part (a), the signal in voxel q will appear as $S_A/4$ and remain at this value for parts (b) and (c) while the noise decreases by $\sqrt{2}$ at each step.

Let ρ_m in the absence of noise be a. If the noise-free phase is $\hat{\phi}$ then the real and imaginary parts, R and I, respectively, of $\hat{\rho}$ are

$$R = a\cos\hat{\phi} + \eta_1 \qquad (15.74)$$
$$I = a\sin\hat{\phi} + \eta_2 \qquad (15.75)$$

where R and I are the real and imaginary parts of the reconstructed complex voxel signal, respectively, and η_1 and η_2 are noise samples from a Gaussian distribution with mean zero and variance σ^2. The mean values of R and I, $\bar{R}$ and $\bar{I}$, respectively, are

$$\bar{R} = a\cos\hat{\phi} \qquad (15.76)$$
$$\bar{I} = a\sin\hat{\phi} \qquad (15.77)$$

Their variances are both equal to σ^2. The magnitude ρ_m of the voxel signal is found from

$$
\begin{aligned}
\rho_m &= (R^2 + I^2)^{1/2} \\
&= (a^2 + 2\eta_2 a \cos\hat\phi + 2\eta_1 a \sin\hat\phi + \eta_1^2 + \eta_2^2)^{1/2} \\
&\simeq a\left(1 + \frac{\eta_2}{a}\cos\hat\phi + \frac{\eta_1}{a}\sin\hat\phi\right)
\end{aligned}
\tag{15.78}
$$

With the approximation made for ρ_m in (15.78), the mean of the magnitude of the voxel signal is, as expected, given by

$$
\overline{\rho_m} = a
\tag{15.79}
$$

To obtain the variance of the magnitude, the noise is taken to be uncorrelated between the real and imaginary channels. Then, from (15.78),

$$
\begin{aligned}
\mathrm{var}(\rho_m) &\equiv \sigma_{\mathrm{mag}}^2 \\
&= \mathrm{var}(\eta_2)\cos^2\hat\phi + \mathrm{var}(\eta_1)\sin^2\hat\phi \\
&= \sigma^2
\end{aligned}
\tag{15.80}
$$

i.e., if the SNR of the magnitude of the voxel signal is much larger than unity, the mean of the magnitude is the true magnitude value, and its variance is the same as the variance in either the real or imaginary part of the voxel signal.

Problem 15.14

An alternate approach can be taken to obtain (15.79) and (15.80) for the case of large SNR. In this limit, the added white noise can be approximated as producing a small error in the measurement of the true magnitude $(\overline{\rho_m})$.

1) The measured voxel signal magnitude ρ_m can then be expanded in a Taylor series around the value $\overline{\rho_m}$ by viewing ρ_m as a function of R and I, the real and imaginary parts of the voxel signal, respectively. With the SNR large, the approximation of its Taylor series up to the linear term is good enough. Using this approximation, write an expression for the error in the measured magnitude, $\delta\rho_m \equiv \rho_m - \overline{\rho_m}$, in terms of the errors in R and I.

2) What is the mean value of $\delta\rho_m$? Assume that $\overline{\delta I} = \overline{\delta R} = 0$.

3) What is the error variance $\overline{(\delta\rho_m - \overline{\delta\rho_m})^2}$? Do you obtain the same result as in (15.80)?

15.7.2 Phase Image SNR

The phase of the signal can be found from

$$
\tan\hat\phi = I/R
\tag{15.81}
$$

Using the approach of differentials on (15.81) to determine the error as in Prob. 15.14 gives

$$\delta\hat\phi\sec^2\hat\phi = \frac{\delta I}{R} - \delta R\frac{I}{R^2} \tag{15.82}$$

Hence, $\overline{\delta\hat\phi} = 0$ and the variance of the phase is given by the mean squared error:

$$
\begin{aligned}
\overline{\delta\hat\phi^2} &= \left(\frac{I}{R}\right)^2\left(\frac{\overline{\delta I^2}}{I^2} + \frac{\overline{\delta R^2}}{R^2}\right)\cos^4\hat\phi \\
&= \sigma^2\cos^4\hat\phi\left(\frac{\rho_m^2}{R^4}\right) \\
&= \frac{\sigma^2}{\rho_m^2}
\end{aligned}
\tag{15.83}
$$

and the standard deviation of the phase $\sigma_{\text{phase}} \simeq (\overline{\delta\hat\phi^2})^{1/2} = \sigma/\rho_m$. This is sometimes written as

$$\sigma_{\text{phase}} = 1/\text{SNR}_{\text{mag}} \quad \text{(units are radians)} \tag{15.84}$$

or in degrees as

$$\sigma_{\text{phase}} = \frac{180°}{\pi(\text{SNR}_{\text{mag}})} \tag{15.85}$$

where SNR_{mag} is the SNR of the voxel signal magnitude. This tells us that at voxels where the SNR of the magnitude is very high, there is a relatively low error in phase measurements. On the other hand, the error is very large if the voxel magnitude has very low SNR.

One of the interesting features of the phase is that if there are artifacts which are of very low magnitude in comparison with the object signal (such as ghosts), the magnitude image does not show these features well. However, these artifacts still have some nonzero phase and even the smallest magnitude effects are highlighted. Such an example is shown in Fig. 15.15.

15.8   SNR as a Function of Field Strength

Finding the optimal field strength for imaging has always been complicated and controversial since many factors affect the outcome. Perhaps the three most important are spin density, T_1, and field inhomogeneity, all of which lead to modifications of SNR and CNR as a function of field strength.

In this section, we will give a prediction of the signal as a function of field strength based on (15.9) and (15.87) and a practical estimate of the ratio of the significance of the two terms in (15.87) at one field strength (the two terms being formed by bulking together the coil and electronics resistances as the sum of electronic resistance R_{coil}, $R_{electronics}$, and the magnetically induced losses due to the presence of the body, R_{body}).

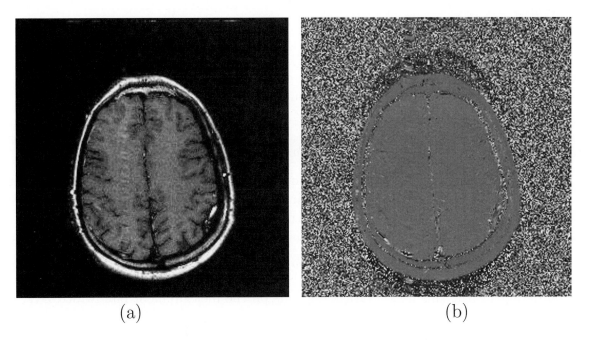

Fig. 15.15: Low amplitude features such as ghosts are typically highlighted in the phase image. Although a shifted ghost is present in the phase encoding direction, (a) it does not show on the magnitude image, yet, it is well depicted in (b) the phase image.

15.8.1   Frequency Dependence of the Noise in MRI

It was observed in Ch. 7 that the induced emf is proportional to $\omega_0 M_0$. Since $M_0 \propto \omega_0$ too, the induced emf increases as the square of the field strength. In a circuit with a frequency-independent resistance, the rms noise voltage is also independent of the frequency (from (15.7)), depending only on the bandwidth of data collection. Unfortunately in MR, the effective resistance 'seen' by the signal-receiving electronics is found to depend on the operating frequency. This dependence causes the rms noise voltage to be frequency-dependent. The resistance of the coil and the electronics can be bulked together as one component contributing to the noise, while the sample resistance corresponds to the other major contributor to the noise voltage. At low frequencies, the coil and electronics resistance dominate over the sample resistance at room temperatures, whereas at high frequencies, the sample resistance of human tissues dominates the coil and electronics resistance.

Let $\omega_{0,mid}$ be some frequency where this transition of noise source dominance begins to occur:

$$R_{eff}(\omega_0) \approx \begin{cases} R_{coil}(\omega_0) + R_{electronics}(\omega_0) & \omega_0 \ll \omega_{0,mid} \\ R_{sample}(\omega_0) & \omega_0 \gg \omega_{0,mid} \end{cases} \tag{15.86}$$

It has been found that the combined coil and electronics resistances have a square-root dependence on ω_0, whereas the sample resistance has an ω_0^2 dependence, i.e.,

$$R_{eff}(\omega_0) \propto \begin{cases} \sqrt{\omega_0} & \omega_0 \ll \omega_{0,mid} \\ \omega_0^2 & \omega_0 \gg \omega_{0,mid} \end{cases} \tag{15.87}$$

and, from (15.7)

$$\sigma_{thermal} \propto \begin{cases} \omega_0^{1/4} & \omega_0 \ll \omega_{0,mid} \\ \omega_0 & \omega_0 \gg \omega_{0,mid} \end{cases} \tag{15.88}$$

since $\sigma_{thermal}^2 \propto R_{eff}$. As a result, when the experiment is designed such that the noise is white noise dominated, the SNR as a function of frequency ω_0 is such that

$$\text{SNR}(\omega_0) \propto \begin{cases} \omega_0^2/\omega_0^{1/4} = \omega_0^{7/4} & \omega_0 \ll \omega_{0,mid} \\ \omega_0^2/\omega_0 = \omega_0 & \omega_0 \gg \omega_{0,mid} \end{cases} \tag{15.89}$$

i.e., at low field strengths, a 7/4 power law improvement in SNR with field strength occurs, whereas at high field strengths, only a linear increase in SNR is obtained. The practical implications of this frequency dependence will be discussed in more detail in Sec. 15.8.2. It suffices to say here that the SNR increases not as ω_0^2 as it would have if $\sigma_{thermal}$ were frequency-independent. It increases only as $\omega_0^{7/4}$ until some transition frequency, after which it increases further slowly for $\omega_0 \gg \omega_{0,mid}$. It is also worth reminding the reader here that at a given frequency, the rms noise voltage depends on the measurement bandwidth BW_{read}.

15.8.2   SNR Dependence on Field Strength

We start with a low field system ($B_{0,low} = 0.065\,\text{T}$), where one expects the noise to be dominated by the electronics. In this case, using a high temperature superconducting surface coil, it has been shown that the noise is reduced by a factor of 2 compared to a conventional coil at room temperature. If one assumes that the remaining noise is from magnetic losses, then it is possible to calculate the ratio of R_{body} to $R_{electronics}$ and predict the SNR increase from 0.065 T to a high field such as 1.5 T, for example. Using the above information in the generalized expression for SNR given the field dependence of R_{eff} in (15.87),

$$\text{SNR}(\omega) = \kappa \frac{\omega^2}{(\omega^2 + a\sqrt{\omega})^{1/2}} \tag{15.90}$$

implies $a = 3\omega_{low}^{3/2}$ where here $\omega_{low}/\gamma = B_{0,low}$ and $\omega = \gamma B_0$ (for simplicity the subscript 0 used in the previous subsection is dropped from ω at this point). The constant κ contains the system scale factor Λ and all other terms on which signal depends. Using the fact that the noise is reduced by a factor of 2, as mentioned above, yields

$$\text{SNR}(\omega) = \text{SNR}(\omega_{low}) \left[\frac{\left(\frac{\omega}{\omega_{low}}\right)^2}{\left(\left(\frac{\omega}{\omega_{low}}\right)^2 + 3\sqrt{\frac{\omega}{\omega_{low}}}\right)^{1/2}} \right] \tag{15.91}$$

Figure 15.16 demonstrates that above 0.5 T, the SNR is linear in ω to within 6.3% of the predicted value and, below 0.04 T, it is proportional to $\omega^{7/4}$ within 37%.

Implications for Low Field Strength Imaging

The possibility of imaging at low fields appears rather dismal from these predictions assuming that the imaging parameters at 1.5 T are ideal. However, at lower fields both T_1 and

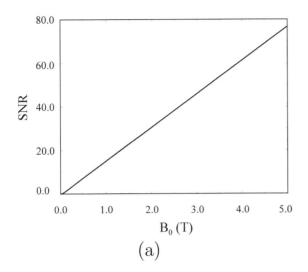
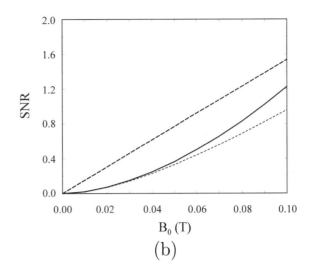

Fig. 15.16: Plot of SNR as a function of field strength. (a) Overall dependence shown over a range of 0.001 T to 5.0 T. (b) Comparison of the dependence with the 7/4 power law (shown as the curve with the short dashed line) and linear behavior (long-dashed line) over a range of 0.001 T to 0.1 T.

susceptibility effects are reduced. For example, it has been empirically shown that

$$T_1(\omega) = 1/(A/\sqrt{\omega} + B) \tag{15.92}$$

This inverse square-root dependence of the longitudinal relaxation rate on the field strength was observed by Escanyé in the article cited in the Suggested Reading found at the end of the chapter. For the tissues evaluated, B was found to be very close to zero, i.e., the relaxation rate was found to vary inversely as the field strength. Recall that for spin echo or gradient echo imaging for short T_R, the signal is proportional to T_R/T_1 so a $\sqrt{\omega}$ decrease in T_1 leads to a $\sqrt{\omega}$ increase in signal.

Problem 15.15

Another estimate for the field dependence of tissue T_1 is

$$T_1(\omega) = a\omega^b \tag{15.93}$$

This power law dependence of T_1 on field strength was proposed by Bottomley in the article cited at the end of this chapter. For gray matter, the values of a and b were found to be 0.00362 and 0.3082, respectively; for white matter, the values are 0.00152 and 0.3477, respectively. For (15.93), plot $T_1(\omega)$ from 1 MHz to 200 MHz for GM and WM. Note that in comparison with the square-root increase in T_1 with field strength described in the text, this predicts approximately a cube root increase in T_1 with field strength. What effects do you expect to see for T_1-weighted scans as the field changes from 1.5 T to 3.0 T?

Also at lower fields, as long as $T_s/2$ is much shorter than T_E at 1.5 T, BW_{read} for a fixed Δx can be reduced proportional to field strength thanks to lower susceptibilities at lower fields and hence reduced signal dephasing and image distortion artifacts. Therefore, down to some field strength where the limiting case is reached, SNR goes up by another factor of $\sqrt{\omega}$. Lo and behold, dependence on ω from the previous SNR argument, under some circumstances, is exactly balanced by the opposite dependence on ω from the two arguments just described.

Problem 15.16

At high magnetic fields, R_2^* of blood becomes a function of field strength. Assume that R_2^* varies directly with magnetic field. Show that the SNR would vary as $\sqrt{B_0}e^{-\alpha T_E B_0}$ for a fixed echo time if the readout bandwidth is also increased to avoid further geometric distortion as B_0 increases. Comment on an optimal choice of B_0 under these conditions.

Suggested Reading

Basic concepts of noise are well described in the following two books:

- C. Kittel. *Thermal Physics.* John Wiley and Sons, Inc., New York, 1969.

- H. L. Van Trees. *Detection, Estimation, and Modulation Theory. Part I.* John Wiley and Sons, Inc., New York, 1968.

The concepts of visibility and detectability are introduced in:

- A. Rose. *Vision: Human and Electronic.* Plenum Press, New York, 1985.

A measure of imaging efficiency is proposed in:

- W. A. Edelstein, G. H. Glover, C. J. Hardy and R. W. Redington. The intrinsic signal-to-noise ratio in NMR imaging. *Magn. Reson. Med.*, 3: 604, 1986.

Issues of contrast and visibility in MR imaging are covered in the following two papers:

- R. T. Constable and R. M. Henkelman. Contrast, resolution, and detectability in MR imaging. *J. Comput. Assist. Tomogr.*, 15: 297, 1991.

- R. Venkatesan and E. M. Haacke. Role of high resolution in magnetic resonance (MR) imaging: Applications to MR angiography, intracranial T_1-weighted imaging, and image interpolation. *Int. J. Imaging Sys. Technol.*, 8: 529, 1997.

The square-root field strength dependence of T_1 was proposed in:

- J. M. Escanyé, D. Canet and J. Robert. Frequency dependence of water proton longitudinal nuclear magnetic relaxation times in mouse tissues at 20°C. *Biochim. Biophys. Acta*, 721: 305, 1982.

The cube root field strength dependence suggested in Prob. 15.15 was observed in:

- P. A. Bottomley, C. J. Hardy, R. E. Argersinger and G. Allen-Moore. A review of ^{1}H nuclear magnetic resonance relaxation in pathology: Are T_1 and T_2 diagnostic? *Med. Phys.*, 14: 1, 1987.

Chapter 16

A Closer Look at Radiofrequency Pulses

Chapter Contents

Summary: The measured spin density is related to the rf fields in terms of the receive coil field, transmit coil field, and the slice selection process. The slice select profile as a Fourier transform of the time-dependent B_1 field is expanded upon. A practical example of slice select sequence design is given which takes into account finite gradient rise times and spoiling. Methods for calibrating the rf transmit amplitude and slice select properties are discussed. Solutions of the Bloch equations for low flip angles are presented which can be used to select an arbitrary 3D region. Spin tagging is introduced in the final section.

Introduction

The image, or measured spin density in an MRI experiment, is not necessarily equivalent to the physical spin density of the object being imaged, even when relaxation and Fourier transform effects are considered. The image is actually a picture of the signal received by the rf receive coil or rf probe. It is, in fact, proportional to the product of the receive coil's field and the transverse magnetization (which itself depends on the transmit coil's field). In

375

this chapter, a study is made of how the applied gradients, transmit rf field, and receive rf field relate to the measured spin density.

In Ch. 10, the notion of using finite bandwidth rf pulses in combination with applied gradients to excite a particular region of spins was introduced. It was assumed there that the rf field was perfectly uniform and that a rectangular spectral excitation could be achieved. The Fourier transform dictates that a rectangular excitation in the frequency domain requires a sinc profile in the time domain extending over all time. In practice, the rf pulse can only last a few milliseconds and, therefore, a perfectly rectangular excitation profile cannot be achieved.

A general introduction relating the applied rf field to the measured spin density will be presented first, and then several sections will explain specific experimental scenarios for rf calibration, specific pulses, and rf power deposition.

16.1   Relating RF Fields and Measured Spin Density

The focus of this section is to understand how variations in the rf field will cause variations in image intensity that are independent of the physical spin density. In Ch. 7, it was shown that the signal measured in an MRI experiment is proportional to the *emf* picked up by the rf receive coil which, in turn, is proportional to the scalar product of the transverse magnetization and the receive rf field (see (7.20)). The signal received from a differential volume element d^3r is

$$ds(\vec{r}) \propto M_\perp(\vec{r})\mathcal{B}_\perp^{receive}(\vec{r})d^3r \tag{16.1}$$

where the time dependence of the signal has been ignored. After Fourier transforming a frequency encoded signal with respect to time, an image is produced which is proportional to the same terms

$$\hat{\rho}(\vec{r}) \propto M_\perp(\vec{r})\mathcal{B}_\perp^{receive}(\vec{r}) \tag{16.2}$$

The reconstructed image is said to represent the physical spin density, although it is seen that other quantities are involved in this expression. Remember that $M_\perp(\vec{r})$ is usually generated when a set of spins is tipped by an rf pulse to create a transverse magnetization. To find the relationship between the measured spin density and the physical spin density, it is necessary to determine how $M_\perp(\vec{r})$ is related to $B_{1,\perp}^{transmit}(\vec{r}, t)$ and the applied slice select gradients.

The magnitude of the perpendicular component of the magnetization, neglecting relaxation and assuming the equilibrium magnetization M_0 is available, is dependent on the flip angle, $\theta(\vec{r})$, at that position, via

$$M_\perp(\vec{r}) = M_0(\vec{r})\sin\theta(\vec{r}) \tag{16.3}$$

The spatial effects of the transmit rf field and applied gradients are reflected in $\theta(\vec{r})$. It is generally assumed in imaging that $\theta(\vec{r})$ is constant over the excited region, but this is the case only if the rf field is perfectly uniform and perfect slice selection occurs. However, neither of these conditions exists in reality (see Fig. 16.1).

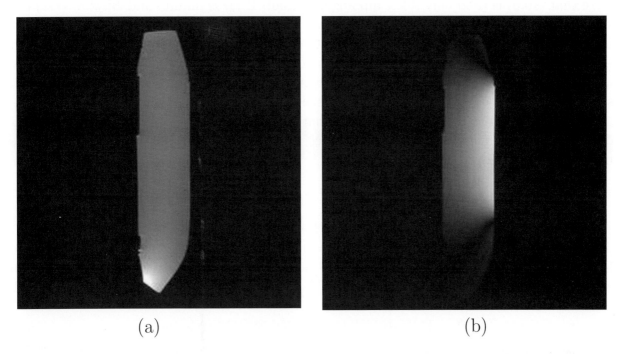

(a)   (b)

Fig. 16.1: A uniform spin density object is placed in two different coils. (a) The first image is acquired with a birdcage coil (see Ch. 27) used for both transmission of the rf pulse and reception of the signal. $B_{1,\perp}^{transmit}(\vec{r})$ produced by this birdcage coil is approximately uniform over the object, and a fairly uniform image results. (b) The same birdcage coil as in (a) was used to tip the spins, but a surface coil was used to receive the signal. The spatial dependence of $\mathcal{B}_{\perp}^{receive}$ leads to a change in intensity of the image as a function of position across the image.

Slice Selection and the Spatial Dependence of B_1

In the following example, the interaction between the spatial dependence of the transmit rf field and slice selection is considered. In a manner similar to frequency encoding of the spins, the rf and the slice select gradient work in tandem to excite spins as a function of frequency (or spatial position). In order to find exactly how the spins behave as a function of the applied rf pulse and slice select gradient, the Bloch equations must be solved (see Sec. 16.4).

In the presence of an applied gradient field, the Larmor frequency in the rotating reference frame is a function of position

$$f(\vec{r}, t) = \gamma \vec{G}(\vec{r}, t) \cdot \vec{r} \tag{16.4}$$

Assuming that this discussion is limited to selecting a transverse slice, only a frequency change along z should be imposed, giving

$$f(z, t) = \gamma G_z(t) z \tag{16.5}$$

The frequency content of a time-dependent rf pulse or the transverse magnetization is found by taking its inverse Fourier transform (see (16.28))

$$M_\perp(\vec{r}, z) = \gamma M_0 \left| \int_{-\tau_{rf}/2}^{\tau_{rf}/2} dt \, B_{1,+}^{transmit}(\vec{r}, t) e^{i2\pi f(z,t)t} \right| \tag{16.6}$$

Note that (16.6) is valid only if the flip angle is small. If τ_{rf} is infinite and $B_{1,+}^{transmit}(\vec{r},t)$ is a sinc pulse, then the transverse magnetization will be a boxcar function. Since the rf pulse is not infinite in time, but truncated, the selectively excited spins will not represent a perfect boxcar along the slice select direction. Further, if the B_0 field or slice select gradient varies as a function of position, the linear relation between z and f will be altered, causing excited slices to be 'distorted' by the field inhomogeneity (see Ch. 20).

The $(\vec{r}, z)$ argument is meant to denote that z-dependence arises from the spatial dependence of both the rf field and the slice select field gradient. Finally, an approximation is used to relate the B_1 field to θ from (3.37)

$$\theta(\vec{r}) = \gamma \int_{-\tau_{rf}/2}^{\tau_{rf}/2} B_{1,+}^{transmit}(\vec{r},t)dt \tag{16.7}$$

Thus, the amplitude of $B_{1,+}^{transmit}(\vec{r},t)$ at $t = 0$ is defined by $\theta(\vec{r})$. When the entire object is excited, i.e., $G_z = 0$, (16.3) and (16.7) show that $\hat{\rho}(\vec{r})$ is proportional to the sine of the integral of the time-dependent rf pulse. It is also proportional to the receive coil field, yielding

$$\hat{\rho}(\vec{r}) \propto M_\perp(\vec{r})\mathcal{B}_\perp^{receive}(\vec{r}) = M_0(\vec{r})\mathcal{B}_\perp^{receive}(\vec{r})\sin(\theta(\vec{r})) \tag{16.8}$$

Since $B_{1,+}^{transmit}(\vec{r})$ is not uniform over all space, there will be some variation of flip angle in the plane of the slice.

Problem 16.1

If the rf field is nonuniform across a slice, the resulting signal in the image will be modified because the excited transverse magnetization is modified.

Consider a typical non-slice select rf/gradient combination where a boxcar pulse is used. The following assumptions are made:

- The rf pulse with amplitude $B_{1,+}^{transmit}(\vec{r},0)$ is turned on from time $-\tau_{rf}/2$ to $\tau_{rf}/2$.

- A uniform sample is being imaged ($M_0(\vec{r}) = M_0$).

- The slice is bounded by z_1 and z_2 with $z_1 < z_2$, $\theta(z_1) = \pi/2$.

- $B_{1,+}^{transmit}(z,t)$ varies linearly in space such that $B_{1,+}^{transmit}(z_1,t) = 2B_{1,+}^{transmit}(z_2,t)$.

- $\mathcal{B}_\perp^{receive}(\vec{r})$ is constant over the region-of-interest.

Plot $\hat{\rho}(z)$ at a fixed (x,y) coordinate across the slice.

16.1.1   RF Pulse Shapes and Apodization

All rf pulses are modulated in time, since they are finite in their time duration, which implies they also have a modified frequency distribution. This situation can be modeled mathematically by multiplying the ideal field $B_{1,ideal}(t)$ by a rect function which effectively represents the act of time truncation

$$B_1(t) = B_{1,ideal}(t) \cdot \mathrm{rect}\left(\frac{t}{\tau_{rf}}\right) \tag{16.9}$$

The inverse Fourier transformation of $B_1(t)$ leads to a frequency response (spatial response for the slice selection process) which is the convolution of the ideal response with a sinc function

$$B_1(f) = B_{1,ideal}(f) * (\tau_{rf}\mathrm{sinc}\,(\pi f \tau_{rf})) \tag{16.10}$$

Strictly speaking, this inverse Fourier transform represents the low flip angle approximation from Sec. 16.4. As the duration of the rf pulse increases, the function $\tau_{rf}\mathrm{sinc}(\pi f \tau_{rf})$ approaches a δ-function (see Prob. 9.3), and $B_1(f)$ approaches $B_{1,ideal}(f)$ but truncation artifacts will still exist, i.e., Gibbs ringing will occur near sharp boundaries.

In practice, an additional apodizing function is used to bring $B_{1,ideal}(t)$ smoothly to zero and reduce truncation effects. Therefore, a more general expression for the time dependence of the field is

$$B_1(t) = B_{1,ideal}(t) \cdot a(t) \cdot \mathrm{rect}\left(\frac{t}{\tau_{rf}}\right) \tag{16.11}$$

where $a(t)$ is an apodizing function and the frequency response of the pulse becomes

$$B_1(f) = B_{1,ideal}(f) * A(f) * (\tau_{rf}\mathrm{sinc}\,(\pi f \tau_{rf})) \tag{16.12}$$

where $A(f)$ is the inverse Fourier transformation of $a(t)$. The convolution theorem can be used to investigate the actual frequency content of the pulse.

An example of the effects of truncation and apodization on an ideal field profile as a function of time and frequency is shown in Fig. 16.2. In Fig. 16.2a, a truncated sinc function is shown, and its associated flip angle profile, $\theta(z)$, is shown in Fig. 16.2b. Figure 16.2c shows the same sinc function after apodization with a Hanning filter (see Ch. 13). The excitation profile shown in Fig. 16.2d demonstrates the smoothing effect which apodization introduces. It is important to reduce the ripples extending past the slice of interest as they either contribute signal from outside the slice of interest for 2D imaging or alias into the images in 3D imaging (see Ch. 12). Filtering the time domain input limits the spatial extent of the excited spins and the excitation profile, but increases the FWHM (Full Width at Half Maximum) relative to the original profile width.

Hard and Soft Pulses

A terminology has developed differentiating between pulses that are spectrally selective and those that excite a large range of frequencies. Short duration, high amplitude pulses generally truncated with a rect function are referred to as 'hard' pulses, since they are approximately an impulse in the time domain. However, their short duration in the time domain leads to a broad excitation profile in the frequency domain. For this reason, hard pulses are also referred to as nonselective pulses. They are generally used for saturation in the absence of gradients, or for spectroscopy where the goal is to excite a large number of frequencies.

Pulses which are lower in amplitude and longer in duration may be used to select a narrow range of frequencies. Pulses which fit this description are often referred to as 'soft' pulses. The rf pulses employed during slice selection are examples of soft pulses.

$\theta_{x,y}$-Pulses

Often, the direction along which B_1 points in the rotating reference frame during the application of the rf pulse is assumed to be irrelevant. However, there are applications where the

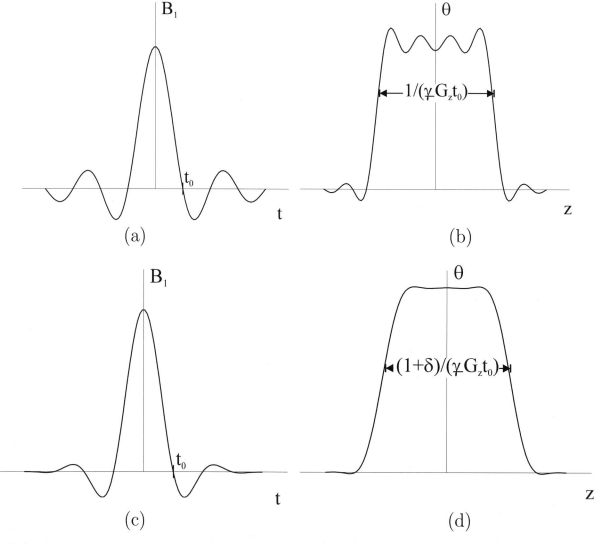

Fig. 16.2: (a) A sinc pulse truncated by a rect filter and (b) its corresponding low flip angle profile, which is contaminated by Gibbs ringing. (c) A smoothly truncated or apodized sinc function (a Hanning filter has been used), and its resulting θ response (d) is spatially smoother than that shown in (b). The differences between (b) and (d) demonstrate how smooth truncation of an rf pulse with an apodizing function can lead to a reduction of Gibbs ringing. The filtered profile is also broader than the original by the fraction δ as shown in (d).

relative phase of the applied B_1 field (i.e., the direction of the applied rf field) is important to the result. In these cases, a convention must be used to describe the axis along which B_1 is applied. The convention used in this text is to subscript the flip angle with the axis along which the pulse has been applied. Whenever θ_x or θ_y appears in a sequence diagram the reader should pay special attention to how the phase of the rf pulse affects the result. If θ is given by itself, it is usually safe to assume that the rf pulse may be applied along any axis.

16.2   Implementing Slice Selection

Slices are excited by applying an rf pulse in the presence of a gradient. However, instantaneously pulsed, square-gradient waveforms are not achievable in practice. In this section, symmetrical trapezoidal gradient waveforms are considered as models of realistic gradient profiles with nonzero ramp-up and ramp-down times. The sequence diagram for slice selection is shown in Fig. 16.3. It is assumed that all transverse magnetization is zero prior to the start of the rf excitation, but as a design measure, G_{ss} is frequently applied prior to starting the rf pulse to dephase any remnant transverse magnetization as well as to stabilize the gradient. The gradient area between t_0 and t_2 ($A+B$ in Fig. 16.3) is adjusted to dephase all spins across the selected slice centered at z_0 (cf. (10.25))

$$\int_{z_0-\frac{TH}{2}}^{z_0+\frac{TH}{2}} dz\, e^{i\phi(z)} = 0 \tag{16.13}$$

where TH is the slice thickness, and it is assumed that the spins in the slice all have the same initial phase. The phase $\phi(z)$ is accumulated by spins at position z during the time between t_0 and t_2, and is linear in z,

$$\phi(z) = -\gamma z \int_{t_0}^{t_2} dt\, G_{ss}(t) \tag{16.14}$$

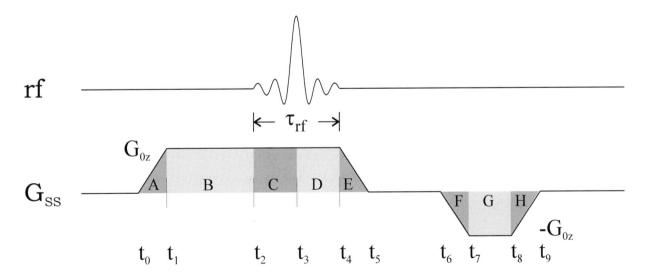

Fig. 16.3: Sequence diagram for the trapezoidal-gradient slice selection.

The dephasing constraint (16.13) will be satisfied if the difference $\phi(z_0+TH/2)-\phi(z_0-TH/2)$ is a nonzero integer multiple of 2π. The minimum area to accomplish this is thereby found to satisfy

$$\gamma(A+B)TH = 2\pi \tag{16.15}$$

(see Ch. 10). Typically, since G_{0z} is fixed by the slice selection process, (16.14) is used to compute $t_2 - t_0$ (see Prob. 16.2).

The rf pulse is assumed to be a truncated sinc pulse, and starts at $t = t_2$ and ends at $t = t_4$. After the rf pulse is turned off, the positive lobe is ramped down to zero and a negative lobe (also of trapezoidal shape) is applied to rephase the spins. For small flip angles, the cancelation of gradient area to rephase the spins requires

$$D + E = F + G + H \tag{16.16}$$

in terms of the areas in Fig. 16.3. This equation is based upon the assumption that all spins are tipped at the exact time center of the rf pulse, and dephase during the remainder of the slice select gradient pulse, which is accurate for the low flip angle approximation (see Sec. 16.4.1 for further details). For a $\pi/2$-pulse, the area $F + G + H$ will be somewhat larger than the area $D + E$ (see Sec. 16.4.2). If the rephasing lobe is symmetric and has the same magnitude (G_{0z}) for its plateau amplitude, (16.16) restricts the timings of Fig. 16.3 according to

$$(t_4 - t_3) + \frac{1}{2}(t_5 - t_4) = t_8 - t_6 \tag{16.17}$$

since $t_9 - t_8 = t_7 - t_6$. Note also that the rf pulse has been assumed to be symmetric about its center, which occurs at time t_3, so the gradient area from t_2 to t_3 is equal to the area between t_3 and t_4.

Problem 16.2

Given $t_0 = 0.0\,\text{ms}$, $t_1 = 0.6\,\text{ms}$, $TH = 2\,\text{mm}$, and $G_{0z} = 23.5\,\text{mT/m}$, find the minimum value of t_2 such that any remnant transverse magnetization is dephased, along the slice select direction, by satisfying (16.13).

Consider a specific imaging example with a low flip angle. Take $\tau_{rf} = t_4 - t_2 = 5.12$ ms and let $t_6 = t_5$ (the negative lobe immediately follows the positive lobe). Assume a slice thickness $TH = 2\,\text{mm}$, $G_{0z} = 23.5\,\text{mT/m}$, and a rise time of 0.6 ms. The bandwidth of the rf pulse is then

$$\begin{aligned} BW_{rf} &= \gamma \cdot TH \cdot G_{0z} \\ &= 2\,\text{kHz} \end{aligned} \tag{16.18}$$

The first zero crossing of the sinc pulse used to generate the slice profile in this case occurs at a time $t_{zc} = \frac{1}{BW_{rf}}$ from the center of the rf pulse, or 0.5 ms. This gives the number of zero crossings in τ_{rf} to be $n_{zc} = 10$ which is usually considered good enough for obtaining well-defined slice profiles, especially after apodizing the rf pulse.

Problem 16.3

Given the slice select parameters $G_{0z} = 23.5\,\text{mT/m}$, $TH = 2\,\text{mm}$, and $\tau_{rf} = 5.12\,\text{ms}$, answer the following questions.

a) If G_{0z} is reduced to $5\,\text{mT/m}$ and BW_{rf} to $390.63\,\text{Hz}$, what is the effect on the slice profile? Discuss the effect in terms of the time of occurrence of the first zero crossing of the sinc function and the number of zero crossings within the rf excitation time, τ_{rf}.

b) Assuming 10 zero crossings are desired in the rf pulse used in (a), what would be the duration of the pulse in (a) if TH remains at $2\,\text{mm}$ and G_{0z} at $5\,\text{mT/m}$? Is your τ_{rf} reasonable for a slice select rf pulse?

16.3 Calibrating the RF Field

When a body is loaded into the rf coil, the amplitude of the rf pulse must be varied until the flip angle reaches a specific value, usually chosen to be 90° or 180° (see Fig. 16.4). Ideally, the rf transmit and receive coils have uniform spatial response. By exciting the whole body and varying the amplitude of the rf pulse, the system can be calibrated as just described. For example, when the rf pulse creates an angle θ which goes through 90°, the transverse

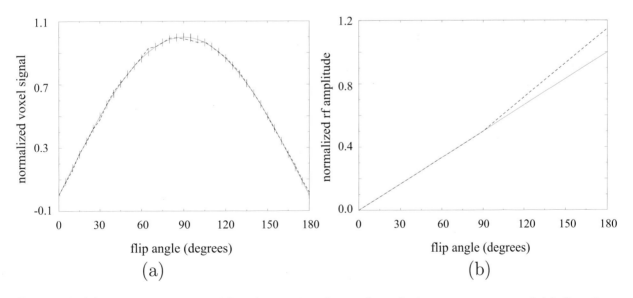

Fig. 16.4: (a) $M_\perp$ as a function of θ with associated error bars during measurement of this function. The dashed line in (a) represents the measurements, and the solid line represents the least-squares fit to the data. Error bars in the plot represent ± 2 noise standard deviations. (b) Plot of the ideal current increase (solid line) and the current amplitude (dashed line) required because of transmitter nonlinearities to generate the correct θ-pulse as a function of θ.

magnetization (and, hence, the measured signal) reaches a maximum; when θ goes through 180°, the transverse magnetization passes through zero (Fig. 16.4). For the signal maximum to occur at $\theta = 90°$ and the correct calibration to be done, the repeat time of the experiment must be large compared to the longitudinal relaxation times of the sample $T_R \gg T_1$ (see Ch. 18 for more details on the effects of non $\pi/2$-pulses when T_R is on the order of, or less than, T_1).

An initial approach to calibrate the rf amplitude might be to find the maximum of the signal and associate this with a 90°-pulse. The problem with this approach is choosing a maximum value for the transverse magnetization ($M_\perp$) in the presence of noise. Fitting $M_\perp(\theta)$ to $\sin \theta$ also helps to reduce the errors due to noise. It is much easier to find the signal zero near 180° where the slope of $M_\perp(\theta)$ is the largest (see Fig. 16.4). The value for B_1 is then chosen for a given θ relative to this value. Actually, since the rf transmitter has a nonlinear response, a calibration curve must be made to obtain accurate values of θ as a function of the input power to the system.

For transmit coils which are inhomogeneous, the choice of which current amplitude or B_1 amplitude applied by the system gives a zero signal will change as the object size and spin density change. For example, if $B_{1,+}^{transmit}$ is homogeneous only over roughly the central half of its volume, then for a small object in the center of the coil, B_1 associated with the 180°-pulse (referred to as $B_{1,180}$) will be correct everywhere. If the object is large compared to the uniform region of the coil, then $B_1 = B_{1,180}$ will not necessarily generate a zero signal. This is due to the fact that for spins not at the coil center, B_1 at those positions will create an angle greater than (or less than) 180° even when B_1 at the center equals $B_{1,180}$. Since the pick-up coil receives an integrated signal, it will take a field at the center smaller than (or greater than) $B_{1,180}$ to generate a 180°-pulse in the outer regions of the phantom. The measured value of 180° will occur when the volume integral of the transverse magnetization is zero.

16.3.1   Checking the RF Profile

It is also necessary to calibrate or measure the effective slice created by the rf transmit pulse, slice select gradient, and rephasing gradient. The slice profile should be calibrated to quote the correct slice thickness and to ensure maximum rephasing. Also, when using fast imaging methods in 2D (see Sec. 18.1.5), the shape of the profile can profoundly affect the results. As discussed earlier, there are many reasons why the rf profile does not match the desired result of a perfect boxcar profile. Fortunately, the rf slice select profile can be measured by an experiment where the read direction is placed along the slice select axis.

A read gradient G_{1z} along the slice select direction can be placed as shown in the region 2B in Fig. 16.5 to generate an echo. Notice that the rephasing lobe may be incorporated into the echo generating gradients (Fig. 16.6). From the Nyquist theorem, the resolution of the slice profile is

$$\Delta ss = \frac{1}{\gamma G_{1z} T_s} \tag{16.19}$$

where T_s is the sampling time. Since G_{1z} can be made large and T_s long, it is possible to acquire many points through the slice. Recall the convention that TH describes the thickness of the excited slice, and $TH = N_{ss}\Delta ss$ where N_{ss} is the number of collected sampling points.

This approach can be used for a single acquisition which then projects the slice profile over all (x, y), it can be run with phase encoding along y at which point the signal is projected only over x, or it can be collected in a 3D mode with phase encoding along both x and y.

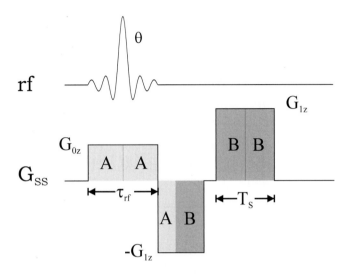

Fig. 16.5: A sequence design for measuring the rf profile along the slice select direction. The slice select gradient G_{0z} is followed by a rephasing gradient $-G_{1z}$. After an echo is formed, this gradient is kept constant and used to dephase the spins after which the spins are rephased again by switching the polarity as shown in the figure. Another echo is formed during the sampling.

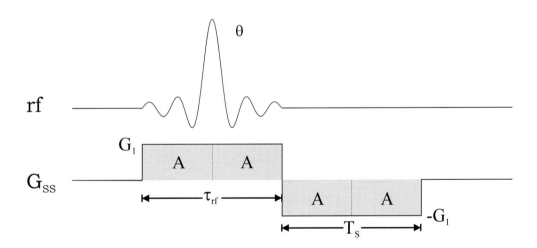

Fig. 16.6: An alternate sequence design for measuring the slice select rf profile.

Problem 16.4

Assume that it is desirable in some situations to measure the rf slice select profile by doubling the time duration of the rephase gradient lobe as shown in Fig. 16.6.

    a) In Fig. 16.5, with the relation between rf bandwidth and slice thickness given in (16.18), find N_{ss} as a function of G_{0z}, G_{1z}, τ_{rf}, T_s, and number of zero crossings n_{zc} used in the rf sinc pulse.

    b) Relate Δss to the slice thickness, and the number of zero crossings in the rf pulse, assuming that a sinc pulse is used to excite the rectangular slice.

    c) Given that an average rf pulse is 3 ms in duration, and a slice thickness of 6.26 mm may be excited with $G_1 = 5$ mT/m, find the number of zero crossings in the rf pulse, and determine Δss. Does this resolution appear to be adequate relative to the slice thickness?

Defining Slice Thickness

The term slice thickness is used to define the thickness of the region along the slice select direction which contributes signal to an MR image. (In 3D imaging, it describes the thickness of a given partition.) Due to the finite time duration of the applied rf pulses, it is not possible to achieve a perfectly rectangular slice excitation, instead the region of spins affected by the rf pulse goes smoothly to zero at the edges of the profile (see Fig. 16.7). As a result, it is necessary to define some criterion for quoting the slice thickness based upon the region where appreciable signal is contributed to the image. In general, the FWHM (Full Width at Half Maximum) of the measured slice select profile is used to define slice thickness as shown in Fig. 16.7. Similar to the use of the FWHM in defining resolution, it is necessary to keep in mind that this definition is somewhat arbitrary. For a slice whose profile approaches the ideal rectangular case, this definition is reasonable since very little transverse magnetization is created beyond the FWHM (see Fig. 16.7) and, therefore, the definition is accurate. If, instead, a Gaussian excitation is chosen, then there may be an appreciable amount of signal created outside of the FWHM of the image profile and, in this case, the FWTM (Full Width at Tenth Maximum) might be a better choice for slice thickness. It is important to remember that the thickness of the image profile is being discussed here. The FWHM of the applied rf pulse does not necessarily match the FWHM of the slice measured in the image (see Secs. 16.1 and 18.1.5). It is the image slice profile that is of interest. Consider two cases where this might be important, 3D imaging and 2D multi-slice imaging. If the z-direction field-of-view is chosen to be TH in a 3D experiment, then there may be a significant amount of aliasing in the image from the spins excited between $TH/2$ and $TH'/2$ (see Sec. 12.3.3). In a 2D multi-slice experiment, if an adjacent slice is imaged right after the scan of the present slice, then there will be 'crosstalk' between slices. Crosstalk refers to the situation where the excitation of one slice significantly affects the signal from a neighboring slice. To avoid excessive crosstalk in 2D multi-slice imaging, the distance between slice centers should be set to TH' outside of which there is essentially no slice excitation.

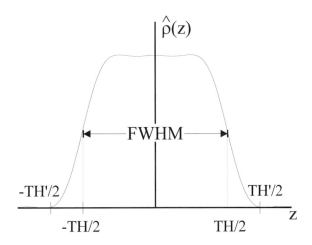

Fig. 16.7: Illustration of the FWHM of a theoretical slice profile generated from an apodized sinc pulse. Although $TH = \text{FWHM}$ is often chosen as the effective slice thickness, clearly information from outside this region is excited as well. Usually, excitation is well-behaved and no further excitation takes place outside the boundaries demarcated by $\pm TH'/2$.

16.4 Solutions of the Bloch Equations

The magnetization was analyzed in the rotating reference frame on-resonance for all spins in Ch. 3. In order to excite a slice, a slice select gradient $\vec{G}$ has to be turned on when the rf field is on. The slice select gradient leads to a fixed range of frequencies being excited that creates a slice whose normal $\vec{r}$ is parallel to $\vec{G}$. All spins inside the desired slice are then tipped from the z-axis by the rf pulse. The equation of motion in the presence of slice select gradients and an rf field over times small compared to the relaxation times is

$$\frac{d\vec{M}}{dt} = \gamma \vec{M} \times \left(\vec{B}_1 + (\vec{G} \cdot \vec{r})\hat{z} \right) \tag{16.20}$$

If the components of the rf field lie in the x-y plane, i.e., $\vec{B}_1 = (B_{1x}, B_{1y}, 0)$, (16.20) can be rewritten as

$$\begin{pmatrix} dM_x/dt \\ dM_y/dt \\ dM_z/dt \end{pmatrix} = \gamma \begin{pmatrix} 0 & \vec{G} \cdot \vec{r} & -B_{1y} \\ -\vec{G} \cdot \vec{r} & 0 & B_{1x} \\ B_{1y} & -B_{1x} & 0 \end{pmatrix} \begin{pmatrix} M_x \\ M_y \\ M_z \end{pmatrix} \tag{16.21}$$

The behavior of a set of spins from these equations can be simulated. Figure 16.8 demonstrates the behavior of the transverse magnetization as a function of time during the rf pulse for spins on-resonance and off-resonance. The solid line in Fig. 16.8 shows $M_\perp(t)$ during an applied sinc pulse for on-resonance spins. When on-resonance, the $\vec{G} \cdot \vec{r}$ term vanishes in the Bloch equation and the solution of $M_\perp$ is the simplified form given in Ch. 3. The dashed line in Fig. 16.8 shows $M_\perp(t)$ during the same pulse for off-resonance spins near the edge of the slice (where the resonance offset is chosen as $\Delta f = BW_{rf}/2$ in which BW_{rf} is the rf excitation bandwidth). Another off-resonance condition with $\Delta f = BW_{rf}$ is also shown for comparison. Recall that the bandwidth is related to the slice select gradient G_{ss} through

$\vec{G} \cdot \vec{r} = G_{ss}TH = BW_{rf}/\gamma$ where TH is the slice thickness. Thus, the desired slice thickness TH is defined by the rf bandwidth and slice select gradients.

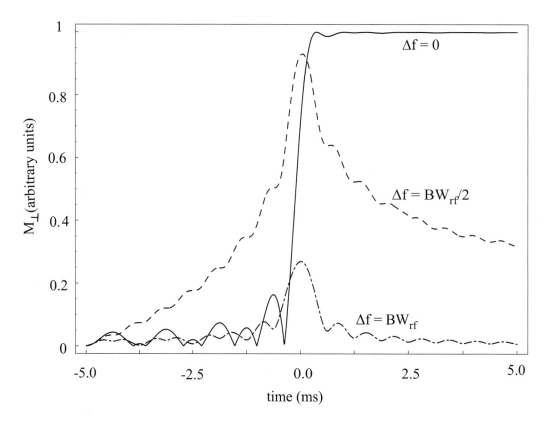

Fig. 16.8: $M_\perp(t)$ during an applied rf sinc pulse for on-resonance and off-resonance spins. When the spins are on-resonance and off-resonance, this figure simulates the transverse signal only from the center of a slice, i.e., $z = 0$. The rf pulse has a total of 16 zero crossings and a bandwidth BW_{rf} of 1.6 kHz in the simulation. Here, Δf is the frequency offset in Hz. The frequency offsets can be translated to the locations of spins. See the Block equation (16.20). For example, when the frequency offset is by one rf bandwidth, spins are actually one slice thickness from the center (which lies outside the excited slice). It is critical for a proper 2D excitation that no spins should be excited at that location at the end of the duration of the rf pulse.

16.4.1   Low Flip Angle Excitation and Rephasing Gradients

A more versatile solution to the behavior of the magnetization in the presence of an applied rf field and gradients can be obtained for the case of low flip angle rf pulses. As a demonstration of the utility of this method, it is used to demonstrate spins dephasing across a slice during slice selection and to show that the area under the rephase pulse must be equal to half of the area under the gradient while the rf field is on. An analysis of the Bloch equations for small tip angles lends insight into the refocusing problem and how oscillating gradients may be used to excite localized regions in 3D.

If only small tip angles are considered such that $\cos\theta \simeq 1$ and $M_z \simeq M_0$, then the transverse and longitudinal equations can be decoupled using arguments similar to those presented in Ch. 4. The resulting equations for M_x and M_y can be combined by choosing

$$M_+ \equiv M_x + iM_y \tag{16.22}$$

and

$$B_{1+} \equiv B_{1x} + iB_{1y} \tag{16.23}$$

then the equation of motion reduces to

$$dM_+/dt = -i\gamma(\vec{G} \cdot \vec{r})M_+ + i\gamma B_{1+}M_0 \tag{16.24}$$

where the explicit spatial dependence of $\vec{G}$ and B_{1+} are left as understood and M_z has been replaced by M_0 in (16.24).

Dephasing and Rephasing across a Slice at Low Flip Angles

A general solution can be used to illustrate the dephasing of the spins across the slice. Assume initial conditions of $M_x(-\tau_{rf}/2) = M_y(-\tau_{rf}/2) = 0, M_z(-\tau_{rf}/2) = M_0$, and that $B_{1+}(t)$ is nonzero over the interval $(-\tau_{rf}/2, \tau_{rf}/2)$. Using, for example, the integrating factor technique, the solution of (16.24) at the end of the rf pulse, $t = \tau_{rf}/2$, is

$$M_+(\vec{r}, \tau_{rf}/2) = i\gamma M_0 \int_{-\tau_{rf}/2}^{\tau_{rf}/2} dt\, B_{1+}(t)e^{-i2\pi\vec{k}(t)\cdot\vec{r}} \tag{16.25}$$

where

$$\vec{k}(t) = \gamma \int_t^{\tau_{rf}/2} ds\, \vec{G}(s) \tag{16.26}$$

For $\vec{G}(s) = \vec{G}$, a constant,

$$\vec{k}(t) = \gamma(\tau_{rf}/2 - t)\vec{G} \tag{16.27}$$

and

$$\begin{aligned} M_+(\vec{r}, \tau_{rf}/2) &= i\gamma M_0 e^{-i\gamma\vec{G}\cdot\vec{r}\tau_{rf}/2} \int_{-\tau_{rf}/2}^{\tau_{rf}/2} dt\, B_{1+}(t)e^{i\gamma\vec{G}\cdot\vec{r}t} \\ &= i\gamma M_0 e^{-i\gamma\vec{G}\cdot\vec{r}\tau_{rf}/2} \mathcal{F}^{-1}\left(B_{1+}(t)\right) \end{aligned} \tag{16.28}$$

where $B_{1+}(t)$ is taken to be zero outside the rf window.

If B_{1x} or B_{1y} is a real and symmetric function, its inverse Fourier transform is also real and symmetric. Therefore, the explicit phase term $e^{-i\gamma\vec{G}\cdot\vec{r}\tau_{rf}/2}$ in (16.28) represents the dephasing across the slice during slice selection. This indicates a need for a 'rephasing gradient' of amplitude G_{rp} after the rf pulse so that the phase it generates cancels the phase term $-\gamma\vec{G} \cdot \vec{r}\tau_{rf}/2 = -\gamma G_{0,z}z\tau_{rf}/2$ in the above equation. Referring to Fig. 16.9, the phase ϕ_{rp} generated at the end of the rephase gradient lobe of amplitude G_{rp} must be

$$\phi_{rp} = \gamma G_{rp}\hat{z} \cdot \vec{r}\tau_{rp} = \gamma G_{rp}z\tau_{rp} \tag{16.29}$$

such that ϕ_{rp} cancels the phase for all $\vec{r}$ in (16.28) and G_{rp} satisfies the equation

$$G_{rp}\tau_{rp} = G_{0,z}\tau_{rf}/2 \tag{16.30}$$

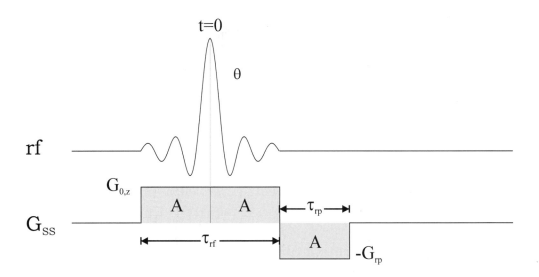

Fig. 16.9: The rf pulse and slice select gradient waveforms (assumed to be along $\hat{z}$). Refocusing occurs thanks to the effect of the negative lobe with amplitude G_{rp}.

i.e., a 50% refocusing pulse should work. If the area $G_{rp}\tau_{rp}$ satisfies (16.30), it brings all spins back into phase along the slice select direction, and shows if $G_{rp} = G_{0,z}$ then $\tau_{rp} = \tau_{rf}/2$ will lead to refocusing. This discussion expands upon the earlier discussion in Ch. 10 where the simple example of an instantaneous rf pulse at $t = 0$ was used to demonstrate that the spins saw only $G_{0,z}$ for $\tau_{rf}/2$. In that case, G_{rp} was required to refocus exactly one-half of the area under $G_{0,z}$. Intuitively, the factor of one-half makes sense if one views the rf pulse as instantaneously exciting the spins at $t = 0$.

16.4.2   Dephasing and Rephasing at Large Flip Angles

The arguments presented in the above subsection only hold true in the low flip angle regime. To find out what happens for larger flip angles, the Bloch equations must be solved numerically. In the examples to follow, a numerical method has been used to solve the Bloch equations during a slice select pulse at several flip angles. It is assumed that $B_{1,+}^{transmit}$ is spatially homogeneous for these simulations and applied along the x-axis in the rotating frame. The solutions obtained also include the effects of dephasing, which occur while the slice select gradient is applied, and rephasing must be performed after the rf pulse is turned off to get an accurate description of the magnetization as it appears just prior to frequency encoding.

Figure 16.10 shows the magnetization as a function of z for a low flip angle pulse which has been rephased with a gradient area equal to half of the slice select lobe. This result shows that the low flip angle approximation is accurate, since the 50% refocusing has eliminated any dephasing (M_x is zero), and the only remnant errors in the profile are due to truncation of the rf pulse. Figure 16.11 shows a $\pi/2$-pulse excitation profile, after refocusing with areas of 50% and 52%, respectively. The presence of a nonzero M_x component introduces a z-dependent phase behavior, if the slice select gradient is along the z-direction. The choice of 50.6% refocusing minimizes the M_x profile. The need for a non 50% refocusing pulse is indicative of the nonlinearities of the Bloch equations. Note that in the simulations, a total of 16 zero crossings of a truncated rf sinc function were used (i.e., $B_1\text{sinc}(\pi t/t_{zc})$, where t is between $-8t_{zc}$ and $8t_{zc}$). In addition, the amplitude of the rf pulse, B_1, was calculated based on the given flip angle and the duration of the rf pulse. If a different value of zero crossings is used, then the refocusing gradient area may be slightly changed in order to minimize the M_x profile.

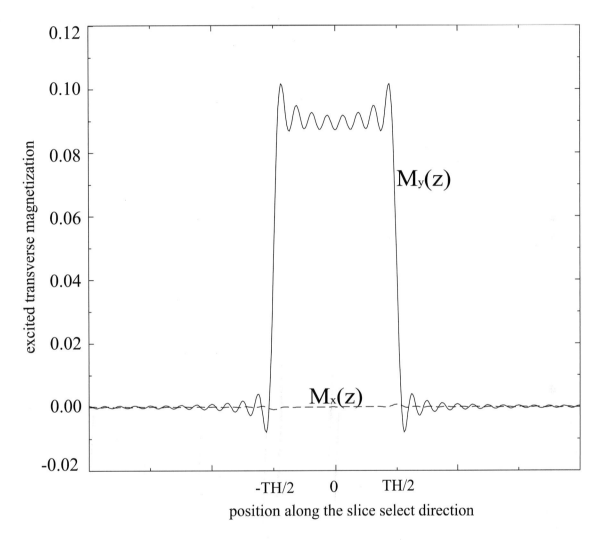

Fig. 16.10: $M_x(z)$ (dashed line) and $M_y(z)$ (solid line) are shown for a 5° sinc pulse, as found by numerically solving the Bloch equations. This result validates the low flip angle approximation that a 50% slice select refocusing gradient should give a maximal response for $M_y(z)$, with a negligible contribution from $M_x(z)$.

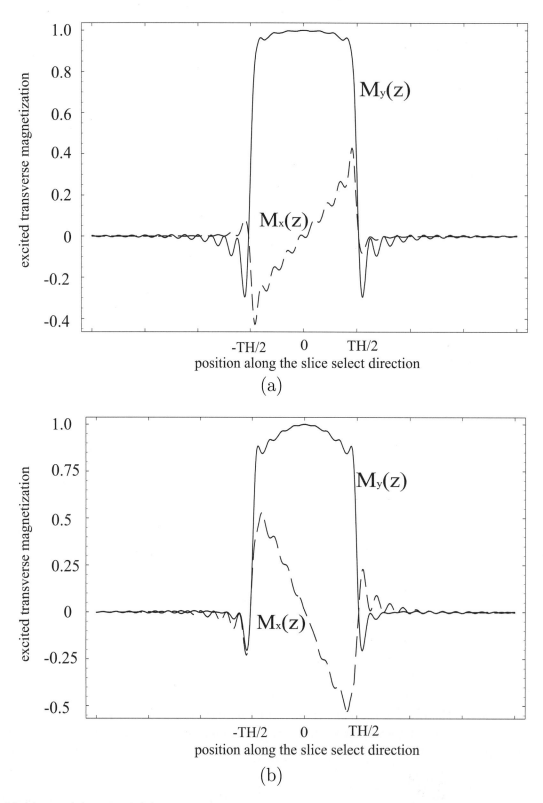

Fig. 16.11: $M_x(z)$ and $M_y(z)$ are shown for a 90° sinc pulse, as found by numerically solving the Bloch equations. The area of the refocusing gradient pulse used in (a) is 50% and in (b) is 52%. The $M_x(z)$ component can be minimized if the refocusing is chosen to be roughly 50.6%.

Problem 16.5

As described in the text, a sinc rf pulse with a total of 16 zero cross sections has been used in several simulations of the Bloch equation. For simplicity, let us consider $\vec{G} \cdot \vec{r} = G_z z$, $B_{1x}(t) = B_1 \text{sinc}(\pi t/t_{zc})$, and $B_{1y} = 0$ in the Bloch equation, where G_z is a constant gradient. The rf pulse is turned on from $-8t_{zc}$ to $8t_{zc}$. When the flip angle θ is given, the amplitude B_1 can be calculated from (3.37):

$$\theta = \gamma \int_{-8t_{zc}}^{8t_{zc}} dt \, B_{1x}(t) \tag{16.31}$$

In addition, the rf bandwidth $1/t_{zc} = BW_{rf} = \gamma G_z TH$ where TH is the desired slice thickness. Now the new dimensionless variables z/TH and t/t_{zc} can be introduced and the Bloch equations can be solved without knowing TH and t_{zc}.

a) Take $\theta = 90°$ and solve the Bloch equation numerically with an initial condition of $M_x(-8t_{zc}) = 0$, $M_y(-8t_{zc}) = 0$, and $M_z(-8t_{zc}) = 1$. With a refocusing gradient area 50.6% of the area under G_z, confirm the results shown in Fig. 16.11.

b) With conditions given in (a), consider the transverse magnetization contributed from one slice (between $-TH/2$ and $TH/2$). Plot the transverse magnetization as a function of time from $-8t_{zc}$ until the end of the rephrasing gradient lobe. Discuss the value of transverse magnetization at $t = 0$. In addition, how can the shape of the curve in the plot be explained from (16.25) or (16.28)? Hint: The M_x and M_y components have to be summed individually within the slice. The inverse Fourier transformation in (16.28) does not depend on spatial parameters.

c) Repeat (a) but let $\theta = 180°$ with no refocusing gradient. Are spins properly inverted at the end of the rf pulse? Is the response of the rf pulse zero outside TH?

d) Analytically solve the Bloch equation with $B_{1x} = B_{1x}(t)$, $B_{1y} = 0$, and $\vec{G} \cdot \vec{r} = 0$. When $\theta = 180°$, are spins properly inverted at the end of the rf pulse?

e) What conclusion can be reached from (c) and (d), if a π-pulse is being applied during a constant gradient but no refocusing gradient is required?

16.5   Spatially Varying RF Excitation

From the previous section, one can excite a limited region of space in 3D. The mathematical details of these excitations, however, can be somewhat laborious. Therefore, an example of how conventional slice select pulses may be used to excite a rectangular region of space is introduced first. Also, as a further introduction to the concepts of slice profile excitations, the 1D example used for selecting a slice will be reintroduced. The notion of varying the time dependence of the gradients while the B_1 field is being applied is considered. Finally, an example of a 2D excitation will be given, where B_1 and two gradients are applied in a time dependent fashion to achieve the cylindrical spatial excitation profile. The reader is reminded that, although usually a gradient along one of the Cartesian axes is used for defining the slice select direction, in general multiple gradients can be applied to generate oblique slices as discussed in Ch. 10.

16.5.1   Two-Dimensional 'Beam' Excitation

It is possible to excite a 'beam' of spins spatially with a spin echo, instead of a slice. This is useful to avoid aliasing when a small FOV in a large object is desired. A sequence diagram for implementing a 'beam' excitation is shown in Fig. 16.12. The first rf pulse and slice select gradient excite a slice in the conventional manner. During the π-pulse, a gradient lobe is placed perpendicular to the original slice select axis. Therefore, the π-pulse rotates spins in a slice perpendicular to the original slice. Only the rectangular set of spins which have experienced both pulses, as shown in Fig. 16.12b, will form a spin echo. The gradients and bandwidths associated with the $\pi/2$- and π-pulses determine the corresponding slice thickness in each direction for the phase encoding or partition encoding steps (see Fig. 16.12). The thickness of the beam will be chosen according to the size of the object being imaged; the thickness usually being greater than the dimension of the object in that direction.

In general, the slice select gradient associated with the π-pulse is placed along the phase encoding direction to reduce the number of phase encoding steps and thus the total imaging time for 2D imaging ($T_T = L_y T_R / \Delta y$) while maintaining or improving resolution. The positioning and shape of the read gradient lobes are also important when employing this method. The slice selective π-pulse acts on all spins in the x-z plane. Although the π-pulse may be very well designed (i.e, creates a sharp magnetization profile), there will always be some spins that undergo only a $\pi/2$-rotation. They can contribute in a detrimental way to the MRI signal. In order to minimize their effect on the image, additional gradients are added to the dephase and rephase gradient lobes (shown as shaded areas in Fig. 16.12). The gradient echo still occurs at T_E where the gradient areas are balanced, but the additional area before data collection dephases spins tipped from the z-axis into the transverse plane by the π-pulse. The additional gradient should be chosen to sufficiently dephase this magnetization before data are collected in a manner similar to that described in Sec. 16.2 for eliminating unwanted magnetization prior to slice selection. The difference is that, in this case, the goal is to ensure that the unwanted magnetization is dephased across a pixel width along the read direction at the echo, and not along the slice select direction.

Other configurations of the gradients are possible as long as they take into account the spins excited by the π-pulse and minimize their effect on the image. For example, one can utilize a similar method to excite a voxel in MR spectroscopy. This approach is even more valuable when 3D imaging must be done, but a limited field-of-view is desired.

Problem 16.6

Draw a sequence diagram designed to excite a cubical volume within a larger physical body by adding an additional π-pulse and gradient to Fig. 16.12.

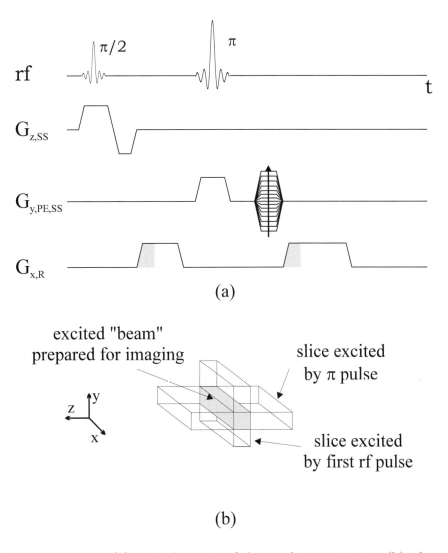

Fig. 16.12: Sequence diagram (a) and schematic of the resulting excitation (b) when a rectangular beam of spins is excited. The number of phase encoding lines needed for the same resolution can be reduced by exciting smaller fields-of-view in two directions. This is achieved for a spin echo sequence, for example, by exciting a plane in one direction during the $\pi/2$-pulse and by exciting a plane perpendicular to the first plane during the π-pulse. In this example, slice selection takes place along z for the $\pi/2$-pulse and along y for the π-pulse. The dephasing and rephasing portions of the read gradient are usually lengthened (see shaded area along $G_{x,R}$) to allow 'crushing' or dephasing of any transverse magnetization which may be created by the π-pulse.

Problem 16.7

In certain applications, imaging of flow, for example (see Sec. 24.2), it is useful to have a slice excitation profile that increases linearly in the direction perpendicular to the plane of the slice (a ramp profile). Using the low flip angle approximation, the slice profile can be determined by two flip angles. The specific utility of this pulse will be described in Ch. 24. Consider the following representation of the variable spatial excitation desired for the refocused $M_+(\vec{r}, \infty)$

$$|M_+(\vec{r}, \infty)/M_0| = \theta_0 \operatorname{rect}\left(\frac{z}{TH}\right) + \theta_1 \cdot z \cdot \frac{1}{TH} \cdot \operatorname{rect}\left(\frac{z}{TH}\right) \qquad (16.32)$$

where θ_0 is the final desired flip angle at the center of the excited region and $\theta_0 \pm \theta_1/2$ are the desired flip angles at the edges of the slice. Show that the Fourier transform of this profile (see (16.28)) leads to the input rf field as a function of time given by

$$B_{1+}(t) = \frac{G_{ss}TH}{2\pi}\left[\theta_0 \cdot \operatorname{sinc}\phi_0 + i\frac{\theta_1}{2\phi_0}(\cos\phi_0 - \operatorname{sinc}\phi_0)\right]$$

$$\text{where} \quad \phi_0 = \pi \cdot TH \cdot \gamma G_{ss}t \qquad (16.33)$$

This input rf and ideal spatial response are shown in Fig. 16.13. It is seen from (16.33) that phase and amplitude control of the rf is necessary to generate a linearly varying slice profile.

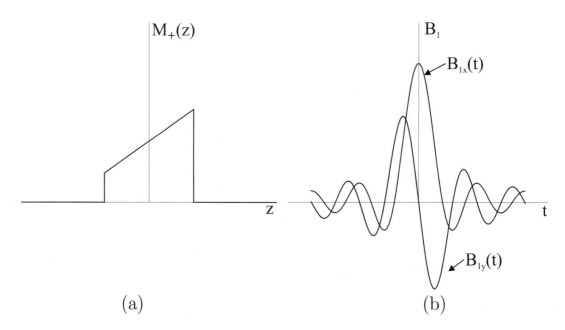

(a)   (b)

Fig. 16.13: (a) $M_+(z)$ for a linearly varying rf pulse slice select experiment. (b) $B_{1x}(t)$ and $B_{1y}(t)$ which produce the slice select profile in (a).

Problem 16.8

Due to the nonlinearities of the Bloch equations, any practical π-pulse also creates a finite amount of transverse magnetization. For phase encoding prior to the π-pulse, this unwanted transverse component always leaks into the sampling window with the same intensity. What is the effect on a conventional 2D spin echo sequence of this extraneous signal? This artifact is often called the 'zipper artifact.' Hint: Recall that the Fourier transform of a constant function is a δ-function.

16.5.2 Time Varying Gradients and Slice Selection

It can be seen from the previous arguments that the spatial region of excitation will be altered if the applied gradient varies during the slice select process. Low flip angle imaging is of particular interest in fast imaging applications (see Ch. 18) and, in this case, reducing the slice select time is often desirable. In these cases, it would be optimal to design the rf and gradient pulse so that the rf is on throughout the application of the gradient, including ramp times for example. Alternately, with extremely powerful gradients, a trapezoidal gradient may be exchanged for a triangular waveform. Therefore, it is desirable to understand how to deal with a time-varying gradient pulse.

Before embarking on a theoretical description, a simple conceptual explanation of the problem is useful. Varying the time dependence of the gradients will not change the fact that $M_+(\vec{r})$ is proportional to the Fourier transform of $B_{1+}(t)$ for a low flip angle approximation. However, when the slice select gradient $G(t)$ is a constant, $B_{1+}(t)dt$ and $B_{1+}(k)dk$ can be related by a simple change of variables since $dk/dt = -\gamma G$ from (16.26). When $G(t)$ varies as a function of time, relating $B_{1+}(t)dt$ to $B_{1+}(k)dk$ is not as easy, although the basic concept is identical. The key is that the quantity of interest is the amount of B_{1+} deposited in a given region of k-space per unit time given by $B_{1+}(k(t))/|dk(t)/dt|$ whether the gradients are time-dependent or not. This quantity, generally referred to as the 'B_1 weighting of k-space,' gives a representation of $B_{1+}(t)$ in k-space. (Note that the k-space here is similar to the 1D k-space described in Ch. 9.)

The following arguments will be restricted to 1D since the interest is in selecting a slice. Consider the general solution for the magnetization in 1D as a generalization of (16.25)

$$M_+(z, \tau_{rf}/2) = i\gamma M_0 \int_{-\tau_{rf}/2}^{\tau_{rf}/2} dt\, B_{1+}(t)e^{-i2\pi k(t)z} \tag{16.34}$$

and $dk(t)/dt$ is not a constant in this case because the applied gradient will vary as a function of time. Using the appropriate Jacobian, this expression can be rewritten in terms of $k(t)$ to recapture the Fourier transform relationship between the spatial excitation and the input $B_{1+}(t)$

$$\begin{aligned} M_+(z, \tau_{rf}/2) &= i\gamma M_0 \int_{-\tau_{rf}/2}^{\tau_{rf}/2} dt\, B_{1+}(t)e^{-i2\pi k(t)z} \\ &= i\gamma M_0 \int_{k(-\tau_{rf}/2)}^{k(\tau_{rf}/2)} dk\, w(k)e^{-i2\pi kz} \end{aligned} \tag{16.35}$$

where

$$w(k(t)) = \frac{B_{1+}(k(t))}{|\gamma G(k(t))|} \tag{16.36}$$

The slice select profile is now the Fourier transform of this quantity which is, as discussed earlier, the B_1 weighting of k-space. As long as $w(k(t))$ is not a multiple valued function, evaluation of (16.35) should be fairly straightforward. This corresponds to using a single positive or negative lobe for slice selection. Problem 16.9 gives an example of how this formalism can be used, and should further clarify why it is a useful tool for slice selection.

Problem 16.9

Assume that in order to minimize eddy currents, and maximize the switching speed of the gradient, a cosine shape might be chosen for the slice select gradient lobe

$$G_{ss}(t) = \begin{cases} G_0 \cos\left(\frac{\pi t}{\tau_{rf}}\right) & -\frac{\tau_{rf}}{2} < t < \frac{\tau_{rf}}{2} \\ 0 & \text{all other times} \end{cases} \tag{16.37}$$

Assume that a Gaussian slice select profile is desired, i.e.,

$$M_+(z) \propto e^{-\alpha_1 z^2} \tag{16.38}$$

Show that the $B_{1+}(t)$ which generates this $M_+(z)$ is

$$B_{1+}(t) \propto \cos\left(\pi t/\tau_{rf}\right) e^{-\left(\gamma G_0 \tau_{rf}(\sin(\pi t/\tau_{rf})-1)\right)^2/\alpha_1} \tag{16.39}$$

Hint: Take the limits in (16.35) to be $-\infty$ to ∞.

16.5.3   An Example of Spatially Selective Excitations in the Low Flip Angle Limit

The previous subsections described how time dependent gradients and rf pulses can be used to obtain different spatial excitation profiles in 1D. Applying all three gradients, certain volume excitation profiles may be obtained.

An example has already appeared in this chapter. Figure 16.12 demonstrates how the combination of a $\pi/2$ and a π-pulse can be used to excite a rectangular region. In fact, this set of pulses has built into it a variable $B_{1+}(t)$ and slice select gradient $\vec{G}(t)$ and helps the reader get a flavor of how rf and $\vec{G}(t)$ can be varied to achieve a specific spatial excitation. If the times separating the pulses and gradients shown in Fig. 16.12 can be reduced to zero, a single composite pulse of gradients and rf designed to excite a volume emerges. Using this example as motivation, the low flip angle solution (16.25) may be developed for selectively exciting 3D volumes.

As mentioned, if $\vec{G}(t)$ is not a constant while the rf is applied, then the convenient Fourier transform relationship between the excited region, and $B_{1+}(t)$ is lost. However, after some analysis, a Fourier transform relationship can be found between the B_1 weighting of k-space as determined by the gradient waveforms and the spatially excited magnetization. The key difference between the slice select case, and the 2D and 3D cases, is that higher dimensional spaces cannot be covered completely, and a path through k-space must be defined. The path must cover a sufficient region of k-space with an adequate density. For example, the k-space can be covered by a spiral coverage with a given desired slice profile in 2D or 3D, such as a Gaussian.

Consider an infinitely long cylinder with a Gaussian profile as the desired excitation,

$$M_+(\vec{r}) \propto e^{-\alpha^2 \rho^2} \tag{16.40}$$

where α is a constant and $\rho \equiv \sqrt{x^2 + y^2}$. Assume that the durations of the rf pulse and slice select gradients are T, then (16.25) can be written as

$$M_+(\vec{r}) = i\gamma M_0 \int_0^T dt \, B_{1+}(t) e^{-i2\pi \vec{k}(t)\cdot\vec{r}} \tag{16.41}$$

If $\vec{k}(t) \cdot \vec{r}$ can somehow be written as a function of ρ, then (16.41) can be simplified as a 1D problem. Although it is obviously impossible to achieve this condition, alternatively, one could allow $\vec{k}(t) \cdot \vec{r}$ to be proportional to ρ in combination with a weak spatial dependence. To accomplish this goal, let us choose

$$
\begin{aligned}
k_x(t) &= A\left(1 - \frac{t}{T}\right)\cos\frac{2n\pi t}{T} \\
k_y(t) &= A\left(1 - \frac{t}{T}\right)\sin\frac{2n\pi t}{T} \\
k_z(t) &= 0
\end{aligned}
\tag{16.42}
$$

such that

$$\vec{k}(t) \cdot \vec{r} = A\left(1 - \frac{t}{T}\right)\rho\cos\left(\frac{2n\pi t}{T} - \phi\right) \tag{16.43}$$

where A is a constant, n is an integer, and ϕ is the azimuthal angle in the cylindrical coordinate system. Note that $\vec{k}(T) = 0$ in order to satisfy (16.26).

Problem 16.10

In order to have a better understanding of what is discussed in the text, the following simulations are considered. Choose $A = 1$, $n = 8$, and $\beta = 2$ (defined below). Define $u \equiv 1 - t/T$.

a) Assume $B_{1+}(u) = \frac{1}{\gamma T}e^{-\beta^2 u^2}$. Simulate contour plots of $|M_+(\vec{r})/M_0|$ in both the Cartesian and polar coordinates. Does the excitation profile match the discussions in the text?

b) Now consider $B_{1+}(u) = \frac{u}{\gamma T}e^{-\beta^2 u^2}$. Repeat the steps in (a). How different is this excitation profile compared to that from (a)?

With the choice of a large n, the ϕ dependence in the integral of (16.41) can be neglected. As a result, $\vec{k}(t) \cdot \vec{r}$ is approximately proportional to ρ. Thus, $B_{1+}(t)$ can be determined from the inverse Fourier transformation of a Gaussian function, which is also a Gaussian function. Furthermore, the FWHM of the Gaussian function controls whether a thicker or thinner cylinder will be excited. Alternatively, the radial excitation profile can be tweaked by tuning $B_{1+}(t)$.

16.6   RF Pulse Characteristics: Flip Angle and RF Power

The previous discussions on rf pulse design for slice selection or saturation have been concerned only with the optimal preparation of the magnetization for imaging. However, when dealing with rf pulses, there are several other practical aspects of the rf pulse design that should be understood. First of all, it is useful to understand how much power must be supplied by the rf amplifiers in order to achieve a given flip angle in a given time for a specified set of slice parameters. A closely related issue of special interest for human imaging is the fact that some of the applied rf power will be deposited in the MRI sample as heat. In human imaging, strict guidelines are set for the SAR (Specific Absorption Rate) of rf power by the body. Therefore, it is important to understand the power and energy characteristics associated with rf pulses. In this section, several symmetric pulses applied during constant gradients are again considered, and the energy and maximum flip angle associated with several potential slice select pulses are found. The power deposited in the body will also briefly be examined here. It will be found that the expressions for the energy associated with a pulse are easier to understand in the spatial domain, rather than the time domain, but since they are proportional to the integral over the square of the field, by Parseval's theorem they are equivalent.

The total energy associated with an rf pulse can be found using a standard electromagnetic formula. A derivation of this formula, however, requires knowledge of Maxwell's equations and general electromagnetic theory which are beyond the scope of this text, so it is presented without proof, and the reader is directed to any college level electromagnetic text for an in-depth derivation. The total energy associated with the rf magnetic field is the time integral over the entire pulse of the power delivered to the system as given by

$$W(\tau_{rf}) = \frac{\omega_0}{2\mu} \int_0^{\tau_{rf}} dt \int d^3r \, B_1^*(\vec{r}, t) B_1(\vec{r}, t) \tag{16.44}$$

The spatial dependence of B_1 is the same for each pulse, and, therefore, the spatial integral in (16.44) is only a scale factor, since it is identical for every rf pulse. The pertinent information for the MRI experiment is contained in the term

$$W_p = \int dt \, B_1(t) B_1^*(t) \tag{16.45}$$

where the spatial dependence is neglected because the field is assumed to be uniform over the region-of-interest. This term will be referred to as 'Parseval Energy' here because Parseval's theorem (Ch. 11) asserts the equivalence of the time integrated 'power' in both the time and frequency domains.[1] From Parseval's theorem, it can also be expressed in the frequency domain as

$$W_p = \int df \, B_1(f) B_1^*(f) \tag{16.46}$$

where $B_1(f) = \mathcal{F}(B_1(t))$. The complex representation of the spatial magnetic field in the two-dimensional transverse plane (Ch. 2) is employed.

Another parameter which is important to the definition of an rf pulse is the angle through which it rotates the magnetization. Here, the flip angle at the center of the BW or position center of the selected slice is used to characterize the flip angle associated with the applied pulse. This reference tip angle θ_0 now requires an integral for its definition

$$\begin{aligned} \theta_0 &= \gamma \int dt \, B_1(t) \\ &= \gamma B_1(f)|_{f=0} \end{aligned} \tag{16.47}$$

Recall that $B_1(f)$ has units of field times time.

16.6.1 Analysis of Slice Selection Parameters

It is useful to look at how the slice select gradient, flip angle, pulse shape, Parseval energy, and applied B_1 field are related during the slice select phase of the MRI sequence. In this discussion, an example where the slice thickness and flip angle are kept constant will be considered, and the effects of varying other parameters will be studied. Several different excitation profiles will be considered here (see Fig. 16.14).

One aspect of the rf pulses that is difficult to determine analytically is the effect of truncating waveforms that are ideally infinite in time. Although these filter effects have been discussed at length, quantifying their effects is difficult. In general, the longer a waveform is, the closer it comes to producing the desired profile. Therefore, in what follows, it is assumed that a characteristic time can be defined for each pulse, and the time duration of the rf pulse is some multiple of this time so that the resulting slice profile is a reasonable approximation of the ideal case.

Sinc Pulse

Consider generating a boxcar slice profile. This implies that a sinc pulse will be applied in the time domain. $B_1(t)$ is then

$$B_1(t) = B_1 \, \text{sinc} \left(\frac{\pi t}{\tau_{\text{sinc}}} \right) \tag{16.48}$$

where $\tau_{\text{sinc}} \equiv t_{zc} = 1/BW_{rf}$ from Sec. 16.2. The thickness of the excited slice associated with this sinc pulse is

$$TH = \frac{BW_{rf}}{\gamma G_{0z}} = \frac{1}{\gamma G_{0z} \tau_{\text{sinc}}} \tag{16.49}$$

---

[1]Notice that, as written, this 'energy' does not have the correct units. It is not a real energy in the physical sense, but represents the relevant terms from the complete energy expression and is easier to deal with logistically.

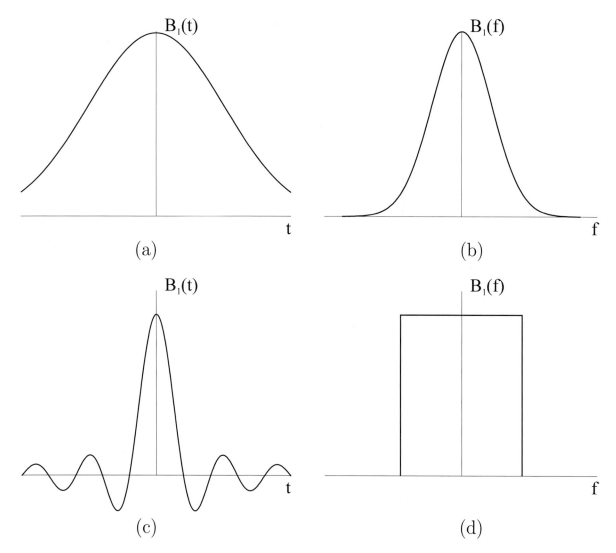

Fig. 16.14: The graphs in (a) and (b) show a Gaussian pulse and its corresponding excitation profile. A sinc pulse appears in (c) and its corresponding excitation profile appears in (d). Alternatively, (d) can be used to represent a rect pulse and (c) can be used to represent its excitation profile.

The characteristic flip angle and Parseval energy for this pulse must also be found. The integrals (16.45) and (16.47) can be computed, for example, by complex contour integration.[2] The Parseval energy is equal to

$$W_p = B_1^2 \int_{-\infty}^{\infty} \frac{\sin^2\left(\frac{\pi t}{\tau_{\text{sinc}}}\right)}{\frac{\pi^2 t^2}{\tau_{\text{sinc}}^2}} dt = B_1^2 \tau_{\text{sinc}} \tag{16.50}$$

where it is assumed that the pulse duration is sufficiently long that it can be approximated by the infinite time result. Equation (16.50) can be verified from the frequency domain

---

[2]Examples of contour integration can be found in any complex analysis text (see the Suggested Reading list, for example).

perspective by a simple integration of (16.46)

$$W_p = B_1^2 \tau_{\text{sinc}}^2 BW_{rf} = B_1^2 \tau_{\text{sinc}} \qquad (16.51)$$

The central flip angle associated with this pulse is

$$\theta_0 = \gamma B_1 \tau_{\text{sinc}} \qquad (16.52)$$

Recall that the Fourier transform of the above sinc pulse is the boxcar function, $B_1(f) = B_1 \tau_{\text{sinc}} \text{rect}(f\tau_{\text{sinc}})$, corresponding to the spread (bandwidth) of frequencies, $BW_{rf} = 1/\tau_{\text{sinc}}$. So all the frequencies between $-1/(2\tau_{\text{sinc}})$ and $1/(2\tau_{\text{sinc}})$ are tipped by the angle θ_0 in (16.52). The B_1 and time dependence of Parseval energy and flip angle will be the same for all pulses, but the factors which multiply this dependence also determine the efficiency of a pulse for giving a certain flip angle within a desired amount of time with minimal energy.

Knowing these parameters by themselves is useful for determining the energy used by the pulse, which is proportional to the energy deposited in the body, relative to the flip angle generated. However, it is also important to understand what happens when these parameters are varied to see what flexibility exists in slice select design (assuming TH and θ_0 remain fixed). In order to minimize T_E, for example, it might be desirable for a given experiment to minimize the time duration of the rf pulse. This will be accomplished if τ_{rf} is fixed to be a multiple of τ_{sinc} and τ_{sinc} is reduced (i.e., the bandwidth of the rf pulse is increased). In this case, if

$$\tau_{\text{sinc}} \to \lambda \tau_{\text{sinc}} \qquad (16.53)$$

and θ_0 and TH are kept constant, then

$$G_{ss} \to \frac{G_{ss}}{\lambda} \quad B_1 \to \frac{B_1}{\lambda} \quad W_p \to \frac{W_p}{\lambda} \qquad (16.54)$$

If λ equals $1/2$, for example, twice the slice select gradient, the B_1 amplitude, and the SAR value must all be physically available for the pulse to be used. Another crucial point is that four times as much rf power must be available from the rf amplifier, since

$$power = \frac{energy}{time} \propto \frac{W_p}{\tau_{rf}} \qquad (16.55)$$

In general, there is an increase in power from the pulse of $1/\lambda^2$. For this reason, very short time duration, larger flip angle pulses may be impossible to use because they require too much rf amplifier power. Of course, it is also possible to look at situations where other parameters are varied or fixed; the above is only an introduction to the topic.

Problem 16.11

Using the given parameters, answer the questions listed below. Assume that a sinc rf pulse excites a $BW_{rf} = 1\,\text{kHz}$ for a boxcar slice profile. In order to get a smooth slice profile with little ringing, assume that $\tau_{rf} = 6\tau_{\text{sinc}}$.

a) If $TH = 3\,\text{mm}$, what value of G_{0z} is required?

b) By what factors are BW_{rf}, B_1, and W_p changed if TH is reduced to $1\,\text{mm}$ or increased to $30\,\text{mm}$, and the flip angle and slice select gradient G_{0z} are kept the same?

Simple Harmonic Pulse

Another example is the finite-time, rect pulse. Consider a sinusoidal pulse on-resonance with ω_0 and applied for a time τ_{rect} with constant amplitude. In the rotating frame,

$$B_1(t) = B_1 \, \text{rect}\left(\frac{t}{\tau_{\text{rect}}}\right) \tag{16.56}$$

The integrations in (16.45) and (16.47) are just the reverse of the previous example, and give

$$W_p = B_1^2 \tau_{\text{rect}} \tag{16.57}$$

and

$$\theta_0 = \gamma B_1 \tau_{\text{rect}} \tag{16.58}$$

Gaussian Pulse

The third example is a Gaussian pulse

$$B_1(t) = B_1 e^{-t^2/(2\tau_{gauss}^2)} \tag{16.59}$$

This pulse decays to e^{-1} of its maximum (at $t = 0$) by the time $t = \sqrt{2}\tau_{gauss}$. The energy and peak angle are now

$$W_p = B_1^2 \int_{-\infty}^{\infty} dt \, e^{-t^2/\tau_{gauss}^2} = \sqrt{\pi}\tau_{gauss}B_1^2 \tag{16.60}$$

and

$$\theta_0 = \sqrt{2\pi}\gamma B_1 \tau_{gauss} \tag{16.61}$$

respectively. Proof of these formulas are left as exercises for the reader. The results derived for the three pulse envelopes are summarized in Table 16.1. One can see that for the same flip angle at the center of the excited slice, the Gaussian pulse has $\sqrt{2}$ less radiated energy than those from the sinc and harmonic pulses (but outside the center, the flip angle varies spatially).

Pulse envelope, $B_1(t)$	Tip angle	Parseval energy
$B_1\text{rect}\left(\frac{t}{\tau_{\text{rect}}}\right)$	$\gamma B_1 \tau_{\text{rect}}$	$B_1^2 \tau_{\text{rect}}$
$B_1\text{sinc}\left(\frac{\pi t}{\tau_{\text{sinc}}}\right)$	$\gamma B_1 \tau_{\text{sinc}}$	$B_1^2 \tau_{\text{sinc}}$
$B_1 e^{-t^2/(2\tau_{gauss}^2)}$	$\sqrt{2\pi}\gamma B_1 \tau_{gauss}$	$\sqrt{\pi}B_1^2 \tau_{gauss}$

Table 16.1: Summary of pulse envelope properties

Problem 16.12

Show by direct calculation that the Parseval energy in both domains is the same for the Gaussian pulse.

Problem 16.13

The slice thickness associated with most pulses is given by the FWHM of their Fourier transform response.

a) Find the thickness of a slice selected with the Gaussian pulse from (16.59), assuming that the slice thickness is defined by the FWHM of the profile of the excitation.

b) Assuming that θ_0 and TH are fixed, what would be the effect on B_1, G_{ss}, W_p for the Gaussian pulse, if $\tau_{gauss} \to \lambda \tau_{gauss}$? Assume that the duration of the pulse is a fixed multiple of τ_{gauss}.

16.7   Spin Tagging

Different combinations of rf pulse and gradient shapes can be used to excite spins with specific frequencies or to track the motion of a particular group of spins. These rf pulse and gradient combinations are generally referred to as spin tagging methods. In this section two special cases are examined, both of which accomplish similar goals.

16.7.1   Tagging with Gradients Applied Between RF Pulses

The application of a series of rf pulses interspersed with gradients has an intriguing effect on the signal (see Fig. 16.15). The simplest example to consider is the case of excitation by two rf pulses, where both pulses are the same except one rotates the spins about $\hat{x}$ and the other about $-\hat{x}$ in the rotating frame (i.e., the rf pulses are applied 180° out-of-phase with respect to each other). From this point forward, the prime will be dropped and it will be assumed that all calculations are done in the rotating reference frame. For an ideal system, all spins will end up back along $\hat{z}$. If a gradient is on between the two pulses, the phase of the spins will spread out as a function of position along the direction of the applied gradient (see Fig. 16.15b). Those spins that end up along $\hat{x}$, for example, will not be affected by the second $\pi/2$-pulse (see Fig. 16.15c). If all of the spins that remain in the transverse plane are then dephased with additional 'spoiling' gradients (see Fig. 16.15d), only those spins that were returned to the longitudinal direction by the second rf pulse will be affected by the slice selective excitation pulse used to create the imaging plane. This results in a spatial modulation of spin density along the direction the spins were dephased in the image (see Fig. 16.15e). The exact behavior of the spin system under the rf pulse sequence $(\pi/2)_x$–$(\pi/2)_{-x}$ is considered next.[3]

If the applied gradient is along the x-direction and of amplitude G_x, then the phase developed over a time τ_x is

$$\phi(x, \tau_x) = -\gamma G_x \tau_x x \qquad (16.62)$$

---

[3]Recall the notation employed to describe these rf pulses is $(\theta)_{axis}$ where θ describes the flip angle, and *axis* tells which axis the $B_1^{transmit}$ is directed along.

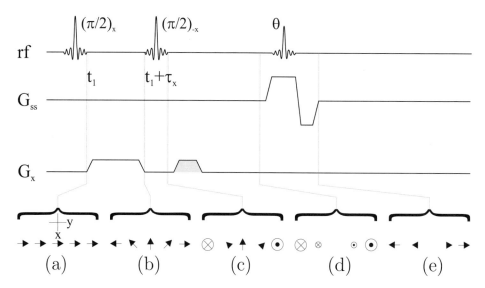

Fig. 16.15: Tagging and slice select design for a spatially modulated spin tagging imaging sequence. The diagrams at the bottom of the figure show the behavior of the magnetization in the transverse plane. (a) shows all spins along z tipped into the transverse plane with a nonselective $\pi/2$-pulse along $\hat{x}$. (b) shows the dephasing of the spins after the application of an additional spatial tagging x-gradient. (c) shows how only some of the spins are affected by the next rf pulse along $-\hat{x}$, as a result of the tagging. (d) demonstrates that the spoiling gradients (those highlighted by shading) dephase all of the transverse magnetization. (e) shows that the final excitation slice selective pulse only tips those spins that were returned to the z-axis into the transverse plane, resulting in spatially modulated tagging along the x-direction. Subsequent to this, the normal phase encoding and read gradients would appear.

Everywhere where $\phi(x, \tau_x)$ is a multiple of π (i.e., at the time of the second pulse, the spins are parallel to the x-direction), the signal will be rotated back along the z-direction. In general, after both pulses have been applied, the remaining transverse magnetization along the x-axis will be

$$M_\perp(x) = |M_0 \sin\left(\gamma G_x x \tau_x\right)| \tag{16.63}$$

This transverse magnetization can be spoiled with additional gradient pulses, leaving the longitudinal magnetization

$$M_z(x) = M_0 \cos\left(\gamma G_x x \tau_x\right) \tag{16.64}$$

If an image is acquired immediately after this sequence of events, a series of dark bands (regions of zero or low signal) will appear in the image. The spacing between the dark bands occurs over a distance of $1/(2\gamma G_x \tau_x)$. The larger G_x or τ_x, the smaller the spacing. From an imaging perspective, the location of the signal zeroes (dark bands) is a type of resolution in the image. If the desired spacing of the zeroes is m pixels, then the relation

$$m\Delta x = \frac{1}{2\gamma G_x \tau_x} \tag{16.65}$$

becomes the appropriate constraint. The size of the gradient required to obtain this spacing relative to the read gradient G_R can be found by using the Nyquist criterion for Δx and yields

$$G_x = \left(\frac{1}{2m}\right)\left(\frac{T_s}{\tau_x}\right)G_R \tag{16.66}$$

The thickness of the bright region of the tag x_w can be estimated as the FWHM of the longitudinal magnetization in (16.64) as

$$\gamma G_x x_w \tau_x = \frac{2\pi}{3}$$

or

$$x_w = \frac{2\pi}{3\gamma G_x \tau_x} \tag{16.67}$$

There will be true signal zeros in the tags only if the θ-pulse is applied immediately after the $(\pi/2)_{-x}$-pulse (see Fig. 16.15). Clearly, the longer the time interval between the $(\pi/2)_{-x}$-pulse and the θ-pulse, the more the spins which were left in the transverse plane after the second pulse have recovered along z and the more nonzero the magnetization becomes.

An example application to a phantom, with spatial modulation applied along two directions, is shown in Fig. 16.16a. The dark bands are angled here (see Prob. 16.15) and are well-defined relative to the excited signal.

Problem 16.14

a) If the full width at one-tenth maximum is used to find x_w in (16.67) instead of the FWHM, what is the expression for x_w?

b) Plot $M_\perp(x)/M_0$ as a function of position with $\gamma G_x \tau_x = 1\,\text{mm}^{-1}$. Discuss why the tags are not sharply defined.

c) Why is it that the tags begin to vanish if the time of application of the θ-pulse after the preparatory tagging pulses becomes greater than the T_1 of the tissue?

Problem 16.15

Draw a sequence diagram that could produce Fig. 16.16a. Hint: Notice the angle the tags make with the x- and y-axes.

16.7.2 Multiple RF and Gradient Pulses for Tagging

As has been shown, rf and gradient pulses, in combination, can be used for more than just exciting a slab for 2D or 3D imaging. In this subsection, a different approach is taken to prepare a set of parallel tags across an object. In fact, this simple concept first espoused for spectroscopy purposes (see the reference for Ernst and Anderson in the Suggested Reading)

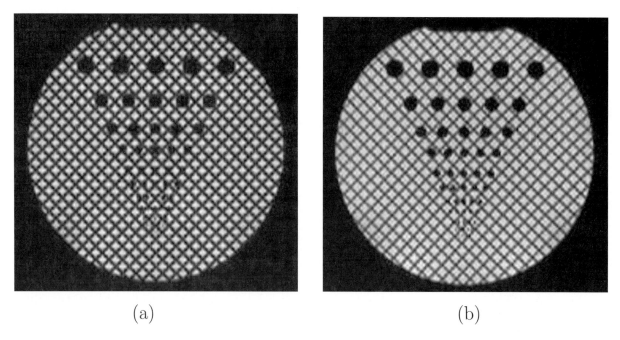

$$(a) \qquad\qquad\qquad\qquad (b)$$

Fig. 16.16: In (a), an image of a phantom with tagging created by applying gradients between rf pulses is shown, and in (b) a similar image of the same phantom is shown, but now collected using multiple rf pulses for tagging. These images demonstrate that either approach can be used to tag a group of spins.

also contains the seeds for a number of rapid imaging methods which use the echo train following a fixed series of rf pulses (see Ch. 18).

The desired excitation is shown in Fig. 16.17a. It is possible to describe this excitation as the convolution of a thin rect function with a comb function, defined as

$$U(x) \equiv \sum_{m=-\infty}^{\infty} \delta\left(x - mx_{tags}\right) \tag{16.68}$$

such that

$$M_{\perp}(x) = M_0 \text{rect}\left(\frac{x}{x_w}\right) * U(x) \tag{16.69}$$

where x_w is the thickness of the tags, and x_{tags} is the distance between their centers. The equivalent convolution is shown in Fig. 16.17b. As described in Sec. 16.4.1, for a low flip angle approximation, the magnetization and rf field of the pulse are related by the Fourier transform. Therefore, using the Fourier transform relation in (16.28), the desired rf input necessary to produce such an excitation can be found with a slice select gradient G_x. This result is shown in Fig. 16.17c and is given by

$$B_1(t) = B_1 u(t) \cdot \text{sinc}\left(\pi \gamma G_x t x_w\right) \tag{16.70}$$

where

$$u(t) \equiv \sum_{m=-\infty}^{\infty} \delta\left(\gamma G_x x_{tags} t - m\right) \tag{16.71}$$

and $B_1 = G_x x_w$. It is seen that the desired input is the product of a comb function and a sinc function. Again, simple Fourier transform concepts, particularly the convolution theorem, have been applied to understand what appears to be a complex mathematical problem. Of course, the rf and slice select gradient pulse duration cannot last for an infinite amount of

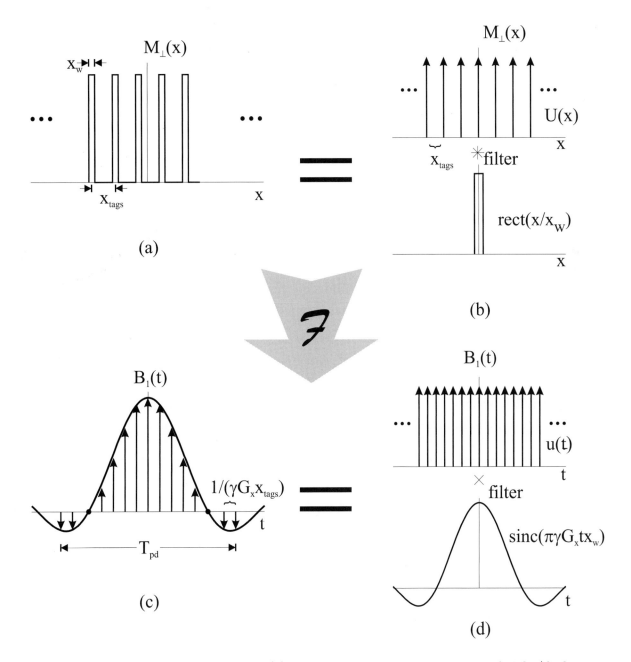

Fig. 16.17: A set of thin excited stripes (a) are desired in an image, to give a bright/dark pattern across the field-of-view. The associated set of rect functions can be described as the convolution of a narrow rect function with a comb function (b). This implies that the input rf (c) should be the product of a comb function and a very broad sinc function (d). Practically, the short hard pulses represented by the arrows in part (c) are of finite duration.

time. Assume that m hard rf pulses (the short duration delta-like pulses in (16.71)) are applied, then the total gradient and rf pulse duration time is

$$T_{pulse\ duration} \equiv T_{pd} = m\frac{1}{\gamma G_x x_{tags}} \tag{16.72}$$

Therefore, the time duration is further filtered by the function $\text{rect}(t/T_{pd})$ whose inverse Fourier transform is

$$g(x) = T_{pd}\,\text{sinc}\,(\pi\gamma G_x T_{pd}\,x) \tag{16.73}$$

To find the blurring this implies for the tags, the convolution of $g(x)$ with $\text{rect}(x/x_w)$ must be performed. Again, after blurring, the FWHM of the tags can be used to approximate their width. Of course, the longer the duration of the gradient and rf pulse combination, the closer $g(x)$ will come to approximating a delta function, and the less blurring will be found. An example of tagging, on a phantom, produced using this method is shown in Fig. 16.16b.

Problem 16.16

If a set of tags with $x_w = 5\,\text{mm}$, and $x_{tags} = 10\,\text{mm}$ is desired and $G_x = 25\,\text{mT/m}$, answer the following questions.

a) Using the given parameters, find the time between the multiple rf hard pulses.

b) For $m = 10$, find T_{pd}.

c) Find the FWHM of $g(x)$ for this pulse, and compare it to x_w. Based upon your answer would you expect that $m = 10$ is a reasonable number to use?

d) Draw a sequence diagram showing the (preparatory) rf tagging pulse, the appropriate imaging gradients and where the data are sampled.

16.7.3 Summary of Tagging Applications

Tagging of this type in imaging is generally used to study the motion of myocardium, CSF, or blood flow, for example. An *in vivo* example of the use of rf tags is shown in Fig. 16.18. In general, the desired tagged lines (or magnetization) should appear in the imaging plane, the slice select excitation will alter the magnetization created by the tags, and the specific modification depends upon the imaging application. An important issue is to make sure that the slice excitation does not alter the magnetization in such a way as to create or destroy magnetization preferentially in the bright or dark region, or the tags will be lost or distorted. Again, if the data are not interrogated immediately after these pulses, M_z will grow back to M_0 and contrast will be lost.

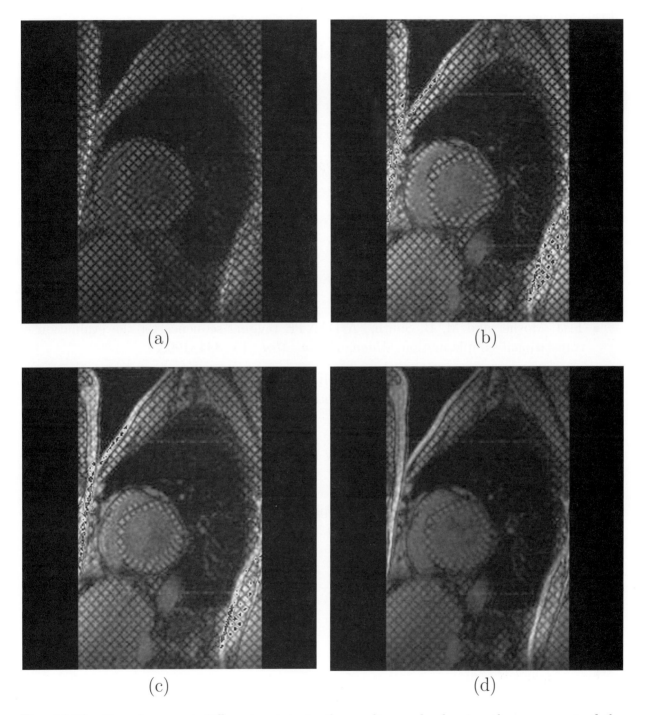

(a)   (b)

(c)   (d)

Fig. 16.18: Four frames at different points in the cardiac cycle showing the movement of the
myocardium via the distortion of the tags using multiple rf pulses. As time evolves going from (a)
to (d), the tags begin to lose their contrast because of longitudinal magnetization recovery.

Suggested Reading

A theory of small tip-angle approximation of viewing slice selection in k-space was developed in this article:

- J. Pauly, D. Nishimura, and A. Macovski. A k-space analysis of small tip angle excitation. *J. Magn. Reson.*, 81: 43, 1989.

The following book is an excellent reference on Complex Analysis. The topic of contour integration is nicely developed in this text:

- R. V. Churchill and J. W. Brown. *Complex Variables and Applications*. McGraw Hill, New York, 1990.

The next three articles are useful introductory references on the applications of the two approaches to spatial tagging in MRI:

- L. Axel and L. Dougherty. MR imaging of motion with spatial modulation of magnetization. *Radiology*, 171: 841, 1989.

- T. J. Mosher and M. B. Smith. A DANTE tagging sequence for the evaluation of translational sample motion. *Magn. Reson. Med.*, 15: 334, 1990.

- E. A. Zerhouni, D. M. Parish, W. J. Rogers, A. Yang, and E. P. Shapiro. Human heart: tagging with MR imaging – a method for noninvasive assessment of myocardial motion. *Radiology*, 169: 59, 1988.

The basic concepts of 'tagging' were actually first evident in the frequency localization described in:

- R. R. Ernst and W. A. Anderson. Application of Fourier transform spectroscopy to magnetic resonance. *Rev. Sci. Instrum.*, 37: 93, 1966.

Chapter 17

Water/Fat Separation Techniques

Chapter Contents

Summary: The basic concepts of separating water and fat, or any two spectrally different components, are discussed. The concept of inversion recovery is reintroduced for water/fat imaging. A description is given for the preferential nulling of specific tissues with spectrally selective rf pulses. A class of chemical shift imaging methods to separate two spectral components is presented.

Introduction

There are many parts of the body that will benefit from good water/fat separation including the optic nerve, bone marrow, the breast, the heart, and knee. Further, any area being imaged by a surface coil (see Ch. 27) will have enhanced signal for tissue near the coil such as the surface layer of fat. Separating water and fat leads to two separate images with improved contrast and a reduction of artifacts caused by the interference of fat and water. Quantification of how much fat or water (i.e., their relative spin densities) is in a given voxel for a given tissue can also be of clinical value. This chapter addresses water/fat nulling techniques and the simplest two-point approach to water/fat separation, followed by a more complex three-point separation method to extract local field inhomogeneity effects. These latter methods represent a marriage of imaging and spectroscopic techniques.

17.1 The Effect of Chemical Shift in Imaging

Even for a perfectly uniform external static field, local fields vary at the molecular level. For example, the protons in water (H_2O) see a different field from those in a lipid-based

413

or fatty compound (which contain CH_2 and CH_3). The former represents the 'water' signal (from water-bearing material or tissue) while the latter represents the 'fat' signal. The fat is shifted to a lower frequency (see Fig. 17.1) so that the difference between their precession frequencies Δf_{fw} is given by

$$\Delta f_{fw} \equiv f_f - f_w = -\sigma_{fw}\gamma B_0 \qquad (17.1)$$

where the suffix w stands for water, f for fat, σ_{fw} (a positive quantity in this case) is the chemical shift between water and fat expressed as a fraction of the field B_0, and Δf_{fw} refers to the frequency shift of fat relative to water.[1] The subscripts w and f denote water and fat in (17.1), but this equation can describe the chemical shift for any two compounds containing the same MR nucleus and the methods outlined in this chapter will work equally well. Most fat in the human body has $\sigma_{fw} \approx 3.35\,\text{ppm}$ ($= 3.35 \times 10^{-6}$), which leads to a frequency shift of 214 Hz at 1.5 T (see Fig. 17.1a). For the remainder of this chapter, the focus will be on imaging objects containing only water and fat.

The spin density of water $\rho_{0,w}$ can be greater than the spin density of fat $\rho_{0,f}$ in healthy tissue. However, the voxel signal from fat for a short-T_R experiment can be significantly larger than the signal from water since fat has a small T_1 relative to most other tissues. Consider a fast, short-T_R, T_1-weighted experiment where $T_R = 40\,\text{ms}$ (such as in Fig. 17.1b) and the flip angle is set to $90°$. The signal from water will be suppressed by T_R/T_{1_w}, and from fat by T_R/T_{1_f}, i.e., the water/fat image intensity ratio is reduced by T_{1_f}/T_{1_w}. Since T_{1_f} is so short, this ratio can be $1/3$ to $1/5$, leading to a significant suppression of the water signal relative to fat (see, for example, Fig. 17.1b). This problem of high signal from fat is further exacerbated when a surface coil is used for signal reception because of the proximity of fat to the coil (see Ch. 27).

17.1.1   Fat Shift Artifact

The fat misregistration will manifest along a frequency encoding direction (read or slice select) since fat is shifted in frequency relative to water.[2] For example, in the rotating frame for water, the precession frequency of fatty tissue in the presence of a read gradient $G_R\hat{x}$ is

$$f_f(x) = \gamma G_R x + \Delta f_{fw}(x) \qquad (17.2)$$

This shift in frequency from the expected value creates a problem in the resulting image if the frequency spread per voxel (or bandwidth per voxel, Δf_{voxel}) is not much greater than Δf_{fw}. In the read and slice select directions, where a spin's position is frequency encoded, this frequency difference causes a 'spatial misregistration' of spins belonging to fatty tissue.

---

[1]Note that this conventional choice of defining chemical shift implies that a positive chemical shift is associated with a lower frequency for fat relative to water. It is typical in NMR spectroscopy to quote all ^{1}H resonance peaks relative to a dilute (volume fraction 1% or less) solution of tetra-methyl silane (TMS) in $CDCl_3$. TMS is chosen because a small amount of it provides a large signal. All biologically common substances, including water, are slightly paramagnetic relative to TMS and, therefore, all other spectral peaks are higher in frequency than this. For example, water and fat are approximately 4.8 ppm and 1.4 ppm higher in frequency than TMS solution, respectively.

[2]The situation is more complicated than this when echo planar imaging is used (see Ch. 19).

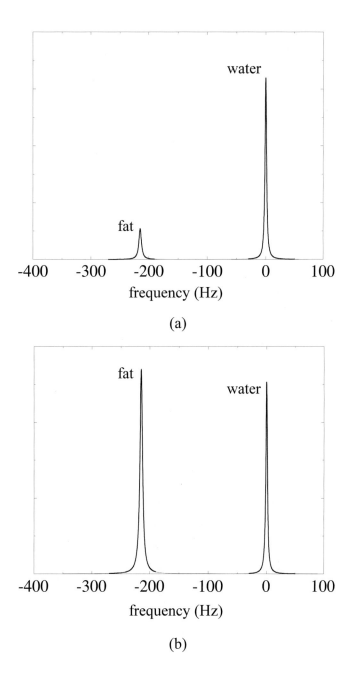

Fig. 17.1: Water and fat frequency components obtained after Fourier transformation of an FID from the marrow of a volunteer. (a) when $T_R = \infty$; and (b) when $T_R = 40\,\text{ms}$. Water in tissue has both a longer T_2 and a narrower spectral peak than fat. Contrary to spectroscopic convention, frequency is shown here increasing from left to right.

For example, when the voxel size $\Delta x = 1\,\mathrm{mm}$ and $G_R = 10\,\mathrm{mT/m}$, $\Delta f_{\mathrm{voxel}} = 426\,\mathrm{Hz}$, recalling that

$$\Delta f_{\mathrm{voxel}} = \gamma G_R \Delta x \tag{17.3}$$

The ratio of the chemical shift frequency to the frequency content per voxel gives the fractional number of voxels the fat is shifted as

$$N_{\mathrm{shift}} = \frac{\Delta f_{fw}}{\Delta f_{\mathrm{voxel}}} \tag{17.4}$$

Hence, the actual physical distance the fat is shifted in the image is

$$\Delta x_{\mathrm{shift}} = N_{\mathrm{shift}} \Delta x \tag{17.5}$$

Consider the example where both water and fat are present in a voxel. Further assume they appear only at the center of the voxel. When the read gradient is sufficiently large so that $N_{\mathrm{shift}} < 0.5$, then all of the fat signal will remain within the same voxel as the water (Fig. 17.2a). For lower gradients, N_{shift} increases and the fat signal begins invading the neighboring voxels (Figs. 17.2b and 17.2c). Equation (17.5) tells us that *the lower the bandwidth per voxel, the worse the spatial misregistration artifact, and the higher the bandwidth per voxel, the less severe the fat shift*.[3] In this example then, only when the bandwidth/voxel is greater than $2\Delta f_{fw} = 428\,\mathrm{Hz}$ does the fat from the center of the voxel get mapped within the right voxel, as shown in Fig. 17.2a for the case when the $BW/$voxel is $500\,\mathrm{Hz}$. Figure 17.3 demonstrates how the spin density is altered for the example where fat and water are uniformly distributed throughout several voxels, and the fat is shifted by 3 voxels relative to water. These idealistic viewpoints must be tempered by the knowledge that each voxel is blurred by the point spread function, and the mix of fat and water in each voxel is unknown.

Problem 17.1

Assume that a voxel centered at x_0 with width Δx contains both water and fat uniformly distributed throughout the voxel.

   a) How large must the read gradient G_R be so that 80% of the fat lies within the same voxel as the water when $\Delta x = 1\,\mathrm{mm}$? Assume that all the fat sits at one frequency with $\sigma_{fw} = 3.35\,\mathrm{ppm}$ and $B_0 = 1.0\,\mathrm{T}$.

   b) In what direction along x is fat shifted?

As an example of the shift artifact, consider a sagittal slice through the leg. The direction of the fat shift will depend on the sign of the read gradient. Figure 17.4a shows an image obtained using a positive read gradient and Fig. 17.4b shows an image acquired with a negative read gradient. The regions where the fat overlaps water are very bright. Regions where fat has shifted away from the tissue now have a black border or interface (illustrated by the arrows in Figs. 17.4c and 17.4d). For example, the regions that contain blood vessels

---

[3]For a detailed discussion of this and other such field inhomogeneity effects, see Ch. 20.

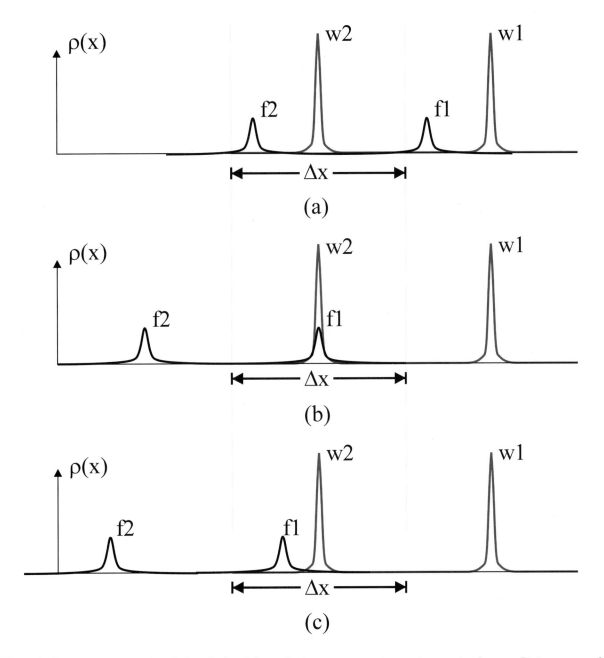

Fig. 17.2: A 1D example of the shift of fat relative to water in an image is shown. It is assumed that a set of samples (acting like point objects) containing a mix of water and fat are positioned at the center of each voxel. The frequency difference between the water and fat components creates a spatial shift of the fat component relative to the water component in the image. Two adjacent voxels are shown, each of which contains water and fat. The voxels are large in size relative to the FWHM of the water or fat spectra. All blurring due to finite sampling is ignored in this example. Assuming that a 1.5 T field is being used for imaging, the following cases are shown: (a) when the BW/voxel is 500 Hz, (b) if the BW/voxel is changed to 214 Hz, exactly the frequency difference between water and fat, the fat signal is shifted by exactly one voxel, (c) a BW/voxel of 172 Hz.

now look like black holes in the shifted fat because their signal did not get displaced. Other artifacts exist due to the changing phase of the fat signal relative to water, but this will be covered in Sec. 17.3. To minimize the fat shift artifact it is necessary to use a high BW which leads to reduced SNR. When a higher SNR is desired and a lower BW is used, methods to eliminate the fat signal (and, hence, fat shift artifacts) are often sought.

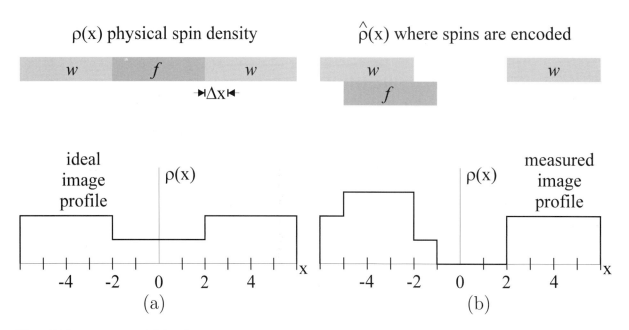

Fig. 17.3: The top of (a) shows a 1D physical spin density where fat is surrounded by some water-bearing tissue. The top of (b) shows where the fat and water will be spatially encoded as a function of their frequency. The fat is assumed to shift three voxels to the left. The lower portion of each figure represents the amplitude which will be seen in the image. The fat is assumed to have a lower signal than the water. (b) demonstrates the effect on the resulting image. The x-axis is marked in intervals of the voxel size Δx.

Problem 17.2

Sketch a figure similar to Fig. 17.3, but in the slice select direction showing which regions of water and fat are excited when a conventional rf slice selective excitation is applied. Assume that no rf pulses have been applied prior to the excitation pulse, and that fat and water are uniformly mixed within the region being excited. Label the distance between the center of the excited fat and water regions in terms of the slice select gradient, and chemical shift between fat and water.

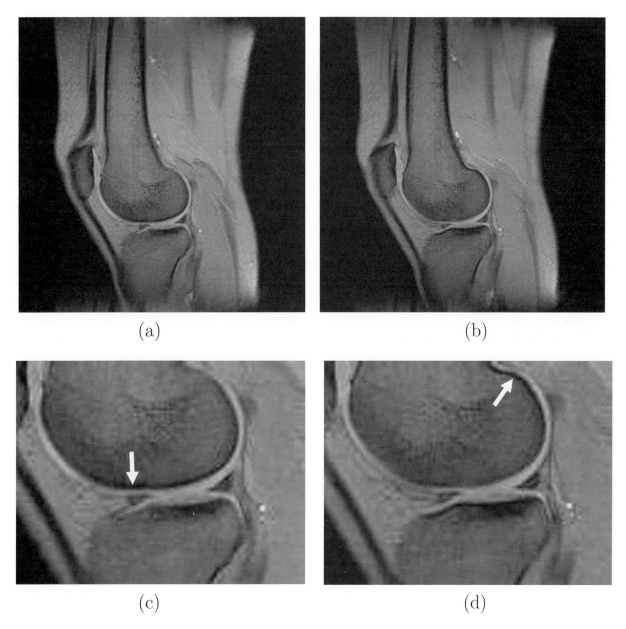

Fig. 17.4: Sagittal images across the human knee obtained with a gradient echo sequence obtained at an echo time where water and fat are in-phase (see for definition, Sec. 17.3.1). In (a), the image was obtained with a positive read gradient and in (b), with a negative read gradient. Notice that the fat has shifted in the opposite direction in the read direction (up/down direction in the image) between the two cases, which is clearly appreciable in the zoomed areas around the knee joint of (a) and (b), shown in (c) and (d), respectively. The read gradient used here gives a BW/voxel of 326 Hz leading to a 0.66 voxel shift.

17.2   Selective Excitation and Tissue Nulling

A number of unique approaches to eliminate signal from either water or fat have been developed. In this section, the concepts of selectively saturating a tissue or selectively nulling a tissue are introduced. A third approach to simultaneously extract information about both tissues is presented in the following section. Each method has its own advantages and disadvantages.

17.2.1   Fat Saturation

Fat and water have different Larmor frequencies, therefore, in a perfectly homogeneous field, a sufficiently narrow band rf pulse can be used to tip either species into the transverse plane. If such a pulse is used to excite fat, for example, then a conventional slice select rf/gradient pulse combination applied shortly thereafter will only tip the water's magnetization into the transverse plane (Fig. 17.5). Since the fat has just been excited, its longitudinal magnetization has not had time to regrow and there is no fat component to tip into the transverse plane. Hence, the resulting signal measurement should be primarily from water. It is said that the first rf pulse has saturated the signal from fat (see also Ch. 16), and this pulse is referred to as a fat saturation pulse. Of course, to image just fat, the roles of water and fat can be reversed.

The difficulty of this method is that poor field homogeneity will cause the fat selective pulse to excite water instead if $\gamma \Delta B = \Delta f_{fw}$. In that case, there will be regions where the water rather than the fat will be saturated. Although static magnetic fields are more homogeneous today, alternate approaches to separate water and fat that succeed independent of the presence of ΔB are desirable. There are other disadvantages of this method: one is that the saturation pulse requires a long duration of the rf pulse (from 5 to 40 ms for an rf bandwidth of 400 Hz to 50 Hz). Second, even for an rf bandwidth of 50 Hz, the spectra of

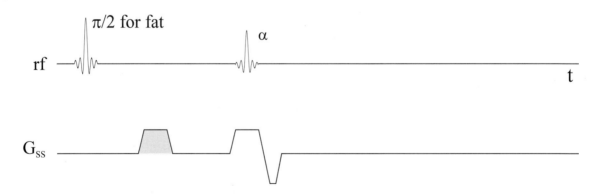

Fig. 17.5: The rf pulse sequence used for imaging one species (say, water). A spectrally selective, fat excitation pulse (90°) is followed immediately (after all transverse magnetization is spoiled) by a spatially-selective pulse to excite water and at the same time saturate fat. The fat signal is dephased prior to water excitation by the spoiling lobe (shown as the shaded region in the figure). Depending on the time between the $\pi/2$ and α-pulses, the $\pi/2$-pulse is usually made somewhat larger in flip angle to account for fat regrowth at the α-pulse.

water and fat could begin to overlap at fields less than 0.35 T. Thus, this method is difficult to apply for fields less than 0.35 T.

17.2.2 Selective Excitation

In Sec. 17.2.1, we referred to the basic concept of selective excitation of fat followed by spoiler gradients as the saturation of fat signal. In this subsection, we discuss two alternate approaches to exciting either water or fat rather than trying to indirectly saturate one or the other. To selectively excite a water or fat signal requires creating a spectral response profile of the rf pulse(s) that has (have) a pass-band at either the water or fat Larmor frequency and a suppression band at the fat or water Larmor frequency. This form of selective excitation can be achieved by using the fact that Δf_{fw} will lead to different magnetization precession between fat and water during or after the rf pulse.

The first method is simply to apply a rectangular rf pulse for a specific duration τ_{rf} with a frequency the same as the water Larmor frequency. In this case, the water is on-resonance and will be excited by B_1 as shown in Fig. 3.3a. The fat will be off-resonance by an amount Δf_{fw} and will see an effective field B_{eff} different from the applied B_1 field that water sees. With a judicious choice of rf pulse duration τ_{rf} such that $\omega_{eff}\tau_{rf} = 2n\pi$, the fat signal can be rotated back to the z-axis. This yields zero transverse signal $M_\perp(\tau_{rf})$, or zero $\alpha(\tau_{rf})$ as determined by (3.54), and yet leaves a nonzero transverse component for water. (See also Prob. 17.3.) The complete expression of the signal response as a function of resonance offset is the subject of Prob. 17.4

$$
\begin{aligned}
M_x(\Delta\omega) &= M_0 \left[1 - \cos\left(\sqrt{(\Delta\omega)^2 + \gamma^2 B_1{}^2}\; \tau_{rf} \right) \right] \frac{(\Delta\omega)\gamma B_1}{(\Delta\omega)^2 + \gamma^2 B_1{}^2} \\
M_y(\Delta\omega) &= M_0 \sin\left(\sqrt{(\Delta\omega)^2 + \gamma^2 B_1{}^2}\; \tau_{rf} \right) \frac{\gamma B_1}{\sqrt{(\Delta\omega)^2 + \gamma^2 B_1{}^2}}
\end{aligned}
\tag{17.6}
$$

Figure 17.6 shows the detectable signal, i.e., $M_\perp(\Delta\omega) = \sqrt{M_x(\Delta\omega)^2 + M_y(\Delta\omega)^2}$, as a function of frequency from (17.6). Since the B_1 field strength of the rf pulse is usually much smaller than the chemical shift frequency difference between water and fat, the nulling points in Fig. 17.6 are insensitive to B_1 (see Prob. 17.4). To selectively excite the fat signal and suppress the water signal, one can tune the demodulated rf frequency to match the Larmor frequency of fat. In this case, fat becomes on-resonance and water resonates at $|\Delta\omega_{fw}| = 2\pi|\Delta f_{fw}|$. As with most selective excitation methods, this method may have excitation leakage to unwanted signals with the presence of inhomogeneous magnetic fields, though practically this problem is alleviated thanks to the highly homogeneous magnetic fields available in most superconducting scanners nowadays (see examples in Fig. 17.7). Finally, as the applied rectangular rf pulse is spatially nonselective, this method only supports 3D imaging. Despite these disadvantages, since both excitation and suppression are accomplished with a single, short, low-power rf pulse, this method is suitable for use in short TR fast imaging sequences even at high field strengths.

Problem 17.3

Ignoring T_1 effects, consider when $\omega_{eff}\tau_{rf} = 2\pi$, at which time fat magnetization returns to the z-axis for the first time at the end of the rf pulse. Determine $\omega_1 = \gamma B_1$ and τ_{rf} in terms of $|\Delta f_{fw}|$, so that the water magnetization experiences a $\pi/2$ excitation. In this way, one can obtain maximum signal from water but no signal from fat.

Problem 17.4

Show that by applying a gradient during the rectangular rf pulse, one can spatially reveal the off-resonance profile, as in Fig. 17.6, along the direction of the gradient. Derive (17.6) and use it to determine the location x at which the signal is zero, in terms of τ_{rf}, B_1, and gradient amplitude G. Also, explain why the profile in Fig. 17.6 deviates slightly from a sinc function for small values of B_1. Hint: Taking $M_\perp = M_0 \sin\alpha$ and assuming a constant $\Delta\omega$, derive $\sin\alpha$ in terms of τ_{rf} and B_1.

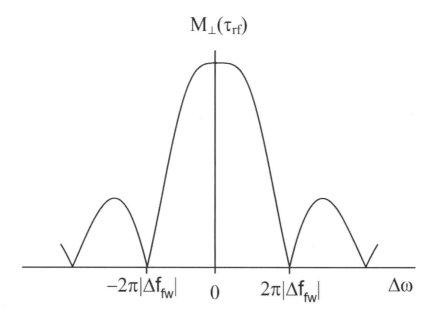

Fig. 17.6: Simulated transverse signal $M_\perp(\tau_{rf})$ as a function of resonant frequency offset $\Delta\omega$, as given by (17.6), with ω_1 and τ_{rf} determined as in Prob. 17.3. If water is on-resonance, the corresponding $M_\perp(\tau_{rf})$ of fat is zero and the corresponding frequency offset is $-2\pi|\Delta f_{fw}|$. On the other hand, if fat is on-resonance, at the frequency offset $2\pi|\Delta f_{fw}|$, the transverse magnetization of water is zero.

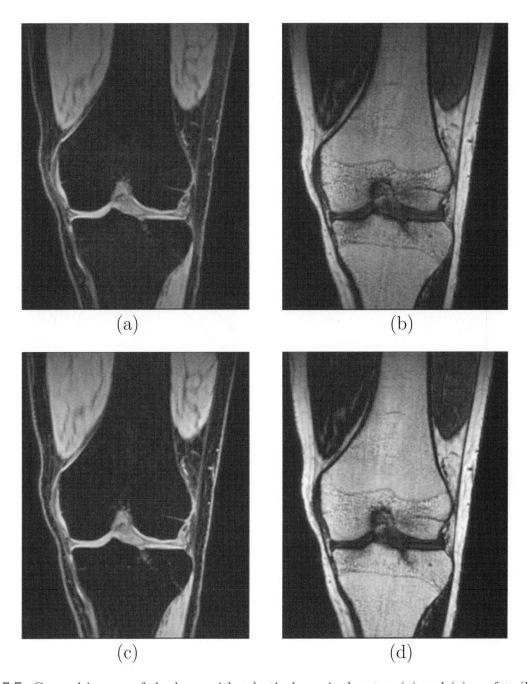

(a) (b)

(c) (d)

Fig. 17.7: Coronal images of the knee with selectively excited water, (a) and (c), or fat, (b) and (d), signal acquired at 3 T using a rectangular rf pulse to excite cases (a) and (b), and the 1-2-1 SPSP pulse to excite cases (c) and (d).

The second method involves using multiple rf pulses as a means to better suppress fat signal by providing a broader nulling region in the frequency domain. This can be useful if there is more than one fat component with slightly different chemical shifts or if there are mild field inhomogeneities present. Consider two rf pulses that have an interval τ between them (Fig. 17.8a). After the first rf pulse along the x-axis tips both fat and water to the y-axis (Fig. 17.8b), a phase difference between water and fat magnetization after time τ develops and is given by $\Delta\phi_{fw}(\tau) = 2\pi|\Delta f_{fw}|\tau$ (Fig. 17.8c). With a demodulated frequency equal to the water Larmor frequency, the water magnetization remains along the y-axis. If the second

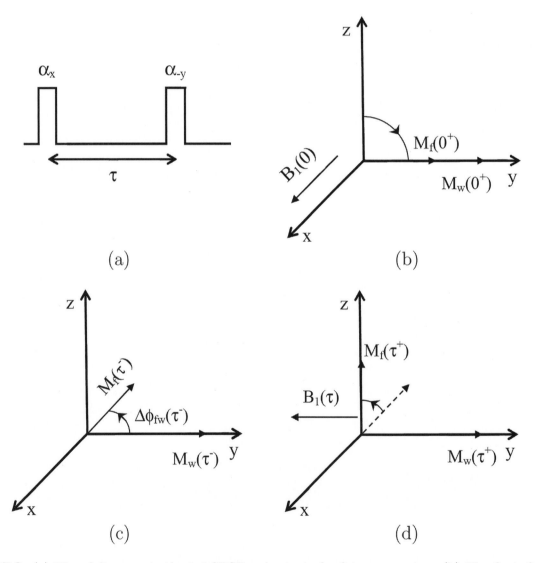

Fig. 17.8: (a) The rf diagram in the 1-1 SPSP pulse train for fat suppression. (b) The first rf pulse along the x-axis excites both fat and water to the y-axis. (c) A phase value of $\Delta\phi_{fw}(\tau) = 2\pi|\Delta f_{fw}|\tau$, relative to the y-axis, in the rotating frame develops for the fat magnetization $M_f(\tau^-)$ at the end of the rf interval, whereas the water magnetization $M_w(\tau^-)$ remains along the y-axis. (d) A second rf pulse applied along the $-y$-axis rotates $M_f(\tau^-)$ back to the z-axis, leaving only $M_w(\tau^+)$ in the transverse plane.

rf pulse, with the same flip angle but along the $-y$-axis, is applied when $\Delta\phi_{fw}$ becomes $\pi/2$, it will rotate the fat magnetization back to the z-axis without affecting the water magnetization (Fig. 17.8d). In this case, water magnetization alone remains in the transverse plane, as if the water signal has been selectively excited. This method is known as the spectral-spatial (SPSP) rf pulse approach, as the multiple rf pulses by themselves can be spatially selective while the combined effect of the pulse train is spectrally selective. This dual pulse scheme, or the so-called 1-1 pulse scheme (i.e., the ratio of flip angles in the rf pulse train is 1:1), is the simplest form of the SPSP pulse. However, it can still be susceptible to field inhomogeneities that may lead to the reduction in both suppression and/or excitation efficiency. To increase the robustness of suppression, multiple pulse schemes such as 1-2-1, 1-3-3-1 or even 1-4-6-4-1 have been developed, applying a train of rf pulses with properly designed τ and B_1 orientation for each rf pulse. However, with longer rf trains, more complicated modulation of τ and B_1 is required to maintain the effectiveness of both excitation and suppression. Sample images of a 1-2-1 SPSP pulse can be found in Figs. 17.7c and 17.7d.

Problem 17.5

Assume that each rf pulse in the 1-1 SPSP design instantly tips all spins. Prove that with the presence of magnetic field inhomogeneities, the water signal decreases while the fat signal increases. Calculate the transverse magnetization for both water and fat spins as a function of an inhomogeneity ΔB when $\Delta\phi_{fw}(\tau) = \pi/2$.

17.2.3   Tissue Nulling with Inversion Recovery

One method of eliminating signal from fat is to take advantage of the differences between T_1 tissue relaxation times by using an inversion recovery sequence. The effectiveness of this approach will not depend upon field homogeneity. By inverting the fat and water longitudinal magnetization and then collecting the data at the zero crossing of the fat signal (Fig. 17.9), the fat signal will be nulled independent of static field variations. (Although the inversion pulse does have some dependence on the local field.) The water component of most tissues has a long T_1 relative to fat so that for short inversion time T_I most of the tissue signal remains large and negative. This inversion recovery sequence (see Chs. 8 and 26) needs a long T_R to allow all tissues to return to M_0 before the next inversion pulse so that the acquisition time is rather long. It is also inefficient because fewer slices are acquired than with a conventional spin echo scan. Nevertheless, with the development of echo planar imaging where the entire brain can be covered in a few seconds, inversion recovery applications become more feasible (see Ch. 19). A comparison between fat saturation and fat nulling using an IR pulse is shown in Fig. 17.10. The former fails behind the knee where the local field inhomogeneity causes a significant shift in background frequency, while the latter is independent of background field.

Problem 17.6

The above discussion suggests the possibility of nulling two tissues if water, fat, and silicon are present in the same voxel. Discuss how you might null water and fat to image silicon using both inversion recovery and saturation techniques. Assume that the chemical shift of silicon relative to water is 4.69 ppm (i.e., it is shifted in the direction of fat, just further along the frequency axis) and its T_1 is the same as the tissue that contains mostly water but is much longer than that of fat.

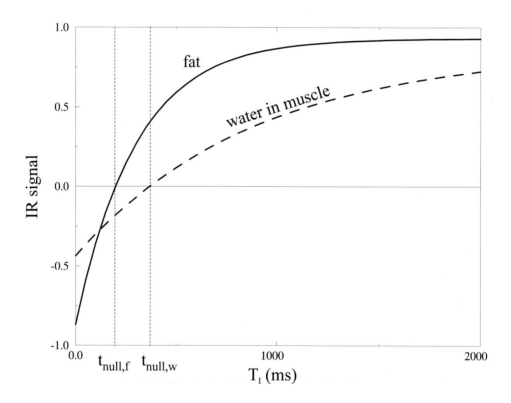

Fig. 17.9: Inversion recovery signal behavior and the choice of the recovery period to null a specific tissue. If data can be collected at the zero crossing (null point) of fat $T_I = t_{null,f}$ or water $T_I = t_{null,w}$ that particular tissue can be suppressed from the image. In this figure, fat and muscle (with essentially no fat component) signals are plotted for an IR sequence using a 1 s T_R. From Ch. 8, the null point for tissues in the finite T_R case is given by $T_{I,null} = T_1 \ln \frac{2}{(1+e^{-T_R/T_1})}$. For T_R much greater than $T_{1,fat}$, $T_{I,null}$ is usually 150 ms to 170 ms for fat at 1.5 T.

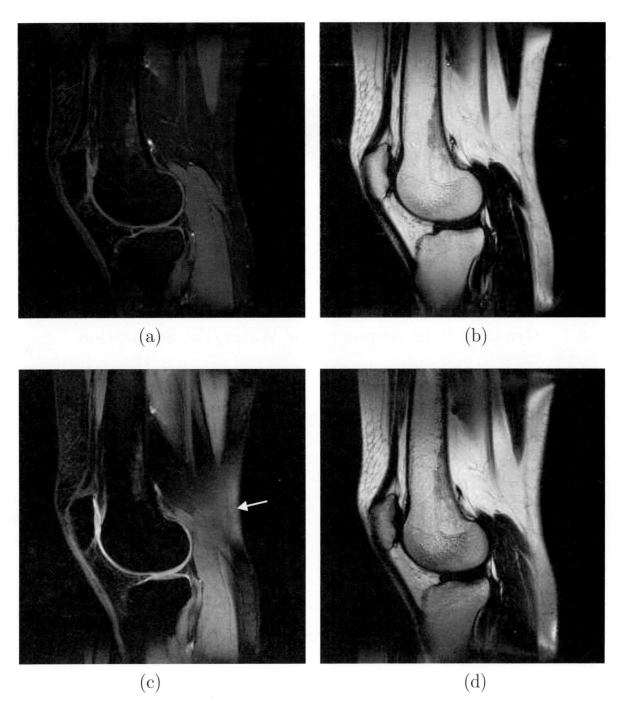

Fig. 17.10: (a) Fat-nulled image obtained using an inversion time (T_I) of 150 ms. (b) Water-nulled image obtained using a T_I of 300 ms. Both IR images were acquired with a T_R of 1 sec. As seen from the curves plotted in Fig. 17.9, $t_{null,w}$ for water in the muscle is about 300 ms. This is what is observed in (b). In (c) and (d), a frequency selective saturation pulse was used. (c) Fat-saturated image, and (d) water-saturated image. In (c) it is apparent that the static field is not uniform behind the knee (arrow) as some of the fat has not been fully saturated (compare with image (a); see also the phase in Fig. 17.18b in the same region).

17.3   Multiple Point Water/Fat Separation Methods

Chemical shift imaging as described in Ch. 10 is a long spectral phase encoding procedure designed for the situation where no, or little, *a priori* knowledge exists about the spectrum. When only two hydrogen-carrying compounds with known chemical shifts are present, the imaging scheme to acquire the requisite information to separate two spectral components is much simplified.

For the water/fat separation techniques of this section, each voxel is modeled using a simple partial volume model (see Ch. 15 for further details) containing some unknown fractional contributions to the voxel signal from water and fat. The fact that the fat signal in a given voxel may have come from a different spatial location becomes irrelevant in this section, since the goal is to separate the water and fat signals. The water/fat separation process determines the relative signal contribution from water and fat, respectively, to each voxel. In this section, modifications of the sequence design are used to collect two or three images with different phase information that can be manipulated to find separate water and fat images.

17.3.1   Gradient Echo Sequence for Water/Fat Separation

For a simple gradient echo sequence, the complex image as a function of time in the presence of water and fat will behave as

$$\hat{\rho}(T_E) = \hat{\rho}_w(T_E) + \hat{\rho}_f(T_E) \tag{17.7}$$

where $\hat{\rho}(T_E)$ represents the complex image obtained at some chosen T_E value, which contains unknown contributions from water and fat. It is assumed that the demodulation frequency is set to the water resonance frequency. In the first few introductory subsections (Sec. 17.3.1 to 17.3.4), it is also assumed that the static field is homogeneous throughout the imaged volume. Using these assumptions it is useful to look at the phase of fat and water during the sampling period[4] to understand the effect of the frequency shift for a specific echo time

$$\begin{aligned} \phi_w(t') &= -2\pi\gamma G_x x t' \\ &= \underbrace{-2\pi k_x x}_{\text{frequency encoding}} \end{aligned} \tag{17.8}$$

and

$$\begin{aligned} \phi_f(t') &= -2\pi\gamma\left(G_x x + \Delta B_{fw}\right)t' &+& -2\pi\gamma\Delta B_{fw}T_E \\ &= \underbrace{-2\pi k_x\left(x + \Delta B_{fw}/G_x\right)}_{\text{frequency encoding}} &+& \underbrace{-\Delta\omega_{fw}T_E}_{\text{additional phase}} \end{aligned} \tag{17.9}$$

where the difference between the frequency encoding terms in (17.8) and (17.9) leads to the frequency encoded fat shift discussed in the previous section. In this section, methods to use the additional phase associated with fat to separate the fat and water signals will be presented. Notice that even if the phase information can be used to separate the fat

---

[4]Recall that $t' = t - T_E$ where $t = 0$ at the center of the rf pulse.

and water signals the fat image will still be spatially shifted along the frequency encoding direction.[5]

Equations (17.8) and (17.9) imply that $\hat{\rho}_w$ is real, while $\hat{\rho}_f$ is complex, having a T_E-dependent phase. The complex voxel signal (17.7) can be rewritten as

$$\hat{\rho}(T_E) = \hat{\rho}_{w,m} + \hat{\rho}_{f,m}e^{-i\Delta\omega_{fw}T_E} \tag{17.10}$$

The subscript m is used to denote the magnitude of the image. In this discussion of water/fat separation, the key issue is the difference in phase generated by the frequency difference between water and fat as a function of T_E. By acquiring images at different values of T_E, the phase information can be used to separate the fat and water signals.

Problem 17.7

As discussed, fat appearing in one voxel may actually come from another location. Show for a gradient echo experiment that the complete expression for the spin density is

$$\hat{\rho}(\vec{r}) = \hat{\rho}_w(\vec{r})e^{-i\gamma\Delta B(\vec{r})T_E} + \hat{\rho}_f(\vec{r}_f)e^{-i\gamma(\Delta B - \sigma_{fw}B_0)T_E} \tag{17.11}$$

with

$$\vec{r}_f = \vec{r} + \frac{\sigma_{fw}B_0}{G_R}\hat{x} \tag{17.12}$$

where the distortion due to $\Delta B(\vec{r})$ has been neglected. The shift from $\vec{r}$ to $\vec{r}_f$ is exactly the same effect that typically causes the spatial shifting of the fat observed in Fig. 17.4 as the BW/voxel changes. The plus sign in (17.12) indicates that the fat signal is from a voxel on the right of the water voxel, if G_R is positive. The high values of G_R generally used limit spatial shifts to a few voxels so that the assumption made by the three-point method in Sec. 17.3.5 that both water and fat experience the same ϕ_0 and ΔB is valid.

Equation (17.10) leads to a beat frequency pattern (see Fig. 17.11, for example) where the water and fat spins are out-of-phase ('opposed phase') at a time when

$$-\Delta\omega_{fw}T_{E,op}(n) = (2n+1)\pi \tag{17.13}$$

and in-phase at a time when

$$-\Delta\omega_{fw}T_{E,in}(n) = 2n\pi \tag{17.14}$$

where n is a non-negative integer; 'op' is used as a short-form for opposed phase, and 'in' for in-phase. The $n = 0$ in-phase condition is achieved with an FID sampling method or, in a symmetric spin echo imaging case, where both water and fat are in-phase at the same time as the occurrence of the $k = 0$ point. For later use, define

$$-\Delta\omega_{fw}T_{E,90}(n) = 2n\pi + \pi/2 \tag{17.15}$$

For the water/fat case, $T_{E,op}(0) = \frac{-1}{2\Delta f_{fw}} \simeq 2.34\,\mathrm{ms}$ and $T_{E,in}(1) \simeq 4.67\,\mathrm{ms}$ at 1.5 T. Different fat components in the body may have different chemical shifts; care should be taken to determine the chemical shift for the region-of-interest.

---

[5]Chapter 20 contains a more in-depth treatment of the relationship between phase variations during sampling, and associated image effects.

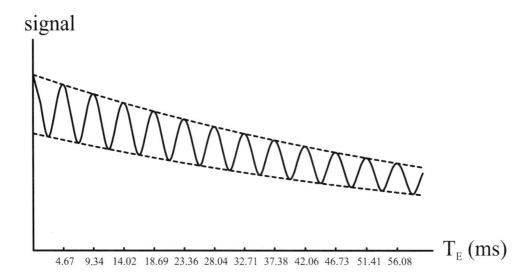

Fig. 17.11: The beating envelope of the combined water and fat signals as a function of time with $\hat{\rho}_{f,m} = 0.2\hat{\rho}_{w,m}$. The T_2^* of water and fat are assumed equal to 80 ms. The markings on the time scale are of special importance in that they represent the times at which water and fat seeing the same field are in-phase at 1.5 T. Note that T_1 effects are neglected, i.e., an infinite T_R is assumed.

Problem 17.8

---

    a) Rewrite (17.10) including T_2^* effects.

    b) Replot Fig. 17.11 for the main static field equal to 0.5 T and 0.1 T assuming T_2^* has not changed.

    c) How do the curves in (b) scale as a function of field strength?

    d) Replot Fig. 17.11 when $T_{2_w}^* = 100$ ms and $T_{2_f}^* = 60$ ms.

    e) Plot $|\hat{\rho}(T_E)|$ as a function of $\phi = -\Delta\omega_{fw}T_E$ for $\hat{\rho}_{w,m} = \hat{\rho}_{f,m}$. Assume the same values of T_2^* given in part (d), and $B_0 = 0.5$ T.

Problem 17.9

For a gradient echo sequence, (17.14) is valid only for $n > 0$. Show that no such restriction exists for a spin echo sequence, but that some negative values of n are also accessible to experiment.

From (17.10), the phase of the fat signal contribution as a function of T_E plays a very important role in determining the summed complex voxel signal. The phase of the voxel signal, on the other hand, additionally depends on the relative signal contributions from the two species. Fig. 17.11 is an illustration of the time progression of the combined water/fat signal. The fat signal contribution to the echo is seen to pass through a progression of phase values relative to water as echo time increases.

As seen earlier, the phase plays a key role in water/fat separation. What role does the T_E-dependent phase of the fat play in a magnitude image? First, we formally define the partial volume model for the voxel signal. If α_f is the relative strength of the fat signal contribution to the voxel signal in magnitude,[6] i.e.,

$$\alpha_f \equiv \frac{\hat{\rho}_{f,m}}{\hat{\rho}_{f,m} + \hat{\rho}_{w,m}} \tag{17.16}$$

then (17.10) can be rewritten as

$$\hat{\rho}(T_E) = (\hat{\rho}_{w,m} + \hat{\rho}_{f,m})((1 - \alpha_f) + \alpha_f e^{-i\Delta\omega_{fw}T_E}) \tag{17.17}$$

In the case when $-\Delta\omega_{fw}T_E$ equals π, the voxel signal is

$$\hat{\rho}(T_E) = (\hat{\rho}_{w,m} + \hat{\rho}_{f,m})(1 - 2\alpha_f) \quad \text{out-of-phase case} \tag{17.18}$$

Clearly, when a fraction of the voxel signal comes from fat, and fat is out-of-phase relative to water, the fat fraction α_f exactly cancels off an equal fraction (α_f) of water, leading to a signal-contributing fraction of $(1 - 2\alpha_f)$, as demonstrated by (17.18).

From (17.10), the magnitude of the voxel signal as a function of echo time T_E is

$$
\begin{aligned}
|\hat{\rho}(T_E)| &= \left((\hat{\rho}_{w,m} + \hat{\rho}_{f,m}\cos\Delta\omega_{fw}T_E)^2 + \hat{\rho}_{f,m}^2\sin^2\Delta\omega_{fw}T_E\right)^{1/2} \\
&= \left(\hat{\rho}_{w,m}^2 + \hat{\rho}_{f,m}^2 + 2\hat{\rho}_{w,m}\hat{\rho}_{f,m}\cos\Delta\omega_{fw}T_E\right)^{1/2}
\end{aligned} \tag{17.19}
$$

where the T_2 decay has been ignored. Fig. 17.12 shows the spin behavior at three different phase angles for water and fat spins. The main theme of this illustration is that water and fat are two different phasors, and their sum is determined by a phasor sum, not a simple scalar sum. It also reminds us that (17.19) is nothing but the magnitude of the vector sum of two vectors which are separated by an angular difference of $\Delta\omega_{fw}T_E$. This magnitude signal is plotted as a function of the volume fraction of fat in Fig. 17.13. When both water and fat occupy the same voxel, and fat is out of phase, signal cancelation will occur. Specifically, when $\alpha_f = 0.5$, total signal cancelation occurs. This almost always happens when the fat shifts more than a voxel away from its actual physical location in an out-of-phase image, since there is likely to be water at the voxel where the fat ends up.

Problem 17.10

Show that (17.19) becomes

a) $|\hat{\rho}(T_E)| = (\hat{\rho}_{w,m} + \hat{\rho}_{f,m})$ for $\Delta\omega_{fw}T_E = 0$, and

b) $|\hat{\rho}(T_E)| = |\hat{\rho}_{w,m} - \hat{\rho}_{f,m}|$ for $-\Delta\omega_{fw}T_E = \pi$.

---

[6]Here, α_f is defined as the relative strength of the fat signal contribution to the voxel signal in the spirit that, although it appears to be the case, α_f is not the fractional voxel spin density; it is only the fractional signal contribution, determined also by the T_1 and T_2 weighting which are, in turn, influenced by the choice of T_R and T_E.

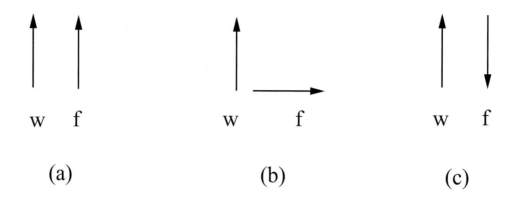

Fig. 17.12: Phasor diagrams representing water and fat spins when they are (a) in-phase, (b) 90°
out-of-phase, and (c) 180° out-of-phase at $T_{E,in}(n)$, $T_{E,90}(n)$, and $T_{E,op}(n)$, respectively.

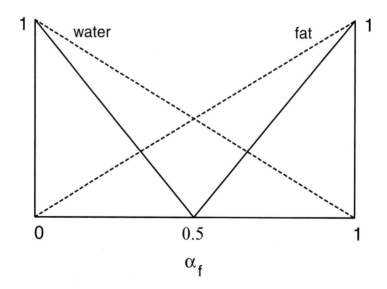

Fig. 17.13: Plot of the magnitude of the signal from a voxel containing both water and fat as
a function of the fraction of fat signal for an opposed-phase image (solid line). There is total
cancelation of signal when $\alpha_f = 0.5$. This lack of signal shows as a black line artifact at fat/water
interfaces in opposed phase images and is observed in a number of the images in this chapter. Shown
in dotted lines (for comparison purposes) are the voxel signal magnitudes of voxels containing only
water or only fat, occupying volume fractions $(1 - \alpha_f)$ and α_f, respectively, in these voxels.

17.3.2 Single-Echo Separation

For a homogeneous field, two pieces of information, the real and the imaginary part, can be obtained from a complex data set. Assume spins start in-phase at $T_E = 0$ (Fig. 17.12) and end up 90° out-of-phase at $T_{E,90}(0) = 1.17\,\text{ms}$ at 1.5 T (from (17.15)). Collecting an image at $T_{E,90}(0)$ gives

$$\hat{\rho}(T_{E,90}(0)) = \hat{\rho}_{w,m} + i\hat{\rho}_{f,m} \tag{17.20}$$

So, the real part of the voxel signal represents the water fraction, while the imaginary part of the voxel signal represents that of fat.

Since sampling does take a finite amount of time, it is not usually possible to obtain a T_E so short that $T_E = T_{E,90}(0)$ when a high resolution image is also desired. The next available echo times where the water signal is real and the fat signal is imaginary occur at the 270° point before the first in-phase point ($T_E = 3.51\,\text{ms}$ at 1.5 T), or the first 90° point after the first in-phase point ($T_E = T_{E,90}(1) = 5.84\,\text{ms}$).

Complex In-Phase and 90° Out-of-Phase Method

For inhomogeneous fields and imaging at 1.5 T with a $T_E = 4.67\,\text{ms} = T_{E,in}(1)$, the in-phase complex image is given by

$$
\begin{aligned}
\hat{\rho}_{in}(n = 1) &= (\hat{\rho}_{w,m} + \hat{\rho}_{f,m})e^{-i\gamma\Delta B T_{E,in}(1)} \\
&= (\hat{\rho}_{w,m} + \hat{\rho}_{f,m})e^{i\phi_{\Delta B}} \quad \text{(in-phase)}
\end{aligned} \tag{17.21}
$$

while the 90° out-of-phase complex image, obtained at an echo time of $T_{E,90}(1) = \frac{5}{4}T_{E,in}(1)$, is given by

$$
\begin{aligned}
\hat{\rho}_{90}(n = 1) &= (\hat{\rho}_{w,m} + \hat{\rho}_{f,m}e^{-i(5/4)T_{E,in}(1)\Delta\omega_{fw}})e^{-i(5/4)\gamma\Delta B T_{E,in}(1)} \\
&= (\hat{\rho}_{w,m} + i\hat{\rho}_{f,m})e^{i(5/4)\phi_{\Delta B}} \quad \text{(90° out-of-phase)}
\end{aligned} \tag{17.22}
$$

where $\phi_{\Delta B} = -\gamma\Delta B T_{E,in}(1)$ is the phase gained due to the presence of magnetic field inhomogeneities for the in-phase image. The $(5/4)\Delta\omega_{fw}T_{E,in}(1)$ term comes from the fact that the second echo is acquired at the $(2\pi + \pi/2)$ relative phase value between water and fat which is at the time $(5/4)T_{E,in}(1)$ of the in-phase image. The phase shift $\phi_{\Delta B}$ can be found from the first image. This can then be used to remove the $\frac{5}{4}\phi_{\Delta B}$ phase term from the second image and then the real and imaginary channels used to obtain water and fat images separate from each other.

The difficulty here occurs when the phase due to field inhomogeneities aliases (because phase is computed only over the range $[-\pi, \pi]$, any value of phase above π wraps back to a negative value and it is not possible to correctly predict the correction $\frac{5}{4}\phi_{\Delta B}$). Another problem can be the presence of a T_E-independent phase shift $e^{i\phi_0}$ where ϕ_0 is position-dependent (this can happen due to rf penetration and the finite, nonzero conductivity of the tissue). These difficulties and other practical issues arising with this method are illustrated in the examples shown in Figs. 17.14 and 17.15.

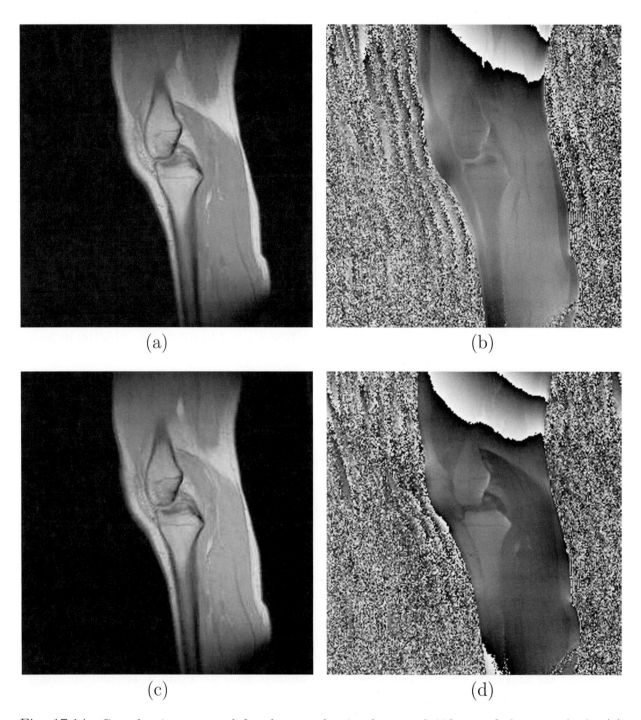

(a)   (b)

(c)   (d)

Fig. 17.14: Complex images used for the complex in-phase and 90° out-of-phase method. (a) In-phase magnitude image, (b) in-phase phase image, (c) 90° out-of-phase magnitude image, and (d) 90° out-of-phase phase image. The read direction is cranio-caudal (the vertical direction). The phase of water and fat are not equal in part (b) because of rf penetration effects; this difference is referred to as ϕ_0 in the text.

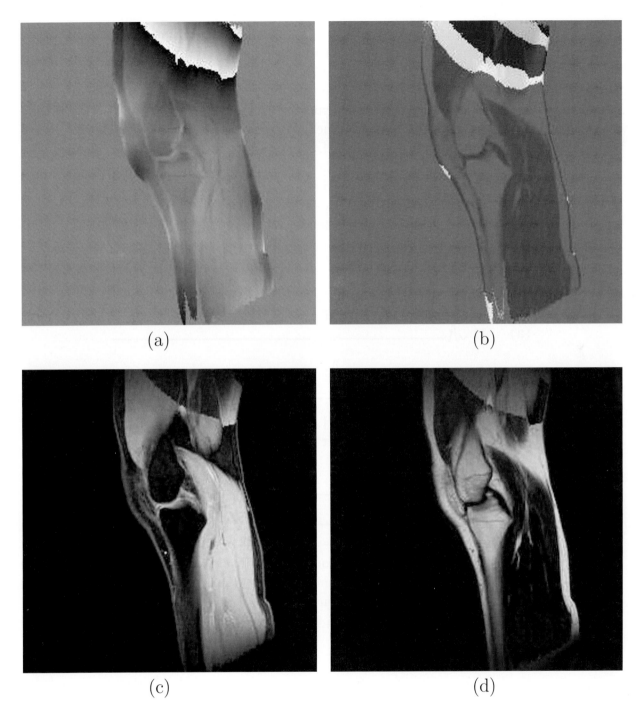

Fig. 17.15: Steps involved in extracting water and fat images from the 90° method are: unwrapping the in-phase phase image and using that to correct the 90° out-of-phase phase image for ΔB effects, and then displaying the real part as the water image and imaginary part as the fat image. (a) Partially unwrapped in-phase phase image. (b) Attempted correction of 90° out-of-phase phase image. (c) Water image. (d) Fat image. The incorrect separation at the top part of the leg occurs because of a large phase wrap (caused by the rapid field variations away from the center of the magnet) that cannot be corrected using only a single phase image for unwrapping.

17.3.3 Spin Echo Approach

One problem with the gradient echo approach is that the image can be acquired only for $n > 0$ (see (17.13) and (17.14)), whether an in-phase image, a 90° out-of-phase image, or an opposed-phase image is required. This causes a problem when either a single-point (see Sec. 17.3.2) or two-point (see Sec. 17.3.4) water/fat separation is performed in the presence of large local field inhomogeneities. This problem can be overcome when a spin echo sequence is used and the π-pulse is shifted toward the $\pi/2$-pulse by a time ϵ (Fig. 17.16). In the presence of a field inhomogeneity ΔB, the rf echo is shifted by $\Delta t = 2\epsilon$ (see Prob. 17.11) relative to the instant when the $k = 0$ sample occurs. This difference in times between the rf echo[7] and the gradient echo acts like a gradient echo T_E since fat magnetization builds up phase relative to water starting from this time-point. Setting $2\epsilon = 1.17\,\text{ms}$ produces the first 90° out-of-phase water/fat image. Setting $2\epsilon = 2.34\,\text{ms}$ produces the first opposed-phase image.

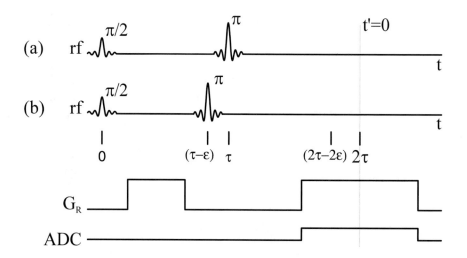

Fig. 17.16: The upper rf trace (a) represents conventional rf pulse timings relative to G_R, while the lower rf trace (b) shows a shifted π-pulse timing. Shifting the π-pulse by an appropriate time ϵ without changing the timing of the read gradient can be used to produce easily the first $\pi/2$ or π out-of-phase point at the time 2ϵ. This time can be made arbitrarily short if field inhomogeneities are large.

Problem 17.11

For the asymmetric spin echo sequence (acquired by shifting the π-pulse earlier in time by ϵ seconds in a sequence designed to acquire an image with a symmetric spin echo) in Fig. 17.16, show that the phase during the ADC data collection window is given for water and fat, respectively, by

---

[7]The rf echo is said to occur at that time-point when all static field inhomogeneities, including chemical shifts, are refocused.

$$\phi_w(t') = -\gamma \Delta B(t' + 2\epsilon) - \gamma G_R x t'$$
$$\phi_f(t') = -\gamma \Delta B(t' + 2\epsilon) + \gamma \sigma_{fw} B_0(t' + 2\epsilon) - \gamma G_R x t'$$

where t' is the time from the center of the readout where $k = 0$ is sampled. Clearly, when $t' = 0$, $\phi(t')$ equals $-2\gamma \Delta B \epsilon$ for water, and $-2\epsilon(\gamma \Delta B - \gamma \sigma_{fw} B_0)$ for fat, assuming the same field inhomogeneities are experienced by both the water and fat fractions.

Although the upcoming subsections focus on the gradient echo sequence, this spin echo approach can always be used instead.

17.3.4 Two-Point Separation

An obvious approach to separating water and fat is to use just two complex gradient echo images; one an in-phase image (obtained at a $T_E = T_{E,in}(n)$), and another, an opposed-phase image ($T_E = T_{E,op}(n)$). The complex voxel signals in these two cases in the absence of any field inhomogeneities are

$$\hat{\rho}_{in}(n) = \hat{\rho}_{w,m} + \hat{\rho}_{f,m} \tag{17.23}$$
$$\hat{\rho}_{op}(n) = \hat{\rho}_{w,m} - \hat{\rho}_{f,m} \tag{17.24}$$

Hence, a first attempt to obtain water and fat images would be to use the simple algorithm

$$\hat{\rho}_{w,m} = \frac{1}{2}(\hat{\rho}_{in} + \hat{\rho}_{op}) \tag{17.25}$$

$$\hat{\rho}_{f,m} = \frac{1}{2}(\hat{\rho}_{in} - \hat{\rho}_{op}) \tag{17.26}$$

Examples of in-phase and opposed-phase magnitude images and their corresponding phase images are shown in Fig. 17.17.

T_2^* effects have been ignored to this point. Since $\hat{\rho}_{in}(n)$ and $\hat{\rho}_{op}(n)$ are acquired at different echo times, (17.23) and (17.24) are not strictly valid, especially for tissues with short T_2^* values such as bone marrow. To reduce possible errors due to T_2^* effects, a third image can be collected to help obtain an in-phase image with approximately the same T_2^* weighting as the opposed-phase image. A third image $\hat{\rho}_{in}(n + 1)$ is collected and averaged with the first in-phase image (two in-phase images surrounding the out-of-phase image in the sequence of three images) to create a new $\hat{\rho}_{in}$, giving both in-phase and opposed-phase images for the calculations in (17.25) and (17.26) with roughly the same T_2^* weighting (see Fig. 17.18).

Problem 17.12

Show that when $(T_{E,in}(n+1) - T_{E,in}(n))/T_2^* \ll 1$ for both fat and water, the last statement in the text is valid. In other words, if $\hat{\rho}_{in}(n)$ is replaced by $\frac{1}{2}(\hat{\rho}_{in}(n) + \hat{\rho}_{in}(n + 1))$ in (17.25) and (17.26), errors due to T_2^* signal changes are removed.

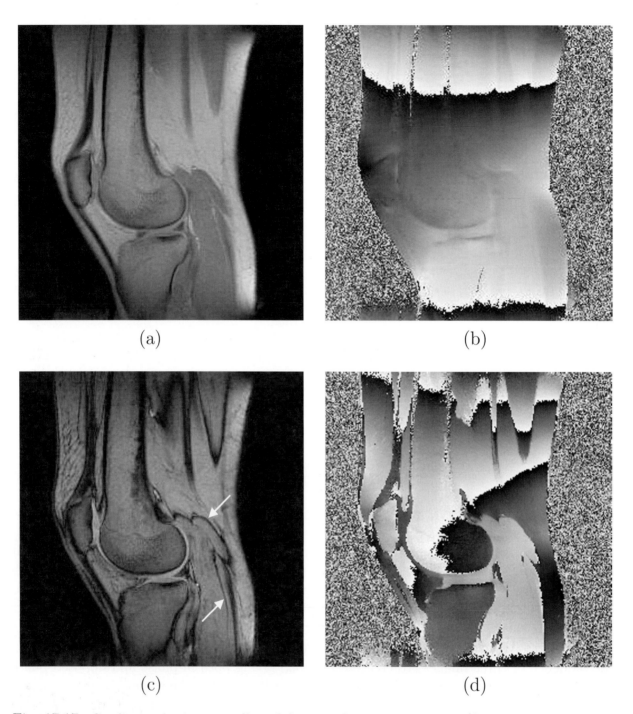

Fig. 17.17: Gradient echo images collected for complex two-point water/fat separation at 1.5 T. These two images were collected at T_E values of 4.5 ms and 6.75 ms, respectively. (a) In-phase magnitude image and (b) in-phase phase image. (c) Opposed-phase magnitude image, and (d) opposed-phase phase image. Note the cancelation artifacts (arrows) at the fat/water boundaries in the magnitude image shown in (c) (see the discussion in Sec. 17.3.1 concerning the effect illustrated in Fig. 17.4).

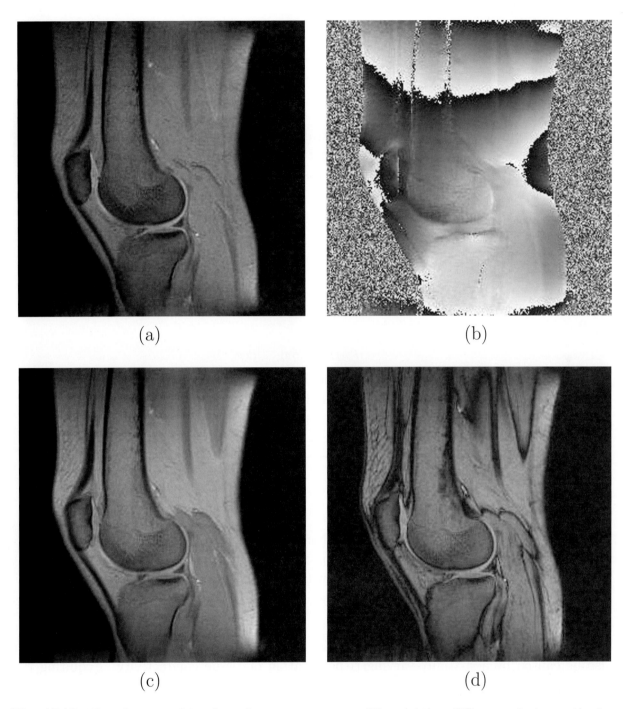

Fig. 17.18: Use of a second in-phase image to overcome T_2^*-weighting differences between the in-phase and opposed-phase images of Fig. 17.17. (a) Second in-phase magnitude image obtained at a T_E of 9 ms, and (b) corresponding phase image. (c) The averaged magnitude image obtained from the two in-phase images. (d) The opposed-phase magnitude image, shown again for comparison purposes. Images (c) and (d) can be used to obtain separate water and fat images using the two-point complex separation method. The in-phase phase image (b) shows some rapid and significant variation behind the knee and in the upper and lower regions of the FOV. The former is caused by the knee itself, the latter can be corrected for, if the background static field variation is known.

Problem 17.13

Assuming perfect magnetic field conditions, if two gradient echo images are collected at different echo times, the resultant magnitude images can be reworked to give a water image and a fat image.

a) To eliminate the effects of any overall phase or systematic errors, magnitude images are often used. Suppose two magnitude images are collected at $T_{E,in}(n)$ and $T_{E,op}(n)$. Write expressions for $|\hat{\rho}_{in}|$ and $|\hat{\rho}_{op}|$ in terms of $\hat{\rho}_{w,m}$ and $\hat{\rho}_{f,m}$.

b) As a naive approach, it is quite possible to attempt to separate water and fat from the magnitude images using the same sum and difference approach applied to a pair of in-phase and opposed-phase images. What do the sum

$$\hat{\rho}_{sum} \equiv |\hat{\rho}_{in}| + |\hat{\rho}_{op}|$$

and the difference

$$\hat{\rho}_{diff} \equiv |\hat{\rho}_{in}| - |\hat{\rho}_{op}|$$

of these two magnitude images yield? Specifically, show that when it is not known whether $\hat{\rho}_{f,m}$ or $\hat{\rho}_{w,m}$ is the larger of the two, there is an ambiguity as to which image, $\hat{\rho}_{sum}$ or $\hat{\rho}_{diff}$, represents fat or water.

17.3.5   Three-Point Separation

In practice, the static field is not perfectly homogeneous, and this can lead to a reversal of water/fat roles again as in the magnitude approach, even for the complex method. Assuming that both water and fat are reconstructed within a voxel and experience the same ϕ_0 and ΔB, then

$$\hat{\rho} = (\hat{\rho}_{w,m} + \hat{\rho}_{f,m} e^{-i\Delta\omega_{fw}T_E}) e^{i\gamma\Delta B T_E} e^{i\phi_0} \tag{17.27}$$

where ϕ_0 is the contribution from an arbitrary global phase shift affecting all voxels and can also be caused by a spatially-varying rf penetration or tissue conductivity. Acquiring two in-phase scans $(\hat{\rho}_{in}(n), \hat{\rho}_{in}(n+1))$ and one opposed-phase scan $(\hat{\rho}_{op}(n))$ makes it possible to find $\hat{\rho}_{w,m}, \hat{\rho}_{f,m}, \Delta B_0$, and ϕ_0. Recall that $\hat{\rho}(x)$ is complex and can be written as

$$\hat{\rho}(x) = |\hat{\rho}(x)| e^{i\phi(x)} \tag{17.28}$$

To avoid the fat's confounding effect on phase, ΔB is determined via the two in-phase images

$$
\begin{aligned}
\phi_{in}(n+1) - \phi_{in}(n) &= -(\gamma\Delta B T_{E,in}(n+1) - \phi_0) + (\gamma\Delta B T_{E,in}(n) - \phi_0) \\
&= -\gamma\Delta B (T_{E,in}(n+1) - T_{E,in}(n)) \tag{17.29}
\end{aligned}
$$

and ϕ_0 from

$$\phi_0 = \phi_{in}(n) + \gamma \Delta B T_{E,in}(n) \qquad (17.30)$$

The next step is to correct the out-of-phase complex image for ϕ_0 and ΔB effects by multiplying $\hat{\rho}_{op}$ by $e^{-i\phi_0 + i\gamma \Delta B T_{E,op}(n)}$ using ϕ_0 and ΔB from (17.29) and (17.30), respectively, and also averaging the magnitude images $\hat{\rho}_{in}(n)$ and $\hat{\rho}_{in}(n+1)$ to get the same effective T_2^* decay as $\hat{\rho}_{op}$

$$\hat{\rho}'_{in} = \frac{1}{2}(|\hat{\rho}_{in}(n)| + |\hat{\rho}_{in}(n+1)|) \qquad (17.31)$$

$$\hat{\rho}'_{op} = \hat{\rho}_{op} e^{-i\phi_0 + i\gamma \Delta B T_{E,op}(n)} \qquad (17.32)$$

In principle, the resulting image $\hat{\rho}'_{op}$ is a real image (however, a magnitude operation still causes a loss of sign, so complex notation should be maintained) and finally

$$\hat{\rho}_{w,m} = \frac{1}{2}(\hat{\rho}'_{in} + \hat{\rho}'_{op}) \qquad (17.33)$$

$$\hat{\rho}_{f,m} = \frac{1}{2}(\hat{\rho}'_{in} - \hat{\rho}'_{op}) \qquad (17.34)$$

The same data used in Fig. 17.17 through Fig. 17.19 are used in this example. The necessary phase images for processing the data are shown in Figs. 17.20a, 17.20b, 17.20c and the resulting ϕ_0 and $\phi_{\Delta B}$ images in Fig. 17.20d and Fig. 17.21a, respectively. The corrected opposed phase image is shown in Fig. 17.21b. Using (17.33) and (17.34), the final water and fat images, corrected for field inhomogeneity effects, are obtained in Figs. 17.21c and 17.21d. As expected, the mixture of water and fat signal behind the knee evident in Fig. 17.19c is gone in Fig. 17.21c.

Problem 17.14

You are interested in quantifying the amount of water and fat in a given voxel, perhaps in bone marrow, for example. You incorrectly judge the first in-phase time to be 4.5 ms instead of 4.67 ms, and all your other times are now appropriate multiples of 4.5 ms rather than 4.67 ms. (Unfortunately, fat in different parts of the body has a variable chemical shift making quantification with a given set of three echoes tenuous unless the chemical shift is known.) Assume $B_0 = 1.5$ T. Take the fat signal fraction to be 80% and water signal fraction to be 20% in a given voxel.

a) Calculate the chemical shift corresponding to an in-phase echo time of 4.5 ms.

b) Neglecting field inhomogeneity effects and T_2^* differences between the tissues, find $\hat{\rho}_{w,m}$ using 4.5 ms as the in-phase image and 6.75 ms as the opposed-phase image.

c) How big is this error relative to the expected value of 80%?

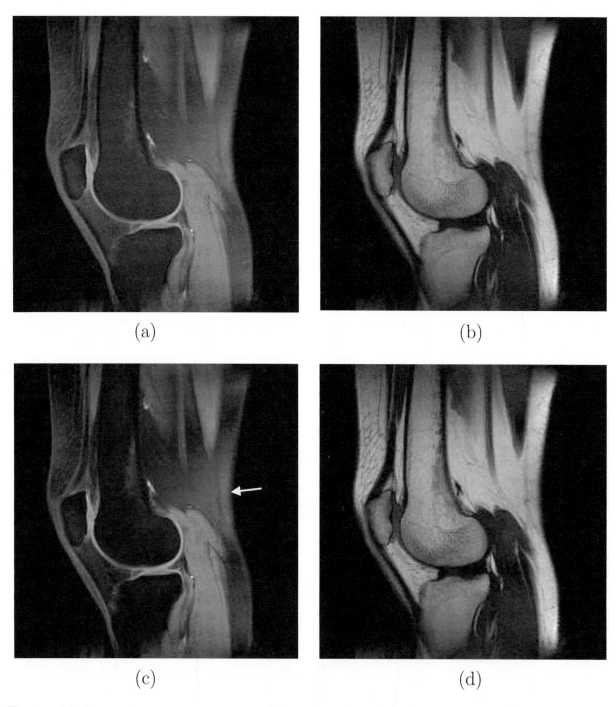

(a)   (b)

(c)   (d)

Fig. 17.19: Two-point water/fat separated images with and without correction for differences in T_2^* weighting. (a) Water image and (b) fat image obtained without correction. (c) Water image and (d) fat image obtained with correction. Artifacts (see arrow) still exist behind the knee caused by the presence of field inhomogeneities (methods of dealing with these are discussed in Sec. 17.3.5).

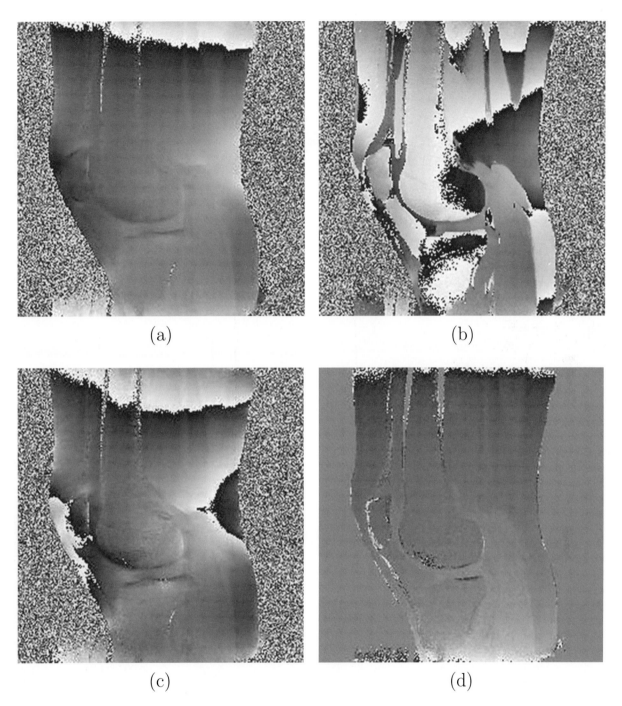

(a)

(b)

(c)

(d)

Fig. 17.20: Different steps involved in the three-point water/fat separation method using gradient echo images. Here, the separation of the different components of the T_E-independent phase difference ϕ_0 is detailed. First, the global, spatially linearly-varying phase due to non-centering of the echo in either direction is determined. Following the removal of this global phase shift, the spatially-variant but still T_E-invariant ϕ_0 phase variation can be determined. Parts (a), (b), and (c) show the echo shifted phase images for the first in-phase image, the opposed-phase image and the second in-phase image, respectively. Part (d) shows the extracted ϕ_0 contribution. Evidently, water and fat have consistently different values of ϕ_0, probably caused by their differences in conductivity.

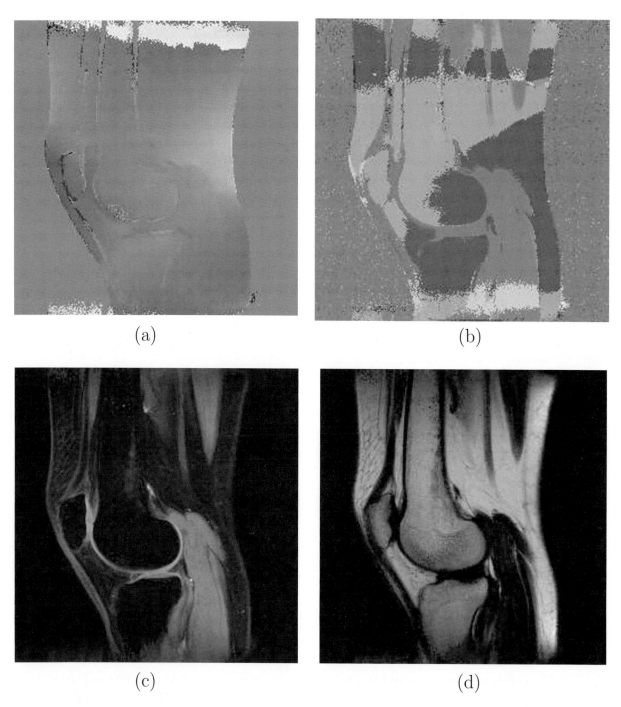

(a)

(b)

(c)

(d)

Fig. 17.21: Remaining steps in the three-point water/fat separation method involve: (a) determination of $\phi_{\Delta B}$, and (b) the correction of the opposed-phase phase image. (c) The water image, and (d) fat image obtained by applying the two-point complex separation method to $\hat{\rho}'_{in}$ and $\hat{\rho}'_{op}$. Local field corrections have successfully removed the artifact behind the knee.

Suggested Reading

Chemical shift imaging was independently introduced in the following three papers:

- T. R. Brown, B. M. Kincaid and K. Ugurbil. NMR chemical shift imaging in three dimensions. *Proc. Natl. Acad. Sci.*, 79: 3523, 1982.

- I. L. Pykett and B. R. Rosen. Nuclear magnetic resonance: *in vivo* proton chemical shift imaging. *Radiology*, 149: 197, 1983.

- R. E. Sepponen, J. T. Sipponen and J. I. Tanttu. A method for chemical shift imaging: demonstration of bone marrow involvement with proton chemical shift imaging. *J. Comput. Assist. Tomogr.*, 8: 58, 1984.

An early two-point chemical shift water/fat separation concept was presented in:

- W. T. Dixon. Simple proton spectroscopic imaging. *Radiology*, 153: 189, 1984.

A review of fat saturation and chemical shift effects appear in:

- E. M. Haacke, J. L. Patrick, G. W. Lenz and T. Parrish. The separation of water and lipid components in the presence of field inhomogeneities. *Rev. Magn. Reson. Med.*, 1: 123, 1986.

Chapter 18

Fast Imaging in the Steady State

Chapter Contents

Summary: This chapter contains an in-depth discussion of the signal behavior when T_R becomes on the order of T_1 and/or T_2. The concepts of incoherent and coherent steady-state signals are discussed, the former leading to a spin density-weighted or T_1-weighted image and the latter a (T_1/T_2)-weighted image. Radiofrequency (rf) spoiling is introduced to show how the steady-state transverse magnetization can be made zero prior to each new rf pulse even if T_R is less than T_2.

Introduction

Fast imaging is perhaps one of the most interesting areas of MRI. Here, and in the next chapter, the foundation for certain basic approaches is laid out, including both short-T_R imaging and echo planar imaging methods. It is intriguing that the limits of continuous rf scanning (which was how the experiments in the early days of NMR were done) are being approached again as repetition times (T_R values) become shorter and shorter. In this chapter, the focus is on understanding the build-up of the magnetization to steady-state and the practical implementation of the simplest forms of imaging in the steady-state. Although it is possible to implement short-T_R spin echo or arbitrary multiple pulse steady-state imaging sequences as well, this chapter focuses on the steady-state built up from conventional, single echo, gradient echo methods.

When a spin system is repeatedly disturbed by a fast repetition of rf pulses and the transverse magnetization available just before each rf pulse is purposefully made zero, the transverse magnetization after each new rf pulse approaches a steady-state value which is

447

smaller than the thermal equilibrium value. The spin system takes a finite number of pulses before this steady-state is reached in a time that depends on both the T_1 of the tissue and the flip angle of the rf pulse.

Sequences utilizing a steady-state approach can be broadly classified as steady-state coherent (SSC) and steady-state incoherent (SSI) sequences. The main difference between the two lies in whether or not the transverse magnetization is allowed to go naturally to steady-state between successive rf pulses. As the nomenclature suggests, the SSI sequences are based on the elimination, or the 'spoiling,' of any remnant transverse magnetization prior to the occurrence of each new rf pulse. On the other hand, in SSC sequences, both transverse and longitudinal magnetization components at the end of a repetition period contribute to the signal in the next cycle, leading to a different magnetization response.

The first two sections in the chapter are dedicated to detailed derivations of expressions for the steady-state magnetization components and their approach to steady-state equilibrium. The final two sections focus on the formation of echoes with multiple rf pulses and their elimination. These discussions lead to insights on coherent steady-state signal formation mechanisms and the understanding of the effectiveness of practical implementations of spoiling.

18.1   Short-T_R, Spoiled, Gradient Echo Imaging

Before an expression for the signal in the spoiled steady-state is obtained, it is worthwhile to see how the signal reaches a steady-state from its initial thermal equilibrium value. For a spin system initially at thermal equilibrium, the longitudinal magnetization is M_0. Let this spin system be acted on by a series of identical rf pulses of flip angle θ. After the first rf pulse, the longitudinal magnetization is given by

$$M_z(0^+) = M_0 \cos\theta \tag{18.1}$$

and the transverse magnetization by

$$M_\perp(0^+) = M_0 \sin\theta \tag{18.2}$$

Between the first and second rf pulses, the longitudinal magnetization grows from the initial value $M_z(0^+)$ toward M_0 according to the Bloch equations (4.21). The longitudinal component has not necessarily reached its thermal equilibrium value by the time of the second rf pulse. At the same time, suppose that the transverse magnetization has been destroyed by some means, a discussion of which is presented in a later section on spoiling mechanisms. $M_z(T_R^-)$ is again transformed into longitudinal and transverse components by the second rf pulse, and this process continues.

After a sufficient number of cycles, the process reaches a steady-state defined by a recurrence of the same magnetization values and identical behavior in each rf cycle. This process is illustrated for one cycle in the steady-state for an arbitrary θ-pulse in Fig. 18.1a. In this steady-state limit, the magnetization is periodic with period T_R. The steady-state values are reached when the loss in longitudinal magnetization due to its tipping by the rf pulse is exactly counterbalanced by its growth due to T_1 recovery during the inter-pulse period. In general, there is an initial transient behavior before the magnetization settles into this periodicity. Notice from Fig. 18.1b that the magnetization reaches steady-state after the second pulse when $\theta = \pi/2$. In general, the number of pulses required to reach steady-state is a function of the flip angle and T_R. The process of achieving steady-state and the dependence on the number of pulses required to reach steady-state are described in detail in Secs. 18.1.1 and 18.1.3.

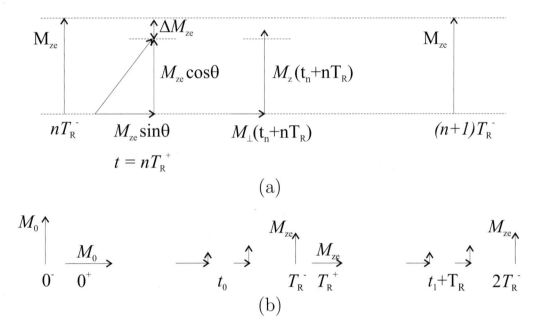

(a)

(b)

Fig. 18.1: Evolution of the magnetization components at successive rf pulse cycles (a) for an arbitrary flip angle θ and one steady-state rf cycle, and (b) for $\theta = \pi/2$ and the first two rf cycles. The evolution in (a) begins at time $t = nT_R^-$ where only the steady-state magnetization M_{ze} is available. The application of a θ rf pulse at $t = nT_R$ creates a new transverse magnetization component $M_{ze}\sin\theta$ while leaving behind longitudinal magnetization $M_{ze}\cos\theta$. The difference between the longitudinal magnetization before and after the rf pulse is represented by ΔM_{ze}. Between the $(n+1)^{st}$ and the $(n+2)^{nd}$ rf pulse, the longitudinal magnetization starts regrowing towards M_0 by T_1 relaxation and the transverse component starts decaying towards zero due to T_2 relaxation. This is depicted by the components $M_z(t_n + nT_R)$ (lengthened) and $M_\perp(t_n + nT_R)$ (shortened in length). The evolution in (b) shows that, when $\theta = \pi/2$, it takes only two rf pulses for the magnetization to reach steady-state. This occurs because each 90°-pulse tips all longitudinal magnetization, and it recovers to the same value $M_0(1 - e^{-T_R/T_1})$ during each subsequent period. For the first rf cycle alone, the initial magnetization is M_0; hence it takes two rf cycles to reach steady-state.

18.1.1   Expression for the Steady-State Incoherent (SSI) Signal

We begin with the simplest concepts that describe short-T_R steady-state incoherent imaging.[1] Consider a gradient echo sequence where $T_R \gg T_2$. This is the situation where $M_\perp(nT_R^-) = 0$, where $t = nT_R$ is the instant of occurrence of the $(n+1)^{st}$ rf pulse. This is a naturally spoiled sequence where all transverse magnetization is essentially zero before the next rf pulse. We wish to find a solution to the steady-state longitudinal magnetization for a given isochromat, for given values of T_1, T_2, T_R, and flip angle θ.[2] The following analysis is valid for an isochromat of spins where there are no T_2^* effects. The macroscopic spin phase effects will be considered after the equilibrium conditions are derived.

The transverse magnetization decays during each evolution period according to (4.32)

$$M_\perp(t_n) = M_\perp(0^+)e^{-t_n/T_2} \qquad 0 < t_n < T_R \tag{18.3}$$

where $M_\perp(0^+)$ is a shorthand notation for $M_\perp(t_n = 0^+)$. The total time from the first pulse is t, and the relative time within each cycle is defined as

$$t_n \equiv t - nT_R \tag{18.4}$$

The regrowth of longitudinal magnetization during this period is

$$M_z(t_n) = M_0(1 - e^{-t_n/T_1}) + M_z(0^-)e^{-t_n/T_1} \tag{18.5}$$

where $M_z(0^-)$ is shorthand notation for $M_z(t_n = 0^-)$. Equations (18.3) and (18.5) can be rewritten by reintroducing the total time:

$$\begin{aligned} M_\perp((n+1)T_R^-) &= M_\perp(nT_R^+)E_2 \\ &= M_z(nT_R^-)\sin\theta E_2 \end{aligned} \tag{18.6}$$

which goes to zero as E_2 goes to zeros and, under these circumstances,

$$M_z((n+1)T_R^-) = M_z(nT_R^-)\cos\theta E_1 + M_0(1 - E_1) \tag{18.7}$$

where E_1 and E_2 are defined by

$$E_1 \equiv e^{-T_R/T_1} \tag{18.8}$$

and

$$E_2 \equiv e^{-T_R/T_2} \tag{18.9}$$

for convenience.

The attainment of the steady-state by the time of the Nth pulse implies that the value of M_z just prior to each subsequent rf pulse is unchanged from cycle to cycle. Define the steady-state equilibrium value of M_z to be M_{ze} so that

$$M_z(mT_R^-) = M_{ze} \qquad m \geq N \tag{18.10}$$

---

[1] These imaging methods are often referred to as FLASH (Fast Low Angle SHot) or spoiled GRASS (Gradient Refocused Acquisition in the Steady-State). We have been reticent to use acronyms in this text but these two are in common usage. In the nomenclature introduced here, they are referred to as short-T_R SSI gradient echo methods.

[2] When the isochromat is replaced by a voxel, T_2 must be replaced by T_2^* for gradient echo imaging.

From (18.7) and (18.10), M_{ze} must satisfy

$$M_{ze} = M_{ze} E_1 \cos\theta + M_0(1 - E_1) \tag{18.11}$$

This yields the steady-state or equilibrium value

$$M_{ze} = \frac{M_0(1 - E_1)}{(1 - E_1 \cos\theta)} \tag{18.12}$$

Plugging in this result into (18.3) gives

$$M_\perp(\theta, t_n) = M_{ze} \sin\theta e^{-t_n/T_2} = \frac{M_0 \sin\theta(1 - E_1)}{(1 - E_1 \cos\theta)} e^{-t_n/T_2} \qquad 0 < t_n < T_R \tag{18.13}$$

under steady-state equilibrium.

   The only changes in (18.13) needed to represent the steady-state signal from a voxel containing several isochromats are the replacements of M_0 by ρ_0 (the voxel spin density) and T_2 by T_2^*. Hence,

$$\hat{\rho}(\theta, T_E) = \rho_0 \sin\theta \frac{(1 - E_1)}{(1 - E_1 \cos\theta)} e^{-T_E/T_2^*} \tag{18.14}$$

Figure 18.2 shows the general behavior of $\hat{\rho}$ as a function of θ for both white matter (WM) and gray matter (GM).[3] The maximum signal occurs for an intermediate angle (less than $\pi/2$) defined as the *Ernst angle* θ_E. The Ernst angle is the subject of Prob. 18.2 and is given in (18.15). Note that (18.14) vanishes at $\theta = 0$ due to the $\sin\theta$ factor (the E_1 dependence cancels out in this limit). But the E_1 dependence in the numerator is not canceled for larger angles, and yields an approximate suppression factor T_R/T_1 for small T_R. In fact, when $\theta = 90°$, the signal is directly proportional to T_R/T_1, as illustrated in Fig. 18.2b.

Problem 18.1

---

a) Plot $\hat{\rho}(\theta, T_E = 0)$ versus θ for $0 \le \theta \le \pi$, with $T_R = 40\,\text{ms}$, for CSF (cerebrospinal fluid), WM, GM, and fatty tissue. Estimates for the associated relative spin density, T_1, and T_2 values at 1.5 T are given in Table 18.1.

b) Show that the crossover point for GM/WM signal plots occurs for $\theta \simeq 17°$ when $T_E = 0$.

---

[3]The gray matter of the cortex of the brain contains the cell bodies of the neurons. The white matter includes the axons which serve as the communication routes from these neurons to other neurons. The neurons are the source of electrical impulses controlling brain and bodily function.

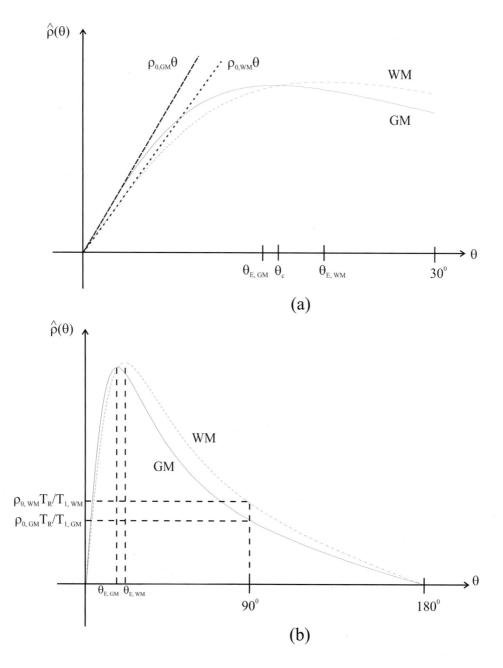

Fig. 18.2: Comparison of the SSI signal behavior of gray matter (GM) and white matter (WM) for the representative values of $T_R = 40\,\mathrm{ms}$ and $T_E = 0\,\mathrm{ms}$. (a) Small flip angle signal behavior. The angles $\theta_{E,\mathrm{GM}}$ and $\theta_{E,\mathrm{WM}}$ denote the Ernst angles of GM and WM, respectively, and θ_c denotes the flip angle at which the two curves cross each other (i.e., the crossover point). (b) SSI signal behavior for the range $0 \leq \theta \leq \pi$.

Tissue	ρ_0	T_1 (ms)	T_2 (ms)
CSF	1.0	4500	2200
WM	0.65	600	80
GM	0.8	950	100
fatty tissue	0.9	250	60

Table 18.1: Estimated NMR properties of cerebrospinal fluid (CSF), WM, GM, and fatty tissue at 1.5 T. Here, ρ_0 is the spin density relative to CSF.

Problem 18.2

a) Show that the maximum SSI signal occurs at the Ernst angle

$$\theta = \cos^{-1} E_1 \equiv \theta_E \qquad (18.15)$$

b) For $T_R \ll T_1$, show that

$$\theta_E \simeq \sqrt{\frac{2T_R}{T_1}} \qquad (18.16)$$

in radians, and

$$M_\perp(\theta_E) = M_0 \sqrt{\frac{(1 - E_1)}{(1 + E_1)}} \simeq M_0 \sqrt{\frac{T_R}{2T_1}} \qquad (18.17)$$

Hence, show that

$$M_\perp(\theta_E) \simeq \frac{1}{2} M_0 \theta_E \qquad (18.18)$$

where θ_E is in radians.

An interesting feature of the SSI sequence is that it is possible to obtain spin-density weighting even for small T_R values ($T_R \ll T_1$). In the low flip angle, short-T_R limit, the SSI signal will be seen to be linearly proportional to ρ_0 and θ, and independent of T_1 and T_2. The linear relationship to flip angle is shown in the plots of Fig. 18.2a. Further, note that the slope is lower for WM which has a lower relative spin density as shown in Table 18.1.

At low flip angles, the expression for $\hat{\rho}$ can be approximated by

$$\hat{\rho}(\theta) \simeq \frac{\rho_0(1 - E_1)\theta}{1 - E_1\left(1 - \frac{\theta^2}{2}\right)} = \frac{\rho_0\theta}{\left(1 + \frac{1}{2}\frac{E_1}{(1-E_1)}\theta^2\right)} \qquad \theta \ll \theta_E \qquad (18.19)$$

If, in addition, $T_R \ll T_1$, the spin density (18.19) can be further approximated by

$$\hat{\rho}(\theta) \simeq \frac{\rho_0\theta}{1 + \left(\frac{T_1}{2T_R}\right)\theta^2} \simeq \frac{\rho_0\theta}{1 + \left(\frac{\theta}{\theta_E}\right)^2} \qquad (18.20)$$

The last approximation comes from the short-T_R result for θ_E obtained in Prob. 18.2b. It is observed in (18.20), that the low flip angle linear approximation is valid to within roughly 1% as long as θ is less than a third of θ_E or so since the nonlinear corrections are second-order in θ/θ_E.

Other features of practical interest are the zero crossing of the SSI signal for all tissues when the flip angle equals 180° and the achievement of T_1-weighted contrast (suppression of long T_1 tissues) past the Ernst angle. This latter feature is seen in Fig. 18.2b where WM has a higher signal than GM (GM has a longer T_1 value; see Table 18.1) for flip angles greater than $\theta_{E,\text{WM}}$. The contrast stays approximately constant past the Ernst angle, a feature which is utilized to obtain T_1-weighted contrast at flip angles much lower than 90°. The important features of SSI signal behavior are demonstrated in the images shown in Fig. 18.3. For $T_R = 20$ ms, $\theta_{E,\text{CSF}} \simeq 5°$, $\theta_{E,\text{GM}} \simeq 12°$, $\theta_{E,\text{WM}} \simeq 15°$, and $\theta_{E,\text{fat}} \simeq 23°$. With these conditions, it is expected that CSF will have the highest signal (highest ρ_0) in a $\theta = 2°$ image, while WM will have the lowest signal as seen in Fig. 18.3a. WM and GM have a signal crossover for $\theta = 10°$, yielding no WM/GM contrast while CSF is T_1-weighted, leading to a heavy suppression of its signal (Fig. 18.3b). For $\theta = 20°$, good T_1-weighted contrast is obtained between GM and WM. CSF is suppressed further and fat now has the highest signal (Fig. 18.3c), all the necessary characteristics of a T_1-weighted image as discussed in Ch. 15. These findings are further illustrated in the plots of the voxel signal as a function of flip angle for these four tissues in Fig. 18.3d.

Problem 18.3

a) Show that from (18.14), (18.20) is more appropriately written as

$$\hat{\rho}(\theta) \approx \rho_0 \theta \frac{(1 - \theta^2/6)}{(1 + (\theta/\theta_E)^2)} \tag{18.21}$$

b) Compare the signal $\hat{\rho}(\theta)/\hat{\rho}(\theta_E)$ when $\theta = \theta_E/3$ using (18.21). What is the fractional loss in signal that occurs with this reduction in flip angle?

c) Consider the case when $T_R = 20$ ms and $T_1 = 1000$ ms. Use (18.16) to estimate θ_E. Use this estimate in (18.21) to find $\hat{\rho}(\theta)/\hat{\rho}(\theta_E)$ when $\theta = \theta_E/3$. Also use the exact form (18.14) to find $\hat{\rho}(\theta)/\hat{\rho}(\theta_E)$ when $\theta = \theta_E/3$. How close is the estimate to the exact value?

Matrix Formulation of Signal Behavior

It is useful to repeat the steady-state analysis of the magnetization in terms of matrices. Let

$$\vec{M}(nT_R^\pm) = \begin{pmatrix} M_x(nT_R^\pm) \\ M_y(nT_R^\pm) \\ M_z(nT_R^\pm) \end{pmatrix} \tag{18.22}$$

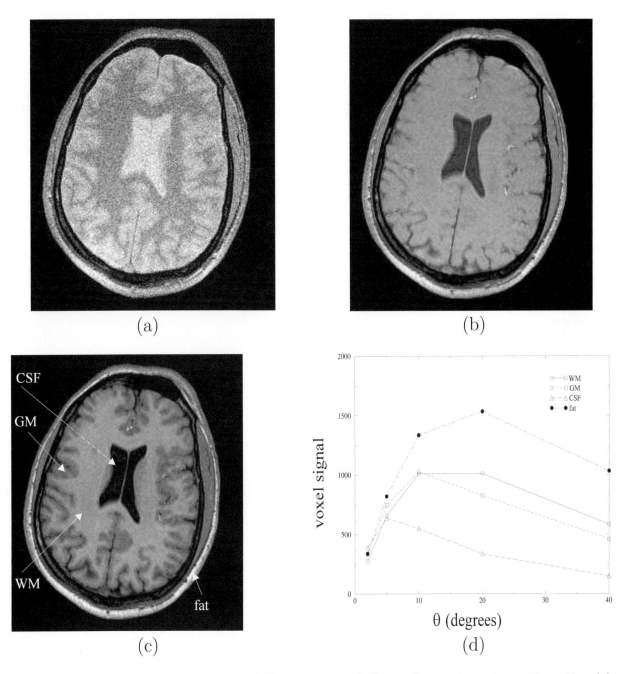

Fig. 18.3: Images obtained with a 3D SSI sequence at different flip angles using a 20 ms T_R. (a) Image for $\theta = 2°$ is spin density-weighted: CSF is the brightest, GM is intermediate, and WM has the lowest signal. (b) Image for $\theta = 10°$ shows the effect due to the crossover between the GM and WM signal curves; note the absence of GM/WM contrast. (c) Image for $\theta = 20°$ is T_1-weighted; the appearance is reversed from that of the spin density-weighted image. (d) The measured image signal $\hat{\rho}$ in arbitrary units as a function of flip angle θ from this data set.

where the time argument is the total time t. Reverting to relative time $t' = t - nT_R$, the Bloch equations with relaxation terms included, (4.22) to (4.24), have the solution

$$\vec{M}_n(t') = D(t')R_x(\theta)\vec{M}_n(0^-) + M_0(1 - E_1)\hat{z} \qquad (18.23)$$

for an on-resonance isochromat. In (18.23),

$$D(t') \equiv \begin{pmatrix} e^{-t'/T_2} & 0 & 0 \\ 0 & e^{-t'/T_2} & 0 \\ 0 & 0 & e^{-t'/T_1} \end{pmatrix} \qquad (18.24)$$

and

$$R_x(\theta) \equiv \begin{pmatrix} 1 & 0 & 0 \\ 0 & \cos\theta & \sin\theta \\ 0 & -\sin\theta & \cos\theta \end{pmatrix} \qquad (18.25)$$

It is recalled from Ch. 2 that $R_x(\theta)$ implies a clockwise rotation through an angle θ about the x-axis. At equilibrium,

$$\vec{M}_{n+1}(0^-) \equiv \vec{M}_n(T_R^-) = \vec{M}_n(0^-) \qquad (18.26)$$

The use of (18.26) in (18.23) gives

$$\vec{M}_n(0^-) = (I - D(T_R)R_x(\theta))^{-1}M_0(1 - E_1)\hat{z} \qquad (18.27)$$

where I is the identity matrix. In the instance when $E_2 \to 0$ (when $T_R \gg T_2$), (18.12) is recovered. If $E_2 \neq 0$, the magnetization behavior is a rather complicated function of T_1 and T_2. An expression for the signal in the coherent steady-state case will be obtained in due course.

Incoherent steady-state methods commonly use T_R values which are short enough that natural spoiling does not occur. These implementations use transverse magnetization spoiling mechanisms which require the knowledge of steady-state free precession. A detailed discussion of these modern implementations is contained in the final section of this chapter. For the time being, it is assumed that spoiling is achieved prior to each new rf pulse even in the short-T_R case, without asking how it is done.

18.1.2   Contrast-to-noise efficiency for small changes in T_1

As illustrated in Fig. 18.3, choosing the right sequence parameters is important for generating good contrast between the tissues of interest. Let us consider the simple case of optimizing the contrast between two different tissues with the same spin density, or between two different acquisition times (say, with and without contrast agent) for the same tissue. Assume these two tissues, or these two different times for the same tissue, are associated with only slightly different values for the longitudinal relaxation time. In the following discussion, let T_1 refer to the first tissue, or the initial value for the same tissue, and $T_1 \pm \delta T_1$ refer to the second tissue, or the later value for the same tissue. (We will often refer to T_1 as the 'initial value.') Contrast-to-noise in either case is calculated (see Sec. 15.3) according to

$$\text{CNR}(\theta) = \frac{\rho(\theta, T_1) - \rho(\theta, T_1 \pm \delta T_1)}{\sigma_0} \qquad (18.28)$$

where the noise σ_0 is taken to be the same throughout. For small δT_1, the first-order expansion of (18.28) for the steady-state case (18.14) yields (see Prob. 18.4)

$$\text{CNR}(\theta) = \frac{\rho_0 E_1 \delta T_1 T_R \sin\theta(1 - \cos\theta)}{\sigma_0 T_1^2 (1 - E_1 \cos\theta)^2}, \qquad \delta T_1 \ll T_1 \qquad (18.29)$$

The flip angle θ_c corresponds to the optimal contrast (the flip angle yielding a maximum of the previous expression) and is given by

$$\cos\theta_c = \frac{2E_1 - 1}{2 - E_1} \qquad (18.30)$$

For small repeat times such that $T_R \ll T_1$, we have

$$\cos\theta_c \simeq 1 - \frac{3T_R}{T_1} \qquad (18.31)$$

or (if $3T_R \ll T_1$)

$$\theta_c \simeq \sqrt{\frac{6T_R}{T_1}} \qquad (18.32)$$

With (18.16), a quick rule of thumb for short T_R is therefore

$$\theta_c \simeq \sqrt{3}\theta_E \qquad (18.33)$$

A more important quantity to consider in a typical clinical setting, where total magnet time is precious, is the contrast-to-noise efficiency for a fixed imaging time (see Sec. 15.2.5). The question then arises: 'How should the data be collected?' The data can be collected with a long T_R, call it $T_{R,max}$ (usually used in 2D gradient echo sequences) or with a shorter T_R (usually used in 3D gradient echo sequences) but with the constraint that $T_R N_{acq} = T_{R,max}$. Under either of these conditions and the limits $T_R \ll T_1$ and $\delta T_1/T_1 \ll 1$, the optimal contrast-to-noise ratio is (Prob. 18.4)

$$\text{CNR} \simeq \frac{3}{8}\sqrt{\frac{3}{2}}\frac{\rho_0}{\sigma_0}\frac{\delta T_1}{T_1}\sqrt{\frac{T_{R,max}}{T_1}} \qquad (18.34)$$

or

$$\text{CNR}(\theta_c) \simeq \left(\frac{3}{16}\frac{\rho_0}{\sigma_0}\frac{\delta T_1}{T_1}\sqrt{N_{acq}}\right)\theta_c \qquad (18.35)$$

Hence, for fixed total imaging time (i.e., for a fixed $T_R N_{acq} = $ constant), the CNR efficiency per unit time, $\text{CNR}/\sqrt{\text{imaging time}}$, is a constant. Figure 18.4a shows the plot of maximum CNR versus $\delta T_1/T_1$ (calculated for general δT_1 by going back to (18.28) and optimizing once again, see (18.4)) for the initial T_1 values of 600 ms and 1500 ms, for a T_R of 20 ms. The change in δT_1 is taken to reduce the initial T_1. As expected, for small δT_1, the contrast is linear and directly proportional to the fractional change in T_1 and the slope is proportional to $1/\sqrt{T_1}$.

Problem 18.4

---

a) Derive (18.29) and (18.30).

b) We are interested in the comparison of the general CNR calculated from (18.28), as a function of flip angle, with the small δT_1 approximation in (18.29). See (18.4a). Show, by plotting CNR versus flip angle, that we get better contrast by replacing initial T_1 with $\overline{T_1} = (T_{1,initial} + T_{1,final})/2$ in (18.29). Assume a T_R of 20 ms, $\rho_0 = 100$, and $\sigma_0 = 1$ and consider a range of values for the fractional change in the initial T_1 given by $\delta T_1/T_1 = 0.1$, 0.2, and 0.3.

c) Ignoring the T_2 component, show that the flip angle for optimal contrast between two tissues with the same spin densities and with $T_1 = T_{1a}$ and $T_1 = T_{1b}$, respectively, is given by

$$\theta_C = \cos^{-1}\left(\frac{-2E_aE_b + E_a + E_b - 2 \pm \sqrt{-3E_a^2 - 3E_b^2 + 4E_a^2E_b^2 - 2E_aE_b + 4}}{2(E_aE_b - E_a - E_b)}\right)$$

(18.36)

where $E_a \equiv e^{-T_R/T_{1a}}$ and $E_b \equiv e^{-T_R/T_{1b}}$.

d) Derive the approximate optimal CNR expression given by (18.34) from (18.29).

In general, even when T_R is on the order of T_1, shortening T_R is compensated by averaging over N_{acq} acquisitions where $N_{acq} = T_{R,max}/T_R$. In this case a factor of $\sqrt{N_{acq}}$ in CNR is recovered despite the loss in CNR due to the reduced optimal flip angle (see Fig. 18.4b). The amount of gain in CNR when considering a long-T_R 2D scan versus a short-T_R 3D scan depends on the relative magnitudes of T_R, $T_{R,max}$, the initial T_1, and δT_1. Note that if the experimental parameters, T_R, T_E, slice thickness, and flip angle, are kept the same between a 2D and a 3D scan, the number of partitions acquired in the 3D scan, N_z, is equivalent to N_z averages; that is, we achieve a $\sqrt{N_z}$ gain in the voxel SNR and hence the same gain in CNR (see Sec. 15.2.4). Figure 18.4 shows the optimal (normalized) CNR as function of T_R (Fig. 18.4b) with no averages, and with N_{acq} averages (Fig. 18.4c), for different values of $\delta T_1/T_1$ and for a fixed $T_{R,max} = T_1$. The plots demonstrate that, when considering small changes in T_1, and when the 2D T_R (i.e., $T_{R,max}$) is comparable to the T_1 of the tissue in question, both 2D and 3D imaging perform comparably. For relatively large changes in T_1, and when $T_{R,max} > T_1$ we gain more with N_{acq}-averaged short-T_R 3D scans. Clearly, when $T_{R,max} \ll T_1$ there is basically no gain in going to a 3D scan as opposed to a 2D scan (see Prob. 18.5). However, the short-T_R 3D experiment offers the further advantages of a relatively homogeneous RF profile across the slices, contiguous volume coverage, and higher slice resolution as compared to the long-T_R 2D implementation (see Chs. 10 and 15 for more details).

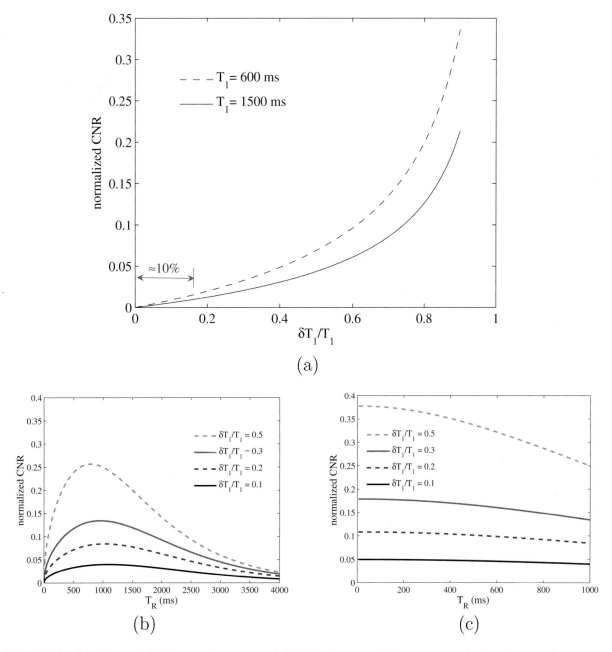

Fig. 18.4: (a) Plot of CNR as a function of $\delta T_1/T_1$ for two different initial T_1 values, 600 ms and 1500 ms. A T_R of 20 ms is assumed and, for simplicity, T_E is set to zero. Note the approximate linearity of the curve (it is within 10% of (18.34) in the region indicated) for small changes in T_1 and the change in slope with the change in initial T_1. (b) Plot of normalized CNR as function of T_R, without $N_{acq} = 1$, for different values of fractional change in T_1. (c) CNR as a function of T_R when collected with $N_{acq} = T_{R,max}/T_R$ for $T_{R,max} = T_1$. In these plots, $T_1 = 1000$ ms, $\sigma_0 = 1$, and $\rho_0 = 1$ have been used and the negative sign has been chosen such that $T_{1,final} = T_{1,initial} - \delta T_1 < T_{1,initial}$.

Problem 18.5

---

a) For small changes $\delta T_1/T_1 \ll 1$, express the optimal CNR as a function of T_R/T_1 and $\delta T_1/T_1$.

b) Using the expression obtained in (a), we can analyze the performance of optimal CNR in a 2D versus a 3D scan. Plot the percent gain in CNR in a short-T_R 3D scan with $N_{acq} = T_{R,max}/T_R$ averages compared to a long-T_R (i.e., $T_{R,max}$) 2D scan, as a function of N_{acq}. Plot the curves for $T_{R,max}/T_1 = 0.1, 0.2, 0.5, 0.7$, and 1.5.

c) Discuss why, even in the limit $T_{R,max} \ll T_1$, it remains preferable to run a 3D scan rather than a 2D scan. Hint: Consider the detrimental bandwidth changes required at very short T_R.

18.1.3   Approach to Incoherent Steady-State

Although equilibrium solutions have been found, the general transient behavior of the magnetization is yet to be evaluated. Some tissues will reach a steady-state equilibrium more quickly than others, depending on their T_1 values. The mathematical description of this approach to steady-state is the goal of this subsection. If the steady-state is reached before data acquisition is started, then there will be no filtering effects in the phase encoding direction. Otherwise, the signal changes from cycle to cycle, and the image quality can suffer. This blurring is reminiscent of the filtering effects in the read direction due to T_2 decay, as discussed in Ch. 13. This is described at the end of the discussion in this subsection.

Let us evaluate how many pulses it takes for a tissue magnetization to approach some fraction of its steady-state value. For convenience, the short-hand notation of $M_z^{\pm}(n)$ is used to denote $M_z(nT_R^{\pm})$. From (18.7), which required that the transverse magnetization just prior to any rf pulse is zero, the longitudinal magnetization at the end of the nth repetition period is given by

$$M_z^-(n) \;=\; M_z^-(n-1)\cos\theta E_1 + M_0(1-E_1) \qquad n \geq 1 \qquad (18.37)$$

A first recursion of this equation in terms of $M_z^-(n-2)$ is

$$M_z^-(n) \;=\; M_z^-(n-2)(\cos\theta E_1)^2 + M_0(1-E_1)\cos\theta E_1 + M_0(1-E_1)$$
$$n \geq 2 \qquad (18.38)$$

Continuing this iteration yields

$$M_z^-(n,\theta) \;=\; \left[\sum_{l=0}^{n-1}(\cos\theta E_1)^l(1-E_1)M_0\right] + M_0(\cos\theta E_1)^n \qquad n \geq 1$$
$$=\; M_0(1-E_1)\frac{(1-(\cos\theta E_1)^n)}{1-\cos\theta E_1} + M_0(\cos\theta E_1)^n \qquad n \geq 1 \qquad (18.39)$$

This expression is most easily evaluated at $\theta = \theta_E$. Using $\cos\theta_E = E_1$ from (18.15), (18.39) becomes

$$M_z^-(n, \theta_E) = M_0 \frac{(1 - E_1^{2n})}{1 + E_1} + M_0 E_1^{2n} \qquad n \geq 1 \tag{18.40}$$

In the new notation, the steady-state value is

$$\lim_{n \to \infty} M_z^-(n, \theta_E) = M_{ze}(\theta_E) = M_0/(1 + E_1) \tag{18.41}$$

The relative error in estimating $M_z^-(n)$ by $M_z^-(\infty)$ at the $(n+1)^{st}$ pulse for the Ernst angle is given by

$$\alpha \equiv \frac{M_z^-(n, \theta_E) - M_{ze}(\theta_E)}{M_{ze}(\theta_E)} = E_1^{2n+1} \tag{18.42}$$

Hence, the number of pulses n_α required to reduce (18.42) to a given α is

$$n_\alpha = \left[-\frac{T_1}{2T_R} \ln\alpha - \frac{1}{2} \right] \tag{18.43}$$

where the square brackets denote the next largest integer of the argument. For the case when $T_R = 40\,\text{ms}$, the approximate values of n_α for $\alpha = 0.01$ and $\alpha = 0.1$ for different tissues are tabulated in Table 18.2. The $T_R = 400\,\text{ms}$ case is tabulated in Table 18.3.

Problem 18.6

Show that $n_\alpha T_R$ for $\alpha = 0.1$ is on the order of the T_1 of the tissue. Assume that $\theta = \theta_E$. Qualitatively argue that this is a reasonable answer. See Fig. 18.5.

	CSF	GM	WM	Fat
$\alpha = 0.01$	250	54	36	16
$\alpha = 0.1$	125	27	18	8

Table 18.2: The pulse number n_α for two α values and different tissues at their respective Ernst angles at 1.5 T when $T_R = 40\,\text{ms}$. See Fig. 18.5a.

	CSF	GM	WM	Fat
$\alpha = 0.01$	26	6	4	2
$\alpha = 0.1$	13	3	2	1

Table 18.3: As in Table 18.2, but for $T_R = 400\,\text{ms}$. See Fig. 18.5b.

The situation in the general θ case is described from (18.39)

$$\begin{aligned} M_z^-(n, \theta) &= M_{ze}(\theta)\left(1 - (E_1\cos\theta)^n\right) + M_0(E_1\cos\theta)^n \\ &= (M_0 - M_{ze}(\theta))(E_1\cos\theta)^n + M_{ze}(\theta) \end{aligned} \tag{18.44}$$

Equation (18.44) describes an exponential decay of $M_z^-(n)$ from M_0 to M_{ze} with a rate determined by the quantity $E_1 \cos\theta$. This means that the approach to steady state is faster if either E_1 or $\cos\theta$ or their product is small. So, shorter T_1 tissues reach steady-state faster as a function of rf pulse number; similarly, all tissues reach steady-state faster for longer T_R values and as θ increases in the range $0 \le \theta \le 90°$.

The plots for magnetization as a function of pulse number n for $\theta = 10°$ are shown for two different T_R values in Fig. 18.5. This figure demonstrates that the steady-state equilibrium longitudinal magnetization can be small compared to the thermal equilibrium value of M_0.

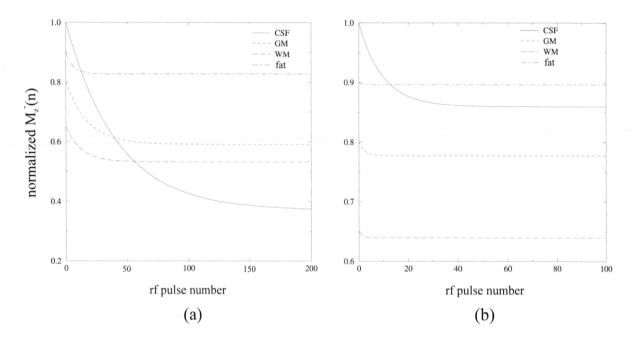

Fig. 18.5: Plot of $M_z^-(n)$ as a function of rf pulse number n for GM, WM, CSF, and fatty tissue at a common flip angle $\theta = 10°$ for (a) $T_R = 40\,\mathrm{ms}$ (b) and $T_R = 400\,\mathrm{ms}$. Note the difference between these data, and Tables 18.2 and 18.3 where the individual Ernst angles are used.

Even though $M_{ze}(\theta_E)$ from tissues with long T_1 values may be small, it is possible to get a rather large signal during the smaller n, pre-steady-state cycles, despite the filtering effect. For example, CSF could appear falsely bright in a T_1-weighted image ($\theta > \theta_E$) if n_α for CSF is greater than the number of phase encoding lines in a 2D scan. Note the small rf pulse number regime in Figs. 18.5a and 18.5b where the CSF signal is much greater than its equilibrium value. To obtain the expected contrast, it is to have reached steady-state before the imaging experiment is carried out. Only after n_α cycles, for $\alpha \ll 1$, can true T_1-weighted data be obtained without filtering effects. This can significantly lengthen the imaging time for a short-T_R 2D scan, but it is less of a problem in a short-T_R 3D scan.

If the k-space data are collected sequentially from $-k_{PE}$ to $+k_{PE}$, a relatively large transient signal does not affect the image very much since the filtering occurs only at high k-space values where the absolute signal is small. In fact, this high pass filtering enhances the edge information in the image and could be quite advantageous in enhancing vessels in MR angiography (see Ch. 24).

Further, by the time the origin of k-space is reached, the signal will generally have reached steady-state and the image contrast is not reversed as in the case briefly discussed in the previous paragraph.

18.1.4 Generating a Constant Transverse Magnetization

Maximizing signal for a fixed T_R by choosing a specific flip angle (the Ernst angle) is important in fast imaging. However, this may not be the most efficient method to obtain high signal if only a limited number of rf pulses is employed to complete the entire imaging experiment.

For short-T_R 2D scans, it is possible to eliminate the filtering effect caused by the variations in magnetization at each new rf pulse during the approach to steady-state equilibrium. Suppose that the transverse magnetization excited by each rf pulse is forced to be equal to that created by the previous rf pulse. That is, the second pulse is designed to return the transverse magnetization to $M_0 \sin \theta_0$, its value after the first pulse. The third pulse is designed to obtain the same transverse magnetization value and so on. By making

$$M_\perp^+(n+1, \theta_{n+1}) = M_\perp^+(n, \theta_n) \tag{18.45}$$

for any n, the filtering effect can be successfully eliminated. Equivalently, the flip angle θ_n is modified from one pulse to the next such that the longitudinal magnetization $M_z^-(n, \theta_n)$ satisfies the condition

$$M_z^-(n+1) \sin \theta_{n+1} = M_z^-(n) \sin \theta_n \tag{18.46}$$

This works as long as (18.46) does not require θ_{n+1} to be larger than $\pi/2$. This results from the fact that if the longitudinal magnetization recovered in a given cycle is less than the desired transverse magnetization, even the maximum rotation of $\pi/2$ is insufficient to recover the correct transverse magnetization. As a result, $\theta_n = \pi/2$ is often used as the terminating condition for this method of producing constant magnetization.

Problem 18.7

From (18.46), show that the longitudinal magnetization just after the nth pulse is $M_0 \sin \theta_0 / \tan \theta_n$ where θ_0 is the starting angle.

a) Using this result, show that

$$E_1 \frac{\sin \theta_0}{\tan \theta_{n-1}} + (1 - E_1) = \frac{\sin \theta_0}{\sin \theta_n} \tag{18.47}$$

Given E_1 and θ_0, this equation can be used to generate θ_n in an iterative fashion.

b) Replicate the result in Fig. 18.6.

The method of changing the flip angle as a function of rf pulse number is typically used in extremely short-T_R 2D SSI imaging applications. A predetermined terminal flip angle is required to occur after a target number of rf pulses p. From the previous problem, it is seen that there is no analytic closed form for θ_n as a function of n. The values for $\{\theta_n\}$ are evaluated numerically; the results of one such simulation are shown in Fig. 18.6.

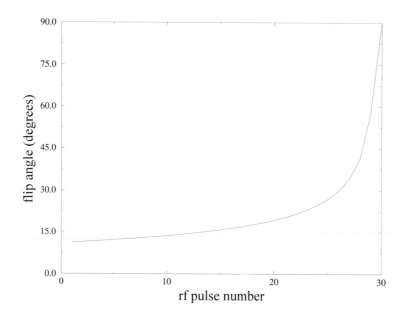

Fig. 18.6: Use of a variable flip angle which increases as a function of rf pulse number in order to force a constant transverse magnetization from one rf pulse to the next. The plot was obtained for a terminal pulse number $p = 30$, with $T_1 = 950\,\text{ms}$ and $T_R = 10\,\text{ms}$.

It is possible to make some general remarks concerning the behavior of θ_n in the above method. Once the spin system is disturbed by the first rf pulse, there is less longitudinal magnetization available for the following rf pulses since T_R is extremely short (see Fig. 18.5). The flip angle must therefore increase with rf pulse number to create a constant transverse magnetization. If θ_0 is too small, the longitudinal magnetization is barely disturbed and almost full magnetization is available for the next pulse(s), and θ_n increases very slowly with n. If the terminal flip angle is 90°, as it is in most 2D imaging applications, this target is reached only after a very large number of pulses. If it is desired that the total number of pulses not be too large, then the value of θ_0 should not be too small. The increase in flip angle with n, which is slow if θ_0 is small and accelerates as θ_n increases, is apparent in Fig. 18.6. The figure shows the case where p is chosen to be 30, corresponding to θ_0 approximately 13° for a tissue with $T_1 = 950\,\text{ms}$ and $T_R = 10\,\text{ms}$.

The advantage of forcing steady-state using variable flip angles is illustrated in Fig. 18.7. An image obtained with fixed flip angle is compared to an image obtained with a flip angle varied to excite constant magnetization at each new rf pulse. The former exhibits more blurring and some ghosting in the phase encoding direction. As discussed before, the blurring in the fixed flip angle case (Fig. 18.7a) is a result of the exponential approach to steady-state as a function of rf pulse number of the excited magnetization, which is then phase encoded. The ghosting is a result of some periodic amplitude inconsistencies created along the phase encoding direction as the k-space data were acquired eight lines at a time with 15° pulses following which the longitudinal magnetization was allowed to relax towards M_0 for roughly a second. (For a detailed discussion of this 'segmented' approach to imaging and reasons for this ghosting, see Ch. 19.)

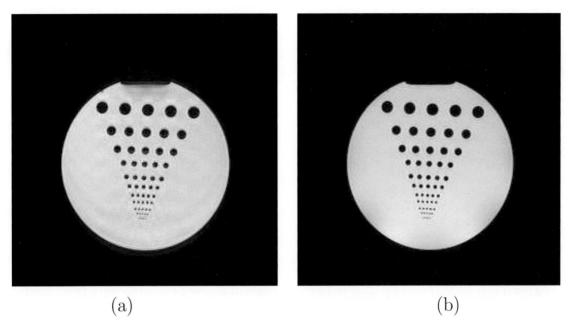

(a)   (b)

Fig. 18.7: A comparison of the use of variable versus fixed flip angle in short-T_R 2D imaging. (a) An image obtained with fixed flip angle appears more blurred in the phase encoding direction than (b) an image obtained according to the method described in Sec. 18.1.4. The blurring occurs in (a) due to the fact that the signal varies with rf pulse number before steady-state has been achieved.

18.1.5   Nonideal Slice Profile Effects on the SSI Signal

It follows from the discussion in the last two subsections that care has to be taken in 2D SSI imaging to ensure that steady-state has been reached. Otherwise, image quality suffers. Two-dimensional SSI imaging also suffers from the effects of signal integration over nonideal rf slice profiles (which lead to spatially varying flip angles along the slice select direction). A discussion of these effects is the focus of this subsection.

An effective spin density for a single 2D slice, with z as the slice select direction, is given by an integration over the rf slice profile,

$$\hat{\rho}_{2D} = \int_{-\infty}^{\infty} dz \, \hat{\rho}(\theta(z)) \qquad (18.48)$$

The flip angle varies over the slice owing to the deviations from a rect function in the slice excitation profile.[4]

---

[4]These variations in flip angle should not be confused with the in-plane and through-plane flip angle variations due to transmit coil inhomogeneities.

The trapezoidal function shown in Fig. 18.8a may be used to model an rf pulse profile. In region I of the figure, the flip angle is linear in z,

$$\theta(z) = \theta_0 \frac{(z+B)}{(B-A)} \quad \text{for} \quad -B \leq z \leq -A \tag{18.49}$$

with θ_0 the maximum flip angle. With a constant profile ($\theta = \theta_0$) in region II and a linearly decreasing angle in region III, the integration in (18.48) gives

$$
\begin{aligned}
\hat{\rho}_{2D,trap}(\theta_0) &= \int_{-B}^{B} \frac{\rho_0(1-E_1)\sin\theta(z)}{1-E_1\cos\theta(z)} dz \\
&= \rho_0(1-E_1)\left\{ \frac{2A\sin\theta_0}{1-E_1\cos\theta_0} + \frac{2(B-A)}{\theta_0}\int_0^{\theta_0} \frac{\sin\theta\, d\theta}{1-E_1\cos\theta}\right\} \tag{18.50} \\
&= 2\rho_0(1-E_1)\left\{ \frac{A\sin\theta_0}{1-E_1\cos\theta_0} + \frac{(B-A)}{\theta_0 E_1}\ln\left(\frac{1-E_1\cos\theta_0}{1-E_1}\right)\right\} \tag{18.51}
\end{aligned}
$$

For comparison, an ideal rect function excitation (constant flip angle θ_0) over a slice of thickness $2B$ yields[5]

$$\hat{\rho}_{2D,rect}(\theta_0) = 2B\rho_0 \frac{(1-E_1)\sin\theta_0}{1-E_1\cos\theta_0} \tag{18.52}$$

Plots of both $\hat{\rho}_{2D,rect}(\theta_0)$ and $\hat{\rho}_{2D,trap}(\theta_0)$ as functions of θ_0 are presented for a trapezoidal slice profile (Fig. 18.8a) are shown in Figs. 18.8c and 18.8d. They contrast ideal SSI behavior with that resulting from an integration over a more realistic rf profile. The shape of the integrated voxel signal as a function of θ is similar to that expected from (18.52), but with an effectively shorter T_1.[6]

Another important point revealed in Fig. 18.8b is how the actual slice thickness should be quoted in terms of the FWHM of the magnetization profile for θ_0 values greater than the Ernst angle. For $\theta_0 > \theta_E$, the magnetization profile $\hat{\rho}_{2D,trap}(z)$ is bimodal in appearance with two local maxima occurring at the two values of z where $\theta(z)$ equals θ_E. Clearly, when the slice thickness is quoted at a given flip angle, it should not be quoted in terms of the FWHM of the slice profile itself; it should be quoted in terms of the FWHM of the signal profile. For example, FWHM$_2$ as measured for θ_0 greater than the Ernst angle is larger than FWHM$_1$, that measured at $\theta_0 < \theta_E$ (Fig. 18.8b).

Problem 18.8

Reproduce Fig. 18.8c and add curves for white matter using the values of ρ_0 and T_1 from Table 18.1. Hence conclude that the contrast between GM and WM as a function of flip angle has changed in comparison with the ideal results illustrated in Fig. 18.2.

---

[5]This result is obtained assuming that ρ_0 is the relative spin density value obtained for a unit slice thickness.

[6]The results quoted for T_1 values at 1.5 T in Table 18.1 for GM and WM are based on 2D measurements and may be significantly lower than their actual values. Nevertheless, they do correctly predict the signal behavior for these scans using similar nonideal rf profiles (see Ch. 22 for more details).

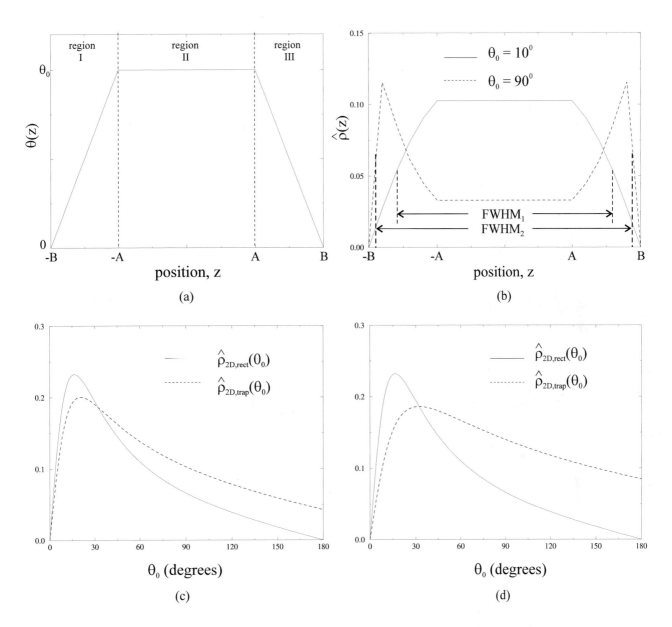

Fig. 18.8: (a) Trapezoidal rf slice profile. (b) SSI signal as a function of position z along the slice select direction in the presence of a trapezoidal rf profile with $A = B/2 = 0.5$ for gray matter. The signal response is shown for $T_R = 40$ ms for values of $\theta_0 = 10°$ (less than the Ernst angle; solid line curve) and $90°$ (greater than the Ernst angle; dashed line curve). (c) $\hat{\rho}_{2D,trap}(\theta_0)$ and $\hat{\rho}_{2D,rect}(\theta_0)$ as functions of θ_0 for the same values of A and B as in (b). (d) Same as (c), except now A equals zero, so the profile is triangular rather than trapezoidal.

The plots in Fig. 18.8 and the results in Prob. 18.8 demonstrate that the contrast can be significantly affected by integration across the slice profile. The main aspect to be noted is the flattening of the signal response as a function of θ_0 as seen in Figs. 18.8c and 18.8d for gray matter, leading to a reduction of contrast between GM and WM, for example. On the other hand, in 3D imaging, where individual 3D partitions are thin relative to changes in rf profile (or spatial flip angle variations), the effective spin density is well approximated by $\hat{\rho}_{2D,rect}(\theta_0)$. This effect is demonstrated in Fig. 18.9, where the GM/WM contrast seen in a single 3D partition from a T_1-weighted acquisition is reduced in the corresponding 2D image obtained for the same flip angle.

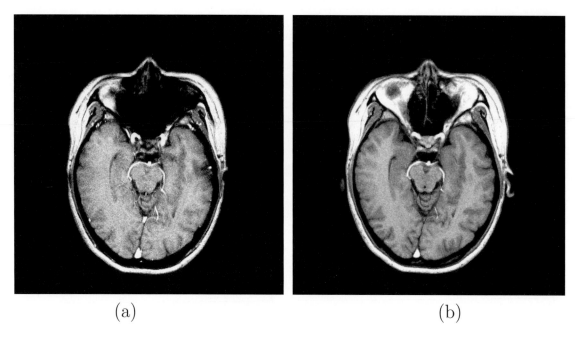

(a)   (b)

Fig. 18.9: Reduced T_1-weighted contrast in 2D imaging due to slice profile integration. Although both (a) the 2D image and (b) the 3D image shown were obtained with the same flip angle of 20°, there is reduced T_1-weighted GM/WM contrast in the 2D image. The signal loss in the region of the nasal sinuses (in the top half of the image) in the 2D image is due to T_2^* dephasing over the 4 mm thick 2D slice. This is not evident in the 3D case which is a sum over four 1 mm thick magnitude images (the reasons for the absence of signal loss in the 3D case are discussed in detail in Ch. 20).

18.2   Short-T_R, Coherent, Gradient Echo Imaging

When T_R is on the order of, or less than, T_2 and no attempt is made to spoil the transverse magnetization, there will be a coherent build-up of signal towards a steady-state value which is a mixture of longitudinal and transverse components present at the initial state. This dependence on the initial magnetization is illustrated in Figs. 18.10 and 18.11 by assuming two different initial conditions. In Fig. 18.10, it is assumed that equal magnetization exists along both y- and z-axes, while in Fig. 18.11 it is assumed that equal magnetization components exist along all three axes.

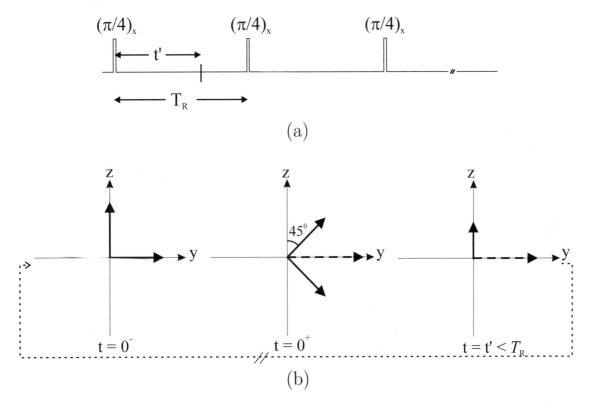

(a)

(b)

Fig. 18.10: Demonstration of coherent steady-state formation. (a) Sequence diagram showing an rf pulse repetition example which leads to a steady-state. (b) The case when equal magnetization is available along the y- and z-axes at the beginning of a free precession period, and a $45°$-pulse is applied along the x-axis. The effective z magnetization after the rf pulse is zero. Assume that the magnetization considered here is from a resonant isochromat of spins. Their precession angle in the rotating frame is zero, leaving them all along $\hat{y}$ throughout the evolution period. It is now easy to visualize that, depending on the T_R value, the y magnetization decays due to T_2 decay while the z magnetization recovers towards M_0 and, at the end of the evolution period, the magnetization state returns to the value it had just before the previous rf pulse, leading to a steady-state.

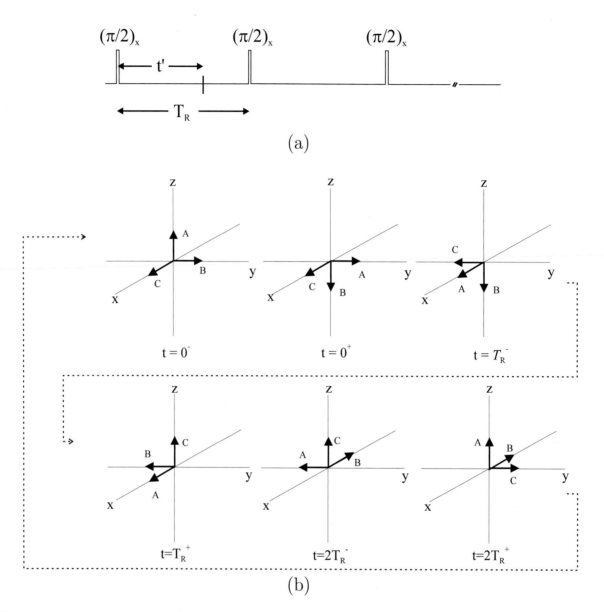

(a)

(b)

Fig. 18.11: (a) Sequence diagram showing a second rf pulse repetition example which leads to a
different steady-state. (b) Steady-state formation with equal x, y, and z components just before
the first rf pulse. The presence of a B_0 inhomogeneity is assumed to cause a $\pi/2$ precession of
transverse magnetization during the evolution period. Following the second rf pulse, the third free
precession period leads to the initial condition (at $t = 0^-$), thereby creating the required periodicity
to reach steady state. This is indicated by the arrow going from the state at $t = 2T_R^+$ to the state
at $t = 0^-$. It is also assumed that T_R is so short that all relaxation effects can be neglected.

From Figs. 18.10 and 18.11, it is also seen that the steady-state magnetization components depend on the field seen by the isochromat of interest. That is, two isochromats seeing different static fields will reach different steady-state values after free precession. In an imaging experiment, different gradients are used from one rf pulse to the next. These cause additional magnetic field inhomogeneities during the transverse magnetization evolution period, which can also affect the steady-state signal. As before, we consider an isochromat of spins where there are no T_2^* effects.

Problem 18.9

a) Starting with the same initial magnetization vector as in Fig. 18.10, show the build-up to steady-state when the precession angle per T_R is π.

b) Starting from thermal equilibrium conditions (i.e., $M_z(0^-) = M_0$, $M_x(0^-) = M_y(0^-) = 0$), show that steady-state is reached after the first free precession period for a $45°_{-x}$-$[90°_x, 90°_{-x}]_{repeat}$ sequence when the precession angle of the transverse magnetization per T_R is zero. Assume that T_R is short enough to also ignore all relaxation effects.

From Figs. 18.10, 18.11, and Prob. 18.9, it is seen that the steady-state magnetization depends on the flip angle, the initial magnetization components, and T_R. Further, in Figs. 18.10 and 18.11, the events that were followed carefully were the initial condition existing just before an rf pulse, the immediate effect of the rf pulse, and the final condition created at the end of the free precession period without paying much attention to the details of how the final condition was achieved. It seems that the steady-state magnetization is determined by the total precession angle of the transverse magnetization components during each T_R, i.e., the steady-state magnetization depends on the quantity

$$\beta_{\text{total}}(T_R) = \gamma \Delta B T_R + \gamma \vec{r} \cdot \int_0^{T_R} \vec{G}(t) dt \qquad (18.53)$$

where the two terms are the static and gradient field inhomogeneity-induced resonance offset angles, respectively. The quantity β_{total} is referred to as the resonance offset angle. To let all isochromats contained in the imaged volume reach steady-state free precession (SSFP) equilibrium depending only on the 'free' precession angle (the precession angle with no gradients on; in this case, the background field inhomogeneities, ΔB, are the source of resonance offset), all the gradients used must have zero zeroth moment over each repetition period, i.e., they should all be 'balanced' over each repetition period. Such a balanced gradient coherent steady-state sequence implementation is shown in Fig. 18.12.[7] For the rest of the discussion in this section, it is assumed that all imaging gradients used in the sequence are balanced, thereby the resonance offset angle depends only on the static field inhomogeneities. For this reason, the subscript 'total' is dropped from β_{total} for the remaining part of this section.

---

[7]It is common to use the term 'SSFP sequence' in the MR imaging literature to loosely mean a balanced gradient coherent steady-state sequence. The terms SSC sequence and SSFP sequence are interchangeably used in this sense in the text too.

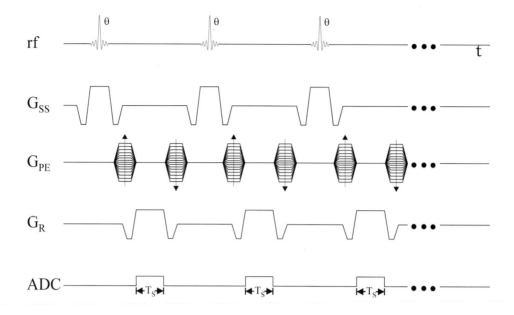

Fig. 18.12: A typical SSC imaging sequence implementation. Note the balancing of all imaging gradients to let all isochromats evolve under equivalent free precession conditions over each repetition period unaffected by a particular phase encoding or read gradient structure.

18.2.1   Steady-State Free Precession: The Equilibrium Signal

In this section, the equilibrium solution will be found under a variety of conditions which affect the phase of the transverse magnetization. Let $\beta(t) = \Delta\omega \cdot t$ with $\Delta\omega = \omega_0 - \omega = \gamma\Delta B$. Here, $\Delta\omega$ is referred to as the *resonance offset frequency*, and $\beta(T_R)$, the *resonance offset (angle)*. For $nT_R \leq t \leq (n+1)T_R$, $t' = t - nT_R$, and the argument n representing the time nT_R,

$$M_x(n,t') = [M_x^+(n)\cos\beta(t') + M_y^+(n)\sin\beta(t')]e^{-t'/T_2} \tag{18.54}$$

$$M_y(n,t') = [-M_x^+(n)\sin\beta(t') + M_y^+(n)\cos\beta(t')]e^{-t'/T_2} \tag{18.55}$$

$$M_z(n,t') = M_z^+(n)e^{-t'/T_1} + M_0(1 - e^{-t'/T_1}) \tag{18.56}$$

For a clockwise rotation about $\hat{x}$, the matrix representation for (18.54)–(18.56) is found using

$$R_x(\theta) = \begin{pmatrix} 1 & 0 & 0 \\ 0 & \cos\theta & \sin\theta \\ 0 & -\sin\theta & \cos\theta \end{pmatrix} \tag{18.57}$$

with

$$D(t') = \begin{pmatrix} e^{-t'/T_2}\cos\beta(t') & e^{-t'/T_2}\sin\beta(t') & 0 \\ -e^{-t'/T_2}\sin\beta(t') & e^{-t'/T_2}\cos\beta(t') & 0 \\ 0 & 0 & e^{-t'/T_1} \end{pmatrix} \tag{18.58}$$

With these definitions,

$$\vec{M}^+(n) = R_x(\theta)\vec{M}^-(n) \tag{18.59}$$

and

$$\vec{M}^-(n+1) = D(T_R)\vec{M}^+(n) + M_0(1-E_1)\hat{z} \qquad (18.60)$$

Now, $\vec{M}^-(n+1)$ can be set equal to $\vec{M}^-(n)$ to find the steady-state value.

An alternate approach is to use the equation (18.59) and the identity

$$\vec{M}^-(n) = D(T_R)\vec{M}^+(n-1) + M_0(1-E_1)\hat{z} \qquad (18.61)$$

and then set $\vec{M}^+(n) = \vec{M}^+(n-1)$ to solve for the steady-state value for $\vec{M}^+$.

The solutions are quite simple and compact in matrix form. From (18.59) and (18.60), as n approaches ∞,

$$\vec{M}^-(\infty) = (I - D(T_R)R_x(\theta))^{-1}M_0(1-E_1)\hat{z} \qquad (18.62)$$

while, from (18.59) and (18.61),

$$\vec{M}^+(\infty) = R_x(\theta)(I - R_x(\theta)D(T_R))^{-1}M_0(1-E_1)\hat{z} \qquad (18.63)$$

The tedious part is to find the vector components of $\vec{M}$ from the compact results of (18.62) or (18.63). Writing out the individual components of the magnetization vectors $\vec{M}^-(\infty)$ and $\vec{M}^+(\infty)$:

$$M_x^-(\infty) = M_0(1-E_1)\frac{E_2\sin\theta\sin\beta}{d} \qquad (18.64)$$

$$M_y^-(\infty) = M_0(1-E_1)\frac{E_2\sin\theta(\cos\beta - E_2)}{d} \qquad (18.65)$$

$$M_z^-(\infty) = M_0(1-E_1)\frac{[(1-E_2\cos\beta) - E_2\cos\theta(\cos\beta - E_2)]}{d} \qquad (18.66)$$

and

$$M_x^+(\infty) = M_x^-(\infty) \qquad (18.67)$$

$$M_y^+(\infty) = M_0(1-E_1)\frac{\sin\theta(1-E_2\cos\beta)}{d} \qquad (18.68)$$

$$M_z^+(\infty) = M_0(1-E_1)\frac{[E_2(E_2-\cos\beta) + (1-E_2\cos\beta)\cos\theta]}{d} \qquad (18.69)$$

where $E_2 \equiv e^{-T_R/T_2}$ and

$$d = (1-E_1\cos\theta)(1-E_2\cos\beta) - E_2(E_1-\cos\theta)(E_2-\cos\beta) \qquad (18.70)$$

Problem 18.10

From (18.62), derive (18.64) through (18.66). From your results, verify (18.67) through (18.69) using (18.59).

Problem 18.11

---

a) Show that for $\theta = \theta_E$, the Ernst angle, $M_y^+(\infty)$ collapses to the expression in (18.13) evaluated at $t = 0$.

b) Show that for β such that $\cos \beta = E_2$, $M_y^+(\infty)$ again collapses to the expression in (18.13) evaluated at $t = 0$.

c) What is $M_x^+(\infty)$ in parts (a) and (b)? Is $M_+^+(\infty)$ in part (a) equal to that in part (b)? Show that $|\int_{-\pi}^{\pi} \vec{M}_+^+ d\beta| = |\int_{-\pi}^{\pi} M_y^+ d\beta|$. The steady-state obtained by integrating over the entire range of β values is also known as the 'resonance offset averaged steady-state.' It is a useful extension of the SSFP limit, whereby a β-independent signal which equals the SSI signal value is obtained under two conditions: either the flip angle must equal the Ernst angle, or β must equal $\cos^{-1} E_2$. It is integration across β which incorporates variations in the local magnetic field.

Clearly, the SSFP signal is a complicated function of θ, E_1, E_2, and β. The dependence on θ and β is summarized for different tissues in Fig. 18.13 for a choice of $T_R \ll T_2$ of all the tissues. These plots show that for small flip angles (for example, see curves for $\theta = 10°$), a large signal response is achieved only when β is close to $0°$ or $360°$. On the other hand, for large flip angles (for example, see curves for $\theta = 70°$), a uniformly high signal is obtained for a range of β values centered around $\beta = 180°$.

Since the static field varies as a function of position, β varies as a function of position within the image and, typically, this leads to signal variation for SSC images of homogeneous objects. However, $\Delta B(\vec{r})$ does not usually vary over a single voxel. As a result, each voxel can be considered an isochromat whose signal expression is defined based on (18.64)–(18.69). Practically, if there is a significant field variation across the object, this will lead to a changing $\beta(\vec{r})$ and the dependence of the magnetization components on the resonance offset angle (see Fig. 18.13) means that uniformity will be degraded in the reconstructed image. The measured signal in a voxel for a given echo time will be found by integrating $M_+^+(\infty)e^{-T_E/T_2}$ over the physical distribution of β values present in that voxel (see Sec. 20.4). Up to this point, all field dependence is carried by β and, therefore, E_2 should not be replaced by E_2^* even though this is a gradient echo experiment. *The above mentioned integration is what may eventually lead to e^{-T_E/T_2} being replaced by e^{-T_E/T_2^*} in the voxel.*

However, if β remains close to $180°$, this is not problematic as long as the variation in β across the object is small. This is typically achieved by shimming the field well, and keeping T_R as short as possible. On the other hand, if $\beta(\vec{r})$ ranges in the neighborhood of $0°$ or $360°$, the signal variation is drastically enhanced.

The question arises at this point as to how $\beta(\vec{r})$ can be biased around π to obtain a homogeneous image. An additional means to change the resonance offset angle other than using an unbalanced gradient is to make the rf phase a function of rf pulse number, typically by incrementing the phase linearly.[8] The linear rf phase increment is represented by the

---

[8]In any multi-pulse experiment such as in imaging, it is assumed that the demodulator and the rf transmitter are in phase for each readout despite the linear rf phase increment. This requires the demodulator phase to be incremented the same way as the rf pulse.

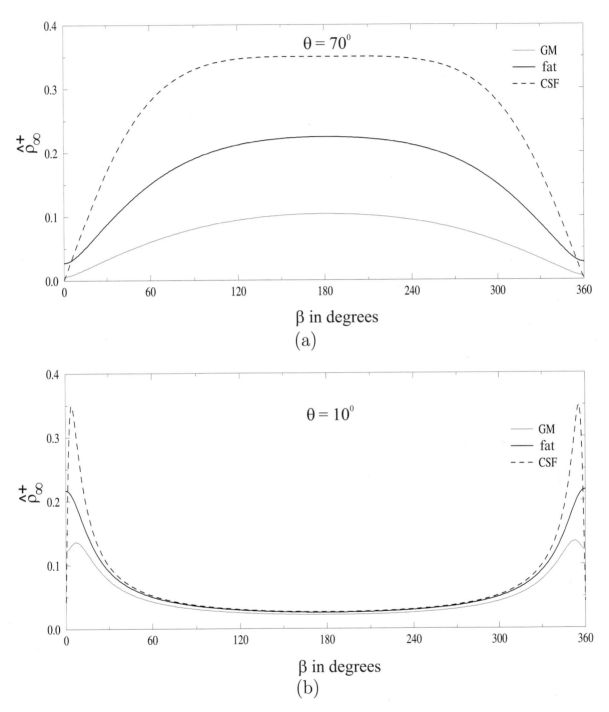

Fig. 18.13: Plot of the magnitude of the steady-state voxel signal, $\hat{\rho}_\infty^+$, as a function of β for different tissues for (a) $\theta = 70°$ and (b) $\theta = 10°$. A T_R of 10 ms and a T_E of 0 ms were assumed.

quantity β_{rf}. (Recall that the term 'rf phase' is used to refer to the angle of the axis about which the rf pulse is applied.) Although the steady-state magnetization in the presence of a linear rf phase increment does not conform to the solutions of (18.64)–(18.69), in the general case, it can be shown that the steady-state magnetization satisfies these equations when β_{rf} equals 180°, with β effectively replaced by $(\beta + \pi)$. Now, signal uniformity can be preserved for large flip angles by keeping $\gamma \Delta B T_R$ small. These effects and the contrasting signal behavior as functions of β for small flip angle versus large flip angle excitation are summarized in the imaging results obtained on a homogeneous phantom shown in Fig. 18.14. As seen from the panels (a)–(d) of this figure, these images show peak signal on the low flip angle images (c and d) only where the signal in the corresponding rf alternated large flip angle image (a and b) is at its lowest. Similarly, note the transformation of low signal areas into peak signal areas between the non-alternated (a and c) and alternated rf (b and d) image acquisitions.

Problem 18.12

a) Show that when an rf pulse with a phase ϕ (clockwise angle with respect to $\hat{x}$) and flip angle θ is applied, $\vec{M}^+ = R_x(\theta)R_z(-\phi)\vec{M}^-$. Hint: First, write the transverse components of $\vec{M}^-$ in terms of components along and perpendicular to the rf axis.

b) Rewrite the steady-state vector equations (18.59) and (18.60) for the rf alternated case, i.e., for $\beta_{rf} = 180°$.

c) Hence show that the steady-state magnetization components satisfy (18.64)–(18.69) with $\beta \to \beta + \pi$.

18.2.2   Approach to Coherent Steady-State

As in the case of incoherent steady-state, the magnetization takes a finite time to reach steady-state in the coherent or unspoiled case as well. For two arbitrary initial magnetization vector conditions, this was qualitatively shown to vary depending on the resonance offset angle and flip angle in Figs. 18.10 and 18.11. A further look at the steady-state magnetization components defined in (18.64)–(18.69) tells us that the approach to steady-state also depends on T_1, T_2, and T_R. The complicated dependence of the SSC signal on these quantities makes an analytical writing of the approach to steady-state along lines similar to the SSI case very complicated. For this reason, an understanding of the dependence on these parameters can be obtained only by Bloch equation simulation for a fixed set of values of β, T_R, and θ for a given tissue of interest. A plot showing the multi-parameter dependence of the approach to steady-state for different tissues (i.e., different E_1 and E_2 values) is given in Fig. 18.15. The approach to steady-state is also changed by changing the flip angle or β. As in the SSI case, the different magnetization components reach steady-state in a time which is on the order of T_1.

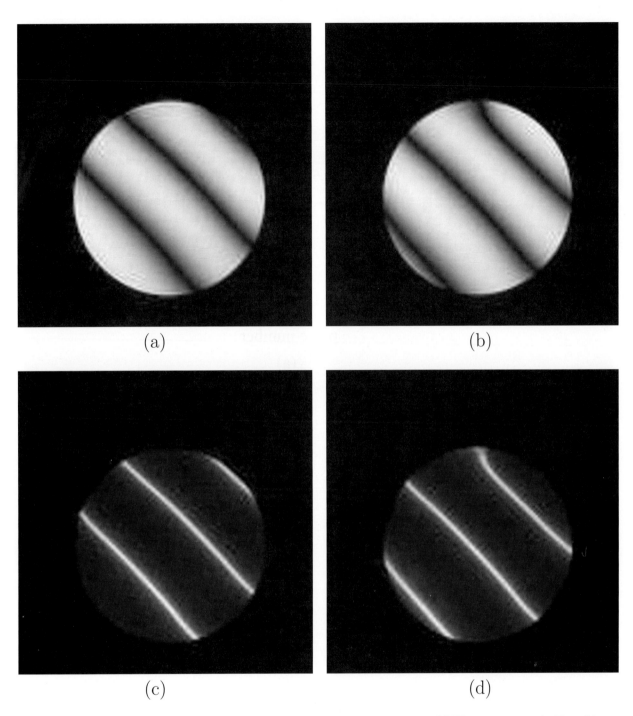

Fig. 18.14: Images of a homogeneous phantom obtained using an SSFP sequence. A T_R of 7 ms was used to image the phantom which had a T_1 of 350 ms and T_2 of 200 ms. Images (a) and (b) were obtained using non-alternating ($\beta_{rf} = 0$) and alternating ($\beta_{rf} = \pi$) rf pulses, respectively, at a flip angle of 90°. Images (c) and (d) were obtained with a flip angle of 2° also with non-alternating and alternating rf pulses, respectively. The background field homogeneity was changed by adding a gradient offset of 0.004 mT/m along both the read and phase encoding directions, resulting in a linearly varying resonance offset along a 45° angle as displayed by the valleys and peaks in the signal in these images.

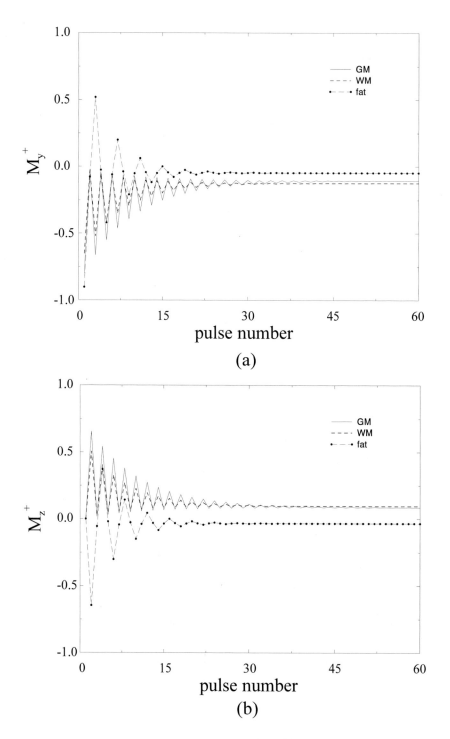

Fig. 18.15: Approach to steady-state of M_y^+ and M_z^+ for three different tissues at a T_R of 20 ms for $\theta = \pi/2$ and $\beta = 180°$. (a) M_y^+ as a function of rf pulse number n. (b) M_z^+ as a function of rf pulse number n. M_x^+ is not shown for this case since the above plots were generated by assuming thermal equilibrium initial conditions and, for this particular initial condition, M_x^+ is zero throughout the experiment. The additional chemical shift-induced resonance offset angle for fat is assumed to be 8π, so that the effective (total) resonance offset angle for fat in the plot is 9π.

18.2.3   Utility of SSC Imaging

Steady-state coherent imaging is of practical interest despite its complicated signal behavior. To appreciate this, it is instructive to examine the limit $T_R \ll T_2, T_1$ with β set to either zero or π. In either case, $M_x^+ = 0$. When $\beta = \pi$,

$$
\begin{aligned}
M_y^+(\infty) &= \frac{M_0(1 - E_1)\sin\theta}{(1 - E_1\cos\theta) - E_2(E_1 - \cos\theta)} \\[2mm]
&\simeq \frac{M_0\sin\theta}{\left(\frac{T_1}{T_2} + 1\right) - \cos\theta\left(\frac{T_1}{T_2} - 1\right)}
\end{aligned}
\tag{18.71}
$$

as both E_1 and E_2 can be approximated with $\left(1 - \frac{T_R}{T_1}\right)$ and $\left(1 - \frac{T_R}{T_2}\right)$, respectively. Therefore, the contrast obtained with an SSFP sequence is essentially T_2/T_1-weighted, which is yet another form of contrast available in MRI.

   The optimal signal as a function of flip angle for a fixed β can be shown to occur at the flip angle θ_{opt} such that

$$
\cos\theta_{opt} = \frac{E_1 + E_2(\cos\beta - E_2)/(1 - E_2\cos\beta)}{1 + E_1 E_2(\cos\beta - E_2)/(1 - E_2\cos\beta)}
\tag{18.72}
$$

In the case when $\beta \simeq \pi$, i.e., the alternating rf case for the short-T_R limit, the above expression approximates to (see Prob. 18.13)

$$
\cos\theta_{opt} \simeq \frac{T_1/T_2 - 1}{T_1/T_2 + 1}
\tag{18.73}
$$

with the peak signal being proportional to

$$
M_y^+(\infty)|_{\theta=\theta_{opt}} \simeq \frac{1}{2}M_0\sqrt{\frac{T_2}{T_1}}
\tag{18.74}
$$

From (18.74), we observe that tissues whose T_2-to-T_1 ratios are high have high signal. For example, a tissue such as CSF, whose T_1-to-T_2 ratio is roughly 2 (see Table 18.1), θ_{opt} equals 70°. At this flip angle, the peak signal for $\beta = \pi$ is found from (18.74) to be roughly $0.35\,M_0$ (see also Fig. 18.13b). That is, a signal which equals 35% of the highest signal that can ever be attained for CSF (remember that, in the infinite T_R limit, the signal is given by ρ_0; see Chs. 8 and 15) is obtained at the shortest possible T_R. Another interesting phenomenon which is noted in Fig. 18.13b is that CSF has the same peak signal response (roughly $0.35\,M_0$) even in the low flip angle regime. This leads to a very interesting high signal regime: if the background static field can be designed such that all isochromats experience a ΔB which leads to the unique value of β where this peak value occurs, a large signal is obtained at short-T_R values with small flip angle excitation.

Problem 18.13

Derive (18.72) and show that (18.73) holds exactly when $\beta = \pi$. Both θ_{opt} and $M_y^+(\theta_{\text{opt}})$ are determined by the ratio (T_1/T_2) when $\beta \simeq \pi$. Both values are independent of T_R, and this is of utmost interest.

The nature of the T_2/T_1 dependence is illustrated in the images of the brain shown in Fig. 18.16. Since CSF has the highest T_2-to-T_1 ratio (see Table 18.1), it has the highest signal. On the other hand, GM and WM appear about the same because of their comparable T_2-to-T_1 ratios. This effect is further demonstrated by comparing this different contrast mechanism with the more common T_1 and T_2-weighted contrast (see Figs. 18.16c and 18.16d). An additional important point is the complementarity of images acquired with non-alternating rf and alternating rf (Figs. 18.16a and 18.16b). It is seen that if the local ΔB value causes the signal to be low in one image, the same inhomogeneity causes the signal to be high in the other image (see the structure indicated by the filled arrow and the blood vessel indicated by the open arrow, for example). Evidently, a homogeneous image can be obtained by choosing the higher of the two voxel signal values on a pixel-by-pixel basis.

Equation (18.74) shows that SSC imaging represents the most efficient way to collect data for a given tissue using as short a T_R as possible. This T_R independence of the SSC signal leads to a T_R independent SNR as long as T_R can be reduced without a concomitant

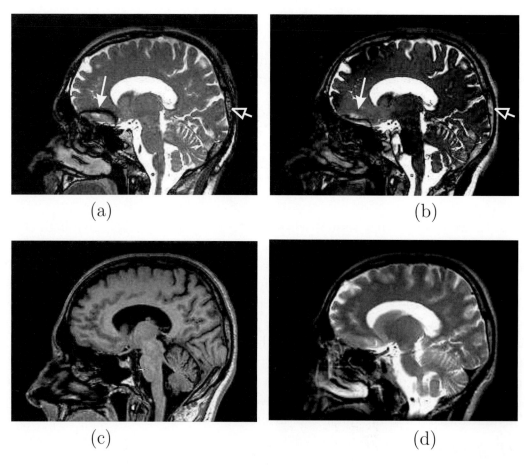

(a)   (b)

(c)   (d)

Fig. 18.16: Images obtained with a fully-balanced 3D SSC imaging sequence for $\theta = 35°$ and T_R = 7.3 ms: (a) non-alternating rf (i.e., $\beta_{\rm rf} = 0$) (b) alternating rf (i.e., $\beta_{\rm rf} = \pi$). (c) A T_1-weighted image and (d) a T_2-weighted image at the same slice location are shown for comparison. The T_2-weighted image in (d) is a thicker slice (5 mm thick in comparison with 2 mm thick slices for the others). Hence, the slight difference in anatomical depiction from the other three images.

decrease in T_s and increase in the noise (since BW must be increased). In comparison, the signal at the optimal flip angle for SSI imaging (i.e., $\theta = \theta_E$) is proportional to $\sqrt{T_R}$ for short T_R (Prob. 18.2b). The T_R independence of the SSC signal has been untapped until now for several reasons. One relates to available gradient strengths and the other to the background field inhomogeneity. For example, if $T_R = 10\,\text{ms}$ (which is easily achievable on commercial scanners for $1\,\text{mm}^3$ voxels in 3D imaging), only a ΔB of about $0.75\,\text{ppm}$ is required to create a resonance offset range of π at $1.5\,\text{T}$. As discussed earlier, this leads to image signal inhomogeneity and also a T_R dependence of the signal. The shorter T_R can be made, the less of a problem ΔB will be. Overall, as magnet homogeneity improves, with better shimming and faster gradient switching capability, there will be an increasing number of applications of extremely short-T_R SSC imaging.

18.3 SSFP Signal Formation Mechanisms

In this section, a purely classical treatment of SSFP signal formation principles is developed using the concept of spin-coherence pathways. It is important to state that, since the presentation is classical, the usage of the word 'spin' in spin phase pathway is, for the purposes of this section, synonymous with 'isochromat magnetization,' i.e., the treatment is of a spin population, not a single spin. It is worthwhile to note that a parallel and more complete quantum mechanical treatment exists for the probabilities of evolution of a spin's phase after being acted upon by a multitude of rf pulses. This treatment requires the usage of spin operator arithmetic which is not treated in this text. It is in keeping with the spirit of one-to-one equivalence of the two theories that, in the treatment given here, spin phase pathway 'probabilities' are replaced with 'observable signal amplitudes' and/or 'fraction of isochromat population,' which is a measure of the population probability along a phase pathway.

18.3.1 Magnetization Rotation Effects of an Arbitrary Flip Angle Pulse

First, the effect of an arbitrary flip angle rf pulse on any prior magnetization is considered. For this purpose, only the magnetization just following the rf pulse is of interest. From the Bloch equations, the magnetization response to an on-resonance θ-pulse applied along the x-direction in the rotating frame is described by

$$\vec{M}^+ = R_x(\theta)\vec{M}^- \tag{18.75}$$

if relaxation effects can be neglected during the rf pulse (i.e., the rf pulse is assumed to be instantaneous). Expanding (18.75) into its component equations gives

$$M_x^+ = M_x^- = M_x^- \left(\cos^2\left(\frac{\theta}{2}\right) + \sin^2\left(\frac{\theta}{2}\right) \right) \tag{18.76}$$

$$M_y^+ = M_y^- \cos\theta + M_z^- \sin\theta = M_y^- \left(\cos^2\left(\frac{\theta}{2}\right) - \sin^2\left(\frac{\theta}{2}\right) \right) + M_z^- \sin\theta \tag{18.77}$$

$$M_z^+ = -M_y^- \sin\theta + M_z^- \cos\theta = -M_y^- \sin\theta + M_z^- \left(\cos^2\left(\frac{\theta}{2}\right) - \sin^2\left(\frac{\theta}{2}\right) \right) \tag{18.78}$$

Using the notation $M_+ = M_x + iM_y$ for the complex transverse magnetization established earlier in (4.29), (18.77) and (18.78) can be combined to give

$$M_+^+ = M_+^- \cos^2\left(\frac{\theta}{2}\right) + \left(M_+^*\right)^- \sin^2\left(\frac{\theta}{2}\right) + iM_z^- \sin\theta \qquad (18.79)$$

$$M_z^+ = M_z^- \cos^2\left(\frac{\theta}{2}\right) - M_z^- \sin^2\left(\frac{\theta}{2}\right) - \frac{i}{2}((M_+^*)^- - M_+^-)\sin\theta \qquad (18.80)$$

In the above expressions, the isochromat populations M_+ and M_+^* are counter-rotating partners. Since only the y-component of the transverse magnetization is rotated by the θ-pulse applied along $\hat{x}$, these two counter-rotating isochromat populations are used to represent M_y during free precession periods. Switching back to the notation of M_+ and M_- in (4.29) and (4.34), instead of the cumbersome notation of M_+ and M_+^*, (18.79) and (18.80) can be rewritten as

$$M_+^+ = M_+^- \cos^2\left(\frac{\theta}{2}\right) + M_-^- \sin^2\left(\frac{\theta}{2}\right) + iM_z^- \sin\theta \qquad (18.81)$$

$$M_z^+ = M_z^- \cos^2\left(\frac{\theta}{2}\right) - M_z^- \sin^2\left(\frac{\theta}{2}\right) - \frac{i}{2}(M_-^- - M_+^-)\sin\theta \qquad (18.82)$$

Two Views of Thinking about the Population Represented by M_-

One needs to stop and consider what isochromat population M_-^- represents. One way to think of it is as a 'fictitious, non-observable' representation of the tipped transverse magnetization which precesses in a direction opposite to the natural direction (the natural direction is clockwise in a positive field offset from resonance). In this framework, the y-component of the transverse magnetization is made up of an observable and a non-observable component during the free precession period. Additionally, (18.81) shows that any arbitrary flip angle rf pulse ($\theta \neq 0$) is capable of converting the non-observable magnetization (M_-^-) into observable magnetization by converting $\sin^2(\theta/2)$ of it into M_+ following the rf pulse (second term in (18.81)). In effect, there is a change in the sense of precession of this magnetization, exactly the same effect as a 180°-pulse would have had on observable transverse magnetization. It now seems necessary to include a third equation representing the fate of the non-observable population created by the rf pulse (obtained by complex conjugate of (18.81)):

$$M_-^+ = M_-^- \cos^2\left(\frac{\theta}{2}\right) + M_+^- \sin^2\left(\frac{\theta}{2}\right) - i(M_z^-)^* \sin\theta \qquad (18.83)$$

In other words, there are two parallel existences for the isochromat population, one as an observable sub-population and another as a non-observable sub-population, the rf pulse acting to mix the two populations and later leading to echoes. *To state this behavior concisely, any rf pulse automatically creates both fresh observable (the third component of (18.83)) and non-observable transverse magnetization (third component of the complex conjugate version of (18.81)) from z-magnetization components. On prevailing transverse magnetization, the rf pulse partly converts from observable to non-observable magnetization and vice versa as well as partly preserving the population type.*

In a second view, which is purely classical with no quantum mechanical undertones, the explanation is based on the use of just (18.79) and (18.80). Here, the population $\left(M_+^-\right)^*$ is interpreted as an isochromat population which precesses normally during the free precession period and whose phase is inverted instantaneously by the rf pulse. *In this viewpoint, the rf pulse achieves an instantaneous complex conjugate of a sub-population of the prevalent transverse magnetization.* This is the interpretation used in the remainder of this section.

Interpretation of (18.79) and (18.80)

Equation (18.79) reveals that the fraction $\cos^2(\theta/2)$ of the population of spins originally in the transverse plane maintain their precession phase as it was before the rf pulse. From (18.80), the same fraction of the population of spins originally in the longitudinal direction stay there. Since this isochromat sub-population remains unaffected by the rf pulse, it appears as though it has been effectively acted upon by a 0°-pulse.

The fraction $\sin^2(\theta/2)$ of the spin population originally in the transverse plane stay there after having their precession phase instantaneously inverted at the time of occurrence of the rf pulse. A similar fraction of any prior longitudinal magnetization is also inverted by the rf pulse. This part of the spin population appears to have been acted upon by an ideal 180° pulse.

Finally, $\sin\theta$ of the original y-magnetization is converted into negative z-magnetization (see (18.78)) and the same fraction of the original z-magnetization is converted into magnetization in the y-direction after the pulse. This spin-population has effectively been acted upon by a 90° pulse. *This discussion demonstrates that a single rf pulse appears to act as a weighted combination of three components: a 0° component of amplitude $\cos^2(\theta/2)$, a 90° component of amplitude $\sin\theta$, and a 180° component of amplitude $\sin^2(\theta/2)$.*

Further, the y-magnetization that is converted into negative z-magnetization by the 90° component of the rf pulse consists of two sub-populations: half of this population maintains its phase prior to the rf pulse (fourth term in (18.80)) and the other half has its phase inverted prior to the end of the rf pulse (third term in (18.80)). Since all phase history is remembered by spins, these two sub-populations will reappear with opposite phases when they are reconverted to transverse magnetization by a later rf pulse.

We summarize next the effects of the 0°-pulse, the 90°-pulse, and the 180°-pulse on the precession phase of the magnetization after the rf pulse. The 0°-pulse does nothing to the magnetization; phase development of isochromats in the transverse plane continues in the same sense as before the pulse and longitudinal magnetization stays in that direction recovering towards M_0. The 180°-pulse, on the other hand, causes phase rewinding following the rf pulse by inverting the accumulated phase of transverse magnetization prior to the pulse. This leads to a refocusing of all static magnetic field inhomogeneities, and spin echoes are produced. In similar fashion, it also inverts any previously present longitudinal magnetization. The 90°-pulse creates transverse magnetization out of longitudinal magnetization and original transverse magnetization turns into longitudinal magnetization. The transverse magnetization converted to new longitudinal magnetization after the pulse remembers its phase history, i.e., its total accumulated phase up to that time-point; this process is usually termed 'phase storage.' *It is important to note that (18.80) states that the 90° component converts half the free-precessed transverse magnetization directly into longitudinal magnetization*

whereas another half has its phase inverted before this phase is stored. These observations
are summarized in Table 18.4.

Flip angle	Effective amplitude	Effect on	
		prior transverse magnetization	prior longitudinal magnetization
$0°$	$\cos^2(\theta/2)$	stays as transverse magnetization; continues to evolve later	stays as longitudinal magnetization; continues regrowth towards M_0
$90°$	$\sin\theta$	tipped to longitudinal axis; storage of accumulated phase and inverted phase in equal numbers ($\frac{1}{2}\sin\theta$) during the following free precession period	tipping of fresh and stored magnetization to transverse plane
$180°$	$\sin^2(\theta/2)$	phase inverted; rephased later	magnetization inversion

Table 18.4: Summary of the effect of an arbitrary flip angle rf pulse.

18.3.2   Multi-Pulse Experiments and Echoes

As a result of any arbitrary rf pulse acting as a combination of $0°$-, $90°$-, and $180°$-pulse
components as discussed in Sec. 18.3.1, any repetitive sequence of rf pulses acting on a spin
population leads to various combinations of echoes. In this section, the discussion focuses
on the development of echoes in arbitrarily time-spaced multi-pulse experiments leading
eventually to an interpretation of the SSFP signal as a combination of a multitude of echoes.
This understanding is achieved by looking at the limiting case of an experiment containing
an infinite number of periodically repeated rf pulses acting on some initial magnetization.
The discussion progresses from a presentation of the formation of echoes in two- and three-
pulse experiments to arbitrarily spaced n-pulse experiments which lead to the SSFP limit.
Certain terminologies and pictorial representations which aid in the determination of echo
locations and echo amplitudes are developed from the results of Sec. 18.3.1.

Echoes from $90°$-τ-$90°$ Pulse Sequences: Hahn Echoes

In Ch. 8, the formation of a spin echo following a $90°$-$180°$ rf pulse pair was described. In
this section, we will see how a partial spin echo is formed even when a $90°$-$90°$ rf pulse pair
is applied (Fig. 18.17).

Let us start with all magnetization along the z-direction (Fig. 18.18a). Assume that both
$90°$ pulses are applied along the x-direction as shown in Fig. 18.17. The second pulse occurs
at time τ after the first pulse (Fig. 18.17). The first pulse tips all magnetization down to
the transverse plane (Fig. 18.18b). At time τ after the first pulse, it is assumed that the
isochromats are dephased and are uniformly distributed over the unit circle (Fig. 18.18c)
because they experience a linear gradient as shown in Fig. 18.18a. The second $90°$-pulse
(occurring at $t = \tau$) rotates these isochromats spread over a unit circle lying in the x-y plane

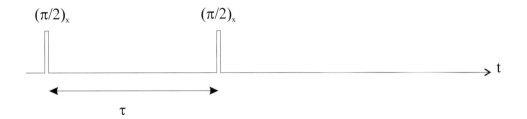

Fig. 18.17: A $90°$-τ-$90°$ pulse sequence.

into the x-z plane, with the x-components preserved and the y-components converted to negative z-components (Fig. 18.18d). Assume that almost no longitudinal recovery occurs in the time τ. Starting at time $t = \tau^+$, the isochromats 2, 3, 4, 6, 7, and 8 with nonzero x-components just after the second $90°$-pulse ($t = \tau^+$) start precessing again, precessing by the same angle in the x-y plane as they did in the free precession period following the first pulse. As a result, at time τ after the second pulse, all these isochromats end up on one side of the y-axis (Fig. 18.18e). This leads to a partial refocusing of magnetization along the negative y-axis, and is called the 'Hahn echo.' Of course, since two of the eight isochromats (1 and 5) have been converted to longitudinal magnetization, the spin echo obtained has a smaller magnitude than the $90°$-$180°$ spin echo.[9] It is for this reason that it is referred to as a partial echo.

On the other hand, the quantitative reduction of the echo amplitude is easily obtained by looking at the population of spins in the transverse plane after the first $90°$-pulse which were acted upon by the $180°$-like component of the second $90°$-pulse. For a general θ-degree pulse, this population is given by $\sin^2(\theta/2)$; for $\theta = 90°$, the echo amplitude is therefore half the magnetization that was tipped into the transverse plane by the first $90°$-pulse (refer to (18.79)), a result which is required to be shown pictorially in an involved fashion in Prob. 18.14.

Problem 18.14

Redraw with accompanying detailed captions Fig. 18.18 for the case when the magnetic field shown in part (a) has a sign change. This problem is given as an exercise to ensure that the reader appreciates the difficulties involved in arriving at the final result using the vector model which uses a spin phasor pictorial representation.

---

[9]For those interested in the complete spin picture including the z-components when the partial echo occurs, imagine a figure eight wrapped around a unit sphere's surface with the point of intersection of the two loops of the figure eight positioned at the point $(0, -1, 0)$ (the contour defined by the equation $\phi = \pm\theta$). This contour defines the locus of vectors originally uniformly distributed in the x-y plane.

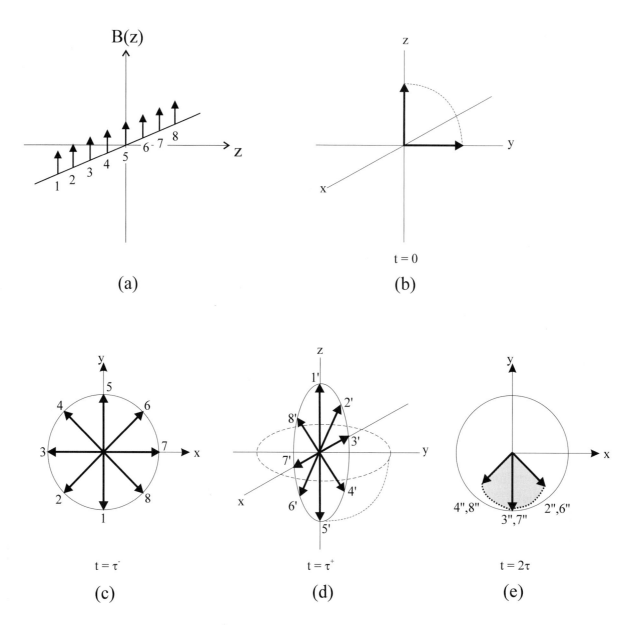

Fig. 18.18: Illustration of the refocusing of magnetization after two 90° pulses. (a) Magnetic field seen by eight isochromats in the rotating frame. Isochromat 5 is on-resonance. (b) The first 90°-pulse tips all z-magnetization into the y-axis. (c) Free precession in the presence of a gradient as shown in (a) occurs for the next τ seconds; a set of of eight isochromats with phases uniformly spread over the unit circle at time τ after the first pulse is considered. This is caused by the dephasing action of the field gradient shown in (a). Remember that our convention is that the isochromats precess clockwise in the presence of a positive field offset in the rotating frame. This makes the isochromats attain the positions shown in (c). (d) The second 90°-pulse rotates the eight isochromats by 90° with respect to the x-axis and puts them in the x-z plane. (e) Isochromats with nonzero x-components after the second pulse precess by the same precession angle as they did in the first free precession period. Hence, τ seconds later, all of these spins end up with negative y-components; this creates the Hahn echo.

Problem 18.15

Based on the discussion about the effects of arbitrary flip angle rf pulses on the magnetization, it is easy to visualize the formation of a weak echo in a sequence based on the generalization of the flip angles of the two rf pulses in the Hahn echo sequence to be arbitrary flip angles θ_1 and θ_2.

   a) What is the amplitude of this echo for a single pulse pair experiment?

   b) For $\theta_1 = 10°$ and $\theta_2 = 180°$, what is the amplitude of this echo relative to a 'full' spin echo?

   c) How does the echo amplitude change when θ_2 is changed to 60°? How does this change when $\theta_1 = 60°$ and $\theta_2 = 180°$? This part of the problem is useful in redesigning short-T_R spin echo sequences for improved T_1-weighted contrast.

Problem 18.16

A problem closely related to Prob. 18.15 leads to a very interesting and important result which has some practical implications for spin echo imaging.

Here we consider a conventional spin echo sequence using a $(\pi/2)$-π pulse pair. Even in well-designed rf transmit coils, it is very difficult to create a homogeneous B_1 field over a large volume comparable to the coil's dimensions.

In such a case, in areas within the coil excitation volume where there are B_1 field inhomogeneities, the $\pi/2$-pulse acts like a θ-pulse (θ arbitrary) and the π-pulse acts like a pulse with flip angle 2θ. What is the relative amplitude of the spin echo signal obtained in such a region in comparison with a region where the B_1 field is correct so that a full echo is obtained? The computation of this relative amplitude would not have been as straightforward as it turns out here if one were to attempt this calculation without using the formulas and interpretation derived in Sec. 18.3.1.

This reduced signal (assuming $\theta \leq \pi$) exacerbates the B_1 inhomogeneity and is a hindrance when the goal is to obtain a uniform signal response over the volume of the coil. One such example is illustrated in Fig. 18.19.

The Three-Pulse Experiment, Phase Memory, and Stimulated Echoes

The previous discussion focused on the mechanism of formation of an echo following two $\pi/2$-pulses (or any two arbitrary flip angle rf pulses). The addition of more $\pi/2$-pulses to this pulse sequence will lead to multiple echoes. For example, a total of five echoes can be observed with three 90° pulses (see Fig. 18.20). To understand the formation of these five echoes, it is necessary to discuss phase memory, spin phase pathways, and coherence levels in detail. These and two examples for the three-pulse experiment are addressed below.

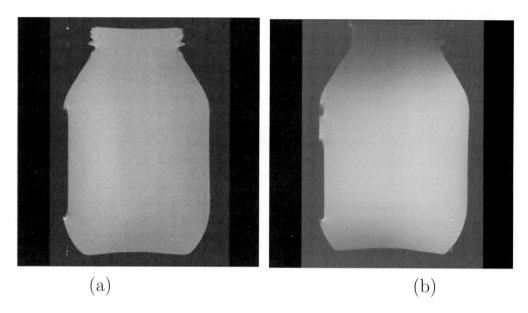

(a)   (b)

Fig. 18.19: Signal drop-off in spin echo imaging due to rf field inhomogeneity. (a) Image of a uniform object when the object sees a homogeneous rf transmit field. (b) Image of the same object when it is imaged in a coil whose volume of transmit field homogeneity is smaller than the object dimension in the up-down direction. This shows the signal drop-off due to an inhomogeneous rf transmit field. As expected, the signal drops off as $\sin^3 \theta$.

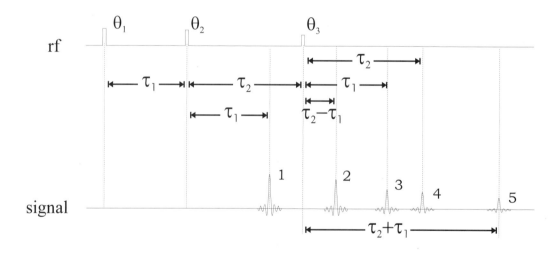

Fig. 18.20: Pulse sequence for a generalized three-pulse experiment.

i) Phase memory

Phase memory is the phenomenon by which isochromats with a history of having been in the transverse plane during previous free precession periods remember their phase accumulated in the past. For example, any transverse magnetization which was recently converted to longitudinal magnetization remembers its earlier accumulated phase value with the same or opposite sign with equal probability. This phase is stored by the isochromats, and the stored phase will reappear when a second rf pulse reconverts them back to transverse magnetization.

ii) Extended spin phase diagrams, spin phase pathways and spin configurations

In the previous discussion, even while following just eight isochromats, it was already becoming difficult to keep track of each isochromat at the end of two pulses and a free-precession period following it. A new pictorial representation which is more intuitively appealing and less complicated is therefore developed to understand echo formation in multi-pulse experiments. We are interested in two aspects: locating the occurrence of echoes, and determining their amplitudes. Echo locations in time can be determined by following the phase of each transverse component and keeping track of the phase memory of any longitudinal component. The phase evolution of a given component between rf pulses is represented by so-called spin phase pathways which plot a non-dimensional quantity which reflects the phase development of several different isochromats as a function of time. Echo amplitudes can be determined by keeping track of the fraction of the magnetization based on (18.79) and (18.80) for the pathway leading to the echo of interest. To create the multitude of spin phase pathways, an initial transverse magnetization is allowed to evolve in phase along each possible phase evolution path by the action of rf pulses. This leads to what are called 'extended spin phase diagrams.'

To remain exact, the time evolution of amplitudes along each pathway between rf pulses should be relaxation-weighted as well. *First, longitudinal magnetization pathways with phase memory have a T_1-dependent exponential decay during their stay along the longitudinal axis. Second, fresh longitudinal magnetization will grow exponentially towards the thermal equilibrium value. Third, T_2 decay of transverse magnetization occurs in addition to the free precession which occurs in the period between rf pulses. These relaxation properties can be used to one's advantage in devising imaging schemes with special weighting mechanisms.*

Some terminology and descriptions about extended spin phase diagrams need to be established. First, the 'spin phase diagram' is a tree of the evolving phase of a starting spin-population as a function of time as it is acted upon by multiple rf pulses; each branch of this tree represents a 'spin configuration' and each sub-pathway represents one particular fraction of the starting spin population, and is called a 'spin phase pathway.' Second, each rf pulse is a branching point for a spin configuration; there are either three or four branches (three branches originate from each longitudinal configuration and four branches originate from each transverse configuration) corresponding to new configurations created by the 0°-like, the 90°-like, and the 180°-like components of the θ pulse (see Fig. 18.21). Each branch has an associated weight that specifies the fraction of the magnetization which goes off into a given branching configuration. Third, an echo is said to occur along a spin pathway whenever there is a zero crossing by a particular configuration along that pathway.

The vertex diagrams of Fig. 18.21 need to be understood first. As mentioned in the previous paragraph, each rf pulse acts as a branching point for a pathway. Let us first look at the four possible branches emanating from transverse configurations (Fig. 18.21a). Suppose this configuration has dephased only during the free-precession period prior to the rf pulse. This isochromat population is split into four possible sub-populations: one which continues to dephase (by the 0° component; solid line in Fig. 18.21a), one whose accumulated phase is inverted by the rf pulse and will form an echo (by the 180° component; dashed line in Fig. 18.21a), one which is converted to M_z which stores the phase accumulated prior to the rf pulse (by the 90° component; dot-dashed line in Fig. 18.21a), and one which is converted to M_z where the prior phase accumulation is inverted prior to storage (by the 90° component;

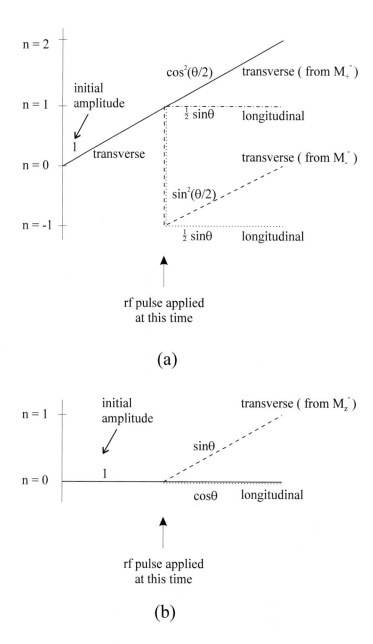

Fig. 18.21: Vertex diagram at an arbitrary rf pulse for (a) a transverse configuration, and (b) a longitudinal configuration. The corresponding fractions of the population prior to the pulse which belong to a given branch are also marked in the vicinity of each newly created configuration. Here, n represents the number of dephasing cycles a given configuration has undergone and is referred to as the 'coherence level.' The numbers along the pathways represent the amplitude reductions.

dotted line in Fig. 18.21a). Associated fractions of the population along each branch are given in the figure. Three branches are similarly created from each longitudinal configuration, one acted on by the $0°$ component which continues to stay along $\hat{z}$ (solid line in Fig. 18.21b), a second by the $90°$ component which is converted to transverse magnetization (dashed line in Fig. 18.21b) and a third by the $180°$ component which puts it along $-\hat{z}$ (dotted line in Fig. 18.21b). Since two sub-populations coincide along $\hat{z}$, it is convenient to take their sum (yielding a fraction $\cos\theta$) and consider only two branches emanating from any longitudinal configuration prior to an rf pulse.

iii) Coherence levels

One of the interesting notions which results from the vertex diagrams of Fig. 18.21 is that of a coherence level. To introduce the concept of a coherence level, let us consider a periodically repeated rf pulse experiment. Suppose we are interested in the magnetization at the end of the $(N-1)^{st}$ repetition period. Let a single $90°$ pulse be placed arbitrarily at the end of one of the repetition periods in this cycle and a single $180°$-pulse be placed at the end of the Nth repetition period. The rest of the rf pulses are $0°$ rf pulses. Let the $90°$-pulse occur after m repetition periods, where $0 \leq m \leq (N-1)$. Now, consider the $180°$-pulse at the end of the Nth repetition period. Prior to the π-pulse, the transverse magnetization would have gone through n dephase periods where n ranges from N to 1 corresponding to $m = 0$ to $m = (N-1)$, respectively. The π-pulse creates rephasing of the transverse magnetization, whereby the $n = 0$ in-phase condition is reached only after $(N - m - 1)$ further repetition periods following the π-pulse.[10] It must be remembered that each repetition period following the π-pulse adds unity to the number of dephase periods a spin configuration has seen. Clearly, n must be negative immediately after the π-pulse for the $n = 0$ condition to be reached later, the value of n being given by $(N - m)$ and the possible values ranging from $-N$ to -1.

From the previous discussion, it is seen that the number n qualitatively describes the condition of the isochromat population: 'dephased' $(n > 0)$, 'rephasing' $(n < 0)$, or 'fully-rephased' $(n = 0)$. This description of an entire sub-population of isochromats is achieved without necessarily delving into the details of how each individual isochromat's phase has evolved (which depends on ΔB and T_R). Because of the quantized integer nature of this qualitative description of the phase evolution of the isochromats, the quantum number n is called a 'coherence level' representing isochromats experiencing different fields, but all of which can be coherently moved to another level by a new rf pulse. Since the coherence level represents the condition of the isochromats on a time scale which is quantized in terms of an artificially-introduced, fixed repetition period and the spin phase continues to evolve linearly with time, the magnetization state at any intermediate time-point is described by a linear increase from one coherence level to the next (upper) coherence level during each free precession period. Let this ΔB-independent quantity representing the coherence level occupied by a particular configuration viewed as a continuous function of time be denoted by $q(t)$. To get the actual phase $\phi(t)$ of some isochromat experiencing a static field inhomogeneity of

---

[10]Here n is used to symbolize the number of dephase periods experienced by a spin configuration and the adjective 'in-phase' symbolizes that each isochromat represented by a configuration has a phase which equals its starting phase value when it was first converted to transverse magnetization.

ΔB, the resonance offset angle per repetition period, $\gamma \Delta B T_R$, is multiplied by $q(t)$, that is,

$$\phi(t) = -\gamma \Delta B T_R \cdot q(t) \tag{18.84}$$

iv) Two specific examples of echo amplitude computation for the three-pulse experiment

Using an extended spin phase diagram, the five echo forming pathways for the three-pulse sequence shown in Fig. 18.20 can be obtained. The extended spin phase diagram for this sequence is shown in Fig. 18.22. The times of occurrence of the five echoes are easily determined from this diagram. This diagram also provides the amplitudes of the individual echoes as described in the next few paragraphs. Of all the five echoes, one of them (echo number 3 in Fig. 18.20) is the most interesting. Unlike the rest, all of which echo through the refocusing action of the 180°-pulse component of the θ-pulse while being in the transverse plane, this echo is formed from the refocusing action of the 90°-like component of the θ-pulse acting on a fraction of longitudinal magnetization which has stored phase history. This echo is called a 'stimulated echo,' and requires the concept of phase memory to describe its formation.

Echo amplitudes are easily obtained. Indexed transverse magnetization vectors M are used to represent different configurations. An index 0 indicates phase storage (occupying a nonzero, positive coherence level) or regrowing longitudinal magnetization (occupying the zero coherence level); an index 0* indicates storage of inverted phase (occupying a nonzero, negative coherence level); an index 1 indicates continued dephasing of transverse magnetization; and an index –1 indicates rephasing because of phase inversion. As a spin population experiences multiple pulses, more indices are added to each configuration in chronological order (see, for example, Fig. 18.22).

For example, the pathway $M_{0,1,-1}$ represents a spin configuration which stayed in the longitudinal plane after the first rf pulse, then got tipped to the transverse plane by the second rf pulse, dephases in the period between pulses 2 and 3 (coherence level 1), is inverted instantaneously by the second rf pulse (instantaneous jump to coherence level -1), and then rephases during the second free precession period to form an echo (echo SE4 in Fig. 18.22) τ_2 seconds following the third pulse (coherence level 0). See Fig. 18.23a for calculation of the echo amplitude. Starting with unit longitudinal magnetization, $\cos \theta_1$ stays as longitudinal magnetization, $\sin \theta_2$ of that fraction is converted to transverse magnetization, and finally $\sin^2 (\theta_3/2)$ of this fraction forms the echo of interest. The echo amplitude is therefore given by $\cos \theta_1 \sin \theta_2 \sin^2 (\theta_3/2)$.[11]

Similarly, $M_{1,0^*,1}$ represents a spin pathway with an isochromat sub-population which was converted from longitudinal to transverse magnetization by the first pulse, gained phase between pulses 1 and 2 (coherence level 1), got stored as longitudinal magnetization at the second pulse with its phase inverted (coherence level -1), and got reconverted to transverse magnetization which rewinds its earlier phase after the third pulse and echoes (coherence level 0). This sub-population would therefore echo following the third pulse after a time equal to the period between the first and the second pulse equaling the dephasing time duration. Refer to Fig. 18.23b for computation of this echo's amplitude. Starting with

---

[11] Relaxation effects are neglected here, but the results with relaxation effects included for all five echoes are given in Table 18.5.

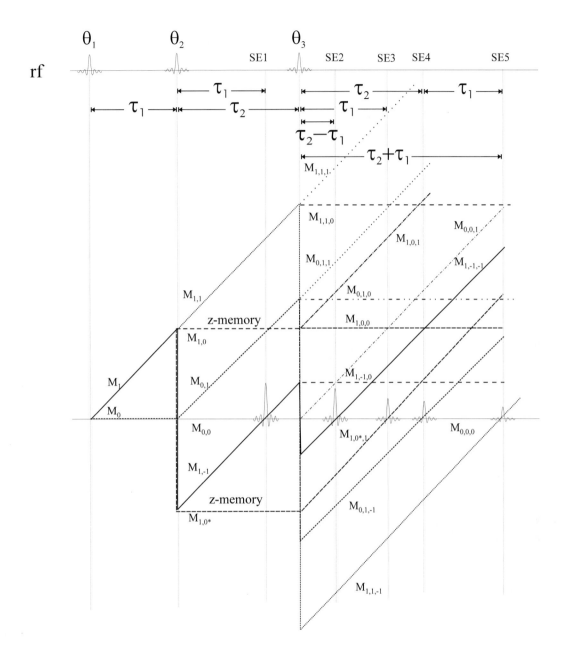

Fig. 18.22: Extended spin phase diagram as a function of time for an arbitrary-angle three-pulse experiment. The abscissa is time and the ordinate is phase. Note that the spin populations under consideration along any diagonal pathway have phase changes, whereas those forming the horizontal pathways have no phase changes during the free precession period. It should be noted that the configurations labeled M_0, $M_{0,0}$, and $M_{0,0,0}$ are the least interesting as these represent the spin population growing towards thermal equilibrium and have experienced no prior dephasing. The three pathways $M_{1,-1,1}$, $M_{0,0,1}$, and $M_{1,0,1}$ are not shown since they do not contribute to any further echoes after θ_3 in this three-pulse sequence.

unit magnetization before pulse 1, $\sin\theta_1$ of that population gets converted to transverse magnetization (from (18.79)); $\frac{1}{2}\sin\theta_2$ of this population then gets stored as longitudinal magnetization with its phase inverted; and $\sin\theta_3$ of this population gets converted into transverse magnetization, which rewinds to form the stimulated echo. The echo amplitude is therefore given by $\frac{1}{2}\sin\theta_1\sin\theta_2\sin\theta_3$.

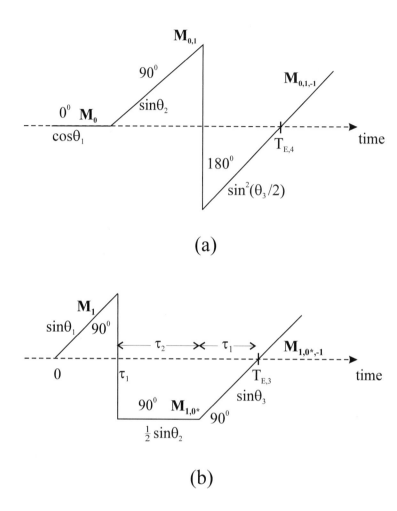

Fig. 18.23: Two particular pathways from Fig. 18.22 with the fraction of spin population associated for each of the free precession periods indicated. (a) Pathway ($M_{0,1,-1}$) involved in the formation of the echo SE4. (b) Pathway ($M_{1,0*,1}$) involved in the formation of the stimulated echo (SE3).

Problem 18.17

Show that when relaxation effects are included in the calculation of the relative stimulated echo amplitude for the $M_{1,0*,1}$ configuration (echo number 3 in Fig. 18.20) is $\frac{1}{2}\sin\theta_1\sin\theta_2\sin\theta_3 e^{-2\tau_1/T_2}e^{-\tau_2/T_1}$ where τ_1 and τ_2 are defined in Fig. 18.20. How does this expression change when the signal is the resultant of a few different isochromats, and T_2^* effects have to be considered? Hint: Remember that there is T_1 decay of the stored magnetization during the period τ_2.

Echo	Time of echo	Amplitude
SE1	$T_{E,1} = 2\tau_1$	$\sin\theta_1 \sin^2\left(\frac{\theta_2}{2}\right) e^{-T_{E,1}/T_2}$
SE2	$T_{E,2} = 2\tau_2$	$\sin\theta_1 \sin^2\left(\frac{\theta_2}{2}\right) \sin^2\left(\frac{\theta_3}{2}\right) e^{-T_{E,2}/T_2}$
SE3	$T_{E,3} = 2\tau_1 + \tau_2$	$\frac{1}{2}\sin\theta_1 \sin\theta_2 \sin\theta_3 e^{-\tau_2/T_1} e^{-2\tau_1/T_2}$
SE4	$T_{E,4} = \tau_1 + 2\tau_2$	$\left[1 - (1 - \cos\theta_1)e^{-\tau_1/T_1}\right] \sin\theta_2 \sin^2\left(\frac{\theta_3}{2}\right) e^{-2\tau_2/T_2}$
SE5	$T_{E,5} = 2(\tau_1 + \tau_2)$	$\sin\theta_1 \cos^2\left(\frac{\theta_2}{2}\right) \sin^2\left(\frac{\theta_3}{2}\right) e^{-T_{E,5}/T_2}$

Table 18.5: Amplitudes and times of occurrence of the five echoes in the three-pulse arbitrary flip angle experiment.

Echo	Description	Pathway forming echo
SE1	Hahn partial echo	$M_{1,-1}$
SE2	virtual echo	$M_{1,-1,-1}$
SE3	stimulated echo	$M_{1,0^*,1}$
SE4	echo from pulse 2	$M_{0,1,-1}$
SE5	echo from pulse 1	$M_{1,1,-1}$

Table 18.6: Descriptions of, and pathways forming, the five echoes in the general three-pulse experiment.

Problem 18.18

Based on the pathways given in Table 18.6, verify the amplitudes of the five echoes SE1, SE2, SE3, SE4, and SE5 as given in Table 18.5. How do these respective amplitudes change if T_2^* dependence is considered? Discuss why SE2 is referred to as a virtual echo and does not exist for certain pulse timings. Hint: Consider the case when τ_2 is less than τ_1.

Maximum Number of Echoes in a Stopped-Pulse Experiment

The spin phase diagram can easily be extended to arbitrary multi-pulse sequences. A stopped-pulse experiment is one where a set of rf pulses spaced arbitrarily from each other is stopped abruptly after a number of rf pulses. The two-pulse and three-pulse experiments discussed before are just specific examples of stopped-pulse experiments. Once the rf pulses are stopped, no phase inversion of transverse configurations can occur; nevertheless, the phase of any transverse configurations already created continues to evolve. As a result of this phase evolution, those pathways occupying negative coherence levels following the last pulse will echo at later time instants.

The maximum number of echoes that can be obtained at the end of a train of n pulses needs to be determined. For this purpose, the maximum possible number of transverse configurations following the nth pulse (T_n) needs to be determined first. T_n can be determined iteratively using mathematical induction. It must be remembered that T_n has contributions from the longitudinal configurations present prior to the nth pulse (Z_{n-1}, say). Iterative, inter-dependent expressions will next be obtained for T_n and Z_n.

i) Iterative determination of T_n

There are T_{n-1} transverse configurations created by the $0°$-like component and the $180°$-like component of the nth pulse acting on the previous transverse magnetization. A single new transverse configuration is created from fresh longitudinal magnetization by the $(n-1)^{st}$ pulse. Finally, Z_{n-1} transverse configurations are created from longitudinal magnetization occupying nonzero coherence levels. (Z_{n-1} is defined as the number of longitudinal configurations occupying a nonzero coherence level following the $(n-1)^{st}$ pulse.) Therefore,

$$T_n = 2T_{n-1} + Z_{n-1} + 1 \tag{18.85}$$

Similarly,

$$Z_n = 2T_{n-1} + Z_{n-1} \tag{18.86}$$

With $T_0 = Z_0 = 0$, applying the above two formulas iteratively gives $T_n \equiv 3^{n-1}$ as seen in Prob. 18.19.

Problem 18.19

___

In this problem, we derive the result that $T_n = 3^{n-1}$.

  a) First, show from (18.85) and (18.86) that T_n satisfies the recursive equation $T_n = 3T_{n-1}$.

  b) Hence, obtain the result that $T_n = 3^{n-1}$ by applying the initial condition.

___

ii) Maximum number of echoes

Except for the one newly formed transverse configuration, the remaining configurations are equally distributed amongst positive and negative coherence levels after the nth pulse. Amongst these configurations, only those occupying negative coherence levels will echo at a later time. This implies that the maximum number of echoes E_n which occur after the nth pulse equals

$$E_n = \frac{(3^{n-1} - 1)}{2} \tag{18.87}$$

which equals the number of negative coherence level transverse configurations. This maximum number can be achieved only if the timings between the n pulses are designed carefully so that none of these echoes overlap in time. In essence, rf pulse timing is a crucial determinant of whether the number of echoes increases only linearly with the number of pulses (as occurs when the inter rf pulse period is a constant), or reaches the maximum limit of (18.87). For example, in a three-pulse stopped-pulse experiment, $E_n \equiv E_3 = 4$. Remember that E_n

represents only the number of echoes which occur at the end of the rf pulse train, and the additional multiple echoes which occur in between adjacent rf pulses are not counted. These echoes are considered to be 'virtual' echoes, as they are not utilized in such stopped-pulse experiments. It is worthwhile to note that the E_n echoes are formed by pathways which go through both possible echo formation mechanisms, either due to the refocusing effect of a given rf pulse (the 180° component) acting on dephased transverse configurations, or due to the stimulated echo formation mechanism.

The utility of a stopped-pulse approach is that, if these echoes are well-separated, a complete image may be obtained by phase encoding each echo differently to cover the k-space required for image reconstruction. For example, a 7-pulse experiment leads to a maximum of $(3^6 - 1)/2$ echoes; this provides the number of echoes needed to obtain 365 phase encoding steps, provided that there is enough separation between successive echoes to allow the application of the phase encoding gradient and to allow coverage of the required k-space sampling window in the read direction.

Problem 18.20

---

a) What is the number of echoes for an n-pulse stopped-pulse experiment when the spacing between the rf pulses is equal?

b) Many other echoes (as given by E_n) are formed. Where do they appear?

c) Can each echo therefore be considered the sum of several echoes?

The answers to the questions in this problem provide the basis of the explanation behind the formation of the coherent steady-state signal.

SSFP Signal as a Sum of Multiple Echoes

The motivation for the detailed discussion of multi-pulse experiments was to lead the reader to understand the formation of multiple echoes in arbitrary multi-pulse experiments. The ultimate aim is to understand the constituent parts of the coherent steady-state signal which is obtained in the infinite pulse number limit.

The SSFP experiment is actually a rather easy-to-visualize version of the arbitrary multi-pulse experiment. Here, the rf pulse separation is fixed (to be T_R) so that, in steady-state, multiple overlapping echoes occur in a periodic fashion, concurrent with each new rf pulse. As we have seen, half of the transverse spin configurations following an rf pulse will form echoes some time later. The free precession period of any configuration is an integer multiple of T_R. Therefore, multiple spin phase pathways created by previous rf pulses and occupying coherence level –1 following the previous pulse converge to form echoes at the instant of occurrence of each new rf pulse. When the spin system reaches steady-state, each of these echoes, aptly named 'rf echoes,' are formed by an infinite sum of echoes created from an infinitely large collection of pathways, each pathway having different relaxation weighting factors and, hence, different amplitudes. After the rf pulse ends, yet another new free precession period begins, all possible configurations are created, and an FID is produced.

In summary, the SSFP signal is composed of an rf echo which coincides with each new rf pulse's occurrence and an FID during the following free precession period. A plot of the SSFP signal from one rf pulse to the next will therefore consist of a decaying envelope (the FID) just after the rf pulse which rises to a maximum at the next rf pulse (the rf echo). This is illustrated in Fig. 18.24.

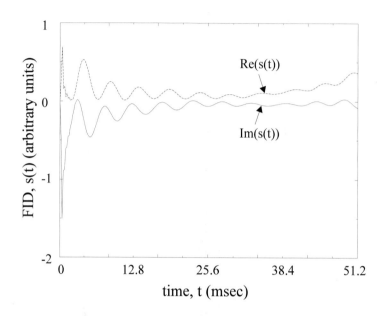

Fig. 18.24: The signal collected after one rf pulse up to the next following the establishment of coherent steady-state. The FID was collected on a water/fat phantom, which is the reason for the periodic modulation of the real and imaginary parts of the FID. Note the initial decaying part, the FID, and the increasing envelope towards the end of the free precession period to form the rf echo.

18.4 Understanding Spoiling Mechanisms

A detailed discussion of spoiling using mechanisms other than the natural T_2 signal loss in cases where T_R is comparable to T_2 has been postponed till now since understanding the process requires some of the concepts discussed in the previous section. This section discusses, from basic principles, the means by which the signal in a short-T_R experiment can be made to approach the SSI limit using external spoiling mechanisms.

18.4.1 General Principles of Spoiling

When T_R is on the order of or less than T_2, a coherent steady-state magnetization with nonzero transverse components occurs prior to each rf pulse as long as the resonance offset angle for any isochromat is independent of rf pulse number. As discussed at the end of Sec. 18.3, the characteristic of this SSFP buildup is that several pathways add together coherently at each new rf pulse to create a refocusing or 'echo' at the instant of each new rf pulse.[12] Of course, there are several other pathways with transverse configurations which do not contribute to the echo, and still contribute to the signal following the current rf pulse. However, these configurations are vulnerable to dephasing due to T_2' mechanisms and the presence of gradient waveforms with nonzero moments that are applied during the current free precession period. To create SSI equilibrium means that all transverse magnetization configurations within each voxel must be forced to have zero contribution to the signal by the end of each free precession period.

It is easy to achieve dephasing just before each new rf pulse for the configurations not forming echoes. The presence of some fixed gradient waveform $\vec{G}(t)$ between each pair of adjacent rf pulses which satisfies

$$\gamma \int_{voxel} d^3r \int_0^{T_R} dt\, \vec{r} \cdot \vec{G}(t) = 2\pi \tag{18.88}$$

for each repetition cycle ensures that

$$\int_{voxel} d^3r\, e^{-i\gamma\vec{r}\cdot\int_0^{T_R} dt\vec{G}(t)} = 0 \tag{18.89}$$

i.e., all these configurations within a voxel are completely dephased. On the other hand, *this rf pulse number independent gradient waveform $\vec{G}(t)$ behaves like a static field inhomogeneity, and its effect is 'refocused' for all echo forming pathways. As a result, their coherent build-up towards rf echo formation is undisturbed.* To eliminate the contribution of the various echoing pathways to the voxel signal, their phases need to be scrambled in such a manner that they add together in a destructive fashion and do not, in effect, contribute to the signal following the rf pulse. *This phase scrambling is achieved by making the resonance offset angle a function of rf pulse number.* There are two ways of achieving this: one is to use an rf pulse number dependent rf phase, and the second is to use variable gradients whose strengths vary as a function of rf pulse number, i.e., by using unrefocused gradient tables between rf pulses. The first is known as 'rf spoiling' and the second as 'gradient spoiling.'

Problem 18.21

Consider a voxel where an extraneous gradient $\vec{G}'$ is present in addition to the dephasing gradient $\vec{G}$. Let $|G'| \ll |G|$. Discuss why the use of $\vec{G}$ such that it distributes isochromats within a voxel over a large integer multiple of 2π in phase is recommended in this case.

18.4.2   A Detailed Discussion of Spoiling

In an imaging experiment, the aim of spoiling is to eliminate the contribution of any prior transverse magnetization to each voxel's signal following a new rf pulse. It should be remembered that in the absence of any gradients, the magnetization in each voxel can be considered

---

[12]The echoing pathways are comprised of only those isochromats with transverse configurations in coherence level -1 or longitudinal configurations in coherence level 0^* immediately after the previous rf pulse.

to be formed by one set of isochromats because $\Delta B(\vec{r})$ is usually a slowly varying function of $\vec{r}$. *In the ensuing discussion, it is critical to realize that we need to be considering a set of isochromats within an imaging voxel which see a variation in resonance offset angle from* $-\pi$ *to* π*. This variation is necessary to force the vector sum of the transverse magnetization components generated by certain pathways to zero.* We will see that spoiling is achieved by a combination of a dephasing gradient and an rf pulse number dependent addition to the free precession resonance offset. The former serves the purpose of dephasing the non-echo forming configurations, and the latter serves the purpose of creating a pathway-dependent phase at a given rf pulse such that all echo forming pathways vectorially add to zero just before each new rf pulse, achieving the conditions necessary for SSI steady-state formation.

Spin Phase Diagram Explanation with Examples

The effects of dephasing gradients and a pulse number dependent additional phase on different pathways are best illustrated with spin phase diagrams. (From Figs. 18.25–18.28, the ordinate represents the phase of the spin isochromats.) Let us consider the three pathways shown in Fig. 18.25 with transverse configurations prior to the fifth rf pulse. In the freely precessing case, two of these pathways (pathways 1 and 2 in Fig. 18.25) end up with zero phase (creating a partial echo) while the third pathway (pathway 3 in Fig. 18.25) ends up with a nonzero phase. In general, this leads to a complex voxel signal after rf pulse number 5.

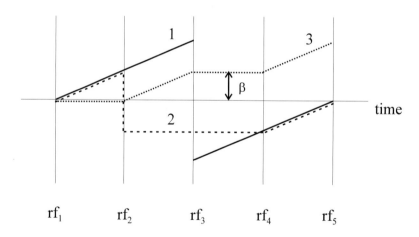

Fig. 18.25: Different spin pathways add together to create the SSFP signal and the rf echo. β is the resonance offset angle.

Gradient Effects

With a constant gradient introduced between each adjacent pair of rf pulses, several isochromats with position-dependent precession frequencies are formed within the voxel. The population amongst these isochromats which evolve along phase pathways 1 and 2 still rephase fully just before the fifth rf pulse and form an rf echo (see Fig. 18.26a). However, the isochromats evolving along pathway 3 develop different phase values and are dephased by the presence of the gradient (see Fig. 18.26b). The amount of dephasing and hence these isochromats' contribution to the signal following the fifth rf pulse depends on both the strength and duration of the gradient. With this in mind, we ignore pathway 3 for the next discussion, assuming that it contributes very little or no signal at the end.

Effects of RF Pulse Number Dependent Phase

With the inclusion of an additional phase to each pathway which is a function of the rf pulse number n, say $\varphi(n)$, the pathways 1 and 2 do not add together in phase anymore (see Fig. 18.27). However, the effects of any magnetic field inhomogeneity which is independent of the repetition period number are still refocused in these pathways. This includes the presence of the constant gradient summoned in Fig. 18.26 to dephase the non-echo forming pathway 3. Because of their different phases, the combined contribution to the signal of pathways 1 and 2 following rf pulse 5 is reduced.

Generalization and Extension to Multiple Spin Phase Pathways

In all the scenarios discussed before, only two broad classes of generalized spin phase pathways were considered: the echo forming pathways and the non-echo forming pathways. Let $\{p_{ij}\}$ be the indices representing the state of the spin population forming pathway i's configuration during the jth free precession period (for example, see Fig. 18.28). For example, since pathway 1 corresponds to $M_{1,1,-1,1}$ (using the notation of Fig. 18.22), $p_{11} = 1$, $p_{12} = 1$, $p_{13} = -1$ and $p_{14} = 1$.

Assume that ΔB does not change within the voxel, i.e., the voxel can be considered an isochromat. Each isochromat's phase is therefore incremented in any evolution period by $\gamma \Delta B T_R$ as long as p_{ij} does not equal 0. At the rf pulse, the phase accumulated prior to the rf pulse is either maintained (for the cases $p_{ij} = 0$ or 1) or is inverted ($p_{ij} = -1$ or 0^*). Therefore, the phase of isochromats forming pathway i just before the $(n+1)^{st}$ pulse satisfies the relation:

$$\phi_i(n+1) = \begin{cases} p_{in}\phi_i(n) + \beta & p_{in} \neq 0 \\ \phi_i(n) & p_{in} = 0 \\ -\phi_i(n) & p_{in} = 0^* \end{cases} \qquad (18.90)$$
$$\equiv l\beta$$

where l is an integer ranging from $-(n-2)$ to n.[13] Amongst the multitude of possible pathways, only those with transverse configurations satisfying $\phi_i(n) = 0$ (i.e., pathways with same number of periods of precession before and after phase inversion) form the so-called 'rf echo' at the nth rf pulse. The non-echo pathways, representing isochromats whose phase values span the whole range of $-(n-2)\beta$ to $n\beta$, have a partially reduced contribution to the signal following the nth rf pulse. The reason that their contribution is only partially reduced is because the fractions of the population contributing to each pathway (and the relative amplitude of a given pathway's contribution to the signal) are still different from one

---

[13] $l = -(n-2)$ corresponds to that pathway where there is a continuous evolution of phase up to the nth pulse, where a phase inversion occurs. The isochromats precess for another T_R, picking up an extra β. On the other hand, $l = n$ corresponds to the complete continuous phase evolution case.

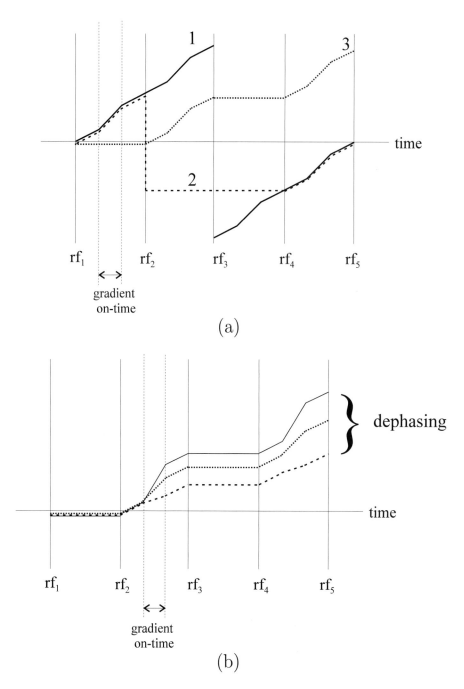

(a)

(b)

Fig. 18.26: (a) Presence of a constant gradient between each rf pulse does not damage the formation of SSFP equilibrium. Again, echoing pathways come together in phase at different rf pulses while non-echoing pathways become dephased. (b) The presence of a gradient of fixed strength occurring every repetition period creates many isochromats within a voxel. The spin population within each isochromat (defined by all spins corresponding to a given position $\vec{r}$) which evolve along a non-echo pathway such as pathway 3 gain different phase values. This leads to their complete dephasing when the phase of the different isochromats ranges from $-\pi$ to π. The end result is that these pathways do not contribute to the FID following each new rf pulse.

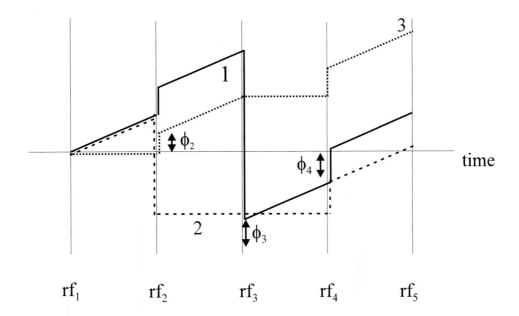

Fig. 18.27: Introduction of extraneous phase which is a function of the rf pulse number makes the phase of a given configuration depend on the pathway it goes through to reach the rf pulse. This prevents constructive interference of different configurations and promotes destructive interference of different configurations just before the next rf pulse.

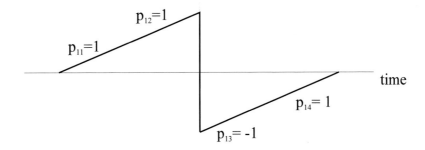

Fig. 18.28: Illustration of the use of spin phase pathway indices using the example of pathway 2. Hence, i equals 2, and j varies for each T_R.

another. Luckily, there are some special cases where the combined signal essentially sums to zero.

With a constant gradient turned on for some fixed time in every repetition period, the phase accumulated up to pulse n additionally becomes a function of position $\vec{r}$. However, it is still independent of n. That is, the accumulated phase still obeys (18.90) with $\phi_i(n+1)$ replaced by the phase accumulated in the presence of gradients, $\phi_{\text{grad},i}(\vec{r}, n+1)$, and β by $\beta(\vec{r}) \equiv \gamma \Delta B T_R + \gamma \vec{r} \cdot \int_0^{T_R} dt \vec{G}(t)$.[14] The effect on echo forming pathways remains the same. These pathways continue to form echoes which add together coherently. The gradient causes isochromats from different locations within each voxel to go to a different SSFP equilibrium magnetization because of the spatially varying resonance offset. When the gradient is such that it causes a 2π phase shift across a voxel, the voxel signal is a resonance offset averaged steady-state signal. One distinction is that, unlike SSFP, the non-echoing pathways are dephased, and they do not contribute to the signal, unlike in the free precession case.

With an rf pulse number dependent extraneous phase $\varphi(\vec{r}, n)$ added, the total accumulated phase $\phi_{\text{total},i}(\vec{r}, n+1)$ in the most general case is given by

$$\phi_{\text{total},i}(\vec{r}, n+1) = \phi_{\text{grad},i}(\vec{r}, n+1) + \varphi_i(\vec{r}, n+1) \qquad (18.91)$$

where $\varphi_i(\vec{r}, n+1)$ is the phase accumulated by pathway i due to this extraneous phase. As reasoned before, the non-echo pathways are ignored for this discussion too. For all the isochromats evolving along the different echo forming pathways, the contribution from the first term in the above sum goes to zero. The second term creates a pathway-specific phase accumulation for the originally echo forming pathways such that there are equal number of positive and negative rf phase terms added to obtain this value. Hence

$$
\begin{aligned}
\varphi_i(\vec{r}, n) &= \phi_{\text{total},i}(\vec{r}, n) \qquad \text{for all echoing pathways} \\
&= \sum_{k=1}^{K} \varphi(\vec{r}, n - m_k) - \sum_{l=1}^{K} \varphi(\vec{r}, n - m_l) \qquad (18.92)
\end{aligned}
$$

where $\{m_k\}$ and $\{m_l\}$ represent those rf pulse numbers relative to pulse number n at which there is either continued phase evolution, or phase inversion, respectively. The number $2K$ ($\leq n-1$) represents the total number of free precession periods for which the spin population along pathway i stays in the transverse plane.

If the fraction of the spin population (or their corresponding amplitudes) forming each of these pathways is the same, the simple requirement to spoil the signal would be to let $\varphi(\vec{r}, n)$ span the entire range of phase values ranging from $-\pi$ to π so that they will be dephased. Their relative amplitudes not being the same, however, means that the form for $\varphi(\vec{r}, n)$ needs to be obtained numerically.

18.4.3   Practical Implementation of Spoiling

As briefly mentioned before, there are two ways of adding an rf pulse number dependent phase to the transverse magnetization: variable rf phase, and varying gradients. In the first

---

[14]Here, $\vec{r}$ is the position inside a voxel and ΔB is assumed to be constant inside a voxel and, consequently, contains no $\vec{r}$ dependence.

case, there is no spatial dependence on φ, and is replaced by $\varphi_{\mathrm{rf}}(n)$. *The use of a variable gradient table for spoiling, on the other hand, creates a position dependence of φ.* This means that spin populations evolving along the same pathway but at different positions in the image will be spoiled to different degrees, creating signal inhomogeneities. This aspect becomes more apparent after a discussion of rf spoiling, since the gradient spoiling method creates a spatially-varying continuum of rf pulse number dependent phase values while the rf spoiling method creates a spatially constant phase. Hence, gradient spoiling is understood by a simple extension of the rf spoiling method.

RF Spoiling

All that needs to be determined here is a simple function for a variable phase $\varphi_{\mathrm{rf}}(n)$ which, in the steady-state, will create an effective signal which equals the SSI signal. This method of spoiling by varying the phase of the rf pulse as a function of rf pulse number is called 'rf spoiling.'

One observation is crucial to understanding the form of the function $\varphi_{\mathrm{rf}}(n)$. At steady-state, the same combinations of different echo forming pathways with the same amplitude add together at each new rf pulse. Therefore, the phase of each such echo forming pathway $\{i\}$ with rf spoiling should be independent of rf pulse number for the attainment of steady-state by the magnetization, i.e.,

$$\sum_k \varphi_{\mathrm{rf}}(n - m_k) - \sum_l \varphi_{\mathrm{rf}}(n - m_l) \equiv \text{independent of } n \qquad (18.93)$$

The condition (18.93) is satisfied only by a linearly varying function of rf pulse number. Hence $\varphi_{\mathrm{rf}}(n)$ must be of the form

$$\varphi_{\mathrm{rf}}(n) \equiv n\epsilon_1 + \epsilon_0 \qquad (18.94)$$

ϵ_0 can be made equal to zero without any loss of generality because a constant rf phase only adds a constant phase to the reconstructed image. Determination of ϵ_1 is done numerically, as briefly mentioned before. This numerical procedure is described next.

The time evolution of a set of isochromats with resonance offset values covering the entire set of phase values from $-\pi$ to $+\pi$ is simulated using the Bloch equations with relaxation terms included. These isochromats are supposed to represent the entire set of spins within a voxel which experience a constant gradient $\vec{G}$ during each precession period, creating the required resonance offset distribution within the voxel. To each isochromat's position-dependent resonance offset, a position-independent but linearly increasing rf pulse number-dependent phase $n\epsilon_1$ is added during each precession period. The steady-state signal is estimated as the magnitude of the complex sum of the transverse components of these isochromats after an evolution time of about $3T_1$ (by which time it is assumed that the spins have reached steady-state as described in Sec. 18.1.3). It is found that a value of ϵ_1 of $117°$ or $123°$ makes the steady-state rf spoiled signal equal to the ideal SSI equilibrium value for all values of $E_1, E_2,$ and θ of practical interest. One such example steady-state signal as a function of ϵ_1 is plotted for gray matter ($T_1 = 950\,\mathrm{ms}$ and $T_2 = 100\,\mathrm{ms}$) for a T_R of $15\,\mathrm{ms}$ (which is much shorter than the T_2's of different tissues in the brain) in Fig. 18.29. This plot shows

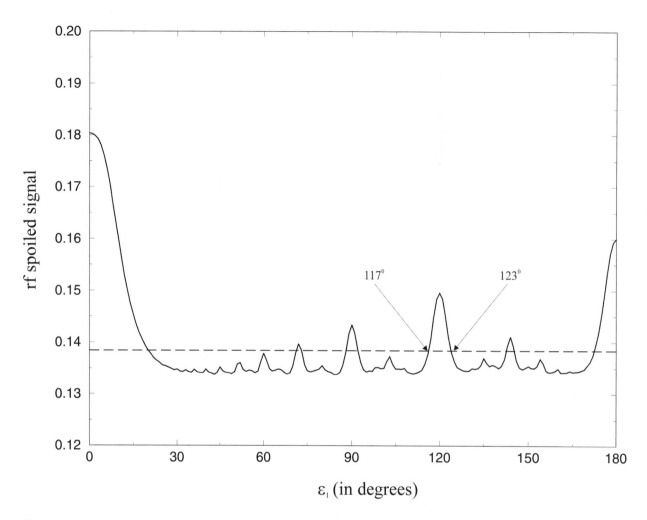

Fig. 18.29: Plot of rf spoiled signal as a function of ϵ_1 for gray matter at a T_R of 15ms. The ideal SSI equilibrium signal for each tissue is plotted as a dotted line to indicate the equality of the two signals when ϵ_1 is either 117° or 123°. A similar equality of the rf spoiled signal and ideal SSI signal is found to occur for other tissues too.

that the use of an ϵ_1 value of either 117° or 123° is successful in achieving the SSI signal at steady-state.

The same rf spoiled signal for $\epsilon_1 = 117°$ is plotted as a function of flip angle in Fig. 18.30, and compared with the ideally expected SSI equilibrium signal as a function of flip angle at a T_R of 25 ms. The close matching of the two curves shows the success of rf spoiling even at extremely short T_Rs when $\epsilon_1 = 117°$. A similar result is obtained for $\epsilon_1 = 123°$.

Gradient Spoiling

The presence of a linearly increasing unbalanced gradient table in each precession period also satisfies the condition (18.94) at each position along the direction of application of the gradient table. However, the phase increment, ϵ_1, takes on all possible values as a function of position. As seen in Fig. 18.29, there are multiple ϵ_1 values where the steady-state signal

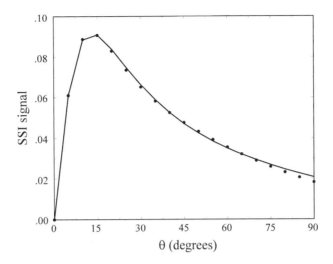

Fig. 18.30: Comparison of rf spoiled signal (solid line) as a function of flip angle for gray matter with the ideal SSI signal (dashed line) at a T_R of 25 ms, and $\epsilon_1 = 117°$. Note the close matching of the two curves for all flip angles, indicating the success of rf spoiling. Similar results are obtained for other tissues as well.

differs from the ideal SSI signal significantly. At positions which experience this ϵ_1 value, the signal is overwhelmingly large and different from the signal at other positions. That is, the gradient-spoiled signal will be spatially varying. This effect is observed when images of homogeneous objects are obtained using large flip angles, where the coherent steady-state signal can be quite large in comparison with the SSI signal when certain special conditions are met.

Problem 18.22

The spatial inhomogeneity of a gradient-spoiled image can be taken advantage of to measure ϵ_1. This problem introduces this application of a gradient-spoiled sequence structure.

a) As seen from Fig. 18.29, the spoiled signal is a maximum when ϵ_1 equals zero. For a 2D imaging sequence with an unbalanced phase encoding gradient (with the component of the sequence labeled (B) removed from the sequence shown in Fig. 18.31) and no rf phase increment, is there a position along the phase encoding direction which satisfies this? If so, which position?

b) Show that the position where this signal maximum occurs is shifted in the phase encoding direction when a constant rf phase increment ϵ_1 is introduced additionally. Relate this shift to ϵ_1.

c) How much is this position shift in number of voxels for $\epsilon_1 = 117°$?

18.4.4   RF Spoiled SSI Sequence Implementation

This subsection serves as a summarizing point for explaining the special features of a typical implementation of an rf spoiled SSI sequence shown in Fig. 18.31. The salient features of interest are labeled and highlighted in Fig. 18.31. As shown in the figure, a dephasing gradient (labeled (A)) is applied in every repetition period and the rf phase (labeled (C)) in the rotating frame is incremented by 117° or 123°. Further, all phase encoding gradients are refocused (the refocusing lobes being labeled (B)). Feature (B) ensures that no spatial inhomogeneity of signal as in a gradient-spoiled experiment is seen. Feature (A) dephases all the non-echoing pathways during each precession period. For example, when used in the read direction, this dephasing gradient lobe $G_{\text{dephase}}(t)$ must satisfy the first moment condition

$$\int_0^{T_R} (G_{\text{dephase}}(t) + G_R(t))dt \equiv mGT_s \tag{18.95}$$

where m is any positive integer and G is the frequency encoding read gradient amplitude.

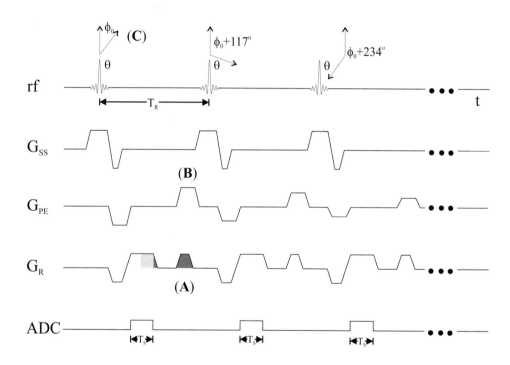

Fig. 18.31: An rf spoiled implementation of an SSI imaging sequence. Note that the areas under the read gradient during the second half of sampling and the rest of the read gradient waveform (shown with denser shading) are the same.

Suggested Reading

The following article covering both the coherent and incoherent steady-states gives expressions for flip angles which maximize the signal (hence the name 'Ernst angle'):

- R. R. Ernst and W. A. Anderson. Application of Fourier transform spectroscopy to magnetic resonance. *Rev. Sci. Instrum.*, 37: 93, 1966.

Using just classical Bloch equation solutions, the following paper first described the action of any arbitrary rf pulse as a composite of $0°$, $90°$, and $180°$ pulses in its action on magnetization:

- D. E. Woessner. Effects of diffusion in nuclear magnetic resonance spin echo experiments. *J. Chem. Phys.*, 34: 2057, 1961.

Spin-phase diagrams to locate echoes and determine their amplitudes when a set of rf pulses act on a population of spins are described in:

- R. Kaiser, E. Bartholdi and R. R. Ernst. Diffusion and field-gradient effects in NMR Fourier spectroscopy. *J. Chem. Phys.*, 60: 2966, 1974.

A method for phase encoding rf echoes resulting from a stopped-pulse experiment to obtain images was first described in:

- J. Hennig and M. Hodapp. Burst imaging. *MAGMA*, 1: 39, 1993.

A specific solution to the rf spoiling problem is given in:

- Y. Zur, M. L. Wood and L. J. Neuringer. Spoiling of transverse magnetization in steady-state sequences. *Magn. Reson. Med.*, 21: 251, 1991.

The next three articles listed here are modern reviews of the field of steady-state, fast imaging methods:

- E. M. Haacke, P. A. Wielopolski and J. A. Tkach. A comprehensive technical review of short T_R, fast magnetic resonance imaging techniques. *Rev. Magn. Reson. Med.*, 3: 53, 1991.

- J. Hennig. Echoes – how to generate, recognize, use or avoid them in MR-imaging sequences. Part I: Fundamental and not so fundamental properties of spin echoes. *Concepts Magn. Reson.*, 3: 125, 1991.

- J. Hennig. Part II: Echoes in imaging sequences. *Concepts Magn. Reson.*, 3: 179, 1991.

The following four papers proposed different short T_E, fast imaging methods:

- G. M. Bydder and I. R. Young. Clinical use of the partial and saturation recovery sequences in MR imaging. *J. Comput. Assist. Tomogr.*, 9: 1020, 1985.

- A. Haase, J. Frahm, D. Matthei, W. Hannicke and K.-D. Merboldt. FLASH imaging: Rapid imaging using low flip angle pulses. *J. Magn. Reson.*, 67: 256, 1986.

- A. Oppelt, R. Graumann, H. Barfuss, H. Fischer, W. Hertl and W. Schajor. FISP: A new fast MRI sequence. *Electromedica*, 3: 15, 1986.

- P. van der Muelen, J. P. Croen and J. J. M. Cuppen. Very fast MR imaging by field echoes and small angle excitation. *Magn. Reson. Imag.*, 3: 297, 1985.

Chapter 19

Segmented k-Space and Echo Planar Imaging

Chapter Contents

Summary: Methods of phase encoding between gradient echoes to reduce the number of rf pulses required to create a 2D image are developed. This concept is extended to allow a single shot acquisition referred to as echo planar imaging or EPI. Both conventional and spiral EPI methods are introduced. These concepts are extended to phase encoding between π-pulses to allow for rapid T_2 weighted spin echo imaging.

Introduction

This chapter introduces the reader to alternate forms of rapid imaging, as compared to the short-T_R methods discussed in the previous chapter. The concept of k-space segmentation is discussed, and two examples of methods where multiple k-space lines per rf excitation are phase encoded between gradient echoes or spin echoes are given. Different methods of

511

echo planar imaging (EPI) are introduced, including conventional EPI, spiral EPI, and square-spiral EPI. Technical limitations of each method are reviewed. The thrust for such single shot acquisitions has been driven by cardiac imaging, functional imaging and diffusion weighted imaging applications. These studies require rapid temporal acquisition over 3D volumes. One form of EPI that exists in the above-mentioned list includes collecting multiple lines of data by phase encoding between spin echoes to allow for rapid T_2-weighted data acquisition. Since T_2-weighted imaging has high clinical utility, reduction of the usually long scan times is critical. This is achieved using phase encoding between spin echoes, different variants of which are discussed in the last section of this chapter.

19.1   Reducing Scan Times

As an introduction to reducing imaging time, a review of what leads to long or short scan times is useful. The total scan or acquisition time T_T in MRI is determined by the repeat time T_R, the number of phase encoding steps N_y, the number of partition encoding steps N_z, and the number of acquisitions N_{acq}, giving

$$T_T = N_{acq} N_z N_y T_R \tag{19.1}$$

How can scan time be reduced? In the previous chapter it was demonstrated that T_R could be reduced and yet T_1-weighting or T_1/T_2-weighting could be maintained when large flip angles ($\theta > \theta_E$) are used. In the following discussion, the role of each term in (19.1) in reducing T_T and their resulting effects on contrast will be considered.

19.1.1   Reducing T_R

One way to reduce T_T is to shorten the repetition time. Bear in mind, however, as $T_R \to \lambda T_R$ with $\lambda < 1$, that there is a concomitant change in signal-to-noise such that, at best (at the Ernst angle defined in Ch. 18), SNR $\to \sqrt{\lambda}$SNR. There is no escaping the limit imposed by nature that SNR $\propto \sqrt{time}$. For a simple spin echo scan, where the first pulse is a $\pi/2$-pulse, SNR $\to \lambda$SNR since the signal is directly proportional to T_R/T_1 when $T_R \ll T_1$. Of course, as T_R changes, contrast also changes, and if it changes for the worse, the short T_R scan may not be useful.

19.1.2   Reducing the Number of Phase/Partition Encoding Steps

Another way to reduce T_T is to cut back on the number of phase encoding or partition encoding steps. This approach is useful because contrast is unchanged, although partial volume effects will become worse (see Ch. 15). There are two ways to accomplish this. First, assume L_y and L_z remain fixed. Then, for $N_y \to \lambda N_y$ with $\lambda < 1$, the acquisition time is reduced by a factor λ, but the resolution becomes a factor λ worse (i.e., $\Delta y \to \Delta y/\lambda$). See Figs. 19.1a and 19.1b. On the other hand, SNR is increased by a factor $\frac{1}{\sqrt{\lambda}}$. (Recall that the signal goes up by $1/\lambda$, but the noise standard deviation goes up by only $\frac{1}{\sqrt{\lambda}}$.) If resolution is too important to be sacrificed, then this is a poor strategy for reducing scan time.

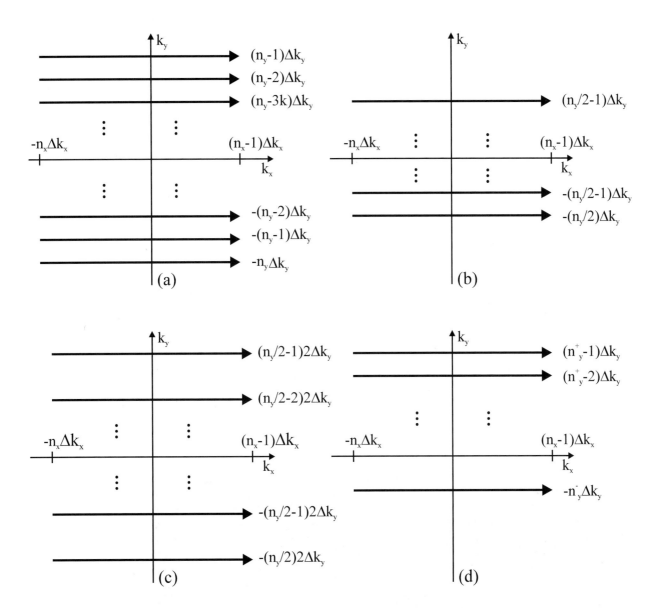

Fig. 19.1: (a) Conventional 2D k-space coverage with $\Delta x = L_x/N_x$ and $\Delta y = L_y/N_y$. (b) Reducing N_y by a factor of two (from $2n_y$ to n_y) by sampling only the central part of k-space increases the pixel size Δy by a factor of two ($k_{y,max}$ is now cut in half). (c) Reducing acquisition time while maintaining the same resolution. In this case, $k_{y,max}$ is not changed but Δk_y has become $2\Delta k_y$ (L_y has become $L_y/2$), n_y has become $n_y/2$, so that Δy remains invariant. (d) Example of k-space coverage for a partial Fourier method. In the case shown, standard MRI sampling is taking place in the read direction, but less data is collected in the phase encoding direction to reduce imaging time. The k-space data are collected from $-n_y^- \Delta k_y$ to $(n_y^+ - 1)\Delta k_y$ where n_y^- is usually chosen to be small relative to n_y^+. The missing negative k_y-space data are reconstructed using the partial Fourier reconstruction method discussed in Ch. 13.

The second method maintains resolution by reducing N_y and L_y by the same factor of λ, thereby keeping Δy fixed (see Fig. 19.1c). Now $T_T \to \lambda T_T$ but SNR is reduced to $\sqrt{\lambda}$SNR. This loss in SNR is unavoidable when smaller fields-of-view are used. In order to avoid aliasing, the object size A_y in the y-direction must be larger than λL_y.

19.1.3 Fixing the Number of Acquisitions

A third method to reduce scan time is to keep $N_{acq} = 1$, which is feasible if there is sufficient SNR. Using a small field-of-view has been seen to be very inefficient, causing a reduction by at least $\sqrt{\lambda}$ in SNR when $T_T \to \lambda T_T$. By using better rf coil designs such as smaller coils or a set of multiple coils,[1] SNR can be increased (see Ch. 27). Better SNR also allows a shorter T_R to be used. Hence, even rf coil design can be considered part of a faster imaging strategy. If SNR is not a limiting factor, the proposed short-T_R methods of the previous chapter, or those described in this chapter, will be more practical.

19.1.4 Partial Fourier Data Acquisition

A fourth approach is to force N_{acq} to be effectively less than unity. This is possible, thanks to the complex conjugate property of the Fourier transform of real objects and the associated reconstruction method called *partial Fourier reconstruction* (see Ch. 13). In this method, only λN_y ($0.5 \leq \lambda \leq 1.0$) lines are collected which reduces T_T to λT_T. Imaging schemes that employ other methods for speeding up the process can be further accelerated using this capability. The reduction is by at most a factor of 2, the maximum referring to the ability to relate one half of 2D k-space to the other half. Also, due to the reduction in the number of data points collected for similar imaging parameters, the signal-to-noise ratio of the partial Fourier data is reduced by $\sqrt{\lambda}$.

Problem 19.1

Of the methods discussed so far to reduce imaging time, which ones leave the contrast unchanged? Is CNR also kept constant in those cases where the contrast is unchanged?

19.2 Segmented k-Space: Phase Encoding Multiple k-Space Lines per RF Excitation for Gradient Echo Imaging

Section 19.1 constitutes a review of methods employed in previous chapters. The main focus of this chapter involves the concept of collecting multiple lines of k-space data after a single

---

[1] A set of multiple rf coils used to collect data simultaneously in the same experiment is often referred to as a phased array coil.

rf excitation. In this section, an example is studied where two lines of k-space are acquired after one rf pulse. The approach of collecting more than one line of k-space after a single echo is a form of 'segmented k-space coverage.' However, a more general definition of segmented k-space coverage would be the collection of multiple k-space lines in a set, each set being collected in a given order, but not constituting a complete coverage of k-space until all of the sets are merged together. It is then possible to collect one line of k-space for each rf pulse and yet still create a segmented k-space coverage. For example, if the even lines $-n_y, -(n_y-2), -(n_y-4), \dots$ are collected using single echo sequences during one cardiac cycle and odd lines $-(n_y-1), -(n_y-3), -(n_y-5), \dots$ during the next, then this is referred to as a two-segment coverage of k-space relative to the cardiac cycle. In a sense, the conventional 2D Fourier transform coverage of k-space requiring N_y phase encoding steps is an N_y-segment coverage. However, since it is in such common use, this adjective is never used in practice.

19.2.1 Conventional Multiple Echo Acquisition

The double gradient echo[2] is a good introduction to collecting more than one line of k-space data after a single rf excitation. The double gradient echo experiment can be used in two ways. One is to collect two images with different contrast levels by collecting the same line of k-space with different values of T_E. The second is to employ phase encoding between the two gradient echoes, thereby collecting multiple lines of k-space data to create a single image in half of the total imaging time. The sequence diagrams for the two cases are shown in Fig. 19.2 and the k-space coverages appear in Fig. 19.3.

Assume that the double gradient echo is to be used to collect two images. The single-image case is discussed in the next subsection. In the double-image case, the k-space lines covered for each echo per rf excitation will be the same but, as shown in Fig. 19.3a, the direction of traversal through k-space in the read direction is opposite for the two echoes. The reason it may be desirable to collect two echoes in this way is to get images with different T_2^* or flow contrast (see Sec. 24.3 on phase contrast imaging in Ch. 24) in the same time. Consider, for example, an experiment with a relatively long T_R. This experiment could be used to generate a spin density weighted image if $T_E \ll T_2^*$, or a T_2^* weighted image if $T_E \simeq T_{2,average}^*$. However, using the double gradient echo, and making proper choices of $T_{E,1}$ and $T_{E,2}$ both images can be acquired in half of the time than if the scan were run twice with a different T_E each time.

More gradient echoes may be employed after the single rf pulse; their number is limited only by T_R, the available gradient strengths and rise times, and the T_2^* of the object. Such procedures are referred to as multi-echo image acquisitions.

---

[2]In review, recall that a gradient echo occurs at any time after the application of the first read gradient lobe where the accumulated phase due to the read gradient is zero for all stationary spins. Gradient echoes are also referred to as field echoes or gradient field echoes in the MRI literature. A gradient echo should not be confused with a spin echo which is an rf echo that occurs when all of the phase accumulated by stationary spins due to static field variations is refocused to zero. This double gradient echo scan is also referred to as a two echo, multi-gradient echo scan.

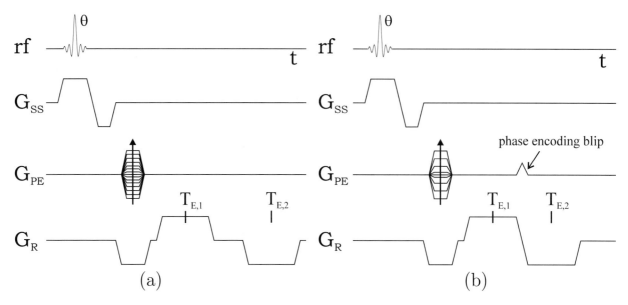

Fig. 19.2: The read and phase encoding gradient waveforms with an arbitrary flip angle θ for (a) a simple double gradient echo sequence, and (b) a segmented k-space double gradient echo sequence. Note that a small phase encoding gradient blip waveform has been added between the two gradient echoes in (b). This encodes the next line in 2D k-space for the second echo. The stepped phase encoding table covers all even k-space lines (assuming n_y is a multiple of 2) in the first echo while the odd lines are generated after the short phase encoding gradient (shown as a triangular waveform) and are collected in the second echo. This constitutes a simple form of segmented k-space coverage.

Problem 19.2

    a) Draw a sequence diagram for an experiment where two images with different contrast are collected (no phase encoding between the echoes). The first acquisition (first echo) follows a $\pi/2$ excitation pulse and the second acquisition (second echo) follows a π pulse. Design the sequence such that the first echo provides data for a T_2^*-weighted image, and the second echo provides data for a T_2-weighted image.

    b) Assuming an experiment is performed with $T_R \gg T_1$, modify the sequence diagram in part (a) to employ three echoes. Design the timings of the experiment such that one of the resulting images is spin density weighted, one is T_2^* weighted, and one is T_2 weighted.

    c) Show that data acquired with the simple double gradient echo acquisition illustrated in the right-hand side of Fig. 19.3a leads to a spatially reversed second image unless the data are reordered (i.e., put in the order shown in the left-hand side of Fig. 19.3a).

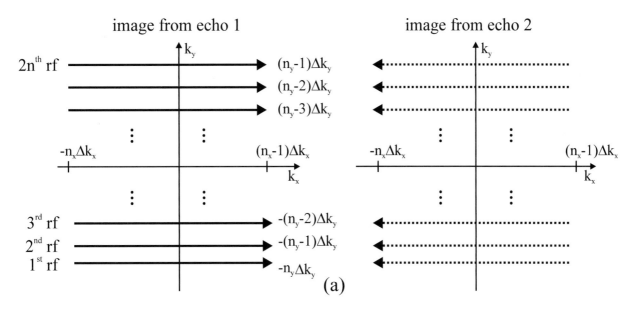

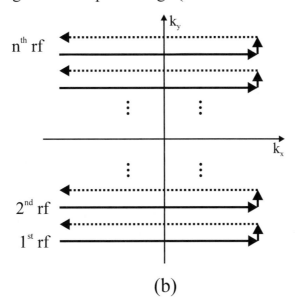

Fig. 19.3: Part (a) depicts the 2D k-space coverage of the double gradient echo sequence when it is used to collect two images and the same line of k-space is covered twice after each rf excitation. The left-hand side of (a) shows the k-space coverage for the image collected from the first echo, and the right-hand side of (a) shows the k-space coverage for the image collected from the second echo. Shown in (b) is the temporal coverage of k-space when additional phase encoding is applied between the two echoes. The upward arrow in (b) indicates the movement in k-space due to the application of the triangular gradient blip in the phase encoding direction. The dashed lines represent the reversed k-space order in which the data are temporally collected. Notice that only half as many rf excitations are needed to cover the same region of k-space and that the return pathway in k-space from the second gradient echo is running from right to left.

19.2.2   Phase Encoding Between Gradient Echoes

The previous application of the conventional double gradient echo experiment did not allow the collection of a single image in less time. Although several images could be collected in the same time as one, the time needed to collect one image did not change. The primary goal of this chapter is to show how to collect a single image in a much shorter period of time than that given by (19.1). This may be accomplished by acquiring more than one line of k-space after a single rf excitation. In other words, a full 2D, and possibly a 3D region of k-space may be acquired after each rf excitation, instead of just a line. Phase encoding can be introduced between the two gradient echoes so two lines of k-space are acquired in the double gradient echo experiment. The k-space structure is shown in Fig. 19.3b. By phase encoding between two echoes, a factor of two in time can be saved over that of normal k-space coverage. The phase encoding is accomplished by applying a short gradient pulse or 'blip' of the phase encoding gradient between the sampling times (the triangular waveform added to the phase encoding gradient waveform in Fig. 19.2b). In terms of k-space coverage,

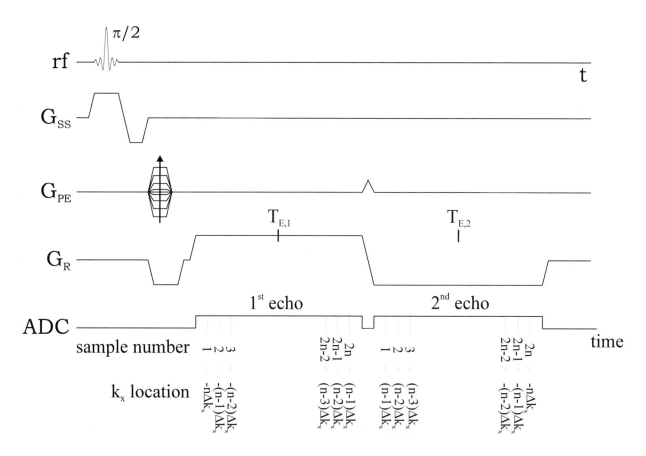

Fig. 19.4: The ADC line explicitly demonstrates that the ordering of k-space data relative to the sampled points varies between the two echoes. Note that the k-space traversal is reversed in time along k_x for the second echo. When multiple gradient echoes are used, such data must be reordered before data reconstruction takes place. Specifically, the even echoes must be time reversed before being placed at their respective k-space points.

every odd line from the second echo is interleaved between every even line from the first to create a hybrid or *segmented k*-space. Factors of two can be quite significant in terms of time saved, especially for rather long sequences.

Reordering the Data

In previous experiments dealing with single echoes, the direction of traversal in k-space was identical for each repetition of a cycle. However, when multiple gradient echoes are collected after a single excitation, this is not always the case. An examination of the data collected during the double gradient echo experiment is a useful introduction to how data must often be rearranged after collection before being used to reconstruct an image (see Fig. 19.4). The $2n$ sampled points ($n \equiv n_x$) from the first echo running from 1 to $2n$ correspond to the k-space data beginning at $-n\Delta k_x$ and ending with $(n-1)\Delta k_x$. The $2n$ sampled points from the second echo from 1 to $2n$ correspond to k-space data at the next phase encoding line beginning at $(n-1)\Delta k_x$ and ending with $-n\Delta k_x$. The first point collected in the first echo corresponds to a negative k-space point, but the first point from the second echo corresponds to a positive k-space point. In fact, the data collected from the second echo are ordered exactly opposite to the k-space ordering of the first echo. Before the data can be reconstructed, the even echo data must be reordered (time reversed) so that the final data matrix represents the correct coverage in k-space.[3] *Specifically, data from every other line of k-space must be reversed from the order in which it was collected before being reconstructed.*

Problem 19.3

There is an image artifact associated with segmented data collection due to T_2^* filtering. The possibility that the k_y data points may be collected at different times following a single excitation pulse leads to a discontinuity in the effective magnitude of the data sampled along k_y at every other point (see Fig. 19.5). This can be modeled by a changing magnitude of the k-space sampling function. In effect, the time-reversal of data collection relative to k-space causes this discontinuity to be a different function of k_x for the odd and even lines. Consider the product of the signal in the absence of relaxation and an exponential representing the effects of transverse relaxation

$$s(k_x, k_y) = s_0(k_x, k_y)e^{-t(k_x,k_y)/T_2^*} \tag{19.2}$$

a) Show that for the case of the double gradient echo, the signal at the even k_y points is given by

$$s(r\Delta k_x, 2p\Delta k_y) = s_0(r\Delta k_x, 2p\Delta k_y)e^{-(T_{E,1}+r\Delta t)/T_2^*} \tag{19.3}$$

where r represents the index in k-space (not the index of the sampled point; see Fig. 19.4) $-n \le r \le (n-1)$ and $-n/2 \le p \le (n/2-1)$.

---

[3]Almost all of the methods discussed in this chapter cover k-space differently in comparison with conventional methods discussed in other chapters. The data from each of these methods must be time reversed or reordered, in general, before images can be reconstructed.

b) Show that for the odd lines, the T_2^* filter is different and is given by

$$s(r\Delta k_x, (2p+1)\Delta k_y) = s_0(r\Delta k_x, (2p+1)\Delta k_y)e^{-(T_{E,2}-r\Delta t)/T_2^*} \quad (19.4)$$

Take special note of the time-reversal in the exponent.

c) Finally show that the k dependence of the time given in (19.2) follows from

$$
\begin{aligned}
t(r\Delta k_x, 2p\Delta k_y) &= T_{E,1} + r\Delta t \\
t(r\Delta k_x, (2p+1)\Delta k_y) &= T_{E,2} - r\Delta t
\end{aligned}
\quad (19.5)
$$

It should be observed that even for infinitely short sampling times (when the term $r\Delta t$ goes to zero) there still exists a discontinuity in the even and odd line k-space signals determined by $(T_{E,2} - T_{E,1})$.

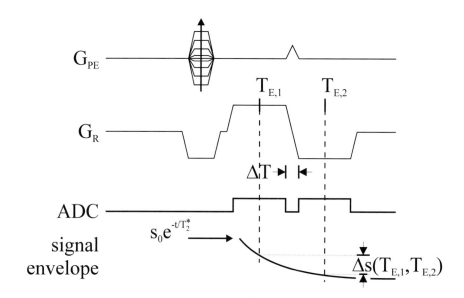

Fig. 19.5: The k-space discontinuities caused by differences in the T_2^* decay envelopes between corresponding points along k_x in successive lines of k-space. These discontinuities lead to aliasing artifacts. The read and phase encoding gradients are shown above the T_2^* decay envelope to provide a time reference. The signal discontinuity Δs is shown to indicate the signal difference at the two echo times $T_{E,1}$ and $T_{E,2}$.

Filter Effects and $N/2$ Ghosting

A ubiquitous problem that occurs with phase encoding between echoes is due to T_2^* or T_2 decay during sampling from one echo to the next (see Fig. 19.5). An efficient way to model the effect the decay in signal amplitude will have on the resulting images is to consider the two-dimensional data as a summation of two interleaved data sets, corresponding to odd and even echoes, respectively. The relevant sampling function centered around the first echo is given by

$$u_{first\ echo}(k_x, k_y) = \Delta k_x \Delta k_y \sum_{r=-n}^{n-1} \sum_{p=-n/2}^{n/2-1} e^{-T_{E,1}/T_2^*} e^{-r\Delta t/T_2^*} \delta(k_x - r\Delta k_x)\delta(k_y - 2p\Delta k_y) \quad (19.6)$$

where the magnitude of the sampling function has been normalized to its ideal value at the center of the first echo. The magnitude of the sampling function during the second echo is further reduced by the effects of transverse relaxation

$$u_{second\ echo}(k_x, k_y) = \Delta k_x \Delta k_y \sum_{r=-n}^{n-1} \sum_{p=-n/2}^{n/2-1} e^{-T_{E,2}/T_2^*} e^{+r\Delta t/T_2^*} \delta(k_x - r\Delta k_x)\delta(k_y - (2p+1)\Delta k_y)$$

$$(19.7)$$

The total sampling function for the experiment is the sum

$$u(k_x, k_y) = u_{first\ echo}(k_x, k_y) + u_{second\ echo}(k_x, k_y) \quad (19.8)$$

Suppose the exponents $\pm r\Delta t/T_2^*$ are very small in magnitude compared with unity and with respect to $\Delta T_E/T_2^*$ (where $\Delta T_E \equiv (T_{E,2} - T_{E,1})$) for all values of r. If ΔT_E is also small compared to T_2^*, the sampling function at the second echo is simply that at the first echo scaled by $1 - \zeta$ where

$$\zeta \simeq \frac{\Delta T_E}{T_2^*} \ll 1 \quad (19.9)$$

After a Fourier transformation along k_y, the discontinuity in the signal envelope (see Fig. 19.5) will lead to aliasing, or an $N/2$ ghost (a ghost which is shifted by exactly half an FOV or $N/2$ points from the actual image), in the phase encoding direction, of amplitude $\zeta/2$ and it would appear to reduce the amplitude of the central image by a factor of $1 - \zeta/2$ (see Sec. 12.4 in Ch. 12). (See Fig. 19.8 for a visual example of this phenomenon.)

Problem 19.4

Investigate the validity of the above statements regarding ghosting by considering a 1D Fourier transform of the data along the phase encoding direction for a 2D boxcar function. The sides of the boxcar function are parallel to the Cartesian axes. Assume that relaxation effects along the read direction can be neglected.

a) Write the sampling function along a line in the phase encoding direction for a fixed value of r in (19.6)–(19.7).

b) Describe qualitatively the resulting image using the formalism developed in Sec. 12.4 of Ch. 12.

c) Assume that T_2^* for the box being imaged is 40 ms. What will be the magnitude of the $N/2$ ghost, if $T_{E,1} = 10$ ms and $T_{E,2} = 20$ ms, relative to the ideal value from the center of the first echo?

This situation is actually more complicated because the magnitude of the sampling function depends on k_x. This leads to filtering of the image in the x-direction because of the exponential decay of transverse magnetization during sampling (see Sec. 13.5 in Ch. 13). In general, however, the sampling time $(2n\Delta t)$ is small compared to T_2^* and this effect may often be ignored. The effects of T_2^* filtering are perhaps best seen by simulating the data for an object of known geometry and putting in the correct temporal behavior such as that in (19.6) and (19.7) for the two-echo case.

19.3   Echo Planar Imaging (EPI)

The above segmented double gradient echo method lends itself to a more general procedure of phase encoding between multiple gradient echoes. The collection of all the data necessary to reconstruct a reasonable image using one set, or 'train,' of echoes after a single rf excitation with a short phase encoding gradient pulse (a blip) between each echo is referred to as echo planar imaging or EPI. The sequence diagram and corresponding k-space coverage for a standard 'blipped' EPI imaging sequence are shown in Figs. 19.6 and 19.7, respectively.

The total acquisition time T_D to collect the k-space data is shown in Fig. 19.6 and represents the time associated with all read and phase encoding gradients, excluding preparatory

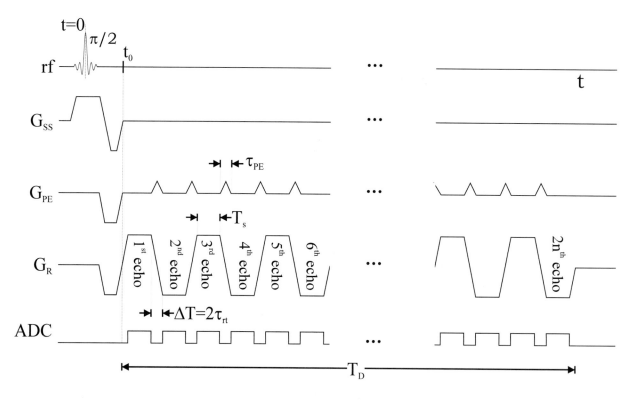

Fig. 19.6: Sequence diagram showing the phase encoding and read gradient waveforms for an EPI sequence.

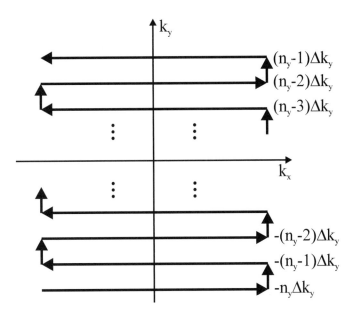

Fig. 19.7: Temporal order of the 2D k-space coverage in EPI.

pulses,

$$\begin{aligned} T_D &= N_y(T_s + \Delta T) \\ &= N_x N_y \Delta t + N_y \Delta T \end{aligned} \tag{19.10}$$

where $\Delta T \equiv 2\tau_{rt}$ is defined as the time to take the read gradient from peak to opposite peak between echoes, as shown in Fig. 19.6. With additional time parameters also defined in that figure, the minimum total time to complete an experiment is seen to be

$$T_T = \tau_{rf}/2 + t_0 + T_D \tag{19.11}$$

In this case, T_T denotes the total imaging time for an EPI experiment where all of the data is collected following one rf pulse, and the experiment is not repeated. Therefore, T_R is not a relevant parameter and the total time is the sum of the time needed for rf excitation, preparatory gradient lobes, and data sampling.

Since EPI collects a full set of 2D information during the time T_D with just one rf excitation, the contrast is governed by spin density and T_2^* alone, with no T_1 dependence. T_1-weighted contrast can be obtained by repeating the EPI experiment at intervals of T_R, in which case T_T becomes

$$T_T = N_{acq}T_R \tag{19.12}$$

Practically, EPI experiments are often run with $T_R \gg T_1$ (in humans, $T_R = 3$ s meets this criterion at 1.5 T for all tissues, except CSF) and if the data are collected only once then T_R is not a factor in the contrast. Under these circumstances, the images are T_2^*-weighted since the effective echo time ($T_{E,\vec{k}=0}$) is quite long ($t_0 + T_D/2$), so that it becomes comparable to T_2^* (see Fig. 19.8).

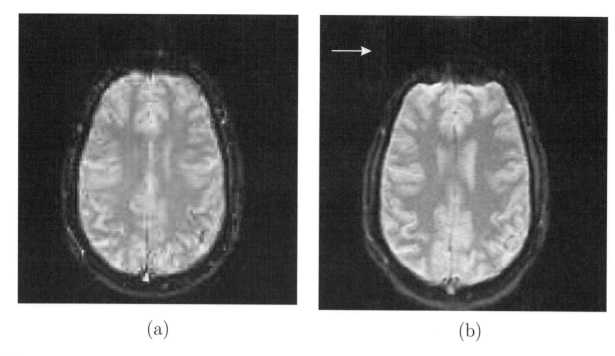

(a)   (b)

Fig. 19.8: (a) A low resolution conventional 2D gradient echo image. (b) A low resolution 2D EPI image. Generally, the image quality of the EPI image is good in the center of the brain where there are no strong local gradients. However, image distortion is visible near the sinuses (top, anterior part of the brain). The worse distortion in (b) is due to the fact that the bandwidth is lower in the vertical direction in comparison with (a) (see Ch. 20 for a detailed explanation of bandwidth dependence of the distortion phenomenon). Also, some low amplitude $N/2$-ghosts are visible in (b), one of which is indicated by the long white arrow.

The $k = 0$ Point

Much of the signal comes from the sampling of data near the center of k-space or the $k = 0$ point. This is especially true for low spatial frequency structures. Due to the use of multiple echoes, the minimum echo time in EPI must be longer than the standard short-T_R gradient echo sequences. The central field echo time in EPI is defined to be the time from the beginning of the read gradient to the central echo (defined to occur at the instant in time when the 2D k-space origin is sampled) and is given by

$$T_{E,\vec{k}=0} = \frac{N_y + 1}{2} N_x \Delta t + (N_y + 1)\tau_{rt} + t_0 \tag{19.13}$$

where τ_{rt} is the rise time.

Excluding filtering effects, for a $\pi/2$ excitation pulse, the EPI image intensity for a single excitation pulse, or the first pulse of a repeated sequence is approximated by

$$\hat{\rho}(\vec{r}) = \rho_0(\vec{r})e^{-T_{E,\vec{k}=0}/T_2^*(\vec{r})} \tag{19.14}$$

Conventional T_1-weighted contrast occurs for EPI if the experiment is repeated, i.e., for the $\pi/2$-excitation

$$\hat{\rho}(\vec{r}) = \rho_0(\vec{r})e^{-T_{E,\vec{k}=0}/T_2^*(\vec{r})} \left(1 - e^{-T_R/T_1(\vec{r})}\right) \tag{19.15}$$

The coverage of k-space can be reordered so that $T_{E,\vec{k}=0}$ occurs at a different time than that given in (19.13). This is done by varying the amplitude of the negative lobe along the phase encoding direction at the beginning of the sequence which determines the starting position along k_y. Equation (19.13) is only accurate when k_y is covered sequentially from $-k_{y_{max}}$ to $k_{y_{max}}$. Different expressions would have to be developed for segmented, partial Fourier, reordered, or other k-space coverages (see Sec. 19.4). Centric k-space, for example, would give the shortest effective T_E using the above argument. As usual, the choice of T_E will determine how heavily T_2^*-weighted the image is, despite the long sampling times (recall that central k-space data carries the bulk of the signal for low spatial frequency information).

Problem 19.5

It is also possible to create an inversion recovery EPI sequence. This is particularly useful when trying to null the CSF signal, for example.

a) Draw an inversion recovery EPI sequence diagram.

b) Write an expression for $\hat{\rho}(\vec{r})$ for an inversion recovery EPI sequence with a single $\pi/2$-excitation.

c) What should T_I be to null the signal from CSF?

19.3.1 An In-Depth Analysis of the EPI Imaging Parameters

The implementation of EPI is limited by how quickly the data can be acquired with a given value of gradient strength, gradient rise time and sampling rate. A straightforward analysis of the Nyquist conditions is all that is needed to determine if EPI is viable for a given set of parameters. It will be shown that it is important to carefully keep track of all imaging parameters and that each choice of an imaging parameter fixes one or several others.

A step-by-step determination of the imaging parameters will be considered in the following discussion. A numerical example will be developed based on the parameters fixed in each step.

Sampling Rate

First, it is important to determine the limitations imposed by sampling along the read direction. Usually, the field-of-view will be given by physical conditions (such as the size of a human organ) and the gradient strength by the system's maximum available gradient strength. As usual, the sampling time is determined by the Nyquist criterion

$$\Delta t = \frac{1}{\gamma G_x L_x} \qquad \text{for constant read gradient} \tag{19.16}$$

If the data are to be collected as fast as possible (i.e., T_s is minimized to keep T_T small; see (19.10) and (19.11)), then G_x must be the maximum available gradient strength. The numerical example to follow will be seeded with the convenient values $L_x = 256\,\text{mm}$ and $G_x = 25\,\text{mT/m}$, leading to a value of $\Delta t = 3.67\,\mu\text{s}$.

Resolution along the Read Direction

Given a desired resolution Δx, the number of sampled points per echo is

$$N_x = \frac{L_x}{\Delta x} \tag{19.17}$$

For $\Delta x = 2\,\mathrm{mm}$, $N_x = 128$ points, and this gives the sampling time per readout of a single read gradient lobe, $T_s = 0.470\,\mathrm{ms}$.

Phase Encoding Step Amplitude

As before, the object size will determine L_y. In standard short-T_R, gradient echo imaging sequences, the choice of τ_{pe} (time duration of the phase encoding gradient) is made based on how much time is taken to apply the dephasing lobe of the read gradient. The phase encoding in an EPI sequence is different from a conventional phase encoding table. From L_y and τ_{pe}, the zeroth moment of the phase encoding gradient blip waveform $\Delta G_y(t)$ is seen to be

$$\int_t^{t+\tau_{pe}} dt'\, \Delta G_y(t') = \frac{1}{\gamma L_y} \tag{19.18}$$

If $\Delta G_y(t)$ is a triangular waveform with a peak value of ΔG_{y_0}, then (19.18) yields

$$\Delta G_{y_0} = 2/(\gamma L_y \tau_{pe}) \tag{19.19}$$

In EPI sequences, τ_{pe} is usually $2\tau_{rt}$ (where τ_{rt} is the rise time of each readout gradient lobe) to minimize scan time since the echo reversals take $2\tau_{rt}$ (see Fig. 19.6). This leads to

$$\Delta G_{y_0} = 1/(\gamma L_y \tau_{rt}) \tag{19.20}$$

For $L_y = L_x = 256\,\mathrm{mm}$, $\tau_{rt} = 0.3\,\mathrm{ms}$, (19.20) leads to $\Delta G_{y_0} = 0.31\,\mathrm{mT/m}$. (Actually, these blips can be applied much more quickly than $0.3\,\mathrm{ms}$ since a peak gradient strength of $25\,\mathrm{mT/m}$ or higher is typically available and it typically takes about $0.3\,\mathrm{ms}$ to rise to $25\,\mathrm{mT/m}$. Since the read gradient needs to switch from $-25\,\mathrm{mT/m}$ to $+25\,\mathrm{mT/m}$ or vice versa during the application of this blip waveform, each of which takes τ_{rt}, it is typical to use $\tau_{pe} = 2\tau_{rt}$.)

Phase Encoding Resolution

The next question concerns the maximum number of phase encoding steps. The only factor that limits how many lines can be covered in k-space (and, hence, the spatial resolution in the y-direction) is T_2^*. The exact amount of time that can be used for sampling depends upon the goals of the experiment and how the data are collected, but is ultimately limited by transverse relaxation driving the signal to zero. A reasonable rule to follow is to assume it is possible to move from one k-space line to the next until the total data sampling time T_D becomes comparable to T_2^*. The number of lines covered in a time $T_D = T_2^*$ or T_2 (depending on whether a gradient echo or spin echo version of EPI is run) determines the maximum number of phase encoding steps $N_{y,max}$ based on the relation

$$N_{y,max} \simeq \frac{T_2^*}{N_x \Delta t + 2\tau_{rt}} \tag{19.21}$$

This maximum then fixes the best spatial resolution along y to be

$$\Delta y_{min} \simeq \frac{L_y}{N_{y,max}} \qquad (19.22)$$

for a conventional single-shot EPI experiment. If $T_2^* = 100$ ms, based upon the above choices, $N_{y,max} = 93$. The data are customarily zero filled to allow a 128 point Fourier transform in y as well as x and the image will be displayed on a 128×128 grid. Notice that (19.21) is only a guideline, representing a realistic balance between resolution loss due to filtering, signal loss due to transverse relaxation, and adequate sampling time for the EPI experiment already introduced; hence the approximate sign in (19.22). However, as found in Ch. 13, changing the imaging methodology can alter the filter effects. Therefore, the determination of the maximum available sampling time for each of the EPI methods introduced in the remainder of this chapter should be considered individually for each designed sequence. Also, segmentation offers a potential way to circumvent the sampling time constraints on resolution by collecting a fraction of the total number of k-space lines per excitation. Unfortunately, a segmented experiment takes longer and finite-T_R effects are invariably introduced.

Summary of Considerations

The previous considerations warrant a review. The following array of formulas summarizes the aforementioned relations that must be considered when developing an EPI sequence.

$$
\begin{array}{cl}
(a) & \Delta t = 1/\left(\gamma G_{x,max}L_x\right) \\[4pt]
(b) & \Delta x = L_x/N_x \\[4pt]
(c) & \Delta G_{y0} = 1/\left(\gamma L_y \tau_{rt}\right) \\[4pt]
(d) & N_{y,max} \simeq T_2^*/\left(N_x\Delta t + 2\tau_{rt}\right) \\[4pt]
(e) & \Delta y_{min} \simeq L_y/N_{y,max}
\end{array}
\qquad (19.23)
$$

Problem 19.6

Consider a gradient coil with a 50 mT/m maximum gradient strength, a rise time of 200 μs to 50 mT/m, a desired resolution of $\Delta x = 1$ mm, and equal fields-of-view, $L_x = L_y = 256$ mm. Find N_x, T_s, ΔG_{y0}, and $N_{y,max}$ for a tissue whose T_2^* is 100 ms. It is good practice to design EPI sequences with as short a T_D as possible for a given required $N_{y,max}$. For a fixed $N_{y,max}$, T_D is dependent only on T_s and τ_{rt}. To a good approximation, the rise time is proportional to the gradient amplitude, which, for this example suggests:

$$\tau_{rt} = 4G \qquad (19.24)$$

where G is in mT/m and τ_{rt} is in μs. Also, for fixed Δx, T_s is also dependent only on G. The optimal choice of T_D is therefore given by an optimal choice of G obtained by solving a minimization problem for the given set of system limitations such as G_{max} and τ_{rt}.

19.3.2   Signal-to-Noise

In Ch. 15, we learned that SNR is determined both by the bandwidth $BW_{read} = 1/\Delta t$ (see (15.27), for example) and by $T_{E,\vec{k}=0}/T_2^*$. Since there is no need to repeat the experiment for a single-slice or multi-slice EPI experiment, the full magnetization (M_0) can be interrogated without T_1-saturation effects. In the following discussion, a comparison will be made between 2D EPI and 3D short-T_R gradient echo imaging at the same spatial resolution.

3D Volume Coverage: 2D Multi-Slice EPI Versus 3D Incoherent Steady-State Imaging

The obvious question facing EPI imaging is whether or not it is really more efficient[4] than conventional methods. Here, a conventional method for covering a 3D volume is compared with an EPI method for covering the same volume. For a field-of-view L_z in the z-direction, a slice thickness Δz would require $N_z = L_z/\Delta z$ individual 2D slices to be acquired with multi-slice EPI. The methods being compared are assumed to be the optimal approaches in their respective categories for these applications. The SNR for the 2D EPI scan is

$$\text{SNR}_{EPI-2D} \propto \frac{\rho_0 e^{-N_y T_s/2T_2^*}}{\sqrt{BW_{read}}} \cdot \sqrt{N_y} \tag{19.25}$$

The same fields-of-view (L_x, L_y, and L_z) and resolution can be achieved using a 3D SSI experiment with N_z partitions instead of slices. The 3D experiment would take a time $N_y N_z T_R$ to acquire. For a short-T_R 3D SSI (described in Ch. 18) scan at the Ernst angle, the SNR is

$$\text{SNR}_{GE-3D} \propto \rho_0 \sqrt{N_y N_z} \sqrt{\frac{T_R}{2T_1}} e^{-(t_0 + \tau_{rt} + n_x \Delta t)/T_2^*} / \sqrt{BW_{read}} \tag{19.26}$$

using the same sequence structure for a conventional blipped EPI sequence up to the first echo ($T_E = t_0 + \tau_{rt} + n_x \Delta t$). The shortest T_R that can be used in this type of gradient echo sequence is

$$T_{R_{min}} \simeq \tau_{rf} + 4\tau_{rt} + 2N_x \Delta t \tag{19.27}$$

since the read gradient is kept on after data acquisition for spoiling. Both $2\tau_{rt}$ and $N_x \Delta t$ are about 1 ms and τ_{rf} is usually about 1 ms for a 3D scan (i.e., all three times are roughly equally long). Therefore, in this numerical example, $T_{R_{min}} \simeq 5N_x \Delta t$ and SNR becomes

$$\text{SNR}_{GE-3D} \propto \rho_0 \sqrt{\frac{5N_x N_y N_z \Delta t}{2T_1 BW_{read}}} e^{-T_E/T_2^*} \tag{19.28}$$

In order to cover the same volume with multi-slice 2D EPI, the total acquisition time is $N_z T_D$ where

$$T_D \simeq N_y T_R = 2N_y N_x \Delta t \tag{19.29}$$

again assuming $2\tau_{rt} \simeq N_x \Delta t$. The time to run 30 slices for EPI will be only 2.4 s compared to 6 s for the 3D scan to cover the same region.

---

[4]By 'efficient,' we mean the largest SNR in the least imaging time.

For the same total acquisition time ($T_R \rightarrow T_R/2.5$), the ratio of the two SNR values is

$$\frac{\text{SNR}_{GE-3D:T_R \rightarrow T_R/2.5}}{\text{SNR}_{EPI-2D}} \simeq \sqrt{\frac{N_z T_s}{T_1}} e^{N_y T_s/2T_2^*} = \sqrt{\left(\frac{T_{tot}}{T_D}\right)\left(\frac{T_s}{T_1}\right)} e^{N_y T_s/2T_2^*} \qquad (19.30)$$

where the long echo time of the EPI scan is assumed to dominate (i.e., we consider $T_E \ll T_2^*$ and neglect the e^{-T_E/T_2^*} factor in the 3D case).

Problem 19.7

a) For a single shot 2D EPI sequence, show for a fixed N_y that

$$\text{SNR} \propto \sqrt{\frac{T_s}{N_x}} e^{-N_y T_s/2T_2^*}$$

b) Show that the optimal SNR for EPI for fixed N_x and N_y occurs when

$$T_s = \frac{T_2^*}{N_y}$$

c) It is useful to determine for what number of slices EPI is more efficient than SSI imaging, and vice versa. Given that $T_1 = 1\,\text{s}$, $T_2^* = 100\,\text{ms}$, $\Delta t = 4\,\mu\text{s}$, $N_x = N_y = 100$, determine the value of N_z for which the SNR for 2D multi-slice EPI surpasses 3D SSI gradient echo.

Problem 19.8

A variant of the gradient echo EPI sequence is the spin echo EPI sequence where lines of phase encoded data are collected symmetrically about the rf echo. The sequence diagram for this experiment is given in Fig. 19.9.

a) Draw the k-space diagram corresponding to the sequence diagram given in Fig. 19.9.

b) Given $G_{max} = 20\,\text{mT/m}$, $\tau_{rt} = 0.2\,\text{ms}$, $T_2^* = 40\,\text{ms}$, $T_2 = 80\,\text{ms}$, $\Delta x = 2\,\text{mm}$, and $L_x = L_y = 25.6\,\text{cm}$, find how many phase encoding lines may be reasonably acquired. Assume that $T_D \leq 2T_2^*$ so that the image is relatively free of significant filtering due to transverse relaxation. (This choice of $2T_2^*$ is somewhat arbitrary, but represents the point where roughly one tenth of the signal remains from T_2^* effects.) To what resolution does this correspond in the phase encoding direction?

c) Write expressions for the k-space filters due to transverse decay along the phase encoding direction for both the gradient echo and spin echo experiment.

While EPI is well-suited to spin density or T_2^*-weighted scans, rapid 3D imaging with short T_R requires $\theta \ll \theta_E$ to achieve spin density weighting (Ch. 18). This reduces the SNR dramatically for the latter case, in comparison with EPI. If $\theta \to \frac{\theta_E}{4}$, then N_z should go to $4N_z$ to recover the factor of 2 loss in SNR in comparison with the previously considered imaging at the Ernst angle for the 3D SSI method. On the other hand, the long sampling time in EPI produces some T_2^* filter artifacts (Ch. 13) and signal loss as discussed above, and later, in this chapter.

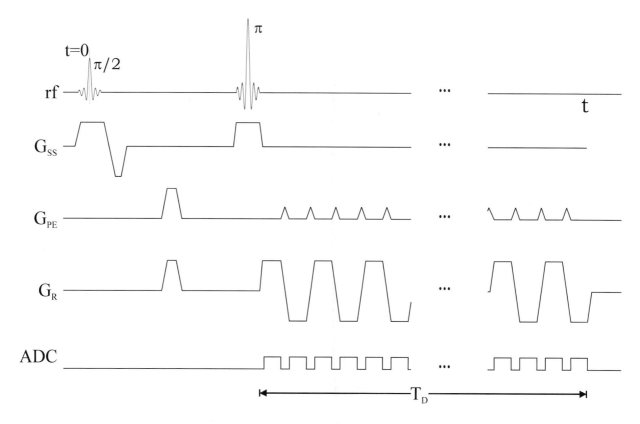

Fig. 19.9: A spin echo EPI imaging sequence.

19.4   Alternate Forms of Conventional EPI

The previous discussion of EPI represents the conventional approach to obtaining a regular Cartesian grid of points covering the required region of k-space after a single rf excitation. The following EPI schemes give alternate ways of covering large areas of k-space after a single rf excitation. If the sampled points do not lie on a regular Cartesian grid, the data must be manipulated (reordered and interpolated) before a conventional discrete Fourier transform can be used to obtain an accurate image. In some cases, the methods lend themselves well to alternate reconstruction methods such as projection reconstruction.

19.4.1 Nonuniform Sampling

A feature of these EPI implementations is that they involve sampling during the application of time-varying gradients. This implies that data sampled at uniform spaced time points will no longer give a uniform distribution of points in k-space. For instance, nonuniform (in time) sampling may be necessary to obtain uniform sampling density in k-space. The necessary tools to understand nonuniform sampling have already been introduced (Sec. 12.4 in Ch. 12), but a brief introduction to the subject will be presented. The optimal implementation of data sampling and manipulation for each method should be treated on an *a priori* basis.

The term nonuniform sampling implies that data are sampled nonuniformly in time in order to get a uniform density of sampled points in k-space. In other words, for the conventional 1D discrete Fourier transform, adjacent sampled points in k-space must be separated by an equal distance Δk. The constant k-space separation of two sampled points in terms of the applied gradient and the times at which they are sampled (t_{r-1}, t_r) is given by

$$\Delta k = \gamma \int_{t_{r-1}}^{t_r} dt\, G(t) \tag{19.31}$$

If $G(t)$ is not constant as a function of time, the time t_r must be calculated for each point during readout for a given gradient waveform to guarantee the Nyquist criterion is always satisfied. If $G(t)$ is a constant then $t_{r-1} - t_r$ must also be constant, and a uniform sampling interval Δt is used.

Alternatively, it is possible to oversample in k-space by defining a sampling rate based upon the maximum applied gradient, i.e.,

$$\Delta t \leq \frac{1}{\gamma G_{max} L} \tag{19.32}$$

If this sampling rate is used, the Nyquist criterion will not be violated. However, the resulting data will still not be uniformly spaced in k-space if G varies with time, and the data should be interpolated before being reconstructed. This approach is useful if the available hardware is not flexible enough to implement nonuniform sampling times, but the method does require more data storage and processing (data interpolation). The latter step is imperfect and subjects the image to possible ghosting. The main advantage with the use of nonuniform sampling, as seen later in Sec. 19.4.5, is the ability to collect the necessary k-space data more efficiently over time as it allows sampling during gradient ramp-up and ramp-down.

19.4.2 Segmented EPI

The simplest alternative to conventional EPI is to use the same method but to cover smaller regions of k-space after each excitation, and combine the resulting k-space data to form a complete k-space data set. The double gradient echo sequence is a simple example of this type of k-space coverage, and could be referred to as an $N/2$ segment EPI experiment. This is a useful approach when the available hardware and SNR make it difficult to obtain all of the necessary k-space data before transverse relaxation eliminates the MR signal.

The reader is reminded that segmentation refers to breaking the entire k-space data set into subsets to highlight some logical decomposition of the collected data. These subsets can refer to multiple lines of data collected after a single rf excitation. Alternatively, segmentation may refer to groups of data collected during different cardiac cycles, for example.

Simple Offset Segments

In the previous section, it was shown that T_2^* limits N_y to some maximum value. This may limit the region of k-space which can be covered after a single rf excitation for a given resolution along the read direction, as shown in Fig. 19.10a. However, the experiment can be run twice, once with a large k_y offset and once with a zero offset. The corresponding regions of k-space covered by these two sequences are shown in Fig. 19.10b as shaded regions. The upper shaded region in Fig. 19.10b represents the k-space region covered by a conventional EPI sequence with zero k_y offset. This approach effectively doubles N_y and, therefore, improves resolution by a factor of two. Care must be taken to properly match (or phase correct) the two segments. This method will also suffer from T_2 discontinuities. Segmenting the acquisition also allows T_1 weighting to be added to EPI along with the benefit of improved resolution.

Problem 19.9

---

a) Suppose the time-spacing between the acquisition of the two segments (T_R) is such that $T_R \simeq T_1$ but is greater than T_2^*. Why does the first segment need to be collected twice to avoid a large jump in signal when a $\pi/2$-pulse is used to create the transverse magnetization?

b) If the rf pulse is less than $\pi/2$, are two acquisitions enough to reach steady-state?

Interleaved Segments

One way to avoid periodic modulation of the signal in k-space, as discussed in Sec. 19.2, is to collect the data in a segmented and interleaved fashion. Here, a sequence is considered where three lines of k-space (with a jump in k_y between each of them) are collected after each rf excitation as shown in Fig. 19.11a. The signal discontinuity due to T_2^* occurs only twice (see Fig. 19.11b) for this three-gradient echo multi-segment sequence. By appropriately stepping through the phase encoding, the aliasing artifacts discussed earlier are largely avoided as the remaining discontinuities in k-space approaches a smooth filter. The signal modulation for each gradient echo is shown in Fig. 19.11b. (In general, the actual point spread function of the filter will depend on how the segmentation is implemented.) The disadvantage of this method is that the k_y distance to be covered by the phase encoding blip must be significantly greater than in conventional EPI. This requires a large area of the phase encoding gradient and the full $2\tau_{rt}$ will usually be needed to accomplish this, thereby reducing the data acquisition efficiency. Of course, other modulations of the k-space signal can be obtained using this approach, such as employing an arbitrary number of echoes or segments, and different interleaving schemes.

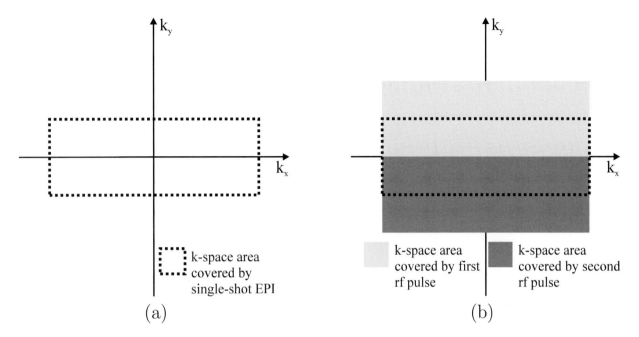

Fig. 19.10: (a) The k-space area covered by *single shot* EPI. (b) Segmented k-space coverage for EPI with two rf pulses. During the first rf pulse, no k_y-offset is used, while for the second rf pulse, a large negative k_y-offset is used. These two k-space coverages can be merged into one as shown here to get effectively better spatial resolution along the y-direction.

Problem 19.10

a) Determine whether $\Delta T = 600$ μs is long enough in time to allow a phase encoding jump of $N_y/3$ in k-space if $\Delta x = \Delta y$, $L_x = L_y = 256$ mm, and $G_{max} = 25$ mT/m.

b) What problems can be caused by turning a large gradient on and off? How would the resulting data and reconstructed image be affected?

c) Combine the segmentation and interleaving ideas presented in this section to develop a three-gradient, echo planar sequence that gives symmetric filtering in the k_y direction with maximum signal modulation at $k_y = 0$. Draw the necessary sequence diagrams for your proposed sequence. Draw the associated k-space coverage for your sequences. Find the point spread function for this filter. Give several reasons why this method is desirable.

Nevertheless, collecting three echoes at once does save a factor of three in time over conventional methods and if artifacts do not appear and SNR remains high enough, this can prove quite useful. An example set of phantom images is shown in Fig. 19.12. There is still some problem with matching k-space at the boundaries of these sets correctly (especially near field inhomogeneities). These k-space discontinuities lead to ringing in the image in the phase encoding direction (compare Figs. 19.12a and 19.12c). Switching the directions of read and phase encoding shows a very different response (Fig. 19.12b) since phase errors in the one direction are less of a problem. The following problem asks the reader to develop an alternate approach for the three echo case.

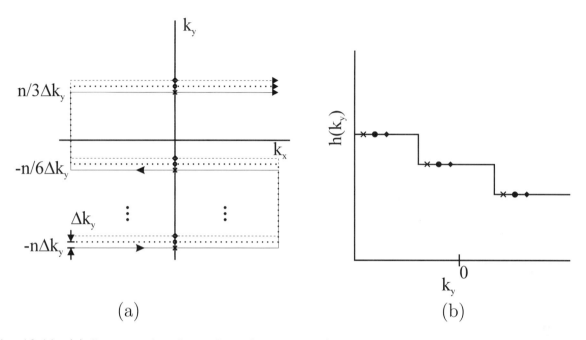

(a)   (b)

Fig. 19.11: (a) Segmented and interleaved coverage of k-space. The three sample k-space trajectories shown are repeated with different k_y offset values until all of k-space is covered. (b) Signal as a function of k_y at the gradient echo ($k_x = 0$) for the segmented and interleaved sequence shown in (a) (this behavior changes for $k_x \neq 0$). The symbols shown represent different cycles. In (b), the cross, the dot, and the solid diamond denote the solid line, the dotted line, and the dashed line, respectively. The size of the step discontinuity depends on the time between gradient echoes and on T_2^*. The change in amplitude of the signal as a function of k_y is denoted by $h(k_y)$. The Fourier transform of the filter $h(k_y)$ gives the point spread function associated with the T_2^* effects of the segmented acquisition.

19.4.3   Angled k-Space EPI

Another EPI method is to use a constant phase encoding gradient (see Fig. 19.13) rather than blips. The sequence diagram for this EPI experiment is shown in Fig. 19.13 and leads to k-space coverage of the form shown in Fig. 19.14. It is obvious from this picture that the sampled points in k-space will not be uniformly distributed. Consider the case where the phase encoding gradient covers $2\Delta k_y$ during the period of the trapezoidal oscillating read gradients (i.e., two successive read intervals) to give the k-space trajectory shown in Fig. 19.14a. Notice that at a constant value of k_x, the sampled k_y points are not evenly distributed (see the points marked by ×'s and ∘'s in Fig. 19.14a). Further, depending upon the choice of k_x, it is seen that the k_y spacing of the samples is clearly nonuniform ($0 < \Delta k_y(k_x) < 2\Delta k_y$). In order to avoid ghosting, the data must be processed using the Fourier transform shift theorem.

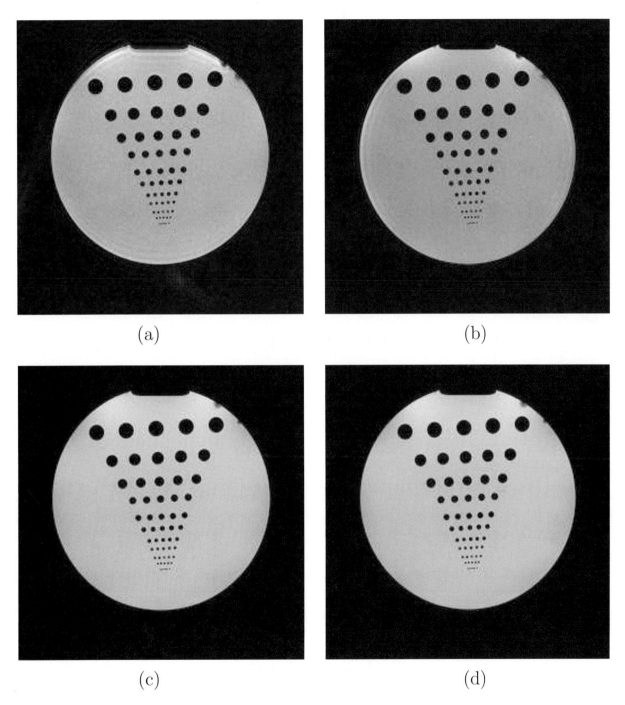

(a)

(b)

(c)

(d)

Fig. 19.12: The first two images (a) and (b) are collected with the segmented scheme. A comparison of a three-segment EPI sequence with a conventional 2D gradient echo acquisition. In (a) the read direction is horizontal, and in (b) vertical. The second two images (c) and (d) are collected with a single echo (the shortest echo time of the three-segment sequence). The read directions are horizontal and vertical in (c) and (d), respectively. This single-echo gradient echo image took three times longer to collect than the segmented acquisition scheme.

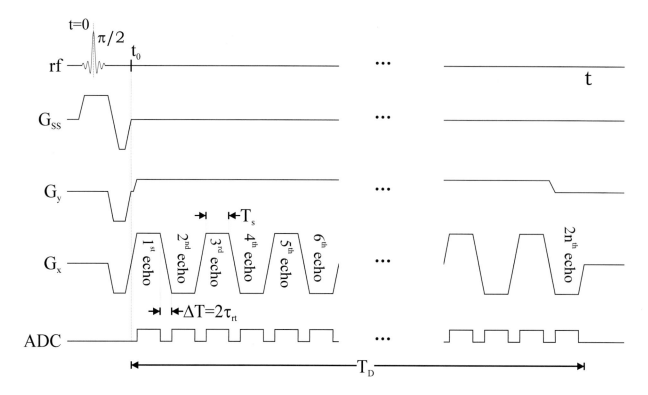

Fig. 19.13: An alternative, angled k-space EPI sequence. The phase encoding gradient waveform remains constant during the gradient oscillations and yields the k-space coverage shown in the next figure.

Avoiding Ghosts with Angled k-Space EPI

It is possible to get a more uniform distribution of points in the k_y direction by only using lines in which k_x is traversed in the same direction (dashed lines only or solid lines only in Fig. 19.14). Using this approach in Fig. 19.14a, the FOV is cut in half (Fig. 19.14a) or, if the frequency of the read gradients is doubled (Fig. 19.14b, which loses $\sqrt{2}$ in SNR), the FOV can be maintained in the same total sampling time. The second approach requires more rapid gradient rise times, but if they are available, it is a robust approach for artifact-free image reconstruction. The solid lines and dashed lines can be reconstructed separately (all points in k-space are used). The two data sets (solid lines and dashed lines) are sheared versions of the normal Cartesian coverage, but with spacing along k_y of $2\Delta k_y$. If an image is reconstructed prior to undoing this shear in k-space, the resulting image is also sheared. In order to reconstruct the image properly, a 1D Fourier transform of the data is performed at each value of k_x, and these 1D images are phase shifted to put them onto a Cartesian grid before performing the Fourier transform along the x-direction at each y-point. Finally, the two images (obtained from the dotted and solid lines) can be added together after applying the Fourier transform shift theorem (see Ch. 11) in the image domain to recover $\sqrt{2}$ in SNR. It is as if the data were collected on the same Cartesian grid in two separate experiments.

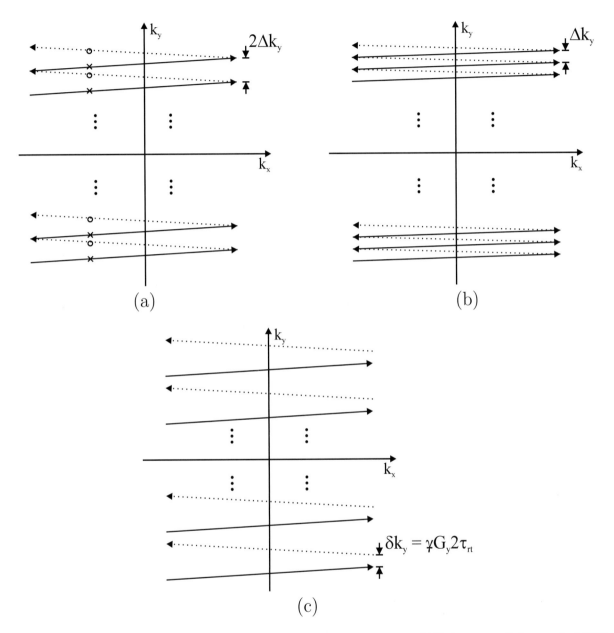

Fig. 19.14: The ideal ($\tau_{rt} = 0$) triangular waveform-like coverage of 2D k-space of the angled EPI sequence for (a) a k-space sampling interval of Δk_y and (b) a k-space sampling interval of $\Delta k_y/2$. Taking every even line or odd line, an image without $N/2$ ghosts can be created similar to that in (a) but without artifacts due to nonuniform sampling. Note that the left arrowhead refers to the acquisition direction of the dotted line. (c) A more realistic coverage of k-space when $\tau_{rt} \neq 0$ where there is a space between the endpoints of adjacent k-space lines. Nevertheless, there is still uniform coverage along k_y.

Problem 19.11

a) Assume angled k-space EPI is performed on a square object, so $L_x = L_y$ and $\Delta k \equiv \Delta k_x = \Delta k_y$. If G_x and G_y are held constant during the time T_s, the k_x distance covered in order to satisfy the Nyquist criterion is $N_x \Delta k$, and the k_y distance covered is Δk (neglect the effect of the ramp times). Neglecting the k_y distance covered during the ramp times of G_x, show that

$$G_y = \frac{G_x}{N_x} \qquad (19.33)$$

Notice that if $G_x = 25\,\text{mT/m}$ and $N_x = 256$, then $G_y = 0.1\,\text{mT/m}$. Results like this make it easier to understand why external field anomalies pose serious difficulties for EPI, causing significant image distortion.

b) Complete Fig. 19.14c by sketching the k-space coverage during the ramp times of the x-gradient.

c) Figure 19.14c demonstrates that there is additional k_y distance covered during the ramp times because the y-gradient stays on. Considering this finite ramp time, show that the relation between G_y and G_x is given by

$$G_y = \frac{G_x T_s}{N_x(T_s + 2\tau_{rt})} \qquad (19.34)$$

if adjacent points along k_y at the gradient echo are to be separated by a k-space distance Δk.

d) Find the phase shift $\phi(k_x)$ of each k_x for the solid lines in Fig. 19.14b. This information is needed to create a relatively artifact-free image.

e) Show that an accurate image is found from

$$\hat{\rho}(x,y) = \mathcal{F}_x^{-1}\left[e^{-i\phi(k_x)}\mathcal{F}_y^{-1}\left[s(k_x,k_y)\right]\right]$$

if the solid lines (only) are used to reconstruct the image.

Read and Phase Encoding

In conventional single echo sequences, the difference between the read and phase encoding directions is clear cut. The read direction is defined by the gradient applied during the period the ADC is on, and the phase encoding directions are encoded when the ADC is off. However, in many forms of EPI imaging, the distinction is not as clear. For example, in the angled k-space method just described, the x- and y-gradients were both applied during the acquisition of data, causing readout to occur at an angle in k-space. It is somewhat conventional to choose the read axis along which adjacent k-space points were collected closer in time, and the perpendicular axes are then chosen to be either phase or partition encoding. However, for certain segmentation schemes even these conventions may not adequately separate the axes (see Sec. 19.4.4). In fact, in some EPI methods, the x- and y-gradients are applied with similar amplitudes and time dependencies, so it is virtually impossible to define a read and phase encoding direction. Therefore, it is necessary to establish the conventions that are being used when an EPI sequence is described, keeping in mind that read and phase encoding may not be relevant terms.

19.4.4   Segmented EPI with Oscillating Gradients

An EPI method similar to the angled k-space just discussed can be found if the trapezoidal gradients are replaced by sinusoidally varying gradients. When a sinusoidally oscillating read gradient is used in place of trapezoidal waveforms, the gradient timings, sampling, and SNR change. In this section, the oscillating gradient is switched to the y-axis (see Fig. 19.15), and the data are segmented along y also (see Fig. 19.16). In this case, the phase encoding direction is generally taken to be y, and x is referred to as the read direction.

If the oscillating gradient applied along the y-direction is

$$G_y(t) = G_0 \sin \omega_{osc}(t - t_0) \tag{19.35}$$

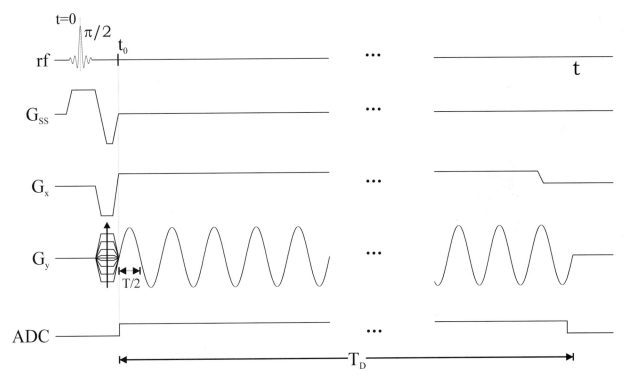

Fig. 19.15: Sequence diagram for an oscillating-gradient EPI experiment. The choice of the phase encoding dephasing and read gradient dephasing is usually made so that k-space is symmetrically covered.

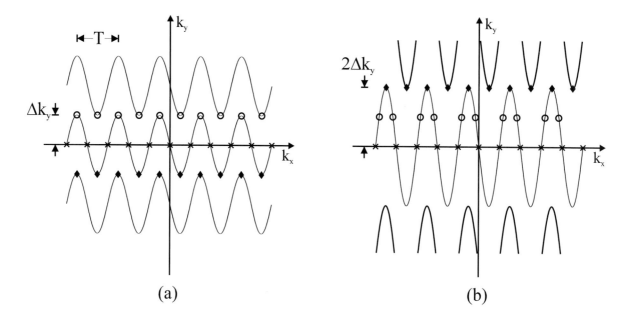

(a)   (b)

Fig. 19.16: Sampling of k-space coverage for an $N/2$-segmented version of the oscillating k-space EPI experiments. A $q = 1$ experiment is shown in (a) and a $q = 2$ case is shown in (b). The diamonds, circles, and crosses represent sampled points at given values of k_y. Notice that the k-space data do not always fall on a uniformly sampled Cartesian grid (although all points lie along k_x-lines evenly spaced in k_y), and some data at the same value of k_y are collected in different cycles. This implies that data from this experiment must be reordered and shifted before an image can be reconstructed with a Fourier transform.

then the k_y step covered in any quarter period is

$$
\begin{aligned}
q\Delta k_y &= \gamma G_0 \int_0^{T/4} dt \, \sin \omega_{osc} t \\
&= \gamma G_0 / \omega_{osc}
\end{aligned}
\tag{19.36}
$$

where $T = 2\pi/\omega_{osc}$ is the period of oscillation, Δk_y is determined by the Nyquist criterion, and $\pm q$ points are to be covered in the k_y direction relative to the initial k_y offset during each repetition of the sequence. The offset for the central coverage is set to $-\Delta k_y$. The k-space coverage for the cases where $q = 1$ and $q = 2$ are shown in Fig. 19.16. In order to complete coverage of k-space, at least $[2n_y/(2q + 1)]$ different segments must be collected with different k_y offsets.

The integral under the x-gradient during a half period determines the step size in k_x, and should be equivalent to the step size determined by the Nyquist criterion

$$
\Delta k_x = \gamma \int_0^{T/2} dt \, G_x(t) = \frac{\gamma G_x T}{2}
\tag{19.37}
$$

since the x-gradient is constant during data acquisition. This implies that if $L_x = L_y$, then $\Delta k_x = \Delta k_y$, and

$$
G_x = \frac{G_0}{\pi q} \qquad \text{for } L_x = L_y
\tag{19.38}
$$

Notice that G_x is inversely proportional to q, which implies that as q becomes large the x-gradient can become very small, especially if G_0 (usually chosen to be G_{max}) for the scanner is not large. Also, the data must be sampled nonuniformly in time to make the closest approximation to a Cartesian (rectangular) grid coverage of k-space.

Problem 19.12

---

a) If $L_y = 256\,\text{mm}$, $G_0 = 25\,\text{mT/m}$, and $T = 1.2\,\text{ms}$, then show $q_{max} \simeq 50$ and $\Delta y \simeq 2.5\,\text{mm}$.

b) Assume that $G_{max} \equiv G_0 = 10\ \text{mT/m}$ for a given scanner, n_y is chosen to be 256, and $L_x = L_y$. What is the value of G_x if segmented oscillating EPI is used to collect the data, and $q = 2$, $q = n/2$, and $q = n$?

Problem 19.13

---

a) Comparing segmented EPI with oscillating gradients (Fig. 19.15) with a blipped EPI sequence (Fig. 19.6), if $q = n_{x,trap}$, $L_{osc} = L_{trap}$, and $BW_{osc} = BW_{trap}$, show $T = \pi T_s$. Here, T is the period of the oscillation and T_s is the total sampling time during the constant gradient part of the trapezoidal waveform and the suffix '$trap$' is used to indicate parameters describing the oscillating trapezoidal read gradient in the blipped EPI sequence.

b) Why is it reasonable to take $G_0 \simeq G_{x,trap}$ for $q = n_{x,trap}$?

c) Draw a picture of what these two waveforms look like. Label all timings and gradient amplitudes.

d) Which is longer, T or $2(T_s + 2\tau_{rt})$ for $G_0 = G_{x,trap} = 25\,\text{mT/m}$, $\Delta x = 1\,\text{mm}$, and $\tau_{rt} = 300\,\mu\text{s}$.

e) Discuss how the Fourier transform shift theorem can be used to create a uniform grid coverage of k-space in Fig. 19.16b and, therefore, a ghost-free reconstructed image can be obtained.

19.4.5 Trapezoidal Versus Oscillating Waveforms

In the limit of $q = n_x$, segmented EPI with oscillating gradients covers k-space completely. It looks as if Fig. 19.14 has been turned on its side. In this limit, what is called the read gradient becomes the equivalent of the phase encoding in the trapezoidal case. The distinction between read and phase encoding has essentially vanished and the artifacts, such as chemical shift, can be understood in the more conventional sense with the format described by the method in this section.

Sampling Considerations

The choice of one method over another depends on the available hardware (i.e., gradient coil performance) and sampling capabilities, and the ease of reconstruction. Up to this point, it has always been assumed that sampling only occurred during the flat portion of the trapezoidal waveform. However, when rise times are long, nonuniform sampling can be used to increase the resolution by increasing the number of points covered in the k_x direction. The extra number of points is found from the ratio of the areas of the flat portion to the total area as follows:

$$\left.\left(\frac{N_x}{N'_x}\right)\right|_{trap} = \frac{\int_{T_{E,p}-n\Delta t}^{T_{E,p}+n\Delta t} dt\, G_x(t)}{\int_{T_{E,p}-n\Delta t-\tau_{rt}}^{T_{E,p}+n\Delta t+\tau_{rt}} dt\, G_x(t)}$$

$$= \left(\frac{T_s}{T_s + \tau_{rt}}\right) \tag{19.39}$$

where N_x is the total number of sampled points during the period of constant gradient, and N'_x is the number of points sampled during the entire gradient, including rise times. The fractional increase in the number of points is then

$$\frac{\Delta N_x}{N_x} \equiv \frac{(N'_x - N_x)}{N_x} = \frac{\tau_{rt}}{T_s} \tag{19.40}$$

Bandwidth Considerations

To make a comparison between a sinusoidal and a trapezoidal waveform requires fixing either the rise time or the area over half an oscillation (hence, voxel size). In order to compare identical images, consider the second approach. The same resolution will be obtained if the area under the two gradients is the same, i.e.,

$$2(G_0/\omega_{osc}) = G_{trap}(T_s + \tau_{rt}) \tag{19.41}$$

Using $\omega_{osc} = 2\pi/T$ and assuming both the sinusoidal and trapezoidal gradients have the same period, i.e.,

$$T/2 = T_s + 2\tau_{rt} \tag{19.42}$$

then

$$\frac{G_{trap}}{G_0} = \frac{2}{\pi}\left(\frac{T_s + 2\tau_{rt}}{T_s + \tau_{rt}}\right) \tag{19.43}$$

In order to get uniform coverage of k-space, both waveforms must be sampled nonuniformly in time, as discussed earlier.

The analog filter BW is set to the maximum frequency bandwidth in the image. For the trapezoidal gradient

$$BW_{trap} = \gamma G_{trap} L_x \tag{19.44}$$

while for the sinusoidal case where G_x is on at the same time

$$BW_{osc} = \gamma L_x \sqrt{G_0^2 + G_x^2} \tag{19.45}$$

The ratio of these two gives (for large q)

$$\frac{BW_{trap}}{BW_{osc}} = \frac{G_{trap}}{\sqrt{G_0^2 + G_x^2}} \simeq \frac{G_{trap}}{G_0}$$

$$\simeq \frac{2}{\pi}\left(1 + \frac{\tau_{rt}}{T_s}\right) \tag{19.46}$$

For $T_s = 1\,\text{ms}$ and $\tau_{rt} = 300\,\mu\text{s}$, as a representative example, the value of BW_{trap}/BW_{osc} is $2.6/\pi$ for which the trapezoidal approach gives better SNR.

19.5 Artifacts and Phase Correction

Image reconstruction for EPI is often not straightforward. The k-space coverage is rarely uniform, implying that some special Fourier transform methods must be used. Even when the right reconstruction is used, the coverage of k-space may be distorted and quite different from the desired coverage because of eddy currents (see Ch. 27), field inhomogeneities (see Ch. 20), or chemical shifts (see Ch. 17).

19.5.1 Phase Errors and Their Correction

Consider the simple example of a global background gradient $G' < 0$ applied along the read direction (in a blipped EPI sequence) throughout the sampling. The cumulative area from this gradient gives a k-space shift at the qth gradient echo of[5]

$$\Delta k_{\text{shift},q} = (-1)^q \gamma G' T_{E,q} \tag{19.47}$$

The odd echoes have a negative k-space shift because the actual read gradient is negative, and the data need to be time reversed prior to image reconstruction (see Fig. 19.17). This oscillating phase error (from positive to negative phase) in k-space leads to strong $N/2$ ghosting in the reconstructed image.

These phase errors can be corrected by estimating the echo shifts and correcting for their effects. In the absence of any phase encoding, the presence of the k-space shift $\Delta k_{\text{shift},q}$ associated with a given echo leads to a linear phase in a reconstructed 1D image of the object according to the Fourier transform shift theorem (see Ch. 18). If the 1D image for the qth line is $\hat{\rho}_{1D,q}(x)$, then

$$\hat{\rho}_{1D,q}(x) = \rho(x)e^{-i2\pi\Delta k_{\text{shift},q}x} \tag{19.48}$$

Assuming that the background gradient G' is the only source of phase error in the data collection, applying the inverse of the phase of the qth image removes this phase error. Just a 1D phase correction is enough in this case, since the source of phase error, G', is assumed to be along the read direction.

The shifted echoes can be demonstrated in k-space in real data by turning off the phase encoding blips (Fig. 19.18). The sources of G' are from either 1D eddy currents or local field

---

[5]See Ch. 20 for a detailed discussion of this k-space shift effect.

inhomogeneities. The latter cannot be corrected fully with the above approach when the field changes along y. This remains a distressing source of error with EPI. This correction does not also address time-dependent gradient sources induced by the phase encoding gradient blips.

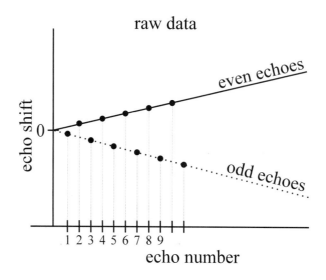

Fig. 19.17: Behavior of the phase due to a static background gradient for even and odd echoes in an EPI sequence prior to phase correction.

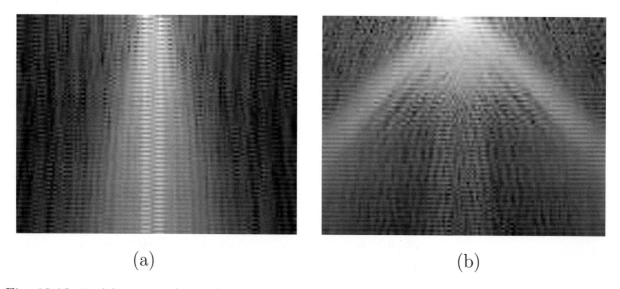

Fig. 19.18: In (a) k-space (or raw) data are shown in the absence of the phase encoding gradient blips. In (b) the same data are shown, but in a more inhomogeneous field, before reordering of the even echo data. The bad field in (b) causes the echoes to shift from the center more rapidly than in (a).

19.5.2 Chemical Shift and Geometric Distortion

As has been discussed in Ch. 17, the chemical shift artifact causes signal from one chemical species to be spatially shifted from another because of the base frequency difference between the two chemical species. The shift takes place only along the read direction for conventional gradient echo or spin echo imaging. The situation changes, though, when multiple phase encoding steps are applied. For the standard EPI sequence, where all data are collected after one rf pulse (i.e., it is a non-segmented sequence), a phase shift develops in time from phase encoding step to phase encoding step. Here, let us consider a blipped EPI sequence. The phase shift between any two adjacent k_y points at the same value of k_x is given by

$$\phi_\sigma(k_x, (p+1)\Delta k_y) - \phi_\sigma(k_x, p\Delta k_y) = \gamma \Delta B_\sigma \Delta \tau_{pe} \qquad (19.49)$$

where $\Delta \tau_{pe} \equiv T_s + 2\tau_{rt}$ is the time separation between two successive phase encoding gradient blips. Remember that the Fourier transform shift theorem (Sec. 11.2.2 in Ch. 11) stipulates that every 2π variation in phase across k-space (from k_{min} to k_{max}) leads to a single pixel shift in the image. Therefore, the total number of pixels 'shifted' due to the chemical tissue difference is

$$n_{\sigma,pe} = \frac{N_y(\phi_\sigma(k_x, (p+1)\Delta k_y) - \phi_\sigma(k_x, p\Delta k_y))}{2\pi}$$
$$= N_y \gamma \Delta B_\sigma \Delta \tau_{pe} \qquad (19.50)$$

and similarly,

$$n_{\sigma,r} = N_x \gamma \Delta B_\sigma \Delta t \qquad (19.51)$$

The shift in the read direction can also be written as

$$n_{\sigma,r} = \frac{\gamma \Delta B_\sigma}{\Delta f/pixel}$$
$$= \frac{\gamma \Delta B_\sigma}{\gamma G_x \Delta x}$$
$$= \frac{\Delta B_\sigma}{G_x \Delta x} \qquad (19.52)$$

The ratio of these two shifts

$$R_{cs} = \frac{n_{\sigma,pe}}{n_{\sigma,r}}$$
$$= \frac{N_y}{N_x} \cdot \frac{\Delta \tau_{pe}}{\Delta t} \qquad (19.53)$$

Consider $B_0 = 1.5$ T. For $\Delta B_\sigma = 1$ ppm, $G = 25$ mT/m, and $\Delta x = 1$ mm (so $G\Delta x = 50/3$ ppm) the pixel shift along the read direction is only 3/50 of a pixel. For $N_y = 128$ and $\tau_{rt} = 0$, R_{cs} collapses to N_y and the shift along the phase encoding direction is roughly 8 pixels. Similar chemical shift effects will take place in all echo planar methods where the whole of 2D k-space is covered in a single shot. In segmented EPI, or angled EPI, the chemical shift can be periodic in its effect in k-space and may lead to ghosting. The oscillating gradient case with a constant low amplitude read gradient is identical to the phase encoding direction in the conventional EPI case, but no matter what it is referred to as, *the effects of the most severe shifts occur physically along the direction associated with the lowest gradient amplitude.*

Since fat can be shifted significantly from its true position, fat saturation is often used to avoid the shift artifact since the resulting signal interferes with other tissue. See Fig. 19.19.

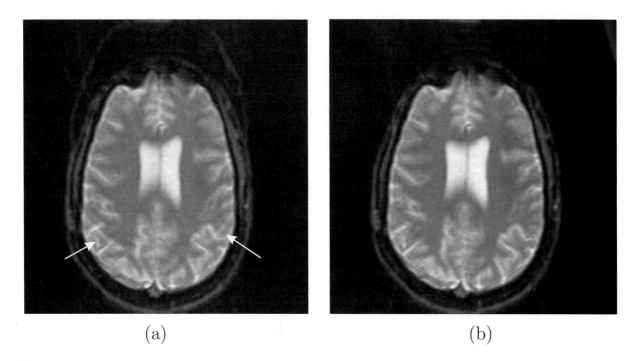

(a)   (b)

Fig. 19.19: (a) Fat shift demonstrated in a conventional EPI experiment. The effective low bandwidth in the vertical direction (phase encoding direction) causes the 220 Hz fat chemical shift relative to water to manifest itself as a large spatial shift of the fat in the image. The arrows indicate a false structure created within the brain by the overlap of the shifted fat on the brain tissue. (b) Fat saturation (see Sec. 17.2.1 in Ch. 17) significantly reduces this artifactual structure.

19.5.3   Geometric Distortion

Similar to chemical shift effects, the presence of background fields and background gradients will lead to position shifts and distortions of the image (see Figs. 19.20 and 19.21). This effect is not as severe in the read direction for conventional EPI, but the physical shift of information can be quite significant in the phase encoding direction (or the direction associated with the lowest effective gradient). For a detailed discussion of the distortion effects in imaging, see Ch. 20.

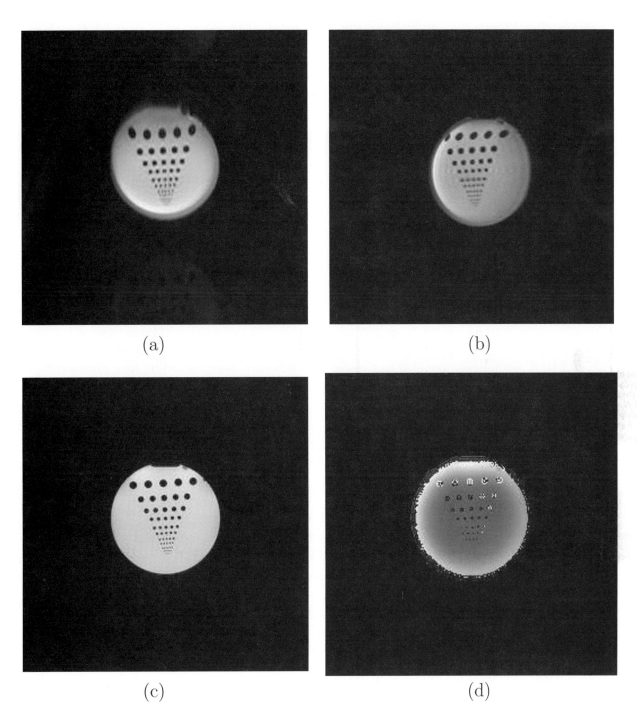

Fig. 19.20: Phantom images demonstrating geometric distortion in EPI images. In (a), the oscillating gradients are in the horizontal direction and in (b), they are applied along the vertical direction. The effects of the bad field are also evident in the $N/2$ ghosts that were not eliminated despite the application of the global phase correction discussed before. Image (c) is a conventional 2D gradient echo image acquired with the same FOV to show the lack of distortion when a large read gradient is used. In (d), the phase image of the phantom in (c) is shown to reveal the low spatial frequency field distortion that permeates the imaging volume.

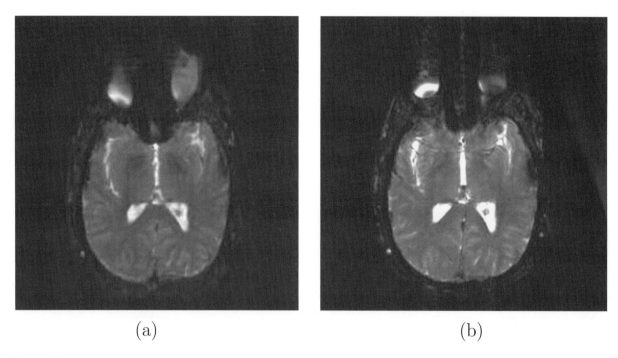

(a)   (b)

Fig. 19.21: A second example of image distortion, this time near the orbits and sinus cavities in a human head. The bad field near the eyes leads to significant distortion in the EPI image in (a). Image (b) is a long-T_E gradient echo image collected at the same T_E as the EPI image. However, the gradient echo image suffers from motion artifacts because of the longer echo time, as seen from the ghosting of the eyes due to eye movement during the acquisition.

19.5.4 T_2^*-Filter Effects

The collection of the data over a long sampling time will cause the term e^{-t/T_2^*} to significantly modulate the signal amplitude. Even if the k-space data are reordered so that the filter behaves as $e^{-\alpha|k_y|}$, spatial resolution will be limited by the FWHM of the Fourier transform of $e^{-\alpha|k_y|}$. From Ch. 13, the blur or extra effect on spatial resolution is given by

$$\Delta y_{T_2^*} \equiv \mathrm{FWHM}_{T_2^*} = \frac{\alpha}{\pi} \tag{19.54}$$

For a blipped gradient EPI sequence reordered so that the k_y maximum occurs at the origin $\alpha = 2\Delta\tau_{pe}/(T_2^* \Delta k_y)$ and

$$\Delta y_{T_2^*} = \left(\frac{2\Delta\tau_{pe} L_y}{\pi T_2^*} \right) = \left(\frac{2\Delta\tau_{pe} N_y}{\pi T_2^*} \right) \Delta y \tag{19.55}$$

Apart from this blurring phenomenon, the actual signal present will depend on the spatial frequencies of the object. For example, a low spatial frequency object will have significant signal only near $\vec{k} = 0$. For the blipped EPI case, this would imply a signal dominated by T_E at the $\vec{k} = 0$ sampling point. On the other hand, the edges of objects and small objects (which have significant high spatial frequencies; see Sec. 13.4 in Ch. 13) will suffer the blurring effect given above.

19.5.5 Ghosting

A number of different problems can manifest themselves as ghosting either in EPI or segmented EPI. One such example was discussed in Sec. 19.2 where every other point had an amplitude modulation due to T_2^* decay between the two encoded echoes. Any periodic variations that occur in the phase or amplitude of the method will also manifest themselves as ghosting. The most common effect is $N/2$ ghosting which can arise when an oscillating gradient is employed together with a constant low gradient in the other in-plane direction such that signals deviate, in every other line, from their correct values in the presence of background field inhomogeneities and eddy currents.

19.6 Spiral Forms of EPI

A rather different approach to acquiring EPI data is to apply oscillating gradients with different timings and amplitudes such that a 'spiraling out' in k-space results. This method offers the advantages of a better T_2^* filter behavior, less motion artifacts, and the need for less powerful gradients.

19.6.1 Square-Spiral EPI

As mentioned throughout the previous discussions, the filtering effects of transverse relaxation on multiple echo sequences can produce undesirable image artifacts. Using a spin echo to produce a more 'symmetric' filtering of the data (see Sec. 13.6) can alleviate this problem, but the time needed to prepare the rf echo lowers the overall signal by roughly doubling the effective echo time for a symmetric echo acquisition, and leaves even less time to acquire the necessary data. Therefore, it would be desirable to find another method which allows for collection of the data immediately after the rf excitation pulse and which has an approximately symmetrical filtering by the transverse relaxation decay e^{-t/T_2^*}. One method with such properties is spiral EPI.

In spiral EPI methods, data are collected by starting at the k-space origin at $t = t_0$, and spiraling out to larger values of $|\vec{k}|$ as time increases. This type of k-space coverage leads to a smooth signal decay along the entire k-space trajectory. It has the approximate k-space form

$$h_{T_2^*}(k_x, k_y) \simeq e^{-a\sqrt{k_x^2 + k_y^2}/T_2^*} \equiv e^{-ak_r/T_2^*} \tag{19.56}$$

where a depends on the timing of the gradients. Although small jumps in signal amplitude still occur along a given line in k-space, they do not oscillate from one k_r point to the next such as in blipped EPI, and no ghosting occurs.

The sequence diagram for a square spiral sequence is shown in Fig. 19.22 and its corresponding k-space coverage appears in Fig. 19.23. Notice, from Fig. 19.22, that there is no well-defined read or phase encoding direction in spiral scanning. The corresponding k-space coverage is similar to the radial k-space coverage method described in Ch. 14. This implies that most motion artifacts will cause a blurring, rather than an aliasing (see Ch. 14). In the 2D example shown, the x- and y-gradients will both be referred to as read gradients.

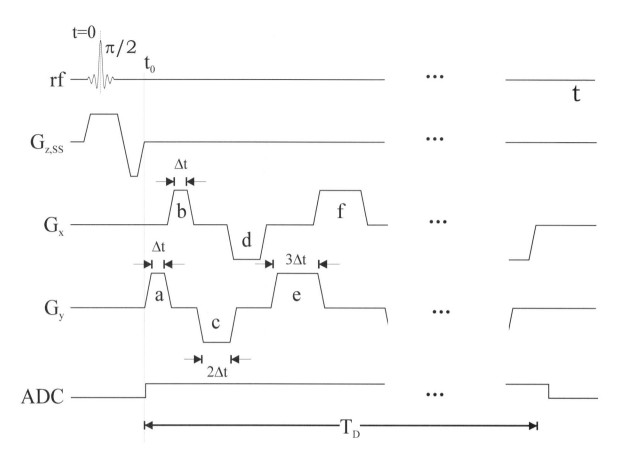

Fig. 19.22: Sequence diagram for a square spiral EPI experiment. The corresponding k-space coverage for the labeled gradient lobes is found in the following figure. It is seen that G_x is just a delayed version of G_y such that only one of the two gradients is on at a given point in time.

In order to obtain a uniform coverage of k-space with the square spiral method, each successive read gradient lobe must contain an increment Δk_x or Δk_y in area from the previous gradient pulse applied along that direction. For the example given in Fig. 19.22, this implies the following conditions on the area of the rth gradient pulse for either the x- or y-gradients

$$\gamma \int_{\text{time duration of } r^{th} \text{ gradient pulse}} dt G_{x,y}(t) = r\Delta k_{x,y} \tag{19.57}$$

Suppose the gradient amplitudes at the flat-tops on the trapezoidal lobes are kept the same throughout sampling. Then, (19.57) implies that the gradient lobe flat-top durations need to be equally incremented from the duration in the previous pulse (by Δt, say) if the same rise time is used for each lobe.

An even number $2n$ of each of the two sets of k_x and k_y lines will be collected. This progression of the areas of the read gradients leads to a uniform coverage of k-space in both directions. For equal Δt in k_x and k_y, the total data sampling time is given by

$$T_D = 2n(2n + 1)\Delta t + 4n\tau_{rt} \tag{19.58}$$

assuming that points are sampled during the gradient ramp-up and ramp-down, and read

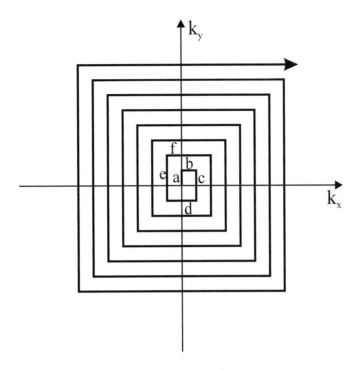

Fig. 19.23: *k*-space coverage for a square spiral imaging scan. Each line of *k*-space is acquired orthogonal to the last. Cartesian sampling is easily implemented. The labels marked a through f on the lines correspond to the applied gradient lobes in the previous figure.

gradient lobes do not overlap as shown in Fig. 19.22. Of course, alternate sampling approaches will require different choices of the area of successive gradient lobes and different data acquisition times. *Finally, the k-space data acquired from the square spiral scan must be properly placed in k-space and interpolated to a uniformly sampled Cartesian grid before a conventional 2D discrete Fourier transform is applied to the data.*

Problem 19.14

a) Can the *k*-space coverage shown in Fig. 19.23 still be realized if the time duration of each gradient lobe in Fig. 19.22 is fixed, and its amplitude is varied instead?

b) How would (19.57) be rewritten in this case?

c) What ramifications does this have for image resolution inclusive of the filter effects due to T_2^* decay during data sampling?

Problem 19.15

It is useful to make a comparison of square spiral and conventional EPI imaging. Assume that $\tau_{rt} = 100\,\mu s$, $G_{max} = 15\,\text{mT/m}$, $N_x = N_y = 128$, and $L_x = L_y = 25\,\text{cm}$.

a) Find T_D for a conventional EPI sequence given the above parameters.

b) Find T_D for a square spiral scan using the given parameters and compare your result with that found in (a).

c) Assume that a trapezoidal waveform is used for the square spiral scan. Find the number of k-space points that can be covered during the rise and fall of each gradient lobe.

d) Based on all of your imaging knowledge, make a comparison of conventional EPI and square spiral EPI, attempting to summarize the strengths and weaknesses of each method.

e) If the gradient waveforms overlapped during rise and fall times, how would this affect k-space coverage?

f) Approximate the constant a in (19.56) in terms of the sequence timings. What is the FWHM of its Fourier transform and does this relate to the resolution in the image radially?

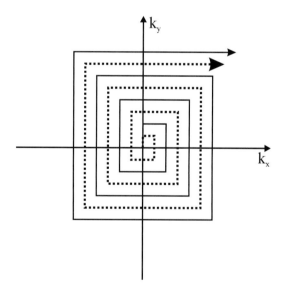

Fig. 19.24: Example of k-space coverage for an interleaved form of segmented square spiral scan where two scans have been combined to give the final k-space coverage. The k-space trajectory for the first scan is shown with solid lines while that for the second scan is shown with dashed lines.

Interleaved Square Spirals

Square spirals can also be interleaved, if the time to collect all of the required data after a single rf excitation is too long relative to the transverse relaxation time. An example of the k-space coverage for an interleaved square spiral scan is shown in Fig. 19.24. To avoid reconstruction artifacts, it must be ensured that the data acquisition starts at $k_x = k_y = 0$ for both segments (i.e., the first sampled point must be identical in both cases). If this is not the case then it can be forced to be the same and the data appropriately adjusted to accommodate that change. For example, a simple change in phase by $\Delta\phi$ is easily corrected by multiplying the entire second segment data by $e^{-i\Delta\phi}$ to correct the phase shift.

Problem 19.16

Assume that the time required to collect square spiral data covering the equivalent of a 128×128 matrix in Cartesian k-space is four times longer than the average T_2^* for the object being imaged. Little signal will be left at the edges of k-space.

a) How does the loss of signal at large $|\vec{k}|$ affect the reconstructed image?

b) Relatively speaking, how much shorter will T_D be for the scan if two spirals are interleaved?

c) Assume that the same problem ($T_D \gg T_2^*$) exists for a conventional EPI scan. By what relative factor is T_D reduced if two conventional EPI scans are interleaved?

d) If the second square spiral (dashed line) coverage is not actually started at the origin, discuss the form of the ensuing artifacts. Hint: Concepts of nonuniform sampling and their effects (discussed in Sec. 12.4 in Ch. 12) need to be invoked here.

19.6.2 Spiral EPI

An alternative to a square spiral is a circular spiral; the latter is commonly used and it is often referred to as simply 'spiral EPI.' In this case, both gradients are applied simultaneously and the data are collected continuously. A sequence diagram for spiral EPI is shown in Fig. 19.25.

While different spiral coverages of k-space exist (such as the square spiral), a linearly increasing sinusoidal form will be considered here. The forms

$$k_x(t) = \gamma\alpha_1 t \sin \alpha_2 t \tag{19.59}$$
$$k_y(t) = \gamma\alpha_1 t \cos \alpha_2 t \tag{19.60}$$

lead to the coverage illustrated in Fig. 19.26, with the origin as the starting point.[6] The gradient waveforms needed to produce this coverage of k-space can be found by differentiation

---

[6]Equations (19.59) and (19.60) are the parametric forms of a circular spiral in (k_x, k_y) space.

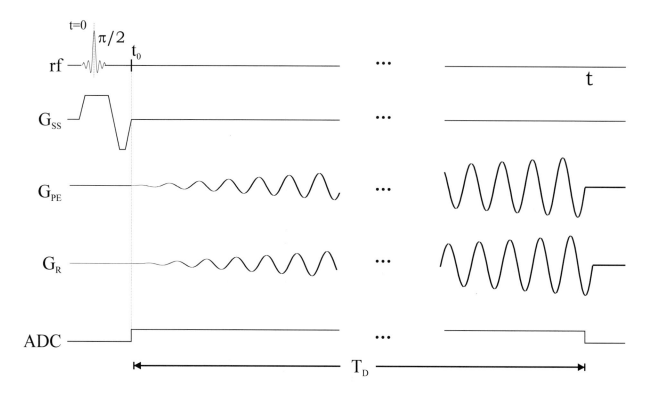

Fig. 19.25: Sequence diagram for the spiral EPI experiment.

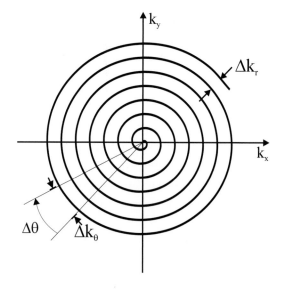

Fig. 19.26: The k-space coverage for the spiral EPI scan.

of the given k-space trajectory:

$$G_x(t) = \alpha_1 \sin \alpha_2 t + \alpha_1 \alpha_2 t \cos \alpha_2 t \tag{19.61}$$
$$G_y(t) = \alpha_1 \cos \alpha_2 t - \alpha_1 \alpha_2 t \sin \alpha_2 t \tag{19.62}$$

Explicit values of α_1 and α_2 can be found by considering the sampling requirements imposed by the Nyquist criterion and choosing an integral number of radial samples. Assume that there are n_θ samples per rotation and n_r samples radially which satisfy the Nyquist criterion (obtained based on the discussion in Sec. 14.1.3 in Ch. 14).

From (19.59) and (19.60),

$$k_r(t) = \gamma \alpha_1 t \tag{19.63}$$
$$\theta(t) = \alpha_2 t \tag{19.64}$$

Hence, it can be seen that α_1 represents a gradient amplitude and α_2 an angular frequency.

Using a simple trigonometric argument, α_2 can be found as follows. The complete angular coverage of one period of the spiral is defined by

$$2\pi = n_\theta \Delta\theta \tag{19.65}$$

The term α_2 is taken as the angular frequency of coverage of k-space. That is, since an angle $\Delta\theta$ is covered in each sampling interval Δt, the angular frequency α_2 is given by

$$\alpha_2 \equiv \frac{\Delta\theta}{\Delta t} = \frac{2\pi}{n_\theta \Delta t} \tag{19.66}$$

From its definition, Δk_r is the distance between two k-space points in the radial direction whose corresponding values of θ are exactly 2π apart. From (19.63) and (19.64), this implies

$$\Delta k_r \equiv k_r(t)|_{t=t'+2\pi/\alpha_2} + k_r(t)|_{t=t'}$$
$$= \gamma \alpha_1 n_\theta \Delta t \tag{19.67}$$

Using the Nyquist relation in the radial direction (see Ch. 14),

$$\Delta k_r = \frac{1}{L} \tag{19.68}$$

where L is the diameter of the circular field-of-view. Now, α_1 is found from (19.67) and (19.68) to be

$$\alpha_1 = \frac{1}{\gamma L n_\theta \Delta t} \tag{19.69}$$

As expected, α_1 has units of a gradient and is not unlike a conventional read gradient. From these results, the total sampling time and maximum required gradient strength can be found. The total sampling time is just the product of the number of sampled points and the sampling interval since data are collected continuously

$$T_D = n_r n_\theta \Delta t \tag{19.70}$$

Since the gradient strength is increasing throughout the experiment, the maximum gradient occurs at the end of the sampling period (when $\alpha_2 t = 2\pi$) and[7]

$$G_{y,max} = \alpha_1 \alpha_2 T_D = \frac{2\pi}{n_\theta \gamma \Delta x \Delta t} \qquad (19.71)$$

The choice of which gradient, G_x or G_y, has the maximum depends upon the specifics of the sampling employed. However, both gradients must have nearly identical capabilities since the maxima only occur a quarter period apart.

Problem 19.17

For a spiral EPI scan, assume that the data will be interpolated onto a Cartesian grid before being reconstructed. The following imaging parameters are required: $\text{FOV}_{x,y} = 25\,\text{cm}$ and $\Delta x = \Delta y = 2\,\text{mm}$. Find values for $G_{y,max}$ and T_D.

Spiral k-space coverage leads to an interesting distribution of the sampled points in k-space. If data are sampled at a constant rate, then points will be sampled much more densely near the center of k-space, and more sparsely at large k-space values similar to the radial k-space coverage method discussed in Ch. 14. Also, if data are to be reconstructed using the conventional 2D discrete Fourier transform, it must be interpolated before being transformed.

If sampling times become too long, a remedy may be found along the lines of previous discussions. In order to improve spatial resolution, two or more spiral scans may be interleaved in a fashion similar to that proposed for square spiral scans. For systems with lower gradient strengths and longer rise times, this is a much more feasible solution. Example spiral images are shown in Fig. 19.27.

The filtering advantages of square spiral k-space coverage are also available with spiral EPI. However, this method has several other potential advantages. First, since the gradients are applied smoothly, dB/dt is kept relatively low which helps to suppress eddy currents, although they are by no means eliminated. Also, sinusoidal waveforms produced by driving the gradients by resonant circuits can lead to a faster gradient response.

19.7 An Overview of EPI Properties

The motivation for any fast imaging method is speed. Some have short T_E as in short-T_R SSFP methods, while others have long T_E such as with EPI. Both require large gradient amplitudes and short rise times to allow for good resolution.

19.7.1 Speed of EPI

Echo planar imaging offers rapid acquisition of a large region-of-interest in a short time period. No other 2D imaging method offers similar variable T_2^* weighting or high SNR spin

---

[7]G_y is at its maximum at the end of sampling, while G_x is at zero. G_x reaches its maximum strength one-quarter of a period earlier.

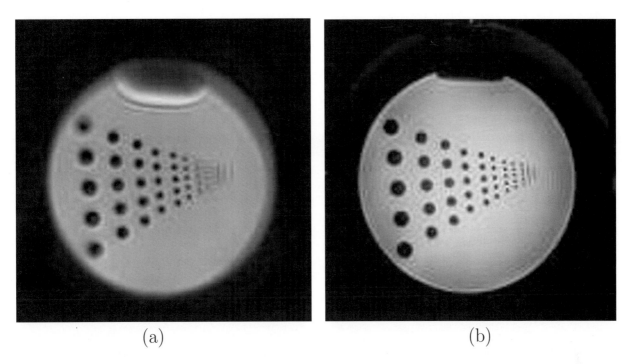

(a)   (b)

Fig. 19.27: (a) An example single-shot spiral EPI scan, and (b) an example of a 16 segment interleaved spiral image. The shorter sampling times associated with the segmented scan and the resulting reduction of resonance offset effects both lead to a much sharper image in (b).

density weighting. In practice, 2D images with reasonable resolution can be collected as quickly as once every 30 ms, allowing coverage of the entire brain volume, for example, in roughly 3 seconds using a multi-slice method. The only limitations on collecting the data this quickly are the gradient duty cycle capability and the data input/output rate. This approach is particularly valuable for studying diffusion weighted imaging, functional brain imaging, or real-time imaging. If improvements in SNR were needed, the entire coverage could be repeated every 3 seconds. A great advantage is that, in each acquisition, motion would be essentially frozen. Example images of the human brain using several of the alternate forms of EPI are shown in Fig. 19.28.

Short-T_R EPI   Echo planar imaging can be run much more quickly than once every 3 seconds. It can be run at a single slice location as a short T_R, optimal flip angle scan where T_R can be chosen much shorter than the period of motion. For example, one 2D image could be collected every 100 ms throughout the cardiac cycle. For most physiological motion, EPI is a dynamic scanning method with great potential.

3D EPI   It is possible to collect 3D EPI by phase (partition) encoding in the slice select direction as is conventionally done for gradient echo imaging. Although T_1 effects will be present with short T_R, 3D EPI offers the advantage of creating thin slice images which can reduce T_2^* effects and give better contiguous slice information. Segmented methods will require multiple rf excitations and multiple data acquisitions and will accordingly take longer to collect.

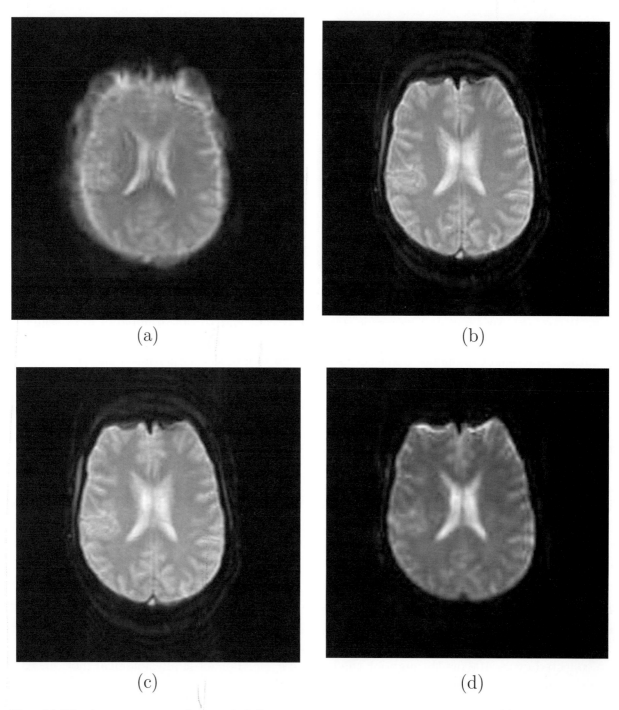

Fig. 19.28: A comparison of several different EPI data acquisition methods: (a) spiral EPI, (b) blipped EPI, (c) EPI using a constant phase encoding gradient, and (d) spin echo EPI. The reader can observe the different artifacts present in each method as discussed throughout this chapter.

19.7.2 Contrast Mechanisms

Echo planar imaging allows very rapid acquisition of data for evaluation of tissue properties such as ρ_0, T_1, T_2, and T_2^*. For example, a set of EPI scans with different $T_{E,\vec{k}=0}$ can be used to evaluate T_2^* in the abdomen in a breath-hold with essentially no motion artifacts. Using T_2^* as input, ρ_0 can then be calculated.

A similar approach to estimate T_1 is also viable by repeating a series of EPI scans. For example, if an EPI scan is run twice, the second time following a rather short wait period of T_R, then two pieces of information are available

$$
\begin{aligned}
\hat{\rho}_1 &= \rho_0 e^{-T_{E,\vec{k}=0}/T_2^*} \\
\hat{\rho}_2 &= \rho_0 e^{-T_{E,\vec{k}=0}/T_2^*} \left(1 - e^{-T_R/T_1}\right)
\end{aligned}
\tag{19.72}
$$

The ratio of these two can be used to find T_1. The reader must be aware, however, that finite slice thickness will affect this T_1 calculation (see Chs. 18 and 22). When a finite T_R is used, it is often very useful to 'cardiac gate' the data,[8] even in the brain.

19.7.3 Field-of-View and Resolution in the Phase Encoding Direction

Although EPI is technically challenging and resolution is often limited, it still has interesting flexibility in terms of available FOV. For example, if the amplitude of the blips in blipped EPI are doubled then Δk_y doubles, the total sampling time stays the same, and the resolution is increased (see Fig. 19.1c).

This offers significant advantages when there is interest in rapid dynamic imaging of small structures such as the wrist or for dynamic contrast enhanced studies of, say, the pituitary gland. If resolution does not need to be increased, then doubling Δk_y will reduce the T_D time by a factor of two allowing for more slices, faster repetition of the experiment, or reduced T_E if T_2^* decay is a serious problem. Returning to the question of image reconstruction when $N/2$ ghosting remains a problem, by reconstructing even and odd lines separately, ghosts can be removed, SNR can be maintained, but the aliasing will still occur unless the object is now half the FOV associated with the original Δk_y coverage. This is easily understood since throwing out every other line is tantamount to having sampled with $2\Delta k_y$ in the first place. Thus, a sequence designed for an FOV $= L$ can also be used for imaging a small object with an FOV $= L/2$ without concern for ghosting artifacts.

Resolution in single shot EPI can be made quite high as seen above, but not without either changing L or lengthening T_D. An alternative, if L and T_D must remain fixed, is to use segmented EPI, but this requires repeating the scan.

---

[8]The data acquisition is synchronized with the cardiac cycle.

19.7.4   EPI Safety Issues

There are a number of safety issues that affect systems with EPI capabilities. First, the resonant gradient systems themselves require huge voltages to create short rise times (see Ch. 27). The rapid rise time to high gradients is very demanding on electrical/mechanical parts of the gradient coil and can lead to 'spikes' appearing in the data. These can destroy the utility of an image.

Second, the rapid switching causes a high frequency mechanical pulse to be generated from the coil/enclosed coil system which makes this one of the most expensive speakers in the world. Driving the system at 1 kHz, for example, creates a squeal that requires wearing ear protection (either ear plugs or acoustic damping headsets).

Third, the rate of change of the magnetic field can induce a current in the body which can stimulate nerves, causing muscles to twitch. Today, both dB/dt and the maximum field strength that can be applied at a given frequency, $B_{max}(f)$, are considered to be measures of possible stimulation. A value of $dB/dt = 50$ T/s can be run safely while for frequencies less than 2 kHz a peak value of 6 mT is considered safe.

Problem 19.18

Consider a gradient coil 50 cm in length. Assume the peak values are 25 mT/m and the rise time is 300 μs. A current loop of radius 25 cm can be established in the body for the y-gradient. Assume that both coils do not produce significant fields outside their enclosing volume.

a) Find $dB/dt|_{max}$. Is it less than 50 T/s?

b) Find B_{max}. Is it less than 6 mT? Is this a safe set of values to use?

c) You plan on designing a new head gradient coil 20 cm in length with a rise time of 100 μs and a peak gradient amplitude of 50 mT/m. Can it be used safely at full capacity for EPI imaging?

d) How could the coil in part (c) improve EPI image quality?

19.8   Phase Encoding Between Spin Echoes and Segmented Acquisition

A natural extension to phase encoding between gradient echoes is to phase encode between spin echoes. This allows the effects of magnetic field inhomogeneities to be dramatically reduced. The coverage of k-space as shown in Fig. 19.1a can be equivalently generated using a spin echo train of π-pulses as shown in Fig. 19.29. Although the k-space coverage is identical to conventional imaging, it must be kept in mind that there will be filter effects associated with the data due to T_2 effects during data collection. The discussion of these filter effects would be similar to that already presented for EPI.

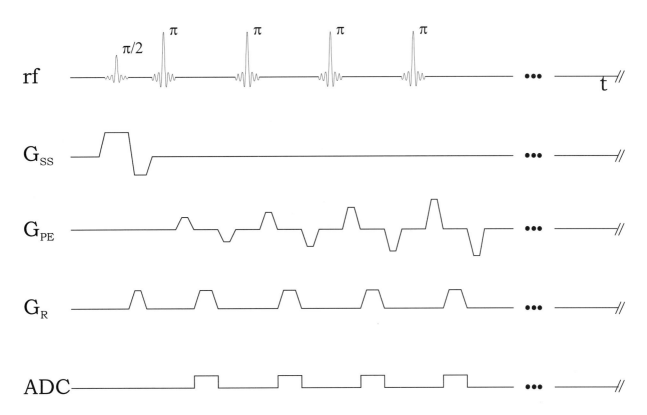

Fig. 19.29: Sequence diagram for an experiment covering k-space by repeated acquisition of spin echoes. Each phase encoding lobe is rewound before the end of the rf cycle and the area of the phase encoding gradients is set up to increment by an amount which increments k_y by Δk_y from one refocusing pulse to the next. The reason for using such a scheme instead of using a constant phase encoding blip waveform as in Fig. 19.15 is because a constant gradient such as a blip is refocused by the π-pulse and, consequently, no phase encoding is achieved.

A major limitation is how many π-pulses can be applied, while keeping power deposition within the SAR (Specific Absorption Rate) limit. For this reason, usually between 8 and 32 rf pulses are applied. This leads to a segmented acquisition with the use of several excitation pulses, a finite T_R, and a small number of refocusing pulses per T_R.

Another method can be used to overcome this limitation. Here, multiple gradient echoes can be added between π-pulses to increase the number of phase encoding steps possible within a given echo train. In either case, the data acquisition will, in general, be segmented in order to obtain N_y phase encoding lines of data. A simple example is given in Fig. 19.30 to demonstrate the k-space coverage when two π-pulses are used. Usually, for purposes of obtaining better spatial resolution, 6, 12, or 24 π-pulses would be used when 5 gradient echoes are collected between π-pulses.

Conventional, long T_R spin echo imaging has always been the bane for T_2-weighted acquisitions in the body. However, phase encoding between echoes (say, for example, 16) keeps even high resolution T_2 weighted imaging to a few minutes. The T_R can be kept quite long (in this case, on the order of 10 seconds) so that enough slices can be acquired, despite the increase in effective sampling time. A comparison with other T_2 weighted methods is

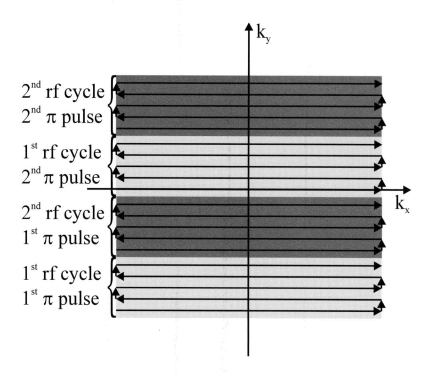

Fig. 19.30: The k-space coverage for a sequence where two π pulses follow each excitation, and five gradient echoes have been employed between the π-pulses to speed up acquisition of the k-space data while reducing the number of rf pulses and, hence, the rf energy deposited in the object being imaged. The coverage shown here is only an illustrative example where 20 lines have been collected along k_y following two excitation pulses.

presented in Fig. 19.31. The single slice gradient echo acquisition suffers from local field inhomogeneities and the concomitant loss of signal associated with them, but still has bright CSF. With these imaging parameters, a total of 25 slices can be obtained in 6.5 minutes. For the single shot EPI sequence, one slice can be acquired roughly every 300 ms (so it takes only about 8 seconds to collect 25 slices). This high resolution EPI scan clearly shows well-delineated CSF in the sulci. It too will suffer badly from field inhomogeneity effects. The conventional spin echo sequence yields the sharpest image. The best scan in terms of having spin echo properties and being fast is the sequence using phase encoding between echoes. This scan allows for a longer T_R for better signal recovery and more slices than the conventional spin echo. Here, the acquisition time was less than 4 minutes for acquiring 42 slices.

Generally, when multiple rf pulses are used, problems in SSFP buildup of signal can occur. Radiofrequency spoiling can alleviate these difficulties. Long sampling causes a limit in terms of available resolution and small objects may be lost (i.e., have insufficient contrast or resolution to be resolved from the surrounding tissue). If m π-pulses are each separated by a time 2τ, the total sampling will occur over a time $2\tau m$. As discussed earlier, this will cause image blurring (see also Ch. 13).

Problem 19.19

---

a) Draw a sequence diagram for the k-space coverage shown in Fig. 19.30. Comment on the filter effects that might be present for this sequence.

b) If an rf spacing of 20 ms is possible, how many gradient echoes can be encoded between the π pulses if $G_{max} = 25\,\text{mT/m}$, $L = 256\,\text{mm}$, $N_x = 256$, and $\tau_{rt} = 300\,\mu\text{s}$?

c) If 8 π-pulses are used, how quickly can this combined spin echo, gradient echo method be collected if 256 phase encoding steps are desired and $T_R = 1\,\text{s}$?

d) If $T_2 = 100\,\text{ms}$, how many rf pulses should be applied? Repeat this question, assuming $T_2 = 200\,\text{ms}$.

e) Repeat part (d) for $T_2 = 2\,\text{s}$. Considering that CSF and water have such long T_2 values, this method can be used to acquire very high resolution images of water-filled structures such as CSF spaces or the urinary bladder in a single shot.

19.9 Mansfield 2D to 1D Transformation Insight

Reconstructing an image from different k-space paths can be a tricky issue. Consider the case of diagonal sampling of k-space (Fig. 19.32a). In this instance we want to be able to construct $\rho(x, y)$ as if the data had been collected on the usual Cartesian grid. To accomplish this, it requires multiple applications of the Fourier transform shift theorem in the k_y direction.

19.9.1 Application of the Fourier Transform Shift Theorem

Denoting the angled k-space data as $s_a(k_x, k_y)$, how can we transform this data to obtain the correct $\rho(x, y)$? Applying the usual 2D DFT yields an image sheared along the x-direction. The first step is to find the shift in k_y at each k_x. If all the readout lines make an angle θ to the x-axis, then

$$\delta k_y = k_x \tan \theta \tag{19.73}$$

and for lines that rise to $\frac{1}{2}\Delta k_y$ at k_{max}, this becomes

$$\begin{aligned} \delta k_y &= k_x \Delta k_y/(2k_{x,max}) \\ &= k_x \Delta x \Delta k_y \\ &= u \Delta k_y/N_x \end{aligned} \tag{19.74}$$

where $k_x = u\Delta k_x = u/L_x = u/(N_x\Delta x)$. The data points marked by x can be placed into a Cartesian grid by applying the Fourier transform shift theorem. First, we correct the data by

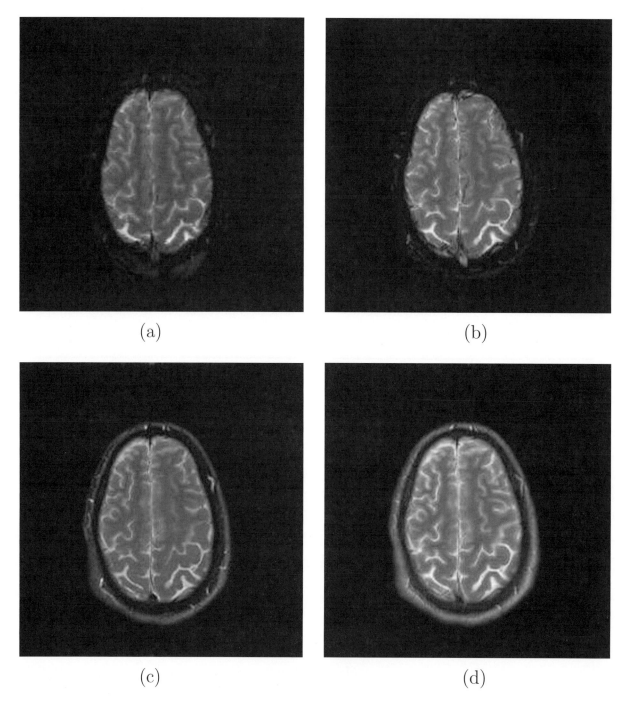

(a)

(b)

(c)

(d)

Fig. 19.31: A comparison of different fast imaging T_2-weighted methods with the conventional spin echo method in the brain. A single slice gradient echo image from a 20 slice 2D data set with $T_R/T_E = 2\,\mathrm{s}/68\,\mathrm{ms}$ in (a) is similar to that in the conventional gradient echo EPI image ($T_D/T_E = 270\,\mathrm{ms}/68\,\mathrm{ms}$) shown in (b). The conventional spin echo image ($T_R/T_E = 2\,\mathrm{s}/120\,\mathrm{ms}$) in (c) has less bright fat and less contrast than the very long T_R, phase encoding between spin echoes scan ($T_R/T_E = 6\,\mathrm{s}/90\,\mathrm{ms}$ with 5 π-pulses per T_R) shown in (d). The contrast for GM and CSF in the phase encoding between spin echoes scan is the best because of its long T_R of 6000 ms.

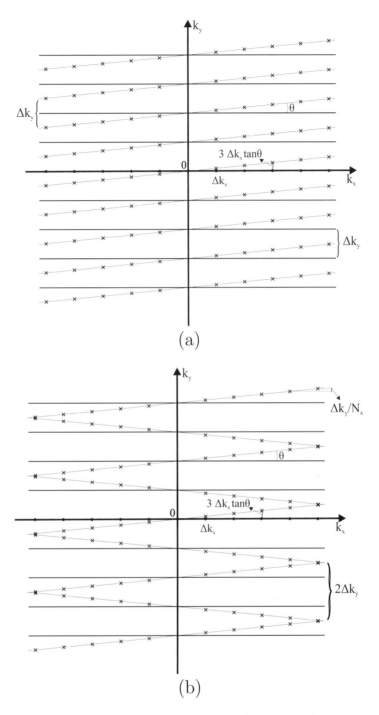

(a)

(b)

Fig. 19.32: Two variations of diagonal k-space coverage for two different echo planar acquisition schemes. (a) Sheared k-space coverage with a linear shift as a function of k_x. This type of coverage occurs when we throw away the signal from the odd or even echoes. Note the sampling is offset because time advances as we continue collecting the data. (b) Keeping both odd and even echoes, but with each having a temporal advancement opposite to the other, creating two separate and opposite diagonal like coverages of k-space. This problem is a little more difficult to deal with than the first case, but quite easily handled when the problem is posed as a 1D Fourier transform.

performing the Fourier transform over k_y transform and then multiplying the intermediate (k_x, y) space data $\tilde{s}_a(k_x, y)$ by $e^{i2\pi\delta k_y y}$

$$\tilde{s}(k_x, y) = \tilde{s}_a(k_x, y)e^{i2\pi k_x \Delta x \Delta k_y y} \tag{19.75}$$

The final step in obtaining $\rho(x, y)$ is to perform the Fourier transformation over k_x

$$\rho(x, y) = \frac{1}{N_x} \sum_{k_x} \tilde{s}_a(k_x, y)e^{i2\pi x k_x} e^{i2\pi k_x \Delta x \Delta k_y y} \tag{19.76}$$

In its discrete form, with $x = p\Delta x$, $y = q\Delta y$, and $k_x = u\Delta k_x$. Equation (19.76) can now be written as

$$\rho(p\Delta x, q\Delta y) = \frac{1}{N_x} \sum_{u} \tilde{s}_a(u\Delta k_x, q\Delta y)e^{i2\pi u(p+q/N_y)/N_x} \tag{19.77}$$

19.9.2   Collapsing the 2D Problem to a 1D Problem

The Fourier transform shift theorem in Sec. 19.9.1 was easy to apply. Our goal in this subsection is to show that the reorganization of the 2D DFT into a 1D DFT actually automatically performs the Fourier transform shift theorem for us without having to indirectly perform the intermediate phase shift step itself.

If we let $\Delta\tilde{k}_y = \Delta k_y/N_x$ (Fig. 19.32b) and $\tilde{y} = \tilde{q}\Delta\tilde{y}$ then the 1D Fourier transform becomes

$$\rho_{1D}(\tilde{y}) = \frac{1}{N_x N_y} \sum_{b} s(b\Delta\tilde{k}_y)e^{i2\pi b\Delta\tilde{k}_y \tilde{y}} \tag{19.78}$$

First let $b = u + N_x v$ (since the index must cover all the k-space points from the bottom to the top of k-space) where $b \in (-N_x N_y, N_x N_y - 1)$. Second, assume that the resulting image is also in a similar fashion but with $\tilde{y} = \tilde{q}\Delta y$ where $\tilde{q} = N_y p + q$. With these assignments, we find

$$\rho_{1D}(\tilde{q}\Delta\tilde{y}) = \frac{1}{N_x N_y} \sum_{u,v} s_a(u\Delta k_x, v\Delta k_y)e^{i2\pi(u+N_x v)(N_y p+q)/N_x N_y} \tag{19.79}$$

where we have used $\Delta\tilde{k}_y\Delta\tilde{y} = (\Delta k_y/N_x)\Delta y = 1/(N_x N_y)$. Now summing over v yields

$$\rho_{1D}((N_y p + q)\Delta y) = \frac{1}{N_x} \sum_{u} s_a(u\Delta k_x, q\Delta y)e^{i2\pi u(N_y p+q)/N_x N_y} \tag{19.80}$$

The term $e^{i2\pi v p}$ plays no role because it is always 1 (since v and p are integers). Clearly (19.77) and (19.80) are identical and we see that the re-sorted ρ_{1D} is equal to a Fourier transform shift corrected original k-space.

Problem 19.20

Show that the uncorrected data leads to a small shear in the x-direction by $\delta x = y/2n$.

Suggested Reading

The concept of echo planar imaging was introduced in:

- P. Mansfield, A. A. Maudsley and T. Baines. Fast scan proton density imaging by NMR. *J. Phys. E: Scient. Instrum.*, 9: 271, 1976.

A scheme for correcting for phase errors occurring because of the presence of global background gradients was discussed in:

- H. Bruder, H. Fischer, H. E. Reinfelder and F. Schmitt. Image reconstruction for echo planar imaging with nonequidistant *k*-space sampling. *Magn. Reson. Med.*, 23: 311, 1992.

The following is a review article of the different approaches to echo planar imaging:

- M. S. Cohen and R. M. Weiskoff. Ultra-fast imaging. *Magn. Reson. Imag.*, 9: 1, 1991.

Echo planar imaging using spiral *k*-space coverage was introduced in:

- C. B. Ahn, J. H. Kim and Z. H. Cho. High speed spiral-scan echo planar imaging. *IEEE Trans. Med. Imag.*, MI-5: 2, 1986.

Phase encoding between echoes was introduced by:

- J. Hennig, A. Nauerth and H. Friedburg. RARE imaging: A fast method for clinical MR. *Magn. Reson. Med.*, 3: 823, 1986.

A detailed review of phase encoding between echoes appears in:

- J. Listerud, S. Einstein and E. Outwater. First principles of fast spin echo. *Magn. Reson. Quart.*, 8: 199, 1992.

Most EPI concepts and applications are covered in the text:

- F. Schmitt, M. K. Stehling and R. Turner, eds. *Echo Planar Imaging: Theory, Technique and Application*. Springer-Verlag, Berlin, Germany, 1998.

Chapter 20

Magnetic Field Inhomogeneity Effects and T_2^* Dephasing

Chapter Contents

Summary: The effects of static field inhomogeneities on the image are considered. Common artifacts of image distortion are analyzed in the linear field approximation. Echo shifting and its effect on image phase are reviewed, and procedures for the reduction of signal loss and distortion are described. Examples of T_2^* signal loss and a means to predict T_2^* from susceptibility producing objects are introduced. Lastly, a method to correct geometric distortion is discussed.

Introduction

A detailed discussion is given in this chapter of image effects due to field inhomogeneities at both the macroscopic level, where their scale is at least voxel sized, and the microscopic regime, where the volumes are much smaller than a voxel. Macroscopic field inhomogeneities modeled by linear gradients lead to two classes of image artifacts. The first artifact is image distortion, which is any misregistration of a spin's position leading to a reconstructed spin density that differs *spatially* from the physical spin density. A background gradient in the read direction causes the spin position to be shifted along that axis in the reconstructed image while those perpendicular to the read direction cause a 'shearing' effect on the image.

The second artifact, 'echo shifting,' pertains to gradient echo imaging, but not to spin echo imaging. The presence of an extra gradient along the read direction means that the gradient echo does not occur at T_E, where the accumulated area under the applied read gradient is zero, but instead occurs at a point T_E', where the area under the read and background gradients is zero. The resulting problems are two-fold. A gradient echo that is not centered in the sampling window leads to signal loss. An unwanted shift in the k-space origin forces an additional phase in the image; this phase changes linearly with position. Other problems include echo shifts in the phase/partition direction produced by background gradients perpendicular to the read direction. Background gradients in the slice select direction can cause the k-space origin to be missed altogether in 2D gradient echo images. These artifacts can arise from external, or global, field anomalies affecting the entire field-of-view, or from local field sources contaminating the image over small scales.

Microscopic magnetic field variations play another important role which is not, however, characterized as an artifact. They lead to shortened transverse relaxation times, an additional subject of this chapter. A description of R_2' is made based upon the assumption that it can be modeled by a distribution of static field inhomogeneities caused by microscopic sources.

20.1   Image Distortion Due to Field Effects

Any field variation beyond the assumed applied linear gradient, and which is present during frequency encoding, causes spins to be spatially encoded at the wrong position. The incorrect spatial localization of a spin during frequency encoding is generally referred to as *image distortion*. Although image distortion effects during frequency encoding are identical for gradient echo and spin echo images, it will be seen later that anomalous field variations generally have greater impact on gradient echo images. The differences for gradient echo and spin echo images will be discussed briefly at the end of this section, and in the next section on echo shifting.

Although the general spatial dependence is complex, a linear gradient approximation can be used to model both the external background and the local field variations. The former is considered to be accurate over the entire field-of-view and the latter over scales on the order of a voxel. The local variations may be generated by small structures, such as water/air boundaries, embedded in the object of interest that, due to differences in their internal magnetic susceptibilities (Ch. 25), perturb the surrounding magnetic field.

20.1.1   Distortion Due to Background Gradients Parallel to the Read Direction

Following the above remarks, it is assumed that it is reasonable to write the field at a point $\vec{r}$ in the region of a point $\vec{r}_0$ as

$$B(\vec{r}) \approx B_0 + \vec{G}'(\vec{r}_0) \cdot (\vec{r} - \vec{r}_0) \tag{20.1}$$

The region about the point $\vec{r}_0$ over which this expression is valid depends upon what is creating the field variation. In this chapter, $\vec{G}'$ is assumed to be a static[1] background gradient due to field inhomogeneities, rather than an applied (imaging) gradient.

Consider a 1D imaging example as an introduction to field distortion effects, where a background gradient $\vec{G}'_x$ parallel to the read direction exists across the entire field-of-view. The effect of the background gradient on the measured signal during the sampling window can be found by looking at the phase behavior of the spins during this period:

$$
\begin{aligned}
\phi(t') &= -2\pi\gamma\left(G_x x + G'_x x\right)t' \\
&= -2\pi\gamma G_x t' x \left(1 + \frac{G'_x}{G_x}\right) \\
&= -2\pi k_x x \left(1 + \frac{G'_x}{G_x}\right)
\end{aligned}
\tag{20.2}
$$

where G_x and G'_x are the amplitudes of $\vec{G}_x$ and $\vec{G}'_x$, respectively. Equation (20.2) implies that the spins residing at position x will be encoded at position x' in the reconstructed image, where

$$
x' = x \left(1 + \frac{G'_x}{G_x}\right)
\tag{20.3}
$$

The presence of the background gradient causes spins to be shifted parallel to the read direction. Of course, this distortion affects the distance between spins in the reconstructed image changing the effective spin density $\hat{\rho}(x)$, as well as the actual positioning of objects. It is obvious from (20.3) that the only way to reduce the distortion caused by the background gradient is to increase the applied read gradient G_x. One consequence of increasing the read gradient is a decrease in SNR/voxel because of the increased bandwidth/voxel (see Ch. 15).

An alternative way to consider the distortion caused by a background gradient over the entire FOV is to return to the Nyquist relation. For an FOV of L, a read gradient G_x, and a sampling interval of Δt, the Nyquist relation gives

$$
\gamma |G_x| \Delta t L = 1
\tag{20.4}
$$

The presence of the constant background gradient inhomogeneity G'_x across the entire field-of-view means that the FOV changes to

$$
L' = \frac{1}{\gamma |G_x + G'_x| \Delta t} = \left|\frac{G_x}{G_x + G'_x}\right| L \equiv \lambda L
\tag{20.5}
$$

When G'_x has the same sign as G_x, the field-of-view is reduced and the coverage of k-space is increased due to distortion (see Fig. 20.1a). This leads to a smaller effective voxel size $\Delta x'$ which equals $\lambda \Delta x$ where Δx is the voxel size if no inhomogeneity were present and λ is less than unity. This distortion effect leads to an incorrect estimate of the size of the entire object, or of any feature within the object. If A is the physical size of the imaged object,

---

[1] The term 'static' refers to constancy in time.

the number of voxels representing the object changes from $A/\Delta x$ to $A/\Delta x'$. Alternately, the observed length of the object is changed

$$A_{observed} \equiv A' = \frac{A}{\lambda} \tag{20.6}$$

As a result, the object seems to be stretched in length (or compressed in the case when G'_x has a sign opposite that of G_x) in the read direction as shown in Fig. 20.1b.

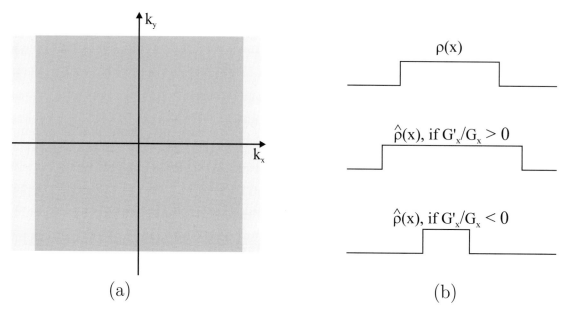

Fig. 20.1: In (a) the ideal 2D k-space region covered is shown by the darkly shaded region, but the actual region covered is the lightly shaded area when a background gradient G'_x parallel to G_x, the read gradient, exists. In (b), a 1D example of the effect that a global background gradient parallel and anti-parallel to the read gradient G_x has on the reconstructed image of a uniform rectangular object. In this graphical visualization of the change in field-of-view, the overall amplitudes of each $\hat{\rho}(x)$ are not shown to scale (i.e., they are not representative of what would physically appear in the actual reconstructed image).

The image distortion effect is not necessarily disadvantageous if the distortion can be corrected, but then G'_x needs to be known throughout all space. In practice, global gradient inhomogeneities, which exist across the entire FOV, are removed by correcting the static field with the first-order shims.[2] As long as $G'_x/G_x > 0$ and hence $L' < L$, the resolution has improved, and such a correction is possible; on the other hand, if $G'_x/G_x < 0$, the object collapses, i.e., $A' < A$, and correction is not possible. If $G'_x = -G_x$, for example, no read gradient exists during sampling and all spins contributing to the transverse magnetization, no matter what their location, collapse to a single point. This leads to a false impression from the image that all spins are at the origin. If the original adjacent pixels which combine have image intensities ρ_1 and ρ_2, respectively, the final result is then $\rho_{12} = \rho_1 + \rho_2$. Given

[2]Shimming is the adjustment of the main magnetic field used to reduce low spatial frequency field inhomogeneities. See Ch. 27 for further details on shimming.

this distorted image, now just a point, it is impossible to restore the original signals from different spatial locations. To make G'_x/G_x positive, for a G'_x of unknown sign and magnitude, two images are acquired: one with a positive read gradient and another is acquired with a negative read gradient. It will then be possible to estimate G'_x both in sign and magnitude by estimating λ from the two images.

Problem 20.1

Assume that a local background gradient G'_x exists over the interval $x_1 < x < x_2$ such that, in the absence of the applied read gradient, G_x, the field is given by

$$B_z(x) = B_0 + G'_x(x - x_0) \qquad\qquad x_1 < x < x_2 \qquad\qquad (20.7)$$

where $x_0 = (x_1 + x_2)/2$. Show that the spins in the interval $x_1 < x < x_2$ will appear at

$$x' = x\left(1 + \frac{G'_x}{G_x}\right) - x_0\frac{G'_x}{G_x} \qquad\qquad (20.8)$$

in the image. Note that this distortion is local to a specific population of spins within an image. Such local distortions often occur around structures with different magnetic susceptibilities. Since gradients over the entire FOV can generally be corrected by external sources, it is local gradients that cause most of the uncompensated distortion effects observed in images.

Local Gradients and Image Distortion: An Example

Although the above discussion centered around the effects created by a global gradient, the results are equally valid if the gradient is local, except the effects discussed only occur over the spatial extent of the field disturbance. The distortion effect due to a simplified version of a local field inhomogeneity is illustrated in Fig. 20.2.

The simple argument made above can be extended to understand why some regions in an image which should be uniform in response have higher signal and some have lower signal in the presence of local field inhomogeneities. This can occur for an object in the body such as the pituitary gland or when a foreign body such as a diamagnetic clip is present. This effect can be understood with a simplified physical example. Assume a 1D object has spin density $\rho_0 = 100$. It is one pixel wide and generates a gradient $+G'_x$ across the pixel to the left, and a gradient $-G'_x$ across the pixel to its right (see Fig. 20.2a). The neighboring two pixels contain a different tissue, but one which has the same spin density as the center pixel. These three regions defining the spatial variations of the local gradient will be referred to as L (left), C (center), and R (right), respectively. For simplicity, also assume $G'_x = G_x$ (see Fig. 20.2b). The spins in region L see a stronger gradient (Fig. 20.2b) and the object is stretched, with the spatial interval (x_1, x_2) mapped to the interval (x_1, x_3) since the frequency spread over this region is twice that which would have been present if there had been no local gradient (Fig. 20.2c). The spins in region C see the intended gradient behavior but with a frequency offset corresponding to a distance mapping of Δx along the positive x-direction, i.e., the

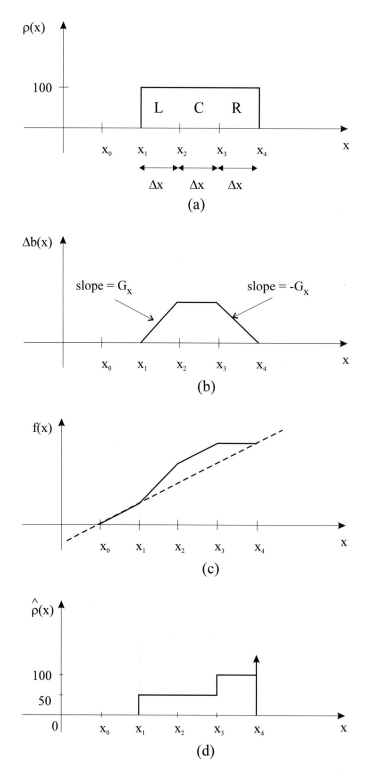

Fig. 20.2: Field inhomogeneity distortion effects in the read direction. For the spin density model shown in (a) and the background field deviation from B_0 as a function of position, $\Delta b(x)$ in (b), the demodulated frequency as a function of position, $f(x)$, is shown in (c), and the resulting image, $\hat{\rho}(x)$, is shown in (d). Note all information from x_3 to x_4 in (a) has been mapped to the point x_4 in (d).

interval (x_2, x_3) is mapped to the interval (x_3, x_4). All the spins in region R precess at a fixed frequency and are mapped to a single point determined by the field at x_3; this implies that spins in the interval (x_3, x_4) are mapped to the single point x_4. Of course, the signal that gets pushed from the interval (x_3, x_4) to x_4 gets spread out over several pixels in practice due to the finite point spread function in the reconstructed image. In summary, local gradients cause local distortion. These distortions can lead to stretching in certain parts of the image and shrinking in other parts, if they occur over distances comparable to several voxels.

Problem 20.2

Consider a specific example with $\Delta B(x) = G'_x x$, where G'_x is a constant gradient with the same sign as the read gradient G_x, $\rho(x) = \rho_0$ for $0 \le x \le A$ and the field-of-view is L.

a) Show that $\rho_0 \to \rho'_0 = \lambda \rho_0$ and draw a profile showing the image (neglecting Gibbs ringing effects) when $G'_x = G_x$. Note that the measured object size, A', changes when $\lambda \ne 1$.

b) Redo part (a) for $G'_x = -G_x$.

c) If it were not possible to avoid having a field gradient G'_x, would it be preferable to have $G'_x/G_x > 0$ or $G'_x/G_x < 0$, and why? Hint: Assuming G'_x is known, think in terms of correcting for the effects of G'_x after the image has been reconstructed.

20.1.2 Distortion Due to Gradient Perpendicular to the Read Direction

The previous 1D examples were useful for introducing distortion, but it is necessary to understand what occurs in 2D and 3D imaging where an arbitrary background gradient may be present. In the following discussion, phase accumulated prior to data readout is disregarded, so distortion becomes the theme of concentration. The accumulated effects of background gradients on an image, and particularly the difference between how spin echo and gradient echo methods are affected, are discussed later.

Any field variation present during data readout will alter the frequency at which spins precess. This leads to a misregistration of the spins' spatial location because a particular one-to-one relationship between a spin's position and frequency is the basis for spatial localization in MRI. Here, background gradients in the y- and z-directions (perpendicular to the read direction) are considered.

Background Gradient along the Phase Encoding Direction

When data is being read out, spins along x are associated with a particular frequency, and the introduction of a gradient perpendicular to the x-direction does not encode data in that direction during readout. Instead the additional gradient causes spins to be shifted along the x-axis as a function of their position in the y-direction (see Fig. 20.3). This can be seen explicitly by looking at the phase behavior during data readout in the presence of a background y-gradient

$$
\begin{aligned}
\phi(t') &= -2\pi\gamma(G_x x + G'_y y)t' \\
&= -2\pi\gamma t' G_x(x + (G'_y/G_x)y) \\
&= -2\pi k_x \left(x + \frac{G'_y}{G_x}y\right)
\end{aligned}
\tag{20.9}
$$

where

$$
x' = x + \frac{G'_y}{G_x}y
\tag{20.10}
$$

and the position where spins are encoded varies as a function of y. This effect is illustrated in Fig. 20.3b. The k-space coverage for this experiment is also shown in Fig. 20.3a.

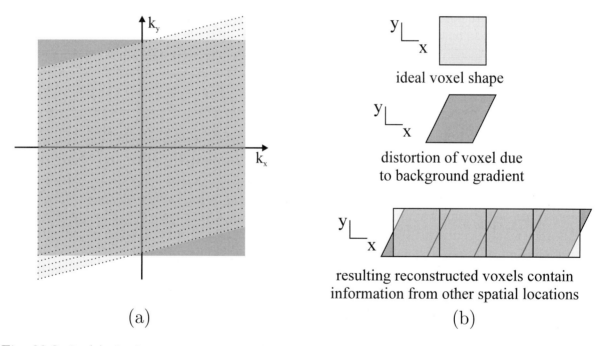

(a)   (b)

Fig. 20.3: In (a) the k-space coverage in the presence of a background gradient in the y-direction is shown for a spin echo experiment. The ideal k-space coverage is the dark shaded region, but the actual coverage is shown by the lighter shaded region (with the dotted lines representing the sampled data along the affected k_x-lines). Notice that the read axis is not parallel to k_x. In (b), the distortion of a single voxel is shown. The reconstructed image still consists of squares. The effect of the distortion will be to shift the information from one voxel into adjacent voxels. The same discussion holds true for k_y replaced by k_z (see also the next section).

Background Gradient along the Partition Encoding Direction

As in the above discussion, the phase for a background z-gradient is

$$
\begin{aligned}
\phi(t') &= -2\pi\gamma(G_x x + G'_z z)t' \\
&= -2\pi\gamma t' G_x (x + (G'_z/G_x)z) \\
&= -2\pi k_x \left(x + \frac{G'_z}{G_x} z \right)
\end{aligned}
\tag{20.11}
$$

where, similar to the background y-gradient case it is possible to define

$$
x' = x + \frac{G'_z}{G_x} z
\tag{20.12}
$$

and, in this case, the position where spins are encoded varies as a function of z.

If a background G'_z gradient exists during a 3D experiment, then a z-position-dependent pixel misregistration in the x-direction will result as revealed in (20.12) (see Fig. 20.4). Similarly, a y-dependent pixel misregistration in the x-direction is the result of a background G'_y gradient as revealed in (20.10). This implies, for example, that a blood vessel which is parallel to the z-direction would not appear this way in the resulting image. Instead, it would appear parallel to a line with an x- and z-component. A further point to note is, if a stack of successive 2D images are acquired at different z-positions, the vessel will appear parallel to the z-direction, but distortion of the form shown in Fig. 20.3 (with z replacing y) will still exist in each slice.

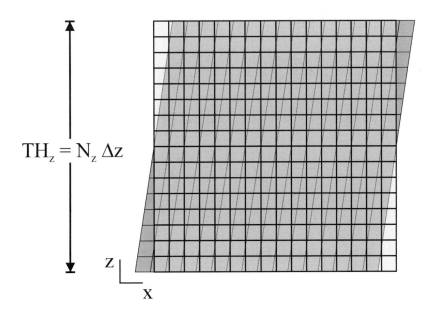

Fig. 20.4: This figure demonstrates image distortion due to a background gradient parallel to the partition encoding direction. The positions where spins are frequency encoded are shown by the darkly shaded grid. The undistorted image grid is shown as the lightly shaded region. The Δx-Δz voxel is distorted in the x-direction and a shift of the voxel center occurs along the x-direction. This can lead to errors in through-plane registration of objects in a 3D image.

Finally, it is seen that if $G_x \gg G_y'$ or G_z' the distortion will be reduced. This shows that a large read gradient also reduces distortion due to gradients along orthogonal directions. However, it is necessary to keep in mind that increasing the read gradient for the same resolution and FOV_x leads to a reduction in SNR.

20.1.3 Slice Select Distortion

Up to this point, the slice selection process has been ignored. Background gradients in the slice select direction do lead to distortion, however, and should be considered. Two things happen during the slice select process in the presence of a field variation when a slice selective rf/gradient pulse is used, as in a 2D or 3D imaging experiment. First, the slice will be distorted and, second, the ideal slice refocusing will fail to give maximum signal. The refocusing problem will be discussed in the next section on echo shifting, and only the slice distortion effects are considered here.

The slice distortion effect can be understood following the discussion about readout distortion effects since both are frequency encoding processes. If a background z-gradient G_z' is present, a thicker or thinner slice than desired will be excited. If a background field shift also exists, the center of the slice will be spatially shifted as illustrated schematically in Fig. 20.5. In the presence of G_x', or any background gradient perpendicular to the slice select direction, instead of the $\hat{z}$ direction such as shown in Fig. 20.5, the slice select gradient becomes $\vec{G}' = G_z\hat{z} + G_x'\hat{x}$. This causes the excited plane to be rotated (see also Ch. 10).

These slice select distortions are often not evident in an image since the contributing

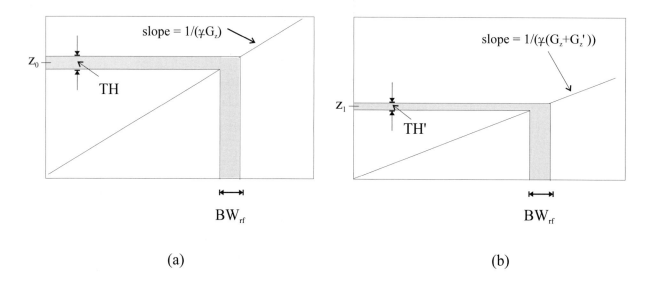

(a)   (b)

Fig. 20.5: Distortion effects due to a local background gradient G_z' in the slice select direction. The local background field can lead to a slice thickness different from the designed value and a shifted slice center. (a) With only G_z present, a slice of thickness TH is excited. (b) With the inhomogeneity along z producing an additional background gradient G_z' and a background field shift, the slice thickness is modified to TH'. At the same time, the slice center is shifted from position $z = z_0$ to $z = z_1$.

spins still come from an excited slice but not the desired slice.

Background Gradient Effects on 1D Spin Echo Imaging

In Ch. 8, it was shown that the spin echo sequence refocuses any time invariant field inhomogeneity at the echo. Therefore, there is no signal dephasing effect for instantaneous sampling at the echo time. However, the distortion effect persists since data sampling in a frequency encoded readout is not instantaneous and G'_x is still present during sampling. To understand this effect, we revisit the expression for the signal measured from a 1D spin echo imaging experiment in the presence of a background gradient. As seen in Ch. 9, the phase term due to all static gradients (imaging gradients and background gradients alike) must become zero at the echo time. For all times $t' = (t - T_E)$ defined during sampling, the measured spin echo signal is given by

$$s(t') = \int dx\, \rho(x) e^{-i2\pi\gamma(G_x + G'_x)xt'} \tag{20.13}$$

Using $k = \gamma G_x t'$ gives

$$
\begin{aligned}
s(t') &= \int dx\, \rho(x) e^{-i2\pi k(1 + G'_x/G_x)x} \\
&= \int dx\, \rho(x) e^{-i2\pi k' x}
\end{aligned}
\tag{20.14}
$$

where the scaled k-space variable k' is defined as

$$k' \equiv \left(1 + \frac{G'_x}{G_x}\right) k = \frac{k}{\lambda} \tag{20.15}$$

What is the implication of this scaled k-space variable? From the scaling property of the Fourier transform (see Table 11.1), this leads to a reciprocal scaling of the spatial variable x on the image, and the image signal is also scaled by the reciprocal of the scaling factor in k-space. Hence,

$$\rho'(x) = \lambda\rho(\lambda x) \quad \text{(due to scaling of } k_x) \tag{20.16}$$

and distortion occurs in the image ($\rho'(x)$ is the distorted image) which cannot be corrected unless G'_x is known.

Note that there is no phase dispersion within a voxel due to the presence of the background gradient, only distortion. This means that the distortion of $\rho(x)$ to $\rho'(x)$ does not affect the integrated magnetization over any spatial scale, whether it is over a voxel or if the entire object is disturbed. Therefore,

$$\int dx'\, \rho'(x') \equiv \int dx\, \rho(x) \tag{20.17}$$

when integrated over all space. Therefore, the total signal from a distorted object will be the same (within SNR limitations) as that which would have been obtained from the undistorted object. Another interpretation of this observation is that all distortion does is map the signal over a distorted grid of points while conserving the total integrated signal, independent of the size of the object. This is easily understood as long as the frequency shift never causes the object to alias out of the field-of-view since the aliased part of the object has a nonzero phase associated with it. Stated precisely, (20.17) is strictly true only if $\rho(x)$ is positive definite (which is not the case if aliasing occurs).

The property of integrated signal conservation in the presence of inhomogeneities is unique to the spin echo experiment since the T_E-dependent phase dispersion across finite distances is absent in the spin echo experiment. This is taken advantage of in spectroscopy where quantitative metabolite concentrations are obtained by integrating under different spectral peaks. Also, although a 1D example is presented here, the result is true for a background gradient along any direction.

Problem 20.3

---

a) Prove (20.17).

b) Is this expression valid if the limits of integration cover just the field-of-view?
   Hint: Consider both the case when aliasing is present and when there is no aliasing.

20.2   Echo Shifting Due to Field Inhomogeneities in Gradient Echo Imaging

The last section concentrated on distortion effects in the read and slice select directions. The basis of the dephasing effects in a gradient echo imaging experiment due to the accumulated phase behavior from static field variations was only briefly mentioned. As will be shown below, dephasing due to phase dispersion created by the presence of background gradients can be easily conceptualized as being due to an echo shift, whether it is in the read direction, the slice select direction, or any phase encoding direction in a gradient echo experiment.

The Echo Shift Effect in Gradient Echo Imaging

Consider a 1D gradient echo imaging experiment. The main conceptual difference between the gradient echo experiment and the spin echo experiment is the absence of a refocusing of the phase dispersion imposed by background gradients at the echo. The measured signal in the presence of a constant linear background gradient G_x' parallel to the read direction can be written as

$$
\begin{aligned}
s(t') &= \int dx\, \rho(x) e^{-i2\pi\bar{\gamma}G_x x t' - i2\pi\bar{\gamma}G_x' x(t' + T_E)} \\
&= \int dx\, \rho(x) e^{-i2\pi\bar{\gamma}G_x t'\left(1 + \frac{G_x'}{G_x}\right)x - i2\pi\bar{\gamma}G_x' x T_E}
\end{aligned}
\tag{20.18}
$$

There is the usual scaling of the k-space variable that leads to distortion and an additional position-dependent phase term

$$
\phi(x) = -2\pi\bar{\gamma}G_x' x T_E
\tag{20.19}
$$

This phase depends linearly on T_E and leads to a phase spread across a distance d given by

$$\Delta\phi(d) = -2\pi\gamma G_x' d T_E \tag{20.20}$$

The most appropriate spatial distance to consider is the voxel size Δx. Assuming that each voxel contains a homogeneous distribution of spins, the effect of a phase distribution $\Delta\phi$ which ranges from $-\frac{\Delta\phi}{2}$ to $+\frac{\Delta\phi}{2}$ across the voxel (Fig. 20.6) leads to a reconstructed voxel signal of reduced magnitude, i.e., signal dephasing occurs. This dephased signal is given by[3]

$$\hat{\rho}(x) = \rho_0 \left[\frac{1}{\Delta\phi} \int_{-\Delta\phi/2}^{\Delta\phi/2} e^{i\phi} d\phi \right] \quad \text{(due to phase dispersion across the voxel)}$$

$$= \rho_0 \text{sinc}(\Delta\phi/2) \tag{20.21}$$

where ρ_0 is the homogeneous spin density value. Equation (20.21) shows that the voxel signal vanishes when the phase dispersion becomes equal to any nonzero integer multiple of 2π. In general, it is an oscillatory function whose envelope dampens inversely as the phase spread (see Fig. 20.7).

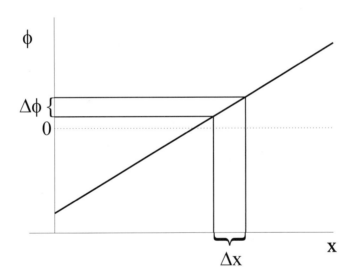

Fig. 20.6: This figure demonstrates that a linear phase change in an image leads to a finite phase dispersion $\Delta\phi$ across each voxel. The phase dispersion across a voxel implies a reduction of image intensity.

Although static field (B_0) inhomogeneities exist across the object, they can be easily reduced to the order of a fraction of a ppm across the entire useful volume of the bore of the magnet. In any case, the effect of such a 'global background gradient' is usually minimal in terms of signal loss (although, as seen from (20.20) and (20.21), this will depend on echo time). The major effect of these slow field changes is the bulk phase shift due to the term $-2\pi\gamma G_x' x T_E$ or generally $-2\pi\gamma\Delta B T_E$ (see Fig. 20.7).

---

[3]The effect of the point spread function $h_w(x)$ has been neglected in the derivation of (20.21).

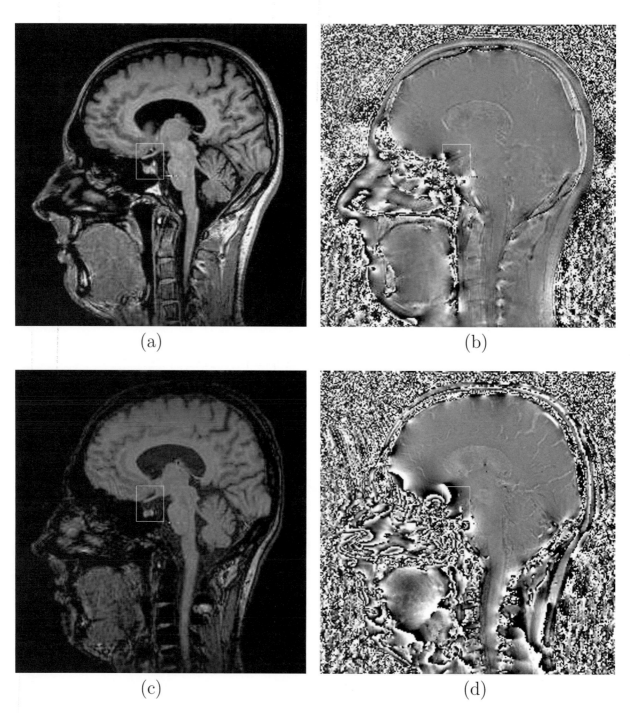

Fig. 20.7: Magnitude (a) and phase (b) images from a gradient echo acquisition with $T_E = 5\,\text{ms}$ are shown. Magnitude (c) and phase (d) images from the same slice for $T_E = 15\,\text{ms}$. The generally slow spatial variation of the B_0 field is evident in the phase images. Increased signal loss in the magnitude image (c) due to phase dispersion across a voxel at the longer T_E can be seen in the region of the pituitary gland (this is in the lower half of the box). The areas of rapid phase change in (d) reveal where greater signal losses are expected. The phase images are contaminated with nonzero phase from moving blood since the sequence was not velocity compensated (see Ch. 23).

Problem 20.4

A static field is usually shimmed across a given distance. Today it is not unreasonable to obtain a field variation of only 1 ppm across the head (assume $L_x = 256$ mm). What would be the signal loss at 1.5 T for a voxel size of (a) 1 mm, (b) 1 cm, and (c) 10 cm if the T_E is 10 ms? Model this 1 ppm field variation as a linear field gradient across the head to find G'_x. The signal loss for a given field inhomogeneity is clearly dependent on the voxel size. Note that this global signal loss usually goes unnoticed on the magnitude image. (d) For part (a), will dephasing become the same as in (b) if T_E is 100 ms for part (a) but still 10 ms for part (b)?

20.2.1   Echo Shift in Terms of Number of Sampled Points

In general for an extraneous gradient in some arbitrary direction present during data sampling, the echo is shifted from its designated position in k-space, and the effective read axis is rotated (see Ch. 10 or Sec. 20.1.3). It is quite easy to understand the echo shifting effect of a background gradient. The echo is said to occur at that instant when the phase imposed by the (effective) read gradient is refocused, i.e., when the zeroth moment of the effective read gradient becomes zero. Picture the typical read gradient structure which leads to a gradient echo (Fig. 20.8). A negative gradient lobe followed by a positive lobe on during the sampling period T_s is the typical structure for the read gradient. Consider a background gradient G'_x. Suppose $G'_x < 0$ as shown in Fig. 20.8. The effective dephasing gradient in

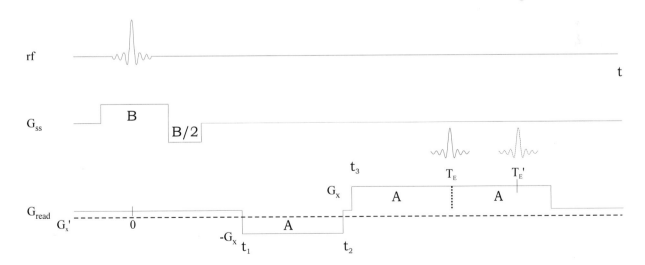

Fig. 20.8: Echo shifting in the presence of a background gradient. A negative background gradient is used here to demonstrate how the echo shifts to the right within the sampling window. The ideal echo is shown above the read gradient centered around the ideal echo time T_E, while the shifted echo is shown as a dashed line centered around the shifted echo time T'_E.

this case is $-(G_x + G'_x)$, i.e., the effectiveness of the dephasing lobe is increased. During the readout, the effective read gradient is $(G_x - G'_x)$. This decreases the rate of rephasing, and as a result of these two effects (the more effective dephasing and the slower rephasing) the echo occurs later than $t = T_E$, i.e., the echo is shifted temporally to the right (to $t = T'_E$) within the sampling period. On the other hand, the echo is shifted to the left within the sampling period if $G'_x > 0$.

Problem 20.5

Describe why the echo is shifted to an earlier time (i.e., temporally to the left in Fig. 20.8) in the $G'_x > 0$ case.

This echo shifting effect is analyzed in detail next. The analysis follows the situation depicted in Fig. 20.8. The echo takes place at $t = T'_E$ such that

$$\int_0^{T'_E} dt\, G_x^{total}(t) = 0 \tag{20.22}$$

Let

$$T'_E \equiv t_3 + n'\Delta t \tag{20.23}$$

be the time of occurrence of the shifted echo, i.e., $n'\Delta t$ is the time from the beginning of the sampling period to where the echo occurs in the presence of G'_x. For the case considered here, (20.22) leads to the equality

$$-G_x n\Delta t + G_x n'\Delta t + G'_x(t_3 + n'\Delta t) = 0 \tag{20.24}$$

where n is half the total number of sampling points. Solving for n' from (20.24) yields

$$n'\Delta t = \frac{G_x n\Delta t - G'_x t_3}{G_x + G'_x} \tag{20.25}$$

for $|G'_x| < G_x$, from which T'_E is given by

$$\begin{aligned} T'_E &= \frac{G_x n\Delta t - G'_x t_3}{(G_x + G'_x)} + t_3 \\ &= \frac{G_x}{(G_x + G'_x)}(t_3 + n\Delta t) \\ &= \frac{G_x}{(G_x + G'_x)}T_E \\ &= \lambda T_E \end{aligned} \tag{20.26}$$

Problem 20.6

In terms of an echo shift, let n_{shift} be the number of sampled points by which the echo is shifted to the right (or left) of the ideal echo time.

a) Show that

$$
\begin{aligned}
n_{\text{shift}} \Delta t &= \Delta T_E \equiv T_E' - T_E \\
&= -\frac{G_x'}{G_x + G_x'} T_E
\end{aligned}
\tag{20.27}
$$

b) If $G_x' \to -G_x'$ does $|n_{\text{shift}}|$ remain the same?

20.2.2 Echo Shift Due to Background Phase/Partition Encoding Gradients

The effect which leads to image distortion in conventional imaging methods is the continuous variation of the phase generated by the static field inhomogeneity as data are being sampled (as described by the phase term $2\pi\gamma G_x' x t'$ in (20.13) and (20.18) in the case when the inhomogeneity is in the form of a local gradient). On the other hand, the presence of an inhomogeneity in either phase encoding direction in a conventional imaging experiment creates an extraneous phase which is constant from one k-space line to the next. Such a constant phase leads to a shift in the k-space origin of the collected data and a resulting dephasing effect due to phase dispersion in the gradient echo experiment. Simply put, *there is technically no distortion in the phase encoding direction.* The distortion associated with the background gradient during readout which causes the slant in the k-space coverage shown in Fig. 20.3 leads to a shift of the spins parallel to the read direction. Also, this distortion varies as a function of position along the phase encoding direction in the reconstructed image. As a result, to the end observer, some form of geometric distortion does seem to occur in the phase encoding direction in conventional imaging methods where the read direction is frequency encoded (see for example Fig. 20.3a).

As mentioned above, a position-dependent phase is generated in the phase encoding direction. This phase is given by

$$
\phi_{\text{pe}}' \equiv -\gamma G_y' y T_E
\tag{20.28}
$$

What this phase offset does is shift the origin of k-space in the $\hat{k}_y$ direction. In the current case, the $k_y = 0$ line now occurs at that line at which there is complete cancelation of this phase by a particular phase encoding gradient step, i.e., it occurs at line m which satisfies

$$
\gamma m \Delta G_y y \tau_y + \gamma G_y' y T_E = 0
\tag{20.29}
$$

Hence, m is given by

$$
m = -\frac{G_y' T_E}{\Delta G_y \tau_y} = -\gamma G_y' L_y T_E
\tag{20.30}
$$

Again, as in the read direction, the rule of thumb to avoid total signal loss is to ensure that m is less than $N_y/2$.

20.2.3   Echo Shift Due to Background Gradients Parallel to the Slice Select Direction

The ideal refocusing lobe assumes no background inhomogeneity, and any local gradient within the slice locally disturbs the refocusing effect of the rephasing lobe. As a result, the rephasing can be incomplete at the end of the rephasing lobe and there may be a local reduction in the slice integrated signal. The misadjustment of the rephasing lobe due to the presence of gradients can be thought of as creating a time-shifting of the echo along the z-direction (see Fig. 20.9). In practice, the rephasing lobe amplitude is varied until the peak signal is formed (which is fine for global G'_z) but this does not help correct for local G'_z (see Secs. 20.3.4 and 20.3.5 for a method that leads to a recovery of this signal). These slice select background gradients can be a major problem for 2D gradient echo imaging, because the complex signal has to be integrated over the slice (see (20.21)) and it leads to a signal loss. In the presence of the G'_z inhomogeneities, there is no mechanism for refocusing the phase due to background gradients during the imaging sequence, so the k-space origin may be missed altogether, as shown in Fig. 20.9, and signal may be significantly reduced. Background gradients along the read and phase encoding gradients cause echo shifts that are usually refocused somewhere within the sampling window, but since no further gradients are applied along the z-direction in a 2D experiment, no shift compensation occurs.

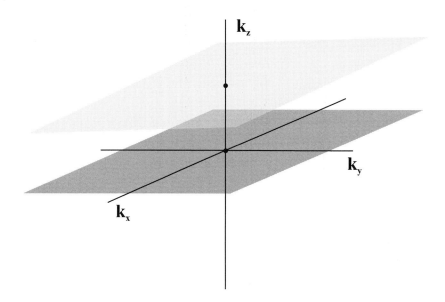

Fig. 20.9: The k-space coverage for a 2D imaging experiment when a background z-gradient is present. The ideal coverage is shown by the darkly shaded region, and the lightly shaded area shows the actual coverage. In this case, the k-space origin is missed altogether and the resulting signal will be reduced (recall that the signal is a maximum for 2D imaging when $k_z = 0$). This effect will occur for both gradient echoes and spin echoes, but the magnitude of the shift will be greater in the gradient echo case. In the case of 3D imaging this echo shift will lead to a k-space shift along the partition encoding direction.

20.2.4 Echo Shift Due to Background Gradients Orthogonal to the Slice Select Direction

The presence of a background gradient orthogonal to the slice select direction creates two effects. First, the selected slice will be rotated from the ideal orientation (see the section in Ch. 10 on selecting an arbitrarily oriented slice for a general discussion of this phenomenon). Second, the refocusing gradient lobe will not refocus phase accumulated across the slice due to these gradients. In the spin echo case, the phase due to this gradient will be refocused at the echo, and only distortion during readout will occur. In the gradient echo case, background gradients orthogonal to the slice select direction lead to an echo shift along their respective direction and distortion along the read direction.

20.3 Methods for Minimizing Distortion and Echo Shifting Artifacts

This section is used as a summarizing point in reviewing the effects of field inhomogeneities in different gradient echo imaging scenarios. Since the discussion focuses on gradient echo rather than spin echo imaging methods, focus is on a logical progression towards higher dimensional imaging methods which minimize all distortion effects and reduce signal loss. Since imaging in higher dimensions leads to longer imaging times, some of the proposed methods might not have practical uses at present. Such considerations apart, the general underlying theme in the methods discussed here is the use of progressively higher resolution, both spatially (in all three dimensions) and spectrally. Resolution requirements are specified based on the echo time required, or achievable, in the intended application according to (20.36). The other underlying message is that with the encoding of more and more dimensions, 'collapsing' a higher dimensional image to a lower dimensional image or an image with higher spatial resolution to one with lower spatial resolution by spatial filtering (a simple example is one of averaging of the signal from immediate spatial neighbors to improve SNR) allows the visualization of the perturbing field inhomogeneities. It will also be shown that if 3D CSI is used, averaging images from all frequencies (spectral projection) allows the creation of gradient echo images with all spatial information mapped correctly to the right physical location.

20.3.1 Distortion Versus Dephasing

Something interesting happens as $G_x \to \infty$. Distortion doesn't occur (since $\lambda \to 1$), but echo shifting still does. This can be seen by rewriting (20.27) from Prob. 20.6 as

$$|n_{\text{shift}}| \approx \left|\frac{G'_x T_E}{G_x \Delta t}\right| = |\gamma G'_x L_x T_E| \tag{20.31}$$

Note that this approximation is equally valid for the case when G'_x is negative or positive as long as $|G_x| \gg |G'_x|$. *In summary, a large read gradient relative to local gradients caused by field inhomogeneities will reduce distortion but not dephasing.* Of course, as $G_x \to \infty$,

T_E can be reduced to minimize dephasing, but if a fixed T_E is desired for contrast reasons, increasing G_x does not reduce dephasing.

Problem 20.7

a) Show that n_{shift} for $G'_x = G_0$ is less than $|n_{\text{shift}}|$ for $G'_x = -G_0$ where G_0 is a positive quantity.

b) How many sample points is the echo shift if $T_E = 50\,\text{ms}$, $\Delta t = 20\,\mu s$, $G_x = 3\,\text{mT/m}$, and $G_0 = 0.1\,\text{mT/m}$?

c) What is L in the above example?

d) For the case when $G_x \gg G_0$, explain why the phase shift at T_E is independent of a doubling of G_x with Δx unchanged. Hint: See Fig. 20.10 and review the discussion behind (20.31).

e) Why is it either difficult or undesirable to use too large a G_x?

Part (d) of Prob. 20.7 has a very important implication for gradient echo imaging in the presence of B_0 field inhomogeneities. A large read gradient can be used to reduced geometric distortion, but it will not reduce signal loss due to dephasing. Therefore, the read gradient G_x cannot be increased without a concomitant loss in SNR for a fixed voxel size, field-of-view, and T_E. So, it should be increased only to such a value at which the distortion is tolerable and yet the SNR is acceptable.

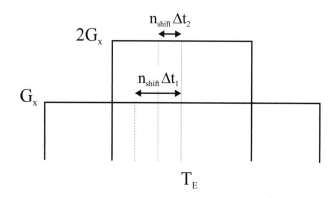

Fig. 20.10: Obtaining an image using twice the read gradient strength reduces the distortion effect but has no effect on the echo shift as long as $|G'_x| \ll G_x$. The area between the dashed and dotted lines is proportional to the shift in k-space for the read gradient G_x caused by G'_x. Likewise, the area between the dashed and dotted lines under the gradient $2G_x$. Here Δt_1 is the sampling interval when the read gradient G_x is used, and $\Delta t_2 = \frac{1}{2}\Delta t_1$ is the sampling interval when the read gradient $2G_x$ is used (Δx constant). Note that the shifted echo occurs at a time $n_{\text{shift}}\Delta t_1$ to the left of the ideal echo time in the lower gradient case and at time $n_{\text{shift}}\Delta t_2$ in the higher gradient case, which, in terms of the number of sampled points, is the same in each case.

20.3.2 High Resolution and Phase Dispersion

It is easy to understand qualitatively that signal is lost as the echo shifts outside the sampling window. On a more quantitative basis, the effect can be explained from a signal processing perspective. Recall that an echo shift by $n_{shift}\Delta t$ in time corresponds to a shift in k-space by

$$k_{shift} \equiv \gamma G n_{shift}\Delta t = n_{shift}\Delta k \qquad (20.32)$$

Also, recall from the Fourier transform shift theorem that a shift in k-space of $s(k)$ to $s(k + k_{shift})$ causes a phase dispersion across a voxel in the image of

$$\Delta\phi = -2\pi k_{shift}\Delta x = -2\pi n_{shift}/N_x \qquad (20.33)$$

When $|n_{shift}| \geq N_x/2$, the echo is completely outside the sampling window. This leads to a uniform phase dispersion of at least π across a voxel and, according to the discussion surrounding (20.21), the voxel signal will be reduced significantly or vanish.

Problem 20.8

---

a) Using the Fourier transform shift theorem, show that the phase shift across a voxel as given in (20.33) can also be equivalently written as

$$\Delta\phi = \phi(x + \Delta x) - \phi(x) = -2\pi n_{shift}\frac{\Delta x}{L_x} \qquad (20.34)$$

b) What is the signal loss for an object of uniform spin density but only one pixel wide when $n_{shift} = 4$ points and $N_x = L_x/\Delta x = 128$?

c) Assume that the dephasing gradient lobe before the sampling window is mistakenly doubled in time. Such a mistake will cause the echo shifted by $N_x/2$ points such that the echo is at the edge of the sampling window. Consider an object of uniform density and equal in size to the FOV. Neglecting the signal loss within one voxel as it was considered above, show that the signal at the center of the object can be approximated by the integral of half a sinc function and is roughly half of its original signal when the echo was properly refocused at the center of the sampling window. If the echo is shifted by $(N_x/2+1)$ points so the echo is just outside the sampling window, show that the signal at the center of the object is now only roughly 9% of its original signal. Although complete signal loss within a voxel does not occur unless n_{shift} equals to a multiple of N_x, this additional signal loss suggests that $n_{shift} \leq N_x/2$ be used in the design of gradient echo imaging techniques for human imaging in which objects are generally smooth without many sharp signal transitions.

High Resolution Advantage and Use in Long-T_E Imaging

For a homogeneous collection of spins experiencing a uniform field distribution (i.e., all fields within a finite range of values are equiprobable), suppose the resolution is improved in the read direction with the read gradient held fixed so that the frequency shift per unit distance remains fixed. Choosing Δx smaller by a factor β (i.e., going to higher resolution) reduces phase dispersion across the voxel. In the case, where the phase is already spread from 0 to 2π, the phase dispersion is reduced from 0 to $2\pi/\beta$. As β gets large, the phase dispersion across a voxel gets smaller and signal loss is reduced. Therefore, high resolution can actually improve SNR in the local region affected by the presence of local field inhomogeneities.

There are certain applications which require the acquisition of gradient echo images at long T_E values. In such cases, it takes only a proportionally smaller background gradient value to cause complete voxel signal loss for a given Δx value. The general rule is that as the echo time increases, for a given high resolution voxel size, robustness of acquisition to avoid signal dephasing can be achieved only for proportionately smaller G_x' values. As a closing comment to the previous discussion of the utility of high resolution to overcome signal loss, a conservative upper limit on the voxel size can be determined from (20.31) to limit signal loss for a given G_x' value as T_E varies. A useful rule of thumb is to limit the number of sample points by which the echo is shifted to be less than or equal to $N_x/2$. Using (20.31) leads to an upper limit on Δx for a given G_x' and T_E given by

$$\Delta x_{max} = \frac{1}{|2\gamma G_x' T_E|} \quad \text{fixed } T_E \text{ case} \tag{20.35}$$

Problem 20.9

In order to obtain a better understanding of the effects of a result such as (20.35), it is often useful to express it in terms of a particular set of units. Therefore, show that the following expressions are correct, where the background gradient has been expressed in terms of field variation per millimeter, T_E is milliseconds, and Δx_{max} is given in millimeters. Assume that δB_0 is the background inhomogeneity measured over a distance of $\Delta x'$ mm. If $\Delta x'$ is arbitrarily set to 1 mm and $\delta' \equiv \frac{\delta}{\Delta x'}$ in ppm/mm (i.e., $\delta' B_0$ is effectively a field gradient), show that (20.35) becomes

$$\Delta x_{max} \simeq \left(\frac{8}{\delta'} \frac{1.5}{B_0} \cdot \frac{1}{T_E} \right) \text{ mm} \tag{20.36}$$

when normalized to the above mentioned units (i.e., B_0 in tesla, δ' in ppm/mm, and T_E in ms). In these long-T_E applications, it is typical to acquire the data under low bandwidth conditions to optimize the SNR/voxel, which suffers because of the lower signal at long T_E values.

This high resolution approach will usually work if the echo is shifted to the right (Fig. 20.8) and out of the sampling window. The sampling window can eventually be extended in order to incorporate the echo. However, it will not always work for negative shifts because the sampling window may not be extended to the left. In that case, the data must be collected a second time with the polarity of the read gradient reversed (now that inhomogeneity will cause a shift of the echo to the right).

Multi-Echo, High Bandwidth Versus Single Echo, Low Bandwidth Acquisitions

Instead of acquiring a single image with a long T_s value (Fig. 20.11a), which is known to suffer from several limitations, it is advantageous to acquire images at multiple echo times (say N_{echo} times) in the same time period by using an alternating read gradient structure (see Fig. 20.11b), each of which is acquired with a read bandwidth which is N_{echo} times larger. The utility of this method lies in the possibility of computing the signal envelope, characterizing it, and then using it to optimally sum the magnitude images of this multi-echo data to create an equivalent long T_E image with essentially the same SNR as the long T_s acquisition, but with less distortion and resolution loss as in the long T_s acquisition. The price to pay for this approach is larger reconstruction times and potentially more data storage if all images are kept. Finally, it is important to realize that this is one of several approaches which demonstrates one aspect of the non-commutativity (nonlinear) behavior in MRI. Although the total acquisition and sampling times in this approach are the same, the resulting images are not.

Phase Shifts

As a final comment along these lines, note that an off-center asymmetric echo which remains within the sampling window (as would be the case for areas experiencing background gradients and the sequence is designed for a symmetric echo acquisition in the case when $n_{shift} \leq N_x/2$) leads to an image which obeys the Fourier transform shift theorem leading to

$$\hat{\rho}_{ae}(x) = e^{-i2\pi n_{shift}\Delta k_x x}\hat{\rho}(x) \tag{20.37}$$

when the echo is shifted by n_{shift} samples and the suffix 'ae' refers to 'asymmetric echo.' Taking the magnitude yields

$$|\hat{\rho}_{ae}(x)| = |\hat{\rho}(x)| \tag{20.38}$$

If $\Delta x \to 0$ (as resolution is improved), there is essentially no phase dispersion and no signal loss. Only a bulk phase shift remains, indicating the presence of local field inhomogeneities. The magnitude image could then be filtered to create a lower resolution image to overcome the SNR degradation normally associated with a higher resolution image.

20.3.3 2D Imaging

Conventional 2D imaging suffers from all the problems considered in this chapter. It suffers from distortion in the read and slice select directions, and also from nonorthogonality of the three encoded directions in the presence of arbitrarily directed field inhomogeneities. In addition to these problems, the slice thickness is limited by the available slice select gradient capability and SNR limitations. As a result, there is not as much flexibility to achieve high resolution in the slice select direction and dephasing across the slice can occur. These

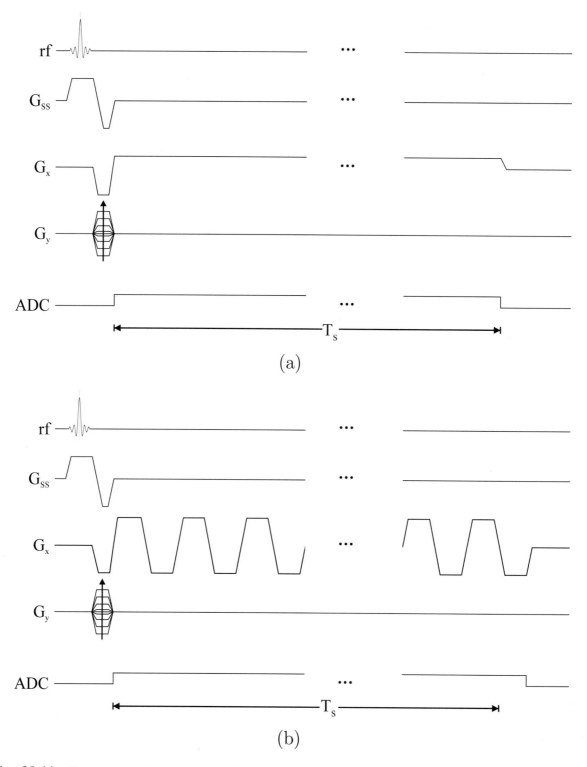

(a)

(b)

Fig. 20.11: Two acquisition strategies for acquiring long-T_E image data in the presence of local static field inhomogeneities. (a) Single-echo acquisition with a long T_s. (b) Multi-echo acquisition of N_{echo} echoes using a high bandwidth alternating read gradient structure.

combined effects can be differentiated by comparing a pair of 2D images from spin echo and gradient echo acquisitions. It is assumed that the same slice select gradient, the same rf bandwidth, the same read gradient, the same echo time, and the same resolution were used for these two acquisitions. In that case, the spin echo example is likely to suffer only from the distortion effects (whether it is in the slice select direction or the read direction) while the gradient echo example suffers from signal loss due to phase dispersion in addition. A comparison of the two images then differentiates the distortion effect from the dephasing effect. This is illustrated in Fig. 20.12, where a 2D spin echo image and a gradient echo image in the area surrounding the maxillary sinus are shown, whereby the use of a rather long T_E of 45 ms has caused complete signal loss in the area surrounding the maxillary sinus despite the use of high in-plane spatial resolution (0.5 mm × 1.0 mm) because of the rather thick (8.0 mm) slice thickness. Note also the complete loss of structural detail in the nasal cavity.

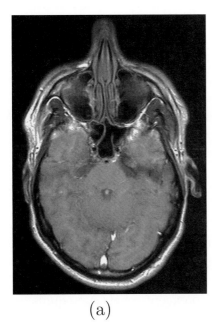 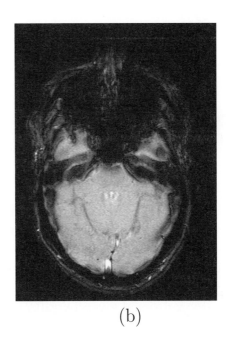

(a)   (b)

Fig. 20.12: Gradient echo and spin echo 2D imaging comparison in the area near the maxillary sinus at a rather long T_E of 45 ms. (a) Spin echo image, and (b) 2D gradient echo image, each collected with a slice thickness of 8 mm. It is worthwhile to remember here that only slice distortion (including slice center shift) occurs in the spin echo, while signal loss due to dispersion occurs in the 2D gradient echo image because of the large slice thickness.

20.3.4   2D Imaging with Variable Rephasing Gradients

Since signal loss in the slice select direction in 2D imaging is perpetrated by the imperfect slice refocusing mechanism, this loss can be overcome by varying the slice refocusing gradient strength centered around the ideal value. The expectation is that there exists a refocusing gradient step which can cancel the dephasing caused by the gradient inhomogeneity. This occurs when

$$\Delta G_{rp}\tau_{rp} + G'_z T_E = 0 \qquad (20.39)$$

These ΔG_{rp} steps are applied effectively as partition encoding steps (see Fig. 20.13).

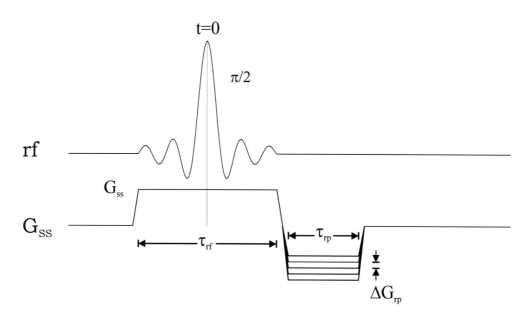

Fig. 20.13: Slice select sequence diagram depicting the application of variable rephasing gradients.

If a spectrum of inhomogeneities is present or if the magnitude of the inhomogeneity present in the area of interest is unknown, then a variety of different ΔG_{rp} will be needed and the experiment will need to be repeated N_{refocus} times. The hope is that these images can be summed in magnitude to overcome signal loss in regions affected by background gradients. A note of caution is that the individual images obtained with each value of the refocusing gradient can contain nonzero voxel signal even if that gradient value does not satisfy (20.39). The incomplete refocusing leads to a phase dispersion $\Delta\phi$ across the voxel, leading to an integrated voxel signal given by (20.21) which is nonzero except when $\Delta\phi$ equals an integer multiple of 2π. Fig. 20.14 shows the use of such a variable refocusing gradient experiment where it was found that the maxillary sinus was rephased with the use of a positive step away from the ideal refocusing lobe amplitude showing that a negative gradient was created by the sinuses (whose value can be calculated from (20.39)) in the slice select direction, causing some of the dephasing. It will be shown next that the appropriate analysis comes from a Fourier inversion of a set of 3D images, not the summed magnitude as suggested above.

20.3.5   3D Imaging

The 3D imaging experiment is conceptually similar to stepping through various ΔG_{rp} values as discussed in Sec. 20.3.4. In this case, the gradient table is used to phase encode the excited slice. The main conceptual difference between the two methods is that now a Fourier transform is performed along the slice select dimension. The resultant images lead to partitions (individual slices of the 3D data set) of size $\Delta z = TH/N_z$. As before, one of the phase encoding gradient steps cancels the phase dispersion created by the background gradient. Although this leads to an echo shift and an associated phase dispersion across the voxel in the reconstructed image, the resulting phase dispersion is minimal because of the higher spatial resolution obtained in the slice select direction with 3D imaging. As seen in Sec. 20.2.2, use of the thinner 3D partitions leads to improved SNR in areas suffering from echo shift mechanisms in the slice select direction. This is illustrated in Fig. 20.15a, where a single partition from a 3D data set obtained with 0.5 mm × 1.0 mm × 0.5 mm voxel dimensions is shown.

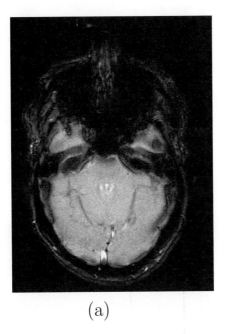
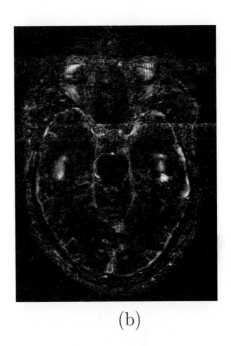

(a)   (b)

Fig. 20.14: Use of variable rephasing gradients in the slice select direction allows the visualization of structures which are influenced by background gradients by nulling the effect of this gradient exactly. (a) The 2D gradient echo image shown in Fig. 20.12b is repeated here for comparison purposes. Although this slice includes the maxillary sinuses (which can be characterized as an air-tissue interface), the long T_E of 45 ms leaves the signal completely dephased in the area surrounding this sinus area. (b) With the use of a positive gradient offset to the slice select rephase lobe, this lost signal in the maxillary sinus area is recovered. However, this dephases the signal in the other areas which were visualized with the ideal rephasing lobe. Hence, different regions of the object influenced by background gradients of different strengths are best visualized by using different rephasing gradient amplitudes.

Magnitude Averaging or 'Collapsing' of 3D Images

Sometimes, although the minimal dephasing effect found in a high resolution 3D image is desirable, lower SNR can make the overall image quality poor. One way to utilize this data is to 'collapse' it, i.e., create fewer N_z 2D slices from the 3D data set by averaging the magnitude of several slices to create a single thicker slice, with increased SNR, and minimal phase dispersion. Magnitude averaging can be performed over N_z slices or a subset $\mathcal{N}_z$ (see Fig. 20.16), partitions to obtain an image of the same slice thickness as a 2D slice but with less signal loss due to through-plane dephasing. The operation of collapsing data is just one

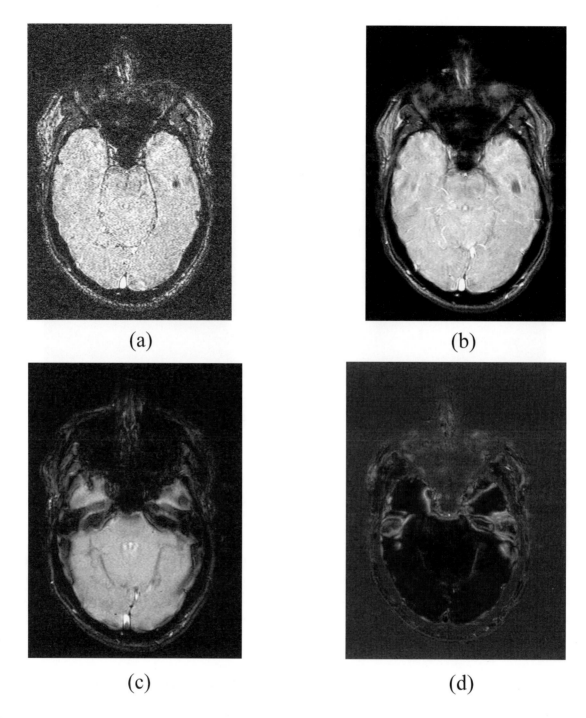

(a)   (b)

(c)   (d)

Fig. 20.15: Utility of high resolution in all three dimensions in recovering signal loss while maintaining SNR. (a) A single 3D partition from a data set collected with a 0.5 mm partition thickness. Two things are immediately apparent: first, the SNR in a single partition is very poor; and second, signal is recovered in the area surrounding the maxillary sinuses. (b) The recovered SNR in areas influenced by local gradients can be taken advantage of by averaging 16 magnitude images to create an equivalent 8 mm thick slice. Signal is recovered in comparison with a 2D gradient echo image (with $TH = 8$ mm) shown in (c) for comparison purposes. The regions of the image which are affected by background gradients are highlighted by (d) the difference image obtained by subtracting the image in (c) from that in (b). Note that the long T_E of 45 ms in (a) has caused total signal cancelation in the nasal cavity despite the very high spatial resolution.

of averaging data or projecting a 3D data set onto a 2D space to create a new image, i.e.,

$$\hat{\rho}_{2D \leftarrow 3D}(m\Delta x, n\Delta y; TH_{2D} = \mathcal{N}_z\Delta z) = \frac{1}{\mathcal{N}_z} \sum_{j=-\mathcal{N}_z/2}^{\mathcal{N}_z/2-1} |\hat{\rho}_{3D}(m\Delta x, n\Delta y, j\Delta z)| \qquad (20.40)$$

This method is illustrated in Fig. 20.15b, where most of the signal lost in the area around the maxillary sinuses is recovered in comparison with the 2D gradient echo image shown again for comparison purposes in Fig. 20.15c. The areas where signal has been recovered in Fig. 20.15b in comparison with Fig. 20.15c is depicted by subtraction of the two images, as shown in Fig. 20.15d. However, both methods still suffer from distortion in the read direction because of the finitely sampled frequency encoding process occurring in this direction.

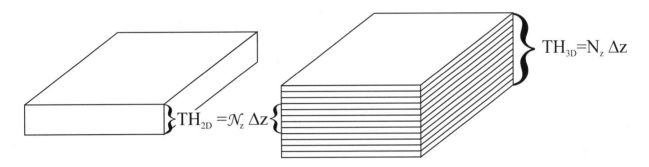

Fig. 20.16: A depiction of a subset of slices from a 3D data set used to construct a single 2D slice of effective thickness $\mathcal{N}_z\Delta z = TH_{2D}$. If (20.42) is used to create this 2D slice, the resulting image will have less signal loss due to echo shifting than using (20.41) or exciting a 2D slice of thickness TH_{2D}.

A Formalism for Collapsing Images

The filtering which helps overcome most of the signal loss due to phase dispersion, as described in the context of this section, can be formally described using operators. If M is the operation of taking the magnitude of the operand and C represents the averaging operation, the magnitude of a complex averaged image is represented by the combined operation MC,

$$MC\left[\hat{\rho}_{3D}(m\Delta x, n\Delta y, j\Delta z)\right] = \left|\frac{1}{\mathcal{N}_z} \sum_{j=-\mathcal{N}_z/2}^{\mathcal{N}_z/2-1} \hat{\rho}_{3D}(m\Delta x, n\Delta y, j\Delta z)\right| \qquad (20.41)$$

and an averaging of magnitude images can be represented by the operation CM.

$$CM\left[\hat{\rho}_{3D}(m\Delta x, n\Delta y, j\Delta z)\right] = \frac{1}{\mathcal{N}_z} \sum_{j=-\mathcal{N}_z/2}^{\mathcal{N}_z/2-1} |\hat{\rho}_{3D}(m\Delta x, n\Delta y, j\Delta z)| \qquad (20.42)$$

Operator order is important, and the two images (MC- and CM-operated) are different in areas experiencing field inhomogeneities. Hence, the difference operator ($MC-CM$), a 'commutator' operation, delineates regions suffering from field inhomogeneities, as in Fig. 20.15d. In this particular case, a spatial collapsing was done in the through-plane direction, and the commutator image depicts those regions which experience through-plane background gradients.

Visualizing Background Gradients by Fourier Transformation of 3D Data Sets

A set of 2D images with several slice select refocusing gradients (Fig. 20.13) can be reconstructed from a complete set of 3D images (see Fig. 20.16). The basic assumptions here are that both magnitude and phase (i.e., complex) 3D images $\hat{\rho}(x,y,z)$ are already collected and the signal loss in each 3D slice has been neglected. In essence, the 3D data set is treated as the 'perfect model' because of its truly high spatial resolution. In the simple case when the background gradients do not exist and the slice select refocusing gradient intended to be used in acquiring 2D images is not varied, each 2D slice with a thickness TH_{2D} will be the complex sum of $\mathcal{N}_z$ slices of the 3D images, with the slice thickness Δz and the relation $TH_{2D} = \mathcal{N}_z \Delta z$.

Since the background gradients usually exist in images, instead of varying the slice select refocusing gradient in the 2D method, the combination of the slice select refocusing gradient and the partition encoding gradients in the 3D method can be used to compensate the background fields such that the lost signal due to the background fields can be recovered and the tissue structure affected by the background fields can be seen. The partition encoding gradients control the phase values in k-space. As a result, such a process is similar to the 1D Fourier transformation (or weighting) of 3D images in the slice select direction.

In order to formulate the above complicated descriptions, consider a 3D slab with thickness TH_{3D} and N_z slices such that

$$TH_{3D} = N_z \Delta z \qquad (20.43)$$

and $N_z \geq \mathcal{N}_z$. The reconstructed (or desired) 2D data in the z-direction are

$$\hat{\rho}_{2D,TH_{2D}}(x,y,z_0,m)$$
$$= \frac{1}{TH_{2D}} \int_{z_0-TH_{2D}/2}^{z_0+TH_{2D}/2} dz\, \hat{\rho}_{3D}(x,y,z) \cdot e^{-i2\pi \dot{\gamma}(m\Delta G_{rp}\tau_{rp})z}$$
$$= \frac{1}{TH_{2D}} \int_{-TH_{2D}/2}^{TH_{2D}/2} dz\, \hat{\rho}_{3D}(x,y,z+z_0) \cdot e^{-i2\pi \dot{\gamma}(m\Delta G_{rp}\tau_{rp})z - i2\pi \dot{\gamma}(m\Delta G_{rp}\tau_{rp})z_0}$$
$$\simeq \frac{\Delta z}{TH_{2D}} \sum_{n=-\mathcal{N}_z/2}^{\mathcal{N}_z/2-1} \hat{\rho}_{3D}(x,y,n\Delta z+z_0) \cdot e^{-i2\pi \dot{\gamma} mn\Delta G_{rp}\tau_{rp}\Delta z} \cdot e^{-i2\pi \dot{\gamma}(m\Delta G_{rp}\tau_{rp})z_0} \quad (20.44)$$

where z_0 is the center position of the desired 2D slice, $\Delta G_{rp}\tau_{rp}$ is the intended phase change in the slice select refocusing gradient of the 2D method, and m is an integer that controls the step of the phase change. With a given value m, a specific background gradient field in the desired 2D slice can be compensated. The quantity $\Delta G_{rp}\tau_{rp}$ can be defined as $2G_{z,max}\tau_z/\mathcal{N}_z$ with $G_{z,max}$ being the maximum partition encoding gradient value and τ_z being its associated duration used in the collection of the 3D data set. Note that here the denominator $\mathcal{N}_z$ can be replaced by any number not larger than N_z. Under these definitions and the Nyquist theorem, the reconstructed 2D images are

$$\hat{\rho}_{2D,TH_{2D}}(x,y,z_0,m) = \frac{1}{\mathcal{N}_z}\left[\sum_{n=-\mathcal{N}_z/2}^{\mathcal{N}_z/2-1} \hat{\rho}_{3D}(x,y,n\Delta z+z_0) \cdot e^{-i2\pi mn/\mathcal{N}_z}\right] e^{-i2\pi mz_0/TH_{2D}} \quad (20.45)$$

The set of images created with this process represents 2D images of thickness TH_{2D} collected using additional slice refocusing gradients of value $m\Delta G_{rp}$. In the mth image of a given 2D slice at z_0, the refocused local gradients are those which exactly cancel in phase with the phase generated by the mth refocusing gradient lobe, $m\Delta G_{rp}\tau_{rp}$. That is, the background gradient G_z' is refocused if there exists some integer m such that

$$m\Delta G_{rp}\tau_{rp} + G_z' T_E = 0 \tag{20.46}$$

or

$$
\begin{aligned}
G_z' &= -\frac{m\Delta G_{rp}\tau_{rp}}{T_E} \\
&= -\frac{m}{\gamma TH_{2D}T_E}
\end{aligned}
\tag{20.47}
$$

Only after transforming the 3D data back to a set of thicker 2D images can the operation discussed in the last subsection (Sec. 20.3.4) be accomplished. Fig. 20.17 shows the results of Fourier transformation of the eight partitions which cover the same spatial region as covered by the 2D image in Fig. 20.12b. The $m = 0$ image, which is nothing but the complex average of the 8 partitions and which is expected to be the same as the 2D slice, is very different in appearance from the 2D image. This is due to the fact that the eight partitions used here came from a much larger 64 partition data set covering 32 mm which allowed for the use of a much larger rf bandwidth than was possible with the 2D imaging method and a reduction of slice distortion. Such a concept of complex sum can be generalized to visualize background gradients acting over distances larger than the measured voxel size in any direction including the read and in-plane phase encoding directions.

Visualizing Background Gradients Using Phase Images

Gradient echo phase images can also be used to determine local gradients acting over a few voxels since these phase images themselves represent field maps in the high resolution case. Hence, gradients can be mapped by taking spatial derivatives of the phase images, i.e., G_x' can be determined from $\phi(x,y,z)$ by obtaining the spatial derivative map $\partial\phi(x,y,z)/\partial x$ and likewise for y and z. Prior to performing this operation the phase data will need to be unwrapped.

20.3.6 Phase Encoded 2D and 3D Imaging with Single-Point Sampling: A Limited Version of CSI

As seen in Secs. 20.1.1 and 20.1.2, distortion and nonorthogonality of the different imaged voxel dimensions occur because of the finite time it takes for frequency encoding in the read direction in conventional imaging methods. This effect can be overcome by phase encoding that dimension as well. This is very similar to the CSI method discussed in Ch. 10. To reconstruct an image without any distortion effect then requires the sampling of only one time-point. Let us revisit the reason why no distortion occurs in this case. Going back to the background gradient inhomogeneity case considered in Sec. 20.1.1, a scaling of the

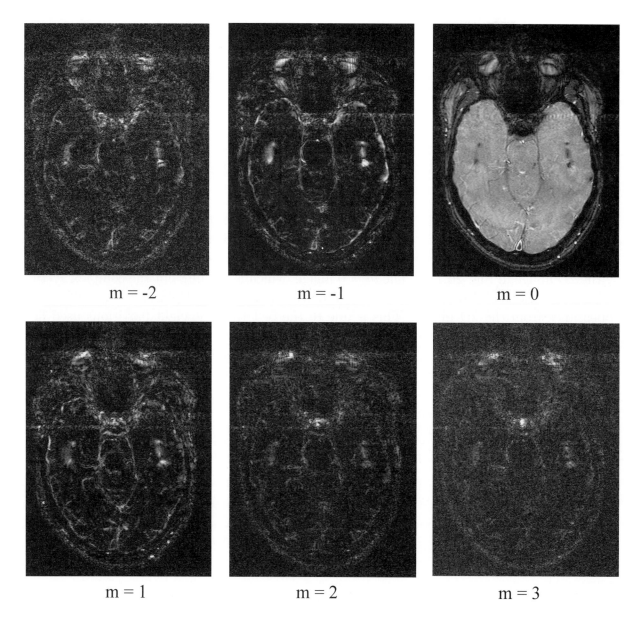

m = -2   m = -1   m = 0

m = 1   m = 2   m = 3

Fig. 20.17: Fourier transformation of the same 16 partitions using the complex image data from each 3D partition gives images which are conceptually the same as having done a 2D imaging experiment with 8 mm slice thickness with a large slice select gradient with the images acquired with different rephasing gradient values. Note that the local gradient value that is refocused at a given m is given by $-\dfrac{m}{\gamma T H_{2D} T_E}$. The appearance of the pituitary gland in the $m = +3$ image implies that a local gradient of about 0.2 mT/m must be present.

k-space variable was what led to distortion. Relative to the single time-point sample that is measured in the present method, only a phase dispersion independent of k-space sample number occurs. No scaling of the k-space variable occurs, hence, no distortion. The result of getting a final undistorted image is that all spatial information is mapped correctly.

The phase encoded 2D imaging method still suffers from signal loss due to the poor spatial resolution achievable in the slice select direction. This effect is overcome only by phase encoding the slice select direction as well, i.e., performing 3D single point phase encoding imaging.

20.3.7   Spectrally Resolved 2D and 3D Imaging

The approach taken toward creating a gradient echo imaging method insensitive to field inhomogeneities has been to increase the spatial resolution and reduce distortion. The underlying assumption has been that there is only a single chemical species within the voxel. If there were different chemical species within the voxel, which have different chemical shifts, this can lead to some integrated signal loss as well. The best approach to take is to spectrally resolve these components and then add them up in magnitude. This is achieved by extending the single-point scheme to become a CSI method by sampling multiple time points after all the spatial encoding is over. As discussed in the last few sections, the CSI phase encoding tables lead to distortion-free images. The reciprocal of the sampling interval, $1/\Delta t$, defines the total spectral bandwidth available (and, hence, the analog low pass filter cutoff frequency, i.e., BW_{read}) and, similarly, $1/T_s$ defines the spectral resolution.

There is an interesting question here related to sampling the FID after phase encoding, if there are no field inhomogeneities present. It should be possible to sample the data infinitely quickly and averaging all of the data or all of the images (ignoring T_2^* effects) will create an image with infinite SNR. This does not work, of course, because the data must be filtered to reduce noise. For example, for a $BW_{read} = 1\,\text{kHz}$, the smallest sampling possible without correlation of noise is $1\,\text{ms}$. That is, an image created by using a point sampled $0.5\,\text{ms}$ after the first would not be significantly different than the original image. After $1\,\text{ms}$, however, the noise will no longer be correlated and averaging will improve SNR. If field inhomogeneities are present leading to a spectral BW of $1\,\text{kHz}$, then this should be the filter BW of choice. Sampling can take place at the rate of $1/BW$ and continue as long as desired to enhance the spectral resolution.

20.3.8   Understanding the Recovered Signal with Spectral Collapsing

This subsection serves as a summarizing point for the discussion carried out in this section. The spin density function as a function of position, $\rho(x)$, which actually equals $\int df\, \rho(x, f)$, is shown in Fig. 20.18a. The only difference is that the impulse functions are now replaced by boxcar functions. In Fig. 20.18b, the spin density is shown as a function of frequency, $\rho(f)$. The complete picture is contained only in a plot of spin density as a function of both position and frequency, $\rho(x, f)$. This is shown in Fig. 20.18c. Accordingly, the three species are distributed in this 2D space-frequency plot in such a way that although they occupy the same position, they have different frequency components. In addition, these components also pick up an extra T_E-dependent phase in a gradient echo experiment.

Consider the first two simple cases shown in Fig. 20.18a and Fig. 20.18b, where there is no spectral resolution or spatial resolution, respectively. In the first case, the voxel signal is reduced from 2 units to $(1 + 0.5e^{i\phi_1} + 0.5e^{i\phi_2})$ which, on taking the magnitude, yields $\sqrt{(1 + 0.5\cos\phi_1 + 0.5\cos\phi_2)^2 + (0.5\sin\phi_1 + 0.5\sin\phi_2)^2}$ which is less than or equal to 2. In Fig. 20.18b, there is no knowledge of where they came from spatially; however, they are correctly represented spectrally. If the spatial dimension x in Fig. 20.18a is frequency encoded rather than being phase encoded, the frequency axis in Fig. 20.18b can be replaced by x, modulo a constant. Fig. 20.18b, in combination with Fig. 20.18a, shows that different chemical species are spatially incorrectly mapped along frequency encoding directions, while this does not occur along phase encoding directions. Spectrally resolved imaging resolves $\rho(x, f)$ in both dimensions and can overcome both a loss of integrated signal due to spectral phase dispersion as well as spatially map the species correctly.

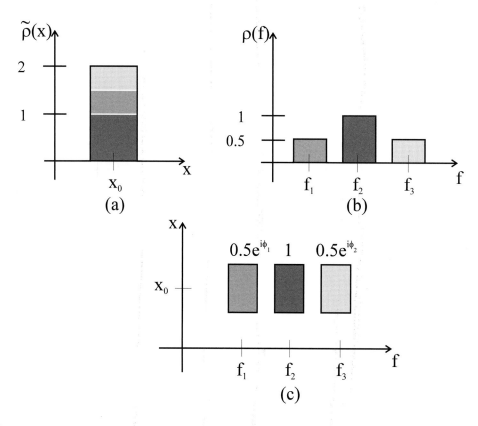

Fig. 20.18: An object consisting of three 1D boxes each of which resonates at a slightly different frequency represented as (a) a function of position, x, (b) frequency, f, and (c) in the f-x plane. As represented, there exists an object centered at the position x_0 containing three substances each of different resonant frequency (f_1, f_2, and f_3). These three frequency components pick up a T_E-dependent phase of ϕ_1, 0, and ϕ_2, respectively.

20.4 Empirical T_2^*

Macroscopic sources of magnetic field disturbance have been the only ones of concern so far in this chapter. There are, of course, other smaller or microscopic sources of disturbance. The taxonomy of sources as microscopic or macroscopic is dependent on the distances of effectiveness of their field disturbances versus the spatial resolution in the image. Sources which are capable of acting over typical voxel dimensions are classified as macroscopic. Their effect is to create some kind of deterministic field distribution and, hence, phase dispersion across the voxel in a gradient echo experiment. Typically, on the other hand, essentially a multitude of microscopic sources are present, their geometries are usually random, and they are also spatially randomly distributed. Some biologically interesting microscopic sources are the capillary network of blood vessels and trabeculae in bone, for example. These intricate, randomly distributed geometries create a complex distribution of field variations within the voxel. As we see later in this section, the shape of the signal envelope around a spin echo is determined by the Fourier transform of this field distribution.

20.4.1 Arbitrariness of T_2^* Modeling of Gradient Echo Signal Envelopes

It is common to write the phenomenological transverse relaxation rate as a sum of the intrinsic rate R_2 and the external decay rate due to the field contribution R_2' (Ch. 4), i.e.,

$$R_2^* = R_2 + R_2' \qquad (20.48)$$

or, in terms of relaxation times,

$$\frac{1}{T_2^*} = \frac{1}{T_2} + \frac{1}{T_2'} \qquad (20.49)$$

Equation (20.49) assumes that the transverse relaxation behaves exponentially. It is very common to write $1/T_2'$ as being given by $\gamma \Delta B$. As we see next, this is true only for a hypothetical case.

Consider a scenario that would lead to the additive term R_2' in R_2^*. Assume an object has a Lorentzian spin density

$$\rho(x) = N_0 \frac{2b}{b^2 + 4\pi^2 x^2}, \quad \text{with} \quad b = 2\pi \Delta x \qquad (20.50)$$

where $2\Delta x$ is the FWHM of the distribution and N_0 is the total number of spins. That is, the object has a spatially smeared spin density, with most of the spins being contained within a voxel of size Δx. If a background gradient G_x' exists over all space, then the signal (and the voxel signal in an approximate sense) is

$$\tilde{\rho}(T_E) = \int_{-\infty}^{\infty} dx\, \rho(x) e^{-i\gamma G_x' x T_E} \qquad (20.51)$$

The right-hand side in (20.51) is a well-known Fourier integral for the form of $\rho(x)$ given in (20.50). Estimating this Fourier integral gives

$$\tilde{\rho}(T_E) = N_0 e^{-T_E/T_2'} \quad \text{where} \quad T_2' = 1/(\gamma b |G_x'|) \qquad (20.52)$$

In terms of an average field inhomogeneity ΔB defined by the inhomogeneity across a voxel,

$$\Delta B \equiv G_x' \Delta x = b G_x'/2\pi \tag{20.53}$$

the expression for T_2' from (20.52) is $T_2' = 1/(\gamma |\Delta B|)$, which leads to

$$\frac{1}{T_2^*} = \frac{1}{T_2} + \gamma |\Delta B| \tag{20.54}$$

Note that this is valid only for a gradient echo experiment.

Analysis of more realistic models for field variations typically experienced by a system of spins are found to lead to exponential decays with relaxation rates which are determined by

$$\frac{1}{T_2^*} = \frac{1}{T_2} + \kappa \gamma |\Delta B| \tag{20.55}$$

where κ is not necessarily unity and ΔB is the field inhomogeneity across some distance characterizing the geometry and spatial distribution of the sources creating the field disturbance. Not all models lead to an exponential decay, some lead to a Gaussian or other form for the decay. The constant κ depends both on the field inhomogeneity across the characteristic distance and on the form of the spin density function.

Problem 20.10

a) For a given value of Δx and an object with $\rho(x) = \rho_0 \text{rect}\left(\frac{2x}{\Delta x}\right)$, find the first zero crossing of the signal as a function of T_E. This is an example of a homogeneous object experiencing a gradient inhomogeneity. This example shows how arbitrary an exponential decay shape is. The signal loss is characterized by the type of field inhomogeneity and analytical form of the spin density function.

b) The time found in (a) is a good first-order guess of T_2' for this situation. Is there a corresponding value for κ?

c) What is κ if the FWHM of the Lorentzian in (20.50) is Δx instead of $2\Delta x$?

20.4.2   The Spin Echo Signal Envelope and the Magnetic Field Density of States

It was briefly mentioned in the introduction to this section that the signal envelope in a spin echo experiment is determined by the Fourier transform of the field distribution within the object of interest. This relation is formally derived in this subsection.

Because of the linearity of the Fourier transform, the field inhomogeneity effect on each voxel can be studied independently. Each voxel can be thought of as contributing to the echo, this contribution being termed a 'voxel echo.' In a gradient echo experiment, each individual voxel can be thought of as having an echo which is shifted in time by an amount determined by the gradient inhomogeneity experienced by the spins within that voxel. In the case of a spin echo experiment, there is no voxel echo shifting; as a result, there is no phase dispersion across the voxel. The background gradient just leads to distortion (see Sec. 20.1.1).

Inasmuch as the phenomenology of treating the total measured k-space signal as being the sum of voxel echoes is allowed, a single voxel can be treated as being the entire imaged volume. This simply means that for the quantities described, spatial scale can be arbitrarily chosen, and analyzed using the usual reconstruction tools. The signal dependence obtained by frequency encoding the information across a voxel in a spin echo experiment is given by

$$s(t') = \int d^3r \, \rho(\vec{r}) e^{-i2\pi\gamma B(\vec{r})t'} \tag{20.56}$$

where $B(\vec{r})$ is the field imposed at different positions $\vec{r}$ within the voxel by the imaging gradient as well as the background gradients. As usual, t' is the time variable defined relative to the echo time.

The signal $s(t')$ in (20.56) can be thought of as the time-dependence of the 'voxel echo.' In as much as the spin density is a function of $\vec{r}$, and $B(\vec{r})$ is an invertible function of $\vec{r}$, the variable of integration $\vec{r}$ can be replaced with B, and $\rho(\vec{r})d^3r$ can be replaced with $\rho_0 V p(B) dB$ where $p(B)$ is found from the integrated volume over which a given value of B occurs divided by the total volume and normalized so that $\int dB \, p(B) = 1$.[4] Therefore, $\rho_0 V$ is used as a normalizing constant where V is the volume of the object being imaged. Hence, $s(t')$ can be written as

$$s(t') = \rho_0 V \int dB \, p(B) e^{-i2\pi\gamma Bt'} \tag{20.57}$$

where $p(B)$ is called the 'density of states.' The normalized signal envelope is clearly proportional to the Fourier transform of the density of states. A physically more realistic case to consider than that in the previous section, which also leads to an exponential decay, is to assume that $p(B)$ rather than $\rho(x)$ is Lorentzian (see Fig. 20.19). For example, let

$$p(B) = \frac{2b}{b^2 + 4\pi^2 B^2} \tag{20.58}$$

where the FWHM of the distribution is b/π and $s(t') = s(0)e^{-\gamma b|t'|}$. Again, a 'cusp-like' symmetric exponential decay is obtained centered around the spin echo as in the artificial case of a Lorentzian spatial form for the spin density.

20.4.3 Decaying Signal Envelopes and Integrated Signal Conservation

As seen in Secs. 20.4.1 and 20.4.2, both spin echo and gradient echo sequences have decaying k-space signal envelopes due to T_2^* signal loss during data sampling. Superficially, the main difference seems to be that, in the spin echo case, the envelope is symmetric about the origin of k-space while it is asymmetric in the gradient echo case. Yet, why is it that the integrated

---

[4]Note that $p(B)$ is a density function. A density function represents the number of events $p(B)\,dB$ occurring in a given interval $(B, B + dB)$.

signal is preserved only in the spin echo case as seen briefly in Sec. 20.1.3 (see (20.17)) and not in the gradient echo case? How can this seemingly paradoxical property of the symmetric k-space signal envelope which conserves integrated signal in one domain while there is signal loss in the other domain (independent of the spatial variation of field inhomogeneities) be reconciled?

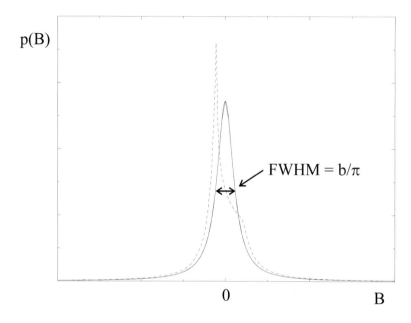

Fig. 20.19: Plot of $p(B)$ versus B for the Lorentzian field distribution. The dashed line represents $p(B)$ for the dipole pattern for a sphere (see Ch. 25 for details). In theory, the density of states can be measured from an FID experiment by evaluating the spectral response of the signal.

Conservation of Signal in the Presence of Chemical Species

As an illustrative example showing this property, consider a voxel containing three different chemical species, one at the resonant frequency and having unit spin density, and two others at $\pm\Delta\omega$ relative to ω_0 and having spin density of half each (see Fig. 20.20a). The measured spin echo signal envelope (neglecting imaging gradient effects which are taken care of by the Fourier inversion) is then given by

$$s(t') = 1 + \frac{1}{2}e^{-i\Delta\omega t'} + \frac{1}{2}e^{i\Delta\omega t'} = 1 + \cos\Delta\omega t' \quad \text{(spin echo case)} \qquad (20.59)$$

In a finitely sampled case with $T_s = \frac{\pi}{\Delta\omega}$, the signal envelope starts at the integrated signal level (of 2 units) and decays symmetrically to one at the edge of the sampling window (see Fig. 20.20b), a form of T_2' decay. Neglecting the smearing effect of the finite point spread function imposed by the finite sampling, the above envelope leads to an image upon inversion of

$$\tilde{\rho}(x) = \delta(x) + \frac{1}{2}\left(\delta\left(x - \frac{\Delta\omega}{\gamma G}\right) + \delta\left(x + \frac{\Delta\omega}{\gamma G}\right)\right) \qquad (20.60)$$

and despite the apparent suppression of signal the total integrated signal is conserved in the image domain (see Fig. 20.20c). The only effect is an incorrect spatially shifted mapping, a spatial misregistration of the chemical species, which is also a form of distortion.

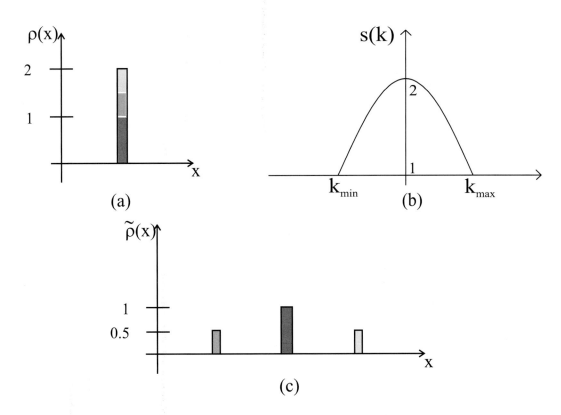

Fig. 20.20: An example frequency distribution illustrating signal loss in k-space but conservation of integrated signal in the image domain. (a) The spin density function $\rho(x)$ consists of three different chemical species distinguished by different levels of shading. (b) The k-space signal envelope obtained in the special case when $T_s = \frac{\pi}{\Delta\omega}$ shows a decaying envelope which passes through one at the two edges of the sampling window. This filter multiplies the data that would have been obtained if there had been no chemical shift. (c) The reconstructed image $\tilde{\rho}(x)$ still conserves the integrated signal. Note that the delta functions are represented here with boxcar functions.

In the case of a gradient echo experiment, the only difference is that t' is replaced by $(t' + T_E)$, as the dephasing of the three isochromats begins at $t = 0$ or $t' = -T_E$. Hence,

$$
\begin{aligned}
s(t') &= 1 + \frac{1}{2}e^{-i\Delta\omega(t'+T_E)} + \frac{1}{2}e^{i\Delta\omega(t'+T_E)} \\
&= 1 + \cos\Delta\omega(t' + T_E) \quad \text{(gradient echo case)} \\
&= 1 + \cos\Delta\omega t' \cos\Delta\omega T_E - \sin\Delta\omega t' \sin\Delta\omega T_E
\end{aligned}
\tag{20.61}
$$

and the reconstructed image is given by

$$
\begin{aligned}
\tilde{\rho}(x) = \delta(x) &+ \frac{1}{2}\cos\Delta\omega T_E \left(\delta\left(x - \frac{\Delta\omega}{\gamma G}\right) + \delta\left(x + \frac{\Delta\omega}{\gamma G}\right) \right) \\
&+ \frac{i}{2}\sin\Delta\omega T_E \left(\delta\left(x + \frac{\Delta\omega}{\gamma G}\right) - \delta\left(x - \frac{\Delta\omega}{\gamma G}\right) \right)
\end{aligned}
\tag{20.62}
$$

In this case, the integrated signal is conserved only when T_E is chosen to be

$$T_E = m\frac{2\pi}{\Delta\omega} \qquad (20.63)$$

where m is any positive integer. These kinds of field inhomogeneity effects caused by the presence of different chemically shielded species are considered in detail in Ch. 17.

Problem 20.11

Discuss why signal is conserved when $T_E = 2\pi m/\Delta\omega$. Extend this argument to the case of many chemical species.

Signal Conservation for Random Microscopic Sources

At the other end of the spectrum of field inhomogeneities are those created by a richness of microscopic sources within a voxel. For a Lorentzian density of states, the spread of fields leads to a symmetrical, exponentially decaying signal envelope of the form $e^{-R_2'|t'|}$. This type of signal decay was shown (in Ch. 13) to create a real (i.e., zero imaginary part) blur in the image domain (this blur can be thought of as a more generalized form of image distortion). Convolution of two real signals ($\rho(x)$ and the 'real' blur function in this case) again leads to a conservation of integrated signal.

What property is it that ensures this conservation of integrated signal in the image domain? The first and foremost property of the signal in the spin echo case to note is that all the envelopes that have been considered had complex conjugate symmetry. Multiplication in time (and equivalently in k-space) by an envelope which has complex conjugate symmetry leads to convolution in the image domain of the ideal image by a real blurring function. The definition of a blur function is that it takes each point in the ideal image and smears it across a finite width, and each point in the resultant image is obtained as the integral (or finite sum) of the smeared values from each point in the ideal image. When the blurring function is real, the smeared values from all points add up in phase as they do in the absence of the smearing effect. As a result, the integrated signal is preserved.

We next formalize these arguments mathematically. As described before, the ideal k-space signal envelope $s_{\text{ideal}}(k)$ (that which is determined by the imaging gradients alone) is multiplied by the Fourier transform of the density of states, say, $f(k)$.[5] The measured spin echo k-space signal is therefore

$$s_m(k) = s_{\text{ideal}}(k) \cdot f(k) \quad \text{(symmetric spin echo case)} \qquad (20.64)$$

where $f(k)$ is defined as

$$f(k) \equiv \int dB\, p(B)e^{-i\alpha Bk} \qquad (20.65)$$

---

[5]This is strictly valid only when the local field effects have the same effect at all pixel locations.

where α is the constant which relates time t' to k, i.e.,

$$\alpha = \frac{2\pi}{G_x} \tag{20.66}$$

from (20.57). There is a great advantage gained in writing out the effect of any field disturbance in this manner. Once the density of states is computed, its Fourier transform multiplies the ideal k-space function. That is, once the density of states is determined, all field inhomogeneity effects due to finite sampling can be predicted.

Since $p(B)$ is a probability density function, $f(k)$ must also satisfy the identity $f(0) = 1$. This means that

$$\int dx\, \hat{\rho}(x) \equiv s_m(0) = s_{\text{ideal}}(0) \equiv \int dx\, \rho(x) \tag{20.67}$$

which implies that the integrated signal is preserved independent of the shape of $p(B)$. Next, the reconstructed image is given by

$$\hat{\rho}(x) = \rho(x) * F(x) \tag{20.68}$$

where $F(x) \equiv \int dk\, f(k)e^{i2\pi kx}$ is the blurring function. Using $\alpha B = 2\pi x$, i.e., $B = \frac{2\pi x}{\alpha}$ in (20.65) gives

$$f(k) = \frac{2\pi}{\alpha} \int dx\, p\left(\frac{2\pi x}{\alpha}\right) e^{-i2\pi kx} \tag{20.69}$$

The blur function can now be written as

$$F(x) = \beta p(\beta x) \tag{20.70}$$

where β is defined by $\beta \equiv \frac{2\pi}{\alpha} = G_x$. Hence, $F(x) = G_x p(G_x x)$, i.e., $F(x)$ is also a normalized density function and, therefore, is real. For $\rho(x) = \delta(x)$, $\hat{\rho}(x) = F(x)$ and the total signal $\rho_T = \int dx\, \hat{\rho}(x) = 1$. Once again, the integrated signal is conserved.

20.4.4 Obtaining a Lorentzian Density of States: A Simple Argument

It is possible to understand how, for a specific system of particles with some random spatial and magnetic properties, an exponential decay can be predicted, i.e., a Lorentzian density of states can be achieved. Let us first examine a rather geometrically simple source of field variation such as due to a sphere embedded in a surrounding medium (tissue), with a susceptibility difference $\Delta\chi$ from the material in the sphere to the medium. The change in field dependence in the medium outside the sphere is then dipolar in nature (see (25.21)), i.e.,

$$\Delta B_{z,out}(\vec{r}) = \frac{\Delta\chi}{3} B_0 \left(\frac{R}{r}\right)^3 (3\cos^2\theta - 1) \tag{20.71}$$

where R is the radius of the sphere and θ is the solid angle made by the point of observation to $\hat{z}$. Note also that the field behavior is normalized to the value at $r = R$. The $p(B)$ created by this dipolar field is asymmetric, but not so dissimilar to a Lorentzian in shape (see Fig. 20.19). Upon averaging over magnetization and over dipole location as would be created by a random distribution of an infinite number of such spheres within the voxel, we expect to see some smoothing out (averaging) of this plot, leading to a Lorentzian-like $p(B)$ shape. We will see in Sec. 20.5 that, for long times relative to a characteristic time, the decay is truly exponential.

20.4.5 Predicting the Effects of Arbitrary Field Inhomogeneities on the Image

The important implication of Sec. 20.4.4 lies in the prediction of the effect of some arbitrary field inhomogeneity on an image acquired with a spin echo or gradient echo sequence. According to the earlier discussion, complete knowledge of the density of states produced by the given inhomogeneous field is sufficient for predicting all effects due to a spatially varying magnetic field. Also, from the previous discussion, the density of states is obtained by Fourier transforming the spin echo signal envelope. The spin echo signal envelope can be obtained on a pixel-by-pixel basis by measuring the signal at different time points about the echo time. This can be accomplished using a multi-echo experiment (see Fig. 20.21) to sample the voxel signal at different time points (the different echo times) before, at, and after the spin echo. A Fourier transformation of the complex data points on a voxel-by-voxel basis then maps the density of states within each voxel. If it happens to be Lorentzian, then the resulting set of images can be used to find T_2 and T_2' (see Sec. 20.5 and Ch. 22). Practically, the number of gradient echoes which can be acquired prior to the occurrence of the spin echo ($t = T_E$) is limited by the available gradient strength. For imaging the brain, where T_2 is roughly 100 ms, a T_E of 100 ms will still offer good SNR for a reasonable spatial resolution. With current gradient capabilities of at least 25 mT/m and 200 μs rise times, it is feasible to collect an echo every ms, allowing for at least 32 images before T_E. The number collected after T_E can be set to 32 or depend on T_2.

Problem 20.12

Given the above example with 64 total gradient echoes

a) What is the spectral resolution possible?

b) What is the spectral bandwidth after which aliasing will occur?

c) Why should sampling not continue too long after T_E?

d) How are these spectral results related to the density of states?

To reiterate, fitting such multi-echo data to an exponential assumes a Lorentzian density of states. As illustrated by the argument in the previous subsection, this situation is satisfied only in special circumstances. The presence of a single nearby macroscopic source, on the other hand, creates a highly asymmetric field distribution across a voxel. In this case, it is meaningless to fit the voxel signal to an exponential; rather, the signal behavior is determined by the combined density of states imposed by the internal (to the voxel) microscopic and external macroscopic sources acting at a distance. Again, mapping the density of states is

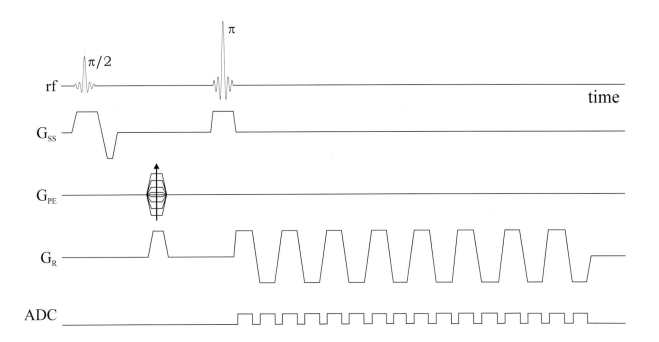

Fig. 20.21: An example 16 echo, multi-echo sequence for mapping the density of states on a voxel-by-voxel basis. A Fourier transform (i.e., spectral analysis) of each voxel's signal as a function of echo time yields the density of states within each voxel.

more informative rather than simply extracting a single number, the relaxation rate. It contains information about the local variety of chemical species, about nearby macroscopic field disturbances, about bulk field shifts, and about relaxation rates induced by local microscopic sources.

20.5 Predicting T_2^* for Random Susceptibility Producing Structures

There is significant interest in indirectly determining either the properties or volume of an infiltrate in an otherwise homogeneous tissue. In this section, the signal loss associated with a set of spheres (the infiltrate) embedded in the substrate (the homogeneous tissue) will be considered for a gradient echo sequence with a short sampling time. By collecting a set of multiple echo images and calculating T_2^*, it may be possible to extract the volume fraction and/or the magnetic moment of the spheres.

The presence of a sphere in the form of a small air bubble or ferrite microsphere in a tissue will affect the local magnetic field (see Ch. 25). From (20.71), the local change in magnetic field for a sphere located at the origin is given by

$$b(\vec{r}) \equiv \Delta B_{z,out}(\vec{r}) = \frac{\mu}{r^3}(3\cos^2\theta - 1) \qquad \text{for } r > R \qquad (20.72)$$

with

$$\mu = \frac{\Delta\chi}{3} B_0 R^3 = \frac{\Delta\chi}{4\pi} V_\mu B_0 \tag{20.73}$$

where $\Delta\chi$ is the magnetic susceptibility between the sphere and background, B_0 is the uniform background magnetic field, R is the radius of the particle, and V_μ is the volume of the sphere.

For a gradient echo experiment, the signal as a function of T_E for a uniform object of spin density ρ_0 and volume V_0 can be approximated by[6]

$$
\begin{aligned}
\tilde{\rho}(T_E) &\simeq \rho_0 \int_{V_0 - V_\mu} d^3r \, e^{-i\gamma b(\vec{r})T_E} \\
&= \rho_0 \int_{V_0 - V_\mu} d^3r \left((e^{-i\gamma b(\vec{r})T_E} - 1) + 1 \right) \\
&= \rho_0 (V_0 - V_\mu) - \rho_0 \int_{V_0 - V_\mu} d^3r \left(1 - e^{-i\gamma b(\vec{r})T_E} \right)
\end{aligned}
\tag{20.74}
$$

For a zero echo time or for $b(\vec{r}) = 0$, the signal reduces to $\rho_0 (V_0 - V_\mu)$. The volume-normalized signal, the voxel signal, is defined to be the usual effective spin density

$$
\begin{aligned}
\hat{\rho}(T_E) &= \frac{\tilde{\rho}(T_E)}{V_0} \\
&= \rho_0 \left(1 - \frac{V_\mu}{V_0} \right) - \frac{\rho_0}{V_0} \int_{V_0 - V_\mu} d^3r \left(1 - e^{-i\gamma b(\vec{r})T_E} \right)
\end{aligned}
\tag{20.75}
$$

The key here is to evaluate the dephasing effect represented by

$$
\begin{aligned}
I &= \int d^3r \left(1 - e^{-i\gamma b(\vec{r})T_E} \right) \\
&= \int_0^{2\pi} \int_0^\pi \int_R^\infty dr \, d\theta \, d\phi \, r^2 \sin\theta \left(1 - e^{-i\gamma\mu(3\cos^2\theta - 1)T_E/r^3} \right) \\
&= 2\pi \int_0^\pi \int_R^\infty dr \, d\theta \left(1 - e^{-i\gamma\mu(3\cos^2\theta - 1)T_E/r^3} \right) r^2 \sin\theta \\
&= \frac{4\pi}{3} \gamma\mu T_E \underbrace{\int_0^1 \int_0^{\omega_d T_E} \frac{dx}{x^2} dy \left(1 - e^{-ix(3y^2 - 1)} \right)}_{f(\omega_d T_E)}
\end{aligned}
\tag{20.76}
$$

where $\omega_d = \gamma\mu/R^3$, $x = \gamma\mu T_E/r^3$, and $y = \cos\theta$. Note that $f(\omega_d T_E)$ does not depend on either μ or R except through ω_d. With $I \equiv V_\mu \omega_d T_E f(\omega_d T_E)$ and $g(\omega_d T_E) \equiv \omega_d T_E f(\omega_d T_E)$, (20.75) becomes

$$\hat{\rho}(T_E) = \rho_0 \left(1 - \frac{V_\mu}{V_0} (1 + g(\omega_d T_E)) \right) \tag{20.77}$$

Imagine now that there is a set of N identical, non-interacting spheres so that each acts independently of the other on the phase and each produces a signal loss of $\frac{V_\mu}{V_0}(1 + g(\omega_d T_E))$.

---

[6]In fact, this formula is valid only when the sampling time is essentially zero (i.e., the read gradient is very large relative to any gradient caused by $b(\vec{r})$).

With $\eta \equiv \frac{NV_\mu}{V_0}$, the volume-normalized signal then becomes

$$
\begin{aligned}
\hat{\rho}(T_E) &= \rho_0(1 - \eta - \eta g(\omega_d T_E)) \\
&= \rho_0(1 - \eta(1 + g(\omega_d T_E)))
\end{aligned} \tag{20.78}
$$

Problem 20.13

---

   a) Discuss why (20.78) remains of the same form even if all spheres are of different sizes, have different values of susceptibility, or are located at random locations throughout the substrate. This result demonstrates that there can be a wide variety of values of susceptibility and locations of the infiltrate which will not affect the form of the signal decay.

   b) Show that $\hat{\rho}(T_E) = \rho_0(1 - \eta)e^{-\eta g(\omega_d T_E)}$ collapses to (20.78) when η and $\eta g(\omega_d T_E)$ are small. Empirically, the MR data appears to follow this exponential decay in the presence of an infiltrate.

A simple form for the function $g(\omega_d T_E)$ can be written when the argument $\omega_d T_E$ is either small or large

$$
g(\omega_d T_E) = \begin{cases} \frac{2}{5}(\omega_d T_E)^2 & \omega_d T_E \ll 1 \\ a_1 \omega_d (T_E - t_s) + i a_2 \omega_d T_E & \omega_d T_E \gg 1 \end{cases} \tag{20.79}
$$

where

$$
a_1 = \frac{2\pi}{3\sqrt{3}} \simeq 1.21 \tag{20.80}
$$

$$
a_2 = \frac{2}{3}\left(\frac{1}{\sqrt{3}} \ln \frac{(\sqrt{3}+1)}{(\sqrt{3}-1)} - 1\right) \simeq -0.16 \tag{20.81}
$$

and

$$
t_s = (a_1 \omega_d)^{-1} \tag{20.82}
$$

If the signal, in fact, decays as an exponential, then it suggests that the density of states is Lorentzian as discussed in Sec. 20.4.2. Empirically, the signal decay in the presence of such spheres is exponential. In that case, putting (20.78) in a more conventional form gives

$$
\hat{\rho}(T_E) = \rho_0(1 - \eta)e^{-R_2'(\eta, T_E)T_E} \tag{20.83}
$$

where

$$
R_2'(\eta, T_E) = \eta g(\omega_d T_E)/T_E \tag{20.84}
$$

and, using (20.73),

$$
\begin{aligned}
\omega_d &= \gamma\mu/R^3 \\
&= \frac{1}{3}\gamma\Delta\chi B_0
\end{aligned} \tag{20.85}
$$

When t_s is close to zero, R_2' loses its dependence on T_E and can be written as

$$
\begin{aligned}
R_2' &= \eta a_1 \omega_d \\
&= \frac{2\pi}{9\sqrt{3}} \eta \gamma \Delta\chi B_0
\end{aligned} \tag{20.86}
$$

The linear behavior of R_2' on both volume fraction and change in susceptibility are now evident. The following problem reveals how measuring either R_2' or, better yet, the shape of the signal decay can lead to information about either the product $\eta \Delta\chi$ or a separate extraction of η and $\Delta\chi$ depending on whether (20.84) or (20.86) is used.

Problem 20.14

a) Using a Taylor series expansion to second order in the integral for $g(\omega_d T_E)$, validate (20.79) when $\omega_d T_E \ll 1$. Hint: When $\omega_d T_E \gg 1$, take $\omega_d T_E$ to be infinity first to get (20.80) and (20.81), and then calculate (20.82) when $\omega_d T_E$ is a large number but not infinity. To calculate the imaginary part of $f(\omega_d T_E)$, integrate over x in (20.76) from a small positive number ϵ to infinity, change variables from x to $x(3y^2 - 1)$ (be careful about the sign of $3y^2 - 1$), use the asymptotic form of this integral as $-\ln(\epsilon|3y^2 - 1|)$, and then integrate over y. The terms containing ϵ will cancel.

b) Show graphically or numerically that an $\omega_d T_E$ value of 1.5 is a good crossover point between $\omega_d T_E \ll 1$ and $\omega_d T_E \gg 1$.

c) Does the term $ia_2\omega_d T_E$ make sense for the expected phase term in the presence of a field inhomogeneity?

d) Show for a spin echo sequence that T_E is replaced by $|t'|$ in (20.79) where $t' \equiv t - T_E$ is the time at which the image is collected about the echo time.

Problem 20.15

Until recently, the switch from quadratic to linear dependence of $g(\omega_d T_E)$ has not been observed. Usually, $R_2^* = R_2 + R_2'$ has no time dependence (although it can have a dependence on η). This can be understood by examining the sampling rate, how R_2^* is usually calculated, and when t_s is small. For ferrite microspheres, $\Delta\chi$ can be as large as 10^4 or 10^5 ppm, while, for changes in blood oxygenation levels, it can be as small as 0.1 ppm. Ironically, the larger changes lead to a very small t_s so that the signal decay looks like a conventional exponential decay. On the other hand, the smaller changes have long t_s values, on the order of milliseconds, and should be observable with conventional MR imaging techniques in use today.

a) Find ω_d and t_s when $\Delta\chi = 10^5$ ppm, $\Delta\chi = 0.1$ ppm, and $\eta = 0.1$, with $B_0 = 1.5$ T.

b) Plot (20.83) for $\Delta \chi = 3.77$ ppm against T_E (this value represents local field changes in the bone marrow).

c) What can be discovered from the fit to (20.83) as a function of T_E? Can both η and $\Delta \chi$ be extracted from this information?

20.6 Correcting Geometric Distortion

As seen in earlier sections, the presence of local magnetic field inhomogeneities leads not only to signal loss but also geometric distortion. It is instructive to examine this problem in more detail for a 1D imaging experiment using an FID readout. Assume that the rf pulse is instantaneous. In the presence of a general inhomogeneity, $\Delta B(x)$, the NMR signal is

$$s(t') = \int dx \, \rho(x) e^{-i\gamma G_x \left(x + \frac{\Delta B(x)}{G_x}\right) t'} \tag{20.87}$$

Here the time origin is centered at the echo. This integral can be simplified back into a more conventional Fourier transform. To see this, let

$$x' \equiv x + \frac{\Delta B(x)}{G_x} \tag{20.88}$$

and

$$G_x'(x) = \frac{d}{dx} \Delta B(x) \tag{20.89}$$

Here, x' represents the spatial variable in the distorted image created by $\Delta B(x)$. The distortion is viewed here as a one-to-one mapping, taking point x in the object domain to point x' in the distorted image domain. Using the definitions of (20.88) and (20.89)

$$dx = \frac{dx'}{1 + \frac{G_x'(x)}{G_x}} = \lambda(x) dx' \tag{20.90}$$

where $\lambda(x)$ is now the spatially dependent dilation factor of the elemental distance dx in the object domain given, as before, by

$$\lambda(x) = \frac{G_x}{G_x + G_x'(x)} \tag{20.91}$$

As promised, the expression for $s(t')$ in (20.87) can be rewritten in distorted image coordinates as the Fourier transform over a modified spin density function $\rho'(x')$ via

$$s(t') = \int dx' \, \rho'(x') e^{-i\gamma G_x x' t'} \tag{20.92}$$

where

$$\rho'(x') \equiv \rho \left(x' - \frac{\Delta B(x(x'))}{G_x}\right) \cdot \lambda \left(x' - \frac{\Delta B(x(x'))}{G_x}\right) \tag{20.93}$$

is now the reconstructed image. Implicit to the existence of a relation as in (20.93) is the requirement that the mapping from x to x' be both analytic and invertible. The conclusive message is that the presence of a general field inhomogeneity causes the spatial information to be mapped incorrectly (as seen from the first term which shifts the object in the reconstructed image) while also affecting the signal amplitude (through the second term) leading to geometric and signal distortion. Other than these two pointers, there is very little intuition that can be generally obtained about the effects of an inhomogeneous field from (20.93). However, the situation is both simplified and instructive when $G_x'(x)$ is a constant gradient. Such a case is the subject of the forthcoming problem.

If $\Delta B(x)$ is known, then x' can be found, as can $\lambda(x')$ and the shifted distance in (20.93). Geometric distortion correction can then be made. Analytically, the corrected image is found from the expression

$$\rho\left(x' - \frac{\Delta B(x(x'))}{G_x}\right) = \frac{\rho'(x')}{\lambda\left(x' - \frac{\Delta B(x(x'))}{G_x}\right)} \tag{20.94}$$

For a background field gradient inhomogeneity G_x' independent of x with λ defined as in (20.91),

$$\Delta B(x(x')) = (1 - \lambda)G_x x'/\lambda^2 \tag{20.95}$$

the corrected image, $\rho(\lambda x')$, is given by

$$\rho(\lambda x') = \frac{\rho'(x')}{\lambda} \tag{20.96}$$

Problem 20.16

Since $\rho'(x')$ is known on a pixel-by-pixel basis, how would you go about finding the corrected image $\rho(x)$ on the same grid points as $\rho'(x')$ is known for the case where $\Delta B(x) = G_x' x$? Hint: Consider interpolation of the pixels of $\rho'(x')$ back onto $\rho(x)$. For example, a gradient G_x' of the same sign as that of the read gradient G_x will cause a stretching of the object and a reduction of voxel signal. The stretched image is sampled at a $\Delta x' = \lambda \Delta x$. In principle, if $\lambda(x')$ is constant across $\Delta x'$, then (20.96) is valid to place the signal from $\Delta x'$ into a voxel of size Δx of increased voxel signal $1/\lambda$, although regridding still occurs at the voxel size $\Delta x'$.

Suggested Reading

The effects of background gradients in gradient echo imaging are reviewed in:

- J. R. Reichenbach, R. Venkatesan, D. A. Yablonskiy, M. R. Thompson, S. Lai and E. M. Haacke. Theory and application of static field inhomogeneity effects in gradient-echo imaging. *J. Magn. Reson. Imag.*, 7: 266, 1997.

A theory of NMR signal behavior in the presence of arbitrary static magnetic field disturbance source geometries is presented in this article:

- D. A. Yablonskiy and E. M. Haacke. Theory of NMR signal behavior in magnetically inhomogeneous tissues: the static dephasing regime. *Magn. Reson. Med.*, 32: 749, 1994.

An algorithm for overcoming geometric distortion in spin echo imaging is discussed in:

- H. Chang and J. M. Fitzpatrick. A technique for accurate magnetic resonance imaging in the presence of field inhomogeneities. *IEEE Trans. Med. Imag.*, 11: 319, 1992.

- K. Sekihara, M. Kuroda and H. Kohno. Image restoration from nonuniform magnetic field influence for direct Fourier NMR imaging. *Phys. Med. Biol.*, 29: 15, 1984.

Chapter 21

Random Walks, Relaxation, and Diffusion

Chapter Contents

Summary: Brownian motion models are analyzed for the phase effects due to both the fluctuations in the local field experienced by a spin and in the spatial position of the spin (diffusion effects). Mechanisms for the suppression of diffusion phase accumulation are discussed for both gradient echo and spin echo sequences. The additional term required for diffusion in the Bloch equation is presented, along with a treatment of diffusion sensitive gradients. Results for diffusion weighted images are shown.

Introduction

In the first section of this chapter, we develop a random-walk model in the presence of local field inhomogeneities for the intrinsic spin-spin decay with which the familiar exponential decay expression can be derived. A model for the additional dephasing brought about by the diffusive motion of, for example, protons in water is presented in the second section. This again leads to exponential decay but now with different time dependence in the argument of the exponent. This time dependence reflects important signal loss, for longer times, due to proton motion through larger and larger external field variations. A well-known procedure for recovering the signal in this case, and an improvement to this method, are described in the next two sections.

Diffusion is revisited in the framework of the Bloch differential equation in the fifth section, and velocity compensated gradients are also discussed therein. *In vivo* examples of diffusion weighting in the brain and the potential contrast available are described in the final section.

21.1   Simple Model for Intrinsic T_2

A simple molecular model is considered in which the basic exponential-decay time dependence e^{-t/T_2} for spin-spin relaxation can be derived. Additional spin evolution properties and effects can be understood, subsequently, from the same kind of modeling. Only a classical discussion is necessary, but the quantum framework laid out in Ch. 5 is entirely consistent with the model.

The intrinsic T_2 relaxation arises from the rapid, random fluctuations in the local magnetic field vector experienced by spinning nuclei making up the magnetization of interest. These lead to a dephasing of the signal from an isochromat of spins. The variations are due to both the Brownian motion of the neighboring atoms and molecules, and the spin itself. Electric quadrupole moments are neglected, and the picture is essentially the interaction between a given magnetic moment and the surrounding magnetic moments.

Consider the ith moment in a magnetization population that has been tipped by an rf pulse onto the y' axis. Since the random variations in the local fields are so much more rapid than the Larmor precession frequency, we can develop the model in either the rotating or laboratory reference frames. The torque on the moment fluctuates quickly and persistently, and the tip of the moment proceeds to walk randomly over a sphere with a radius defined by its constant magnitude $|\vec{\mu}_i|$, as shown in Fig. 21.1. An ensemble of such vector moments dephases by this meandering over the sphere. The statistical evaluation of this and similar random phenomena is discussed next to demonstrate the ubiquitous presence of exponential decay in these situations. Our goal in each case will be to find the decay constant in terms of the relevant microscopic variables.

21.1.1   Gaussian Behavior for Random Spin Systems

The central limit theorem in statistical analysis can now be applied to the accumulated phase distribution. Suppose that each of, say, N steps, in the accumulation of the phase ϕ_i for the ith moment, is independent and random over all the nuclei, though dictated by the same probability distribution. From the central limit theorem, the phase is normally distributed around its average value. Since the average value of each step is zero over all nuclei, the probability of finding spins with total phase ϕ is the centered Gaussian

$$P(\phi) = \frac{e^{-\phi^2/(2<\phi_i^2>)}}{\sqrt{2\pi <\phi_i^2>}} \qquad (21.1)$$

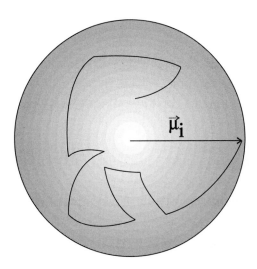

Fig. 21.1: The random walk of a magnetic moment over the surface of a constant magnitude sphere. The steps can arise from fluctuation both in the local fields and in the spatial position of the spin (diffusion).

Hence, the average over the nuclear ensemble of the complex magnetization (4.29) is

$$M_+ = \frac{M_0}{\sqrt{2\pi <\phi_i^2>}} \int_{-\infty}^{\infty} d\phi\, e^{i\phi} e^{-\phi^2/(2<\phi_i^2>)} \qquad (21.2)$$

The integration can be carried out by completing the square in the exponent and noting that, by construction, the normalization is chosen in (21.1) such that the integral over $P(\phi)$ is unity. The result is

$$M_+ = M_0 e^{-<\phi_i^2>/2} \qquad (21.3)$$

It is important to observe that a random average of the purely imaginary phase factor $e^{i\phi}$ has led to a real exponential form with negative exponent.

21.1.2 Brownian Motion and T_2 Signal Loss

For convenience, the imaging sample can be considered homogeneous. Each spin is assumed to change orientation on the average once every τ_2 seconds. If a given spin i sees a local field $\vec{B}_i$, its precession frequency around the z-axis is $\gamma B_{i,z}$ and, after N time steps over different local fields, its accumulated phase is

$$\phi_i(N\tau_2) = -\sum_{j=1}^{N} \gamma B_{i,z,j}\tau_2 \qquad (21.4)$$

The intrinsic field component at the jth position has been denoted by $B_{i,z,j}$. Its average value for the ensemble, or isochromat (Ch. 4), of nuclei that experience the same external field, is zero, i.e., $<B_{i,z,j}>= 0$. Thus $<\phi_i>= 0$, and the cross terms vanish in the average over ϕ_i^2 yielding

$$< \phi_i^2(N\tau_2) > = \gamma^2 \tau_2^2 \sum_{j=1}^{N} < B_{i,z,j}^2 > \qquad (21.5)$$

Since there is no preferred direction singled out by the microscopic fields, the averages over the squares of different components of the local magnetic fields should be the same and equal to one-third of the square of their magnitude. Therefore, with j suppressed,

$$< B_{i,x}^2 > = < B_{i,y}^2 > = < B_{i,z}^2 > = \frac{1}{3} < B^2 > \qquad (21.6)$$

in terms of a generic nuclear field magnitude B. Equations (21.5) and (21.6) lead to

$$< \phi_i^2 > = \frac{1}{3} \gamma^2 \tau_2^2 N < B^2 > \qquad (21.7)$$

Equation (21.7) and the total time $t = N\tau_2$ combine with (21.3) to give

$$M_+ = M_0 e^{-\gamma^2 \tau_2 < B^2 > t/6} \qquad (21.8)$$

This is the expected exponential decay for the spin-spin relaxation. A formula for the intrinsic decay time in terms of the average fluctuation period, the average local field (squared), and the nuclear gyromagnetic ratio follows from (21.8),

$$T_2 = \frac{6}{\gamma^2 \tau_2 < B^2 >} \qquad (21.9)$$

Problem 21.1

Consider a 1D random walk with the displacement after the ith step given by $x_i = \sum_{j=1}^{i} \epsilon_j \delta$ where δ is the step size and ϵ_j takes its values $\epsilon_j = \pm 1$ completely randomly.

a) Find the average values for $< x_i >$ and $< x_i^2 >$ after N steps.

b) Find the probability $P(x)$ for finding the random walker at the displacement x after N steps.

21.2   Simple Model for Diffusion

The spin echo method described in Ch. 8 is a procedure to recover the loss of signal due to inhomogeneities in the external static field B_z. While the T_2' effects are reduced in this way, there is another effect arising from the same inhomogeneities that can cause signal loss. 'Self-diffusion' of molecules through inhomogeneous external fields can rival and even dominate the intrinsic irreversible T_2 spin-spin relaxation time, especially in liquids and gases. While a $\pi/2$-π sequence can correct the dephasing due to the variations in the external field experienced by different molecules at different positions, the dephasing due to the change in position of a given molecule (because of diffusion) is a different story. In this section, the diffusion effect is modeled in a simple way. In the next section, a method for reducing this effect is detailed.

The spread in the Larmor magnetic field values B_z can be considered fairly narrow for the small molecular meandering leading to diffusion. The rotation of the magnetization into the transverse plane by a $\pi/2$-pulse is unchanged by such inhomogeneities, since their mean square deviation can be taken to be much less than the rf excitation, B_1. Diffusion may be analyzed in the rotating reference frame where the transverse magnetization precesses clockwise with frequency $\gamma(B_z - B_{0_z})$.

Brownian motion of the magnetic moment arises from the random transport of the proton from one region to another where the applied field has slightly changed. The picture in Fig. 21.1 is again pertinent, because the spin will undergo random-walk fluctuations in its position and, hence, in its phase, due to the rapid changes in the field it experiences. Assume one spatial dimension, for simplicity. A spin at a given position x is said to jump to a new position $x + \epsilon_i \delta$, as in the previous problem, every τ_d seconds. The step size δ is small and fixed, and ϵ_i takes on the values ± 1 randomly. The variations in the external field relevant to precession (call it $B_z \equiv B(x)$) can be approximated by a constant linear gradient in the x direction, $dB/dx \simeq G$. Therefore, the spin sees the new field $B(j\tau_d) = B(0) + G\delta \sum_{i=1}^{j} \epsilon_i$ after j steps.

The precession frequency thus changes step by step. Define the field change $\Delta B(j\tau_d) = B(j\tau_d) - B(0)$. After the first step, there is a change in phase given by $-\gamma \Delta B(\tau_d)\tau_d$. After the second step, the accumulated phase change is $-\gamma \Delta B(2\tau_d)\tau_d - \gamma \Delta B(\tau_d)\tau_d$. After N steps, the total phase change for a particular nucleus is

$$
\begin{aligned}
\phi &= -\sum_{j=1}^{N} \gamma \tau_d \Delta B(j\tau_d) \\
&= -G\delta \gamma \tau_d \sum_{j=1}^{N} \sum_{i=1}^{j} \epsilon_i \\
&= -G\delta \gamma \tau_d \sum_{p=1}^{N} p \epsilon_{N+1-p}
\end{aligned}
\tag{21.10}
$$

The last step is achieved by changing summation variables and constitutes the following problem.

Problem 21.2

Illustrate with a picture that the lattice of points described by $1 \leq i \leq j, 1 \leq j \leq N$ is equally well covered by $1 \leq i \leq N, i \leq j \leq N$. Thus show by a change of variable that the second line reduces to the third in (21.10).

The central limit theorem can be called upon again. The average over an isochromat of m nuclear spins leads to

$$< \phi_k >= 0 \tag{21.11}$$

where $1 \leq k \leq m$, inasmuch as the mean of ϵ_k vanishes for all k. The mean square phase calculation follows the derivation of (21.7), except that the resulting double summation reduces to a sum of p^2 terms (see Ch. 5). The leading term for the large-N limit of this sum is $N^3/3$ leading to

$$< \phi_k^2 >= \frac{1}{3}G^2\delta^2\gamma^2t^3/\tau_d \tag{21.12}$$

where the time is $t = N\tau_d$. Though slightly different than the intrinsic case, the distribution (21.1) still applies to this system of random walks, and the integration (21.3) carries over to produce

$$M_+(\text{diffusion}) = M_0e^{-\gamma^2G^2\delta^2t^3/(6\tau_d)} \tag{21.13}$$

The full decay from both local and diffusion effects is obtained by combining (21.13) and the spin-spin exponential. Noting that the standard diffusion constant D is related to the average step parameters in this model by $D = \delta^2/(2\tau_d)$, we have

$$M_+ = M_0e^{-t/T_2}e^{-\gamma^2G^2Dt^3/3} \tag{21.14}$$

It is observed that the diffusion exponential dominates the intrinsic decay in (21.14) for larger times. For shorter time intervals, there is less opportunity for significant phase evolution and the diffusion effect is significantly reduced. In practice, it is common to rewrite (21.14) in the form

$$M_+ = M_0e^{-t/T_2}e^{-bD} \tag{21.15}$$

where

$$b = \gamma^2G^2t^3/3 \tag{21.16}$$

This signal loss is over and above that caused by the usual spin dephasing across a voxel in the presence of a background or applied gradient. Throughout the text it has been noted that the application of gradients leads to dephasing between spins located at different spatial locations. The difference now is that, while gradient dephasing of the stationary spins can be refocused with a negative gradient lobe to form a gradient echo, the signal loss due to the diffusion of the spins during the application of the gradient cannot be recovered. This will be demonstrated in explicit detail in the next section.

21.3 Carr-Purcell Mechanism

A series of π-pulses can be inserted to suppress the diffusion effects (the Carr-Purcell method). The idea is to use spin flips to prevent the build-up of phase accumulation for a given spin random walk. The following discussion is relevant for any background or applied gradient that is present throughout the entire duration of the experiment.

The sequence involves the following rf pulses, all with respect to the same axis (say, x). Start with a $\pi/2$-pulse at time $t = 0$, and uniformly insert n π-pulses, one for every time step $\Delta t \equiv N\tau_d/n$, starting with $t_1 = \Delta t/2$ and ending with $t_n = N\tau_d - \Delta t/2$. (The echoes occur at multiples of $\Delta t = T_E$, $t = m T_E$, $m = 1, 2, \ldots n$.) Each π-pulse reverses, in turn, the sign of the previous phase accumulation. Within an overall sign, the total phase becomes

$$\phi = G \delta \gamma \tau_d \sum_{j=1}^{N} \epsilon'_j \sum_{i=1}^{j} \epsilon_i \tag{21.17}$$

with $\epsilon'_j = 1$ ($\epsilon'_j = -1$) for $0 < j \le N/(2n)$, $3N/(2n) < j \le 5N/(2n)$, $7N/(2n) < j \le 9N/(2n)$, etc. (for $N/(2n) < j \le 3N/(2n)$, $5N/(2n) < j \le 7N/(2n)$, $9N/(2n) < j \le 11N/(2n)$, etc.). This implies that there are two sets of independent sums arising in (21.17). It can be shown that the total phase can be written in terms of n sums of the form $\displaystyle\sum_{j=1}^{N/(2n)} j \alpha_j$

and n sums of the form $\displaystyle\sum_{j=1}^{(N/(2n))-1} j \beta_j$ where the two sets $\{\alpha_j\}$ and $\{\beta_j\}$ together belong to the set of $\{\epsilon_j\}$ variables. A demonstration that this is true is left for Prob. 21.3.

Problem 21.3

Show how n of each kind of sum, $\displaystyle\sum_{j=1}^{N/(2n)} j \alpha_j$ and $\displaystyle\sum_{j=1}^{(N/(2n))-1} j \beta_j$, arises in the double sum of (21.17). Hint: Consider the cancelation of adjacent elements in j of width $N/(2n)$ as ϵ'_j changes sign, then use Prob. 21.2.

The phase remains normally (Gaussian) distributed in view of the sum over the random variables, again with zero mean. The mean square variation is now proportional to the term $n \left(\displaystyle\sum_{j=1}^{N/(2n)} j^2 + \sum_{j=1}^{(N/(2n))-1} j^2 \right)$ which has the limit of $N^3/(12 n^2)$ for large N. For data sampled at $t = N \tau_d$,

$$< \phi_k^2 > = G^2 \gamma^2 D t^3 / (6 n^2) \tag{21.18}$$

Using (21.3), the transverse magnetization becomes

$$M_+ = M_0 e^{-t/T_2} e^{-\gamma^2 G^2 D t^3 / (12 n^2)} \tag{21.19}$$

It is evident in (21.19) that now the diffusion exponent is inversely proportional to $1/n^2$. The diffusion effect is suppressed as n is increased for fixed t. The decay of the signal would then be dominated by the linear exponent from the intrinsic spin-spin dephasing. (The above formulas, while they have been derived in simple 1D models, are more general.)

If the time T_E were to be fixed instead of the total time t, the modified diffusion exponent has a different n dependence. Consider first a simple spin echo experiment corresponding to $n = 1$ in (21.19). The effective b-value at the single echo ($t_1 = T_E$) is given by

$$b(1) = \gamma^2 G^2 T_E^3 / 12 \tag{21.20}$$

This is four times smaller than (21.16), which is essentially the gradient echo case, because the phase accumulation clock was modified at $T_E/2$. (Consider the value of (21.16) at the time $t/2$ and then double that value to arrive at (21.20).) For a multi-echo experiment, the time at the last echo is $t_n = nT_E$. The diffusion exponent b in (21.19) now becomes

$$b(n) = n\gamma^2 G^2 T_E^3/12 = nb(1) \tag{21.21}$$

Thus the entire exponent in the signal decay is linear in time t_n (or n, the total echo number)

$$M_+(n) = M_0 e^{-t_n/T_2} e^{-t_n/T_{2,diff}} = M_0 e^{-nT_E/T_{2,diff}^*} \tag{21.22}$$

where

$$T_{2,diff} = \frac{12}{\gamma^2 G^2 T_E^2 D} \tag{21.23}$$

and

$$\frac{1}{T_{2,diff}^*} = \frac{1}{T_2} + \frac{1}{T_{2,diff}} \tag{21.24}$$

The envelope in Fig. 21.2 exhibits the decay expected from (21.22). It traces the peaks of every echo in the Carr-Purcell series of π-pulses in that figure.

Problem 21.4

Diffusion effects are often ignored in practical MR imaging. Consider a conventional spin echo sequence with $T_E = 100\,\text{ms}$. Human brain tissue has a diffusion value of roughly $10^{-3}\,\text{mm}^2/\text{sec}$. Assume that a read gradient of $5\,\text{mT/m}$ is used and is kept on at all times except during the instantaneous rf pulses.

a) How much signal loss occurs over and above the usual T_2 decay?

b) If a second scan is run in the usual fashion (where a simple bipolar dephase/rephase read gradient is used) where diffusion effects can be neglected, how can D be found?

21.4   Meiboom-Gill Improvement

The large number of π-pulses used in the Carr-Purcell method gives rise to another kind of problem. A given 'π' pulse will deviate, at different spatial locations, from producing an exact 180° spin flip. This leads to a reduced transverse magnetization after each subsequent π-pulse. Consider the first flip shown in Fig. 21.3, for a 'π' pulse of less than 180°, for example. The spin is left slightly lifted off the transverse plane, and after the next flip, it is left lifted by twice the angle (2α), and so forth, leading to a reduced available transverse magnetization.

A solution to this problem has been proposed by Meiboom and Gill. The key is to use a different axis for the initial $\pi/2$ excitation. Specifically, choose the negative y' axis for this initial pulse, and the x' axis for all subsequent 'π' pulses. The demonstration that the spins are put back into the transverse plane is left as Prob. 21.5. This approach is referred to as the CPMG method.

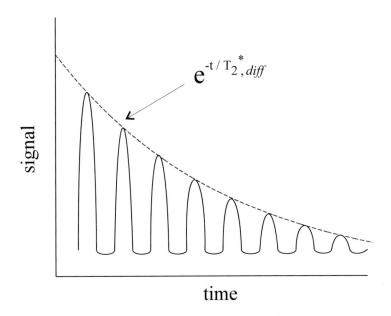

Fig. 21.2: The recovered signal for each echo after implementation of an 8-echo Carr-Purcell sequence. The envelope appears to have a conventional exponential decay (characterized by $T^*_{2,diff}$) despite the cubic dependence on T_E found in b.

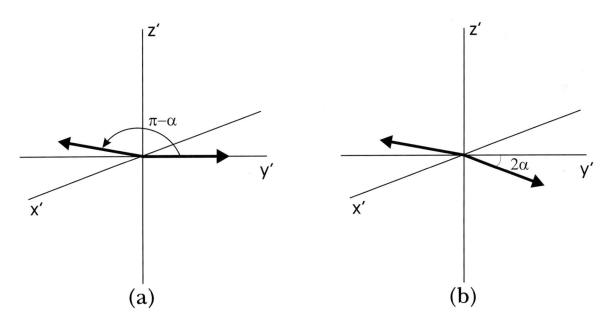

Fig. 21.3: (a) The result of a 'π' pulse giving less than a 180 degree flip. (b) The accumulated error after two such 'π' pulses.

Problem 21.5

Show that there is no longer a cumulative error for the series of 'π' pulses if the Meiboom-Gill procedure is followed.

21.5   The Bloch-Torrey Equation

The process of self-diffusion is associated with random Brownian motion of molecules in a material (such as a liquid) that has on average a uniform temperature and no bulk changes in concentration of its constituents. Referring to the Suggested Reading, we learn that conservation of mass leads (in the rotating frame) to an additional, diffusion term in the Bloch equation

$$\frac{\partial \vec{M}(\vec{r},t)}{\partial t} = \gamma \vec{M}(\vec{r},t) \times \vec{B} + D\nabla^2 \vec{M}(\vec{r},t) \tag{21.25}$$

Note that the relaxation terms have been neglected in (21.25). In order to solve this partial differential equation, set $\vec{B} \equiv \vec{G} \cdot \vec{r}\hat{z}$. The problem is again diagonalized (Ch. 4) by

$$M_+(\vec{r},t) = M_x(\vec{r},t) + iM_y(\vec{r},t) \tag{21.26}$$

such that

$$\frac{\partial M_+(\vec{r},t)}{\partial t} = -i\gamma(\vec{r} \cdot \vec{G})M_+(\vec{r},t) + D\nabla^2 M_+(\vec{r},t) \tag{21.27}$$

where $\vec{G}$ is independent of position. When $D = 0$, the solution is

$$M_+(\vec{r},t) = Ae^{-i\gamma\vec{r}\cdot\int_0^t \vec{G}(t')dt'} \tag{21.28}$$

with A constant. For $D \neq 0$, it is sufficient to consider $A \rightarrow A(t)$, (this is equivalent to a spatially invariant diffusion effect). The substitution of (21.28) into (21.27) yields

$$\frac{\partial A(t)}{\partial t} = e^{i\gamma\vec{r}\cdot\int_0^t \vec{G}(t')dt'} D\nabla^2 M_+(\vec{r},t) \tag{21.29}$$

or

$$\frac{\partial}{\partial t} \ln A(t) = De^{i\gamma\vec{r}\cdot\int_0^t \vec{G}(t')dt'}\nabla^2 \left[e^{-i\gamma\vec{r}\cdot\int_0^t \vec{G}(t')dt'}\right] \tag{21.30}$$

Therefore

$$\ln A(t) = -D\gamma^2 \int_0^t dt'' \left[\left(\int_0^{t''} \vec{G}(t')dt'\right) \cdot \left(\int_0^{t''} \vec{G}(t')dt'\right)\right] + \ln A(0) \tag{21.31}$$

The constant term $\ln A(0)$ is ignored from this point forward by assuming $A(0) = 1$. As before, this implies an additional exponential factor, but one that is a more complicated function of $\vec{G}(t)$.

21.5.1 The Gradient Echo Case for a Bipolar Pulse

As a first example of how the presence of gradients can affect the measured signal, consider the usual gradient echo sequence but with a bipolar pulse sandwiched between the rf excitation pulse and the read gradient.

For a simple bipolar pulse of duration $2\tau_b$ (i.e., of amplitude G for $0 \leq t < \tau_b$ and amplitude $-G$ for $\tau_b \leq t < 2\tau_b$),

$$\int_0^{t''} G(t')dt' = \begin{cases} Gt'' & \text{for } t'' < \tau_b \\ -G(t'' - 2\tau_b) & \text{for } \tau_b < t'' < 2\tau_b \end{cases} \tag{21.32}$$

For $t = 2\tau_b$, (21.31) becomes

$$\ln A_{bi}(2\tau_b) = -D\gamma^2 \int_0^{\tau_b} G^2 t''^2 dt'' - D\gamma^2 \int_{\tau_b}^{2\tau_b} G^2(t'' - 2\tau_b)^2 dt'' \tag{21.33}$$

The change to $u = 2\tau_b - t''$ for the second integration variable just leaves twice the first integral as the answer

$$\ln A_{bi}(2\tau_b) = -\frac{2}{3}D\gamma^2 G^2 \tau_b^3 \tag{21.34}$$

Therefore, over and above the usual T_2 decay, there is a signal loss from diffusion governed generally by the square of the gradient and the cube of a temporal parameter (here, τ_b).

Note that the reversed gradient causes the spins to reset their dephasing clock at the echo similar to the effect of the π-pulse in the spin echo case. The resulting signal loss is not the same as if the gradient had kept the same sign over the full time period of $2\tau_b$.

Applying the bipolar pulse along any of the x-, y-, or z-axes prior to the read gradient, the signal is proportional to

$$M_+(T_E) \propto e^{-\frac{2}{3}D\gamma^2 G^2 \tau_b^3 - T_E/T_2} \tag{21.35}$$

For a fixed echo time, varying the diffusion gradient amplitude from scan to scan can be used to extract D. Expression (21.35) is particularly useful in imaging, and an example of producing diffusion weighting in an image is presented in the next section.

21.5.2 The Spin Echo Case

We can rederive the Carr-Purcell result in the present framework. Assume the presence of a gradient G that is constant in time. When a single π-pulse is applied at a time τ, it will reset the phase clock at the echo so that

$$M_+(t > 2\tau) = A_1(t - 2\tau)A_1(2\tau)e^{-i\gamma z G(t-2\tau)-t/T_2} \tag{21.36}$$

where a simple calculation gives

$$\ln A_1(2\tau) = -\frac{2}{3}D\gamma^2 G^2 \tau^3 \tag{21.37}$$

For the multi-echo case, the signal loss at the nth echo $(t_n = nT_E = 2n\tau)$ is given by

$$
\begin{aligned}
A_n &= (A_1(2\tau))^n = e^{-\frac{2n}{3}D\gamma^2 G^2 \tau^3} \\
&= e^{-nD\gamma^2 G^2 T_E^3/12} = e^{-D\gamma^2 G^2 t_n^3/(12n^2)}
\end{aligned}
\tag{21.38}
$$

This is the same factor as in (21.19).

Problem 21.6

Use (21.31) to show that the conventional Stejskal-Tanner pulse sequence in Fig. 21.4 with a gradient pair yields

$$
\ln A_{ST} = -D\gamma^2 G^2 \delta^2 \left(\Delta - \frac{1}{3}\delta\right)
\tag{21.39}
$$

Neglect the strength of the intermediate, positive gradient lobe under the π-pulse. It is evident that (21.39) consistently reduces to (21.37) when $\Delta = \delta = \tau$.

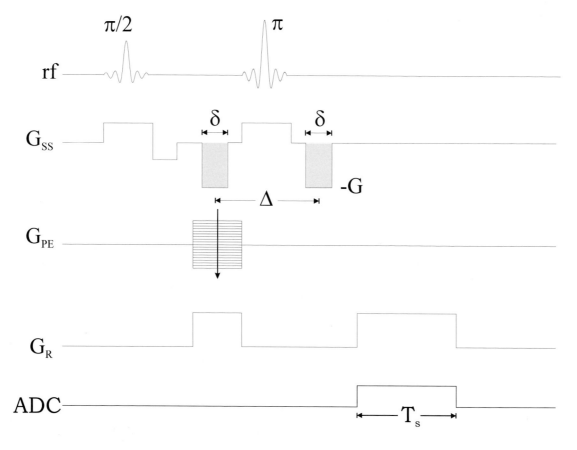

Fig. 21.4: A conventional 'Stejskal-Tanner' spin echo pulse sequence with slice select and diffusion sensitive gradients applied along one physical dimension (shown shaded).

21.5.3 Velocity Compensated Diffusion Weighted Sequences

The large phase spread generated by these bipolar pulses causes a problem when bulk motion and/or flow is present (see Ch. 23). To avoid such problems, a time-reversed pair of bipolar pulses can be used as shown in Fig. 21.5 (see also Ch. 23 for a detailed description of velocity compensation).

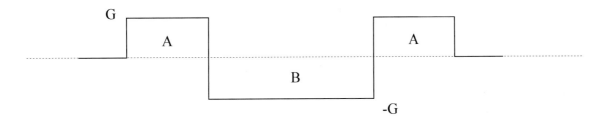

Fig. 21.5: A velocity compensated gradient waveform can be used as a diffusion weighting gradient. The area $B = 2A$.

Using (21.30), $\ln A(\tau)$ is seen to change by $-\frac{1}{3}D\gamma^2G^2\tau^3$ for each gradient of amplitude G and duration τ and by $-\frac{2}{3}D\gamma^2G^2\tau^3$ for the negative lobe of amplitude G and duration 2τ. The total diffusion argument for the waveform in Fig. 21.5 is then

$$\ln A(t)_{\text{velocity compensated}} = -\frac{4}{3}D\gamma^2G^2\tau^3 \qquad (21.40)$$

If the conventional bipolar lobe had been used so that the bipolar pulse were of the same duration (i.e., 4τ), then

$$\ln A(t)_{\text{bipolar}} = -\frac{16}{3}D\gamma^2G^2\tau^3 \qquad (21.41)$$

Problem 21.7

A rapidly oscillating multi-echo read gradient similar in design to that shown in Fig. 21.5 (with vanishing zeroth moment) builds up little diffusion-related signal loss compared to a bipolar gradient pulse of the same length.

a) Specifically, show that for $p \geq 3$ lobes ($p - 2$ are of duration 2τ)

$$\ln A(p\tau) = -\frac{2}{3}(p-1)\gamma^2G^2\tau^3 D \qquad (21.42)$$

b) Calculate $\ln A(p\tau)$ for $p = 31$, $G = 25\,\text{mT/m}$, $\tau = 1\,\text{ms}$, and $D = 10^{-3}\,\text{mm}^2/\text{sec}$.

c) Are the values of p, G, and τ reasonable for a conventional gradient echo sequence?

21.6   Some Practical Examples of Diffusion Imaging

As already described here, the contrast in MRI associated with diffusion of water in tissue comes from additional dephasing accumulated by randomly moving spins in the presence of an applied gradient. Therefore, the diffusion weighting in an MR image reflects random motion along the direction of the applied gradients. Contrast variations in the white matter, of a healthy human subject, seen when the direction of the applied diffusion weighted gradients is changed, are assumed to be related to variations in the free diffusion of water parallel and perpendicular to the myelinated sheaths in white matter. Water is assumed to diffuse more freely parallel to the tracts (bundles), and have its motion restricted perpendicular to the tracts. Therefore, white matter tracts running parallel to an applied diffusion gradient should have their signal suppressed, and tracts perpendicular to the applied gradient will be unaffected and appear brighter in the image. Other variations in diffusion weighted contrast are usually associated with disease. For example, in regions affected by stroke,[1] the diffusion of water is often decreased, and these regions appear bright on diffusion weighted images.

All of the images shown in this section were collected using a 192×256 matrix size SE-EPI sequence. A bipolar gradient pulse of total length 62 ms and amplitude of up to 40 mT/m was applied before the π-pulse to generate diffusion weighted contrast. The combination of overall signal suppression due to diffusion weighting and long echo times (120 ms to 140 ms) led to a low signal-to-noise ratio (SNR) in the individual acquisitions collected to obtain these images. As a result, to improve the SNR in the final images presented here, 80 individual magnitude images were averaged. Using a T_R of 2 s, it took 2 min 40 s to collect the images.

Problem 21.8

Cerebrospinal fluid (CSF) moves at a rate of up to 1 cm/s. How much will the CSF dephase for a b-value of

   a) $300\,\text{s/mm}^2$

   b) $1200\,\text{s/mm}^2$

   c) $2100\,\text{s/mm}^2$?

Hint: Find the v_{enc} value in terms of b and τ (see the discussion on flow quantification in Ch. 24 for a definition of v_{enc}) for each case.

The loss of signal due to motion leads to a much more rapid signal loss for CSF which, in turn, leads one to predict a higher value for D than is appropriate. For this reason, the measured *in vivo* D is referred to as an 'apparent diffusion coefficient' or ADC for short (beware of the possible confusion with the analog-to-digital-converter acronym).

In Figs. 21.6a–c, a series of $b = 1200\,\text{s/mm}^2$ images demonstrating the directional anisotropies in diffusion coefficients in the human brain are demonstrated. When different

---

[1]Stroke is caused by a lack of blood supply to the tissue. Cells have less access to oxygen, and if not quickly resupplied with blood, can stop functioning and die.

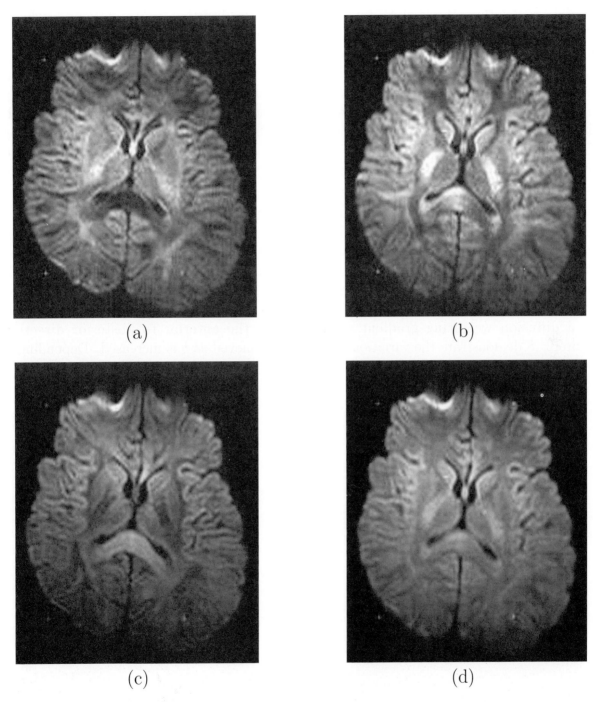

Fig. 21.6: A set of images collected with the diffusion weighting gradient pulses placed along different directions, and a trace image showing isotropic diffusion weighting. (a) $\vec{G}_{diff}$ along the horizontal direction, (b) $\vec{G}_{diff}$ along the vertical direction, (c) $\vec{G}_{diff}$ along the slice select direction (through-plane), and (d) averaged image which provides more isotropic diffusion weighting. Many anatomical structures can be seen in (a), (b), and (c).

gradients are applied along the direction where diffusion effects are significant, the tissue will appear dark because the signal has been suppressed. In Fig. 21.6a, white matter tracts running in the through-plane or anterior to posterior direction appear bright, as do the white matter tracts running in the through-plane or left to right direction in Fig. 21.6b. In Fig. 21.6c, where the gradient is applied along the slice select direction in the brain, white matter tracts in the plane of the image appear bright in the image, and tracts traveling along the slice select direction are dark. In a similar fashion, numerous other structures visible in Figs. 21.6a–c can be seen to change their intensities significantly as a function of the direction of the applied diffusion weighting. From this, one can deduce important directions of diffusion in these structures. Figure 21.6d is an image representing a summation of the images in Figs. 21.6a–c. This image gives an example of isotropic diffusion weighting with respect to spatial direction of the diffusion.

Figure 21.7a is a $b = 0$ image, or conventional T_2-weighted image of the brain, which can be used as a baseline image, against which to make calculations of the ADC (referring to the apparent diffusion coefficient, as noted in the above problem) observed by the MRI scan. An ADC map is calculated by normalizing all images with $b > 0$ with the $b = 0$ image and taking the logarithm of each image pixel value. The ADC value is found by fitting each new pixel series to $-bD$ and finding D. Figure 21.7b represents an ADC map obtained using Fig. 21.8a–d for a diffusion weighting gradient applied along the anterior to posterior direction. Figure 21.8 demonstrate the variation in contrast achieved as b is increased. Depending on

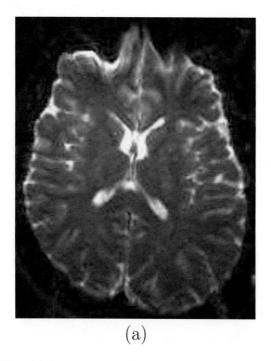
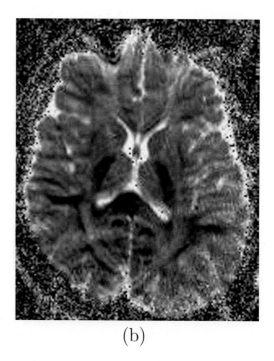

(a)   (b)

Fig. 21.7: Example images demonstrating changing contrast with increasing diffusion weighting, and an ADC map calculated from the diffusion weighted images. The diffusion weighting gradient pulse was applied along the vertical direction (anterior-posterior) in these images. (a) $b = 0$ and (b) ADC map.

the goal, b may be chosen to highlight regions of low diffusion without suppressing signal from other anatomy (as in Figs. 21.8a–b), or b may be increased (as in Figs. 21.8c and 21.8d) so that only large white matter tracts are visualized.

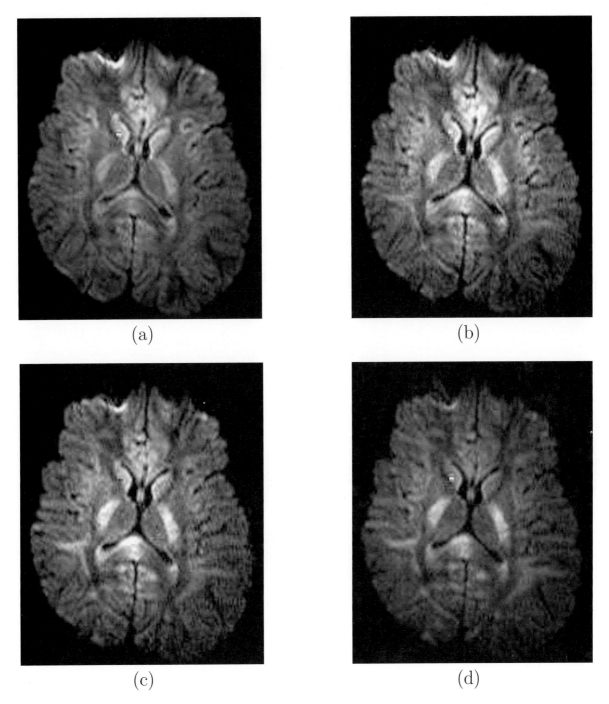

Fig. 21.8: Continuing from Fig. 21.7, more example images demonstrating changing contrast with increasing diffusion weighting. The diffusion weighting gradient pulse was applied along the vertical direction (anterior-posterior) in these images. (a) $b = 800\,\text{s/mm}^2$, (b) $b = 1200\,\text{s/mm}^2$, (c) $b = 1600\,\text{s/mm}^2$, and (d) $b = 2100\,\text{s/mm}^2$.

Suggested Reading

The pioneering paper in the application of MR for measuring diffusion is:

- E. O. Stejskal and J. E. Tanner. Spin diffusion measurements: Spin echoes in the presence of a time-dependent field gradient. *J. Chem. Phys.*, 42: 288, 1965.

An excellent overview of the technical aspects of diffusion in MR imaging is given in:

- P. T. Callaghan. *Principles of Nuclear Magnetic Resonance Microscopy.* Oxford Press, New York, 1991.

The basic mechanisms of how diffusion depends on inter-pulse spacing is introduced in:

- H. Y. Carr and E. M. Purcell. Effects of diffusion on free precession in nuclear magnetic resonance experiments. *Phys. Rev.*, 94: 630, 1954.

An important modification to the multiple π-pulse Carr-Purcell approach appears in:

- S. Meiboom and D. Gill. Modified spin echo method for measuring nuclear relaxation times. *Rev. Sci. Instrum.*, 29: 668, 1958.

Chapter 22

Spin Density, T_1, and T_2 Quantification Methods in MR Imaging

Chapter Contents

Summary: Different methods for the quantification of relative spin density (ρ_0), T_1, and T_2 are described. Starting with methods that are based on simplistic signal models, more efficient data collection schemes are later presented. For each method, the optimal choice of relevant imaging parameters that minimize the percent error in the estimate induced by additive white noise in the individual data points is given. Some of the common nonidealities that one has to deal with in the estimation of these tissue parameters are presented. Finally, the relevant properties of some materials commonly used for calibrating a given estimation method are given.

Introduction

As seen in Ch. 15, spin density and the relaxation times, T_1 and T_2, provide the three most basic, intrinsic contrast mechanisms in MR imaging. It is of interest in the MR imaging community to measure these parameters for a variety of reasons: one is to help predict SNR and CNR for a given sequence and the other is that the resulting measured values could be used for tissue characterization, not just for detecting disease. Characterization of tissue as normal tissue or lesion and differentiation between malignant and benign tumors, for example, is of great interest in the medical community. In addition, for an objective diagnostic decision to be made based on some quantitative methodology, such as relaxation time measurements, it needs to be shown that these measurements correlate well with relevant clinical, biochemical, and histopathological data. In this sense, quantitation of these parameters also makes it possible to understand contrast mechanisms better, thereby allowing appropriate imaging methods which are optimized for efficient pathological tissue discrimination.

There is a variety of factors that can affect the accuracy of tissue parameter measurements. To complicate matters, these factors are found to vary from experiment to experiment. One major problem is the ubiquitous partial volume effect. The mixture of two tissue types in one voxel implies that the experiment needs to be designed so that the extraction of the tissue property is based on a two-compartment model. Partial volume averaging can result from poor spatial resolution or the presence of two or more chemical species within a single voxel. A second concern is that tissue properties can be sensitive to field strength and temperature. For example, it is easy to quantitate the effects of field strength and temperature on the spin density. This is the topic of interest in the following problem. Some of these problems are mentioned en route to a solution to the simpler methods of extracting tissue properties while some of the more important ones are discussed in detail in Sec. 22.5 on practical issues.

Problem 22.1

Although relative spin densities do not change, the actual effective spin density, ρ_0, as we use it in this book does change.

  a) How does ρ_0 vary with field strength?

  b) How does ρ_0 vary with temperature? What is the percent change in ρ_0 if temperature changes from $37°$ to $40°$ C?

The chapter closes by examining the effects of doping materials and contrast agents.[1] Understanding changes in relaxation times due to the injection of a contrast agent in the bloodstream is useful in studying lesion enhancement, MR angiography, and MR perfusion. In these studies, knowing T_1 or T_2 of the blood helps to optimize the sequence design and imaging parameters. Some examples of contrast changes using these agents have been given in Ch. 15 and will be seen in Ch. 24. In this chapter, some discussion of extracting the relaxivities after doping the phantom, or blood for that matter, is given.

22.1   Simplistic Estimates of ρ_0, T_1, and T_2

As a means of review, the spin echo signal as a function of ρ_0, T_1, and T_2 for $T_R \gg T_E$ is:

$$\hat{\rho}(T_R, T_E) = \rho_0 e^{-T_E/T_2}(1 - e^{-T_R/T_1}) \tag{22.1}$$

---

[1] Doping a phantom implies mixing a chemical (such as NaCl) along with the substrate (water) to change its NMR properties.

This simple expression will be used as the starting point to extract values for the tissue parameters. Three scans will be considered to extract these values.

Some problems arise with spin echo imaging experiments conducted at short repetition times from a buildup of steady-state effects. To avoid this, rf spoiling must be applied. As a result, when T_R is required to be much less than T_1, it is typical to use what is called a 'saturation recovery' experiment (SR experiment, for short). The SR experiment is nothing but a 90° SSI gradient echo experiment with T_2 replaced by T_2^* in (22.1).

22.1.1 Spin Density Measurement

In the limit of $T_E \to 0$ and $T_R \to \infty$,

$$\lim_{T_R \to \infty, T_E \to 0} \hat{\rho}(T_R, T_E) = \rho_0 \tag{22.2}$$

Of course, because of physical limitations, neither $T_E = 0$ nor very long T_R values can be achieved. The necessary practical choices are obtained by choosing T_R and T_E such that $T_R \gg T_1$ and $T_E \ll T_2$, based on a first guess of the true T_1 and T_2 values, i.e., an approximate estimate of ρ_0 is given by

$$\hat{\rho}_0 = \hat{\rho}(T_R \gg T_1, T_E \ll T_2) \qquad \text{(scan 1)} \tag{22.3}$$

As a result of these practical choices, the measured spin density has some resultant T_1 weighting and T_2 weighting.

Problem 22.2

Suppose $T_R = 3T_1$ and $T_E = 0.1T_2$. What is the percent error in the estimated spin density due to the partial T_1 and T_2 weighting?

22.1.2 T_1 Measurement

Once ρ_0 is obtained, it is then possible to measure both T_1 and T_2 by acquiring the signal at a T_R on the order of T_1 and usually less than T_1 at a T_E comparable to but usually less than T_2, respectively. For example, in the limit of extremely short T_R relative to T_1, i.e., when $T_R \ll T_1$,

$$\hat{\rho}(T_R \ll T_1, T_E \ll T_2) \simeq \rho_0 \frac{T_R}{T_1} \qquad \text{(scan 2)} \tag{22.4}$$

The estimate of T_1 is obtained from the voxel signal measurements in scans 1 and 2 via

$$\begin{aligned} \hat{T}_1 &= \frac{\rho_0 T_R}{\hat{\rho}(T_R \ll T_1, T_E \ll T_2)} \\ &= T_R \cdot \frac{\hat{\rho}(T_R \gg T_1, T_E \ll T_2)}{\hat{\rho}(T_R \ll T_1, T_E \ll T_2)} \end{aligned} \tag{22.5}$$

The practical problem here is that SNR for scan 2 is very low and multiple acquisitions is often required to obtain a good SNR for T_1. Coupled with the long T_R requirements to extract ρ_0, total scan time can be rather long.

22.1.3 T_2 Measurement

Next, T_2 is obtained from a third signal measurement using a long T_E which is comparable to the T_2 being measured (usually with $T_R \gg T_1$, but this restriction is not necessary). In these limits,

$$\hat{\rho}(T_R \gg T_1, T_E \simeq T_2) = \rho_0 e^{-T_E/T_2} \qquad \text{(scan 3)} \tag{22.6}$$

Then an estimate of T_2 can be obtained from

$$
\begin{aligned}
\hat{T}_2 &= T_E \left/ \left(\ln \frac{\rho_0}{\hat{\rho}(T_R \gg T_1, T_E \simeq T_2)} \right) \right. \\
&= T_E \left/ \left(\ln \frac{\hat{\rho}(T_R \gg T_1, T_E \ll T_2)}{\hat{\rho}(T_R \gg T_1, T_E \simeq T_2)} \right) \right.
\end{aligned}
\tag{22.7}
$$

To avoid any possible contamination by remnant T_1 effects, the T_R for both scans 1 and 3 are chosen the same. Clearly, equivalent arguments hold for measuring T_2^* as well.

Problem 22.3

Suppose ρ_0 was estimated from the same parameters as in Prob. 22.2. Let T_1 and T_2 be estimated from (22.4) and (22.6), respectively. What are the percent errors in the estimated T_1 and T_2 values if T_R in (22.4) equals $0.1T_1$ and T_E in (22.6) equals $0.2T_2$, respectively (i.e., $T_{E_1} = 0.1T_2$ and $T_{E_2} = 0.2T_2$)?

22.2   Estimating T_1 and T_2 from Signal Ratio Measurements

There is an inherent advantage to using a ratio of signal measurements to estimate either T_1 or T_2. Since a ratio of two measurements is used, ρ_0 is eliminated from the picture, and both T_1 and T_2 are estimated independent of ρ_0 (the use of either (22.5) or (22.7) leads to a concomitant error in the estimate of T_1 and T_2 when there is an error in the estimate for ρ_0).

It can be easily shown that the error in measuring ρ_0 as in the previous simplistic methods can be reduced to less than 1% only when a combined T_R of about $5T_1$ and an ultrashort T_E of $0.001T_2$ is used. Otherwise, the accuracy of the estimated T_1 and T_2 values will also suffer. These inaccuracies can be eliminated by using signal ratios to estimate both T_1 and T_2 and then using these two estimates to determine ρ_0. In the process, it then becomes possible to avoid the long T_R requirement and, as long as there is adequate SNR, the acquisition time can be shortened considerably.

22.2.1 T_1 Estimation from a Signal Ratio Measurement

As suggested by the last comment in Sec. 22.1.2, it is impossible to achieve either the $T_R \ll T_1$ limit (for SNR reasons) or the $T_R \gg T_1$ limit (for scanning time purposes), especially in the case when a large range of unknown T_1 values needs to be measured. Therefore, an estimation method based on a prediction of T_1 from a ratio of two signal measurements is a common choice for obtaining a first guess of the T_1 value.

In keeping with the previous discussion, consider the estimation of T_1 from a ratio of two spin echo signal measurements. Using a short T_E to maintain good SNR, let the two signal measurements be done at T_R values of T_{R_1} and T_{R_2}, respectively. If ρ_1 and ρ_2 are these two voxel signal magnitude measurements,

$$
\begin{aligned}
\rho_1 &= \rho_0(1 - e^{-T_{R_1}/T_1})e^{-T_E/T_2} & (22.8) \\
\rho_2 &= \rho_0(1 - e^{-T_{R_2}/T_1})e^{-T_E/T_2} & (22.9)
\end{aligned}
$$

Hence, the ratio R of ρ_1 to ρ_2, assuming that $T_{R_1} > T_{R_2}$ (thereby $R > 1$), is given by:

$$
R \equiv \frac{\rho_1}{\rho_2} = \frac{(1 - e^{-T_{R_1}/T_1})}{(1 - e^{-T_{R_2}/T_1})} \tag{22.10}
$$

Note the cancelation of the T_2 effect by taking a ratio of the signal measurements so that any T_E value that is practically achievable and useful can be chosen.

The rather simple expression for R in (22.10) requires a careful analysis to determine how best to extract T_1 with good SNR. This is the topic of discussion in the next two subsubsections.

R as a Function of T_1

Usually there is a fixed amount of time available for imaging with one type of contrast. In that case, if the goal is to measure T_1, the SNR of the T_1 estimate must be optimized given an upper limit on the total imaging time T_{total}, where

$$
T_{\text{total}} = N_{acq_1}T_{R_1} + N_{acq_2}T_{R_2} \tag{22.11}
$$

Here, N_{acq_1} and N_{acq_2} are the number of acquisitions used for improving the SNR of the images at the two respective T_R values by averaging the N_{acq} acquisitions. Again, T_{R_1} is taken to be greater than T_{R_2}. For the rest of the discussion, it is assumed that N_{acq_1} and N_{acq_2} are unity unless specified otherwise.

There are no simple analytic means for extracting T_1 from R (unless T_{R_1} and T_{R_2} are related by an integer ratio of 2 or 3; see Prob. 22.4), and a look-up table is used instead. Figure 22.1 shows that there is a one-to-one mapping from R to T_1. Hence, a unique $\hat{T}_1$ can be found given a measured value of R. A plot of R as a function of T_1 for different values of T_{R_1} for $N_{acq_1} = N_{acq_2} = 1$ and a fixed total time constraint, for a range of T_1 reveals regions where R changes most rapidly as a function of T_1 which is where T_1 is expected to be the most precisely determined. Only $T_{R_1} > T_{\text{total}}/2$ is needed to extract T_1.

Note from Fig. 22.1 how an error made in the measurement of R propagates to the T_1 estimate. For example, for the case where T_{R_1} and T_{R_2} are comparable, the change in R as a function of T_1 is very gradual. Therefore, in the presence of added noise, the inverse mapping from R to T_1 becomes highly ill-posed, i.e., appears like a many-to-one mapping rather than the true one-to-one map.

Problem 22.4

In some special cases, it is possible to obtain an analytic solution for T_1 from a measured value of R. We consider such an example here. Let $T_{R_1} = 3T_{R_2}$. Derive an analytic form for estimating T_1 from R. Hint: If $x = e^{-T_{R_2}/T_1}$, then it is possible to write an analytic expression for T_1.

Error Propagation from the Signal Measurements into R

R has an error dependent on the noise in the measured signal and leads to an error in the T_1 estimate. In this subsubsection, an expression for the standard deviation, σ_R, of the error in R is determined. Some general comments can be made about the error in, or the expected SNR of, the T_1 estimate based on the behavior of σ_R as a function of T_{R_1} and T_{R_2}.

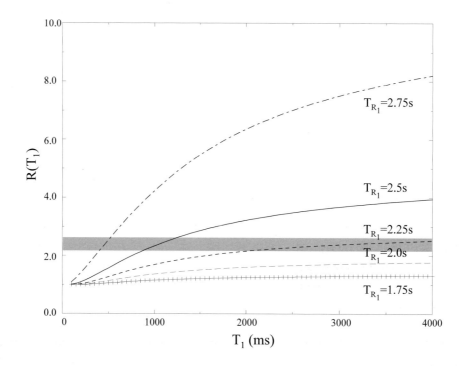

Fig. 22.1: A plot of the signal ratio R as a function of T_1. This plot shows the strictly increasing nature of the mapping and its one-to-one nature, taken advantage of in the estimation of T_1 from a measurement of R. The total repetition period T_{total} is 3 s. The shaded area represents a possible two standard deviation range of R values for an actual measurement based on an assumed T_1 of 1 s. For error bounds in the experimental determination of R indicated by the shaded region, the bounds on the estimated T_1 are expected to be 2.4 s and 4 s for a T_{R_1} value of 2.0 s and a true T_1 value of about 3.2 s. On the other hand, the bounds are 0.9 s to 1.1 s for a T_{R_1} of 2.5 s and a true T_1 value of about 1 s.

To find the variance of R, σ_R^2, consider two noisy signal measurements $\hat{\rho}_1$ and $\hat{\rho}_2$ such that

$$\hat{\rho}_1 = \rho_1 + \epsilon_1 \tag{22.12}$$
$$\hat{\rho}_2 = \rho_2 + \epsilon_2 \tag{22.13}$$

where ϵ_1 and ϵ_2 are independent Gaussian zero mean random variables with equal variance σ^2. Assume

$$\mathrm{SNR}_1 \equiv \frac{\rho_1}{\sigma} \tag{22.14}$$
$$\mathrm{SNR}_2 \equiv \frac{\rho_2}{\sigma} \tag{22.15}$$

are on the order of 10:1 or better. In this limit, the measured ratio $\hat{R}$ can be approximated with a Taylor series by

$$\hat{R} \equiv \frac{\hat{\rho}_1}{\hat{\rho}_2} \simeq R\left(1 + \frac{\epsilon_1}{\rho_1} - \frac{\epsilon_2}{\rho_2}\right) \tag{22.16}$$

Assuming that the noise is independent in each measurement, it is straightforward to show from (22.16) that the mean value of $\hat{R}$, $\bar{\hat{R}} = R$ and that

$$\frac{\sigma_{\hat{R}}^2}{R^2} = \sigma^2\left(\frac{1}{\rho_1^2} + \frac{1}{\rho_2^2}\right) = \frac{1}{\mathrm{SNR}_1^2}(1 + R^2) \tag{22.17}$$

This implies that

$$\mathrm{SNR}_R = \frac{\mathrm{SNR}_1}{\sqrt{1 + R^2}} \tag{22.18}$$

Note from Fig. 22.1 that when R is viewed as a function of T_1, for each T_{R_1} choice there exists small localized ranges of T_1 values where the behavior is almost linear. That is, each curve is piecewise linear with steep slopes for certain range of T_1 values. When the error in R, as determined by (22.17), is much smaller than the region of linearity in the locality of the true T_1 value being measured, the SNR of the T_1 estimate must equal that of R as given by (22.18). In other regions where R changes very gradually as a function of T_1, it becomes impossible to estimate T_1 in the presence of even small errors.

In summary, for fixed values of T_{R_1} and T_{R_2}, R takes on the value of unity for those values of T_1 that are much shorter than T_{R_2} while it takes on progressively increasing values for a certain range of T_1 values comparable to both T_{R_1} and T_{R_2}. However, R again becomes unity for values of T_1 that are much longer than T_{R_1}. As R approaches unity, the T_1 estimation problem becomes ill-posed and large errors in the T_1 measurement ensue. For the intermediate range of T_1 values, the measured T_1 has an SNR very similar to that of R, and SNR_{T_1} decreases as T_1 increases in this range. In effect, this description leads to the conclusion that each choice of T_{R_1} and T_{R_2} will lead to an optimal SNR value for a certain single T_1 value where SNR_{T_1} is maximized as a function of T_1. This type of behavior is shown to occur in numerical plots of the theoretical variance of the error propagated from the signal measurements into the T_1 estimate which is derived in the next subsubsection.

Error Propagation from the Signal Measurements into the T_1 Estimate

The whole argument provided above assumes that the inverse function relating T_1 to R is known. Since this function is not known analytically, an analytic expression for the SNR of the estimated T_1 value cannot be obtained from a knowledge of $\sigma_{\hat{R}}$. However, an analytic expression can be derived for $\mathrm{SNR}_{\hat{T}_1}$ from simple first-order error propagation calculations.

From basic error analysis principles, the standard deviation of the error in the T_1 measurement, σ_{T_1} viewed as a function of ρ_1 and ρ_2 is given by

$$\sigma_{\hat{T}_1}^2 = \sigma^2 \left[\left(\frac{\partial T_1}{\partial \rho_1} \right)^2 + \left(\frac{\partial T_1}{\partial \rho_2} \right)^2 \right] \tag{22.19}$$

where it is assumed that both ρ_1 and ρ_2 are two noisy, independent signal measurements. Using

$$E_1' \equiv \frac{\partial}{\partial T_1}(1 - E_{11}) = -\frac{T_{R_1}}{T_1^2} e^{-T_{R_1}/T_1} \tag{22.20}$$

$$E_2' \equiv \frac{\partial}{\partial T_1}(1 - E_{12}) = -\frac{T_{R_2}}{T_1^2} e^{-T_{R_2}/T_1} \tag{22.21}$$

gives the final result for the mean squared error value in T_1 of

$$\sigma_{\hat{T}_1} = \frac{\sigma}{\rho_0} \left| \frac{\sqrt{(1 - E_{11})^2 + (1 - E_{12})^2}}{(1 - E_{12})E_1' - (1 - E_{11})E_2'} \right| \tag{22.22}$$

where $E_{11} \equiv e^{-T_{R_1}/T_1}$ and $E_{12} \equiv e^{-T_{R_2}/T_1}$.

Problem 22.5

---

a) Derive the expression in (22.19) by using a first-order Taylor series expansion of T_1 written as a function of two variables ρ_1 and ρ_2.

b) Derive the expression shown in (22.22) from (22.19). Hint: To obtain the partial derivatives of T_1 relative to the two signal measurements ρ_i, use the chain rule,

$$\frac{\partial T_1}{\partial \rho_i} = \frac{\partial T_1}{\partial R} \cdot \frac{\partial R}{\partial \rho_i} \tag{22.23}$$

Evaluation of the partial derivatives of R with respect to ρ_i is straightforward. $\frac{\partial T_1}{\partial R}$ can be evaluated using the identity

$$\frac{\partial T_1}{\partial R} = \left[\frac{\partial R}{\partial T_1} \right]^{-1} \tag{22.24}$$

To evaluate the partial derivative of R with respect to T_1 requires the explicit expression of R as a function of T_1. For this purpose, use (22.10).

c) Suppose the true T_1 value of a tissue is 500 ms and this tissue's T_1 is estimated from the ratio of two signal measurements done with repetition times of 500 ms and 1500 ms. What is the relative percent error $(\sigma_{T_1}/T_1 \times 100)$ made in this measurement if $\rho_0/\sigma = 200{:}1$? How does this relative error change if the true T_1 value were (i) 100 ms and (ii) 1000 ms?

The observations summarized at the end of the previous subsubsection can be verified by computing the SNR of a T_1 measurement $(\mathrm{SNR}_{\hat{T}_1} \equiv T_1/\sigma_{\hat{T}_1})$ from (22.22) for a fixed set of T_{R_1} and T_{R_2} values (see Fig. 22.2, which is a plot of T_1/σ_{T_1} evaluated from (22.22)). To this effect, SNR_{T_1} is plotted as a function of T_1 for different values of T_{R_2} given that T_{total} is fixed at 2 sec. Note that each curve has a clearly defined T_1 value at which the SNR is maximized. This maximum SNR value decreases as T_{R_1} decreases. Note also that the shorter T_{R_1} becomes, the higher the T_1 value at which the SNR reaches a maximum.

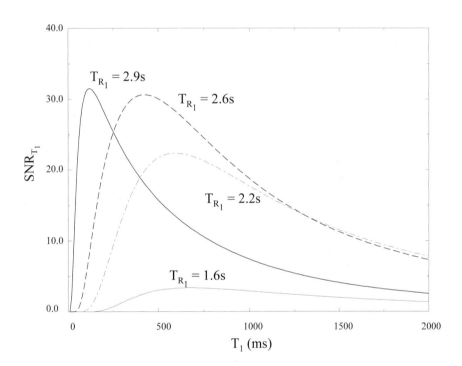

Fig. 22.2: Plot of the SNR_{T_1} as a function of T_1 for four values of T_{R_1} given that T_{total} equals 3 s and that ρ_0/σ is 100:1. No value for $T_{R_2} \geq T_{\mathrm{total}}/2 = 1.5$ s is shown since it is impossible to determine T_1 when $T_{R_2} = T_{\mathrm{total}}/2$.

Another plot of practical interest is one showing the expected behavior of the SNR of estimates of T_1 of different tissues as a function of T_{R_1} for a fixed T_{total} (see Fig. 22.3). This allows the determination of an optimal choice of T_{R_1} for an expected range of expected T_1 values for the tissues of interest.

Other dependencies of $\sigma_{\hat{T}_1}/T_1$ such as on T_{total}/T_1, given that both T_{R_1} and T_{R_2} can be related to T_{total}, can be studied. These allow the examination of how the SNR can be further improved for a range of T_1 values of interest when the SNR increase as a function of T_{total} for $N_{acq_1} = N_{acq_2} = 1$ becomes invariant.

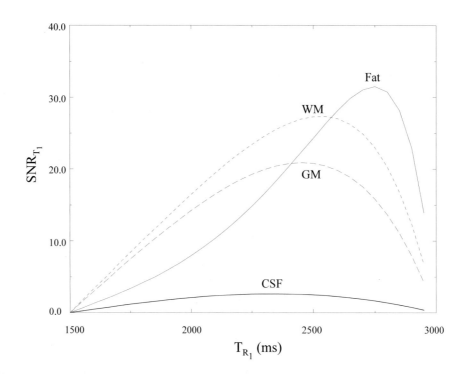

Fig. 22.3: Plot of the SNR of the estimated T_1 value as a function of T_{R_1} for different tissues given that T_{total} equals 3 s and ρ_0/σ is 100:1. Note that the choice of T_{R_1} equal to four times the average T_1 value between GM, WM, and fat (about 600 ms) and T_{R_2} value equal to the average T_1 value yields a comparable SNR for all the T_1 estimates for all three tissues.

The SNR behavior of the estimated T_1 for just one method, the ratio method, is considered in such detail in this chapter. However, the tools used in examining and deriving the dependencies on different parameters can be extended to estimation with any other method. Such an analysis for other methods will be highly instructive for the first-time reader.

22.2.2 T_2 Estimation

T_2 can be estimated similar to T_1 from a ratio of two signal measurements. However, estimation of T_2 from a signal ratio is much easier as described in (22.7) in Sec. 22.1. Suppose two signal measurements ρ_1 and ρ_2 are made with a spin echo sequence using two different echo times T_{E_1} and T_{E_2} and $T_{E_2} > T_{E_1}$. Then

$$\rho_1 = \rho_0 e^{-T_{E_1}/T_2}\left(1 - e^{-T_R/T_1}\right) \tag{22.25}$$
$$\rho_2 = \rho_0 e^{-T_{E_2}/T_2}\left(1 - e^{-T_R/T_1}\right) \tag{22.26}$$

T_2 is then estimated from the expression

$$\hat{T}_2 = \frac{(T_{E_2} - T_{E_1})}{\ln\left(\frac{\rho_1}{\rho_2}\right)} \tag{22.27}$$

The SNR for $\hat{T}_2$ is found from

$$\frac{\sigma_{\hat{T}_2}}{T_2} = \frac{\sigma}{\rho_0} \cdot \frac{T_2}{(T_{E_2} - T_{E_1})} \cdot \left[\frac{\sqrt{(e^{-2T_{E_1}/T_2} + e^{-2T_{E_2}/T_2})}}{e^{-(T_{E_1}+T_{E_2})/T_2}} \right] \tag{22.28}$$

As expected, as T_{E_2} approaches T_{E_1}, the T_2 estimation problem becomes ill-posed.

Problem 22.6

The purpose of using two measurements for T_2 estimation is to eliminate other associated parameters (in this case, ρ_0 and T_1).

a) Derive the expression in (22.28).

b) For $r \equiv T_{E_1}/T_{E_2}$ and $T_{E_1} + T_{E_2} = 100\,\mathrm{ms}$, numerically compute and plot the SNR of $\hat{T}_2$ for T_2 values ranging from 0 to 500 ms for $r = 2$, 5, and 10. Assume that $\rho_0/\sigma = 200{:}1$.

c) Explain the behavior of these SNR curves for the three different values of r over the range of T_2 values considered for part (b).

22.3 Estimating T_1 and T_2 from Multiple Signal Measurements

From the discussions in the previous section, it appears that, to achieve at least some preset level of percent precision in T_1 and T_2 over a range of values, signal measurements will have to be performed at multiple rather than just two T_R or T_E values. By measuring at more than just two points, it is expected that the steeply peaked and steeply falling nature of the SNR as a function of T_1 or T_2 can be changed into a more gradually varying function with a broad peak. The explanation for this behavior is that each pair of T_R or T_2 values will have an SNR response curve with its own characteristic SNR maximum. By choosing properly spaced data point intervals, the SNR maxima of each pair can be made to occur in such a way that a smooth transition will occur and lead to a broadly maximized SNR curve.

22.3.1 Parameter Estimation from Multiple Signal Measurements

A more powerful statistical approach is to estimate a set of two parameters (ρ_0 and T_1 or ρ_0 and T_2) from a set of N signal measurements where $N > 2$. Then the parameter estimation problem is to find that set of parameter values which best fits the N data points to the signal equation described by the imaging parameters. It is typical in such overdetermined problems to use a least-squares approach to determine the parameter values.[2] See Appendix B for a brief discussion about the basis of least-squares estimation.[3]

---

[2]An 'overdetermined' problem is one in which there are more known quantities than there are unknowns.
[3]See the reference for Bevington and Robinson for a nice review of different least-squares solutions.

22.3.2 T_1 Estimation

Let us reconsider the spin (or $90°$ flip angle gradient) echo experiment, where the signal is measured at more than two values of T_R.

Multiple T_R SR Experiments

In this case, the measured data y_i (borrowing the notation of Appendix B) are replaced by ρ_i, the experimental parameter x_i by T_{R_i}, and the underlying signal model expression $y(x; \vec{b})$ by $\hat{\rho}(T_R; \rho_0, T_1)$. Clearly, unless ρ_0 is measured independently by measuring at a $T_R = 5T_1$, there is no way of obtaining a linear relationship between $\hat{\rho}(T_R)$ and T_1. When ρ_0 is known or can be determined, then

$$\frac{\hat{\rho}(\infty) - \hat{\rho}(T_R)}{\hat{\rho}(\infty)} = e^{-T_R/T_1} \tag{22.29}$$

where $\hat{\rho}(\infty) = \rho_0$. Taking the natural logarithm of both sides and rearranging some terms, it can be seen that the variable $R(T_R)$ given by

$$R(T_R) \equiv \ln \frac{\hat{\rho}(\infty) - \hat{\rho}(T_R)}{\hat{\rho}(\infty)} \tag{22.30}$$

is linearly related to the experimental parameter T_R via

$$R = -\frac{1}{T_1} \cdot T_R \tag{22.31}$$

Note that T_1 is then given by the negated reciprocal of the slope of this line. Equation (22.31) can then be used to fit points (T_{R_i}, R_i) to a straight line $y(x) = ax + b$ using a linear least-squares procedure where the slope parameter a will give the value $-1/T_1$ and the intercept parameter b will be forced to be zero.

If ρ_0 is not known from an independent long T_R signal measurement, it is still possible to obtain a least-squares estimate of T_1. In this case, a nonlinear least-squares solution based on the expression for the signal as a function of T_R is sought.

Multiple Inversion Recovery T_1 Measurement

The former method of obtaining T_1 from a linear least-squares fit to R as a function of T_R is also used in inversion recovery T_1 estimation methods. In this case, ρ_0 is estimated from the sign-reversed signal measured at the shortest possible inversion time.

Recall that the IR signal expression for $T_R \gg T_1$ is

$$\hat{\rho}(T_I) = \rho_0(1 - 2e^{-T_I/T_1}) \tag{22.32}$$

Therefore, $\hat{\rho}(T_I)|_{T_I=0} = -\rho_0$, or

$$\hat{\rho}(\infty) = -\hat{\rho}(0) \tag{22.33}$$

Knowing ρ_0, T_1 can then be found. As before, let us define the quantity $R(T_I)$ such that

$$R(T_I) = \ln \frac{-\hat{\rho}(0) - \hat{\rho}(T_I)}{-\hat{\rho}(0)} \tag{22.34}$$

From (22.32) and (22.33), the quantity $R(T_I)$ is given by

$$R(T_I) = -\frac{1}{T_1} \cdot T_I \qquad (22.35)$$

which once again is linearly related to the variable imaging parameter T_I. Once again, T_1 is found from a least-squares fit to the slope of a straight line to the measured paired values $(T_I, R(T_I))$.

22.3.3 T_2 and T_2^* Estimation

For a spin echo sequence acquired using a long T_R, (22.6) can be used to determine T_2 (such as in (22.7)). If a finite T_R is used for time-saving purposes, both ρ_0 and T_2 have to be determined together, and a least-squares solution can be obtained for these two parameters. Taking the natural logarithm on both sides of (22.6) yields

$$\ln \hat{\rho}(T_E) = \ln \rho_0 - \frac{T_E}{T_2} \qquad (22.36)$$

Again, this expression lends itself to a linear least-squares fit to point pairs $(T_E, \ln \hat{\rho}(T_E))$. The fit to the slope then yields the quantity $-1/T_2$, from which an estimate, $\hat{T}_2$, is obtained and the fit to the intercept yields ρ_0.

As understood earlier, the echo time dependent signal decay with a gradient-echo sequence is determined by T_2^*, not T_2. However, the natural dependence on T_2^* is the same as on T_2, being an exponential decay as a function of echo time. Therefore, the results obtained for estimating T_2 are equally valid for T_2^* measurements as well. One major difference, however, is the need for only a single excitation pulse and the acquisition of different echo time images without any associated additional refocusing pulses. This allows for a speed-up in the inter-echo separation. Further, complications occurring in modeling of the signal behavior in the presence of imperfect rf pulse profiles, a topic of discussion in Sec. 22.5.1, are not present as a result of a single-pulse excitation per repetition period.

22.4 Other Methods for Spin Density and T_1 Estimation

Till now, only the conventional, potentially slow methods for spin density and T_1 estimation were considered. The requirement in both the SR and IR methods using multiple signal measurements to accurately estimate the value of M_0 for a linear, least-squares fit to the measured data rather than a numerically less stable nonlinear least-squares fit necessitates the use of at least one acquisition at a long T_R value. There are potentially two different approaches to achieve improved data acquisition efficiency. In one approach, a series of small flip angle rf pulses are used to sample the longitudinal magnetization as it recovers from the effect of an inversion pulse. The aim here is to sample as many points on the inversion recovery curve at different inversion recovery times, all within the same repetition period, making the acquisition of multiple data points very efficient while also allowing the acquisition at long T_R values. In the other approach, based on using multiple flip angle SSI signal measurements, the speed-up is obtained by allowing the acquisition of data with the same SNR as a long-T_R measurement at much shorter T_R values by acquiring the signal with flip angles surrounding the Ernst angle. The first method is the subject of discussion in the first subsection, while the latter is discussed in the second subsection.

22.4.1   The Look-Locker Method

All three methods (spin echo, SR, and IR) mentioned for measuring T_1 have very similar functional dependence on T_1, i.e., an exponential regrowth. Therefore, the signal-to-noise of these methods must have very similar dependencies too. By comparing the SNR expressions for each method, it can be shown that the SNR of the estimated T_1 is directly dependent on the ratio of the signal dynamic range, DR, to image noise standard deviation, σ, i.e.,

$$\sigma_{T_1} \propto \frac{\sigma}{DR} \tag{22.37}$$

The signal dynamic range, DR, is the difference in the limiting values of the signal; hence, the IR experiment has a two-fold advantage because its dynamic range is $2\rho_0$, unlike the spin echo and SR methods which have a dynamic range of ρ_0. This is the reason why the IR method is more popular than the other two methods.

Problem 22.7

---

a) Consider the case where the signal model equation is of the form

$$\hat{\rho}(x) = \eta(\alpha - e^{-\beta x}) \tag{22.38}$$

where η is a constant, $\alpha \leq 1$ and, in a T_1 estimation problem, where x is $1/T_1$, β is either T_I or T_R. Suppose that measurements of $\hat{\rho}(x)$ have additive white noise of standard deviation σ. Show that the SNR of x is dependent on η/σ. Assume two separate measurements of $\hat{\rho}(x)$ are made by varying α or β or both.

b) What are the values for η and α for (i) a short-T_E spin echo sequence, and (ii) an IR sequence?

However, the IR imaging method is a very inefficient method because data is collected immediately following the imaging pulse, but the next inversion pulse is applied only after a very long longitudinal recovery period. This leads to extremely long acquisition times. One method to overcome this problem is to sample the longitudinal magnetization by applying a set of small flip angle (θ) rf pulses during each repetition period. Suppose a separate phase encoding gradient of the same value is used for each θ-pulse and there is no remnant transverse magnetization before each new pulse separated from each other in time by a period τ, then N different points on the longitudinal recovery curve can be sampled in a recovery time of $N\tau$. In the most efficient sampling scheme, $T_R = N\tau$, and there is no time wasted between the inversion pulse and the first θ-pulse. In essence, the N images reconstructed represent samples of the inversion recovery curve (which is slightly disturbed depending on θ and τ) at inversion times T_I of $\{0, \tau, 2\tau, \cdots N\tau\}$. In the problem to follow, it will be shown that the signal measured at the inversion times $T_{I_n} = n\tau$, $n \in \{0, 1, 2, \cdots N\}$ gives a sampling of a generalized exponential recovery curve whose dynamic range and final value both differ significantly from that of a normal inversion recovery curve. Also, the time constant characterizing the exponential recovery is different from T_1.

Problem 22.8

Suppose a perfect π-pulse is applied at the beginning of each cycle, followed a time τ later by a train of $(N - 1)$ θ-pulses separated in time from each other by a time τ (see Fig. 22.4). Assume that the Nth pulse is the π-pulse. Suppose also that there is no remnant transverse magnetization before each new θ-pulse. Let M_n^- be the longitudinal magnetization just prior to the nth θ-pulse, where $n \in \{1, 2, \cdots N\}$.

a) Write an expression for M_n^- in terms of the equilibrium magnetization M_{eq} (instead of the usual M_0 to avoid confusion because of its usage of a numerical subscript) and M_1^-.

b) Hence, obtain an expression for the steady-state value, M_∞^-.

c) Hence show that

$$(M_n^- - M_\infty^-) = (M_1^- - M_\infty^-)(E_1 \cos \theta)^{n-1} \qquad (22.39)$$

d) From (22.39), show that

$$M_N^- = \frac{M_\infty^-(1 - (E_1 \cos \theta)^{N-1}) + M_{eq}(1 - E_1)(E_1 \cos \theta)^{N-1}}{(1 + \cos \theta (E_1 \cos \theta)^{N-1})} \qquad (22.40)$$

in the steady-state. Remember that $M_1^- = -E_1 M_N^- + M_{eq}(1 - E_1)$.

e) Finally, show that the signal measured after the nth pulse is given by

$$\rho_n = \beta \left\{ 1 - DR_{norm} \cdot e^{-(n-1)\tau/T_{1eff}} \right\} \qquad (22.41)$$

where

$$DR_{norm} \equiv \frac{M_1^- - M_\infty^-}{M_\infty^-} = \frac{\cos \theta \left(1 - (E_1 \cos \theta)^{N-1}\right)}{1 + \cos \theta (E_1 \cos \theta)^{N-1}} + 1 \qquad (22.42)$$

$$\beta \equiv M_\infty^- \sin \theta \qquad (22.43)$$

and

$$\frac{\tau}{T_{1eff}} \equiv \frac{\tau}{T_1} - \ln (\cos \theta) \qquad (22.44)$$

Note from (22.41)–(22.44) that for the case of extremely small flip angles $\theta \to 0$, $\tau/T_{1_{eff}} \to \tau/T_1$, $\beta \to \theta M_\infty^-$ and

$$DR_{norm} \to \frac{(1 - E_1^{N-1})}{(1 + E_1^{N-1})} + 1 = \frac{2}{(1 + E_1^{N-1})} \simeq 2$$

The last approximation is valid for $N \gg 1$ since E_1 is a fraction. With these limits, the measured signal variation as a function of the θ-pulse number is

$$\lim_{\theta \to 0} \rho_n \simeq M_\infty^- \theta (1 - 2e^{-(n-1)\tau/T_1}) \tag{22.45}$$

Thus, in the limit of small flip angles, the sequence shown in Fig. 22.4 manipulates the magnetization similar to an IR sequence. In essence, the small flip angles do not perturb the approach to equilibrium of the longitudinal magnetization from inversion by the π-pulse. However, the direct proportionality of the measured signal to the small flip angle θ makes this limit practically less useful as it becomes truly SNR-limited. The potential fast sampling capability of a large set of points on the recovery curve has, however, made this method extremely popular for *in vivo* T_1 measurements.

As a consequence of the behavior of the signal from this sequence in an exponential fashion from one θ-pulse to the next, a nonlinear least-squares fit to the three parameters,

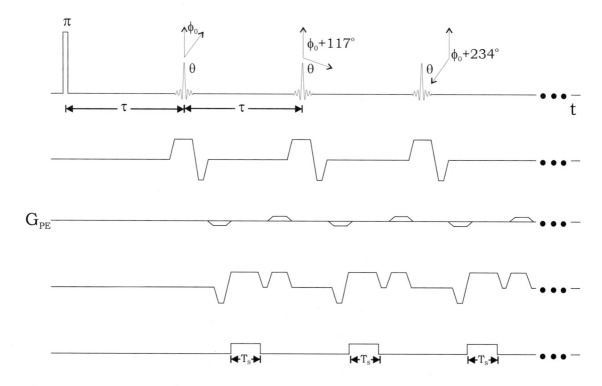

Fig. 22.4: Typical sequence diagram for the fast implementation of an IR sequence where the longitudinal magnetization is sampled several times following a single inversion pulse using small θ-pulses. This sequence is the topic of discussion in extracting T_1 in a more time-efficient manner.

β, DR, and $T_{1_{eff}}$ using the signal expression (22.41) can be done. T_1 can then be estimated from $T_{1_{eff}}$.

On the other hand, if β is previously known, both DR and $T_{1_{eff}}$ can be determined using a linear least-squares procedure. To see this, note that (22.41) can be rewritten in the form

$$R(\tau, n) \equiv \ln \frac{\beta - \rho_n}{\beta} = \ln(DR) - (n-1)\frac{\tau}{T_{1_{eff}}} \tag{22.46}$$

It can now be seen that $T_{1_{eff}}$ and hence, T_1, can be estimated from the slope parameter of a least-squares fit to a line of measured values of point pairs $(n\tau, R(\tau, n))$.

22.4.2 T_1 Estimation from SSI Measurements at Multiple Flip Angles

In this subsection, a method for estimating ρ_0 and T_1 from short-T_R, gradient echo SSI signal measurements at multiple flip angles is presented. The motivation for this method came from the fact that the total measurement time required for their estimation over large volumes-of-interest could be drastically reduced while maintaining the SNR of the estimated variables in comparison with other SE and IR based methods. The time saving is especially significant for tissues with long relaxation times. As the SSI sequence can be used in a fast imaging mode, it is well-suited to 3D imaging and its inherent three-dimensional high resolution capability.

From Ch. 18, the SSI signal as a function of the flip angle θ is given by

$$\hat{\rho}_{\text{ssi}}(\theta) = \rho_0 e^{-T_E/T_2^*} \frac{(1 - E_1)\sin\theta}{(1 - E_1\cos\theta)} \tag{22.47}$$

where $E_1 = e^{-T_R/T_1}$. The two quantities to be determined, ρ_0 and T_1, can be estimated from the signal measured at multiple flip angles at a fixed T_R value by performing a nonlinear least-squares fit to the measured values of $\rho_{\text{ssi}}(\theta)$ as a function of θ.

A computationally easier-to-implement method for estimating both these quantities also exists. Equation (22.47) can be rewritten as

$$\frac{\hat{\rho}_{\text{ssi}}(\theta)}{\sin\theta} = E_1 \frac{\hat{\rho}_{\text{ssi}}(\theta)}{\tan\theta} + \rho_0 e^{-T_E/T_2^*}(1 - E_1) \tag{22.48}$$

From (22.48), it can be seen that a transformation of the points $(\theta, \hat{\rho}(\theta))$ into a plane where the coordinate pairs are

$$(x(\theta), y(\theta)) \equiv \left(\frac{\hat{\rho}_{\text{ssi}}(\theta)}{\tan\theta}, \frac{\hat{\rho}_{\text{ssi}}(\theta)}{\sin\theta} \right) \tag{22.49}$$

transforms the measured points into a straight line with slope E_1 and ordinate intercept of $\rho_0 e^{-T_E/T_2^*}(1 - E_1)$. Shown in Fig. 22.5 are example plots of $\hat{\rho}(\theta)$ versus θ and a replotting of these same points in the transformed $(x(\theta), y(\theta))$ plane, re-emphasizing the linearity of the measured points in the transformed plane. T_1 can then be estimated from E_1, which itself is estimated as the slope parameter from a linear least-squares fit. ρ_0 can be estimated from the ordinate intercept parameter once E_1 is known, assuming that $T_E \ll T_2^*$, so that

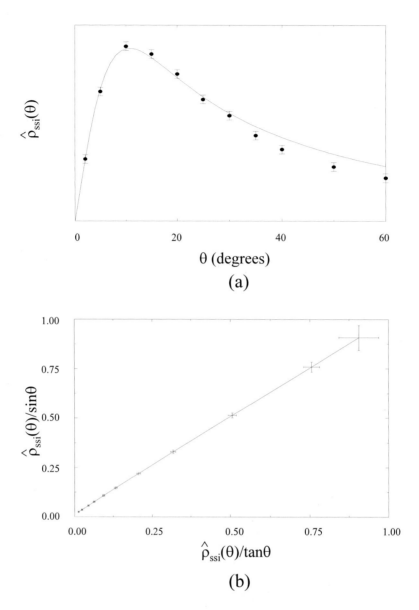

Fig. 22.5: Plot of (a) $\hat{\rho}_{ssi}(\theta)$ versus θ and (b) a replot of the same points in the $(x(\theta), y(\theta))$ plane for a set of signal measurements done on an agarose gel phantom. The phantom has a T_1 value of about 1.5 s and a T_2 of about 250 ms. In (a), the last four points were not used in the fit because the resonance offset increment (as required in short-T_R SSI sequence implementations) used to collect this data was nonideal. This causes the signal at large flip angles to be small in comparison with the expected signal behavior. For tissues in the brain with shorter T_2 values, this deviation at large flip angles is found to be less severe. The fit to $\hat{\rho}_{ssi}(\theta)$ versus θ is shown by the solid line. As seen, the fitted points lie within two standard deviations from the measured points (the error bars show $\pm$ one white noise standard deviation). In (b), the slope of the straight line is E_1 while the ordinate axis intercept is $e^{-T_E/T_2^*}(1 - E_1)$ where we have set ρ_0 to be unity. The fit is again shown by a solid line.

the term e^{-T_E/T_2^*} can be neglected from the ordinate intercept term in (22.48). The other alternative is to acquire signal measurements at multiple T_E values to estimate T_2^* using the method discussed in Sec. 22.3.3 and then eliminating the quantity e^{-T_E/T_2^*} from the intercept estimate of $\rho_0 e^{-T_E/T_2^*}$.

Optimal Choice of Flip Angles

In any estimation problem, the operating points (such as T_R and flip angle in this case) should be chosen so that the sensitivity of the measured quantity relative to the parameter of interest (defined as the partial derivative of the signal expression relative to the estimated parameter) is maximized with respect to the variable of signal measurement (in this case θ). When the sensitivity is maximized, the reciprocal of the sensitivity, which is a measure of how small changes in the signal perturb the estimated value, is minimized. Hence, choosing this as the operating point maximizes the SNR of the estimated variable.

As an example, consider estimating T_1. Assume that ϵ_i, the white noise (with standard deviation σ) added to $\hat{\rho}(\theta_i)$, is such that $\sigma \ll \hat{\rho}(\theta_i)$ for all i. In this limit,

$$\sigma_{\hat{T}_1}^2 = \sigma^2 \sum_i \left(\frac{\partial \hat{T}_1}{\partial \hat{\rho}(\theta_i)} \right)^2 \simeq \sigma^2 \sum_i \left(\frac{\partial T_1}{\partial \hat{\rho}(\theta_i)} \right)^2 \tag{22.50}$$

$$= \sigma^2 \sum_i \frac{1}{\left(\frac{\partial \hat{\rho}(\theta_i)}{\partial T_1} \right)^2} \tag{22.51}$$

Hence, maximizing $\frac{\partial \hat{\rho}(\theta_i)}{\partial T_1}$, the sensitivity of the voxel signal to T_1, maximizes the SNR of $\hat{T}_1$. In the following problem, the question of optimizing the choice of flip angles for maximizing the SNR of the estimated ρ and T_1 values is dealt with.

Problem 22.9

Using SSI signal measurements at multiple flip angles, only two quantities, ρ_0 and T_1, are being estimated. Therefore, if the measured voxel signal behaves according to (22.47), measurement of $\hat{\rho}_{\mathrm{ssi}}(\theta)$ at just two flip angles is required for successfully estimating these two parameters. The choice of the flip angle which maximizes the SNR of $\hat{T}_1$ is the topic of discussion in this problem.

a) Show that the sensitivity of $\hat{\rho}_{\mathrm{ssi}}$ to T_1 as a function of θ is maximized at the flip angle θ_1 given by

$$\cos \theta_1 = \frac{(2E_1 - 1)}{(2 - E_1)} \tag{22.52}$$

b) Hence show that θ_1 is greater than the Ernst angle. Show this result for $T_R \ll T_1$.

The second flip angle is chosen using a different criterion which is discussed following this problem in the text as the sensitivity of the signal to ρ_0 is maximized at the Ernst angle. It is undesirable to use this choice, for there will then be no purely spin density-weighted acquisition.

Since ρ_0 appears in the expression for the signal measured at any flip angle, it will not be possible to measure T_1 without knowing ρ_0. As known from Ch. 18, the SSI signal is spin density-weighted for $\theta \ll \theta_E$, in which limit there is no T_1 dependence. Hence, θ_2, the second optimal flip angle choice, is chosen small enough so that the signal is essentially independent of T_1 and yet, large enough to have adequate SNR. As a result, the two optimal acquisition flip angles are found to be one on either side of the Ernst angle.

Problem 22.10

Interleaved sequences (see Fig. 26.17) are a good means by which to collect data that later need to be subtracted or overlaid one on the other. Interleaved in this case means that any given imaging parameter can be changed from one k-space line to the next where each of these k-space lines has the same phase or partition encoding gradient. As a result, two sets of images from the two different choices of that parameter can be obtained from one sequence. Some example imaging parameters include 1) different flip angles; 2) different echo times; 3) different T_R values; 4) any combination of the above; or 5) exactly the same imaging parameters without changes.

a) Why is it an advantage to run an interleaved sequence? Hint: Patients are not phantoms.

b) Draw a sequence diagram showing one parameter change with the same phase encoding lines.

c) Consider the example with two different rf pulses. If the flip angle of the first rf pulse is θ_1 and the flip angle of the second pulse is θ_2, find the equilibrium longitudinal magnetization $M_{il,ze}$, after each alternate rf pulse. Note that the answer derived from the θ_1 flip angle will be different than that from the θ_2 flip angle. After a sufficient number of rf pulses, show that the equilibrium longitudinal magnetization after the θ_1-pulse is given by

$$M_{il,ze} = \frac{M_0(1 - E_1)(1 + \cos\theta_2 E_1)}{1 - E_1^2 \cos\theta_1 \cos\theta_2} \qquad (22.53)$$

Similarly, the equilibrium longitudinal magnetization after the θ_2-pulse is given by swapping θ_1 and θ_2 in (22.53).

d) Show that when $\theta_1 = \theta_2 = \theta$, $M_{il,ze}$ reduces to (18.12).

e) Plot the contrast between white matter and gray matter at 1.5 T, as a function of θ_1, when θ_2 is equal to either the Ernst angle of the gray matter; a flip angle that is twice the Ernst angle; or 90°. Assume that $T_E = 5$ ms and $T_R = 20$ ms, with tissue properties given in Table 18.1.

The optimization discussed here works for a single tissue with a singular T_1 value. When several tissues are present, the optimization process becomes numerical, with θ_1 and θ_2 chosen as a practical compromise such that σ_{T_1} is within a certain percent of a preset threshold value for the range of T_1 values of interest.

22.5 Practical Issues Related to T_1 and T_2 Measurements

In this section, practical issues relating to T_1 and T_2 estimation in a nonideal setting are considered. One of the main worries in using spin echo sequences relates to the problem of imperfect refocusing pulses. Similar effects of nonideal slice profiles have to be considered even in single excitation (i.e., gradient echo) pulse sequences when a 2D acquisition is utilized, as the 2D image signal is an effective magnetization obtained by integrating over the nonideal slice profile. The other worry relates to how the effects of the random, intravoxel incoherent motion of spins (or diffusion) during image acquisition weight the estimation of T_2 values. Both these effects have to considered along with the issue of minimizing total imaging time.

22.5.1 Inaccuracies Due to Nonideal Slice Profile

This effect plays a central role in introducing inaccuracies in both T_1 and T_2 estimates obtained with estimation methods based on signal measurements with 2D imaging sequences. Voxel signal dependencies in these conventional methods typically make ideal slice profile assumptions, and this is always invalid for 2D imaging experiments. Even with rf pulse excitations with profiles approaching ideality, small deviations from ideality are exacerbated in certain situations which arise in both T_1 and T_2 estimation methods. For example, in T_2 estimation, data must be acquired at a minimum of two echo times using a reasonably long T_R. For reduced imaging time purposes, it is common to use a multi-slice approach which necessitates the use of slice selective excitation and refocusing pulses. Further improvements in efficiency are achieved by acquiring each phase encoding line for multiple echoes following a single excitation pulse. That is, T_2 is most efficiently mapped by acquiring images at different echo times using a multi-slice, multi-echo 2D spin echo sequence. The next discussion focuses on the nonideal refocusing pulses describing their cumulative effects on T_2 estimates using such a multi-echo acquisition. A second discussion following it describes how nonideal rf excitation pulses can affect the accuracy of T_1 estimates.

T_2 Estimation from Multi-Echo Spin Echo Sequences Using Slice Selective $\pi/2$- and π-Pulses

Tissue parameters are often measured with 2D imaging methods. This can cause problems due to nonideal slice profile effects. To see this, assume that the B_1 field imposed by the coil is homogeneous over the entire object. The only B_1 inhomogeneities then imposed are those due to the spatially varying flip angle induced by the nonideal slice profile of the slice selective 90° and 180° rf pulses. Both rf pulses will be taken to have the same shape. For purposes of simplicity, also assume that all non-echoing and stimulated echo pathways are eliminated by careful sequence design.

From Sec. 18.3 in Ch. 18, it is known that the Hahn echo amplitude for a θ-2θ pulse sequence is proportional to $\sin^3 \theta$. Further echoes each have an amplitude reduction by a factor of $\sin^2 \theta$. Hence, the Hahn echo after the nth 180°-pulse has an amplitude which is proportional to $\sin^{2n+1} \theta$. With a distribution of flip angles θ across the slice determined by the slice profile, $p(\theta)$, the signal at the nth echo is given by the slice profile-integrated value (the limits of integration being from $\theta = 0$ to $\theta = \pi/2$), i.e.,

$$\hat{\rho}(n) = \rho_0 e^{-nT_E/T_2} \left[\int d\theta \, p(\theta) \sin^{2n+1} \theta \right] \tag{22.54}$$

where it is assumed that $p(\theta)$ is a normalized slice profile such that $\int d\theta \, p(\theta) = 1$ and that successive echoes are separated in time by T_E. Since $\sin^{2n+1} \theta$ is a more and more localized function of θ around $\theta = \pi/2$ as n increases (approximating the Kronecker delta function $\delta_{\theta,\pi/2}$), the quantity within square brackets, $d(n)$, given by

$$d(n) \equiv \int d\theta \, p(\theta) \sin^{2n+1} \theta \tag{22.55}$$

is a decreasing fractional quantity as a function of n. This signal loss factor after each π-pulse can be approximated with an exponential e^{-nf} where $f > 0$ since a plot of the function $d(n)$ for a typical, time-truncated sinc pulse approximates an exponential decay as a function of n (see Fig. 22.6). Hence $\hat{\rho}(n)$ in (22.54) can be rewritten as

$$\hat{\rho}(n) = \rho_0 \sin \theta e^{-nT_E/T_2} e^{-nf} \tag{22.56}$$

As a result, when $\hat{\rho}(n)$ is fitted to an exponential, only an incorrect 'apparent' (underestimated) T_2 value, $T_{2_{app}}$, is obtained:

$$\frac{1}{T_{2_{app}}} = \frac{1}{T_2} + \frac{f}{T_E} \tag{22.57}$$

Equation (22.57) tells us that the underestimation of T_2 due to a nonideal slice profile is reduced by making the echo time of the first echo, T_E, as large as possible. This makes

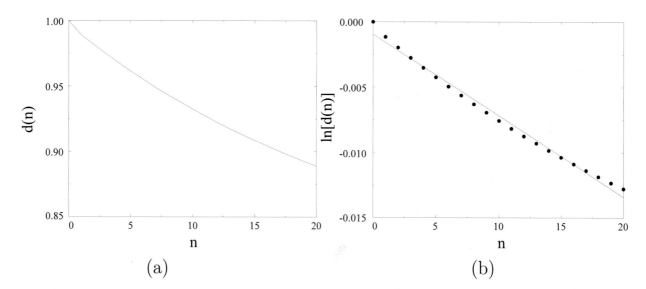

Fig. 22.6: Plot of (a) $d(n)$ and (b) $\ln d(n)$ (points shown using filled circles and evaluated at integer values of n) and a fit to a straight line of $\ln d(n)$ as functions of n for a 10 kHz bandwidth sinc pulse of length 1.28 ms. Both plots verify the approximately exponential decay-like behavior of $d(n)$ as a function of n.

the quantity f/T_E small in comparison with $1/T_2$. In other words, as long as the fractional signal loss at the first echo due to T_2 decay is significantly large in comparison with the fractional signal loss due to the nonideal slice profile, the underestimation of the true T_2 value becomes negligible. However, for purposes of SNR, it is not wise to choose too large a value for T_E. This leads to a practical sequence design for T_2 measurement with multi-echo Carr-Purcell spin echo sequences to compromise between reasonable SNR and a well-defined rf slice profile. For this purpose, it is typical to use either a nonselective 'hard' pulse for the 180° excitation or a selective pulse which excites a slice much larger than the 90°-pulse.[4] Another practical aspect relates to rf transmit calibration and its effect on T_2. Even if a nonselective 180° rf pulse excitation is used, a similar error occurs in the T_2 estimate if the rf pulses are miscalibrated and the 180° pulse now acts like a θ-pulse instead where $\theta \neq 180°$. As a result, care must be taken to ensure the correct calibration of the 180°-pulse amplitude.

Other solutions include the use of a CPMG sequence where the $\pi/2$ and π pulses are 90° out-of-phase with each other and only every other spin echo is sampled. A simpler solution is obtained if time efficiency can be sacrificed. By acquiring the images at different echo times during different repetition periods (following different excitation pulses), the nonideal slice profile effect discussed above factors out commonly in the voxel signal expression for each echo time. T_2 is therefore estimated accurately. In the presence of significant diffusion components, this sequence is however more sensitive to diffusion. Recall from Ch. 21 that the b value in a Carr-Purcell sequence is directly proportional to τ^3. Since the images at different echo times are acquired by varying the value of τ in this method, an additional signal decay effect dependent on τ^3 is additionally present; this might again lead to an underestimation of T_2 similar to the nonideal slice profile effect in a multi-slice, multi-echo sequence. This diffusion effect is reduced in the multi-echo acquisition because it is usual to acquire the multiple echoes with a short inter-echo separation determined by τ.

Slice Profile Effects in T_1 Measurements

In both the gradient echo and spin echo variants of the SR experiment, it was seen that at least one short-T_R acquisition and a long-T_R acquisition were required for keeping the relative error in the measured T_1 small. Both variants of the SR experiment become extremely sensitive to flip angle variations at short T_R values. Making an incoherent steady-state assumption during imaging, for example, it was shown in Ch. 18 that the SSI signal varies in a fashion that it goes through a spin density-weighted domain and then a T_1-weighted domain as a function of flip angle. The point of separation between these two domains is much lower than 90° for short T_R values. As a result, when a 90° excitation pulse with a nonideal slice profile is used, the slice profile-integrated 2D signal is typically much higher than that predicted by the SR signal dependence on T_R (see (22.4)). Recall that this effect was described in Sec. 18.1 in Ch. 18 for the special case where the nonideal slice profile can be considered to be a trapezoidal flip angle variation. A similar nonideal slice profile integration effect is present in the case of the spin echo variant. In the spin echo variant, the spoiled steady-state achieved by a θ-2θ sequence needs to be considered. As will be shown in Ch. 26, this leads to a signal expression as a function of flip angle which is maximized for

---

[4]See Ch. 16 for the definition of a hard pulse.

a flip angle larger than 90° for a θ-π sequence. This flip angle which maximizes the signal as a function of flip angle approaches 180° as T_R becomes shorter and shorter. Here it is assumed that only the spin echo has a significant contribution to the reconstructed voxel signal, leading to an additional $\frac{1}{2} \sin^2 \theta$ factor. Based on a generalization of the result to be obtained in Ch. 26 (see (26.7)), it can be shown that the spoiled steady-state spin echo signal obtained is

$$\hat{\rho}_{\theta\text{-}2\theta}(\theta) = \frac{1}{2}\rho_0 \sin^3 \theta \frac{(1 - 2\sin^2 \theta e^{-(T_R-\tau)/T_1} - \cos 2\theta e^{-T_R/T_1})}{(1 - \cos\theta\cos 2\theta e^{-T_R/T_1})} \tag{22.58}$$

By plotting the above expression as a function of flip angle for $\tau \ll T_R$, it can be seen that the value of θ which maximizes the signal slowly shifts towards 180° as T_R/T_1 approaches zero. It is further clear that for a sequence designed to operate as a 90°-180° spin echo sequence with an imperfect rf pulse will only excite θ-2θ responses for $\theta < 90°$. As a result of these two observations, the overestimation of the true signal value after integration over the nonideal profile is not as accentuated as in the gradient echo SSI limit. The overestimation in comparison with the expected value according to (22.1) at the shorter T_R value leads to an underestimation of T_1 (as suggested by the approximation of (22.4) for T_R values much shorter than T_1).

Problem 22.11

---

a) Derive (22.58).

b) Plot the signal expression for $\hat{\rho}_{\theta\text{-}2\theta}(\theta)$ shown in (22.58) assuming $\tau \ll T_R$ for three different T_R/T_1 values of 0.1, 0.2, and 0.3. Hence, show that the flip angle θ which maximizes the signal slowly shifts towards flip angles larger than 90°.

In both cases, the effect can be generalized by stating that the nonideal slice profile effect can be described as an integration of a function of flip angle over the slice profile. If the incoherent steady-state signal dependence on θ, which also varies with T_R/T_1, is described by a function $f(\theta; T_R/T_1)$ then

$$\hat{\rho}(T_R) = \int d\theta\, p(\theta) f(\theta; T_R/T_1) \tag{22.59}$$

where $p(\theta)$ is the unit-area normalized slice profile as before. Clearly, this integrated signal yields a different answer from that predicted by (22.4), yielding inaccurate estimates for T_1. One commonly used solution to overcome this dependence of the integrated signal dependence on T_R/T_1 can be eliminated by using a ratio method for estimating T_1 from two measurements obtained with the same T_R. To obtain different signal dependencies, it is common to use the ratio of an IR signal measurement to an interleaved SR signal measurement, both acquired with the same T_R.

22.5.2 Other Sources of Inaccuracies in Relaxation Time and Spin Density Measurements

The discussion in Sec. 22.5.1 revolved around the important issue of the source of inaccuracy in T_1 and T_2 estimation introduced by the ideal slice profile assumption in modeling the expected signal behavior. Here, inaccuracies introduced by other sources are considered with an aim to improve the modeling of signal dependence on the imaging parameters of interest. Several sources of nonidealities can be postulated as leading to inaccuracies in these measurements

a) rf field inhomogeneities (due to spatial variations of the transmit and receive rf coil sensitivities)

b) rf transmit calibration errors (leading to errors in the specification of flip angles)

c) partial volume averaging

d) Gibbs ringing at tissue boundaries

e) systematic temperature variations

f) Bloch equation nonlinearities (especially in sequences using large flip angle excitation pulses, once again leading to errors similar to rf transmit miscalibration)

g) tissue denaturing effects in measurements in *ex vivo* tissue samples

In the following discussion, the effect of each source is considered and possible methods for either modeling or estimating each nonideality with an aim to correct for or reduce their effects. Whenever the effects and correction strategies are similar, they are discussed under a single heading.

RF Field Inhomogeneities

Radiofrequency field inhomogeneities are the most irksome sources of nonidealities (especially as a result of their omnipresence). As discussed in Sec. 7.4, the spatial variation of the rf field sensitivity of the transmit and receive coils enter the signal expression for any sequence in the form of altering the flip angle at a given spatial location as well as altering the received signal from a spatial location. From a relative point-of-view, the sensitivity variations can be related from $\mathcal{B}^z_{\text{transmit}}(\vec{r})$ and $\mathcal{B}^z_{\text{receive}}(\vec{r})$ to arbitrarily normalized spatial variation of the sensitivities, say $\alpha_{\text{transmit}}(\vec{r})$ and $\alpha_{\text{receive}}(\vec{r})$. Recalling the dependencies,

$$\theta(\vec{r}) = \alpha_{\text{transmit}}(\vec{r})\theta_0 \qquad (22.60)$$
$$\hat{\rho}(\vec{r}) \propto \alpha_{\text{receive}}(\vec{r}) \qquad (22.61)$$

As before, it is the short-T_R signal measurements which suffer most from the spatial variations of flip angle. In the spin density-T_1 estimation method based on multiple flip angle SSI signal measurements, this effect needs to be eliminated; otherwise, large inaccuracies result.

One of the simple ways to eliminate the problem of spatial variation of flip angles is to use a large-volume transmit coil with a homogeneous excitation profile over the volume-of-interest and signal pickup with a small volume pickup coil for high SNR. However, this only ensures that T_1 and T_2 values are estimated correctly. The spin density map still contains the receive coil sensitivity variation and this needs to be mapped and eliminated.

These effects become especially important when tissue parameters are mapped over large volumes-of-interest, in which case the B_1 fields naturally generated by the coils themselves vary across the region-of-interest. They are further significant at higher field strengths, where the generated rf field pattern changes further in the presence of reduced wavelengths inside the human body and the elevated permittivity (ϵ) and conductivity (σ) values at high frequencies. These effects lead to 'rf shielding,' a result predicted by solving the Maxwell's equations given the boundary conditions and ϵ and σ values within each boundary.[5] Correction can be effected by computing $\mathcal{B}(\vec{r})$ for the given coil geometry and modeling the tissue compartments in the body with finite elements and using finite-element solution of the boundary value problem. The more natural way is to map the flip angle as a function of position by imaging the object in a transmit/receive coil, whereby the two different sensitivities reduce to a single effective variation from the reciprocity principle. Using this method also ensures correction for signal variations due to rf shielding.

RF Transmit Miscalibration and Bloch Equation Nonidealities

It is typical on most commercially available scanners to use an automated transmitter calibration by locating a specific flip angle (such as $180°$) using a single, large-volume signal measurement. In the presence of rf and static field inhomogeneities, this is only an approximation to the true calibration voltage required to excite that flip angle. This results in an incorrect specification of the true flip angle even at a chosen nominal level. Further, as discussed in Sec. 16.4.2, the nonlinearity of the Bloch equations should be taken into consideration when nonideal slice profiles are computed for correction of this effect.

Partial Volume Averaging and Gibbs Ringing

Both these effects occur at tissue boundaries, and lead to a violation of the assumption of monoexponential T_1 and T_2 relaxation in voxels at or nearby tissue boundaries. Enough data points have to be collected for the possibility of a two-compartmental modeling of the measured signal behavior without becoming an ill-posed numerical problem in such situations. Another practical solution is to collect high resolution images and then collapse the computed parameter maps to low resolution to achieve the level of precision required for the map as smaller voxel sizes always lead to a reduction of the number of voxels and physical spatial extent of these two effects.

---

[5]A compilation of the Maxwell's equations and other related electromagnetic principles can be found in Appendix A.

Systematic Variations of Temperature

Both the measured spin density and T_1 are temperature-dependent. As the tissue temperature increases, the thermal agitation energy of the spin population increases. This leads to a situation where the spins have a tendency not to align as well as they would at lower temperatures. As a result, there is a lengthening of T_1 values and a reduction in the measured spin density. The temperature must therefore be maintained constant in different experiments for measured T_1 values to make consistent sense.

Although the normal body regulates tissue temperature and maintains it at a constant level, systematic temperature gradients can be set up in different locations under certain pathological and/or abnormal conditions. This can result in a biologically determined broadening of the estimated T_1 distribution.

Denaturing of *Ex Vivo* Tissue Samples

Several relaxation time measurements are made on excised tissue samples. It is typical to preserve these tissue samples in a mild disinfectant such as formalin. Formalin has a denaturing effect on the tissues, leading to a breakdown of the protein make-up of the tissues by soaking in formalin by slow diffusion. As the T_1 of the tissue water content depends on the hydration fraction (the fraction of water molecules weakly held by the protein at its surface) and denaturing of the protein backbone leads to a change in hydration fraction, both T_1 and T_2 are found to change with time. Therefore, care must be taken in experiments with excised samples to avoid time variations post-excision and soaking in formalin.

As a conclusion to this discussion, it must be stressed that, *given the potential utility of these maps in a basic understanding of in vivo physiology, effects of these nonidealities must be modeled and corrected for before significant biological implications can be made from a measurement of tissue parameters.*

22.5.3 Advanced Sequence Design for Relaxation Time and Spin Density Measurements

In this subsection, the focus is on good sequence design practices in imaging MR tissue parameters. In sequences utilizing inversion pulses, it is critical for the inversion pulse slice profile to be as close to ideality as possible. Even with good rf pulse design, whereby the π-pulse is Hanning filtered to avoid ringing of the slices, has enough zero crossings to have good slice definition, and excites a slice of larger thickness than the 90°-pulse, systematic errors are always found to occur in the estimated T_1 value. It is not surprising in multi-slice imaging of T_1 because of the presence of rf inhomogeneities and the ever-present incorrect rf transmit calibration. An inversion pulse which is relatively insensitive to B_1 variations and the nominal preset transmitter voltage is therefore required. *Adiabatic inversion pulses*, which are both amplitude and phase modulated rf pulses, can be used as B_1-insensitive slice selective inversion pulses.

The adiabatic rf pulse is defined in time as

$$B_1(t) = B_{1_0}(\text{sech}(\beta t))^{1+i\mu} \tag{22.62}$$

where sech($\cdot$) is the 'hyperbolic secant' operator. The slice selection bandwidth of this hyperbolic secant pulse is given by

$$\Delta\omega = \pm\beta\mu \qquad (22.63)$$

This pulse has the required properties and is found to be useful in shortening the T_R in IR-based T_1 mapping methods by creating perfect inversion across the slice. However, the time duration of these rf pulses is usually long, and when used for inversion of short T_1 and short T_2 species, is not as effective as an inversion pulse. The power required for the same excited slice is also much higher in comparison with a sinc pulse excitation, which may be a concern especially at high fields. Moreover, the hyperbolic secant pulse cannot be used as a refocusing pulse since it creates a phase dispersion across the slice.

Tissues with high water content which have long T_2 values have the highest signal in the long T_E image collected for T_2 estimation. The Gibbs ringing at sharp boundaries between the long T_2 compartment and other tissues overwhelms the signal contribution from neighboring tissues across the boundary. With this decaying oscillatory contribution from the dominant species, the assumption of monoexponential transverse relaxation is violated. It therefore becomes essential to suppress the signal contribution from the long T_2 species if the T_2 values of nearby tissues can be mapped accurately. The typical method is to use an inversion pulse and a long delay to null tissues with very high water content, which also have longer T_1 values associated with them.

Artifacts occur in multi-echo spin echo experiments using slice selective refocusing pulses because of the presence of the imperfect refocusing action of nonideal π-pulses. This is the subject of a detailed discussion in Sec. 26.3 in Ch. 26. Briefly, most artifacts stem from the fact that the phase encoding table is typically found between the $\pi/2$-pulse and the first refocusing pulse. Good sequence design principles relating to overcoming these artifacts are also presented there, and they are also of importance for obtaining artifact-free T_2 maps computed from the multi-echo data.

22.5.4   Choice of Number of Signal Measurement Points

As shown briefly in the previous section for the SSI method of estimating ρ_0 and T_1, an optimal pair of operating points can be found for any two-parameter estimation problem by maximizing the sensitivity of the voxel signal to the parameter of interest. And, when one of the parameters is an omnipresent parameter such as ρ_0, the operating point is chosen such that it can be measured using that single measurement. In the following problem, we determine such an optimal pair of operating points for a two-point ρ_0, T_2 (or T_2^*) estimation from signal measurements using a spin echo (or gradient echo) sequence.

By doing some numerical simulations, it can easily be shown that the SNR of the estimated parameter, be it ρ_0, T_1, or T_2, is maximized by averaging multiple acquisitions of the signal in a judicious manner at the two operating points chosen in Prob. 22.12 rather than spending time on measuring the signal at any other operating points. Using a two-point method for two-parameter estimation assumes *a priori* that there are only two unknowns and that the noise is white. In practice, this might not necessarily be true because of the presence of systematic errors such as Gibbs ringing at edges, partial voluming (and hence bi-exponentiality), as well as excessive motion artifacts. Therefore, it is generally advisable to obtain signal measurements at multiple points (say N in number), from which a mean squared error variable, $\hat{\chi}^2$, can be determined as

$$\hat{\chi}^2 = \frac{1}{N} \sum_i \left(y_i - y(x_i, \hat{\vec{b}}) \right)^2 \tag{22.64}$$

using the notation of Sec. 22.2.1.

Problem 22.12

a) Show that the sensitivity of $\hat{\rho}$ to T_2 for a spin echo experiment as a function of T_E is maximized at the T_E value of T_{E_1} given by

$$T_{E_1} = T_2 \tag{22.65}$$

b) What is the most judicious practical choice for a second T_E value for determining both ρ_0 and T_2 with optimal SNR values?

In general, such an N-point experiment is conducted once in the beginning to verify consistent signal behavior from point to point. For white, additive Gaussian noise, it can be shown that the variable $\hat{\chi}^2$ is a random variable which is χ^2-distributed with $(N - m)$ degrees of freedom where m is the number of parameters that are estimated. The statistics such as the mean and standard deviation of χ^2 random variables can be easily related to the mean and standard deviation of the underlying Gaussian distribution of the measured voxel signal values. Using simple statistical thresholds, it can therefore be determined if any or all of the signal measurements have skewed or broadened distributions because of systematic errors. Similar statistically determined thresholds can be used to determine and eliminate points which are clear outliers from the fit, thereby decreasing the relative error of the fit.

22.6 Calibration Materials for Relaxation Time Measurements

Calibration materials are usually required for comparing calculated values of tissue parameters using a method of choice with a standard measurement method. It is further required that the relaxation time values of the calibration materials be variable. The need to evaluate the SNR performance of an implemented measurement method over a wide range of T_1 and T_2 values motivates this requirement. Such calibration phantoms are typically made with uniform chemical constituency so that a uniform estimate map can be expected for each calibration tube. Salt solutions of cations such as Ni^{2+}, Cu^{2+}, Mn^{2+}, and Cr^{3+} are common choices for creating these homogeneous phantoms at different concentrations. The reason is that these cations alter the relaxation times of water in the solution such that the change is concentration-dependent. Lanthanide cations such as Gd^{3+} are also widely-used choices as they are capable of altering both T_1 and T_2 quite extensively in comparison with the other cations. A further practical choice for the base material for these phantoms are agarose gels.

It is well-known that the T_1 of water in macromolecular solutions varies when macromolecules which are water-bonding in nature are present in solution. Agarose, being a large molecule, plays the role of protein molecules in human tissues, loosely binding water in 'hydration shells,' thereby shortening the T_1 of the water in the gel. The agarose concentration, when in solution, determines the T_1 shortening but more markedly, a T_2 shortening. To get further shortening of T_1, one of the cations can be added to the agarose solution before gelling by heating. The relaxivities (relaxation rate increase per unit increase in concentration of the cation of interest) of most of these cations are well-documented in the NMR literature. Such a set of values are tabulated for these cations in Table 22.1.

Cation	α_1 (/mM/sec)	α_2 (/mM/sec)
Ni^{2+}	0.5	0.5
Cu^{2+}	0.53	0.56
Mn^{2+}	6.67	50.0
Cr^{3+}	3.13	3.13
Gd^{3+}	5.0	4.5

Table 22.1: Relaxivities induced by different cations when present in solution. These values are B_0-dependent; the tabulated values correspond roughly to a B_0 of 1.5 T. These are values extrapolated from fitted curves for the reciprocals of α_1 and α_2 as functions of Larmor frequency that are given in Morgan and Nolle in the references.

Use of agarose gel phantoms with a relatively low baseline T_1 value before further shortening by addition of one of the cations is of further advantage in estimating relaxivities of different extrinsic contrast agents. This is since it is required in these relaxivity calculations to compute the intrinsic relaxation rate of the solution being used before the relaxivity can be computed and it is advantageous to have to estimate the intrinsic relaxation rate of such a shortened T_1 solution instead of the long T_1 of pure water.

Suggested Reading

An overview of using ratios for estimating T_1 and deriving the relative error in estimating T_1, due to the presence of noise, is given in:

- J. N. Lee, S. J. Riederer, S. A. Bobman, J. P. Johnson and F. Farzaneh. The precision of T_R extrapolation in magnetic resonance image synthesis. *Med. Phys.*, 13: 170, 1986.

For a review of different least-squares solutions, an excellent text is:

- P. R. Bevington and D. K. Robinson. *Data Reduction and Error Analysis in the Physical Sciences*. McGraw-Hill, New York, 1992.

The method of using multiple θ-pulses to sample the recovery of magnetization following the application of a π-pulse was first proposed in the following article:

- D. C. Look and D. R. Locker. Time saving in measurement of NMR and EPR relaxation times. *Rev. Sci. Instrum.*, 41: 250, 1970.

The implementation of the Look and Locker method for an imaging application of mapping T_1 is discussed in:

- I. Kay and R. M. Henkelman. Practical implementation and optimization of one-shot T_1 imaging. *Magn. Reson. Med.*, 22: 414, 1991.

A method for determining T_1 from varied flip angle SSI measurements at a fixed T_R was proposed in:

- R. K. Gupta. A new look at the method of variable nutation angle for the measurement of spin-lattice relaxation times using FT NMR. *J. Magn. Reson.*, 25: 231, 1977.

Problems resulting from the use of slice selective refocusing pulses in multi-slice, multi-echo, spin echo, T_2 estimation methods and possible solutions are presented in:

- C. S. Poon and R. M. Henkelman. Practical T_2 quantitation for clinical applications. *J. Magn. Reson. Imag.*, 2: 541, 1992.

The properties in Table 22.1 were obtained by extrapolation from:

- L. O. Morgan and A. W. Nolle. Proton spin relaxation in aqueous solutions of paramagnetic ions II Cr^{+++}, Mn^{++}, Ni^{++}, Cu^{++} and Gd^{+++}. *J. Chem. Phys.*, 31: 365, 1959.

Measuring the actual flip angle or B_1 field depends on the arrangement of coils. Two early papers on this topic are:

- R. Venkatesan, W. Lin and E. M. Haacke. Accurate determination of spin-density and T_1 in the presence of rf-field inhomogeneities and flip-angle miscalibration. *Magn. Reson. Med.*, 40: 592, 1998.

- V. L. Yarnykh. Actual flip-angle imaging in the pulsed steady state: a method for rapid three-dimensional mapping of the transmitted radiofrequency field. *Magn. Reson. Med.*, 57: 192, 2007.

Chapter 23

Motion Artifacts and Flow Compensation

Chapter Contents

Summary: Effects of motion on local isochromat phase are shown to lead to signal loss and ghosting. A method to bring spins moving with uniform velocity back to zero phase at the echo is introduced. Demonstrations of this velocity compensating concept are presented for motion along each of read, phase encoding, and slice select directions. Lastly, a method to view 3D angiographic data as a projection on to a 2D plane is presented.

Introduction

Throughout the text, it has been implicitly assumed that the object being imaged is at rest. In this chapter, the effects of motion on MR images will be investigated. Two major types of motion are considered in these discussions, and there is some overlap between their effects in MR images. Motion due to flow, as found in blood vessels, is one form of motion that affects the reconstructed MR image. Translational motion of tissue, such as the motion of the chest wall during breathing, is another form of motion that will be considered. If an object moves during acquisition of the data (flow or translational), the image will be blurred, and possibly contaminated with other artifacts depending on the type of motion and image reconstruction used. Most motion artifacts found in MR images are due to a combination of flow and translational motion artifacts. Eliminating these artifacts is different for the two

669

sources of motion even though both generate nonzero phase at the echo. For flow (or motion) through a gradient, by appropriately adjusting the gradient amplitudes and timings along the direction of motion, the phase can be returned to zero at the echo so that it appears as if the imaged spins had been excited just prior to being imaged. On the other hand, translational motion between rf pulses must be accounted for by freezing the motion, or by keeping track of the motion and either correcting for it or only collecting data when the tissue of interest is at one spatial location, effectively freezing it.

Flow can occur along any direction and, to avoid image artifacts, the extraneous phase picked up by the component of the spins flowing parallel to an applied gradient is forced to zero or compensated at the echo. When the effects of motion are considered for a given gradient, it is only that component along the gradient that needs to be evaluated. In this chapter, effects due to flow along each imaging axis are considered separately.

Another interesting aspect of most physiological motion is that it is periodic (both flow and translational). If the period of the motion is on the same order of magnitude as T_R for a conventional MRI experiment, then a number of interesting artifacts may occur along the phase/partition encoding direction. The image artifacts due to periodic motion manifest themselves primarily as replicated images or 'ghosts.' This will be shown to be due to the fact that periodic motion causes an additional periodic phase variation in the collected k-space data.

23.1   Effects on Spin Phase from Motion Along the Read Direction

Through most of this section, the analysis will focus on the effects of motion on spin phase and the signal for flowing spins along the read direction. The effects on the slice select direction are addressed through a problem at the end of the section. The types of flow considered are the less complicated ones such as plug flow or laminar flow. Plug flow is a constant flow where the velocity is independent of position in the vessel. Laminar flow is a more realistic flow representation where velocity varies as a function of position as described later. These two examples are sufficiently instructive to allow a good understanding of signal from flow in MRI.

23.1.1   Spin Phase Due to Constant Velocity Flow or Motion in the Read Direction

We start by examining the phase behavior of the spins during the dephasing and rephasing lobes of the read gradient. The easiest motion to evaluate is simple translational motion of an isochromat of spins during sampling

$$x(t) = x_0 + v_x t \tag{23.1}$$

where x_0 is the initial position at time $t = 0$ and v_x is the uniform velocity within the isochromat. These spins see a changing field as they move through the gradient. The phase behavior during the dephasing lobe of the read gradient (see Fig. 23.1a) is given by

$$
\begin{aligned}
\phi_-(t) &= -\int dt\, \omega(t) = -\gamma \int dt\, B(t) \\
&= -\gamma \int_0^t dt''\, G_x(t'') x(t'') \quad 0 \le t \le \tau \\
&= \gamma G\left(x_0 t + \frac{1}{2} v_x t^2\right)
\end{aligned}
\tag{23.2}
$$

Hence

$$
\phi_-(\tau) = \gamma G x_0 \tau + \frac{1}{2}\gamma G v_x \tau^2
\tag{23.3}
$$

The additional phase accumulated from τ to t during the rephasing of the read gradient is

$$
\phi_+(t) = -\gamma G x_0(t-\tau) - \frac{1}{2}\gamma G v_x(t^2 - \tau^2) \quad \tau \le t \le 3\tau
\tag{23.4}
$$

and the total phase accumulated is given by

$$
\begin{aligned}
\phi(t) &= \phi_-(\tau) + \phi_+(t) \\
&= -\gamma G x_0(t - 2\tau) - \frac{1}{2}\gamma G v_x(t^2 - 2\tau^2) \quad \tau \le t \le 3\tau
\end{aligned}
\tag{23.5}
$$

Using $t' = t - 2\tau$ leads to

$$
\begin{aligned}
\phi(t') &= -\gamma G x_0 t' - \frac{1}{2}\gamma G v_x(t'^2 + 4\tau t' + 2\tau^2) \quad -\tau \le t' \le \tau \\
&= -\gamma G(x_0 + 2 v_x \tau) t' - \gamma G v_x \tau^2 - \frac{1}{2}\gamma G v_x t'^2
\end{aligned}
\tag{23.6}
$$

Rewriting (23.6) in terms of its stationary, s, and velocity, v, components gives

$$
\phi(t') = \phi_s(t') + \phi_v(t')
\tag{23.7}
$$

where

$$
\phi_s(t') = -\gamma G x_0 t'
\tag{23.8}
$$

and

$$
\phi_v(t') = -\frac{1}{2}\gamma G v_x(t'^2 + 4\tau t' + 2\tau^2)
\tag{23.9}
$$

The contribution $-\gamma G v_x 2\tau t'$ can be rewritten as $-4\pi k_x v_x \tau$ and represents a shift in position from x_0 to $x_0 + 2 v_x \tau$ (which is the position of the spin at the echo).

The phase behavior for $\phi_s(t')$ and $\phi_v(t')$ is plotted in Fig. 23.1b, demonstrating that the phase of a stationary spin is zero at the echo, but the phase for a moving spin does not refocus at $t' = 0$ for a conventional gradient echo. Specifically, at the echo in the t' frame, the phase for a constant velocity spin is

$$
\phi_{v0} \equiv \phi_v(0) = -\gamma G v_x \tau^2
\tag{23.10}
$$

Finally, the term $-\gamma v_x t'^2$ acts as a filter on the signal which leads to blurring and signal loss. If the read gradient is the only gradient on, as is usually the case during data sampling, then

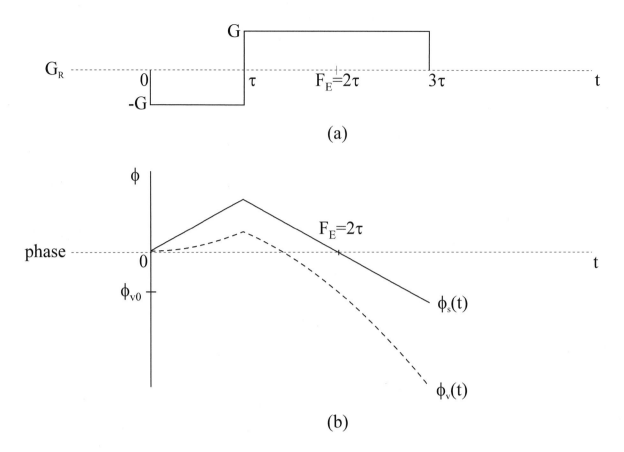

Fig. 23.1: (a) A typical readout gradient waveform whose zeroth moment vanishes at the field echo time F_E. Recall that the first negative lobe is referred to as the dephasing lobe of the read gradient. (b) The phase accumulated as a function of time for stationary spins (solid line) and the additional phase for spins moving with a constant velocity (dashed lines) along the direction of the gradient G accumulate. The actual value of the phase at the echo for the constant velocity case depends on the speed, gradient, and gradient timings.

only v_x plays a role in causing a phase shift. That is, only the projection $\vec{v} \cdot \vec{G}_{read} = v_x G_{read}$ causes the effects described. The effect of spins moving along other axes will be discussed later.

Problem 23.1

Assume $x(t) = x_0 + v_x t + \frac{1}{2}a_x t^2$. Carry through the steps from (23.10) using the gradient waveform shown in Fig. 23.1a and show for constant acceleration, a_x, at the field echo time F_E ($t' = 0$), that $\phi_a = -\gamma G a_x \tau^3$ where ϕ_a is associated with the acceleration term.

23.1.2   Effects of Constant Velocity Flow on the Image

Although it is clear from (23.9) that the phase variation during readout is not linear in time (as is assumed for stationary spins), the effect of the additional velocity dependent phase during sampling will be neglected. It is reasonable to do this for most velocities found in physiological imaging; an analysis of the errors incurred is left as a problem. For finite sampling, the velocity dependent phase in the image will cause blurring along the readout direction. The most significant ramifications are associated with the additional velocity dependent phase at the echo, ϕ_{v0}.

Before these issues can be considered in detail, two different flow scenarios will be defined. First, consider plug flow in a cylindrical vessel where all spins flow at the same velocity (Fig. 23.2a). The term plug flow implies that all of the spins within a given pixel have the same velocity.

Second, consider laminar flow in a cylindrical vessel (Fig. 23.2b), where the velocity as a function of cross-sectional position is defined through the relationship

$$v_x(\vec{r}) = v_{x,max}\left(1 - \left(\frac{r}{a}\right)^2\right) \tag{23.11}$$

where a is the radius of the vessel and v_{max} is the maximum velocity through a longitudinal cross section of the cylinder. For a straight vessel parallel to $\hat{x}$ with phase encoding along y

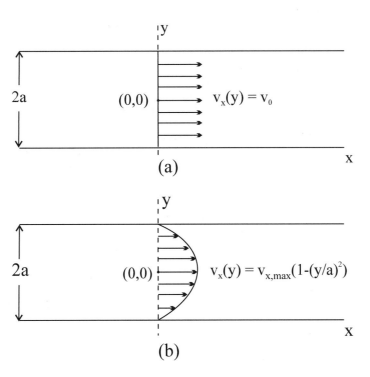

Fig. 23.2: Illustration of (a) a plug flow velocity profile and (b) a laminar flow velocity profile for a cross-sectional cut through a cylindrical vessel.

(assume an infinitesimally thin slice so any variation in $v_x(z)$ can be neglected) then $v_x(y)$ is

$$v_x(y) = v_{x,max}\left(1 - \left(\frac{y}{a}\right)^2\right) \tag{23.12}$$

Consider the simplest case of plug flow, where $v_x(x, y)$ is constant in time for every phase encoding step in a 2D experiment. The more complicated case, where velocity varies from one phase encoding line to the next, is treated in Sec. 23.2. The velocity dependent phase at the echo for a simple bipolar read gradient pulse is a constant and, after the data are Fourier transformed, the image for plug flow in a pixel centered at position (x_0, y_0) is given by

$$\hat{\rho}_v(x_0, y_0) \simeq e^{-i\gamma G v_x(x_0,y_0)\tau^2}\hat{\rho}(x_0, y_0) \tag{23.13}$$

where the 'approximately equal to' symbol is used to signify that other terms present due to velocity dependent phase during sampling have been ignored. Upon taking the magnitude of (23.13), all dependence on phase vanishes and the signal magnitude is recovered as if there had been no motion at all, i.e.,

$$|\hat{\rho}_v(x_0, y_0)| = |\hat{\rho}(x_0, y_0)| \tag{23.14}$$

In addition, the phase from (23.13) could be used to quantify v_x in each pixel, as will be discussed further in Ch. 24. The above treatment for the plug flow case is also valid in the laminar flow case when the spatial resolution is high enough so that there is essentially no significant change in velocity across each voxel.

Signal Dephasing Due to Spatially Varying Constant Velocity Flow

In the case of laminar flow, when the resolution is not high enough to make the plug flow approximation, it is necessary to integrate the spatial variation of the velocity dependent phase over each pixel to understand the effects of signal loss on the reconstructed image. Assuming a uniform spin density $\rho(x, y) = \rho_0$ over a given voxel, centered at (x_0, y_0), containing a spread of constant velocity spins, the reconstructed image is well approximated by

$$\begin{aligned}
\hat{\rho}_v(x_0, y_0) &= \frac{1}{\Delta x \Delta y}\int\int_{pixel} dx\, dy\, \hat{\rho}(x_0, y_0)e^{i\phi_{v0}(x,y)} \\
&= \frac{\hat{\rho}(x_0, y_0)}{\Delta y}\int_{y_0-\Delta y/2}^{y_0+\Delta y/2} dy\, e^{-i\gamma G v_x(y)\tau^2}
\end{aligned} \tag{23.15}$$

If the voxel is small enough so that the velocity variation is approximately linear in y, i.e., $v_x(y) = v_x(x_0, y_0) + \alpha(y - y_0)$ over the voxel, with y integrated from $y_0 - \Delta y/2$ to $y_0 + \Delta y/2$ then

$$\begin{aligned}
\hat{\rho}_v(x_0, y_0) &= \frac{\rho_0(x_0, y_0)}{\Delta y}\int_{y_0-\Delta y/2}^{y_0+\Delta y/2} dy\, e^{-i\gamma G v_x(x_0,y_0)\tau^2}e^{-i\gamma G\alpha(y-y_0)\tau^2} \\
&= \rho_0(x_0, y_0)e^{-i\gamma G v_x(x_0,y_0)\tau^2}\text{sinc}(\gamma\alpha G\tau^2\Delta y/2)
\end{aligned} \tag{23.16}$$

The phase $\phi(y_0) = -\gamma G v_x(x_0, y_0)\tau^2$ is the phase at the center of the voxel and reflects the average velocity of spins in the voxel in this case. The phase at the edge of the voxel is given by

$$\phi(\alpha) \equiv \alpha\gamma G\tau^2 \Delta y/2 \qquad\qquad (23.17)$$

determines the fractional signal loss

$$f(\alpha) \equiv 1 - \text{sinc}\,\phi(\alpha) \qquad\qquad (23.18)$$

Problem 23.2

a) How small does Δy have to be relative to the radius 'a' of a cylindrical vessel to consider the phase across a voxel to be linear (or at least accurate to within 10% say) for laminar flow (see (23.11))?

b) For the carotid artery, $v_{max} \simeq 1\,\text{m/sec}$ and the radius of the vessel is about $1\,\text{cm}$. For a voxel size of $1\,\text{mm}$, is the condition in part (a) met at the voxel at the edge of the vessel? Assume $\Delta t = 20\,\mu s$ and $L = 256\,\text{mm}$.

c) Using (23.18), find the fractional signal loss at the edge voxel.

The dephasing indicated by this formula has important ramifications for understanding flow voids in imaging. For example, Table 23.1 indicates how much signal is lost if the spins are dispersed across various phase intervals. When velocity compensation is not used, the signal from blood is often nonuniform because of the spatial variation of ϕ. Also, the flow pulsatility leads to ghosting as will be discussed later. However, with a flow compensated sequence (see the next section), both of these problems vanish since the phase at the echo is chosen to be zero, independent of velocity, by design.

$\phi(\alpha)$	0	$\dfrac{\pi}{4}$	$\dfrac{\pi}{2}$	$\dfrac{3\pi}{4}$	π
sinc$\phi(\alpha)$	1	$\dfrac{2\sqrt{2}}{\pi}$	$\dfrac{2}{\pi}$	$\dfrac{2\sqrt{2}}{3\pi}$	0
signal loss	0%	10%	36%	70%	100%

Table 23.1: Table describing the dephasing phenomenon due to a spread of velocities across a voxel.

23.2 Velocity Compensation Along the Read and Slice Select Directions

When motion causes phase dispersion across a voxel, or if the phase changes from one T_R to the next, the bipolar gradient waveform is not an ideal design. For this reason, it is necessary to redesign the gradient waveform so that both stationary and moving spins are encoded correctly. These new gradient waveform designs are commonly referred to as velocity compensation techniques.

23.2.1   Velocity Compensation Concepts

One solution to the problem of image degradation due to flow along the read direction is to add another lobe to the read gradient (Fig. 23.3a). The additional gradient lobe is introduced to ensure that the phase at the echo is zero for both stationary and constant velocity moving spins, independent of the velocity of the moving spins. These conditions lead to two equations, one for the zeroth moment of $G_R(t)$ and one for the first moment of $G_R(t)$

$$M_0(F_E) = \int_0^{F_E} G_R(t)dt = 0 \tag{23.19}$$

and

$$M_1(F_E) = v_x \int_0^{F_E} tG_R(t)dt = 0 \tag{23.20}$$

As introduced in Ch. 9, the zeroth moment $M_0(F_E)$ must be zero to get an echo. The first moment, $M_1(F_E)$, must be zero to guarantee $\phi_{v0} \equiv \phi_{v_x}(0) = 0$. The constant velocity v_x is kept in (23.20) to demonstrate that, if these two equations can be solved for a fixed set of timings, the solution will be independent of v_x. The tri-lobed design is used generally for velocity compensation.

Problem 23.3

---

a) Derive an expression for the phase of moving spins as a function of k_x for the gradient structure in Fig. 23.3 that is valid throughout the sampling window.

b) Qualitatively describe the effect of the k_x^2 term on the image. Hint: Use the Fourier transform convolution theorem to describe $\hat{\rho}_v(\vec{r})$ in terms of the convolution of $\hat{\rho}(\vec{r})$ with another function.

Consider an example of velocity compensation. In Fig. 23.3, the amplitudes of the two preparatory lobes G_1 and G_2 need to be found in terms of the physically limited readout gradient lobe of amplitude G. The two moment conditions (zeroth and first moments) lead to the following equations involving unknown gradient amplitudes and the timings shown in Fig. 23.3

$$G_1\tau + G_2\tau + G\tau = 0 \tag{23.21}$$

i.e.,

$$G_1 + G_2 + G = 0 \tag{23.22}$$

and

$$\frac{1}{2}G_1\tau^2 + \frac{1}{2}G_2(4\tau^2 - \tau^2) + \frac{1}{2}G(9\tau^2 - 4\tau^2) = 0 \tag{23.23}$$

or

$$G_1 + 3G_2 + 5G = 0 \qquad (23.24)$$

Solving these equations yields

$$G_1 = G \quad \text{and} \qquad (23.25)$$
$$G_2 = -2G \qquad (23.26)$$

This set of conditions creates a nulling of phase at the echo $\phi(T_E) = 0$, independent of the speed of flow, known as velocity compensation (see Fig. 23.3). Velocity compensation avoids intravoxel spin dephasing and maintains constant phase at the echo independent of v_x. Of course, depending on the FOV and resolution, it may not be possible to attain a value of $2G$, in which case, the gradient amplitudes must be reduced, and the timings varied.

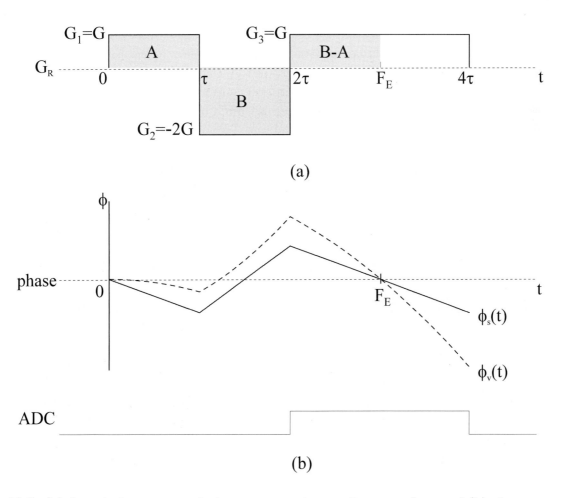

Fig. 23.3: (a) A typical constant velocity compensating gradient waveform and (b) phase accumulated by stationary spins (solid line) and constant velocity spins (dashed line) as functions of time during the presence of such a readout gradient. The shaded gradients sum to zero as required to cause stationary spins to form an echo. The 1:−2:1 ratio of the gradient lobe areas leads to velocity compensation. The ADC on time is shown to remind the reader that sampling occurs only at the second gradient echo during the ADC on period.

Problem 23.4

The minimum FOV is often chosen via the Nyquist relation given a minimum sampling interval Δt.

a) How do (23.25) and (23.26) limit the FOV in the read direction?

b) Does velocity compensation lead to an increase in the minimum achievable value of T_E, relative to that found for a conventional gradient echo experiment?

Generally, in designing velocity compensated sequences, it is important to minimize the echo time because of T_2^* signal loss and the presence of background magnetic field gradients induced by the body itself (see Chs. 20 and 25). In addition, it is important to keep the field echo time as short as possible to avoid higher order flow effects such as those caused by acceleration or flow through such a background gradient. In any case, the application of velocity compensation can make a dramatic difference in the image quality for flowing blood, a prerequisite for good MR angiographic imaging. Such an example is shown in Fig. 23.4.

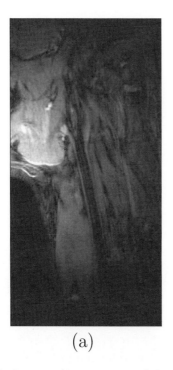 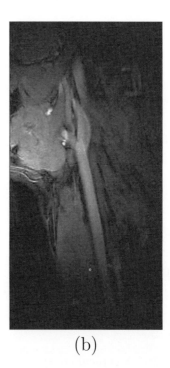

(a)   (b)

Fig. 23.4: Images from a sagittal data set in the neck showing the importance of velocity compensation to overcome signal loss from intravoxel dephasing due to laminar flow in the read direction. (a) The intravoxel dephasing effect and consequent signal loss of the blood are well-demonstrated with an uncompensated acquisition. (b) This dephasing effect is absent in a velocity compensated image acquisition.

Problem 23.5

It is possible to add more lobes and compensate for higher-order effects such as acceleration as well.

a) How does the acceleration phase, ϕ_a, vary with F_E at the echo time? Is the gradient waveform in Fig. 23.3a acceleration compensated? For $\tau = 2.5\,\text{ms}$, $G_{read} = 5\,\text{mT/m}$ and $a = 10^4\,\text{cm/sec}^2$, what is ϕ_a? Will this phase cause signal loss if there is a distribution of acceleration values? What would happen if τ is cut in half and G is doubled (so the FOV is maintained)? What disadvantage exists when doing this?

b) Another variant on read gradient design is to compensate for acceleration but not velocity and to use the remnant phase information to measure velocity. Design such a read gradient.

It is important to remember that, if motion compensation is performed up to and including the nth order flow, the $(n + 1)^{st}$ and higher-order effects are not generally compensated (except in some special symmetry cases where some of the later echoes are by design compensated as discussed in the even echo rephasing subsubsection).

A demonstration of how velocity compensation affects the phase of flowing spins is shown in Fig. 23.5 where a cylinder containing flowing spins passes through an otherwise uniform phantom. The phase of the spins in Fig. 23.5a is clearly distorted within the cylinder when velocity compensation is not applied. However, when velocity compensation is applied (Fig. 23.5b) the phase of the flowing spins is the same as that for the stationary tissue.

Even Echo Rephasing

It is an interesting result that when a series of multiple gradient echoes are generated following a single rf excitation, all of the even gradient echoes may be velocity compensated. This phenomenon is referred to as even echo rephasing. For example, the structure in Fig. 23.3a can be considered a double echo, gradient echo sequence. Sampling could take place during the negative lobe of amplitude $-2G$ as well as during the third lobe of amplitude G. This is an example of even echo rephasing which in turn represents the property that a time-reversed symmetric gradient is velocity compensated. To see this, assume that $G(F_E - t) = G(t)$ (i.e., this is a symmetric function about the time $F_E/2$) and that the sequence is compensated for stationary spins, i.e., the zeroth moment of $G(t)$ vanishes. The time origin is set to the onset of the first gradient lobe. Then the first moment is

$$M_1(F_E) = \int_0^{F_E} dt\, t G(t)$$
$$= \int_0^{F_E/2} dt\, t G(t) + \int_{F_E/2}^{F_E} dt\, t G(F_E - t)$$

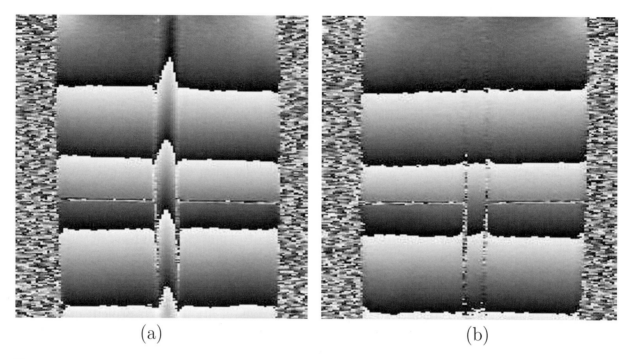

(a)   (b)

Fig. 23.5: Phase images of a phantom containing a cylinder with flowing spins. The velocity profile of the spins in the cylinder is laminar. The cylinder is in the image plane, oriented parallel to the read direction (vertical). (a) Phase image obtained from an uncompensated read gradient structure in the presence of laminar flow demonstrates how phase is affected by velocity within the cylinder. (b) Phase image of the same object now obtained with a velocity compensated structure shows the image phase is velocity independent. The striping in the vertical direction represents phase changing linearly from $-\pi$ (black) to π (bright). This feature makes it possible to view the laminar phase profile clearly. It was induced by shifting the echo by four points off the center of the data matrix in the vertical direction. (Recall the Fourier transform shift theorem (Ch. 11) to understand why four phase wraps occur in the images.)

$$
\begin{aligned}
&= \int_0^{F_E/2} dt\, tG(t) - \int_{F_E/2}^0 du\,(F_E - u)G(u) \\
&= \int_0^{F_E/2} dt\, tG(t) - \int_0^{F_E/2} du\, uG(u) + F_E \int_0^{F_E/2} du\, G(u) \\
&= F_E \int_0^{F_E/2} du\, G(u)
\end{aligned}
\tag{23.27}
$$

If the first echo occurs at $F_E/2$, that is, the zeroth moment is zero there, then $M_1(F_E) = 0$ as postulated.

Problem 23.6

---

a) Redraw Fig. 23.3a with the second lobe (referred to as the dephasing lobe) of amplitude $-2G$ and duration τ changed to amplitude $-G$ and duration 2τ.

b) Show by direct computation that the (second) gradient echo, now at $F_E = 4\tau$ for this double echo, gradient echo sequence, is still velocity compensated.

Importance of Time-Origin in Moment Calculations

Suppose there is a general gradient waveform $G(t)$ with no special properties. Suppose that we want to calculate the nth moment of this gradient waveform at time t_1. Assume that the gradient waveform starts at time t_0 and is zero prior to this time. Then,

$$M_n(t_0, t_1) = \int_{t_0}^{t_1} dt\, t^n G(t) \tag{23.28}$$

by definition. Shifting origins so that $t' = t - t_0$

$$M_n(t_0, t_1) = \int_0^{t_1-t_0} dt'\, (t' + t_0)^n G(t' + t_0) \tag{23.29}$$

Expanding $(t' + t_0)^n$ in a binomial expansion gives

$$
\begin{aligned}
M_n(t_0, t_1) &\equiv \int_{t_0}^{t_1} dt\, t^n G(t) \\
&= \int_0^{t_1-t_0} dt' \left((t')^n + \binom{n}{1} t_0(t')^{n-1} + \binom{n}{2} t_0^2(t')^{n-2} + \cdots + t_0^n \right) G(t' + t_0)
\end{aligned}
\tag{23.30}
$$

From (23.30), it is clear that $M_n(t_0, t_1)$ is the same as $M_n(0, t_1 - t_0)$, i.e., the nth moment is independent of time-origin, if and only if

$$\int_0^{t_1-t_0} dt'\, (t')^{n-1} G(t' + t_0) = \int_0^{t_1-t_0} dt'\, (t')^{n-2} G(t' + t_0) = \cdots = \int_0^{t_1-t_0} dt'\, G(t' + t_0) = 0 \tag{23.31}$$

In conclusion, *the time-origin in a general n^{th} moment calculation can be arbitrarily chosen only when all lower order moments of that gradient waveform are zero at the point of interest; otherwise, moment calculations must be with respect to a particular time (for example, T_E).* This will have important consequences for studying velocity compensation for the phase encoding gradient.

23.2.2   Velocity Compensation along the Slice Select Direction

Flow or motion which occurs along the slice select direction during the slice select process can also lead to signal loss and image degradation. Velocity compensation in the slice select direction is critical to obtaining an artifact-free image in the presence of motion. Motion compensation along the slice select direction is achieved by adding an additional slice select gradient lobe, using an analogous method to that employed in the read gradient case. Gradient lobes are chosen such that the zeroth and first moment of the slice select gradients are zero at the end of the slice select process ($t = t_1$) as demonstrated in Fig. 23.6.

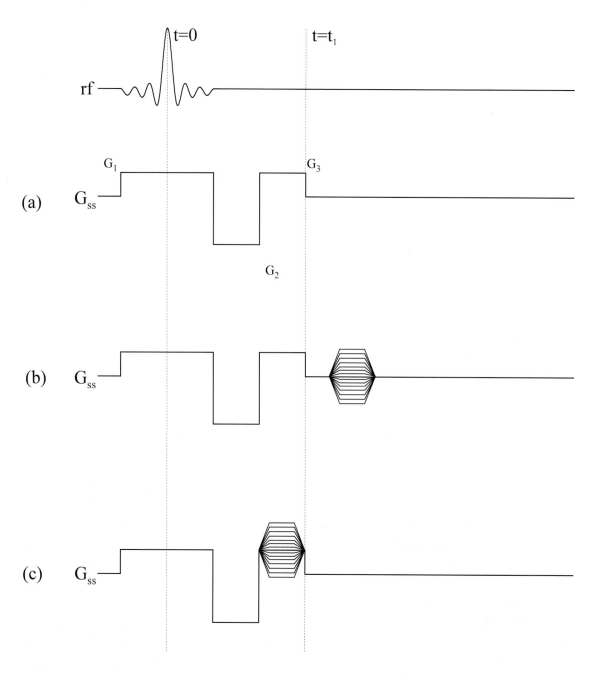

Fig. 23.6: Velocity compensated slice select configurations for (a) a 2D imaging sequence, (b) a 3D imaging sequence, and (c) a 3D sequence with a shorter echo time. Superimposing the phase encoding table on the third lobe of the compensated slice select gradient allows a shorter T_E but at the expense of the resolution achievable in that direction. In the 3D examples shown in (b) and (c), the partition encoding tables are not velocity compensated.

The approximation is generally used that the center of the rf pulse is the time when spins are tipped into the transverse plane ($t = 0$) which is accurate for low flip angles, at least. To demonstrate the design, the analogous structure from Fig. 23.3 is shown in Fig. 23.6 for the slice select direction in a 2D (Fig. 23.6a) and a 3D (Fig. 23.6b) sequence.

Note that the phase encoding in a 3D sequence can be done separately if a short T_E is not required (Fig. 23.6b). This also allows a higher resolution in the slice select direction. Combining the third lobe with the phase encoding table allows the echo time to be shortened (Fig. 23.6c).

23.3   Ghosting Due to Periodic Motion

An interesting flow artifact is found if the effect of some motion on the readout data varies from one T_R to the next with a given periodicity. Regardless of the direction of the flow, or translational motion, the artifacts it creates will manifest themselves along the phase encoding direction as ghosts (see Ch. 12). A discussion of how ghosting would occur for the case of uncompensated flow is presented. Fortunately, using velocity compensation techniques from the previous section, these ghosts can be minimized. An analytical treatment of the ghosts associated with periodic translational motion is also made, because they are not reducible by simple velocity compensation.

23.3.1   Ghosting Due to Periodic Flow

In practice, flow rates in blood vessels change during the cardiac cycle (of period T) due to the pulsatile nature of the flow. For example, for $T_R = T/2$, all even k_y steps will have phase ϕ_1 at $t = 0$ such that $\phi_1 = -\gamma G v_1 \tau^2$ and all odd k_y lines will have phase ϕ_2 such that $\phi_2 = -\gamma G v_2 \tau^2$. Here v_1 is the plug flow velocity along the gradient direction during the first repeat time, during which even lines are acquired, and v_2 is the plug flow velocity during the second repeat time, during which odd lines are acquired. The gradient G is the amplitude of a simple bipolar pulse which occurs either in the read (Fig. 23.1a) or slice select directions. This phase variation leads to aliasing of the vessel, as discussed in Ch. 12. In general, if $T_R = T/n$, there will be n multiple images (ghosts) across the field-of-view L_y in the phase encoding direction, each separated from the other by a distance of L_y/n (see Fig. 23.7). Note that the image is not affected in the read direction except in phase. The above discussion helps understand the positioning of the ghosts but does not give a prediction of their amplitudes. Fortunately, in this case, where only flow is assumed to be involved, velocity compensation as discussed in the last section will eliminate the phase differences between different phase encoding lines, and the ghosts will largely be eliminated.

23.3.2   Sinusoidal Translational Motion

Instead of flowing spins, consider macroscopic motion as found in the motion of the chest wall, for example. Velocity compensation will eliminate the phase due to the motion of the spin during frequency encoding (while the gradients are on), but will not address the change in the initial position of the spins x_0 between repetitions of the experiment. In what follows,

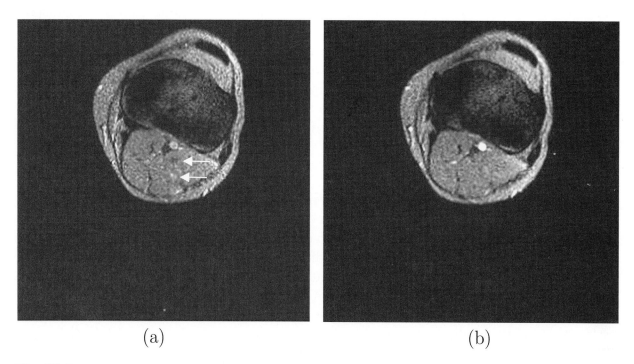

(a)   (b)

Fig. 23.7: Velocity compensation in the slice select direction. Transverse image of the knee obtained with (a) an uncompensated slice select gradient structure and (b) a compensated slice select gradient structure. The uncompensated image acquisition shows ghosting (arrows) as well as some dephasing and consequent signal loss (as discussed in Sec. 23.1.2) whereas both these effects are removed by velocity compensation. The cancelation of signal from the ghosts in some cases (rather than coherent addition to the background) occurs because the phase of that particular ghost is negative (relative to the background).

the effect of motion during frequency encoding will be neglected; instead, the effect of the shift in x_0 will be the focus. Assume that the motion is sinusoidal in time such that each spin oscillates with the same angular frequency ω_m about some equilibrium position x_0 according to (here $\omega_m = 2\pi/T$ where T is the period of the respiratory motion)

$$x(t') = x_0 + \alpha \sin(\omega_m t') \tag{23.32}$$

Here, t' represents the time from application of the first phase encoding step (where $G_y/\Delta G = -n_y$) to the current step

$$
\begin{aligned}
t' &= (G_y/\Delta G + n_y)T_R \\
&= (k_y/\Delta k_y + n_y)T_R
\end{aligned}
\tag{23.33}
$$

This implies that $\rho(x,y)$ is actually a function of time. For a 2D experiment, the measured signal would then be given by

$$s(k_x, k_y) = \int \int dx\, dy\, \rho(x(t'), y) e^{-i2\pi(k_x x(t') + k_y y)} \tag{23.34}$$

However, if a change of variable is made to eliminate the time dependence of the spin density, i.e., $x' = x - \alpha \sin \omega_m t'$, then the signal can be rewritten as

$$s(k_x, k_y) = \int \int dx'\, dy\, \rho(x', y) e^{-i2\pi k_x (x' + \alpha \sin(\omega_m t'))} e^{-i2\pi k_y y} \qquad (23.35)$$

By using the relationship

$$\exp\left\{-(ia \sin \omega_m t')\right\} = \sum_{p=-\infty}^{\infty} J_p(a) e^{-ip\omega_m t'} \qquad (23.36)$$

where $J_p(a)$ is a Bessel function of order p and substituting for t', (23.35) becomes

$$s(k_x, k_y) = \sum_{p=-\infty}^{\infty} \int \int dx\, dy\, \rho(x, y) J_p(2\pi \alpha k_x) e^{-i2\pi(k_x x + k_y y) - ip\omega_m(k_y/\Delta k_y + n_y)T_R} \qquad (23.37)$$

This form for the raw data is sufficient to understand much about the resulting images. An important point to recognize is that motion along $\hat{x}$ determines the amplitude of the ghosts along $\hat{y}$. Notice also that for $k_x = 0$, all amplitude weights $J_p(2\pi \alpha k_x)$, except for $p = 0$, are zero. This indicates that the $k_x = 0$ point in each line is left unaffected only for the central image. Since the k-space weighting factors $J_p(2\pi \alpha k_x)$ modulate the k-space data that would have been obtained in the absence of the periodic motion, these can be thought of as filter coefficients for their respective ghosts. The ghosts are therefore high pass filtered and can be expected to contain only predominantly high spatial frequency (edge) information.

Problem 23.7

a) Write a program to simulate (23.34) and reconstruct the image. Assume that the object is 5 cm × 5 cm with $\rho_0 = 1000$ units. Take $\theta = 90°$, $\Delta x = \Delta y = 1$ mm, $N_x = N_y = 256$, $L_x = L_y = 256$ mm, $\alpha = 5$ mm (the peak sinusoidal displacement), and $T = 10\, T_R$.

b) Assume the motion is in y instead of x and repeat part (a).

c) Discuss the result in the context of ghost location, shape, amplitude, and phase.

The time origin has been chosen so that when $k_{y,min} = -n_y \Delta k_y$ for the first phase encoding step then $t' = 0$. From (23.37), the total phase associated with a given k_y is proportional to $k_y y + p k_y T_R/(T \Delta k_y)$. Equating this term to $k_y(y + \Delta y)$ yields

$$\Delta y(p) = \left[p\left(\frac{T_R}{T}\right) L_y \right] \text{modulo } L_y \qquad (23.38)$$

The modulo L_y behavior is present because the ghosts alias back into the image. The image amplitude is determined by the inverse 2D FT over k_x and k_y and the phase of the pth ghost is $-i2\pi n_y p T_R/T$. The phase of the upper ghost ($p = 1$) is of opposite sign to that for the lower ghost ($p = -1$). Although these ghosts may seem well-behaved, the final image is

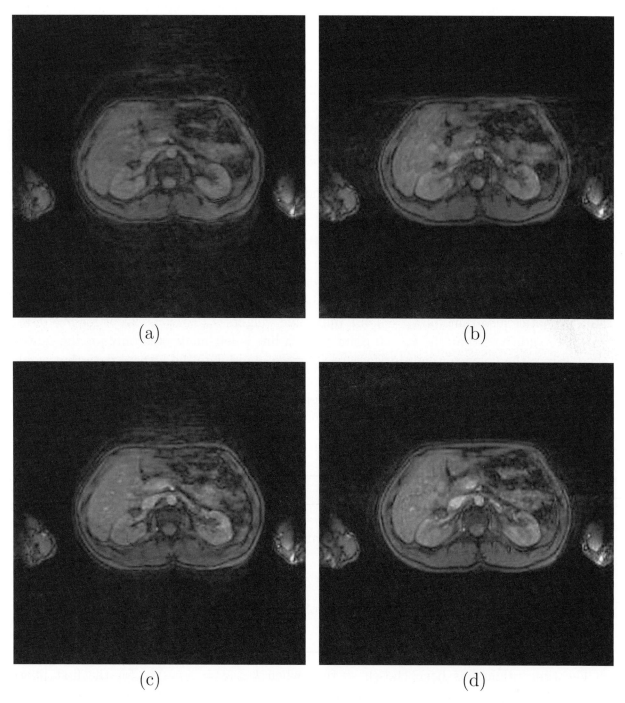

(a)   (b)

(c)   (d)

Fig. 23.8: Simple periodic translational motion, such as that in respiration, leads to ghosting. A gradient echo sequence compensated in both read and slice select directions still exhibits ghosting. Images (a) and (b) were collected with a T_R of 400 ms while images (c) and (d) were collected with a T_R of 200 ms. Images (a) and (c) were acquired with the phase encoding direction in the vertical direction along which chest wall motion occurs during respiration. Images (b) and (d) are acquisitions of the same 2D slice with the read direction now along the direction of motion. In both cases, the ghosts appear along the phase encoding direction and their positions are determined according to (23.38).

not. The ghosts usually overlap the original object in the image domain and, since they have different phases, they can either constructively or destructively add to the central image (see Figs. 23.8b and 23.8d).

For motion along the phase encoding direction, similar ghosts will occur and they follow the same general characteristics and are in the same direction (the phase encoding) as those caused by motion along $\hat{x}$ (see Figs. 23.8a and 23.8c).

As T_R becomes very short so that nT_R is roughly T, then, only a blur of the image will occur. The spatial extent of this blur is equal to the motion during the acquisition (Fig. 23.9a). When the total acquisition is about 15 seconds or less, a breath-hold image is possible (Fig. 23.9b). In this case, no motion from respiration remains and an excellent image is obtained. Ideally, ghosting will vanish with velocity compensation.

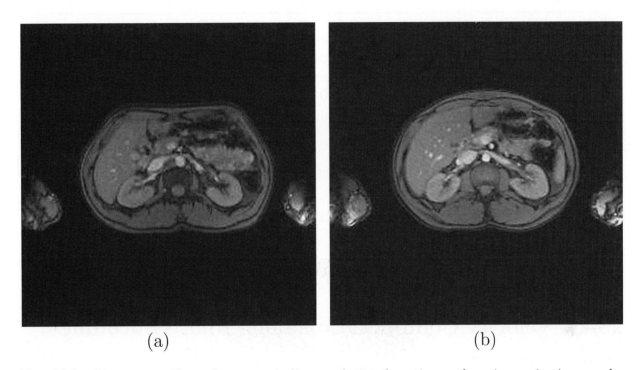

(a)   (b)

Fig. 23.9: Ghosting artifacts due to periodic translational motion such as in respiration can be eliminated either by acquiring over a short period of time or by avoiding the motion. (a) When a T_R of 50 ms is used to acquire the same slice as in Fig. 23.8, the acquisition time is on the order of only three breaths, and the ghosting artifact is imperceptible. Instead, it is replaced by a small blur of the edge features where motion occurs. (b) With a breath-hold, the chest wall motion is avoided. Using the same T_R of 50 ms, the entire slice can be acquired in a short breath-hold period (in this case, about 13 sec). Now, there are no ghosting artifacts or blurring, although subject co-operation is required.

23.3.3   Examples of Ghosting from Pulsatile Flow

Even with velocity compensation, ghosting can still occur due to flow. For example, if $\rho(x, y)$ becomes a periodic function of time due to varying inflow (see Ch. 24 for a detailed description of inflow effects) then the measured k-space signal will vary from one phase encoding line to the next, leading to ghosting (see Fig. 23.10).

If each given phase encoding line is acquired twice for purposes of averaging, then the ghosts will behave as if the T_R in (23.38) were effectively twice the actual value, i.e., $T_{R,eff} = 2T_R$. If 3D imaging is performed, $T_{R,eff} = N_z T_R$ should be used to compute the ghost positions with N_z, the number of 3D partitions acquired. Ghosting from pulsatile (time-varying, but periodic) flow will be dramatically reduced if $T_{R,eff}$ equals the period of the flow variation (physiologically, the pulsatile flow period is determined by the cardiac cycle). In other words, if the signal variation is periodic, as $T_{R,eff}$ increases, the ghosts get farther apart and eventually vanish for $T_{R,eff} = T$ (see (23.38)).

Problem 23.8

The effects of motion (spin dephasing and ghosting), as just described, are most dramatic in 2D slice selective imaging because of the large slice select gradients used for thin slices. An example of the ghosting for a short-T_R gradient echo imaging sequence is shown in Fig. 23.10 for two different T_R values to illustrate the dependence of both the ghost amplitude and position on T_R relative to T, the period of the motion.

a) Explain the location of the artifacts which appear in the images and why they are worse in Fig. 23.10c.

b) Explain why the ghosts in Figs. 23.10b and 23.10d are spaced twice as far apart as those in Figs. 23.10a and 23.10c.

23.4   Velocity Compensation along Phase Encoding Directions

In the phase encoding direction, say y (as well as for the slice select or partition encoding direction for 3D imaging), the effects of motion are different from those in the read-direction. For this section, constant plug-like flow will be assumed since the results obtained here can be extended easily to the more general laminar flow and pulsatile flow cases. The vessel is also assumed to be in-plane so there is no flow along the slice select direction.

23.4.1   Effects of Constant Velocity Flow in the Phase Encoding Direction: The Misregistration Artifact

The main effect of flow parallel to the phase encoding direction is one of spatial misregistration. Spins along each axis in the reconstructed image appear at the location where they were at the time they were encoded by the associated gradient. If they continue to move before the data are collected, they will still appear at the position where they were encoded.

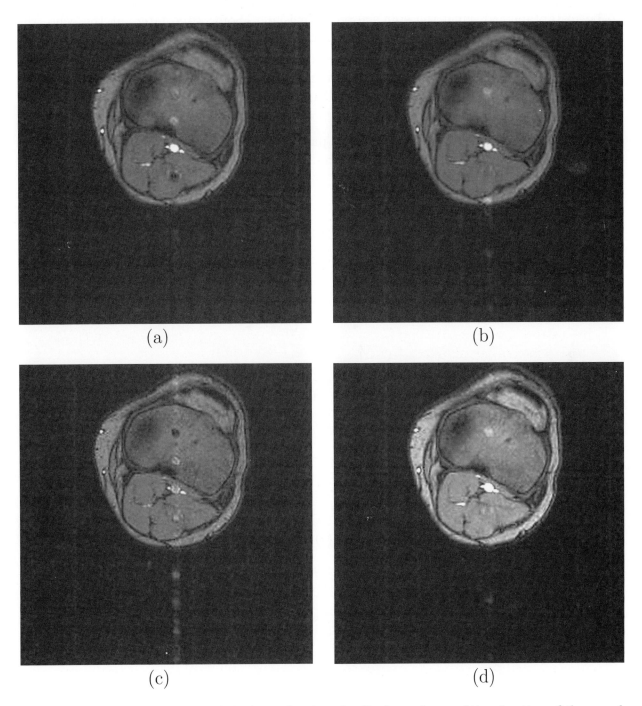

Fig. 23.10: Transverse images of the knee showing the T_R dependence of the ghosting of the vessel signal in the phase encoding direction due to through-plane flow. (a) $T_R = 14\,\mathrm{ms}$, $N_{acq} = 1$, (b) $T_R = 14\,\mathrm{ms}$, $N_{acq} = 2$, (c) $T_R = 14\,\mathrm{ms}$, $N_{acq} = 1$, with no velocity compensation (all other images shown here are velocity compensated), and (d) $T_R = 28\,\mathrm{ms}$, $N_{acq} = 1$. For long T_E, where the background tissue tends to be suppressed, but arterial blood remains bright (see Ch. 24), one can afford to go to even smaller flip angles, making the image more and more spin density weighted and less prone to ghosting artifacts.

For example, consider phase encoding a moving spin at a time t_{pe} (assume phase encoding to be instantaneous) when the spin's y-position is y_{pe}. Some time later, at the echo, the MRI data for the same spin are collected, but the spin has moved to a new position y_{TE}. In the reconstructed MRI image, the spin will appear at the y-position y_{pe} where it was encoded. This can lead to a spatial misregistration artifact in the resulting reconstructed image. A common manifestation of this artifact occurs for an in-plane vessel, with velocity components along the x- and y-axes as shown in Fig. 23.11.

In Fig. 23.11b the physical location of a particular spin is plotted at different times. It is seen that the spin is phase encoded at the position y_{pe}, at a time t_{pe}. Its x-position is

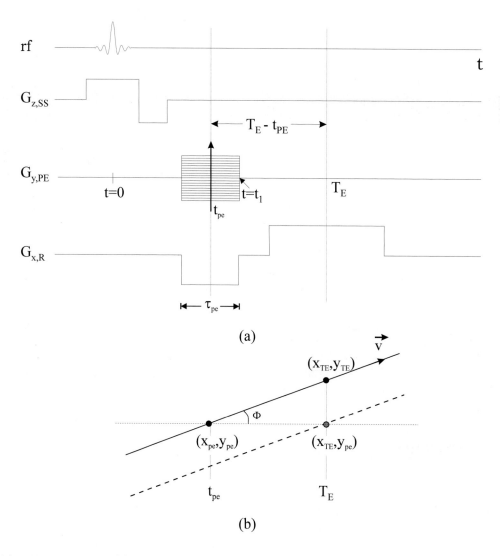

Fig. 23.11: Illustration of (a) the time difference $(T_E - t_{pe})$ between the effective time when phase encoding occurs and the echo time, and (b) the misregistration artifact due to oblique flow. The solid line represents the physical path of the spins. The dashed line is where the same spins appear in the MR image. Spins at the physical location (x_{TE}, y_{TE}) appear at their encoded position (x_{TE}, y_{pe}) in the resulting image.

encoded later at the echo, when data are collected at the position x_{TE}. Therefore, in the resulting image, the spin appears at the point (x_{TE}, y_{pe}), at the location where information for each axis was encoded, but a location that the spin never physically occupies.

Usually, it is assumed that the spin should appear in the image at the physical location it occupies at the echo, but the spin is shifted from its physical location in the y-direction because it moves between the time it is phase encoded and the time the data are read. Given a spin with a constant y-velocity, the shift of the spin along y in the image can be calculated from

$$\Delta y_v = -v_y(T_E - t_{pe}) \tag{23.39}$$

The direction of the shift is dependent on the direction of flow but independent of the point along a vessel (see Fig. 23.12). For plug flow, the whole vessel is shifted or misregistered in the image. If flow is in the reverse direction to that shown in Fig. 23.11, the shift is up instead.

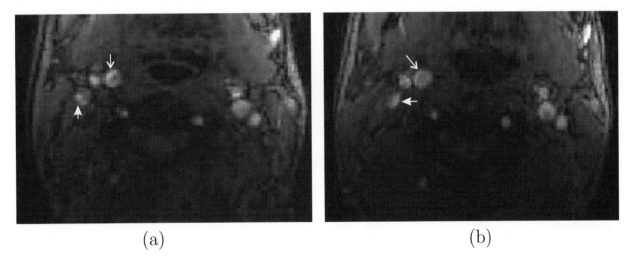

(a)   (b)

Fig. 23.12: Images showing an oblique vessel obtained with a normal phase encoding gradient structure. In (a), the read direction is in the left-right direction while in (b) it is in the up-down direction. Note the misregistration artifact (as shown by the arrows) changes its direction as the phase encoding direction changes.

23.4.2   Phase Variation View of the Shift Artifact

A signal processing view of the misregistration problem adds further insight into this vessel-shifting effect. Recall from the Fourier transform shift theorem that such a constant shift occurs in the image if the k-space data has a linear phase shift proportional to the shift in the image domain. The correct y-position of the isochromat at $t = T_E$ (the time of spatial encoding in the x direction and data measurement) was assumed to be

$$y(T_E) = y_{pe} + v_y(T_E - t_{pe}) \tag{23.40}$$

This implies that to find the shift of the vessel coordinates relative to this actual position, the extra phase accumulated by moving spins must be determined relative to a time origin

$t' = 0$ such that $t' = t - T_E$. Time origin matters for the phase encoding gradient first moment calculation because it has a nonzero zeroth moment (see Sec. 23.2.1). The phase accumulated by constant velocity spins needs to be calculated during a phase encoding gradient waveform on a time-scale as shown in Fig. 23.11a. The phase accumulated by a constant velocity isochromat up to a time $t' = 0$ in the presence of a general phase encoding gradient waveform $G_y(t')$ is given by

$$\phi_v(t')|_{t'=0} = -\gamma v_y M_1(t')|_{t'=0} \tag{23.41}$$

where $M_1(t')$ is the first moment of the gradient waveform $G_y(t)$ evaluated at time $t = t'$

$$M_1(t') = \int_{-\infty}^{t'} t G_y(t) dt \tag{23.42}$$

For the phase encoding gradient waveform in Fig. 23.11, using $t'_1 = t_1 - T_E$ to refer to the time of the end of the gradient in the primed time frame, the first moment $M_1(t_1)$ is given by

$$M_1(t'_1) = \frac{G_y}{2} \left(2\tau_{pe} t'_1 - \tau_{pe}^2 \right) \tag{23.43}$$

This implies that the accumulated phase is

$$
\begin{aligned}
\phi_v(t'_1) &= -\gamma v_y G_y \tau_{pe} \left(t'_1 - \frac{\tau_{pe}}{2} \right) \\
&= -2\pi k_y \left[v_y \left(t'_1 - \frac{\tau_{pe}}{2} \right) \right] \\
&\equiv -2\pi k_y \Delta y_v
\end{aligned}
\tag{23.44}
$$

since $k_y \equiv \gamma G_y \tau_{pe}$. The shift term, Δy_v, is then

$$
\begin{aligned}
\Delta y_v &= v_y \left(t'_1 - \frac{\tau_{pe}}{2} \right) \\
&\equiv v_y t'_{pe}
\end{aligned}
\tag{23.45}
$$

where t'_1 is a negative number. The measured k-space signal for the flowing spins viewed as a function of k_y alone, $s_v(k_y)$, is

$$s_v(k_y) = s_s(k_y) e^{i\phi_v(t_1)} \tag{23.46}$$

where $s_s(k_y)$ represents the k-space data for stationary blood. Hence the vessel shifts by an amount Δy_v in the y-direction according to the Fourier transform shift theorem. This solution indicates that, *effectively, the instant at which phase encoding occurs for constant velocity spins is exactly half-way through the phase encoding gradient.*

Problem 23.9

a) Working through similar steps to those given above, show that the shift always appears to take place with respect to the center of the gradient (equivalent to the point t_{pe} in Fig. 23.11a) independent of time origin for the phase encoding gradient waveform in Fig. 23.11.

b) More generally, show that ϕ_v is proportional to M_1, which can be rewritten as $M_0 t_{cent}$ where t_{cent} is the center of gravity of the gradient, i.e.,

$$t_{cent} \equiv \frac{\int dt\, t G(t)}{\int dt\, G(t)} \qquad (23.47)$$

c) Using the trapezoidal waveform shown in Fig. 23.13 and the definition for t_{cent} in (23.47), find t_{cent}.

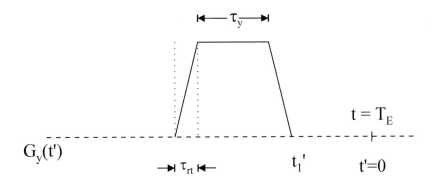

Fig. 23.13: Timings and nomenclature for the trapezoidal gradient lobe moment calculation for Prob. 23.9. Both ramp-up times and ramp-down times, τ_{rt}, are taken to be equal.

23.4.3   Velocity Compensating Phase Encoding Gradients

As shown in the above section, the primary motion effect in the phase encoding direction is a spatial shift of the vessel which occurs because of movement of the isochromat between times t_{pe} and T_E (see Fig. 23.11). The solution to the shift artifact lies in designing a phase encoding gradient which is capable of encoding the position of the constant velocity isochromat at the echo rather than at the center of the phase encoding table (as it occurs in the single phase encoding gradient lobe case). In the signal processing view of this problem, the spatial misregistration was seen to be a manifestation of the extra phase accumulated by moving isochromats because the single-lobed gradient had a nonzero first moment. Therefore, a velocity compensating phase encoding gradient is needed to null the first moment on a time-scale with the echo time as its origin, even though the zeroth moment is not nulled here as it is in the case of a velocity compensating read gradient. Mathematically stated, the two equations which need to be satisfied by a velocity compensating phase encoding gradient waveform are

$$M_0(0) \equiv \int_{-\infty}^{0} \Delta G_y(t)dt = \frac{1}{\gamma L_y} \tag{23.48}$$

and

$$M_1(0) \equiv \int_{-\infty}^{0} t\Delta G_y(t)dt = 0 \tag{23.49}$$

where the time origin is at the echo time T_E. From a physical perspective, when the data are read out using a read gradient, all spins at a given x position (at the echo time T_E) will be measured. They will have come from somewhere else but are all measured at one x value. Therefore, solving for (23.48) and (23.49) will prevent the usual misregistration artifact but only with respect to the time T_E.

Using the experience acquired in velocity compensating the read gradient, consider two pulsed phase encoding gradients, where a second lobe is added to give an additional degree of freedom so that the first moment could be nulled at the echo time as well as satisfying the zeroth moment requirement for phase encoding. The velocity compensated gradient waveform is shown in Fig. 23.14 for a single phase encoding step. The zeroth moment condition reduces to

$$G_+\tau_+ + G_-\tau_- = \frac{1}{\gamma L_y} \tag{23.50}$$

and the first moment condition reduces to

$$\frac{G_+\tau_+}{2}(2t_1' - \tau_+) + \frac{G_-\tau_-}{2}(2(t_1' - \tau_+) - \tau_-) = 0 \tag{23.51}$$

Substituting (23.50) into (23.51), gives

$$G_-(\tau_+\tau_- + \tau_-^2) = \frac{2t_1' - \tau_+}{\gamma L_y} \tag{23.52}$$

and finally

$$G_- = \frac{1}{\gamma L_y \tau_-} \frac{(2t_1' - \tau_+)}{(\tau_- + \tau_+)} \tag{23.53}$$

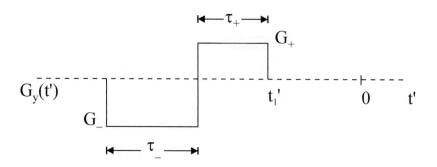

Fig. 23.14: An ideal velocity compensating phase encoding gradient waveform.

Then, G_+ is given by

$$G_+ = \frac{1}{\tau_+}\left(\frac{1}{\gamma L_y} - G_-\tau_-\right) = \frac{(-2t_1' + 2\tau_+ + \tau_-)}{\gamma L_y \tau_+ (\tau_+ + \tau_-)} \qquad (23.54)$$

By identically (and appropriately) scaling both G_+ and G_- based on the Nyquist criterion, the usual phase encoding is accomplished. *The T_E dependence of the velocity compensating phase encoding gradient waveform means that, in a multi-echo sequence, the velocity compensation conditions will be satisfied only for the first echo unless the phase encoding table is modified between echoes.*

Taking a closer look at the problem at hand, there are two equations that must be satisfied; yet, in the above-described procedure, there are four freely variable parameters $(G_-, G_+, \tau_-,$ and $\tau_+)$. This means that there are more degrees of freedom than equations. As a result, this system of equations leads to more than one possible solution. If more constraints are included in the gradient waveform design stage, it may be possible to obtain a unique solution by solving a constrained, nonlinear optimization problem as long as the constraints are reasonable. Possible constraints are field echo time in the readout direction and spatial resolution in the phase encoding direction. The gradient-step waveform thus obtained, and the maximum gradient capability of the system, will then determine the maximum number of phase encoding steps $(N_{y,max})$ and, hence, the spatial resolution along y.

Problem 23.10

Assume that the phase encoding waveform looks like that in Fig. 23.15.

a) Find the zeroth moment, M_0, and first moment, M_1, for each component in Table 23.2 for the gradient waveform shown in Fig. 23.15.

b) Find the ratio G_-/G_+ required to make this a velocity compensated design relative to the origin $t' = 0$ shown in Fig. 23.15. Assume $\tau_+ = \tau_- = 4\tau$ and $t_1 = 8\tau$.

Hint: Use the generalized first-moments for pieces of a trapezoidal gradient waveform shown in Fig. 23.16 and provided in Table 23.2.

Gradient waveform	M_1 at the end of the waveform
(a)	$G_0(3t_0 + 2\tau_{rt})\tau_{rt}/6$
(b)	$G_0(3t_0 + \tau_{rt})\tau_{rt}/6$
(c)	$G_0(2t_0 + \tau_c)\tau_c/2$

Table 23.2: Table for Prob. 23.10. The first moment is calculated here relative to a time origin starting at the left-most side of the gradients shown in Fig. 23.16.

A comparison of a compensated and an uncompensated sequence in the phase encoding direction is shown in Fig. 23.17. The laminar profile generates a marked peak to the left since the rapid center flow shifts a large distance (in this instance, to the edge of the tube) while

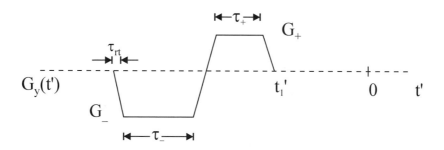

Fig. 23.15: Velocity compensating phase encoding gradient waveform with trapezoidal lobes. All rise and fall times in the waveform are of duration τ_{rt}.

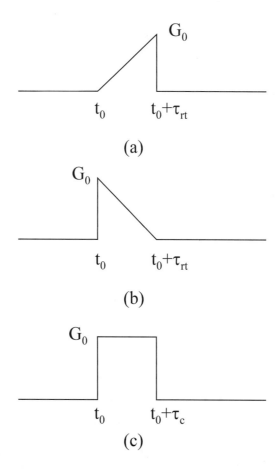

Fig. 23.16: Three pieces which form a trapezoidal waveform referred to in Table 23.2. The ramp-up and ramp-down times are usually the same time. The duration of the flat top, τ_c, is generally different from the ramp times.

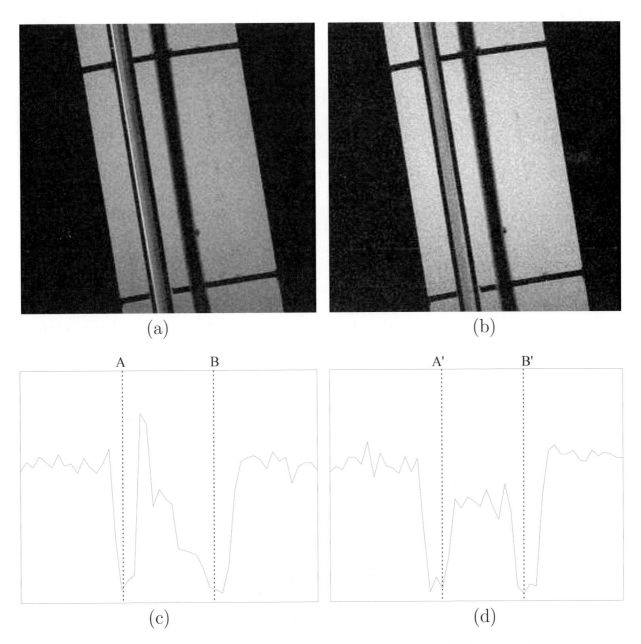

Fig. 23.17: Images showing an oblique cylindrical tube containing flowing material. The flow is upward along the axis of the tube, i.e., in the plane of the image obtained. Images obtained with a short-T_R 2D gradient echo sequence which is uncompensated in the phase encoding direction (image (a)), and with a fully compensated sequence (image (b)). The profiles across the flowing material for these two images are shown in (c) and (d), respectively. The boundaries between the flowing material and the surrounding no-signal region are demarcated as A, B, A′, and B′ in graphs (c) and (d). The large peak in the profile in (c) represents spin signal shifted to the left. The flat profile between A′ and B′ in (d) indicates a successful velocity compensation along the phase encoding (horizontal) direction.

the spins to the left of the center shift less but still tend to fall close to the left edge. The sum total of these shifts gives the profile shown in Fig. 23.17c. The velocity compensated sequence does an excellent job of putting the spins back to where they belong (as evident in the rather uniform profile across the tube in Fig. 23.17d).

23.5   Maximum Intensity Projection

Displaying vascular information can take on many forms. We discuss here briefly just one concept, although numerous others are possible. For a set of slices, it is possible to look through the data at a given angle to see evidence within the 3D volume of vessels. For example, taking the maximum value along a line of sight and writing this value to a point in a 2D display yields a projection image (see Fig. 23.18). This image is referred to as a maximum intensity projection image or an MIP image.

A top-down view of a 3D transverse data set is referred to as a 'zero degree MIP' because the view is taken along the axis running through the volume along the slice select direction (see Fig. 23.19). The images can also be viewed from arbitrary angles, including a sagittal (Fig. 23.19c) and coronal (Fig. 23.19d) view.

By viewing enough angles, a movie can be made of the vessels as if the head were rotating. This is often referred to as a 'ciné' representation of the data set.

The problem with viewing data as a projection is that other bright structures can block or hide the vessels of interest. By cutting out or viewing only a local region-of-interest in each slice and then performing an MIP, this problem can be alleviated. Several examples of these attributes of the MIP will be presented in Ch. 24 after introducing the concepts of MR angiography.

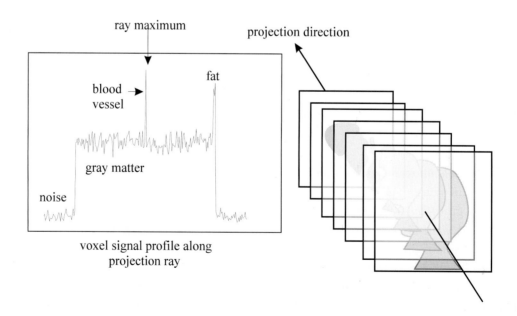

Fig. 23.18: Principle involved in obtaining a maximum intensity projection. The profile shown illustrates the various structures that are typically seen along each projection ray in the head.

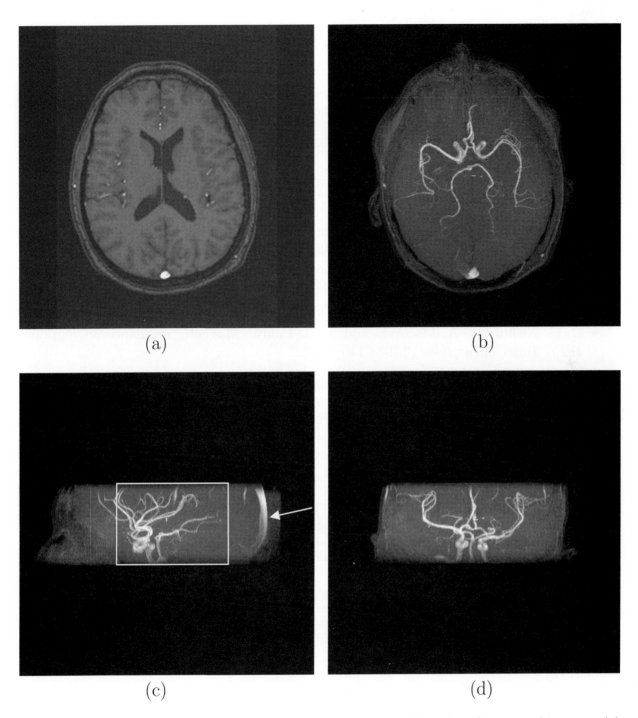

(a)   (b)

(c)   (d)

Fig. 23.19: Maximum intensity projection of large volumes versus MIPs of regions-of-interest. (a) A single transverse image from the collected 3D data set depicts the vessels as bright structures relative to the background. (b) Zero degree transverse MIP from the 3D data set. (c) Sagittal MIP image showing a chosen rectangular region-of-interest which eliminates the bright fatty structures from being projected into the coronal MIP. This allows for better depiction of some vessels which would otherwise be hidden by the bright fat signal and the sagittal sinus (indicated by the arrow). (d) A coronal MIP of the region indicated by the box in part (c).

Suggested Reading

This historical paper introduced phase changes for spins flowing along the direction of the applied magnetic field gradient:

- E. L. Hahn. Detection of sea-water motion by nuclear precession. *Geophys. Res.*, 65: 776, 1960.

These papers describe the concepts involved in velocity compensation:

- L. Axel and D. Morton. MR flow imaging of velocity compensated/uncompensated difference images. *J. Comput. Assist. Tomogr.*, 11: 31, 1987.

- E. M. Haacke and G. W. Lenz. Improving MR image quality in the presence of motion by using rephasing gradients. *Am. J. Roentgenol.*, 148: 1251, 1987.

- G. L. Nayler, D. N. Firmin and D. B. Longmore. Blood flow imaging by cine magnetic resonance. *J. Comput. Assist. Tomogr.*, 10: 715, 1986.

- D. G. Nishimura, A. Macovski and J. M. Pauly. Magnetic resonance angiography. *IEEE Trans. Med. Imag.*, MI-5: 140, 1986.

The concept of even echo rephasing is described in:

- W. G. Bradley. Flow phenomena in MR imaging. *Am. J. Roentgenol.*, 150: 983, 1988.

Periodic bulk motion of the object being imaged and its effects are discussed in the next two articles:

- E. M. Haacke and J. L. Patrick. Reducing motion artifacts in two-dimensional Fourier transform imaging. *Magn. Reson. Imag.*, 4: 359, 1986.

- M. L. Wood and R. M. Henkelman. MR image artifacts from periodic motion. *Med. Phys.*, 12: 143, 1985.

The concept of velocity compensation along the phase encoding direction is described in:

- L. R. Frank, A. P. Crawley and R. B. Buxton. Elimination of oblique flow artifacts in magnetic resonance imaging. *Magn. Reson. Med.*, 25: 299, 1992.

The enhancement of noise when maximum intensity projections are used is described in:

- D. G. Brown and S. J. Riederer. Contrast-to-noise ratios in maximum intensity projection display of MR angiograms. *Magn. Reson. Med.*, 23: 130, 1992.

- H. E. Cline, C. L. Dumoulin, W. E. Lorensen, S. P. Souza and W. J. Adams. Volume rendering and connectivity algorithms for MR angiographic data. *Magn. Reson. Med.*, 18: 384, 1991.

Chapter 24

MR Angiography and Flow Quantification

Chapter Contents

Summary: The enhancement of signal from blood via inflow of fresh spins into a slice of interest via the use of T_1-reducing contrast agents is considered. The extraction of velocity and flow through phase analysis is discussed.

Introduction

The 'flow compensation' of moving spins, as described in the previous chapter, is necessary to visualize blood in MR imaging. In this chapter, we consider the effects of blood flow, in more detail, particularly in the desire for the accurate measurement of the blood vessel lumen (the interior dimensions of the vessel). The imaging of blood vessels (arteries and veins) is often referred to as magnetic resonance angiography (MRA).

In this chapter, we address two major methods to image blood vessels in two or three dimensions. The first is the 'time-of-flight' (TOF) method involving the inflow of blood into the slice being imaged. The TOF MRA sequences are considered to be velocity compensated (the nulling of the first two moments as described in the previous chapter), unless otherwise stated. The second method is based on the information carried by the phase in the image and is called 'phase contrast' or PC MRA. Both of these methods are based on short-T_R, gradient echo methods.

Flow quantification is also considered. This requires knowledge of the cross section of a vessel and the blood's speed at each pixel in the cross section. In simple cases, a quantitative definition of flow is Av, the product of cross-sectional area times speed, which is easily shown to be the same as $V/\Delta t$, the ratio of the volume of blood passing through a cross section divided by the time it takes the volume to pass that point. The latter description lends itself to a measure of 'perfusion' of blood through tissue. The determination of V and Δt and the conditions for which such simple formulas are valid are discussed.

24.1   Inflow or Time-of-Flight (TOF) Effects

In a conventional analysis of imaging sequences, the tissue is assumed to be stationary. As the spins see more and more rf pulses (on-resonance), the longitudinal magnetization approaches the steady-state equilibrium value independent of position within the slice. However, when a blood spin population is flowing in and out of the slice, it may not see the same number of rf pulses and the corresponding longitudinal magnetization approaches steady state in a position-dependent fashion. In this section, the role of inflow of fresh spins into a slice of interest is addressed for short-T_R, gradient echo imaging.

24.1.1   Critical Speeds

Consider plug flow with speed v in a cylinder (Fig. 24.1). If region A with thickness TH is excited with the first rf pulse of a 2D or 3D gradient echo experiment, then a time T_R later, just before excitation by the second rf pulse, the blood in region C, with the same thickness TH, will have completely replaced that in the slice if $z_2 = vT_R > TH$, where z_2 is

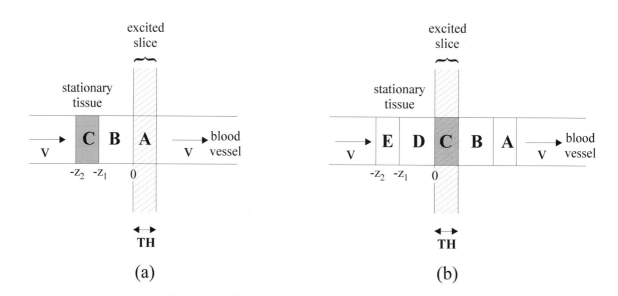

Fig. 24.1: Illustration for explaining TOF in the presence of plug flow with speed v in the z direction. (a) For TH less than vT_R, spins in the blood in region A see one rf pulse and then exit the slice before it is excited again. The spins in region C ($TH = z_2 - z_1$, $z_i > 0$) are not affected by the first rf pulse but (b) see the second one when they enter the slice and occupy the z-region from 0 to TH.

the distance shown in the figure. In general, there is complete refreshment when $vT_R > TH$, or

$$v > v_c \tag{24.1}$$

where

$$v_c \equiv TH/T_R \tag{24.2}$$

To belabor it a bit, the critical speed v_c is that speed at which all blood that enters a region at one rf pulse has left by the next rf pulse. In that case, the z-region between 0 and TH is said to be refreshed by fully 'unsaturated' spins and there has been complete inflow of new blood.[1] The result is a higher signal from blood relative to stationary tissue since the refreshed blood has seen fewer rf pulses and is less saturated.[2] The mechanism which leads to the increased blood signal is sometimes referred to as 'inflow enhancement.'

An important circumstance is the case of smaller speeds. If $v < v_c$, then partial saturation of the blood will begin to take place for distances into the slice greater than vT_R. How this partial saturation manifests itself in an MRA image is considered next.

24.1.2 Approach to Equilibrium

Most MRA methods in use today use short T_R or gradient echo imaging methods. Depending on the flip angle θ, it takes some time for stationary spins in a given isochromat to reach the spoiled equilibrium longitudinal magnetization value of (18.12)

$$M_{ze} = \frac{M_0(1 - E_1)}{1 - q} \tag{24.3}$$

with

$$q \equiv E_1 \cos\theta \tag{24.4}$$

where, as usual, $E_1 \equiv e^{-T_R/T_1}$. For a finite number of rf pulses, the equilibrium value is not yet reached and, just *before* the mth pulse (denoted by m^-), the longitudinal magnetization is instead given by (18.39)

$$M_z(m^-) = M_{ze} + q^{m-1}(M_0 - M_{ze}) \quad m \geq 1 \tag{24.5}$$

Since $|q| < 1$, (24.5) yields (24.3) in the limit, $m \to \infty$. This describes the signal behavior for both stationary spins and moving spins as observed in their moving frame of reference. That is, independent of whether or not a spin is moving, its longitudinal magnetization is found from (24.5) as long as the spin is affected by exactly $(m-1)$ pulses, each of flip angle θ. The relevant transverse magnetization just after the mth rf pulse is found from $M_z(m^-)\sin\theta$. Signal curves for various θ are shown in Fig. 24.2 and exhibit the expected reduction (saturation) with an increase in the number of rf pulses.

---

[1] The adjective 'unsaturated' describes spins whose longitudinal magnetization is at the thermal equilibrium value, M_0.

[2] In this context, a 'fully saturated' set of spins has the equilibrium longitudinal magnetization M_{ze} described in Ch. 18 and reviewed again in this section.

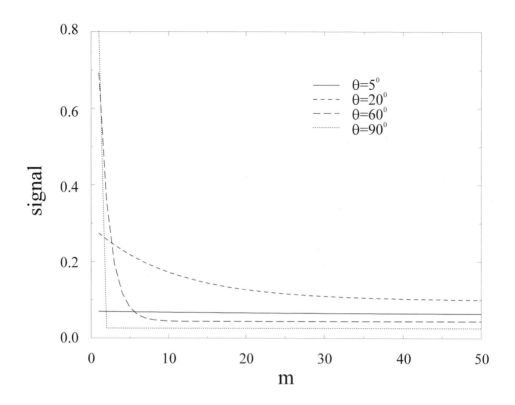

Fig. 24.2: The signal obtained by multiplying (24.5) by $\sin\theta$ is displayed as a function of the number of rf excitation pulses (tip angle θ). The value $T_1 = 1200$ ms has been chosen as relevant to blood at 1.5 T along with $T_R = 40$ ms (or for any experiment with a ratio of $T_R/T_1 = 1/30$). The transverse magnetization is assumed to be zero (i.e., spoiled in some way) at the end of each T_R. Notice the familiar result where the $\pi/2$ pulses reach equilibrium immediately. When motion is considered, the abscissa is linearly related to the distance $d = mvT_R$ that fresh blood has traveled into a 3D volume being imaged during the time of the first m rf pulse cycles. Thus its signal saturates in time, as the moving blood 'velocity segment' sees more and more pulses, fading into the background if the background is stationary tissue with the same T_1. Although the high flip angle examples start off with more magnetization for low m, there is a rapid crossover past which the flip angle giving the highest signal can be associated with the Ernst angle.

24.1.3   2D Imaging

We shall carry through a detailed example with $v < v_c$ for imaging one slice in a 2D imaging experiment where blood flow is perpendicular to the slice as depicted in Fig. 24.3. The experiment consists of a set of p pulses, each a time T_R apart. Consider a subslice or 'velocity segment' defined with thickness vT_R, the distance the blood flows in one repeat time.[3] In different discussions, we may refer either to a moving blood velocity segment (following the spins around) or to a fixed velocity segment through which the blood passes.

Except for edge effects, a fixed or moving velocity segment within the overall slice sees each additional rf pulse administered. For convenience, in the analysis to follow, assume

---

[3]The velocity segment can also be referred to as an imaginary 'bolus' of length vT_R.

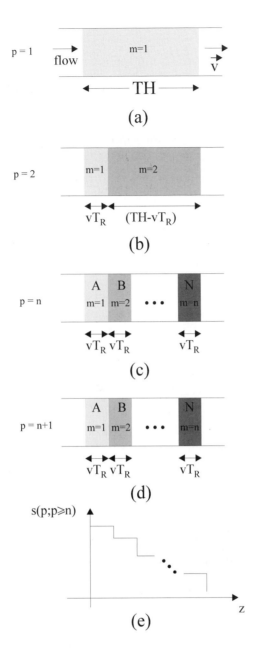

Fig. 24.3: Saturation of spins flowing into a slice is demonstrated in this figure as a function of the number of rf pulses p. (a) At the instant after the first rf pulse, all excited spins have equal transverse magnetization. The index m indicates the number of rf pulses seen in a given velocity segment (and $m-1$ then refers to the number of rf pulses relevant to the evolution of the longitudinal magnetization present in that velocity segment just before the pth pulse). (b) At the instant after the second pulse, a fraction of excited blood has exited and new blood has replaced it. The old (new) blood has experienced 2 rf pulses (1 rf pulse). A steady state is obtained where spins with longitudinal magnetization M_0 freshly enter the slice between rf pulses into the first of the n fixed velocity segments along the direction of flow as illustrated in (c) and (d) for the nth and $(n+1)^{st}$ pulse. The regions with the lower m labels have the higher signal (lighter shading), thanks to the inflow of fresh blood, while the darker shading represents lower (more saturated) signal. The signal behavior as a function of position of the artificially created velocity segments in the direction of flow in the steady state is shown schematically in (e).

that an exact integer n of velocity segments fit into the slice. We have

$$n \equiv (TH/vT_R) \qquad \text{with } n \geq 2 \tag{24.6}$$

(since the $n = 1$ case corresponds to the $v = v_c$ case). For any integer n, all spins in a given fixed velocity segment (and, strictly speaking, provided one of its edges are coincident with a slice edge at some rf pulse instant) will experience the same number of rf pulses as time goes on. This subdivision of the imaged slice makes it possible to follow the signal behavior of the entire slice in the presence of the blood flow. And, in general, for arbitrary, but large values of TH/vT_R, a subdivision according to the nearest integer will lead to a reasonable approximation.

Before any rf pulses, the full thermal equilibrium magnetization value M_0 will be available, and the signal from the slice after the first rf pulse is given by

$$M_\perp(1) = M_0 \sin\theta \tag{24.7}$$

The spins in the slice just before the second rf pulse will have two populations, one which is still inside occupying a fraction $(1 - vT_R/TH)$ of the slice, and the other from incoming blood occupying the remaining fraction vT_R/TH (after one T_R, blood from region A has moved into region B of Fig. 24.3). Hence, the signal from the same slice just after the action of the second pulse is given by the sum of these two contributions. From the $p = 1, 2$ terms in (24.5) rotated through θ

$$M_\perp(2) = \left((1 - \frac{1}{n})(M_{ze} + q(M_0 - M_{ze})) + \frac{1}{n}M_0 \right) \sin\theta \tag{24.8}$$

More generally, the velocity segment of blood that occupied region A just before the first rf pulse, will have moved, just before the pth pulse, an additional distance $(p-1) \cdot v \cdot T_R$. At the instant after the pth pulse, it thus occupies the pth fixed velocity segment of the slice and has experienced p pulses. And at the instant that the nth pulse has occurred, this particular spin population will have experienced a total of n pulses, and occupy the fixed velocity segment labeled N. At the other end, the spin population that moved just prior to section A before the $(n-1)^{st}$ pulse to occupy section A will have experienced only one rf pulse just after the nth rf pulse of the experiment. Altogether, there will be n spin population fixed velocity segments (each of thickness vT_R) experiencing $m = 1, 2, \cdots n$ rf pulses, respectively, the number m increasing with position z in the direction of the flow.[4] By the time the total number p of pulses reaches the total number n of fixed velocity segments, a steady signal is obtained from the blood vessel and is given by a sum over all the velocity segments and their respective contributions derived from (24.5)

$$\begin{aligned} S(p \geq n) &= \Lambda\frac{\sin\theta}{n}\sum_{m=1}^{n}\left(M_{ze} + (M_0 - M_{ze})q^{m-1}\right) \\ &= \Lambda\sin\theta\left(M_{ze} + (M_0 - M_{ze})\frac{1 - q^n}{n(1-q)}\right) \end{aligned} \tag{24.9}$$

---

[4]The mth velocity segment sees m pulses when n rf pulses have been administered to the full slice. Notice that the longitudinal magnetization just before the pth pulse in each segment determines its contribution to the signal just after the pth pulse. Thus the relevant values of the segment magnetization depend on $m - 1$ pulses as seen in the individual terms in the sum in (24.5).

with amplifier gain and other factors represented by Λ.

Problem 24.1

In review, the steady signal behavior for a blood vessel perpendicular to a thick 2D slice with n effective velocity segments is described by (24.9). The steady or equilibrium behavior is reached as soon as the number of rf pulses reaches or exceeds n. Each respective velocity segment has experienced m pulses where $m \in \{1, 2, \cdots n\}$ just *after* the pth pulse for $p \geq n$. Derive (24.9) including the step where the summation is carried out.

A comparison of the saturation of a given velocity segment with that integrated over the whole slice is shown in Figs. 24.4a and 24.4b, respectively. For the saturated or steady behavior of the whole slice, recall that the number p of pulses must be greater than or equal to n, a parameter determined by the velocity of the spins and the slice thickness.

24.1.4 3D Imaging

In 3D imaging, we may be able to obtain spatial information on the scale of the individual velocity segments of a given slab. Recall an advantage of 3D imaging is the ability to obtain thin slices for high resolution imaging and short T_E whereas a thin slice 2D experiment requires a long rf pulse time to create a sharp slice profile and the thickness is limited by the available gradient strength. However, the saturation encountered as the blood propagates into the slab remains an important issue in 3D image contrast.

The analysis of the signal for a velocity segment of the slab is the same as for the 2D slice. Equation (24.3) remains appropriate for the signal from a given segment in a 3D slice where m represents both the velocity segment number and the number of rf pulses experienced by that segment.[5] The segmentation in Fig. 24.3 and the signal plots in Figs. 24.2 and 24.4a apply here as well, and, as the blood moves into the slab, it becomes increasingly saturated. While at large flip angles only a few pulses are needed for saturation, at low flip angles, the signal does not reach the steady-state level even if the spins have experienced as many as 10 rf pulses. The by now familiar point is that the longitudinal magnetization is only slightly tipped for small θ so that it does not need time to recover. Even slow flowing spins are enhanced throughout a 3D region when small flip angles are used.

Consider another perspective for the result that smooth, fast blood flow will tend to produce a larger signal than will slower blood flow or a stationary background (brain parenchyma or muscle, for example). Fig. 24.5 exhibits a realistic spatial velocity distribution for the carotid artery and its bifurcation. The length of each vector represents how far the blood has traveled between each rf pulse and the direction represents the direction of the flow of a spin at that position. For laminar flow, the center or faster flow will see the fewest number of rf pulses and will be brightest at any cross section (see Fig. 24.5b).

---

[5]A series of n pre-pulses, or dummy cycles, may be applied prior to collecting the data so that the blood in each partition has reached the equilibrium condition shown in Fig. 24.3c.

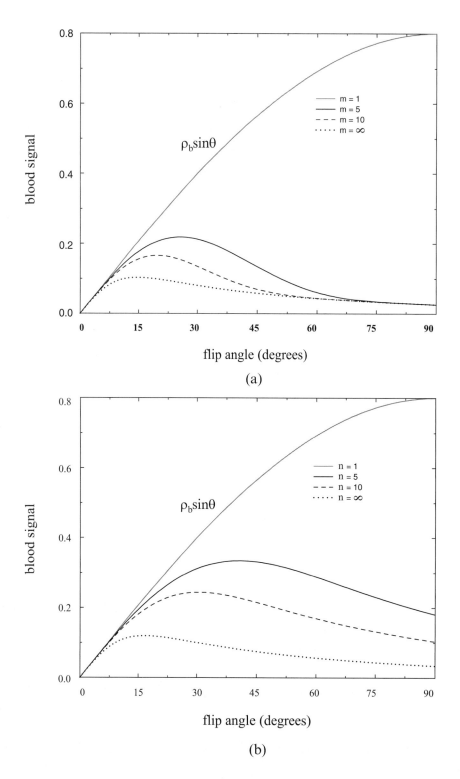

(a)

(b)

Fig. 24.4: Signal from blood as a function of flip angle θ with $T_R = 40\,\mathrm{ms}$ and $T_1 = 1200\,\mathrm{ms}$ for (a) a thin slice (for blood in 2D or 3D or any stationary tissue segment) and (b) the full 2D slice, showing the dependence on the number of pulses. In (a), the number of pulses seen by the thin slice is m and, in (b), the number of pulses administered to the full slice is greater than or equal to n. The slices are perpendicular to the flow. The normalization is such that, for one thin slice and $m = 1$, the signal is $\rho_b \sin \theta$ where ρ_b is stylized as 0.8 relative to the spin density of water.

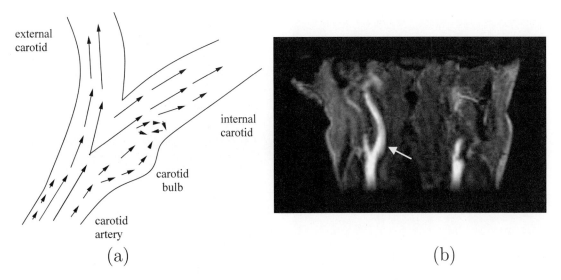

(a)   (b)

Fig. 24.5: (a) Flow pattern seen at some point in a vessel such as that for the carotid artery branching into the internal and external carotids. The carotid bulb area can have vortex flow which is a circulating flow pattern where spins remain longer than those spins flowing straight through the vessel. (b) A coronal slice through the carotid artery of a volunteer showing the 'streamlining' effect where fast flow is bright and slow flow (as in the carotid bulb) is darker.

An example of 3D imaging of blood flowing up through the neck of a pig is shown in Fig. 24.6. The signal remains constant along the blood vessels for low flip angles (faster recovery) in Fig. 24.6a, where the background is suppressed by 'magnetization transfer contrast' illustrated later in this chapter. More saturation is evident in Fig. 24.6b for a larger flip angle and the TOF effect is clearly present. The suppression of smaller vessels, in which the flow is slower, is also observed in this figure.

24.1.5 Understanding Inflow Effects for Small Velocities

The enhanced signal from moving blood may be thought of as mimicking a tissue with a shorter T_1. The goal of this subsection will be to find an expression for a 'pseudo-T_1' or $T_{1,flow}$ behavior of the blood due to inflow in 2D imaging. Note that, as a function of θ, the shape of the curves in Fig. 24.4b is similar to $M_{ze} \sin \theta$ or $\hat{\rho}(\theta)$ in Fig. 18.2b (or the $m = \infty$ case in Fig. 24.4a). Hence, it should be possible to model the behavior of moving blood approximately as a tissue with a shorter T_1, the T_1 shortening depending on the speed of flow.

A simple implementation of this idea is to write a differential equation for $M_{z,flow}(p,t)$, the average longitudinal magnetization over all n velocity segments of the slice for p pulses at time t. Again the flow is assumed to be perpendicular to the slice and the condition $p \geq n$ for a steady signal is assumed. From the increase due to the flow of fresh magnetization into the first segment combined with the decrease due to the flow out of the last segment, the

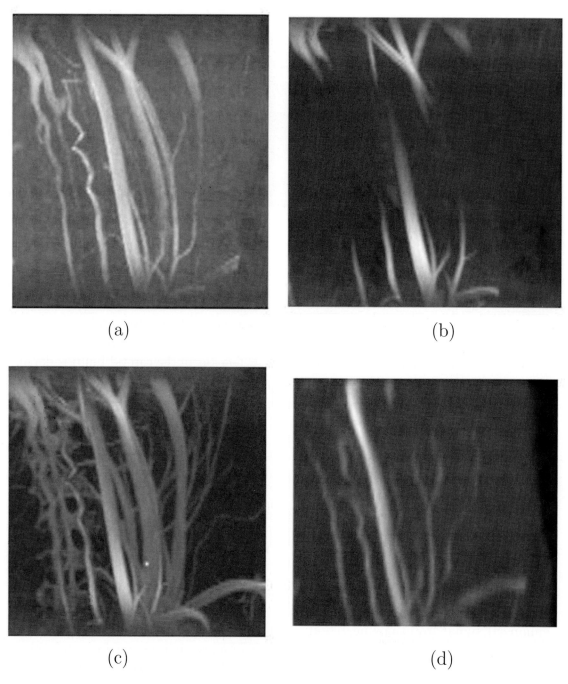

(a)   (b)

(c)   (d)

Fig. 24.6: A short-T_R 3D transverse data acquisition of blood flowing through the neck of a pig. The images shown are constructed by a coronal maximum intensity projection (see Ch. 23) of a stack of the transverse slices. (a) The signal intensity is fairly constant in a low flip angle (15°) acquisition. (b) A powerful demonstration of the saturation effect is obtained when the same region is imaged with a large flip angle such as 55°. Note the decrease in signal of the arteries from bottom upwards and of the veins from top downwards due to spin saturation. Smaller vessels with slower flow are so saturated that they are not even visible on the MIP. (c) A 'post-contrast' MIP of the vessels and (d) a 'pre-contrast' MIP from a 2D MRA acquisition are shown for comparison (see Sec. 24.2 for a discussion of the use of contrast agents to obtain an enhanced vascular signal).

net change is approximated by

$$dM_{z,flow}(p,t) = M_0 \frac{vdt}{TH} - M_{z,flow}(n-1,t)\frac{vdt}{TH} \qquad (24.10)$$

Taking $M_{z,flow}(p,t) \approx M_{z,flow}(p-1,t) \approx M_{z,flow}(n-1,t) \equiv M_{z,flow}(t)$ yields

$$\frac{dM_{z,flow}(t)}{dt} = (M_0 - M_{z,flow}(t))\frac{v}{TH} \qquad (24.11)$$

With the identification

$$T_{1,flow} \equiv \frac{TH}{v} \qquad (24.12)$$

this is seen to have the same form as the T_1 relaxation term in the Bloch equation. The effective T_1 due to the inflow effect is then found from

$$\frac{1}{T_{1,eff}} = \frac{1}{T_1} + \frac{1}{T_{1,flow}} \qquad (24.13)$$

As v becomes small, $T_{1,eff} \to T_1$ and as v becomes large, $T_{1,eff} \to 0$. When $v \geq v_c$, all signal is refreshed and $T_{1,eff}$ is zero.

24.2 TOF Contrast, Contrast Agents, and Spin Density/ T_2^*-Weighting

Now that we understand the behavior of the blood signal as it penetrates deeper into an imaging slice, the next goal is to further increase its signal relative to the background. This can be done by a variety of means. First, the signal can be preferentially enhanced deeper into the slab to offset the TOF saturation as a function of position. This is accomplished by varying the flip angle as a function of position along the slice select direction, typically by linearly increasing the flip angle along the direction of flow (see Figs. 24.7 and 16.13). Second, contrast between blood and background tissue can be increased by using a long T_E scan (see Fig. 24.8). Third, the signal from the background tissue can be suppressed by using 'magnetization transfer saturation.'[6] The MTS pulse suppresses WM and GM leading to enhanced contrast from the blood which is essentially not suppressed (see Fig. 24.9). Fourth, a T_1-reducing contrast agent can be used to increase the signal from blood, the next subject to be discussed.

24.2.1 Contrast Agents

The use of T_1-reducing contrast agents which can be injected into the bloodstream offers the opportunity to selectively enhance signal from blood without altering signal from the surrounding tissue. Reducing T_1 will lead to an increase in SNR for both magnitude and phase

---

[6]Magnetization transfer saturation is a means by which spins residing outside the normal on-resonant frequency are slowly saturated. These spins then exchange into the on-resonant range but now have little signal left. This suppression is best-achieved with specially designed rf pulses whose duration is long enough to cause a significant effect.

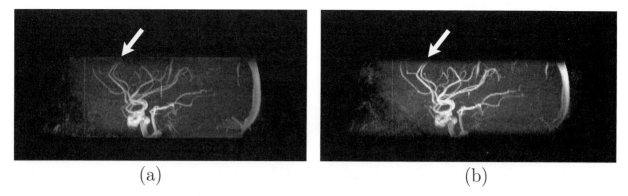

Fig. 24.7: A spatially varying rf pulse acquisition is used to overcome the saturation effect as a function of distance along the slice select direction. Here, flow is assumed to be predominantly occurring in the slice select direction (in the up/down direction here). (a) A thick-slice 3D MRA acquisition shows the saturation effect of the arteries toward the top of the head (arrows) whereas (b) the spatially varying rf pulse acquisition of the same slice shows little visible saturation effect. The arrows in (a) and (b) point to a vessel exiting the top of the slice which is clearly visible in (b), but less so in (a).

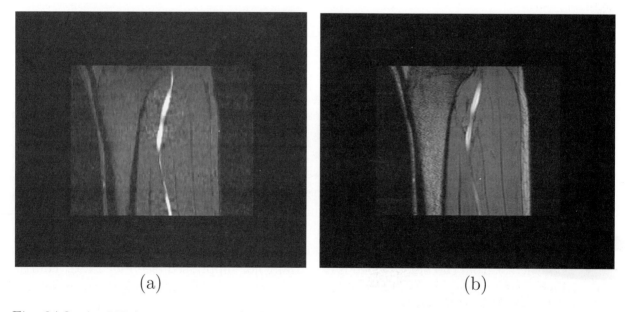

Fig. 24.8: An MRA acquisition in the leg obtained by using a long T_E acquisition utilizing the longer T_2^* of blood in comparison with other surrounding tissues. (a) A conventional 2D MRA sequence which highlights the slow flow, thanks to the TOF effect. (b) A similar suppression of the surrounding tissues in comparison with the blood is obtained by using a long T_E acquisition. Although there is still some time-of-flight effect present, venous blood has a shorter T_2^* than arterial blood and is further suppressed this way. No inflow is required to obtain bright arterial signal relative to muscle when a longer T_E is used. The local MIP shown in (b) was obtained from images that were collected using a T_E of 24 ms, a T_R of 46 ms and a flip angle of $25°$.

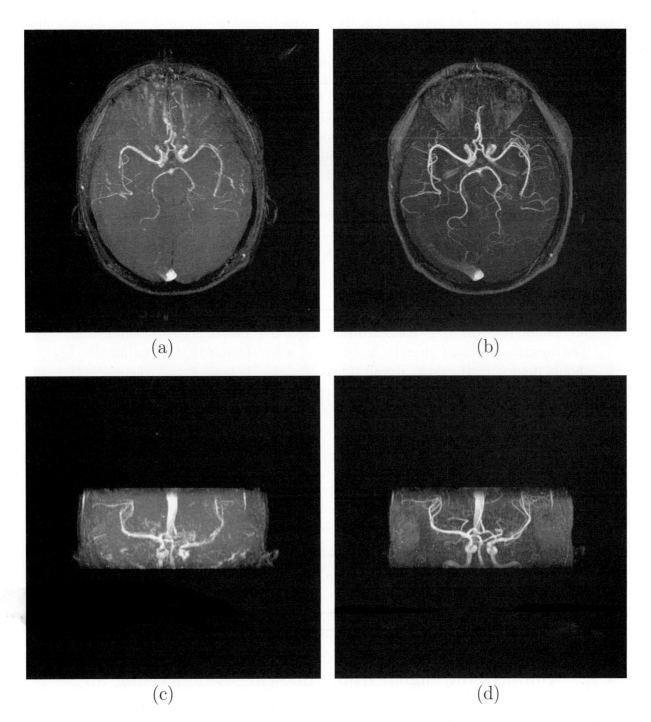

(a)

(b)

(c)

(d)

Fig. 24.9: 'Magnetization transfer saturation' can be utilized to preferentially suppress the background brain tissues to highlight even the more readily saturated small vessels. In this case, a spin density-weighted acquisition can be used to obtain enhanced MR angiograms. (a) Vessels are more easily viewed in a 3D MRA acquisition by performing an MIP. This particular example was obtained using a T_1-weighted sequence. This highlights the large vessels, which have faster flow, while the small vessels are invisible. (b) An MIP from an MRA acquisition using an MTS pulse prior to each excitation pulse now highlights the small vessels as well. Note the suppression of most GM-WM contrast in the background. A coronal view in (c) and (d) also reveals improved vessel visibility with the use of MTS.

imaging. In most imaging applications, the contrast agent is assumed to be intravascular (i.e., it stays within the blood vessel). To appreciate the significance of using a contrast agent for MRA, the signal is plotted as a function of flip angle at steady state for several values of T_1 corresponding to different contrast agent doses (see Fig. 24.10). For example, if the $1/T_1$ relaxivity of the agent is 5 /mM/sec and the concentration in the blood is 0.167 mM in the equilibrium state, then the post-contrast T_1 of blood would be reduced from 1200 ms to 600 ms. With increasing dosage, the T_1 is reduced more and a higher blood signal results for a given flip angle. This reduction in T_1 and the concomitant increase in blood signal is well illustrated in Figs. 24.6c, 24.6d, 24.11, and 24.12, where a large number of blood vessels are enhanced post-contrast injection, and are displayed as bright structures. Even though blood signal is significantly enhanced, and more vessels are apparent on the MIP in Fig. 24.12b than Fig. 24.12a, the MIP operation is still not ideal in that small vessels and low amplitude regions can be significantly suppressed or lost.

Problem 24.2

A common contrast agent concentration injected in people is 0.5 M (moles/liter). The injection is usually given by body weight using the rule that 0.1 millimoles/kg should determine the dose. Recall that $1/T_{1,post} = 1/T_{1,pre} + \alpha[c]$ where α is the relaxivity in units of /mM/sec and $[c]$ is the concentration of contrast agent in mM.

    a) Show that, for a 50 kg person, this implies an injection of 10 cc of the contrast agent.

    b) Assume the blood volume is 5 liters and that half of the contrast agent is 'extravasated' (i.e., it leaves the blood and is taken up elsewhere in the body). What is the concentration of contrast agent now in the blood?

    c) For a relaxivity of 5 /mM/sec, what is the resulting T_1 of the blood?

    d) How much must be injected to reduce T_1 of blood from 1200 ms to 300 ms and 100 ms?

24.2.2   Suppressing Signal from Inflowing Blood Using an Inversion Pulse

The focus up to this point has been to create an image where blood is brighter than the surrounding tissue. Inflow could be used to enhance the signal of blood since the blood from outside the slice has not seen as many rf pulses as has the stationary tissue inside the slice. On the other hand, it is also possible to minimize the signal from the blood by carefully designing the sequence. For example, consider the sequence design in Fig. 24.13. The longitudinal magnetization of all spins in the body (sample) is inverted with a nonselective hard pulse. Then a single region-of-interest is reinverted with a selective rf pulse to restore its longitudinal magnetization. If a delay of $T_I = T_{I,null} = T_{1,blood} \ln 2$ is used between the nonselective

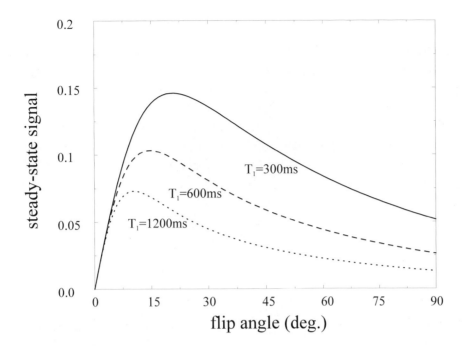

Fig. 24.10: Plot of the blood signal for $m = \infty$, and $T_R = 20\,\text{ms}$ with $T_1 = 1200\,\text{ms}$, $600\,\text{ms}$, and $300\,\text{ms}$. Even blood which sees a large number of rf pulses with $T_1 = 300\,\text{ms}$ still has a signal much higher than that for tissue with $T_1 = 1200\,\text{ms}$. For this reason, T_1-reducing contrast agents play a key role in enhancing vascular information.

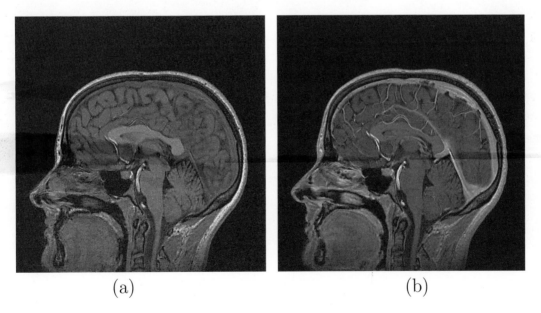

(a)   (b)

Fig. 24.11: Images of the brain pre- and post-contrast injection from a 3D T_1-weighted data set acquired in a sagittal fashion so that there is essentially no inflow effect except in the large vessels. (a) A single 1 mm thick sagittal image showing the saturation effect in the pre-contrast image, and (b) enhancement of the blood vessels in the post-contrast image.

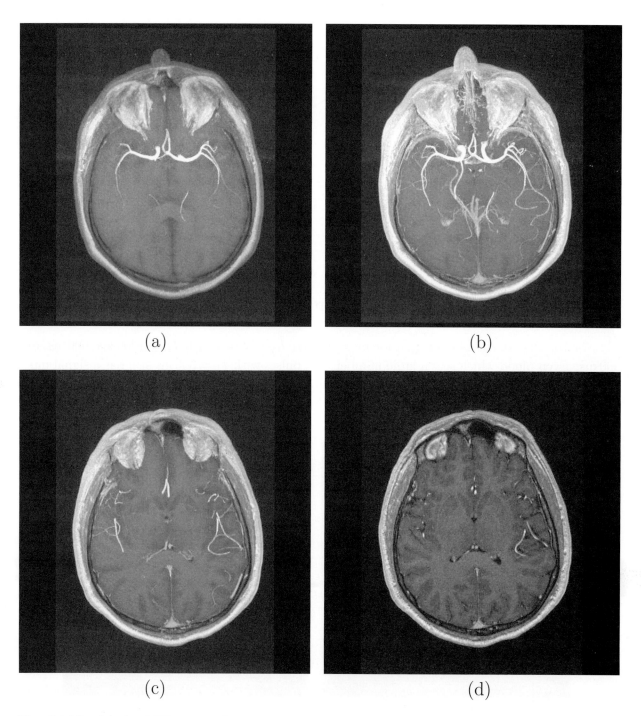

(a)

(b)

(c)

(d)

Fig. 24.12: (a) An MIP image from a pre-contrast 3D data set. In comparison, (b) the post-contrast 3D data set MIP over the entire volume shows an abundance of vascular information. However, projection over a smaller volume as in (c) can also be used to study specific parts of the vascular tree. (d) Examining only a single slice better depicts smaller vessels than in the global MIP image shown in (b). In fact, the vessels look larger in the unprocessed single slices than after the MIP.

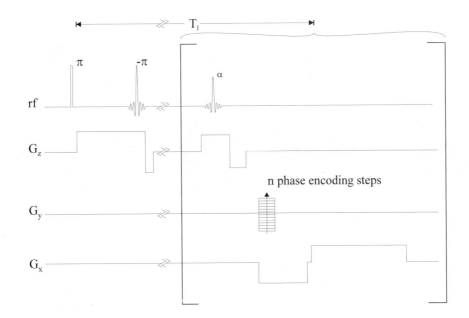

Fig. 24.13: A black-blood TOF sequence used to null inflowing blood. The rf hard pulse is applied along, say, z (for a transverse slice) and then along $-z$ for the soft pulse. This brings the spins back along the z-axis in the slice of interest in preparation for the series of short-T_R α-pulses to follow. T_I is chosen to null the signal from blood that flows into the slice of interest. In general $T_{I,null}$ will be chosen to occur at the $\vec{k} = 0$ point. The repetition of the α-pulses is indicated by the square brackets encompassing all the gradient encoding. This structure is repeated n times as indicated in the figure itself.

inversion and imaging pulse, the signal from any blood which flows into the slice after the first hard pulse will be zero. The signal from blood originally in the slice that was reinverted is assumed to have moved out of the slice before imaging.

Multiple short-T_R pulses are used near the zero crossing ($T_{I,null}$ time) to create a T_1-weighted image for the stationary tissue. For a given k-space acquisition order, the best suppression of blood will occur if $T_{I,null}$ is the time from the first π-pulse to the $k_y=0$ phase encoding step. An example application of both bright and dark blood imaging in the heart is shown in Fig. 24.14 to highlight the blood and myocardium, respectively.

24.2.3 Suppressing Signal from Inflowing Blood Using a Saturation Pulse

The nomenclature 'MR angiography' is usually reserved for imaging of any vessels but often implies imaging arteries (MR arteriography would be more appropriate) whereas MR venography is used when referring to veins. There are situations where it is desirable to selectively image either arteries or veins. Ideally, if resolution were sufficient, separating arteries from veins in a contrast enhanced image would not be difficult. However, in practice, it is easier and more convenient to eliminate the signal from the unwanted component. This can be accomplished by using a saturation pulse upstream from the imaged slice followed shortly

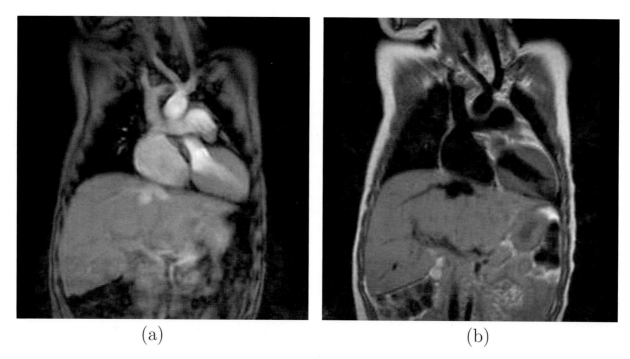

(a)   (b)

Fig. 24.14: (a) A 2D TOF bright-blood MRA data set in the heart. (b) A black blood image acquired at the same slice by pre-conditioning the blood signal to be essentially zero at the time of data acquisition.

before the imaging rf excitation pulse (Fig. 24.15). The time T_{sat} between the saturation and imaging pulse is determined by the velocity of the flowing spins and imaging parameters. When imaging the carotid arteries, for example, the jugular vein signal is minimized by applying a saturation pulse cranial to the excited slice because venous flow is up-to-down (Fig. 24.16).[7] The time between the saturation pulse and signal generating pulse (T_{sat} in Fig. 24.15) is so short that the signal from the veins has no time to regrow and remains essentially zero relative to the surrounding tissue. This capability is demonstrated in Fig. 24.17. Figure 24.18 shows a 3D imaging example while a 2D MRA example is shown in Fig. 24.19. In both cases, venous blood signal contribution was reduced by selectively saturating the venous blood. This selective saturation method is often necessary for 2D TOF MRA because both veins and arteries will otherwise appear bright. As a closing note on the use of saturation pulses, the reader should be aware that the more rf pulses that are applied the larger the rf power deposition (see Ch. 16).

Problem 24.3

---

    a) If the time between the saturation pulse and the usual excitation pulse is T_{sat} as shown in Fig. 24.15, longitudinal regrowth of the saturated magnetization will lead to a signal in the image. This regrowth can be countered by using a saturation flip angle of slightly greater than 90° so that the longitudinal

---

[7]The up-to-down direction is also referred to as head-to-foot or cranio-caudal.

magnetization is zero when the imaging pulse is applied. In terms of T_{sat}, what saturation flip angle needs to be applied so that the signal from the veins is exactly zero? Assume blood has a T_1 of 1200 ms.

b) Does this nulling depend on how quickly the venous blood flows into the slice?

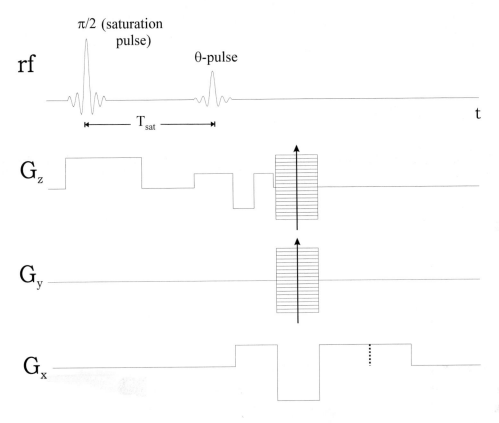

Fig. 24.15: A typical TOF MRA sequence. The slice select gradient applied during the saturation pulse is kept on afterward to spoil the transverse magnetization created by the saturation pulse. The time between the saturation pulse and the θ-pulse, T_{sat}, is usually on the order of 5-10 ms. The saturation pulse thickness can be varied from a few mm to many cm (which is usually the case).

24.3   Phase Contrast and Velocity Quantification

We have shown in Ch. 23 how critical it is to velocity compensate flowing spins when there are either rapid variations in flow or rapid changes in velocity across a voxel, independent of inflow effects. When signal loss due to velocity variations is not large, as in high resolution cardiac gated imaging, it is possible to obtain a good image even if flow affects the phase of the local spins as long as the velocity variation in a pixel is small. Although the discussions in this section are restricted to flow along the read direction, these methods could be applied to the other imaging directions.

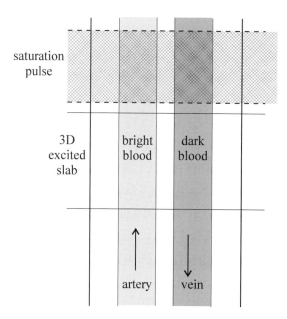

Fig. 24.16: A schematic of the carotid artery and jugular vein. The first pulse used in the sequence shown in the previous figure, often set to 90°, is used to saturate the signal from the veins. The second pulse excites the slab of interest. The resulting images in the next figures show dramatically reduced signal from the veins (see the next three images for an *in vivo* demonstration of these concepts).

Consider the velocity compensated sequence in Fig. 24.20a with positive (solid line) or negative (shaded area) bipolar pulses inserted prior to data collection in the read direction. Spins moving with constant velocity in the read direction will develop a phase

$$\phi_{v\pm} \equiv \phi_{v_x}(T_E) = \mp\gamma G v_x \tau^2 \qquad (24.14)$$

for square bipolar pulses, where the $\mp$ denotes the fact that ϕ_{v_x} changes sign if the negative lobe is applied first, and the positive lobe second. If trapezoidal gradients are applied

$$\phi_{v\pm} \equiv \phi_{v_x}(T_E) = \mp\gamma G_b v_x (\tau + \tau_{rt})(\tau + 2\tau_{rt}) \qquad (24.15)$$

with ramp-up and ramp-down times of τ_{rt}, identical constant gradient periods $\tau_1 = \tau_3 = \tau$, $G_+ = -G_- = G_b$, $\tau_2 = \tau_3$, and $\tau_2 = 0$ (see Fig. 24.20b).[8] The velocity dependent phase generated by the bipolar pulses is not affected by the subsequent velocity compensation gradients, instead it leads to a specific phase corresponding to velocity in the reconstructed phase image.

If this were the only source of phase in an image, then a single image, collected with such a bipolar pulse, would be enough to extract a measurement, at each pixel, of velocity along the read direction. However, other sources of phase errors also exist and must be removed somehow. For this reason, the concept of subtraction of two scans is introduced in the discussions to follow.

---

[8]Note that this value of ϕ was obtained by computing the first moment relative to a time-origin at the beginning of the bipolar lobe.

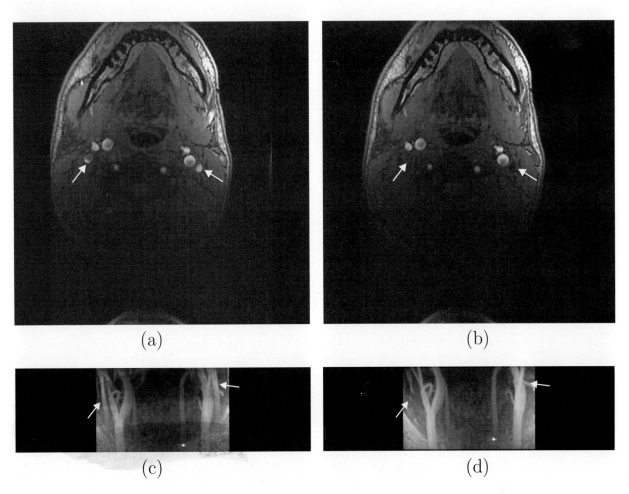

Fig. 24.17: Transverse and coronal planes of a human neck. (a) A transverse image across the neck without a saturation pulse shows a cross section of both the carotid artery and the jugular vein (arrows). (b) After the use of a saturation pulse, the signal from the jugular vein is dramatically suppressed. (c) and (d) are coronally reformatted images obtained from the same 3D transverse data sets used to obtain the images shown in (a) and (b), respectively.

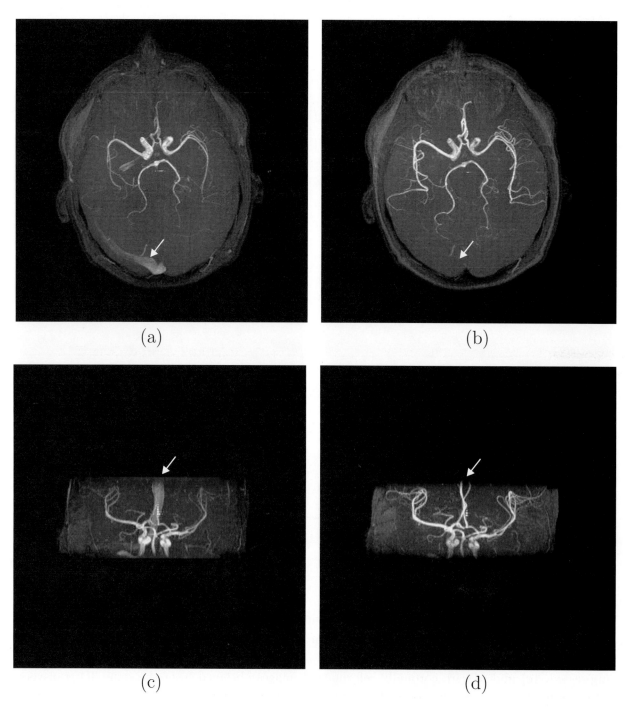

(a)   (b)

(c)   (d)

Fig. 24.18: Comparison between MIP images showing both arteries and veins ((a) and (c)) in the brain and an MR arteriogram (both (b) and (d)) obtained by saturating the venous flow by placing a saturation pulse above the imaging slice (acquired as a transverse 3D slab). (a) and (b) show the comparison in a transverse view while (c) and (d) show the coronal views from the same two data sets, respectively. The transverse sinus (arrows in (a) and (c)) has been successfully suppressed in both (b) and (d).

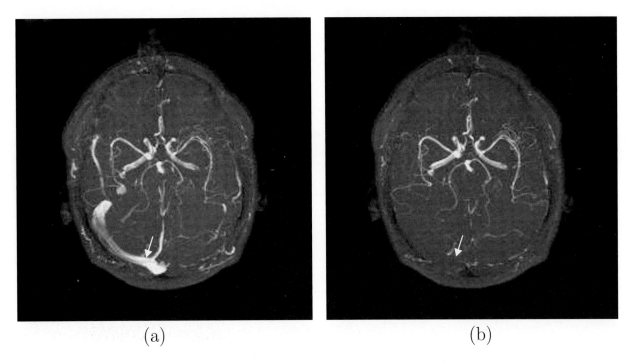

(a)   (b)

Fig. 24.19: Comparison between MIP images obtained (a) without and (b) with the use of a venous saturation pulse obtained from a 2D multi-slice data set with the use of saturation pulse applied before each new 2D slice acquisition. Note the better appearance of small vessels with very slow flow in comparison with the thick slice 3D data sets shown in Fig. 24.18. This is because even slow flow is enhanced in the 2D imaging case in view of the thinner slices. Again, the transverse sinus (arrow) has been suppressed in (b).

Problem 24.4

a) Verify (24.15).

b) Find $\phi_{vx}(T_E)$ if the bipolar gradient lobes are separated by a time τ_2, $\tau_1 = \tau_3$, and $G_+ = -G_- = G_b$.

c) Sketch a sequence diagram which could be used to obtain a phase image with velocity information along the phase encoding direction. Assume that there is flow along the read direction as well, but you only wish to measure v_y (i.e, it is necessary to enforce the condition that $\phi_{v_x}(T_E) = 0$).

24.3.1   Phase Subtraction and Complex Division for Measuring Velocity

Phase images may have spurious errors due to field inhomogeneities (see Chs. 17 and 20) or rf penetration effects (see Ch. 16). These background phases are independent of the bipolar gradient pulse and can be eliminated if two phase images are collected and subtracted. If the

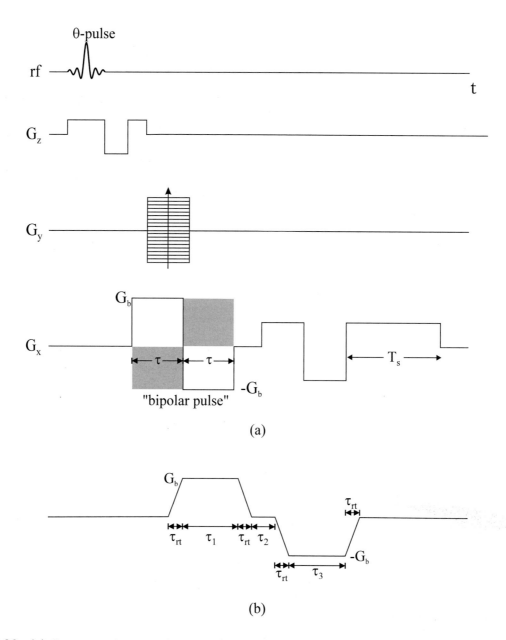

(a)

(b)

Fig. 24.20: (a) Sequence diagram for a fully velocity compensated, in the read direction, sequence where one acquisition is done with a positive bipolar read gradient and the second acquisition is done with a polarity-reversed bipolar read gradient (shaded region). (b) A general ramped trapezoidal bipolar gradient waveform. The lobes can be separated in time and have different amplitude and duration.

polarity or magnitude of the bipolar gradient lobes are changed between two such scans there will be velocity dependent phase information in the subtracted image. For the extraction of flow in one direction, say $\hat{x}$, images are usually acquired with bipolar gradients of equal magnitude and opposite polarity. Subtracting the phase images yields

$$\Delta\phi_{v_x}(\vec{r}) = 2\gamma G v_x(\vec{r})\tau^2 \tag{24.16}$$

and $v_x(\vec{r})$ can be extracted from this phase image. The opposite polarity lobes are used because they lead to the factor of two in $\Delta\phi_{v_x}$ which maximizes the phase change relative to velocity allowing the best separation of velocities for a given gradient strength. Eddy current effects should be minimal with a bipolar pulse (see Ch. 27) and their effects on phase are usually ignored.

Although measuring velocity from the phase is straightforward in concept, there are some practical difficulties. If the phase (24.14) exceeds π in an image, it aliases back to a phase between $-\pi$ and π (see Ch. 17). This will occur for the flow encoding bipolar pulses of Fig. 24.20a when the phase due to the presence of the bipolar pulse, $\phi_{bipolar}$, is such that

$$\phi_{bipolar} = \gamma G_b v_x \tau^2 > \pi \tag{24.17}$$

or equivalently, when $v_x > v_{enc}$ (the value above which aliasing occurs) where

$$v_{enc} \equiv \pi/(\gamma G_b \tau^2) \tag{24.18}$$

There are other possible approaches to extracting v_x. For fast flow (where $v < v_{enc}$), the above method works well, but the available SNR for extracting low velocities (for $v \ll v_{enc}$) is especially poor. From Ch. 15, the SNR for the phase image is given by

$$\begin{aligned} (\text{SNR})_\phi &= \phi(\text{SNR})_m \\ &= \phi\frac{\rho_m}{\sigma} \end{aligned} \tag{24.19}$$

where $(\text{SNR})_m$ refers to the magnitude image. Two important factors are inherent in this expression. First, the SNR of the phase is directly proportional to the signal, hence, for precise measurements of blood velocities the signal from blood should be as high as possible. Second, the larger ϕ_{v_x}, the better SNR_ϕ. Methods of enhancing ρ_m have already been dealt with. To enhance ϕ_{v_x}, the v_{enc} (the velocity encoding anti-aliasing limit) must be lowered and, since there is generally a large spread of velocities within a vessel due to laminar flow, it must be possible to unwrap ϕ_{v_x} from one voxel to the next within a vessel as some velocities may exceed v_{enc}. This would be feasible for a high resolution scan where v changes slowly enough from zero to allow for phase unwrapping (see Ch. 17).

Problem 24.5

As discussed in the text, to improve SNR_ϕ it is desirable to keep v_{enc} small. Given $G_{max} = 20\,\text{mT/m}$, and assuming that there is only 20 ms available during the sequence for velocity encoding, determine the lowest value of v_{enc} that can be achieved. Neglect rise times of the gradient for the purposes of this problem.

Problem 24.6

Each method of extracting velocity will have a unique SNR for velocity. Assume that the only source of ϕ is from flow and is caused by the bipolar gradient.

a) For the two-point method described above, find the standard deviation σ_v for a measured velocity v.

b) If the second scan has no bipolar gradient to encode velocity, what happens to σ_v?

c) What is σ_v if only the velocity encoded (with bipolar gradient pulses to encode velocity) image is acquired?

For vessels partial volumed with neighboring tissue, the phase of the entire voxel will not be the same as that for the flowing spins. Therefore, the subtraction of two phase images will not give the correct velocity measurement, even if all other background phase effects are removed.

Problem 24.7

Partial volume effects can be a significant problem in extracting velocity information.

a) If blood only occupies a fraction λ of the voxel, why is calculating velocity from the phase difference images a poor idea? Hint: Draw a vector diagram of the signal contribution in a voxel.

b) If the signal for the positive (negative) bipolar lobed sequence is ρ_+ (ρ_-) and $|\rho_+| = |\rho_-| = \rho_0$, show that $\Delta\rho = \rho_+ - \rho_+ = 2i\rho_0 \sin(v\pi/v_{enc})$.

c) How would the presence of field inhomogeneity phase shifts affect the calculation of v from $\Delta\phi$?

Problem 24.8

Consider the general problem of a ramped bipolar gradient with timings as shown in Fig. 24.20b.

a) Derive an expression for the phase as a function of G_b, τ_{rt}, τ_1, τ_2, and τ_3.

b) For $\tau_{rt} = 1\,\text{ms}$, $\tau_1 = 10\,\text{ms}$, $\tau_2 = 0\,\text{ms}$, $\tau_3 = 1\,ms$, and $G_b = 25\,\text{mT/m}$, what is v_{enc}?

c) For laminar flow in a vessel of diameter 10 mm with peak flow through-plane of 50 cm/s, how much signal is left at the edge and central pixels when the in-plane resolution is $1 \times 1\,\mathrm{mm}^2$? Assume that the geometric center of the vessel coincides with the center of a pixel, and that pixels at the edge of the vessel are those closest to the edge with no part of the pixel outside of the vessel.

Part of the problem in analyzing the phase data to extract the velocity is phase unwrapping of the data. The previous discussion assumed there was only one velocity component present, but clearly this is not true for laminar flow, nor is it true from vessel to vessel. Hence, the experiment must often be repeated with different v_{enc} values. Further, the phase unwrapping can be done most simply when multiple acquisitions are measured to increase SNR. In that case, the v_{enc} is increased in small steps Δv_{enc} so that any phase difference of the maximum velocity component is made less than π. The scan is repeated n_{scan} times each with a different v_{enc}. That is, the measured phase difference, $\Delta \phi$, from the pth critical velocity step, $v_{enc}(p)$, to the next critical velocity step, $v_{enc}(p+1)$, is less than π where

$$v_{enc}(p) = v_{enc}(0) + p\Delta v_{enc} \qquad (24.20)$$

and $0 \le p \le n_{scan} - 1$. Had the experiment been run n_{scan} times with a fixed v_{enc}, the SNR for estimating the velocity would have been improved by a factor of $\sqrt{n_{scan}}$. Although this increase in SNR is appreciated, the method just described will have a significantly better SNR (see Prob. 24.10).

Problem 24.9

Bipolar gradients are often used to suppress signal from moving blood. Assume a simple bipolar pulse with each lobe of duration τ and maximum gradient amplitude G_{max}.

a) Starting with the Nyquist relation (which defines V_{enc})

$$\gamma G_{max} V_{enc} \tau^2 = \pi$$

Show for diffusion imaging (see Sec. 21.5.1) that

$$b = \frac{2\pi^2}{3V_{enc}^2 \tau}$$

b) What are the values of V_{enc} and b if $G_{max} = 10\,\mathrm{mT/m}$ and $\tau = 10\,\mathrm{ms}$?

c) How does the relation between b and V_{enc} change if the bipolar pulse becomes two unipolar pulses straddled about an instantaneous π-pulse?

Problem 24.10

For the above-described scheme of obtaining n acquisitions, show that the SNR of the measured velocity is increased by a factor

$$v_{enc}(n-1)/v_{enc}(0)$$

Hint: Essentially, with the ability to unwrap the phase, the dynamic range of the phase increases, and this increased dynamic range leads to an increased phase image SNR.

Complex Division Phase Images

A phase difference image can also be created by dividing one complex image on a pixel-by-pixel basis, $(\hat{\rho}_+ = \rho_0 e^{i\phi_{v+}+i\phi_b})$, by the other, $(\hat{\rho}_- = \rho_0 e^{-i\phi_{v-}+i\phi_b})$, where the former is for a positive v_{enc} and the latter for a negative v_{enc}. Here, ϕ_b refers to the background phase errors. The division yields

$$\hat{\rho}_\phi = \hat{\rho}_+/\hat{\rho}_- = e^{i2\phi_v} \tag{24.21}$$

Once again, v_x must be less than v_{enc} to avoid aliasing. This approach is less favored when enhanced SNR is desired since if $v = 2v_{enc}$, then $\phi_{v+} - \phi_{v-} = 0$ and v could just as well be zero. Nevertheless, it is a useful approach when phase unwrapping is performed from one v_{enc} value to the next as in the previous discussion.

Phase measurements for velocity from a single scan can be contaminated by the spatially and temporally dependent eddy current behavior (see Ch. 27). As described above, one way to eliminate these spurious effects is to acquire the data on stationary tissue twice, once with each polarity of the bipolar lobe. Subtracting the phases of the two images yields a phase image which contains eddy current effects only from the bipolar lobes and not from any other applied gradients (since they are the same during both acquisitions).

Problem 24.11

It is often difficult to measure flow in the heart because of its rapid motion. This problem addresses a possible method for doing blood flow measurements in the heart.

a) If flow in end diastole (when the heart is relatively motionless) in the cardiac cycle is constant for 200 ms, how would you use a segmented k-space acquisition with velocity encoding to allow for a breath-hold measurement of through-plane flow?

b) Draw a sequence diagram for your approach.

Problem 24.12

If the phase encoding gradients are removed and a beam of spins is excited, a 1D projection image is obtained. This beam of spins can be used to monitor flow along the readout direction. It may be useful for watching a valve moving in the heart, for example. Consider the following questions to be for such a 1D imaging example.

a) Draw a sequence diagram for an interleaved velocity quantification set of reversed bipolar gradients.

b) For a FOV in $\hat{x}$ of 25 cm, a v_{enc} of 50 cm/sec and $\tau_{rf} = 10$ ms, $G_{max} = 25$ mT/m, and $\tau_{rt} = 600\mu$s, what is the minimum possible T_R? This T_R value then represents the temporal resolution of the velocity quantification.

c) Why is projecting across a beam likely to cause some problems in this method?

24.3.2 Four-Point Velocity Vector Extraction

Rather than collecting two images in each flow encoding direction, there is a more efficient method in 3D. In principle, one image per direction for velocity encoding is theoretically good enough; unfortunately, there is a variety of sources of phase error that make it difficult to get absolute values for velocity. Luckily, most phase errors remain constant when the sign of the bipolar pulse is reversed. Thus, a subtraction yields a more pristine phase image. Using this philosophy, to get velocity information in all three directions requires only four scans, not six.

Problem 24.13

Using six scans is the most straightforward way to get $\vec{v}$.

a) How would you collect the data using six scans?

b) What are the advantages and disadvantages of this method?

The four scans are collected with bipolar pulses in all directions for each scan with the polarities shown in Table 24.1. The phase in x, y, and z corresponding to the different velocity encoding is obtained using a linear combination of the four images. For example, the z-component of velocity v_z is found from

$$2\phi_z = (\rho_3 + \rho_4) - (\rho_1 + \rho_2) \tag{24.22}$$

With all velocity components known, the total speed is found from

$$v = (v_x^2 + v_y^2 + v_z^2)^{1/2} \qquad (24.23)$$

The resulting PC MRA is then a map of $v(\vec{r})$ (for example, see Fig. 24.21). Although this method can do an excellent job of suppressing the background tissue, it still suffers from the above-mentioned problems of ghosting and dephasing.

	x	y	z
1	$-$	$-$	$-$
2	$+$	$+$	$-$
3	$+$	$-$	$+$
4	$-$	$+$	$+$

Table 24.1: Signs of the bipolar waveforms used in each direction for the four scans required for extracting a three-component velocity vector.

Problem 24.14

a) Find ϕ_{v_x} and ϕ_{v_y} in terms of ρ_1, ρ_2, ρ_3, and ρ_4.

b) Find the standard deviation, σ_{v_z}, of flow along $\hat{z}$.

c) Show that the value of v_{enc} for this four-point method is dependent on flow direction.

24.4   Flow Quantification

Physiologically it is often important to know the actual flow through a vessel. This can be found by knowing the cross section of the vessel and the speed of the blood at each pixel. Integrating over the area gives a total blood volume per unit time through that cross section. Using a 2D PC MRA method with through-plane encoding and assuming the vessel is perpendicular to the plane, the flow, F, is calculated to be

$$F = \int v_z \, dA \qquad (24.24)$$

Problem 24.15

Assume that a very high resolution in-plane 2D experiment has been performed.

a) If the vessel is angled to the plane as shown in Fig. 24.22, what is the cross-sectional area now? Hint: A cylinder cut at an angle yields an elliptical cross section.

b) Is (24.24) still valid?

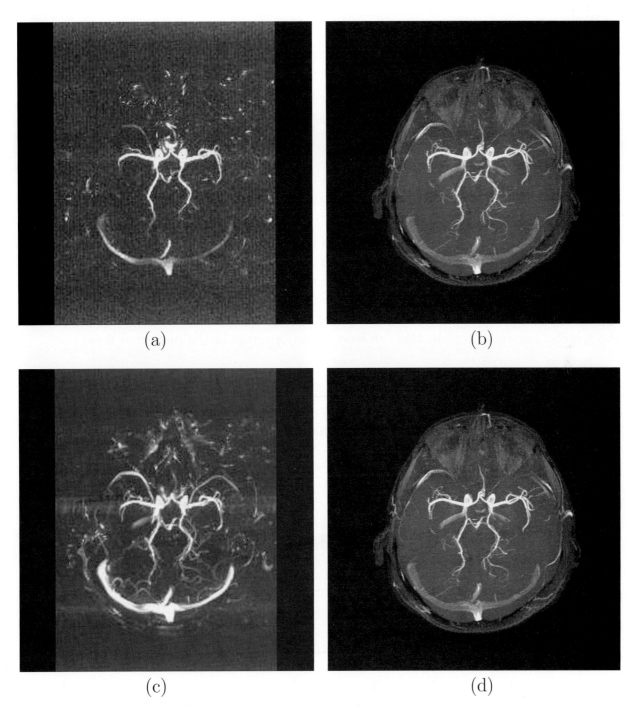

Fig. 24.21: 3D PC MRA images. The image shown in (a) was collected using a v_{enc} value of $100 \, \text{cm/sec}$ while the image in (c) was collected using $v_{enc} = 20 \, \text{cm/sec}$. (a) and (c) are transverse MIP images of the magnitude images. An MIP from a conventional TOF MRA data set is shown in (b) and (d) for the purpose of providing a side-by-side comparison. Image (a), with its high v_{enc} value, highlights only large vessels which have higher velocities. Further, it is seen that the low v_{enc} used to acquire the data set in (c) makes this sequence highly motion-sensitive as shown by the ghosting here.

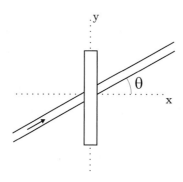

Fig. 24.22: Angled-vessel example for Prob. 24.15.

For a vessel which looks more like a beam with a rectangular cross section A', when it is tilted an angle θ to the x-axis, its cross-section changes to $A' \sec \theta$ and the velocity component along z changes to $v_z = v_z \cos \theta$. It is evident that the product of the two remains invariant at $A'v$. Cross-sectional measurements are critical for accurate flow quantification. Partial volume effects also cause errors in extracting both phase (velocity) and area estimates for the vessels. For small vessels, this can lead to major errors in the measured flow.

Problem 24.16

Assume that the in-plane resolution is $1 \, \text{mm} \times 1 \, \text{mm}$ and the vessel being imaged has a diameter of $5 \, \text{mm}$ and is orthogonal to the slice.

a) Estimate a lower and upper limit of area by examining just those pixels which fit completely within the circular cross section and those which totally encompass it.

b) Assuming a uniform signal response across the vessel (i.e., no TOF effects), how can the partial volume effect be accommodated?

c) How would you finally estimate F?

Problem 24.17

For a cylinder of radius a, the flow at any time is determined by the velocity, $v(t)$, and the area, A, for plug flow via the relation

$$F(t) = Av(t) \tag{24.25}$$

For laminar flow, show that the mean velocity is

$$\begin{aligned} \bar{v} &= \frac{1}{A} \int_0^{2\pi} \int_0^a dr \, d\theta \, r v(r, \theta, t) \\ &= v_0/2 \end{aligned} \tag{24.26}$$

where v_0 is the peak velocity at $r = 0$.

24.4.1 Cardiac Gating

For non-pulsatile (constant) flow, data can be acquired with any T_R. In practice, blood flow is pulsatile and, to accurately measure flow, the data acquisition must be triggered to the cardiac cycle (see Fig. 24.23). If this is done consistently, then no phase variations occur from one phase encoding step to the next, and no ghosting occurs (see Fig. 24.24).

As gradient subsystems become more powerful, it is possible to interleave velocity encoding in all three directions (a total of four T_R intervals) and still keep $4T_R$ short enough that either 3D or 2D ciné acquisitions can be obtained in a reasonable period of time (see Sec. 24.3.2).

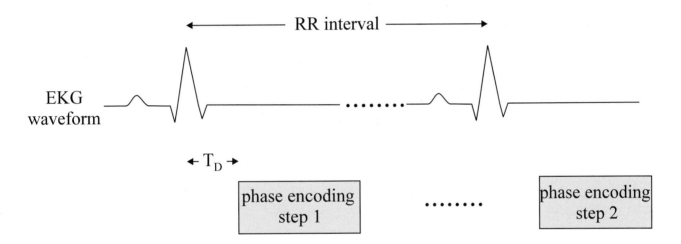

Fig. 24.23: Schematic of a flow quantification sequence insensitive to pulsatile flow during the cardiac cycle. This insensitivity is achieved by gating the acquisition to some point in the electro-cardiogram (EKG) waveform. The PC MRA images are then typically acquired with bipolar gradients superimposed on a velocity compensated sequence structure such as that shown in Fig. 24.20a. Only one phase encoding line is acquired during a given cardiac cycle and, assuming consistency of the cardiac rhythm during acquisition, the data are acquired at a fixed delay time T_D following the peak of the R-wave in the EKG waveform.

Problem 24.18

In cardiac imaging, the shortest possible T_R is desired. This problem looks at the calculation of timings for the velocity encoding and echo times and how this affects the shortest T_R. To obtain a flow encoding of 10 cm/sec, with a gradient strength of

a) 10 mT/m and rise time of 1 ms and

b) 25 mT/m and rise time of 300 μs,

how long must T_R be if T_s equals 5 ms? Assume the rf pulse and the phase encoding gradient are each 2 ms in duration.

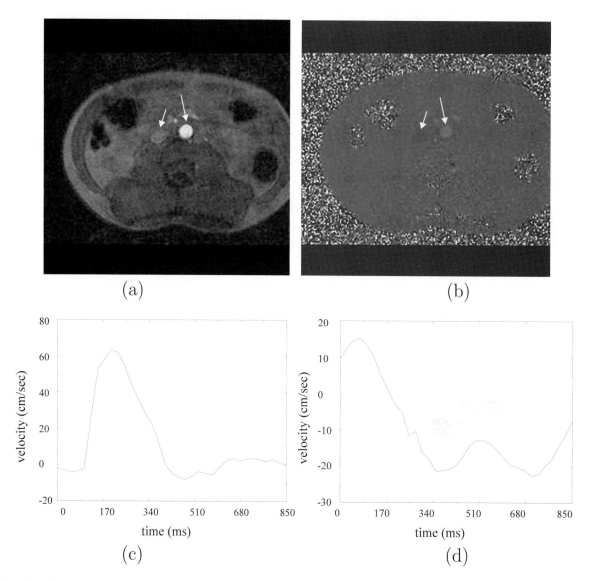

Fig. 24.24: (a) A magnitude image and (b) phase image from a series of transverse images collected during the cardiac cycle. The measured phase profiles across (c) the aorta (see long arrows in (a) and (b)) and (d) the vena cava (short arrows in (a) and (b)). The images were acquired with a cardiac triggered 2D flow imaging method with the velocity encoding gradient applied along the slice select direction. The images were acquired using a segmented k-space acquisition during a single breath-hold period of a few ms.

Fourier Velocity Encoding

The problem with line projections for a fixed velocity encoding is the mixture of numerous velocities in a single voxel (see Prob. 24.12). There is a means to separate out all the velocity spectral components in a single voxel. Assume that in a given voxel centered at position $\vec{r}$, there is a spread of velocities along one axis so that the signal at a pixel is the sum of all spins with different velocities

$$\rho(\vec{r}, k_v) = \int dv\, \rho(\vec{r}, v) e^{-i2\pi k_v v} \tag{24.27}$$

When no bipolar lobe is active, $k_v = 0$. If k_v is varied in steps of intervals Δk_v, then similar to the spatial encoding done to capture the signal $s(\vec{k})$, a signal is obtained for $\rho(\vec{r}, k_v)$. The following problem will carry the reader through the steps necessary to create a 2D image where one dimension is spatial and one is velocity. Both positive and negative components are now naturally separated even when a spread of velocities occupies a single voxel.

Problem 24.19

To successfully extract the fraction of spins within a given velocity interval Δv, and over a range of velocities from $-v_{enc}$ to v_{enc}, a Nyquist condition must be determined. Assume constant duration (2τ) velocity encoding gradient lobes with varying gradients strengths will be employed to encode velocity information, in an analogous fashion to how spatial phase encoding gradients are used.

a) For a given bipolar gradient structure with an amplitude G and total duration 2τ, what is k_v?

b) Using $\Delta k_v = 1/2v_{max}$ and assuming $2n$ gradient steps, what should the size of ΔG be for each step?

c) Show that the velocity resolution is given by

$$\Delta v = \frac{1}{\gamma G_{max} \tau^2} \tag{24.28}$$

d) For $\tau = 10\,\text{ms}$, $G_{max} = 25\,\text{mT/m}$, and $n = 10$, find Δv, the velocity field-of-view, $2n\Delta v$, ΔG, and $G_{max} = n\Delta G$.

Suggested Reading

The basic concepts behind time-of-flight and phase contrast imaging as well as numerous aspects of MR angiography are reviewed in:

- C. M. Anderson, R. R. Edelman and P. A. Turski, eds. *Clinical Magnetic Resonance Angiography*. Raven Press, New York, 1993.

- E. J. Potchen, E. M. Haacke, J. E. Siebert and A. Gottschalk, eds. *Magnetic Resonance Angiography: Concepts & Applications*. Mosby-Year Book, Inc., St. Louis, 1993.

Introductory discussions of blood saturation during 2D and 3D time-of-flight appear in:

- J. H. Gao, S. K. Holland and J. C. Gore. Nuclear magnetic resonance signal from flowing nuclei in rapid imaging using gradient echoes. *Med. Phys.*, 15: 809, 1988.

- E. M. Haacke, T. J. Masaryk, P. A. Wielopolski, F. R. Zypman, J. A. Tkach, S. Amartur, J. Mitchell, M. Clampitt and C. Paschal. Optimizing blood vessel contrast in fast three-dimensional MRI. *Magn. Reson. Med.*, 14: 202, 1990.

The use of magnetization transfer contrast to suppress background tissue was proposed by:

- S. D. Wolff and R. S. Balaban. Magnetization transfer contrast (MTC) and tissue water proton relaxation *in vivo*. *Magn. Reson. Med.*, 10: 135, 1989.

Its use was adopted for MRA by:

- R. R. Edelman, S. S. Ahn, D. Chien, W. Li, A. Goldmann, M. Mantello, J. Kramer and J. Kleefield. Improved time-of-flight MR angiography of the brain with magnetization transfer contrast. *Radiology*, 184: 395, 1992.

- G. B. Pike, B. S. Hu, G. H. Glover and D. R. Enzmann. Magnetization transfer time-of-flight magnetic resonance angiography. *Magn. Reson. Med.*, 25: 372, 1992.

The ability to use contrast agents to enhance vessel visibility was proposed in:

- W. Lin, E. M. Haacke, A. S. Smith and M. E. Clampitt. Gadolinium-enhanced high resolution MR angiography with adaptive vessel tracking: preliminary results in intracranial circulation. *J. Magn. Reson. Imag.*, 2: 277, 1992.

- G. Marchal, H. Bosmans, P. Van Hecke, Y. B. Jiang, P. Aerts and H. Bauer. Experimental Gd-DTPA polylysine enhanced MR angiography: sequence optimization. *J. Comp. Assist. Tomogr.*, 15: 711, 1991.

- M. R. Prince, E. K. Yucel, J. A. Kaufman, D. C. Harrison and S. C. Geller. Dynamic gadolinium-enhanced three-dimensional abdominal MR arteriography. *J. Magn. Reson. Imag.*, 3: 877, 1993.

Blood suppression or black blood imaging using an inversion pulse was suggested in:

- R. R. Edelman, H. P. Mattle, B. Wallner, R. Bajakian, J. Kleefield, C. Kent, J. J. Skillman, J. B. Mendal and D. J. Atkinson. Extracranial carotid arteries: evaluation with 'black blood' MR angiography. *Radiology*, 177: 45, 1990.

- S. J. Wang, B. S. Hu, A. Macovski and D. G. Nishimura. Coronary angiography using fast selective inversion recovery. *Magn. Reson. Med.*, 18: 417, 1991.

The concept of phase contrast and its quantification were described by:

- C. L. Dumoulin and H. R. Hart, Jr. Magnetic resonance angiography. *Radiology*, 161: 717, 1986.

- R. Hausmann, J. S. Lewin and G. Laub. Phase contrast MR angiography with reduced acquisition time: new concepts in sequence design. *J. Magn. Reson. Imag.*, 1: 415, 1991.

- N. J. Pelc, M. A. Bernstein, A. Shimakawa and G. H. Glover. Encoding strategies for three-direction phase contrast MR imaging of flow. *J. Magn. Reson. Imag.*, 1: 405, 1991.

Signal-to-noise issues for PC-MRA were discussed in:

- M. A. Bernstein and Y. Ikezaki. Comparison of phase difference and complex difference processing in phase contrast MR angiography. *J. Magn. Reson. Imag.*, 1: 725, 1991.

- A. T. Lee, G. B. Pike and N. J. Pelc. Three-point phase contrast velocity measurements with increased velocity-to-noise ratio. *Magn. Reson. Med.*, 33: 122, 1995.

Fourier encoding for flow was pioneered by:

- P. R. Moran. A flow zeugmatographic interlace for NMR imaging in humans. *Magn. Reson. Imag.*, 1: 197, 1984.

The virtues of cardiac gating were extolled by:

- G. H. Glover and N. J. Pelc. A rapid-gated ciné MRI technique. *Magn. Reson. Annual*, 299, 1988.

Chapter 25

Magnetic Properties of Tissues: Theory and Measurement

Chapter Contents

Summary: Consideration is given to the magnetic-field contributions from the atomic lattice in the response of a body to an external field. The magnetic properties of body tissue and contrast agents are discussed, along with the influence of such magnetic 'susceptibility' effects on imaging. As an example, the magnetic fields associated with blood and their role in functional imaging are described. Special cases of the field behavior inside and outside of magnetization compartments described by spherical and cylindrical geometries are covered in detail. Applications of these concepts to functional brain imaging and susceptibility weighted imaging are presented.

Introduction

There are numerous sources of magnetic field variation in the body. Some are a nuisance such as those caused by foreign objects such as surgical clips, implants, or even eye shadow (which often contains iron), and internal susceptibility differences between tissues. These can cause image distortion and loss of signal, especially T_2^* losses in gradient-echo imaging. On the other hand, susceptibility is also another intrinsic tissue property and local variations in susceptibility can be useful in identifying special properties or states of the body; this is the

739

focus of the present chapter. These differences will manifest themselves as signal changes in both magnitude and phase images, and can be used to diagnose or extract important information about body function.

We begin by laying out brief descriptions of different magnetic behavior of various material, the 'isms' of para-, dia-, ferro-, antiferro-, ferri-, and superparamagnetism. The magnetic susceptibility and permeability parameters in the field equations are considered next. These parameters can be strong functions of positions, especially at tissue interfaces and in the vicinity of contrast agent particles; thus, objects embedded in the background material are studied in the third section. The full expressions for the local field for both a sphere and an arbitrarily oriented cylinder are presented. The remainder of the chapter is devoted to the blood oxygenation dependent susceptibility in functional MRI.

25.1   Paramagnetism, Diamagnetism, and Ferromagnetism

Inside of a body, a spin is subject to an internal field due to its neighbors, in addition to any external field. The internal field is dominated by the nearby atomic electrons, and individually their contributions can be well approximated by magnetic dipole fields corresponding to the magnetic dipole moments associated with their orbital and spin degrees of freedom. Neighboring nuclear magnetic moments are reduced in importance owing to the inverse-mass dependence first noted in Ch. 2, but the existence and size of the atomic moment is also based on the question of whether there are unpaired constituents, in this case the atomic electrons. The electron magnetic moments are intrinsic or can be induced and, in this section, the classification of materials according to the different kinds of magnetic dipole moments is laid out.

25.1.1   Paramagnetism

The quantum stacking of electrons in an atom or molecule involves a systematic cancelation of spin moments for each pair. An atom with an unpaired electron has a nonvanishing permanent magnetic moment with an associated nonzero dipole magnetic field, and is referred to as 'paramagnetic.' While these moments would be randomly distributed in the absence of outside interactions, they would tend to align with an external magnetic field, producing a bulk magnetic moment and a corresponding macroscopic magnetic field augmenting the external field.

What arises in a paramagnetic material is an atomic magnetization analogous to the nuclear spin magnetization discussed so often in this book. Because the atomic moment is so much larger than the nuclear moment (Ch. 2), the local field inside (and outside, for that matter) can deviate substantially from the applied field value obtained in the absence of material. Much as it does for the proton spins, thermal motion would also reduce the tendency of the atomic moments to line up along an external field.

25.1.2 Diamagnetism

Whether or not there are any permanent magnetic dipole moments, all materials will have induced dipole moments in the presence of time-dependent external (or internal) magnetic fields. The mechanism is the same as that behind Lenz's law, or more basically, Faraday's law. As in the discussion of Ch. 7 concerning the currents induced in detector coils, we can use the analogous picture of induced atomic currents which produce counter magnetic fields, tending to cancel the external field. The microscopic picture is that of slight shifts in the orbital motion of the various electrons of a given atom or molecule.

This is a much weaker effect than paramagnetism, and is called 'diamagnetism.' In those cases where the electrons pair up to cancel their spin magnetic moments, paramagnetism is absent and no longer dominates the omnipresent diamagnetism. In diamagnetism, the macroscopic sum of the induced moments is roughly anti-parallel to the external magnetic field, and its associated macroscopic field opposes (weakly) the external field. Also, the temperature dependence observed in paramagnetism is absent in diamagnetism.

While a fully consistent treatment requires quantum mechanics, it is possible to show how diamagnetism arises in a simple classical model. Consider an electron of charge $-e$ ($e > 0$) and mass m moving at speed v in a circle of radius r around a proton (charge $+e > 0$). The centripetal acceleration inward must be provided by the Coulomb force

$$\frac{mv^2}{r} = \frac{1}{4\pi\epsilon_0}\frac{e^2}{r^2} \qquad (25.1)$$

with the heaviness of the proton justifying the neglect of its motion.

Suppose a differentially small magnetic field dB is turned on perpendicular to the plane of the orbit in a direction given by the right-hand rule with respect to the circulation direction of the electron speed v. The Lorentz force law (see Ch. 2) applied to the electron leads to another term in (25.1)

$$\frac{mv'^2}{r'} = \frac{1}{4\pi\epsilon_0}\frac{e^2}{r'^2} + ev'dB \qquad (25.2)$$

where it is assumed that the electron is moved to a new circle of radius r' and speed v' during the process. In the problem below, Faraday induction is analyzed to show that the radius can be taken as constant, $r = r'$. The comparison of (25.1) and (25.2) yields the differential change $v' = v + dv$ for which

$$dv = \frac{er}{2m}dB \qquad (25.3)$$

The increased speed of the negatively charged electron implied by (25.3) for $dB > 0$ explains diamagnetism. That is, the magnetic moment $\mu = -erv/2$ (see Prob. 2.4) defined along the field direction changes according to

$$d\mu = -\frac{e^2r^2}{4m}dB \qquad (25.4)$$

An increasing external field $dB > 0$ results in an additional magnetic moment (in this case, it is an orbital magnetic moment) opposite to the field. These changes are usually on the order of several ppm of the main field (see Prob. 25.1 and Sec. 25.2.2). As far as MR imaging is concerned, diamagnetic changes in the magnetic field may lead to positive or negative changes in field. For example, the venous blood and calcified tissue are paramagnetic and diamagnetic relative to the surrounding tissue, respectively, which itself is diamagnetic, but whether their induced fields are positive or negative depends on their geometries.

Problem 25.1

We complete the details of the classical model introduced above by showing that the circular orbit of the electron is unchanged when the field change dB is made during time dt.

a) Assume that the radius is in fact changed, $r' = r + dr$. Derive the differential relation

$$mv\, dv = -\frac{1}{8\pi\epsilon_0}\frac{e^2}{r^2}dr + \frac{1}{2}evr\, dB \qquad (25.5)$$

from a comparison of (25.1) and (25.2).

b) Obtain the expression for the electric field induced azimuthally (in the direction defined by the right-hand rule) around the circle at radius r

$$E = -\frac{1}{2}r\frac{dB}{dt} \qquad (25.6)$$

c) Find the change in the kinetic energy dictated by the result in (25.6) and show that it and (25.5) imply that $dr = 0$.

25.1.3   Ferromagnetism

Certain materials have permanent domains of electron spin magnetic moments which conspire to produce very strong macroscopic self-fields existing independently of an external magnetic field. There is this kind of strong 'spin-spin' coupling between nearby atoms in a list of materials that includes iron, nickel, cobalt, gadolinium, dysprosium, and various alloys and oxides. The domains can span distances of millimeters and contain huge numbers of spin moments in a material. Their size is limited by the range of the spin-spin forces.

The domains are randomly distributed throughout the material unless there is an external field. When they are aligned, typically by the temporary application of an external field, a permanent macroscopic magnet is produced. This alignment is called 'magnetic saturation' when it involves essentially all of the domains, producing the maximum magnetic moment density (the familiar magnetization $\vec{M}$). As long as the temperature is not too high (the critical or Curie temperature for iron, for example, is more than $1300\,\mathrm{K}$), there is a 'remanent' magnetization left when the external field is turned off. The dependence of the magnetization on what has happened in the past is the familiar 'hysteresis' effect. There is also 'antiferromagnetic' and 'ferrimagnetic' material where neighboring spins completely and incompletely cancel, respectively.

The importance of contrast agents brings up a special topic. The act of continually subdividing ferromagnetic material eventually leads to particles that are each just one domain. Mixed into a background substance, they behave like a set of very large magnetic moments, producing superparamagnetism. With no external field, their thermal motion leads to vanishing magnetization. With an external field, the alignment of these domain particles can produce a strong self-field, and they can saturate in a manner analogous to homogeneous ferromagnetic materials.

Iron oxide particulates are an example of such superparamagnetic materials. Thanks to the large local fields created, ferric oxide or iron particulates are used as a contrast agent to produce signal loss in regions where they are deposited or to which they have migrated. These particulates vary in size from hundreds of nanometers to several microns, and they behave like a single magnetic domain. The large magnetic moment associated with a particulate has far-reaching effects. A single particle (say, a particulate sphere with a 1-micron diameter) can affect the signal in a volume millions of times the volume of the original particle volume (see Fig. 25.1 and Prob. 25.2).

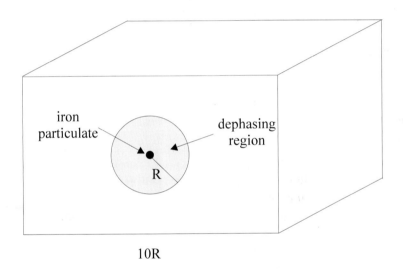

Fig. 25.1: A voxel of volume $1000R^3$ containing a single superparamagnetic spherical particle. The shaded spherical region with radius R can completely dephase in a conventional gradient echo experiment. If hundreds of these spheres were present, the entire voxel signal could be lost.

Problem 25.2

---

a) For a particulate of radius $a = 1$ micron (see Fig. 25.1), find the dipole magnetic field (look ahead at the dipole term in (25.15)) at a point P a distance $100a$ away along the direction of the static magnetic field. Assume the magnetization M in (25.16) is 2.6×10^6 A/m for iron.

b) For an echo time of 10 ms, what phase shift occurs at point P?

c) What do you expect the effects of these phase shifts to be on the magnitude image? Hint: Review Ch. 20 and the concepts behind T_2^*.

25.2   Permeability and Susceptibility: The $\vec{H}$ Field

Important consequences of the preceding discussion are the corrections to the external field due to the dipole fields generated by the electron spin moments. The relevance stems from the basic fact that the precession frequency or, rather, the phase of the local spin density, is determined by the local field.

25.2.1   Permeability and the $\vec{H}$ Field

To parametrize the field changes due to the material's magnetism, a standard quantity called the 'permeability' μ is defined through the 'constitutive' relation between the physical magnetic field $\vec{B}$ and another vector field, called $\vec{H}$. The field $\vec{H}$ is a familiar and convenient vector quantity which would be identical (within a constant universal factor) to $\vec{B}$ if there were no material present and, as such, is closer to the external magnetic field when there is material present.[1]

We shall give a fundamental definition for $\vec{H}$ in a moment, but first consider 'linear' materials where the two fields are proportional. In isotropic materials where no special directions are singled out, they are parallel and the relation is given in terms of the permeability μ as the proportionality constant

$$\vec{B} = \mu\vec{H} \tag{25.7}$$

A relative permeability is defined by $\mu_r \equiv \mu/\mu_0$ where, for empty space, $\mu = \mu_0 = 4\pi \times 10^{-7}$, the aforementioned universal constant. Thus, paramagnetism, diamagnetism, and ferromagnetism correspond to relative permeabilities $\mu_r > 1, < 1$, and $\gg 1$, respectively.

With the magnetic dipole field description as a good approximation over large distances, the magnetization $\vec{M}$ is the macroscopic source of the additional, internal-field contributions due to the material's electron spins. The circulating current to which this magnetization corresponds is its curl (7.5)

$$\vec{J}_M = \vec{\nabla} \times \vec{M} \tag{25.8}$$

It is the combination of the curl terms in Maxwell's equation corresponding to Ampère's law, after the separation of the total current into 'free' current plus the magnetization current (25.8), that gives us a definition for the H field

$$\vec{H} = \vec{B}/\mu_0 - \vec{M} \tag{25.9}$$

25.2.2   Susceptibility

Linear materials are those for which the fields and magnetization are proportional to each other and can be described by a constant magnetic susceptibility χ via the relation

$$\vec{M} = \chi\vec{H} \tag{25.10}$$

---

[1]Although $\vec{H}$ is not equal, in general, to the external magnetic field vector divided by the free-space permeability, the two vectors may be taken as approximately the same in this discussion.

A comparison of this with (25.7) and (25.9) yields the relation between χ and μ

$$\chi = \frac{\mu}{\mu_0} - 1 \quad \text{or} \quad \mu = (1 + \chi)\mu_0 \tag{25.11}$$

and

$$\vec{B} = \frac{1 + \chi}{\chi} \mu_0 \vec{M}(\chi) \tag{25.12}$$

The susceptibility is therefore negative ($\chi < 0$), positive ($\chi > 0$), or zero for diamagnetic, paramagnetic, or nonmagnetic materials, respectively. In the ferromagnetic case, χ can be from $O(0.01)$ to $O(1)$, but it sometimes can be much larger than 1. But in the treatment relevant to human imaging, it is to be kept in mind that the susceptibility is very small, $|\chi| \ll 1$, either because the tissue is diamagnetic or the concentration of paramagnetic contrast agents is very small.

An important issue is the number of different systems of units that are in common usage for the quantities needed in expressing magnetic properties. A partial list of cgs and SI units (recall that the latter is the unit system employed in this book) and their relationships is given for different quantities of interest in Table 25.1. An additional list including different definitions of susceptibility together with conversions from cgs to SI units is given in Table 25.2.

The properties of materials with different types of magnetism discussed in Sec. 25.1 are summarized in Table 25.3. Most tissue in the body is water, which has a susceptibility value of $\chi_{\text{water}} \simeq -9$ ppm. Any paramagnetic changes $\Delta\chi$ in the field in the body will increase the local field so that $\chi_{\text{total}} \simeq \chi_{\text{water}} + \Delta\chi$ but χ_{total} is still usually negative; that is, the tissue is still diamagnetic overall. The values of χ in ppm for each type of magnetism are only to indicate the rough order of the effect. Significant variations about these values can occur and χ will change from substance to substance.

Of paramount interest are phase changes due to 'susceptibility effects.' Moving from one region to another, where the field changes due to variations in susceptibility results in a phase change at the acquisition (echo) time T_E given by

$$\Delta\phi = -\gamma \Delta B T_E \tag{25.13}$$

occurs. It is necessary to calculate the relationship between the field changes and the susceptibility variations

$$\Delta B = f(\Delta\chi) \tag{25.14}$$

With this relationship, we can use phase information to learn about changes in magnetic properties of tissues relative to each other. If all tissue had the same susceptibility (say, that of water), no phase changes would be seen. Models for variations due to simple tissue compartment geometries are the subject of the next section.

25.3 Objects in External Fields: The Lorentz Sphere

We have addressed the shift in the Larmor nuclear spin frequency due to the local magnetism of the molecules being imaged. This has been couched in the language of a susceptibility effect for the tissue material of interest and, as the susceptibility changes from position to position, the shifts must follow suit.

Quantity	Symbol	cgs	SI (MKS)	Conversion factor
length	L	centimeter (cm)	meter (m)	$1\,\mathrm{cm} = 10^{-2}\,\mathrm{m}$
magnetic field	B	gauss (G)	tesla (T)	$1\,\mathrm{G} = 10^{-4}\,\mathrm{T}$
H-field	H	oersted (Oe)	ampere (A)/m	$1\,\mathrm{Oe} = 10^3/(4\pi)\,\mathrm{A/m}$
magnetic moment	μ_m	erg/G	A·m^2	$1\,\mathrm{erg/G} = 10^{-3}\,\mathrm{A \cdot m^2}$
magnetization	M	erg/G/cm^3	A/m	$1\,\mathrm{erg/G/cm^3} = 10^3\,\mathrm{A/m}$
magnetic susceptibility	χ	dimensionless	dimensionless	$1 \to 4\pi$
permeability	μ	dimensionless	weber (Wb)/(A·m)	$1 \to 4\pi \times 10^{-7}\,\mathrm{Wb/(A \cdot m)}$

Table 25.1: Conversion factors from cgs to SI units for different quantities. Tesla is equivalent to Wb/m^2, magnetic susceptibility is sometimes quoted in terms of erg/G^2/cm^3 which is dimensionless, and $\mu_0 = 4\pi \times 10^{-7}$ Wb/(A·m). Even though they have the same cgs dimensions, using different cgs labeling units for B, H, and M helps keep the conversions consistent.

cgs	SI (MKS)	Conversion factor from cgs to SI
$\chi = (\mu - 1)/4\pi$	$\chi = \mu_r - 1$	4π
$\chi_\mathcal{M} = \chi\mathcal{M}/\rho$	$\chi_\mathcal{M} = 4\pi \times 10^{-6}\chi\mathcal{M}/\rho$	$4\pi \times 10^{-6}$
$\chi_m = \chi/\rho$	$\chi_m = 4\pi \times 10^{-3}\chi/\rho$	$4\pi \times 10^{-3}$
$\mu_B = 9.274 \times 10^{-21}$ erg/G	$\mu_B = 9.274 \times 10^{-24}$ A·m^2	10^{-3}

Table 25.2: Here, $\mu_r \equiv \mu/\mu_0$ is the relative permeability, $\mathcal{M}$ is the mass per mole, and ρ is the mass density. Correspondingly, $\chi_\mathcal{M}$ is the molar magnetic susceptibility and χ_m is the mass magnetic susceptibility. The Bohr magneton (Ch. 2) is denoted by μ_B.

Magnetism type	Alignment to B_0	χ in ppm
diamagnetism	anti-parallel	$-O(1)$
paramagnetism	parallel	$O(10)$
superparamagnetism	parallel	$O(10^3)$
ferromagnetism	parallel	$O(10^4)$–$O(10^6)$

Table 25.3: Summary of properties of materials with different types of magnetism. The values given for χ are only orders of magnitude.

The susceptibility change can be important as we move from one tissue to another, the interfacial regions being of particular interest. While a general calculation of the fields over these regions may need to be carried out with complicated (albeit standard) numerical methods, simple geometrical examples are instructive and even quantitatively useful. Blood vessels can be modeled by long cylinders, for example, where the susceptibility takes on different constant values inside the cylinder and outside.

A subtle but sizable effect arises because susceptibility cannot be considered strictly continuous inside compartments, such as biological blood vessels. The atomic or molecular 'granularity' leads to a cancelation of the susceptibility effects on any given nuclear magnetic moment due to its neighbors, a 'Lorentz sphere' phenomenon.

In this section, we consider these changes in external fields over spherical and cylindrical regions whose constant susceptibility differs from that of the background in which the regions are immersed. We also introduce a calculation demonstrating the vanishing of the effective susceptibility in the 'sphere of Lorentz' surrounding a given spin.

25.3.1 Spherical Body

Consider a sphere of radius a and material with constant susceptibility χ surrounded by free space and immersed in a uniform magnetic field $\vec{B}_0 = B_0 \hat{z}$ in the z-direction. One approach in finding the unique solution to this problem is to assume the field outside at position $\vec{r}$ is of the form of a constant field plus a dipole field[2]

$$\vec{B}_{out}(\vec{r}) = B_0 \hat{z} + \frac{\mu_0}{4\pi} \frac{3(\vec{\mu}_m \cdot \hat{r})\hat{r} - \vec{\mu}_m}{r^3} \tag{25.15}$$

where the magnetic dipole moment of the sphere is

$$\vec{\mu}_m = \frac{4\pi}{3} a^3 M(\chi)\hat{z} \tag{25.16}$$

with constant magnetization $M(\chi)$. The sphere is centered at the origin and r is the spherical coordinate. Consistent with (25.12), the field inside is taken to be a constant,

$$\vec{B}_{in} = B_{in}\hat{z} = \frac{1+\chi}{\chi}\mu_0 M(\chi)\hat{z} \tag{25.17}$$

The boundary conditions require that the normal component of the magnetic field $\vec{B}$ and the tangential components of the $\vec{H}$ fields be continuous across the spherical surface, that the limit $\vec{B}_{out} \to \vec{B}_0$ be satisfied far from the sphere, and that the field be finite at the origin. The fact that we can meet these conditions with the above forms guarantees the correct and unique solution. It is verified in the following problem that the conditions are met by a constant magnetization vector inside the sphere

$$\vec{M}(\chi) = \frac{3\chi}{3+\chi}\vec{B}_0/\mu_0 \tag{25.18}$$

_____

[2]A subscript m is added to the magnetic moment symbol to distinguish it from permeability.

The implications for (25.17) and (25.15) are

$$\vec{B}_{out} = B_0 \left(\hat{z} + \frac{\chi}{3+\chi} \left(\frac{a}{r}\right)^3 (3\cos\theta\hat{r} - \hat{z}) \right) \tag{25.19}$$

$$\vec{B}_{in} = 3B_0 \frac{1+\chi}{3+\chi} \hat{z} \tag{25.20}$$

with polar angle θ (see Fig. 25.2 for definitions of the polar coordinates r and θ as used here).

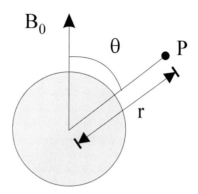

B_0

θ P

r

Fig. 25.2: Polar coordinate system for describing the field at a point P away from a magnetized sphere.

It is thereby seen from (25.19), (25.20), and using $\hat{r} \cdot \hat{z} = \cos\theta$ that the change in the z component of the field due to the presence of the sphere is

$$\Delta B_{z,out} = \frac{\chi}{3+\chi} \left(\frac{a}{r}\right)^3 \left(3\cos^2\theta - 1\right) B_0 \tag{25.21}$$

$$\Delta B_{z,in} = \frac{2\chi}{3+\chi} B_0 \tag{25.22}$$

Equations (25.15) through (25.22) provide the relationship required for the determination of the phase shift (see (25.13)) due to the external field changes, where, in this case, the change in field is governed by the change in susceptibility ($\Delta\chi = \chi$) from outside the sphere to inside the sphere. *Actually, $\Delta B_{z,in}$ as given in (25.22) is only part of the effective (or measurable) local magnetic field. To find the complete result, see the subsequent discussion of the Lorentz correction for molecular structures in Sec. 25.3.3.*

Problem 25.3

---

   a) Show the normal (radial) component of (25.19) matches that of (25.20) at
      $r = a$.

   b) Show that the tangential components of $\vec{H}$ are also continuous at $r = a$.

25.3.2 Infinite Cylindrical Body

Right circular cylinders of constant susceptibility χ can be useful models for blood vessels, and they are fairly simple to analyze when the radius a is much smaller than the length L. In the infinite length limit, the problem is two dimensional and the field solution is complicated only by the question of the external field direction. The solutions can again be found by assuming simple forms that can be shown to satisfy the boundary conditions.

For $\vec{B}_0 = B_0 \hat{z}$ parallel to the cylindrical axis ($\theta = 0$ in Fig. 25.3), the resultant field is equal to the applied field outside and proportional to it inside

$$\vec{B}_{out} = \vec{B}_0 \tag{25.23}$$
$$\vec{B}_{in} = (1+\chi)\vec{B}_0 \qquad \| \text{ case} \tag{25.24}$$

It is clear that $\vec{H}$ is a single constant 'tangential' vector everywhere so that it certainly is continuous at $\rho = a$ where ρ is a cylindrical coordinate defined such that $\rho = 0$ is the cylinder axis. All normal components of all field vectors vanish everywhere.

The case ($\theta = \pi/2$ in Fig. 25.3) in which the field $\vec{B}_0 = B_0 \hat{x}$ is now perpendicular to the cylinder has a solution analogous to that for the sphere. (The z-axis remains parallel to the cylinder.) The field outside is a superposition of the constant external field and a

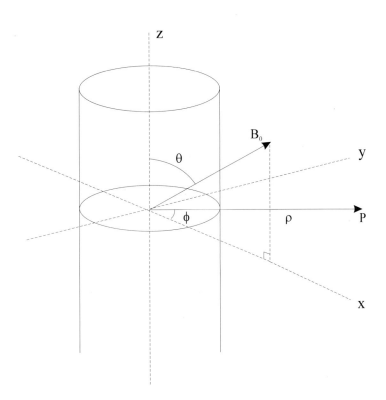

Fig. 25.3: Cylindrical coordinates (ρ, ϕ) for describing the position P relative to a cylinder of magnetic material. The cylinder lies in the x-z plane at an angle θ to the external field $\vec{B}_0$.

two-dimensional dipole field

$$\vec{B}_{out} = B_0 \left(\hat{x} + \frac{\chi/2}{1 + \chi/2} \left(\frac{a}{\rho} \right)^2 (\hat{x} \cos 2\phi + \hat{y} \sin 2\phi) \right) \qquad \perp \text{ case} \qquad (25.25)$$

where $\rho = \sqrt{x^2 + y^2}$ and ϕ is the polar angle in the x-y plane of the observation point relative to the external field (see Fig. 25.3). The field inside is uniform and parallel to $\vec{B}_0$

$$\vec{B}_{in} = \frac{1 + \chi}{1 + \chi/2} \vec{B}_0 \qquad \perp \text{ case} \qquad (25.26)$$

In the following exercise, the reader is asked to show that the field continuity requirements involving the normal components of $\vec{B}$ and the tangential components of $\vec{H}$ are satisfied.

Problem 25.4

Verify that the component normal (radial) to the cylindrical surface of (25.25) matches that of (25.26) at $\rho = a$ and that the tangential components of $\vec{H}$ are continuous there.

The changes in the z-component of the field due to the presence of the cylinder in the parallel case are easily found from (25.23) and (25.24)

$$\Delta B_{z,out} = 0 \qquad\qquad (25.27)$$
$$\Delta B_{z,in} = \chi B_0 \qquad\qquad \| \text{ case} \qquad (25.28)$$

and the perpendicular case from (25.25) and (25.26)

$$\Delta B_{x,out} = \frac{\chi/2}{1 + \chi/2} \left(\frac{a}{\rho} \right)^2 \cos 2\phi \, B_0 \qquad\qquad (25.29)$$

$$\Delta B_{x,in} = \frac{\chi/2}{1 + \chi/2} B_0 \qquad\qquad \perp \text{ case} \qquad (25.30)$$

The general situation of a uniform, external field at an arbitrary angle θ with the axis of the long cylinder (Fig. 25.3), given by

$$\vec{B}_0 = B_0(\sin\theta\hat{x} + \cos\theta\hat{z}) \qquad\qquad (25.31)$$

can be solved by a superposition of the above results to give

$$\vec{B}_{out} = B_0 \cos\theta\hat{z} + B_0 \sin\theta \left(\hat{x} + \frac{\chi/2}{1 + \chi/2} \left(\frac{a}{\rho} \right)^2 (\hat{x} \cos 2\phi + \hat{y} \sin 2\phi) \right) \qquad (25.32)$$

$$\vec{B}_{in} = B_0 \cos\theta(1 + \chi)\hat{z} + \frac{1 + \chi}{1 + \chi/2} B_0 \sin\theta\hat{x} \qquad\qquad (25.33)$$

As before, the imaging quantity of interest is the change, due to the susceptibility, in the component of the field along the original field direction. This component, also as before, is given by $\Delta B \equiv \Delta \vec{B} \cdot \hat{B}_0$, where $\Delta \vec{B} \equiv \vec{B} - \vec{B}_0$. In the limit of small susceptibility, $\chi \ll 1$, which is sufficient for most applications, Prob. 25.5 is to show that

$$\Delta B_{out} \simeq \frac{\chi}{2} B_0 \sin^2 \theta \left(\frac{a}{\rho}\right)^2 \cos 2\phi \qquad \chi \ll 1 \qquad (25.34)$$

$$\Delta B_{in} \simeq \frac{\chi}{2} B_0 (1 + \cos^2 \theta) \qquad \chi \ll 1 \qquad (25.35)$$

These are the ΔB quantities required in (25.13) for the determination of the phase shift due to local susceptibility. In that prescription, the correspondence is $\Delta \chi = \chi$, the change in susceptibility upon entering the cylinder. Again, ΔB_{in} is not the complete contribution to the change in the effective field. *As in the case of the spherical body, note must be taken of the upcoming discussion of the Lorentz correction to the internal field for molecular structures.*

Problem 25.5

Derive (25.35) from (25.33) in the limit of small susceptibility, $\chi \ll 1$.

25.3.3   Local Field Cancelation via Molecular Demagnetization

The discussion to this point has treated the problem of the magnetic field inside of spherical and cylindrical cavities or compartments as sharp interfaces between *continuous* media. But the spin and its immediate neighborhood cannot be considered a continuous distribution of magnetic field sources. There is an important correction, due to a cancelation of the fields of nearby molecules, which defines a 'Lorentz sphere' of influence around the spin.

Recall that the use of a magnetization $\vec{M}$ rests on an average over the dipole fields of the molecular population giving rise to a macroscopic magnetic field

$$\vec{B}_{macro} = \mu \vec{H} \qquad (25.36)$$

such that $\vec{M} = \chi \vec{H}$. The field $\vec{B}_{macro}$ is what has been calculated in the previous spherical and cylindrical configurations. The local field experienced by a spin, however, is

$$\vec{B}_{local} = \vec{B}_{macro} + \vec{B}_{int} \qquad (25.37)$$

where the internal field $\vec{B}_{int}$ is the difference between the net neighboring molecular fields (due to the molecules in a sphere of radius much larger than the intermolecular distance) and their continuous approximation corresponding to the magnetization $\vec{M}$,

$$\vec{B}_{int} = \vec{B}_{near} - \vec{B}_M \qquad (25.38)$$

The nearby field $\vec{B}_{near}$ can be shown to vanish in molecular model calculations

$$\vec{B}_{near} = 0 \qquad (25.39)$$

For example, consider a set $\{\ell\}$ of dipoles, all of which point in the same direction, $\vec{\mu}_\ell = \vec{\mu}_m$. Their total field is

$$\vec{B}_{near} = \frac{\mu_0}{4\pi} \sum_{dipoles\ \ell} \frac{3(\vec{\mu}_m \cdot \hat{r}_\ell)\hat{r}_\ell - \vec{\mu}_m}{r_\ell^3} \tag{25.40}$$

A symmetric distribution of dipoles yields a vanishing sum as observed in the following problem. It is expected that more realistic models would be more random and the sum should *a fortiori* vanish.

Problem 25.6

---

a) Prove that

$$\sum_{\vec{r}} f(r)(\vec{r})_i(\vec{r})_j = \sum_{\vec{r}} \frac{1}{3}r^2\delta_{ij}f(r) \tag{25.41}$$

either by considering a sum over a symmetrical cubic lattice of dipole points or by approximating a sum over spherical shells by an integration.

b) Use the result (25.41) in (25.40) to get (25.39).

The continuous approximation may be taken to be that inside of a continuous sphere (the aforementioned microscopically large but macroscopically small spherical volume) of magnetization $\vec{M}$. From (25.18) and (25.22),

$$\vec{B}_M = +\frac{2\mu_0}{3}\vec{M} \tag{25.42}$$

From (25.38), (25.39), and (25.42),

$$\vec{B}_{int} = -\frac{2\mu_0}{3}\vec{M} \tag{25.43}$$

In essence, (25.43) represents the field expected inside a spherical Lorentz cavity carved out of an otherwise constant background of magnetization $\vec{M}$. The surface magnetization currents on the inner surface of this sphere produce a field in opposition to the magnetization direction.

25.3.4 Sphere and Cylinder Examples Revisited: The Physical Internal Fields

Let us apply the above correction to an example. Consider the answers developed earlier for a cylinder of susceptibility χ immersed in, and at an angle θ with, a constant external field. The exterior is free space. Note that this cylinder refers to a compartment, simulating the inside and outside regions of a blood vessel, for example. The Lorentz sphere is a much smaller region, defined by the molecules surrounding a given spin, whose scale is on the order of several intermolecular distances. The change in the local field (25.37) seen by a spin inside the cylindrical tissue compartment is computed by combining (25.35), which corresponds to the change in $\vec{B}_{macro}$, and (25.43), which reduces to $-\frac{2}{3}\chi\vec{B}_0$ in lowest-order χ. The result is

$$\Delta B_{local,in} \simeq \frac{\chi}{6}B_0(3\cos^2\theta - 1), \qquad\qquad \chi \ll 1 \qquad\qquad (25.44)$$

It is understandable that the same dipolar angular dependence that holds outside a spherical compartment (25.21) applies inside for the Lorentz-corrected cylinder. Outside, where the magnetization vanishes (there is no molecular neighborhood), there is no correction and the external field result in (25.34) remains valid. In the presence of a background tissue with susceptibility χ_e, a Lorentz correction becomes necessary. A summary of the magnetic field shifts in regions with different susceptibility inside and outside spheres and arbitrarily oriented cylinders is given in Table 25.4. The profiles of the expected local field pattern for spheres and cylinders are given in Fig. 25.4 along lines coincident with their diameters.

	Internal field shift = macro + Lorentz correction	External field shift = macro + Lorentz correction
sphere	$\frac{1}{3}\chi_e B_0$	$\frac{\Delta\chi}{3}\frac{a^3}{r^3}(3\cos^2\theta - 1)B_0 + \frac{1}{3}\chi_e B_0$
cylinder	$\frac{\Delta\chi}{6}(3\cos^2\theta - 1)B_0 + \frac{1}{3}\chi_e B_0$	$\frac{\Delta\chi}{2}\frac{a^2}{\rho^2}\sin^2\theta\cos 2\phi\, B_0 + \frac{1}{3}\chi_e B_0$

Table 25.4: Magnetic field shifts where χ_i (χ_e) represents the susceptibility inside (outside) the sphere or cylinder and $\Delta\chi \equiv \chi_i - \chi_e$. The shifts are valid only for small susceptibilities ($\chi_i, \chi_e \ll 1$) and their derivation is the subject of Prob. 25.7. Note that the background shift $\chi_e/3$ (which includes a Lorentz sphere effect) depends on the geometry of the overall (background plus spherical/cylindrical body) system. See Springer in the Suggested Reading list at the end of the chapter for further discussion of the Lorentz sphere corrections.

Problem 25.7

a) Derive the expressions in Table 25.4 valid for small susceptibility. Hint: Replace χ by $\Delta\chi$ in the earlier formulas of this section and superimpose those results with the shift for a uniform background (with susceptibility χ_e and with no body compartment present). Discuss the dependence of your answer on the overall geometry of the background itself.

b) Find the profile for the sphere for a line through its center but orthogonal to $\vec{B}_0$.

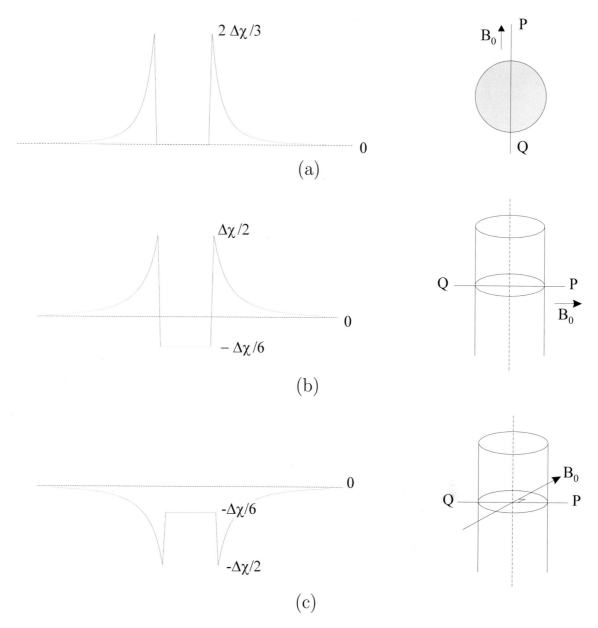

Fig. 25.4: Examples of profiles of the shift in magnetic field due to a spherical or cylindrical body for $\chi_e = 0$ and in units of B_0. (a) Along a diameter of a sphere parallel to $\vec{B}_0$. (b) Along a diameter of a cylindrical body whose axis is perpendicular to the field. The diameter is parallel to $\vec{B}_0$. (c) As in (b) but now along a diameter perpendicular to both $\vec{B}_0$ and the axis of the cylinder. All shifts would be changed by an additive constant if χ_e is not zero.

25.4 Susceptibility Imaging

Measuring local magnetic field variations $\Delta B(\vec{r})$ can be important to obtain tissue properties, to improve sequence design, or to observe effects in the body that change the local field. The flexibility in designing sequences has led to a number of methods to observe and quantify $\Delta B(\vec{r})$. Several of these are addressed below.

25.4.1 Phase Measurements

The presence of local variations in the magnetic field, $\Delta B(\vec{r})$, is known to cause image artifacts. In Ch. 20, we considered both geometric distortion and phase effects. The latter is coupled directly to the signal loss that occurs in gradient echo imaging although its presence alone corrupts the phase image. On the other hand, if there are no other sources of phase error, then the phase images serve as a direct measure of the magnetic field variations (deviations from B_0). The purpose of this section is to introduce the techniques from which phase can be found and, in turn, $\Delta B(\vec{r})$.

The simplest 'gedanken' approach is to acquire a gradient echo image with instantaneous sampling so that there are no phase variations induced by motion and there is no distortion. In that case, the phase should behave according to

$$\phi(\vec{r}, T_E) = -\gamma \Delta B(\vec{r}) T_E \tag{25.45}$$

As long as $\Delta B(\vec{r})$ is small enough for a given T_E that $|\phi| < \pi$, then there is a unique one-to-one map of phase to magnetic field. If not, aliasing occurs (see Chs. 11 and 15) and the phase may appear different than it actually is. This difficulty can be avoided if phase unwrapping is performed (see Prob. 25.9).

This somewhat straightforward, but naive, approach assumes there are no other sources of error. It is true that $\Delta B(\vec{r})$ generates a simple linear dependence of phase on time. However, we have seen that constant velocity flow across a read gradient can generate a quadratic dependence on time (specifically, the time during which the read gradient is on). Further, when gradients are turned on and off, there are often transient field effects which are a function of time and space, $\Delta B(\vec{r}, t)$. Their effect on an image can be quite complicated. Other sources of phase error also exist that are independent of time such as the miscalibration of the echo center.

Problem 25.8

Recall that a single point (Δk_x) positive shift in $s(k_x)$ generates the phase dependence $\phi(x) = 2\pi \Delta k_x x$ in the image. Find the effective constant gradient G'_x across the object that would mimic this phase behavior.

Problem 25.9

For a uniform object with no gaps or signal losses, phase unwrapping can be easily performed. One such algorithm is to take the complex signal $\hat{\rho}(\vec{r} = 0)$ at the origin and use it to renormalize all of its neighbors' signals. The relative spin density to be used in this algorithm is therefore

$$\tilde{\rho}(\vec{r}) \equiv \frac{\hat{\rho}(\vec{r})}{\hat{\rho}(\vec{r} = 0)} \tag{25.46}$$

a) If the phase at $\vec{r} = 0$ is ϕ_0, describe how the phases of the neighboring points will be determined in terms of a phase difference between the two points and ϕ_0. (Assume that the phase does not change by more than $\pm\pi$ between any two points.)

b) How is it that this method of obtaining phase differences prior to estimating the phase is more appropriate than trying to determine whether or not aliasing has occurred from point-to-point using the original phase images?

c) If gaps (zero magnitude signal) are present on the image, how might it cause problems for this algorithm?

d) Is it possible that phase unwrapping may depend on where the unwrapping begins and on the path of the points used? Hint: Consider a cylinder parallel to the field entering a slice in the lower half of the image. Assume the cylinder has a different χ than the background tissue.

Finally, the rf response of an object depends on its local conductivity (and permittivity), which has a direct effect on the phase of the tissue. This can be shown to induce a constant phase offset ϕ_0 independent of time. To account for this effect, the phase must be written as

$$\phi(\vec{r}, T_E) = \phi_0 - \gamma \Delta B(\vec{r}) T_E \tag{25.47}$$

Now, to extract $\Delta B(\vec{r})$, a single scan is not sufficient and two gradient echo scans must be collected, each with a different echo time. If transient field effects are not a problem, then a double echo scan can be used. Otherwise, an interleaved scan can be run where the second echo time has the exact same gradient structure as the first echo (all phase encoding timings relative to the read gradient are kept invariant, that is, both the read and phase encoding gradients are slid along as a group to the desired echo time). The phases from these two echoes are

$$\phi(\vec{r}, T_{E_1}) = \phi_0 - \gamma \Delta B(\vec{r}) T_{E_1} \tag{25.48}$$
$$\phi(\vec{r}, T_{E_2}) = \phi_0 - \gamma \Delta B(\vec{r}) T_{E_2} \tag{25.49}$$

The solutions for $\Delta B(\vec{r})$ and ϕ_0 are:

$$\Delta B(\vec{r}) = \frac{\phi(\vec{r}, T_{E_2}) - \phi(\vec{r}, T_{E_1})}{\gamma(T_{E_1} - T_{E_2})} \tag{25.50}$$

and

$$\phi_0 = \phi(\vec{r}, T_{E_1}) + \gamma \Delta B(\vec{r}) T_{E_1} \qquad (25.51)$$

Problem 25.10

Return to Figs. 17.20d and 17.21a, which represent the phase images for ϕ_0 and $-\gamma \Delta B(\vec{r}) T_{E_1}$.

a) Are there nonlinear phase variations in ϕ_0? If so, what might their origin be?

b) Of all the field variations seen in $-\gamma \Delta B(\vec{r}) T_{E_1}$, discuss why there appears to be a significant effect behind the knee.

Problem 25.11

One of the difficulties with a conventional gradient echo sequence is measuring large $\Delta B(\vec{r})$ effects. This is simply due to the fact that it takes a finite amount of time to generate an rf pulse and collect the data. One means to avoid this is to collect a spin echo data set where first the spin echo and gradient echo both occur at time T_E. Then, shift the π-pulse by a time ϵ toward the origin so that the spin echo now appears at the time $(T_E - 2\epsilon)$. The sampled data then behave as if they were collected as a gradient echo with an effective echo time 2ϵ. (See Sec. 17.3.3 for a more detailed discussion of this type of sequence.)

a) The shift ϵ can be made as small as possible. Why is this an advantage?

b) Why are two scans still necessary?

c) Does the sampling need to be symmetric to correctly extract the phase if the actual echo shift is known?

There is a similar approach one can take with gradient echo imaging by acquiring $T_{E_2} = T_{E_1} + 2\epsilon$.

d) Discuss how performing a complex division of $\hat{\rho}(T_{E_2})$ by $\hat{\rho}(T_{E_1})$ can be made to generate an alias-free phase image for any ΔB for sufficiently small ϵ. Assume that there is sufficient signal at T_{E_2} for the voxel of interest. (For large inhomogeneities, this may not be true because of signal dephasing within the voxel, and the spin echo approach then remains superior.)

To demonstrate that this double echo approach correctly extracts $\Delta B(\vec{r})$, a phantom with a known field effect can be scanned. In this example, a phantom is filled with gel and a cylinder is placed through the gel. The cylinder is empty and this geometry will create the dipolar effect described in various places in the previous section, when the cylinder is placed orthogonal to B_0. Fig. 25.5 reveals the expected signal loss and phase behavior associated with this setup. Fig. 25.6 shows the processed phase images to reveal the phases ϕ_0 and $\gamma\Delta B(\vec{r})(T_{E_1} - T_{E_2})$. The quality of the separation lies in the fact that there are no off-diagonal elements present in the inversion process, i.e., there is no mixing of $\Delta B(\vec{r})$ and ϕ_0 effects. The ϕ_0 map is seen to be almost linear in horizontal phase behavior, indicating that there is a time-independent echo shift associated with the data sampling. Any linear term in ϕ_0 can be removed by shifting $s(k)$ accordingly for one of the echoes (see the discussion on the Fourier transform shift theorem in Ch. 11). This information can also be used to calibrate the sampling so that the shift is no longer present. Finally, if $\Delta B(\vec{r})$ can be found for a known geometry, then $\Delta\chi$ between the two tissues can also be found.

Validation of Bulk Magnetic Susceptibility Theory

Since phase is directly proportional to the local field, we can use it to visualize the field dependence inside and outside of objects embedded in the background and test the theory developed in Sec. 25.3. A cylinder perpendicular to the main field serves to demonstrate the expected field changes as described in Table 25.4. To accomplish this, a cylinder is placed (vertically along $\hat{y}$) in a water phantom so that it is orthogonal to the main field (along $\hat{z}$). The cylinder is doped with a paramagnetic contrast agent. The resulting phase image (Fig. 25.7a) reveals the expected angular behavior as described in (25.25). This has important implications for the measurement of susceptibility changes from tissue to tissue in that geometry must be taken into account.

25.4.2   Magnitude Measurements

In certain cases, it is possible to infer changes in local magnetic field from the magnitude image. Although the pattern of signal loss in Figs. 25.5a and 25.5b is a unique signature for a cylinder, it is dependent on the direction of the read gradient and any underlying distortion along the read direction. Also, there may be a number of different field effects that can lead to signal loss at the pixel level so that the inversion process used to find $\Delta B(\vec{r})$ gives more of an average field change across the voxel. There are two other methods that relate to changes in the image signal associated with the frequency changes $\Delta\omega = \gamma\Delta B(\vec{r})$ which are discussed below.

SSFP: Magnitude Dependence on $\Delta B(\vec{r})$

In Ch. 18, Sec. 18.2, the sensitivity of the SSFP magnitude signal to the resonance offset angle β was discussed. In this subsection, an application of the sensitivity to the local field is turned from being an artifact into revealing something about the local field. For short-T_R and a fully balanced sequence, the resonance offset angle, β, from one rf pulse to the next is simply $\gamma\Delta B(\vec{r})T_R$ plus any purposely impressed rf offset.

According to Fig. 18.12 for a large flip angle scan and β near π, the signal response will be high, while for β near 0, it will be low. (This assumes that the excitation frequency is on-resonance so that $\Delta\omega = 0$. Otherwise, the resonance offset angle becomes $\gamma\Delta BT_R + \Delta\omega T_R$.)

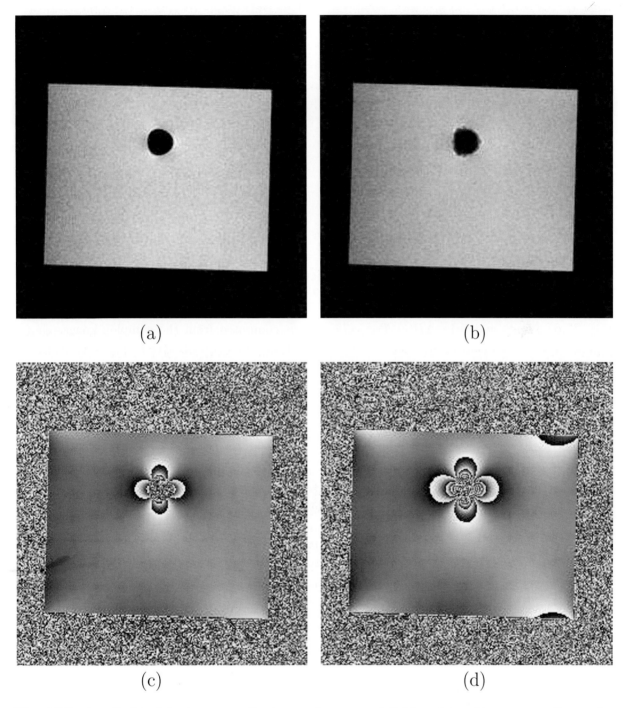

Fig. 25.5: A cylindrical body perpendicular to the external field and its effects on gradient echo magnitude and phase images: (a) magnitude image at T_{E_1}; (b) magnitude image at $2T_{E_1}$; (c) and (d) are the corresponding phase images. Note the dipolar behavior and the increased aliasing of the phase at the longer echo time.

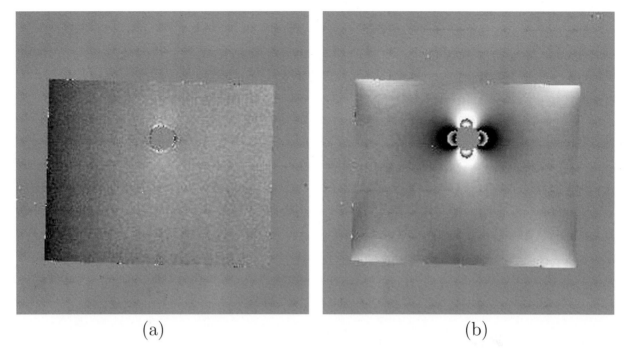

$$(a) \hspace{8cm} (b)$$

Fig. 25.6: (a) ϕ_0 and (b) $\gamma \Delta B(\vec{r})(T_{E_1} - T_{E_2})$ maps computed from the complex images shown in Fig. 25.5. No dipolar field effects from the air-filled tube are observed in (a), indicating a clean separation between ϕ_0 and $\gamma \Delta B(\vec{r})(T_{E_1} - T_{E_2})$. Note the similarity between Fig. 25.6b and Fig. 25.5c. The aliasing is slightly different due to the nonzero result for ϕ_0. In order to avoid the appearance of random phase in regions of noise, the phase values were set to zero whenever the magnitude was less than two standard deviations.

This is demonstrated in Fig. 25.8a. A more dramatic example of this dependence is seen when low flip angles are used. Then, the signal remains high and actually builds up coherence only near $\beta = 0$ (Fig. 25.8b). It is rather astonishing how much coherence builds up even for small flip angles. The resulting stripes of high signal represent regions of constant $\Delta B(\vec{r})$, iso-field lines where $\gamma \Delta B(\vec{r})T_R$ is a multiple of 2π (Fig. 25.8b).

Variable RF Pulse Techniques

In Ch. 16, Sec. 16.7.2, a method was described to excite just thin strips of the object being imaged. The excited strips were spaced at equal frequency intervals. The application to finding $\Delta B(\vec{r})$ is obvious. The effects of the local fields are to bend the lines of constant frequency, again yielding information on $\Delta B(\vec{r})$. Since the frequency of each line is known, shifts in their locations can be used to quantify $\Delta B(\vec{r})$.

25.5   Brain Functional MRI and the BOLD Phenomenon

It is well-known today that as the oxygen content in blood changes so does the local suscep-tibility in the blood. The source of this dependence has been shown to be the unshielded

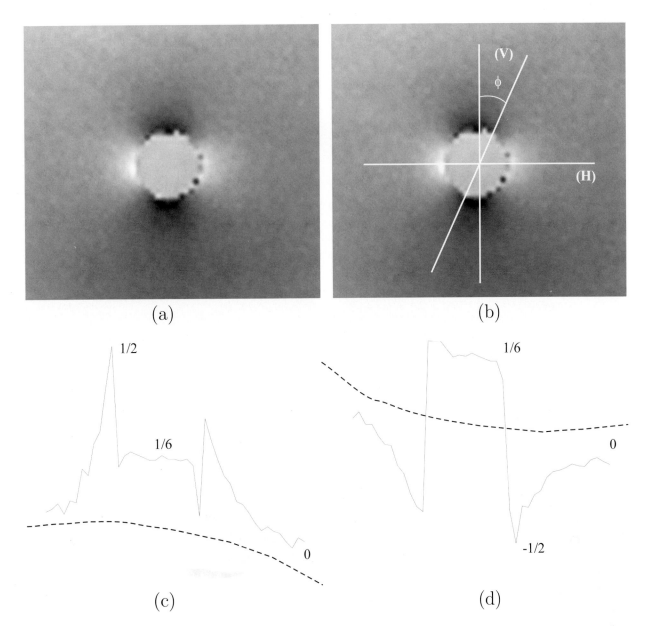

Fig. 25.7: (a) Phase image demonstrating bulk magnetic susceptibility-induced local field variations in the presence of a cylinder whose axis is perpendicular to B_0. The cylinder contains distilled water which is doped with the contrast agent Gd-DTPA (gadopentetate dimeglumine or, equivalently, gadolinium diethylenetriaminepentaacetic acid) to a concentration which creates a noticeable bulk shift in the magnetic susceptibility. (b) The same image as in (a) with the coordinate system overlaid on it showing the two lines (labeled H and V, V is parallel to the external field) across which the profiles of (c) and (d) were respectively obtained. (c) A profile of the phase along the line H, and (d) a profile along the line V. The dashed lines in (c) and (d) represent the estimated baseline in the presence of background static field inhomogeneities. When the drifts are corrected for and Gibbs ringing at the edges is accounted for, these profiles are seen to match, within an overall sign, the expected profiles as suggested in Figs. 25.4b and 25.4c and in Table 25.4.

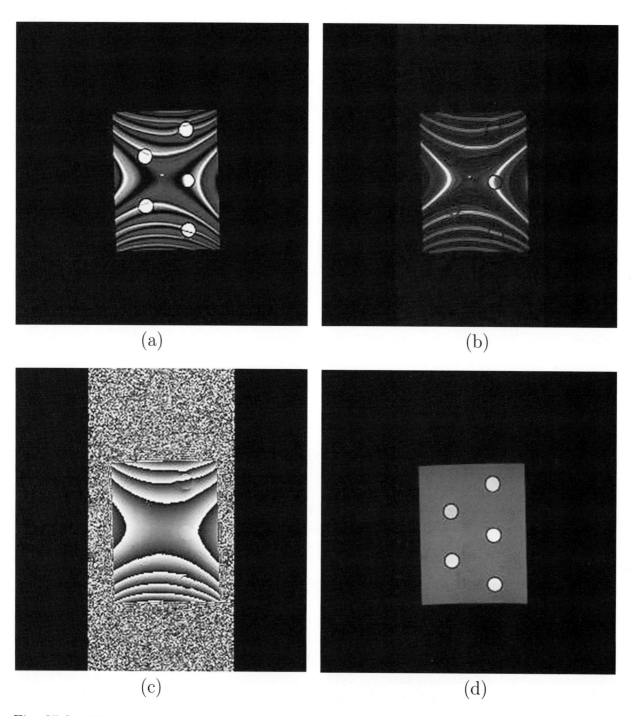

Fig. 25.8: Different methods of visualizing local field changes due to the presence of magnetized objects in the bulk object. (a) A large flip angle ($\theta = 70°$) SSFP magnitude image, (b) a low flip angle ($\theta = 2°$) SSFP magnitude image, both acquired using non-alternating rf pulses ($\beta_{rf} = 0$), (c) a phase image from an SSI sequence with a T_E which equals the T_R (8 ms) used in the SSFP acquisitions, and (d) a magnitude image corresponding to the phase image in (c).

iron in hemoglobin (red blood cells). In this section, we explore the relationship between oxygenation and susceptibility.

Blood can be approximated as a two-compartment system containing both plasma (very water-like) and red blood cells. The fraction of the volume of packed red blood cells to the volume of whole blood is called the hematocrit (Hct), and Hct is typically about 0.4 (40%).[3] It can change at the capillary level where single blood cells course through the tissue. White blood cells are less than 1% of the red blood cells and play little role in our discussion.

Much of the iron in the blood is in the hemoglobin, or more specifically, in one of two states, oxyhemoglobin or deoxyhemoglobin.[4] These two states differ in their magnetic properties. Oxyhemoglobin is diamagnetic with no unpaired electrons. A deoxyhemoglobin molecule has a 'hole' in the structure of the molecule that prevents complete shielding of the iron in its center. That is, there are unpaired electrons (an even number of them) in this relatively complex molecule making deoxyhemoglobin paramagnetic.

25.5.1 Estimation of Oxygenation Levels

If oxygenation of red blood cells is dominated by the formation of oxyhemoglobin, we are led to consider the concomitant change in the red blood cell susceptibility relative to its surroundings. A model for the susceptibility of the total blood system is

$$\chi_{blood} = \text{Hct}\,(Y\chi_{oxy} + (1-Y)\chi_{deoxy}) + (1-\text{Hct})\chi_{plasma} \tag{25.52}$$

in terms of the oxygenation level Y (the fractional oxygenation in the red cells), the susceptibilities of the red blood cell components and the plasma, and the aforesaid fraction of red cells Hct (the fractional hematocrit).

A change ΔY in the oxygenation level shifts the susceptibility according to

$$\Delta\chi_{blood} = -\Delta Y(\chi_{deoxy} - \chi_{oxy})\text{Hct} \tag{25.53}$$

It is evident that the hemoglobin dominance of the oxygenation dependence has led to the susceptibility shift (25.53) given by the difference between the susceptibilities of deoxyhemoglobin and oxyhemoglobin. This approximation also neglects any oxygenation of the plasma component accounting for its absence in this shift.

The change in blood susceptibility from fully oxygenated to deoxygenated blood has been measured to be[5]

$$\begin{aligned}\chi_{do} &\equiv \chi_{deoxy} - \chi_{oxy} \\ &= 4\pi \cdot (0.18)\ \text{ppm per unit Hct}\end{aligned} \tag{25.54}$$

---

[3]The hematocrit can vary significantly and is usually lower for women than men. The value of 40% is closer to the average for women while that for men approaches 45%.

[4]There is also another state called methemoglobin pertaining to clotting. It is an electron paramagnetic substance which leads to a shortening of T_1.

[5]χ_{do} is often expressed as 0.18 ppm in cgs units. More recently, this value is replaced by 0.27 ppm, a change that impacts considerably the expected value of the oxygen saturation Y if the product $\chi_{do}(1-Y)$ remains invariant.

It has been observed that arterial (oxygenated) blood appears to have the same susceptibility as the surrounding tissue. Then, if $\chi_{plasma} \simeq \chi_{oxy}$, (25.52) and (25.54) lead to the practical form

$$\chi_{blood,relative} \equiv \chi_{blood} - \chi_{surr} \simeq \chi_{blood} - \chi_{oxy} = 4\pi \cdot (0.18) \cdot \text{Hct}(1 - Y)\,\text{ppm} \qquad (25.55)$$

relative to the surrounding tissue.

The phase variation in a compartment of blood due to the change in susceptibility induced in turn by the change in oxygenation can be found in models such as the spherical and cylindrical systems considered earlier. An example is the change in the internal field of a long cylinder relative to surrounding tissue (as a model for a blood vessel, say) where the cylindrical axis makes an angle of θ to the external field. From (25.13), (25.44), and (25.55)

$$\begin{aligned} \phi_{blood} &= -\gamma \Delta B_{cyl,in} T_E \\ &= -\gamma \chi_{do}\text{Hct}(1 - Y)(3\cos^2\theta - 1)B_0 T_E/6 \end{aligned} \qquad (25.56)$$

It is seen that phase variations potentially can be used as a source of information about hematocrit or oxygen saturation (percentage oxygen content of blood). If we know the individual susceptibilities of the hemoglobin components and the hematocrit, we can determine the absolute oxygenation level Y from ϕ_{blood}. For the remainder of this chapter, we assume that fully oxygenated arterial blood has the same susceptibility value as the surrounding tissue.

25.5.2   Deoxyhemoglobin Concentration and Flow

Susceptibility artifacts are usually considered a nuisance, but, in the case of blood, the phase plays a key role in visualizing changes in the utilization of oxygen in the brain and in the amount of oxygen in the red blood cells. The susceptibility reflects deoxyhemoglobin levels and, as is shown below, blood flow and cerebral oxygen utilization (the cerebral metabolic rate) affect the deoxyhemoglobin levels. Their joint actions will help determine ϕ_{blood} for a given physiological system. The investigation of this area is referred to as BOLD (Blood Oxygenation Level Dependent) imaging; it was indeed a bold step and is used in the evaluation of brain function, an area often referred to as functional MRI or fMRI.

The fractional oxygen saturation can be written as

$$Y = 1 - \frac{N_{deoxy}}{N_0} \qquad (25.57)$$

where N_{deoxy} is the number of deoxyhemoglobin molecules and N_0 the total number of oxyhemoglobin and deoxyhemoglobin molecules. The change in N_{deoxy} will depend on both the 'flow' and the cerebral 'metabolic rate' (or oxygen utilization). Define the relative change in flow as α and in the metabolic rate as $\beta - 1$ such that the change in N_{deoxy} is given by

$$\Delta N_{deoxy} = \beta N_{deoxy}/(1 + \alpha) - N_{deoxy} \qquad (25.58)$$

(Indeed, $\alpha = 0$ and $\beta = 1$ lead to no change.) This in turn yields

$$\Delta Y = -\Delta N_{deoxy}/N_0$$

$$= \frac{1 + \alpha - \beta}{1 + \alpha} \frac{N_{deoxy}}{N_0}$$

$$= \frac{1 + \alpha - \beta}{1 + \alpha}(1 - Y) \qquad (25.59)$$

When $\beta = 1$ (i.e., there is a decoupling between metabolic rate and flow change), the oxygen saturation shift collapses to

$$\Delta Y = \frac{\alpha}{1 + \alpha}(1 - Y) \qquad (25.60)$$

For instance, with $Y = 0.55$, a 50% increase in flow corresponds to an increase of only 0.15 in Y.[6] Nevertheless, it must be kept in mind that changes in β may mask the effect of the change in flow.

25.5.3 Functional MR Imaging (fMRI): An Example

The sensitivity of both the blood signal and the surrounding tissue signal due to the presence of $\Delta\chi$ caused by deoxyhemoglobin leads to several major effects on the total signal. As T_2^* of the blood changes, so does the signal contribution from blood (see Sec. 25.6). This change together with the phase shift of the blood produces intravoxel signal loss. The extravascular gradients lead to signal dephasing in the tissue surrounding the blood vessels (ignoring the effects of these gradients on other blood vessels).

Functional brain imaging is based on changes in oxygen saturation, ΔY. In the simple case of a volunteer moving a thumb, the signal would increase because the flow increases in a particular vessel (in the primary motor cortex for this example). Fortuitously, the oxygen utilization does not change much ($\beta \simeq 1$) and, hence, ΔY obeys (25.60). This ΔY is then the source of all the signal changes inside and outside of the vessel. The subtracted image yields a representation of where signal changes occurred (see Fig. 25.9).

Problem 25.12

---

a) Estimate the expected change in signal for a blood vessel parallel to the main magnetic field if $Y_i = 0.55$ and $Y_f = 0.70$, where Y_i is the venous oxygen fraction during resting state and Y_f is that during the active state. Assume the venous blood fraction in the voxel, λ_v, equals 0.05, $T_R = \infty$ (i.e., neglect the T_1 and flip angle dependence), and $T_E = T_2^*$(venous blood) $= T_2^*$(background tissue). Hint: Use (25.65).

b) If brain oxygen utilization remains invariant, what is the change in flow needed to effect the change in Y given in part (a)?

---

[6]These numbers have been extracted from phase measurements using the techniques outlined in Sec. 25.4.

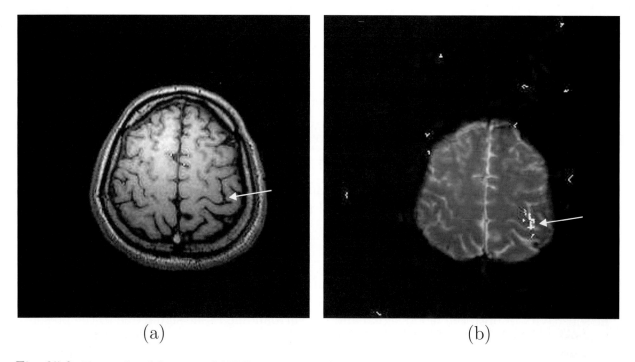

(a)   (b)

Fig. 25.9: Example of functional MRI experimental data on a volunteer during right thumb move-ment. (a) A T_1-weighted image of the brain slice of interest showing excellent anatomical detail. (b) Pixels from the gradient echo images collected during repeated active and resting state cycles which correlated strongly with the cycling in thumb movement or periods of rest are overlaid on one of the original gradient echo echo planar images. Activation is seen to be localized to the left primary motor cortex (arrow).

25.6 Signal Behavior in the Presence of Deoxygenated Blood

In conventional MR imaging, the ideal world is to have all tissues experience the same magnetic field prior to application of the read gradient. This procedure highlights differences in spin density, T_1, and T_2, but purposely neglects chemical shift differences. These were initially thought to be a nuisance, especially as far as fat was concerned. The chemical shift between fat and water is so large that it manifests itself in MR images at short echo times (recall that $\Delta\omega_{fw} = -\sigma_{fw}\gamma B_0$ where σ_{fw} is 3.35 ppm for fat relative to water). Already at $T_E = 2.34$ ms, fat becomes π radians out-of-phase relative to water for $B_0 = 1.5$ T (see Ch. 17).

Now that magnetic fields can be very uniformly created, to roughly 1 ppm across the brain, it is possible to collect long T_E gradient echo images with minimal T_2' dephasing artifacts (see Ch. 20). At long echo times, even small changes in chemical shift or local susceptibility can emerge. Such is the case for a blood vessel parallel to the main field which has an effective maximum frequency shift of $\Delta\omega_{blood} = \gamma\delta_{blood}B_0$ with $\delta_{blood} \simeq 0.3(1-Y)$ ppm for Hct = 0.4. As mentioned before, this frequency shift generates a sensitivity to oxygen saturation.

25.6.1 The MR Properties of Blood

Historically, the MR properties of blood have been measured *in vitro*. In this section, we will deal primarily with the *in vivo* properties of blood.

Spin Density of Blood

In order to appreciate the changes in signal due to changes in local magnetic fields within the venous blood, it is helpful to review the MR properties of blood. Recall that blood contains both plasma and hematocrit (red blood cells) and that plasma is roughly 60% of blood and hematocrit is the other 40%. About half of the latter acts like water, giving an effective spin density of roughly 80% relative to cerebrospinal fluid (CSF) which is essentially water. Blood is highly concentrated in gray matter which has roughly the same spin density, 80% of CSF. Thus, when short echo times are used in a large-volume, spin density weighted, gradient echo scan, small blood vessels in the brain are not usually seen.

T_1 of Blood

The T_1 of blood is quite different from other tissues at 1.5 T. If 2D methods are used, T_1 of blood is often quoted as 1200 ms. However, a full 3D evaluation suggests it is closer to 1400 to 1500 ms. In either case, it is significantly longer than that of other tissues and, unless blood is refreshed, will usually be saturated and appear darker than the surrounding tissue in T_1 weighted scans. To maximize signal from blood relative to other tissues, special choices of flip angle, T_R, and T_E must be made (see Ch. 24).

T_2 and T_2^* of Blood

The measurement of ρ_0 or T_1 is rather simple compared to that of T_2 or T_2^*. The fact that the blood is moving makes it very difficult to estimate accurately either of these two properties (see Ch. 22). The presence of deoxyhemoglobin causes a local gradient to be created, which allows for dephasing from both diffusion (Ch. 21) and conventional static dephasing effects. Since the former depends on the gradient squared and the latter on the gradient, the decay rate must look like

$$R_2 = R_{2,0} + \alpha(1 - Y) + \beta(1 - Y)^2 \tag{25.61}$$

or

$$R_2^* = R_{2,0}^* + \alpha^*(1 - Y) + \beta^*(1 - Y)^2 \tag{25.62}$$

Current estimates for the coefficients are given in Table 25.5.

Clotted Blood

When blood escapes from the vascular system during hemorrhage, its structure is quickly altered. In the early stage, the hemoglobin content can change dramatically from 40% to 90%. This would affect both $\Delta\phi$ and $T_{2,blood}^*$ and lead to significant signal loss in gradient echo images. As blood clots, hemosiderin is formed. Hemosiderin is roughly 25% Fe^{3+} (which has 5 unpaired electrons) and this can cause signal loss on T_2^*-weighted images (from static field dephasing) and on T_2-weighted images (from the presence of gradients, which lead to

Coefficient	$R_{2,0}$, $R_{2,0}^*$	α, α^*	β, β^*
T_2 (a)	3.8	0	13.4
T_2 (b)	3.6	10.7	0
T_2^* (a)	5	14	0
T_2^* (b)	6.6	13.3	0
T_2^* (c)	7.2	1.1	34.7

Table 25.5: Approximate numerical values of the coefficients in (25.61) and (25.62) for T_2 decay and T_2^* decay. For the T_2 decay, the range of Y values measured and fit was from 0.3 to 1.0 for (a) and 0.3 to 0.8 for (b). Part (b) was estimated from the data in Wright *et al.* (see Suggested Reading at the end of the chapter for the complete reference for this article) for a CPMG sequence with an interpulse spacing of 6 ms. For the T_2^* decay, the range of Y was limited to 0.7 to 1.0 in humans for (a) and 0.6 to 1.0 for blood samples (b). For part (c), a more complete range of Y from 0.2 to 1.0 was fit for blood samples (see Li *et al.* in the Suggested Reading).

signal loss from the diffusion process). On T_1-weighted images, the signal goes up because the 5 unpaired electrons lead to a lowering of the T_1. Methemoglobin then forms, which also contains Fe^{3+}. Finally, as red blood cells are broken down, local gradients vanish and signal is less affected (apart from edema still being present throughout this process). Both hemosiderin and methemoglobin are highly paramagnetic.

Problem 25.13

For deoxyhemoglobin, the spin is 2, while for methemoglobin, the spin is 5/2. What is the change in the magnetic moment for methemoglobin versus deoxyhemoglobin and what is the ratio of the susceptibilies of deoxyhemoglobin to methemoglobin?

25.6.2 Two-Compartment Partial Volume Effects on Signal Loss

On a number of occasions, the effects of local magnetic field variations have been considered. In Ch. 20, these field changes were cited as the source for T_2^*. There a discussion was given of how random changes in these fields did, in fact, cause a change in the relaxation rate within a volume for gradient echo imaging through (25.55)

$$\frac{1}{T_2^*} = \frac{1}{T_2} + \kappa\gamma|\Delta B| \tag{25.63}$$

where κ is a geometric factor. However, it was also shown that this form is not always valid and the signal loss associated with a given field distribution need not be exponential.

For example, a linear change in field of ΔB_{voxel} across a voxel (instead of the dipolar field discussed in Secs. 20.4 and 20.5) was shown to lead to a fractional signal loss of (see (20.21))

$$f(T_E) = 1 - \text{sinc}(\gamma \Delta B_{voxel} T_E / 2) \tag{25.64}$$

Two-compartment, partial volume effects have been previously discussed with respect to the chemical shift differences between water and fat. In Sec. 17.3.1, it was shown that mixing water and fat in a single pixel reveals an oscillating signal behavior superimposed on the exponential decay. A similar effect can be expected for a voxel containing both brain parenchyma and venous blood, the latter having a different susceptibility than the former.

Veins Parallel to the Magnetic Field

The easiest example to construct is a voxel containing a vessel parallel to the static field for any of the conventional data acquisition views of transverse, sagittal, or coronal. For a given experiment, let the signal fraction from the blood vessel (veins) be given by λ_v at $T_E = 0$. Then, as the echo time increases, the total signal from, say, brain parenchyma plus venous blood will be

$$\hat{\rho}(T_E) = \rho_0 e^{-T_E / T_2^*} \left((1 - \lambda_v) + \lambda_v e^{i\phi_v(T_E)} \right) \tag{25.65}$$

where $\phi_v(T_E)$ is the phase of the venous blood relative to brain parenchyma at an echo time of T_E. Recall that the signals from blood and brain parenchyma will depend, in general, on the tissue properties and imaging parameters. It has been assumed that brain parenchyma and venous blood have the same T_2^*. With this geometry, there is no gradient created outside the cylinder.

The phase difference between venous blood and brain parenchyma is given by

$$\phi_v(T_E) = -\gamma \Delta B T_E \tag{25.66}$$

where, for a vessel parallel to the static field, (25.56) yields

$$\gamma \Delta B \simeq 40\pi(1 - Y) \tag{25.67}$$

at 1.5 T with $\gamma \Delta B$ given in rad/sec. For $Y = 0.5$ and $T_E = 50\,\text{ms}$, it is expected that maximal signal loss will occur. This is demonstrated in Fig. 25.10 pictorially.

Problem 25.14

The blood volume fraction is often very small, usually about 5% in a given pixel, excluding large vessels. How is it that λ_v might end up being as large as 0.5 when a T_1-weighted acquisition with a short-T_R gradient echo sequence is used? Hint: Consider a 2D plane where blood flow is perpendicular to the plane and T_R is such that $v T_R = T_H$, but otherwise short compared to the T_1 of the brain parenchyma.

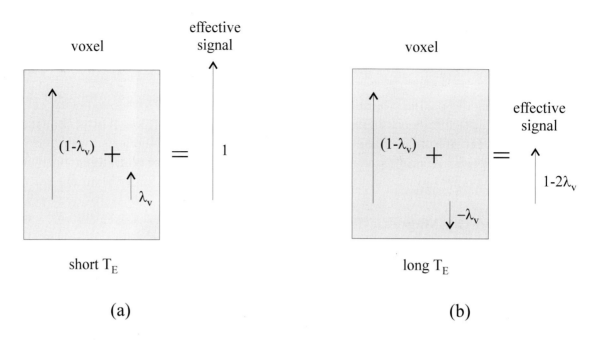

Fig. 25.10: The simplest model to consider the effects of the signal from veins partially canceling with that from surrounding tissue in a voxel. The cylindrical vessel is assumed to be parallel to $\vec{B}_0$. (a) The resulting effective signal for short T_E (normalized to unity). (b) The resulting effective signal for long T_E, where $\phi_v(T_E) = -\pi$ (its normalization is $(1 - 2\lambda_v)e^{-(T_{E,long}-T_{E,short})/T_2^*}$ relative to (a)).

Problem 25.15

a) Consider a field difference ΔB_{voxel} between the edge of the vein (modeled as a cylinder), completely contained in one pixel, and the edge of the adjacent pixel. Assume the field reduces linearly within the pixel from the left-side to the right-side of the pixel. Use the field at $\rho = a$ (where a is the radius of the cylinder) for the left-side of the pixel and $\rho = 3a$ from the right-side. What is the maximum signal loss due to (25.64) if $B_0 = 1.5\,\mathrm{T}$, $Y = 0.7$, and $T_E = 50\,\mathrm{ms}$? Hint: Use the approximation $\phi = 0$ in Table 25.4. This represents the signal loss in the adjacent pixel when no partial volume of the vein exists.

b) Consider a vein parallel to the field but smaller than a voxel. The signal is then given by (25.65). Plot the phase as a function of T_E for a field strength of 1.5 T and for $\lambda_v = 0.1$, 0.2, and 0.5. Assume $Y = 0.7$ and Hct $= 0.4$. The signal behavior shown here represents a non-exponential oscillating form of signal dependence on T_E.

c) For a vein perpendicular to B_0, what modification will be made to (25.65)?

Scale Variance

For certain random systems, the signal loss in a voxel is exponential. The voxel size does not affect the form of the decay. For large voxels, the signal loss from the vascular system may be lumped into this class. However, as voxel size is reduced to the size of a vessel, these assumptions break down and partial volume effects become important. As has just been shown in the previous problem, even a vessel which contributes only a small value of λ_v to the signal may have significant non-exponential effects on the signal loss. This implies that the signal loss behavior is scale variant. Superimposed on this will still be a background T_2^* due to smaller structures which are scale invariant.

As an example, consider the same physical case of a vessel parallel to B_0, and a transverse acquisition. Rather than a large voxel containing one vessel, the resolution is taken to be high enough that at least one voxel fits entirely within the cross section of the vessel (see Fig. 25.11a). For an echo time where the phase of the veins is $-\pi$, the vessel will appear bright in the center, but dark around the edges in a magnitude image. This ring around the vessel occurs because of the partial volume effect in these pixels (see Fig. 25.11b).

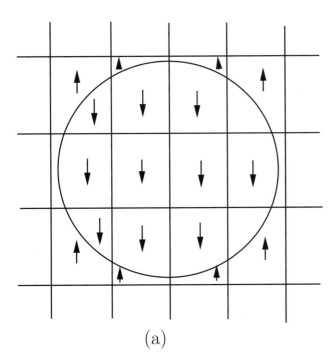
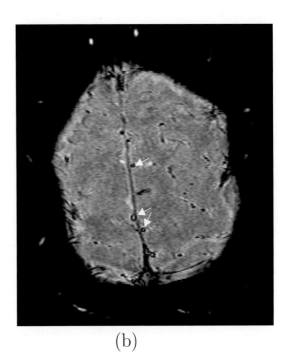

(a)   (b)

Fig. 25.11: (a) A schematic representation of a two-compartment model of a cylindrical vessel sitting in background tissue. Arrows represent the signal contribution from deoxygenated blood (which is inverted for the imaging parameters chosen) or from background tissue (which has zero phase). After taking the magnitude of the image, those voxels that have both terms contributing will have a smaller signal than voxels with no partial volume effects. (b) A long T_E (60 ms) magnitude image extracted from a 3D data set. The vessels encircled by black rings are veins which are significantly larger than a pixel in cross section, some of which are marked by arrows. The other dark structures without rings are also veins but their diameters are on the order of the dimension of the pixel.

MR Densitometry

From the above argument, we see that sub-voxel venous vessels which generate sufficient phase to cause a significant loss of signal can be visualized. Consider the situation where SNR is 100:1 (i.e., there is 1% noise) and λ_v is 4% of the total signal ($\lambda_v = 0.04$). When the phase of the veins is $-\pi$, the signal loss relative to surrounding tissue where λ_v is 0 would be 8%. This is significant in that it is eight times the noise level. This 4% contribution, if it comes from the vessel/voxel volume ratio (and, hence, the ratio of the vessel cross-sectional area to the voxel area) and the vessel is taken to be parallel to B_0 in a transverse slice, would indicate a vessel radius of

$$a = \sqrt{\frac{0.04}{\pi}}\,\mathrm{mm} = 0.113\,\mathrm{mm} \tag{25.68}$$

For a $1\,\mathrm{mm}^2$ voxel size, this implies that a vessel of diameter $0.23\,\mathrm{mm}$ could be seen if there is sufficient CNR.

Despite its sensitivity, MR densitometry is not easy to demonstrate with just small changes in magnitude unless it is enhanced by the associated phase information. This is accomplished, in principle, by creating a mask from the phase image $\hat{\phi}(\vec{r})$ as follows: normalize all phases less than zero by dividing by π and set all phases above zero to zero. This new mask image can be written as

$$g(\vec{r}) = \begin{cases} 1 + \hat{\phi}(\vec{r})/\pi & \text{for } -\pi \leq \hat{\phi}(\vec{r}) \leq 0 \\ 1 & 0 < \hat{\phi}(\vec{r}) < \pi \end{cases} \tag{25.69}$$

The new enhanced densitometric image is given by

$$d(\vec{r}) = |\hat{\rho}(\vec{r})|\, g^p(\vec{r}) \tag{25.70}$$

where p is often chosen to be 4 in practice. Practically, there are other sources of phase error than just the blood in the veins so this approach represents only an idealized situation.

Problem 25.16

---

   a) The filter $g(\vec{r})$ will work as expected for all veins making an angle between 0 and $\theta_m = \cos^{-1}\sqrt{\frac{1}{3}}$ to the static magnetic field $\vec{B}_0$. How should it be modified to enhance vessels perpendicular to the main field?

   b) Given the profile in Fig. 25.4, discuss why the presence of some of the external fields will not be observable in $g(\vec{r})$.

   c) If there exists another source of phase variation in the tissues (such as their own differences in susceptibility), how will this manifest itself in the images?

The resulting venographic images can show exquisite venous detail (Fig. 25.12d) when viewed over a few slices processed with both the above phase masking algorithm and a minimum intensity projection (Fig. 25.13).[7] Since the veins are not the only source of field

---

[7]A minimum intensity projection is the opposite concept to the maximum intensity projection discussed at the end of Ch. 23 and used to produce several images shown in Ch. 24. Here, the minimum (rather than the maximum) voxel signal value is retained for each pixel in the projection plane.

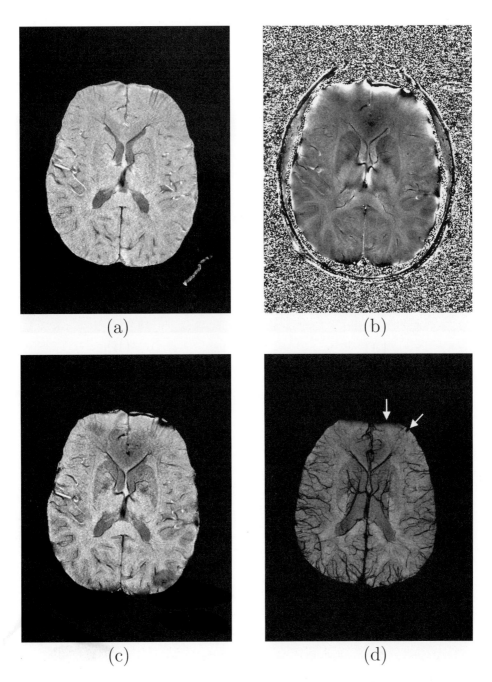

Fig. 25.12: Demonstration of the MR densitometric visualization of venous structures from $3\,T$. (a) An original magnitude image from a high resolution, long T_E acquisition ($T_E = 60\,ms$) 3D SSI data set. (b) Corresponding phase image. (c) Densitometric image created from the same complex image by using a phase mask with p as discussed in (25.70) chosen to be 4. (d) A minimum intensity projection over a $30\,mm$ slab of the densitometric images displays even small venous structures in the brain. Some problems from unwanted macroscopic field effects remain in the anterior portion of the head (arrows).

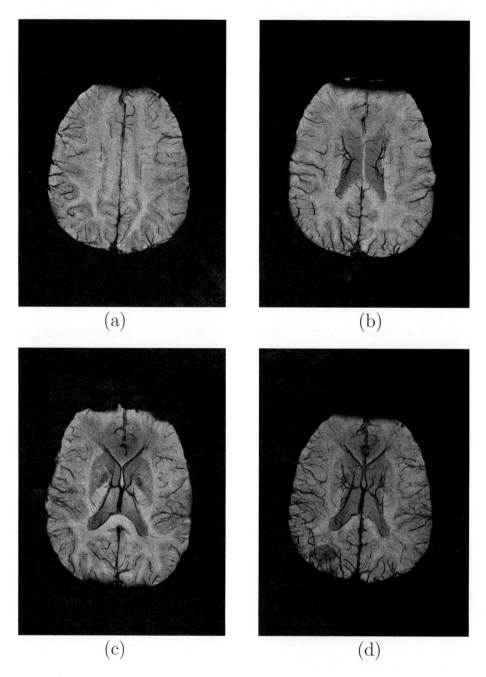

(a)   (b)

(c)   (d)

Fig. 25.13: Second demonstration of the MR densitometric visualization of venous structures from 3 T. (a) A minimum intensity projection over a 10 mm slab of the densitometric images displays even small venous structures in the brain. (b) Projection over the next 10 mm and (c) the following 10 mm of the brain. These three slabs were projected together in Fig. 25.12d to better follow the vascular structures. The projection is repeated here in (d).

inhomogeneity, the above algorithm is affected by extraneous field variations. Although the minimum intensity projection processing better reveals the vessel connectivity, it can also degrade the image quality. The latter occurs because the noise in each slice can reduce the overall background and suppress the contrast of the veins with respect to the background signal.

Suggested Reading

Diamagnetism models, a discussion of near fields that pertain to the Lorentz sphere effect, and a good discussion of units can be found in the following excellent undergraduate and graduate electromagnetism texts:

- D. J. Griffiths. *Introduction to Electrodynamics*. Prentice-Hall, New Jersey, 1989.

- J. D. Jackson. *Classical Electrodynamics*. John Wiley and Sons, New York, 1975.

A good overview of magnetic field phenomena appears in the following two articles (the first being nontechnical while the second is quite technical):

- S. Saini, R. B. Frankel, D. D. Stark and J. T. Ferrucci. Magnetism: A primer and review. *Am. J. Roentgenol.*, 150: 735, 1988.

- J. F. Schenck. The role of magnetic susceptibility in magnetic resonance imaging: MRI magnetic compatibility of the first and second kinds. *Med. Phys.*, 23: 815, 1996.

Understanding local magnetic fields and the Lorentz sphere for a variety of situations is discussed in the following three papers:

- D. T. Edmonds and M. R. Wormald. Theory of resonance in magnetically inhomogeneous specimens and some useful calculations. *J. Magn. Reson.*, 77: 223, 1988.

- P. W. Kuchel and B. T. Bulliman. Perturbation of homogeneous magnetic fields by isolated single and confocal spheroids. Implications for NMR spectroscopy of cells. *NMR Biomed.*, 2: 151, 1989.

- C. S. Springer, Jr. *Ch. 5: Physicochemical principles influencing magnetopharmaceuticals* in *NMR in Physiology and Biomedicine*, 75: 99, Academic Press, New York, 1994.

Several papers dealing with the T_2 and T_2^* dependence on oxygen saturation can be used to further review this area:

- Bodansky. Methemoglobinemia and methemoglobin-producing compounds. *Pharmacol Rev.*, 3: 144, 1951.

- D. Li, Y. Wang and D. J. Waight. Blood oxygen saturation assessment *in vivo* using T_2^* estimation. *Magn. Reson. Med.*, 39: 685, 1998.

- L. Pauling and C. Coryell. The magnetic properties and structure of hemoglobin, oxyhemoglobin and carboxyhemoglobin. *Proc. Natl. Acad. Sci.*, 22: 210, 1936.

- K. R. Thulborn, J. C. Waterton, P. M. Matthews and G. K. Radda. Oxygenation dependence of the transverse relaxation time of water protons in whole blood at high field. *Biochim. Biophy. Acta*, 714: 265, 1982.

- G. A. Wright, B. S. Hu and A. Macovski. Estimating oxygen saturation of blood *in vivo* with MR imaging at 1.5 T. *J. Magn. Reson. Imag.*, 1: 275, 1991.

Using phase to measure susceptibility of blood appears in:

- E. M. Haacke, S. Lai, J. R. Reichenbach, K. Kuppusamy, F. G. C. Hoogenrad, H. Takeichi and W. Lin. *In vivo* measurement of blood oxygen saturation using magnetic resonance imaging: A direct validation of the blood oxygenation level-dependent concept in functional brain imaging. *Human Brain Mapping*, 5: 341, 1997.

- W. M. Spees, D. A. Yablonskiy, M. C. Oswood and J. H. Ackerman. Water proton MR properties of human blood at 1.5 Tesla: magnetic susceptibility, T_1, T_2, T_2^*, and non-Lorentzian signal behavior. *Magn. Reson. Med.*, 45: 533, 2001.

- R. M. Weiskoff and S. Kiihne. MRI susceptometry: Image-based measurement of absolute susceptibility of MR contrast agents and human blood. *Magn. Reson. Med.*, 24: 375, 1992.

Using specially designed variable rf pulse sequences to measure local fields is discussed in:

- S. Li, B. J. Dardzinski, C. M. Collins, Q. X. Yang and M. B. Smith. Three-dimensional mapping of the static magnetic field inside the human head. *Magn. Reson. Med.*, 36: 705, 1994.

Units, paramagnetism and diamagnetism, are reviewed in the following books:

- E. A. Boudreaux and L. N. Mulay. *Theory and Applications of Molecular Paramagnetism.* Wiley, New York, 1976.

- L. N. Mulay and E. A. Boudreaux. *Theory and Applications of Molecular Diamagnetism.* Wiley, New York, 1976.

Chapter 26

Sequence Design, Artifacts, and Nomenclature

Chapter Contents

Summary: Detailed numerical practical sequence design concepts are discussed for spin echo and gradient echo imaging, including a review of some key implementation aspects for short-T_R fast imaging sequences. Several example imaging artifacts and their sources are presented. An attempt at standardizing MR imaging nomenclature is put forward.

Introduction

The heart of magnetic resonance imaging lies in the sequence design and the faithful representation that the image gives for the desired information. Sequences can be designed to investigate simple morphological information using spin density, T_1 or T_2 weighting, functional imaging, flow imaging, and many other applications. This is accomplished by 'massaging' the spin states appropriately and sensitizing the sequence to a specific property, such as flow, for example. In this chapter, we start with an overview of the basic constituents of imaging with some real numerical examples of timings and gradient waveforms.

Historically, spin echo imaging has been the workhorse of clinical MRI as it offers the distinct advantage of limited sensitivity to local field inhomogeneities. The second section covers single slice, single echo spin echo and inversion recovery spin echo imaging. More recent advances in hardware have made it possible to collect high quality short T_E, short-T_R,

779

gradient echo imaging. This approach is covered in the third section. It offers the advantage of very fast single slice acquisition or high resolution, contiguous slice large volume coverage. There are a variety of ways to collect the data in this approach, but two particular classes are of interest: steady state incoherent, where the transverse magnetization is essentially zero prior to any repeated cycle of rf pulses; and steady state coherent, where both the longitudinal and transverse components contribute to the build-up of signal.

Experimental conditions are not always perfect and, for this reason, it behooves us to talk about what can happen when things go wrong. The obvious effect is that the image is imperfect and misrepresents the information; we refer to this as an 'artifacted' image. In the fourth section, some common artifacts are dealt with although this serves only as an illustrative sampling of the problems that can occur; it is by no means an exhaustive list. The chapter closes with a list of adjectives and a proposed MRI vernacular which can be used to communicate the properties of a given sequence.

26.1   Sequence Design and Imaging Parameters

In this section, we consider both 2D and 3D gradient echo sequence constructs to introduce real gradient waveform shapes. For the most part, we have focused on instantaneous pulsed or boxcar gradients. The reader is reminded of the rules in designing each part of the sequence and asked to essentially build one such sequence numerically. Discussions of timings on the sequences for problems found in this section are based on timings marked on Fig. 26.1.

26.1.1   Slice Select Gradient

The first part of most sequence structures is to excite a slice for 2D imaging, or a slab (a thick slice) for 3D imaging. The rf pulse takes a finite amount of time and the shape of the rf field $B_1(t)$ is represented along the rf line (Fig. 26.1). The slice select gradient is usually turned on rather early relative to the rf pulse to stabilize the gradient amplitude (it also causes spin dephasing in the slice select direction which is desired for the elimination of remnant transverse magnetization in most cases). In the linear approximation to the effects of an rf pulse on magnetization, it has been shown (Ch. 16 and Ch. 10) that the zeroth moment of $G(t)$ from the center of the rf pulse prior to sampling the data must be zero, i.e., from Fig. 26.1a,

$$\int_{t_3}^{t_9} G_{ss}(t) = 0 \tag{26.1}$$

For the 3D case, the presence of the gradient table superimposed on the slice select gradient refocusing lobe limits the number of partitions for a given excited slice thickness. If the table can be moved so that it appears after the slice rephasing gradient, a higher resolution in the slice select direction can be obtained.

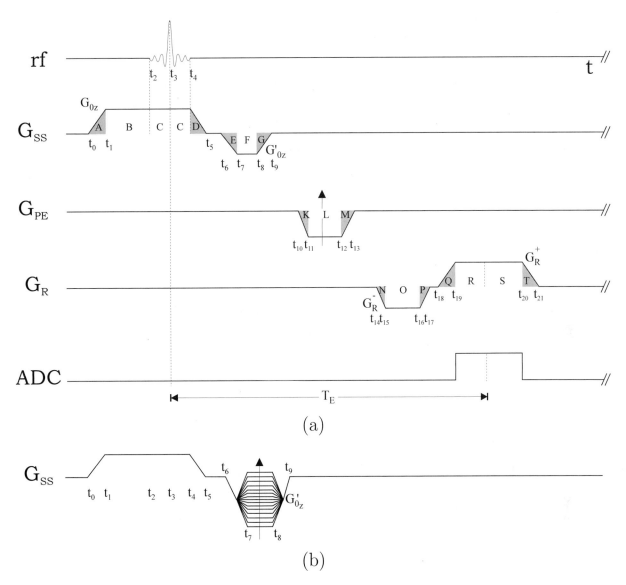

Fig. 26.1: Sequence diagram with necessary timings and realistic trapezoidal gradients for (a) a 2D gradient echo imaging sequence and (b) the modified slice select gradient structure for a 3D gradient echo imaging sequence optimized for keeping the T_E short. Timings are given for each change in gradient structure. Ramped sections are shaded. The capitalized letters A-T represent the area under each gradient section between any two nearest time points. G_{0_z} is the amplitude of the slice select gradient, G'_{0_z} the amplitude of the refocusing lobe of the slice select gradient, G_R^- the amplitude of the dephasing lobe of the read gradient and G_R^+ the amplitude of the read gradient. The phase encoding table is not shown under G_{PE} to allow a clear depiction of the shaded regions K, L, and M although the arrow is still shown to indicate that the gradient should be incremented in steps of ΔG_{PE} as usual.

Problem 26.1

---

a) For $t_1 - t_0 = 1\,\text{ms}$, $t_2 - t_1 = 2\,\text{ms}$, $\tau_{rf} = t_4 - t_2 = 5\,\text{ms}$, and $t_5 - t_4 = 1\,\text{ms}$ find the timings t_7 and t_8 if the ramp times $t_7 - t_6$ and $t_9 - t_8$ are also 1 ms given that $G'_{0z} = -G_{0z}$ and $t_0 = 0$.

b) For an rf pulse with a bandwidth of 1 kHz, and a slice thickness of 2 mm, what is G_{0z}?

c) Is this a good pulse design? If so, why; if not, how would you improve it?

Problem 26.2

For a 3D scan with the same timings as in the 2D case of the previous problem (such as shown in Fig. 26.1b), find the limitation in the spatial resolution Δz in the slice select direction when the initial slab thickness TH is 12.8 cm and the maximum gradient strength is a) $10\,\text{mT/m}$, b) $25\,\text{mT/m}$, and c) $50\,\text{mT/m}$. How much smaller can Δz be made in each case if the partition encoding table is moved after the rephasing gradient but its timings remain the same?

Calibration

The partition encoding gradient table can actually be used to calibrate the rephasing gradient lobe of the slice select gradient. Due to eddy currents or perhaps a design error, signal may not be a maximum. To fine-tune the choice of G'_{0z}, a gradient table can be added to G'_{0z} as in the 3D slice select line in Fig. 26.2 while the phase encoding gradient is not applied. The conventional sampling in the read direction is still performed. The choice of ΔG_z for this table can be made large enough first so that the peak signal lies within the spectra of the $G'_0 + p\Delta G$ window, where p runs from $-n_z$ to $n_z - 1$. Each line of data is then evaluated for its peak magnitude and the line with the largest magnitude determines the required value for G'_z. An alternate approach is to perform the usual 1D Fourier transform on the collected data in the read direction and then evaluate the signal dependence along the phase encoding, now calibration, direction at a given pixel in the object where there is significant signal. A further refinement could be made by choosing $\Delta G_{z_{new}} = \Delta G/2n$ and repeating the scan. The value of G'_{0z} that gives the maximum signal along the phase encoding direction in the reconstructed image will then be used in the final version of the original sequence.

Problem 26.3

Discuss how varying the amplitude of the dephasing lobe of the read gradient could be used to center the echo along the readout direction.

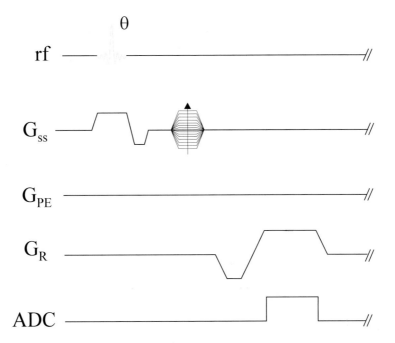

Fig. 26.2: The partition encoding gradient table used in combination with the slice select rephase lobe, as done in 3D imaging sequences, can serve to calibrate the slice select rephasing lobe. Calibration is achieved by reading out the data in the usual fashion, so that a line of projected data is obtained for each partition encoding line. After a 1D transformation of the data in the read direction, the resulting 2D image contains a series of repeated lines, all with slightly different amplitudes. The gradient strength corresponding to that line with the maximum signal is then used as the actual calibrated slice select rephase lobe in further sequence design.

Problem 26.4

There are occasions when a gradient is used to purposefully dephase a signal in 2D imaging. For example, if only narrow structures are desired in the slice select direction, then applying an appropriate gradient along the slice select direction so that the phase across the slice changes from $-\pi$ to π will eliminate the DC signal. These gradients are called 'crusher' or 'twister' gradients. What happens to the signal from narrow objects under these circumstances?

26.1.2   Phase Encoding Gradient

The phase encoding time can be somewhat longer than that for the slice select rephasing (as could the partition encoding time) since, as the slice select gradient is ramped down, the phase encoding can be ramped up (i.e., $t_{10} = t_4$ and $t_{13} = t_9$). For short echo times, when t_{19} equals t_9 and t_{13} equals t_9, there is only a limited time for phase encoding. The voxel size possible along the phase encoding direction will clearly be limited by the echo time which, in turn, limits the repeat time. In the push for faster and faster imaging times, spatial resolution must be sacrificed.

Problem 26.5

Determine the maximum resolution possible in the phase encoding direction given that $t_{11} - t_{10} = t_{13} - t_{12} = 1$ ms and $t_{12} - t_{11} = 1.5$ ms (see Fig. 26.1) when $G_{PE,max}$ is equal to a) $10 \, \text{mT/m}$, b) $25 \, \text{mT/m}$, and c) $50 \, \text{mT/m}$.

26.1.3   Read Gradient

Once the times for the phase encoding are determined, the resolution in the read direction can be fixed. Recall for pulsed boxcar gradients with $L_x = L_y$ that $G_R^+ \Delta t = \tau_{PE} \Delta G_{PE}$ and multiplying by n gives $G_R^+ T_s / 2 = \tau_{PE} G_{max}$ (since $\Delta G_{PE} = 2 G_{max}/n_y$). If $G_R^+ = G_{max}$, then $T_s = 2\tau_{PE}$ and $\Delta x = \Delta y$. However, the read gradient itself has some flexibility since after the phase encoding gradient it can, in principle, stay on for a time limited only by the tissue T_2 value. With $n_x = n_y$ and $T_s \simeq T_2$, G_R^+ can be chosen via

$$G_R^+ = \Delta G_{PE} \tau_{PE} / \Delta t = 2 G_{max} \tau_{PE} / T_s \tag{26.2}$$

Recall that the lower G_R becomes, the lower the readout bandwidth, and the higher the SNR/voxel.

Problem 26.6

The above discussion assumes boxcar gradients. Return to Fig. 26.1, and unless otherwise stated, assume the ramp times are 1 ms and the field-of-view is 256 mm.

a) For $G_{max} = 25 \, \text{mT/m}$, find Δt. Assume that ramp-up occurs by t_{19}.

b) If $T_2 = 100$ ms and $T_s = T_2$, find G_R during data sampling for a 0.25 mm voxel size.

c) What is the readout bandwidth per voxel?

d) If chemical shift (or field inhomogeneity) is 3.35 ppm at 1.5 T, by how many pixels is the tissue shifted in the image?

e) How would you reduce the artifact and how would this affect T_s and SNR/voxel if the spatial resolution in the read direction is maintained constant?

f) Discuss how the concept of partial Fourier imaging could be used to allow for a much shorter echo time.

26.1.4 Data Sampling

Data sampling is fixed by the desired resolution, available gradient strength, $G_x = G_R^+$, and field-of-view, L_x, through the Nyquist relation

$$\Delta t = \frac{1}{\gamma G_x L_x} \tag{26.3}$$

Today, sampling intervals can be easily as short as $4\,\mu s$ and starting times accurate to a few nanoseconds. Despite the accurate timing possible, this does not guarantee an artifact-free image. Only if k-space is uniformly sampled will the data be free from sampling error.

Problem 26.7

Sampling artifacts can manifest themselves in subtle ways. Two examples are considered in this problem. The issues of aliasing have already been addressed in earlier chapters. What effect would you expect to see in the image if

a) The sampling accuracy was not perfect and a small jitter in sampling time occurred about each point?

b) A remnant time-dependent magnetic field gradient in the readout direction of the form $G_{ec}e^{-(t-t_{19})/\tau_{ec}}$ is present during sampling where τ_{ec} is on the order of T_s?

26.2 Early Spin Echo Imaging Sequences

Despite all the numerous developments of new sequences for faster data acquisition and new information, the workhorse of clinical sequences is still the spin echo sequence. In its most widely used form, it appears either as a single echo T_1-weighted sequence (Fig. 26.3) or as a multi-echo spin density and T_2-weighted sequence acquiring two echoes (Fig. 26.4). It is common in these sequences to ensure incoherence by the application of not only rf spoiling but also gradient spoiling, as indicated in Fig. 26.4. The non-shaded portions of the slice select gradient must be balanced to rephase spins along the slice select direction as discussed in Sec. 26.1.1. Variants of the usual spin echo concept exist to speed up data acquisition and these are reviewed in Sec. 26.2.3.

26.2.1 Single and Multi-Echo Spin Echo Sequences

T_1-Weighted

With a single echo, T_R can be kept short (about $600\,\text{ms}$ at $1.5\,\text{T}$) for a multi-slice acquisition to obtain a T_1-weighted image with excellent GM/WM T_1-weighted contrast. Of course, spin density plays a strong role here in determining the optimal choice of T_R since the spin density

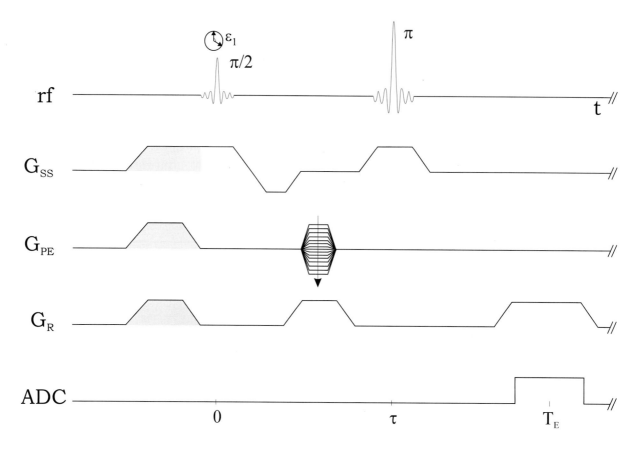

Fig. 26.3: A simple single slice, single echo, spin echo sequence. The shaded regions act as spoilers of remnant transverse magnetization. The wheel symbol, with ϵ_1 representing the rf phase variation from one cycle to the next, is used to indicate rf spoiling.

of GM is so much larger (20%) than that of WM. For this choice of T_R, the $\pi/2$-π rf series is better replaced by a $\pi/3$-π rf series to enhance GM/WM contrast. For short-T_R sequences, it is useful to apply spoiler gradients prior to rf excitation in each repetition (Fig. 26.3).

Problem 26.8

---

a) Show that, for a fixed $T_R = 600$ ms, GM/WM contrast is significantly enhanced if the $\pi/2$-pulse is replaced by a $\pi/3$-pulse. Assume that the transverse magnetization just before each new rf pulse is zero.

b) Will this be true for contrast between any two tissues, or is it tissue-specific and field strength-specific?

T_2-Weighted

The most important contrast clinically is T_2-contrast. Hence the double echo sequence (Fig. 26.4) plays a crucial role in long T_R spin echo experiments. Diseased tissue often

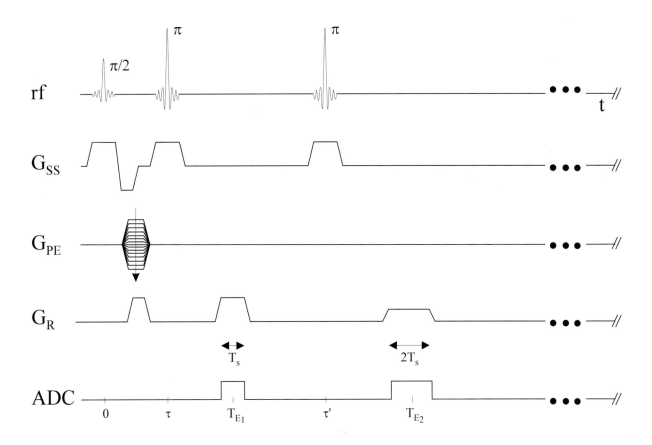

Fig. 26.4: The clinical workhorse sequence using a long T_R and a spin density-weighted short T_E first echo and a T_2-weighted long T_E second echo typically acquired at a lower bandwidth than the first echo. In the example shown, the T_2-weighted image is acquired at half the bandwidth of the spin density-weighted image.

contains more free water than healthy tissue leading to a longer T_2 and, hence, both spin density and T_2-weighted images are sought to enhance its visibility. This dual contrast information is available in a single, long T_R, short T_E (spin density) and long T_E (T_2-weighted) experiment. The second echo is usually acquired with a sampling time of twice that used for the first echo to enhance SNR.

Problem 26.9

---

a) Why is it that the second echo image of a spin density/T_2-weighted double echo scan with $T_R = 2\,\mathrm{sec}$ looks similar to a spin density-weighted scan with $T_R = 20\,\mathrm{sec}$ but with better contrast between GM, WM, and CSF?

b) What is the difference in k-space coverage from the first to the second echo?

26.2.2 Inversion Recovery

Although the inversion recovery sequence provides a method of enhancing T_1 contrast, it has as its major weaknesses long acquisition times and 'crossover' artifact where negative signal from one tissue cancels positive signal from another within the same voxel due to the T_I setting. The ability to invert signal makes it possible to null specific tissues with an appropriate choice of T_I. One such example is using a short $T_I = T_{1_{\text{fat}}} \ln 2$ to null fat and another is using a very long $T_I = T_{1_{\text{CSF}}} \ln 2$ to null CSF. Nulling CSF reduces the dynamic range of voxel signal values in the image and makes non-water tissues with longer than usual T_2 values more obvious. An inversion recovery sequence can be run in a gradient echo mode (Fig. 26.5) or in a more complicated, multi-slice spin echo mode (see also magnetization-prepared sequences in Sec. 26.2.5 and Ch. 15 for a discussion about IR contrast).

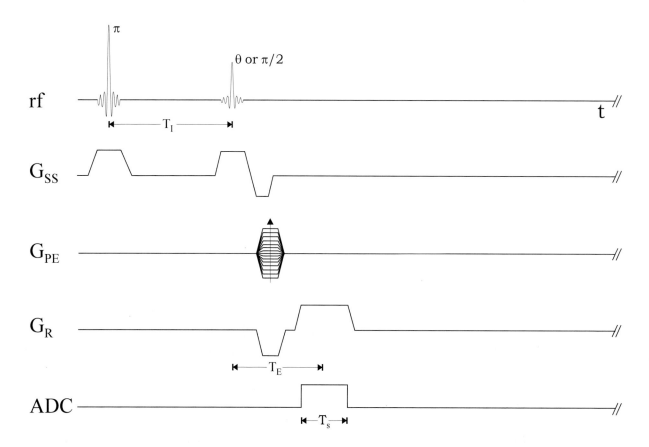

Fig. 26.5: Inversion recovery sequence implemented in a gradient echo mode. T_I is the inversion time between the π and θ pulses.

Problem 26.10

Draw a sequence diagram for an efficient multi-slice IR acquisition. Hint: Carefully consider the order in which the original $\pi/2$- and π-pulses are interleaved.

26.2.3   Spin Echo with Phase Encoding Between Echoes

One approach to speeding up data acquisition is to phase encode between repeated spin echoes (see also Ch. 19). This approach mixes contrast of the different T_2 weighting features of different echoes, but for long T_E scans gives excellent T_2-weighted contrast. Both spin echo (Fig. 26.6) and spin echo interleaved with gradient echo variants (Fig. 26.7) are used.

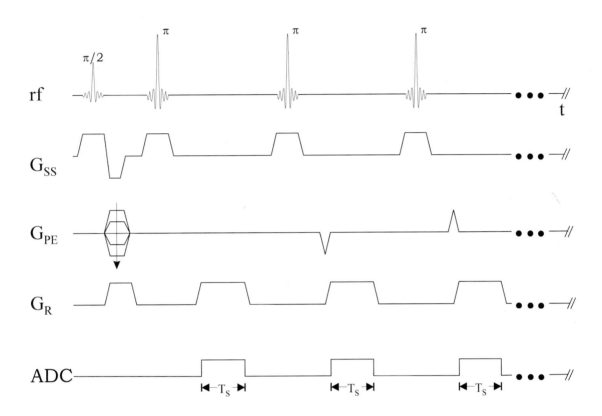

Fig. 26.6: Spin echo variant of sequence with phase encoding between repeated spin echoes. This sequence can also be run as an IR sequence by preceding the above structure with a π-pulse. The gradient table here is shown with a larger step size than usual since m phase encoded echoes are collected after each $\pi/2$-pulse. Hence, $\Delta G_{PE,\text{applied}}$ will be $m\Delta G_{PE,\text{Nyquist}}$.

Problem 26.11

When multiple imperfect π-pulses are applied periodically after a $\pi/2$-pulse, multiple echoes will be produced after the last π-pulse.

   a) How many echoes occur after the last pulse?

   b) What tissue would most likely contribute to the unspoiled echoes?

   c) Should there be spoiling gradients or rf spoiling before the next slice excitation or repetition of the cycle occurs?

   d) Will these spurious echoes create any image artifacts?

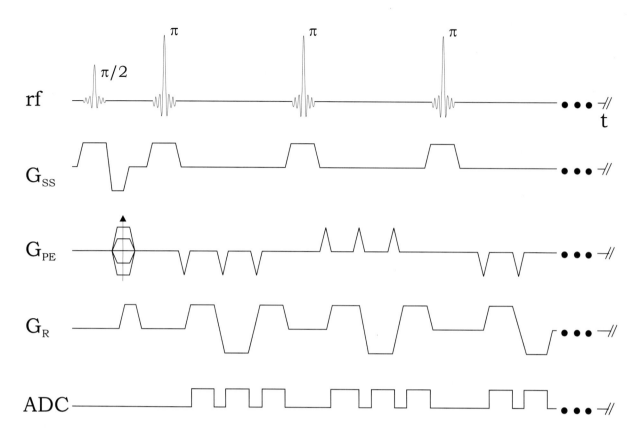

Fig. 26.7: Variant of the sequence in Fig. 26.6 with repeated spin echoes interlaced with gradient echoes. As shown, two gradient echoes are collected over and above each spin echo. For eight π-pulses, this implies that 24 lines of k-space are collected (eight of which are spin echoes and 16 are gradient echoes) for each $\pi/2$-pulse. The steps shown in the phase encoding table just after the $\pi/2$-pulse lead to the collection of a total of 120 lines of k-space when the sequence cycle is repeated five times.

Problem 26.12

Sketch the k-space coverage for one excitation pulse followed by a series of four π-pulses when the phase encoding gradients are applied as in

   a) Fig. 26.6 and

   b) Fig. 26.7.

Assume next that 128 lines of k-space will be covered totally. Recall that T_2 decay takes place during data sampling.

   c) Is there a better way to collect k-space data to avoid sampling (ghosting) artifacts?

26.3   Fast Short T_R Imaging Sequences

Many variants of fast imaging sequences exist. Some are purely gradient echo in nature and some are mixtures which fall between purely gradient echo and spin echo sequences. This section focuses on the concept of short-T_R rapid imaging.

26.3.1   Steady-State Incoherent: Gradient Echo

One of the most common fast imaging approaches is the short-T_R, rf spoiled gradient echo sequence.[1] It can yield a variety of contrast behaviors (Fig. 26.8). For example, with flip angles much less than the Ernst angle, θ_E, the contrast is spin density weighted if $T_E \ll T_2^*$, otherwise, it also contains some T_2^* weighting as well. For flip angles at or above the Ernst angle, the images will be T_1-weighted (on top of the naturally inherent spin density weighting). To properly attain T_1 weighting without extraneous, confounding effects from T_2, for very short T_R, the application of rf spoiling is critical (see Sec. 18.4).

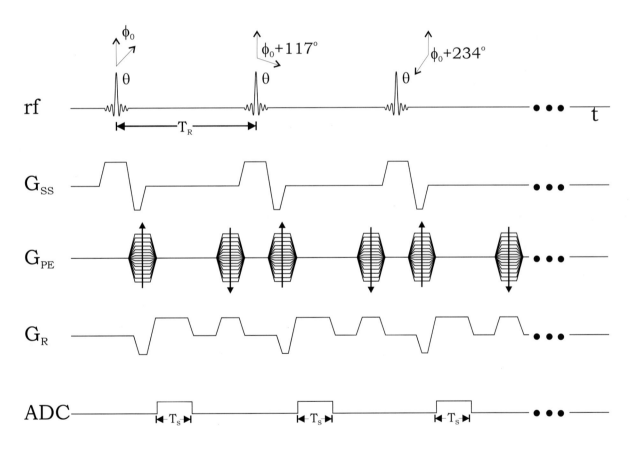

Fig. 26.8: An rf spoiled implementation of the short-T_R gradient echo sequence. The resonance offset is usually incremented by 117° from one rf pulse to the next.

---

[1]This sequence is often called FLASH for 'fast low angle shot' imaging.

Problem 26.13

---

a) Derive an expression for the voxel signal $\rho_{\theta\pi\pi}(\theta)$ as a function of flip angle θ for the θ-π-π sequence in the steady-state. Assume that the transverse magnetization is spoiled prior to any new θ-π-π cycle. Then compare it to the voxel signal from a conventional short-T_R SSI gradient echo experiment which was shown in (18.14) to be given by

$$\rho_\theta(\theta) = \frac{\rho_0 \sin\theta (1 - e^{-T_R/T_1})}{(1 - \cos\theta\, e^{-T_R/T_1})} \tag{26.4}$$

b) Show for echo times short relative to T_R that

$$\rho_{\theta\pi\pi} \simeq \rho_\theta (1 - 2\tau/T_R) \tag{26.5}$$

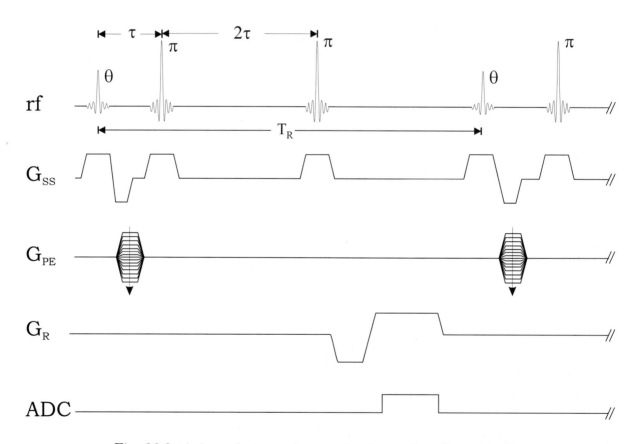

Fig. 26.9: A θ-π-π fast, steady-state incoherent imaging sequence.

26.3.2 Steady-State Incoherent: Spin Echo

By adding two π-pulses after a θ-pulse, it becomes possible to collect two spin echoes rather than one gradient echo and yet maintain the stored magnetization along $\hat{z}$ (Fig. 26.9). The first π-pulse negates the longitudinal component which then slowly regrows until the next π-pulse at a time 2τ later. One might expect that the longitudinal magnetization will be somewhat smaller than that which would have been obtained if neither π-pulse had been applied, by the amount $(1 - 2\tau/T_1)$. This sequence suffers from the need for a longer T_R than is used without the two π-pulses, but is still well-suited for 3D imaging. It could be particularly well-suited for those situations where field inhomogeneities are a problem. Given the larger number of π-pulses applied, the rf power deposition increases and this will also limit how short T_R can be made.

Problem 26.14

The possibility exists for applying just a single π-pulse to obtain a spin echo image, but in that case, the flip angle of the first rf pulse, θ, will need to be larger than 90° to bring the longitudinal magnetization back along the positive z-axis. The advantage is that a shorter T_R can be used, and usually less rf power deposition occurs.

a) Draw a sequence diagram for this θ-π sequence.

b) Show that the longitudinal magnetization just prior to the $(n+1)^{st}$ θ-pulse is

$$M_{n+1} = M_0(1 - 2e^{-(T_R-\tau)/T_1} + e^{-T_R/T_1}(1 - \cos\theta(M_n/M_0))) \qquad (26.6)$$

c) From part (a) show that the equilibrium longitudinal magnetization is

$$M_n = M_0 \left(\frac{1 - 2e^{-(T_R-\tau)/T_1} + e^{-T_R/T_1}}{1 + \cos\theta e^{-T_R/T_1}} \right) \qquad (26.7)$$

d) Show that the flip angle which maximizes the equilibrium signal occurs at that value of θ which satisfies

$$\cos\theta = -e^{-T_R/T_1} \qquad (26.8)$$

e) Find the flip angle needed to optimize (i) the WM signal and (ii) the GM signal at 1.5 T for $T_R = 100\,\mathrm{ms}$ and $T_R = 200\,\mathrm{ms}$.

26.3.3 Steady-State Coherent Imaging

A totally different contrast is available when T_R is shorter than T_2 and no spoiling is used. As discussed in Ch. 18, there is a coherent build-up of signal from all rf pulses which essentially reaches a steady-state for a large number of pulses.

A Fully Balanced SSFP Imaging Sequence

The fully 'balanced' sequence (Fig. 26.10) is one in which all the gradients are 'rewound' so that the zeroth moment of all gradients from the center of one rf pulse to the next is zero. This condition is required to reach a coherent steady-state. If motion is present, then the first moments of all gradients in any one direction should be designed so that their sum is zero from one rf pulse to the next. Interestingly, motion may be beneficial in some circumstances. For example, CSF motion along the read gradient will generate a phase, usually variable over the data acquisition window, which will cause a natural spoiling and, hence, suppression of the CSF signal. This advantage is counterbalanced by the fact that ghosting can also occur if the spoiling is not perfect. The signal of a given tissue obtained with this sequence is also extremely sensitive to field inhomogeneities.

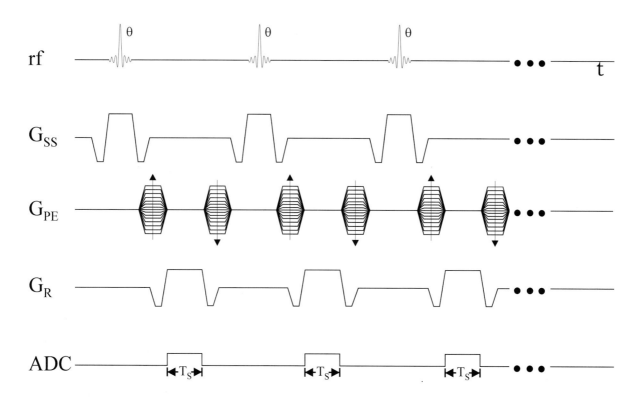

Fig. 26.10: A 'fully balanced' implementation of the SSFP sequence. The read and slice select gradients are not only balanced so that the zeroth moment is zero; they are also velocity compensated so that the first moment is also zero from one rf pulse to the next. In this case, the phase encoding tables are balanced but not velocity compensated.

Resonant Offset Averaged Steady-State Sequence

Any sequence with one or more directions not rewound or balanced but not all three and not rf spoiled has yet a different contrast. This sequence has no sensitivity to field inhomogeneities through resonance offset effects. Unfortunately, it has a very complicated image contrast behavior. If spoiling is applied, it becomes the equivalent of a FLASH sequence.

Delayed Echo Time Sequences

Oddly enough it is possible to create a sequence in which T_E is longer than T_R. This property comes from the presence of multiple pathways which exist during an approach to steady-state or in steady-state sequences. Consider a preparatory gradient applied with the same amplitude as the read gradient and which is on for a time that is $n/2$ times as long as the read gradient (i.e., $B = nA$ for gradient areas A and B defined in Fig. 26.11). At the second pulse following the formation of a new transverse configuration, only that pathway which has the second pulse acting as a π-pulse will be refocused at each acquired gradient echo. Other pathways also lead to echoes, but the larger that B is, the less important these pathways become as a result of relaxation signal loss.

This special sequence (Fig. 26.11) has a complicated signal response, but, thanks to the dephasing from the additional area B, there is essentially no signal left from the FID. It contains the rf echo refocused portion of the signal and can be heavily T_2-weighted. It is very motion sensitive since the gradient waveforms are not velocity compensated at the echo. Large gradients exacerbate the problem so much that even slow flowing CSF dephases.

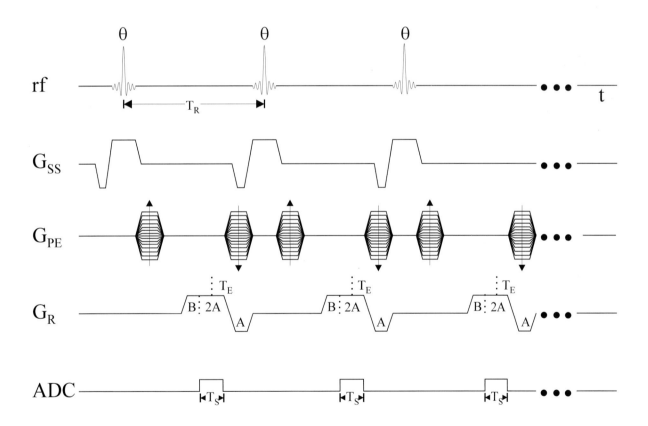

Fig. 26.11: A delayed-echo sequence. Note that the FID part is totally eliminated by not refocusing the slice select gradient while the rf echo part alone is acquired by reversing the read gradient waveform. The read gradient is also usually extended longer than T_s so that the FID part of the steady-state signal is dephased well. In this example, the second θ-pulse acts in part like a π-pulse and creates an echo at T_E after it is applied, this echo having refocused the dephasing from the area $A + B$ (with $B = A$ in this case) after the first pulse.

Problem 26.15

---

     a) Using Fig. 26.11, sketch a few pathways that lead to a refocusing of the signal for $B = A$.

     b) Show that the signal will have a component that varies as $e^{-(2T_R - T_E)/T_2}$.

26.3.4   Pulse Train Methods

One ever-inherent problem with gradient echo sequences is the presence of local field inhomogeneity effects which manifest themselves through T_2^*. With a judicious choice of when to apply the rf pulses, a train of rf pulses can be used to obtain both gradient echo, and spin echo-like images.

Missing Pulse Sequences

One approach to eliminate T_2' effects and obtain just T_2 dependence in an SSFP sequence is to collect the data where an rf pulse would otherwise be applied (see Fig. 26.12). Gradient echoes are created by applying a balanced gradient after each rf pulse and before each even rf pulse (producing echoes 1, 2, and 4 shown in the ADC line in Fig. 26.12). The same structure is also placed after each even rf pulse half way between the even and odd pulses (allowing for sampling of the spin echo components at echo 3 shown in the ADC line in Fig. 26.12). By phase encoding both even and odd pulses separately, four separate images can be collected. These methods may prove very useful for high field imaging (3.0 T and higher for human studies, and 4.7 T and higher for animal and *in vitro* studies).

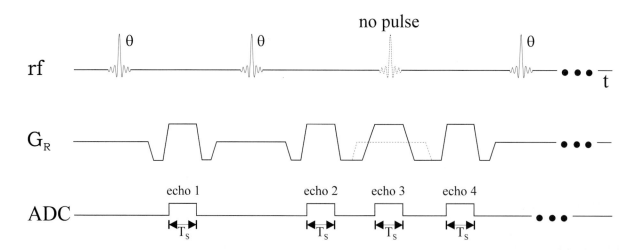

Fig. 26.12: Sequence diagram showing the differences in the rf pulse timings and read gradient waveform between an SSFP sequence and a missing pulse sequence. In the diagram, the missing rf pulse is represented using dashed lines which, in the SSFP sequence, is another θ-pulse. The missing pulse sequence variation in the read gradient relative to the usual SSFP sequence construction (dashed line) is shown as a solid line about echo 3.

Stimulated Echo Acquisition

Applying three pulses allows some interesting combinations of information encoding. Recall that information encoding after the first pulse but before the second pulse gets stored, in part, back along the z-axis. Only after the third pulse is this information brought back into the transverse plane. These pulses also do not need to be equally spaced as in the previous sequences. One can acquire information from just the stimulated echo (Fig. 26.13) or any of the five echoes. During the time between the second and third pulses, while the magnetization along the z-axis is protected from external dephasing effects, there is time to manipulate the transverse signal.

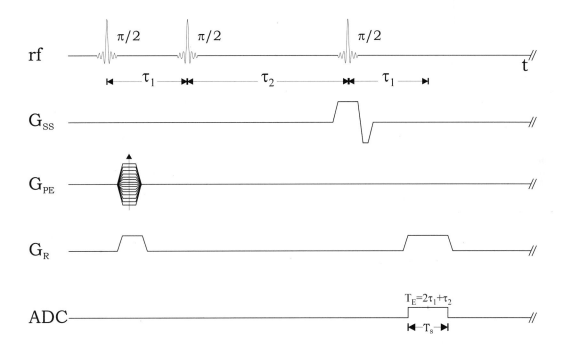

Fig. 26.13: An implementation known as the STEAM sequence, acquiring only the stimulated echo.

26.3.5 Magnetization Prepared Sequences

The order of rf pulses and their timings offer tremendous flexibility in manipulating image contrast. Applying a set of pre-pulses prior to phase encoding offers one avenue to effect a variety of contrast changes (including T_1, T_2, tagging, or other contrast mechanisms).

Inversion Recovery, Short-T_R Gradient Echo Imaging

The simplest example to consider is when a π-pulse is applied to invert the spins. At a time T_I later, a series of rapid rf pulses is applied to collect a 2D data set conventionally. During this transient regrowth, the data are sampled in k_y. The rf pulses modify the regrowth along $\hat{z}$ slightly. For a centrally reordered data acquisition, the signal from the tissue chosen to be nulled will be essentially zero.

3D Magnetization Prepared Short-T_R, Gradient Echo Imaging

The application of a partition encoding loop transforms the 2D approach into a powerful T_1-weighted 3D sequence (see Fig. 26.14). The danger here, as with all inversion recovery sequences, is that signals from some tissue can be sampled when it is negative, causing signal cancelation artifacts or false contrast enhancement. This comes about because of the partial voluming of two tissues in one voxel. Usually, the flip angles are chosen to be near the Ernst angle for WM/GM so that rf spoiling or gradient spoiling will not be needed (see Fig. 26.15).

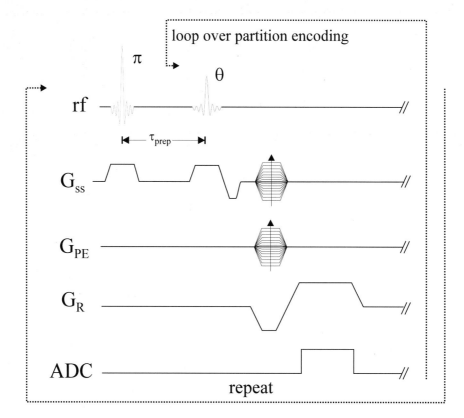

Fig. 26.14: A 3D, magnetization prepared, short-T_R, gradient echo imaging sequence designed for obtaining T_1-weighted images. The θ-pulse is repeated N_z times for each phase encoding step. The whole cycle is then repeated N_y times.

26.4   Imaging Tricks and Image Artifacts

Having studied all the material up to this point, the reader now has an in-depth knowledge of how to design and build a sequence and, in principle, understand the nuances of how it works. This last point is critical because when you first test a sequence, you are likely to run into problems. The object being imaged may appear ghosted, distorted, shifted in the field-of-view, have nonuniform intensity, or not be there at all in the image. Your knowledge

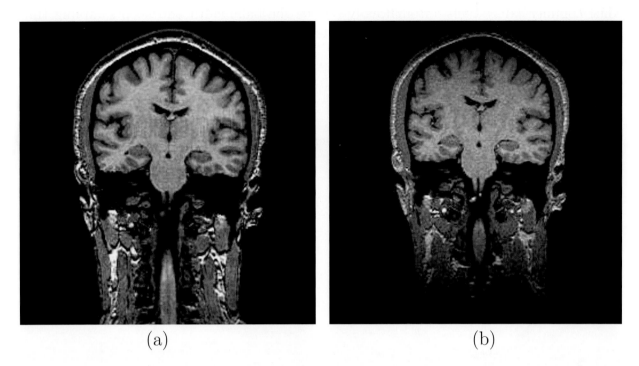

(a)   (b)

Fig. 26.15: A comparison of T_1-weighted coronal images resulting from (a) a 3D SSI imaging sequence and (b) a 3D, magnetization prepared, short-T_R, gradient echo imaging sequence.

of the physics and image reconstruction aspects of MRI will let you determine the problem. Although we do not explicitly talk about artifacts under a separate heading in the book, we have already dealt with many of the most common ones such as ghosting, image distortion, chemical shift effects, and slice profile effects, to name a few.

In working through the basics of each aspect of MRI, we have taken the philosophy that artifacts can be removed by proper acquisition methods or reconstruction methods. In this section, we consider a few other common artifacts associated with the role of bandwidth, gradient structure, interleaving acquisitions, complex subtraction, and phase stability.

26.4.1   Readout Bandwidth

Sequences are usually designed to allow the lowest BW possible. This is particularly true at low fields where susceptibility is not important and SNR is rather low. At high fields, the use of low BW for the read gradient is problematic because of image distortion near regions of susceptibility variations.

Multi-Echo, High Bandwidth Acquisition of Data

Long echo time gradient echo images are often collected with a low bandwidth, BW. Images produced this way often suffer from distortion artifacts. On the other hand, if many echoes are collected with a high bandwidth $BW' = 4BW$, say, each image will have reduced distortion artifacts (see Fig. 26.16). Averaging four of these images together would then be roughly equivalent in SNR to the low bandwidth image. The reader should also recall that some commercial systems automatically reduce the bandwidth and keep sampling time T_s fixed if n_x, the number of sampled points, is reduced to $n_x/2$, from some baseline n_x (usually 256).

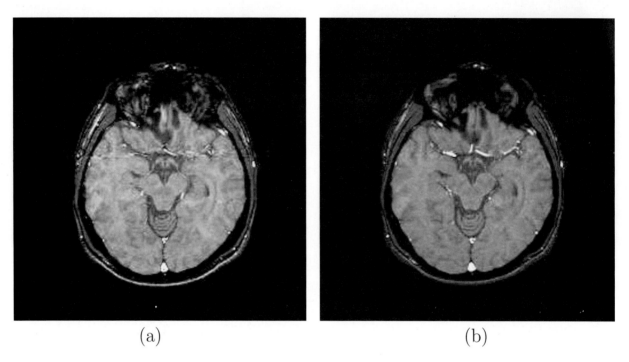

(a)   (b)

Fig. 26.16: A comparison of images obtained with (a) a single echo, low bandwidth, long-T_E acquisition and (b) a magnitude average of images from a five echo, high bandwidth gradient echo acquisition with an average echo time equal to that in (a).

Problem 26.16

If the field variation at the tissue/air interface by the pituitary is $1\,\mathrm{ppm/mm}$, what is the BW/voxel required at $4\,\mathrm{T}$ to keep distortion less than one-fifth of a pixel? Is this likely to be acceptable?

Problem 26.17

A sequence is set to sample the data for $10\,\mathrm{ms}$ with $n_x = 256$ and $L_x = 20\,\mathrm{cm}$.

a) What is the readout bandwidth?

b) What is the BW when the user chooses to collect a 1024 data set in the readout direction keeping T_s fixed?

c) What is the bandwidth per pixel?

d) How has the SNR been affected?

26.4.2   Dealing with System Instabilities

Generally speaking, when two or more tissue properties are being sought so that several scans need to be run, the gradient structures in each acquisition should be identical if possible. In this manner, any artifacts introduced by eddy currents (such as varying phase during sampling) will be the same for each scan. When this is not possible, any additional gradient structures such as those used for diffusion weighting or flow encoding should be oscillatory and fast. This reduces eddy current problems and keeps imaging times short. Alternatively, any new gradient structures should be kept as far away as possible from the read gradient to avoid modifying k-space sampling.

Interleaving Scans

If the design allows it, interleaving scans (Fig. 26.17) is an ideal way to collect data that needs to be subtracted. This concept implies collecting the different modifications of the sequence one after the other, all at the same phase encoding step. Any artifacts that occur from motion will then be essentially the same for each image and they will tend to subtract out if one image is subtracted from the other. This will be true as long as T_R is much shorter than the period of the motion.

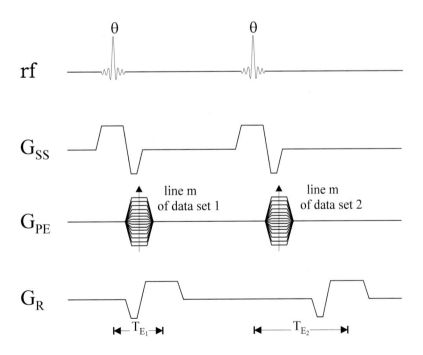

Fig. 26.17: For this sequence, two scans are interleaved. After each of the rf pulses shown, the same phase encoding gradient is applied although echo times may be different or other modifications made to enhance or highlight other desired physical properties.

Phase Locking

As eddy currents are generally present to some degree, the total phase accumulated prior to sampling may change when a sequence is modified. Consider the example of long T_E imaging where the field may change by 0.1 ppm between phase encoding steps or when a variable bipolar pulse for velocity encoding is applied. In both cases, the phase just prior to sampling would change according to

$$\phi(t) = \gamma \Delta B t \qquad (26.9)$$

or, in the general, time-varying field case,

$$\phi(t) = \gamma \int_0^t dt' \, \Delta B(t') \qquad (26.10)$$

If the sequence is designed with the phase encoding table close to the read gradient as in Fig. 26.18, then the phase at time t_1 can be monitored for each phase encoding step. If the phase $\phi(t_1)$ changes, but $\phi(T_E) - \phi(t_1)$ is small, then by phase correcting the signal via

$$s_{\text{corrected}}(k_x, k_y) = s_{\text{measured}}(k_x, k_y) e^{-i\phi(t_1, k_y)} \qquad (26.11)$$

ghosting artifacts can be dramatically reduced. The magnitude of the image can also be similarly monitored and corrected from line to line.

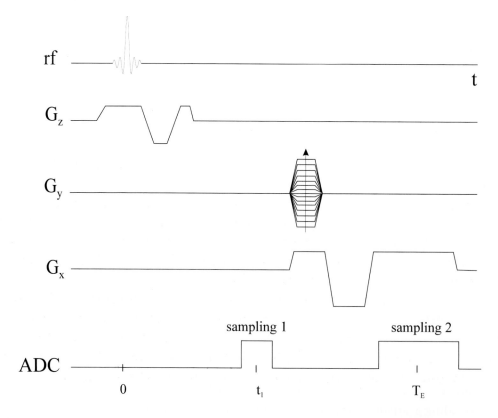

Fig. 26.18: Example sequence using a phase locking technique.

Problem 26.18

Discuss how sampling the signal at more than one time point can be used to estimate the phase correction at time T_E even though it is measured at time t_1. Hint: Consider some form of extrapolating the information to accomplish this.

Testing System Stability

As mentioned above, systems may not be stable, and the data may change in some fashion from one rf pulse to the next. To test stability, a series of scans with no phase encoding gradient can be run to view the projection data. By examining the magnitude and phase of each line, variations in signal or phase dispersion can be observed.

Problem 26.19

What would be a good method to automate the evaluation of stability of the system using the projection method described above? Hint: Consider the role of statistics and the concept of variance.

Monitoring Motion with Navigator Echoes

The concept of monitoring the system can be extended to monitor motion. For this application, projections over too large a region may not be as useful as those over a more narrow beam of excited spins. One means to overcome this weakness is to create a beam of excited spins by applying a $\pi/2$-pulse followed by a π-pulse. The signal from the beam is read out using a read gradient as usual and this readout is referred to as a 'navigator echo.' With this method, information is collected along the beam, i.e., information in the two directions orthogonal to the long axis of the beam is projected along the beam (see Ch. 16, Sec. 16.5 and Fig. 16.12).

This concept makes it possible to monitor motion in one direction, for example. Although this is not a system instability, it is an instability introduced by the imaged subject. It can be used to monitor cardiac or abdominal motion or to monitor translational motion (see Fig. 26.19). The amplitude of the signal near an edge of the object being imaged is monitored to determine position and that position variable is stored in an array corresponding to the phase encoding order. An example set of navigator echo data is shown in Fig. 26.20. When a given phase encoding line is collected p times, the data can be re-sorted so that one phase encoding line is used from this group of lines as close to a fixed position as possible. Averaging over all p lines creates a high SNR but blurred image (Fig. 26.21a), while the re-sorting procedure just discussed leads to a much sharper image (Fig. 26.21b).

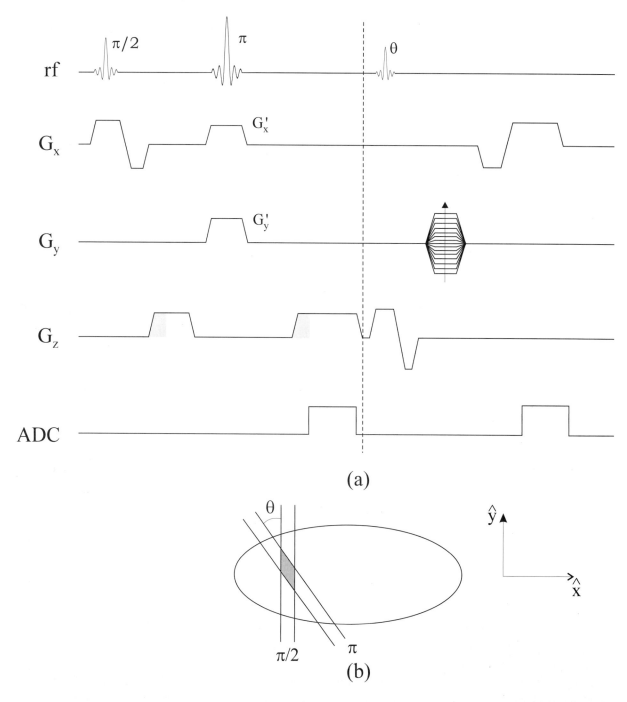

(a)

(b)

Fig. 26.19: A navigator echo design combined with a transverse gradient echo acquisition used to monitor chest wall motion. (a) Sequence diagram for a combined navigator echo gradient echo 2D acquisition. The navigator echo is read out along the direction of a beam excited with a $\pi/2$-π pulse combination. To avoid interference with important features in the transverse slice, it is typical to rotate the π-pulse slice select gradient. As described in diagram (a), the π-pulse slice select gradient is rotated by an angle θ relative to $\hat{x}$ by using two gradients G'_x and G'_y in combination during slice selection where $\theta \equiv \tan^{-1}(G'_y/G'_x)$. (b) Schematic of a cross section to the excited beam. The shaded area contributes to the signal of the navigator echo at each point in $\hat{z}$.

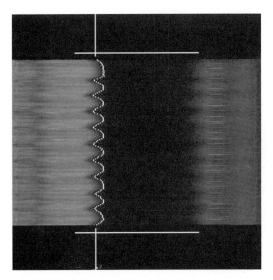

Fig. 26.20: An example set of navigator echo data obtained by exciting a beam that depicts the motion of the diaphragm in a human volunteer. The vertical axis represents time and the horizontal axis the position of the diaphragm along the beam. The changes in edge location of the diaphragm are shown by the vertical dotted line. The darker region is signal from the lung.

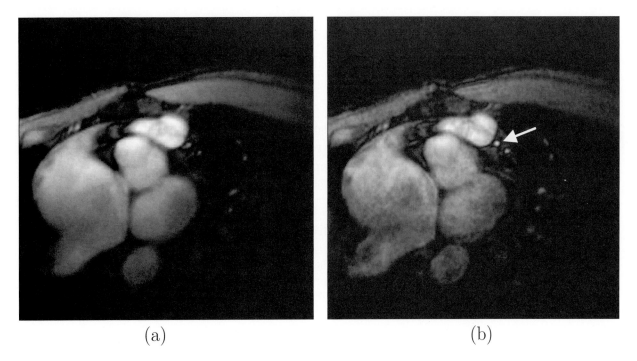

(a)   (b)

Fig. 26.21: By averaging over all oversampled phase encoding steps, a blurred image is obtained as evidenced by lack of edge definition in the coronary vessels (arrow) and most other parts of the image in (a). By including only those lines that fall within a 2 mm window in end expiration based on the navigator echo data, a much sharper image is obtained in (b) (see, for example, the coronary vessel marked by the arrow in (b)).

Problem 26.20

If the motion of the object is purely translational, discuss how the Fourier transform shift theorem can be used to correct the motion back to a reference position for each line of k-space.

Problem 26.21

The beam used to monitor motion will cause an effective loss of signal in the image when implemented as in Fig. 26.19. Discuss why reducing the $90°$-pulse to α and using the resulting α-$180°$ pulse pair to acquire the navigator echo would ameliorate this difficulty.

26.4.3   DC and Line Artifacts

Spurious signals and incorrect signal amplitude settings can cause a variety of problems which are usually correctable. In this section, we detail how knowledge of the artifact and the imaging methodology can be used to redesign the sequence to remove the problem.

DC Offset Error and its Removal

It sometimes occurs that data are recorded with a dc offset (an offset added to each k-space data point) so that

$$s_{m_1}(k) = s(k) + s_0 \qquad (26.12)$$

This problem can be removed by applying a second rf pulse with opposite polarity (i.e., still about x', but now with a negative rotation rather than a positive rotation as in the first pulse). The signal created by this second rf pulse is now

$$s_{m_2}(k) = -s(k) + s_0 \qquad (26.13)$$

Subtracting the latter from the former and dividing by 2 yields

$$s_m(k) = 1/2(s_{m_1}(k) - s_{m_2}(k)) \qquad (26.14)$$

This approach eliminates s_0 and also gives a $\sqrt{2}$ improvement in SNR (although it takes twice as long to collect the required data).

Problem 26.22

If the signal from a single acquisition is corrupted by a noise term $\eta(k)$ with mean zero and standard deviation σ_0, show that the noise in $s(k)$ has zero mean and variance $\sigma_0^2/2$.

To avoid collecting the data twice, an alternate approach is to collect every other line in 2D k-space with an alternating rf pulse. This means every alternating line appears as $\tilde{s}_{\text{odd}}(k_y) = -s(k_y) + s_0$ and when negated, gives $-\tilde{s}_{\text{odd}}(k_y) = s(k_y) - s_0$. The data set $\tilde{s}'(k)$ is given by

$$\tilde{s}'(q\Delta k_y) = \left\{ \begin{array}{ll} -\tilde{s}_{\text{odd}}(q\Delta k_y) & q \text{ odd} \\ \tilde{s}_{\text{even}}(q\Delta k_y) & q \text{ even} \end{array} \right. = \left\{ \begin{array}{ll} s(q\Delta k_y) - s_0 & q \text{ odd} \\ s(q\Delta k_y) + s_0 & q \text{ even} \end{array} \right. = s(q\Delta k_y) + (-1)^q s_0 \tag{26.15}$$

If $\tilde{s}'(k)$ is inverse Fourier transformed, the result is

$$\hat{\rho}(y) = \rho(y) + s_0 \mathcal{F}^{-1}\left((-1)^q \right) \tag{26.16}$$

where it is assumed that y represents the phase encoding direction. On evaluating $s_0 \mathcal{F}^{-1}\left((-1)^q \right)$, two terms

$$\tilde{\rho}_{\text{even}}(y) = \frac{s_0}{2}\left(\delta\left(y - \frac{L}{2}\right) + \delta(y) + \delta\left(y + \frac{L}{2}\right) \right) \tag{26.17}$$

$$\tilde{\rho}_{\text{odd}}(y) = -\frac{s_0}{2}\left(-\delta\left(y - \frac{L}{2}\right) + \delta(y) - \delta\left(y + \frac{L}{2}\right) \right) \tag{26.18}$$

are obtained. So, the corruption to the image from the dc artifact is given by

$$s_0 \mathcal{F}^{-1}\left((-1)^q \right) = \tilde{\rho}_{\text{odd}}(y) + \tilde{\rho}_{\text{even}}(y) = s_0 \delta\left(y - \frac{L}{2}\right) + s_0 \delta\left(y + \frac{L}{2}\right) \tag{26.19}$$

in the reconstructed field-of-view. This pushes the 'dc artifact' from being at the origin (since $s_0 \mathcal{F}^{-1}(1) = s_0 \delta(y)$) to the edges of the FOV.

Imperfect π-Pulses, Their Effects on Spin Echo Images, and Reduction of the Resulting Artifacts

When the π-pulse in a spin echo sequence is imperfect, it creates its own FID signal immediately following the pulse, which an ideal π-pulse does not create. If this FID does not die out naturally, or is not dephased well before the readout occurs, its presence typically leads to an artifact which is very similar to the previously discussed dc artifact, albeit now this constant signal gets added exclusively at the high spatial frequency region of each line. This is easily seen for the spin echo sequence where the phase encoding gradient is present between the 90°-pulse and the 180°-pulse (see Fig. 10.17). In this case, if this FID signal does not die out before the spin echo occurs, it always contributes the same amount of signal to each line of data similar to the effect of an added dc voltage level on the measured signal. The only difference between these two cases is that this FID signal sees the effect of the read gradient, and is frequency encoded in the read direction.

Since this effect contributes a constant signal to each k-space line, it again appears as a bright modulated line along the x-axis (since the Fourier transform of a constant is a delta function at the origin of the y-axis). The only difference between this bright line and the bright line artifact due to the added dc voltage is that the brightness in this case will be position-dependent (because the FID is frequency encoded in the read direction and the brightness as a function of position is representative of the positional variation in the projection along the phase encoding direction) and will be complex in nature (as opposed to the real nature of the dc artifact) because the frequency encoded FID decays in the read direction beginning at the most negative part of k-space. Its complex and spatially varying nature means that, if it appeared on top of some important structure, it could cause signal cancelation as well as signal variation.

There are a number of ways to eliminate this effect. All these methods form the basis of good sequence design criteria for spin echo imaging sequences. The first alternative is to move the phase encoding gradient after the π-pulse (Fig. 26.22a). This ensures the phase encoding of the FID in addition to its frequency encoding. Then again, unfortunately because of its complex signal nature in the image, the signal at each pixel is reduced according to the strength of the contribution to the FID coming from the contents of that pixel. Therefore,

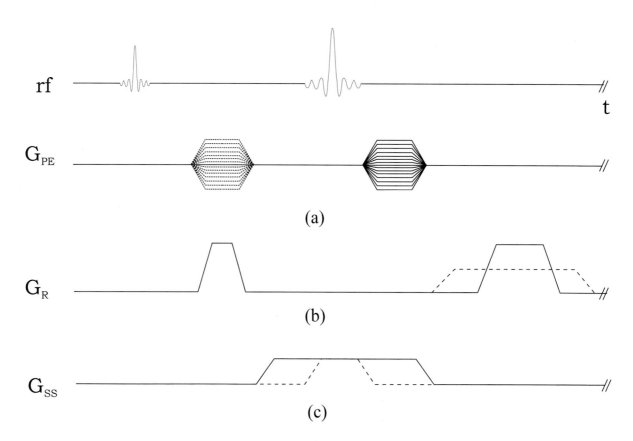

Fig. 26.22: Different methods to eliminate artifacts due to imperfect π-pulses in spin echo imaging sequences. (a) Moving the phase encoding gradient from between the $\pi/2$ and π pulses (dashed phase encoding table) to after the π-pulse (solid lined table) phase encodes the FID signal as well, making the artifact become distributed throughout the image rather than appearing as a bright line at the center of the image. (b) Use of a large read bandwidth (solid line) by using a large read gradient rather than a lower one (dashed line) helps by allowing more time for the FID signal to vanish by natural decay before data sampling begins. (c) Extending the normal π-pulse slice select gradient lobe (dashed line) equally before and after the π-pulse (solid line) preferentially dephases the FID signal contribution while leaving the spin echo part of the signal unchanged at the echo time.

it is a good idea to eliminate the FID signal contribution to the measured signal. There are two methods to achieve this. The first is to use a very high read gradient so that T_s is short enough that the FID decays sufficiently by natural means before data acquisition begins (see Fig. 26.22b). The other more practical method is to extend the slice select gradient as far as possible while also extending its onset and turning-off times equally on both sides from the center of the π-pulse (see Fig. 26.22c). The equal areas under these two extraneous lobes serve the dual purpose of being refocused completely by the spin echo part of the signal at the echo time, while the FID part of the signal is dephased by the part of the gradient lobe which extraneously occurs after the π-pulse. Similar gradients can be applied in the x and y directions as well (although they are not shown in Fig. 26.22). It is also common practice to use an alternating rf pulse in addition to the latter two mechanisms, so that any remnant artifact is moved to the edge of the field-of-view as in the dc artifact case.

Problem 26.23

If two acquisitions of the sequence are collected, detail how phase alternating the π-pulses could be used to eliminate the spurious FID signal.

Data Sampling Error

The reader is referred to Sec. 13.8 for details.

26.4.4   Noise Spikes and Constant-Frequency Noise

Noise Spikes

With the large gradients available today, it is not uncommon to have noise spikes created in the raw data. The causes of these spikes can be due to arcing or loose connections or other electrical/mechanical problems with the system. A noise spike can be modeled as a delta function at some point in k-space

$$s_{\text{spike}}(\vec{k}) = a\delta(k_x - k_{x_0}, k_y - k_{y_0}) \qquad (26.20)$$

The Fourier transform of this yields

$$\hat{\rho}_{\text{spike}}(\vec{r}) = ae^{i2\pi(k_{x_0}x + k_{y_0}y)} \qquad (26.21)$$

When this complex image is added to that for the object itself, the resulting image is

$$\hat{\rho}'(x, y) = \hat{\rho}(x, y) + ae^{i2\pi(k_{x_0}x + k_{y_0}y)} \qquad (26.22)$$

This creates a wave-like pattern in the amplitude of $\hat{\rho}'(x, y)$ as the spike contribution oscillates with amplitude a and a spatial frequency of $k_0 = \sqrt{k_{x_0}^2 + k_{y_0}^2}$.

Figure 26.23 shows a phantom image with a noise spike of amplitude $a = 10$ (one-tenth the value of $\hat{\rho}(x, y)$ in this example) occurring at $k_{x_0} = 0$ and $k_{y_0} = 5$ (Fig. 26.23a) and k_{y_0}

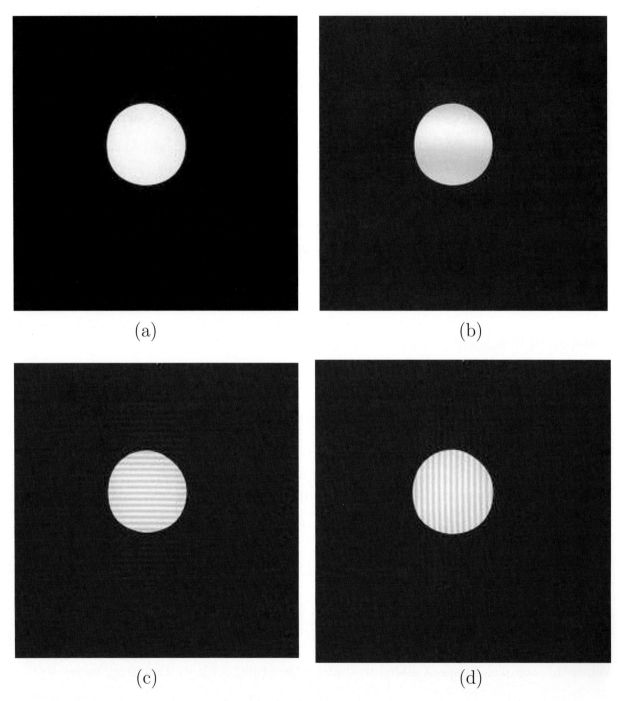

Fig. 26.23: Images showing the effects of a noise spike occurring at different k-space locations. (a) An image reconstructed with no noise spike. Images showing noise spikes in k-space are shown in images (b)–(d). The k-space locations of these spikes are (b) $(0, 5)$, (c) $(0, 50)$, and (d) $(50, 0)$.

= 50 (Fig. 26.23b). The wave-like pattern is evident with a periodicity of once every 256/5 pixels (Fig. 26.23a) or once every 256/50 pixels (Fig. 26.23b) in the $\hat{y}$ direction.

Problem 26.24

Sketch the appearance of the phantom in Fig. 26.23 if the noise spike occurs at $k_{x_0} = k_{y_0} \neq 0$.

Constant-Frequency Noise

When spurious noise of a fixed frequency is picked up by the rf system due to an open door, poor shielding of coaxial cables, or poor shielding in the room itself, the image will have one or many noise lines appearing in the image parallel to the phase encoding axis. An example is shown in Fig. 26.24 (these are the same images as in Fig. 23.7). This artifact actually appeared in several other images earlier in the text in Chs. 23 and 24 that were caused by a poorly shielded coaxial cable in the scanner room.

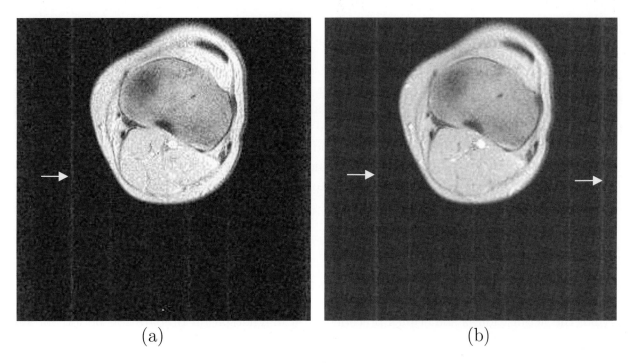

(a) (b)

Fig. 26.24: Images showing constant-frequency (rf) noise artifact. The arrows indicate the location of lines of rf noise.

26.5 Sequence Adjectives and Nomenclature

26.5.1 Nomenclature

In our discussions, we have met examples of most of the existing basic acquisition methods used in MRI. Many other methods exist, but they are generally derivations or combinations of the acquisition methods mentioned so far. The confounding variety of terms and abbreviations used in the description of such MR acquisition methods is a burden to the communication between MR scientists, especially for new-comers in the field. Yet, after writing this book, we have the impression that a step toward a more coherent nomenclature is possible. This step should be helpful in offering, in a short hand format, the essential information for each possible acquisition method. Upon mutual agreement, a similar proposal is given in another textbook on MRI titled: *Magnetic Resonance Imaging: Theory and Practice* by M. Vlaardingerbroek and J. den Boers. We give next a list of terms relevant to the basic aspects of an imaging experiment. Those terms that are different in their text are shown here in square brackets.

Scanning Procedure

Scanning in an MR system is the sum of all actions needed to obtain an image: a scan is specified by its sequence structure, its imaging parameters (which can be adjusted according to the purpose of the scan), the physiological conditions, and the method of reconstruction of the data.

Sequence Structure [Acquisition Method]

The sequence structure describes the entire set of events generated by the MR system to obtain the data necessary for reconstruction. This includes the system initiation for the required scan and the acquisition of the data. The data acquisition process is subdivided into a series of cycles in which all events are repeated, but not necessarily with the same gradient amplitudes (such as the phase encoding gradient strength) or rf pulse flip angles. The combined rf and gradient waveforms in such a period are referred to as an MR sequence cycle (see Fig. 26.25). A sequence diagram often shows only one sequence cycle, but indicates how the cycling occurs.

Sequence Cycle

A sequence always starts with an excitation pulse. In a conventional scan, one line in k-space is acquired per cycle (Fig. 26.25a). If T_R is not much greater than T_1 in a sequence cycle, the acquisition is sometimes preceded by a magnetization preparation period (or set of preparation cycles) to establish a dynamic equilibrium (Fig. 26.25b). In a multiple phase encoding, fast SE or 'multi-shot' EPI or a segmented spiral scan, several lines or trajectories in k-space are acquired in a single cycle (Fig. 26.26a). Sometimes all necessary lines are acquired in a 'single-shot' acquisition; in that case, there is only one cycle (Fig. 26.26b). The repetition time of the cycle is called T_R.

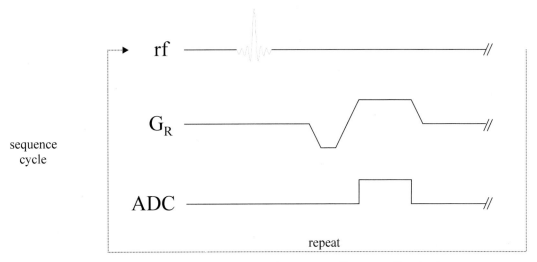

loop over phase encoding amplitude G_{PE}

(a)

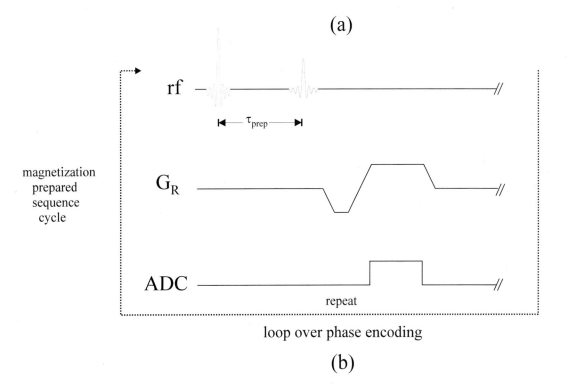

loop over phase encoding

(b)

Fig. 26.25: Various alternatives for a sequence cycle that are used in practice. (a) A conventional single-line acquisition per sequence cycle, where only a single rf pulse is used in a gradient echo acquisition. (b) Sequence cycle for a magnetization-prepared (MP) sequence. A delay τ_{prep} occurs between the MP pulse and the actual signal-producing rf pulse.

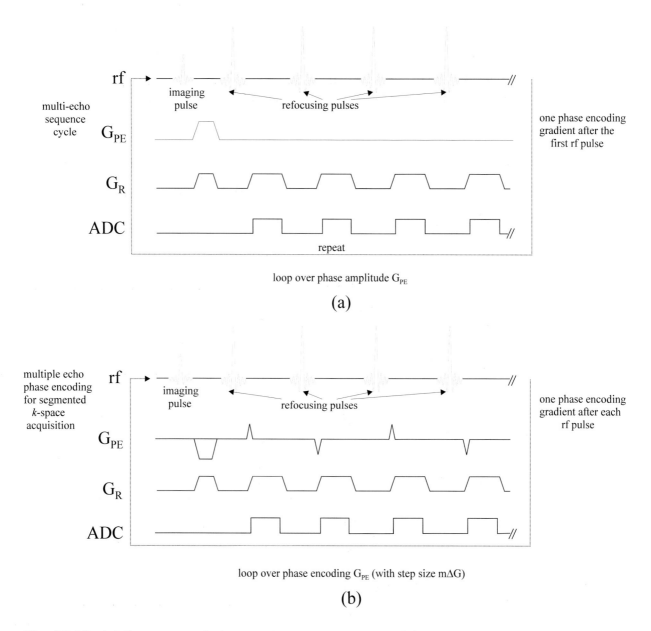

Fig. 26.26: (a) Sequence cycle for a multi-echo acquisition. (b) Sequence cycle for a 'segmented' repeated spin echo acquisition where m phase encoding steps are performed within a given cycle. The same principles can be accomplished with gradient echo sequences as well.

Echoes

The excitation pulse with which a sequence starts generates an FID. Normally this FID is not measured directly, but is transformed into a gradient field echo or a spin echo by applying a π-pulse. We then speak of either gradient echo sequences or spin echo sequences although a mixture of these is also possible. For the simple FID case, the data is sampled during the gradient field echo. For the spin echo case, the measurement usually takes place where the Hahn echo and the echo from the read gradient occur at the same time.

Repeated Echoes

To save acquisition time for a single slice, several echoes are formed and phase encoded after a single excitation pulse. For example, when phase encoding takes place between a series of π-pulses, it would be appropriate to refer to the sequence as a repeated spin echo sequence. In EPI, repeated gradient echoes are acquired. This sequence could just as well have been referred to as a repeated gradient echo experiment. These repeated echo scans can be multi-echo acquisitions or modified to create segmented forms of k-space coverage.

Magnetization State

1. **Steady-State**

   By steady-state, we are implying that the magnetization is the same from cycle to cycle. This condition can be obtained sometimes after one pulse or it can be obtained after many pulses when the system reaches equilibrium.

   (a) **Steady-State Incoherent**

   When the transverse magnetization of the previous cycle does not contribute to the signal, we refer to the results as steady-state incoherent. This can be realized either with long T_R studies where the transverse magnetization is zero prior to applying another rf pulse or by rf spoiling where the magnetization behaves as if the transverse magnetization vanishes prior to the next rf pulse.

   (b) **Steady-State Coherent**

   When the remnant transverse magnetization is not zero prior to each new sequence cycle, the system can still reach equilibration and the equilibrium that is reached is referred to as steady-state coherent.

2. **Transient State**

   Transient state sequences are those in which the magnetization state at the start of each sequence cycle changes, in phase and/or in magnitude. For example, in a short-T_R 2D experiment, where the acquisition cycles run during the transient between the initial magnetization state and the final equilibrium state, we speak of a transient field echo. The initial state may be the equilibrium state, in which at the start of each sequence the longitudinal magnetization is equal to the equilibrium magnetization M_0, or it may be influenced by previous events, such as preparation pulses.

Prepared Magnetization State

In magnetization-prepared (MP) methods, each sequence is preceded by one or more rf pulses and gradient lobes to influence the magnetization state at the start of the sequence. Magnetization-preparation is used to influence the weighting of the resulting images and can make T_1- and T_2-weighting more dominant. Also, other weighting parameters may be influenced (for example, diffusion weighting).

Spoiling

Spoiling (such as by rf phase cycling of the excitation pulses or by gradients) may be applied to minimize the observed coherence in the signal between the contribution of the FID and the transverse magnetization resulting from earlier excitations at the start of each sequence or cycle. This technique plays an important role in some steady-state sequences. In transient state methods, spoiling may also be applied, but its effect is less clear.

Contrast Type

Last, but not least, is the type of contrast which is present. The usual descriptors are spin density-, T_1-, T_2-, and T_2^*-weighted imaging but other types of contrast such as T_1/T_2, diffusion weighted contrast, flow dephasing, etc. also should not be ignored.

The features described above are summarized in Table 26.1.

Descriptor	Descriptor types	
echo type	spin echo	gradient echo
echo number	single echo	multiple echoes
echo encoding	singular phase encoding	encoding between echoes
echo symmetry	symmetric $(n_- = n_+)^2$	asymmetric $(n_- \neq n_+)$
rf type	selective	nonselective
spin state	transient	steady-state
	coherent	incoherent
	unprepared	prepared
number of rf pulses used	single pulse	multi-pulse
phase encoding order	sequential	centrically reordered
spoiling	rf	gradient

Table 26.1: Characterization of scan methods. This table is fairly complete but does not include all possible variants.

$^2 n_-$ is the number of k-space samples collected before and including the $k = 0$ sample. n_+ indicates the number of samples collected after the $k = 0$ sample.

26.5.2 Some Other Descriptive Adjectives and Some Specific Examples

Since MR imaging is primarily governed by a set of linear operations, it is often possible to merge one feature with another in the same sequence. For example, one can acquire flow information or apply a fat saturation pulse or do both simultaneously. Those concepts that can be incorporated separately into a sequence should be used as adjectives to describe the sequence. For example, if we applied a flow encoding gradient and a fat saturation pulse to a conventional spin echo sequence, we should say we are using 'a flow encoded, fat saturated spin echo sequence.' Listed below are a set of adjectives that can be used to describe the features of a sequence.

n-dimensional

The number of directions into which an image can be decomposed.

gradient echo

A method which uses just one rf pulse before reading out a line or multiple lines of data.

spin echo

A method which uses a 90°-pulse followed by at least one 180°-pulse (to minimize field inhomogeneity effects) before reading out a line or multiple lines of data. This can be generalized to an α-β pulse system, although the echo amplitude is accordingly reduced (see Ch. 18).

(rf or gradient) spoiled

A sequence which is designed to dephase or 'spoil' the remnant transverse magnetization so that it is effectively zero prior to the next rf pulse.

nD spatially selective

A description of the type of rf pulse used to excite a slice (1D, hence a slice selective pulse), a cylinder (2D), or a sphere (3D), for example. The spatial selection is effected by applying appropriate time-dependent gradients during the application of the rf pulse.

chemical shift selective pulse

A pulse which excites a chemical species such as water, fat, or silicon, for example (it can be used to invert magnetization, produce a transverse component, or saturate signal from a certain tissue).

magnetization prepared

A term which describes a set of rf pulses and associated gradients used to prepare the spins in a desired state prior to spatial encoding and data acquisition.

magnetization transfer

The application of a magnetization transfer pulse to suppress signal from spins which exchange with or reside in macromolecules. This approach has been applied in tissues such as myocardium or gray matter since it can enhance their contrast with other tissues.

motion enhanced or tagged

A reference to a saturation or tissue-selective pulse or pulses used to preferentially excite spins to follow motion or visualize field effects (also applicable to bolus tagging).

balanced gradients

A reference to a gradient pulse that has zero zeroth moment with respect to time between two successive rf pulses.

order of k-space coverage

A description of the phase encoding order of a sequence, such as sequential, centric or reverse-centric order.

variable flip angle (T_R or T_E)

A reference to the fact that from one rf pulse to the next, the flip angle (T_R or T_E) is modified.

flow (diffusion) sensitive

A reference to a bipolar pulse applied to create a velocity dependent phase (or signal amplitude reduction from diffusion) for moving spins.

flow compensated

A description of the type of motion compensation used for the gradient design which needs to be described as velocity compensated (first moment), acceleration compensated (second moment), or higher order moment compensated.

multi-echo

The acquisition of several data sets after a single rf pulse from multiple gradient recalled echoes or spin echoes.

shared echo

The use of the same k-space line twice, once in each of two reconstructions. This is usually implemented in cardiac gated images where segmented k-space is acquired. Since this usually reduces the temporal resolution, echo sharing can regain some of the lost time.

segmented k-space

The acquisition of a fraction of k-space in a given cycle or given fraction of time in a periodic event such as collecting part of k-space during one cardiac cycle and part during another to speed up acquisition by using the time between the excitation pulses (i.e., within a cycle) to encode between multiple (repeated) echoes.

contrast enhanced

An adjective which describes the use of a contrast agent to enhance the signal (or enhance the loss of signal). The contrast enhancement usually occurs between blood and surrounding tissue when the agent is intravascular. Tissues can enhance if there is a breakdown of the vascular wall that normally acts as a barrier to large molecules such as the contrast agent molecule and prevents their entry into the surrounding tissues.

reconstruction type

A reference to the type of image reconstruction used such as fast Fourier transform, projection reconstruction, partial Fourier image reconstruction, or parallel imaging, for example.

echo symmetry

The asymmetry or degree of asymmetry in sampling the data relative to a symmetric acquisition is given by $2m/N$ where m is the number of points away from the center of the sampling window that the echo occurs and N is the total number of sampled points. This can also be written as $(n_+ - n_-)/N$ where n_+ is the number of points sampled after the echo, n_- is the number of points sampled before and including the echo. For example, a 256 point sampling scheme with 31 points before the echo (i.e., $n_- = 32$) is said to be 75% asymmetric. This same concept as used for the read direction is identical for the phase encoding direction if the echo center $k_x = 0$ is replaced by the $k_y = 0$ line.

imaging parameters

Those variables that must be set to determine imaging time, contrast, signal-to-noise ratio, etc. These include, but are not limited to, T_R, T_E, flip angle, etc. For a more extensive list of these parameters, see Appendix C.

imaging conditions

These can specify coil type, audio/visual equipment, cardiac gating and monitoring equipment, for example.

initiating a scan and patient consent

If a person is being imaged, he/she is interviewed to determine if it is safe for him/her to go in the magnet and is asked to sign a consent form agreeing to the scanning procedure if the images are being acquired for research. This form will have to be pre-approved by the local IRB (Institutional Review Board) for research purposes.

The scanning procedure itself begins by placing the object or person on the patient table and centering the ROI in the center of the rf coil being used. The table is moved into the magnet and the loaded coil is then tuned (see Ch. 27). The static magnetic field may be fine-tuned at this point by shimming the system to ensure optimal field homogeneity. The appropriate sequence is then loaded and signal attenuation levels are automatically calibrated and set to ensure a proper reconstruction of the data.

an example description of the scanning

The sequences used will depend on the clinical situation and whether it is an anatomical and/or pathological problem. The choice of sequence(s), orientation, coils, etc. are referred to as the 'protocol' and there are many different protocols in clinical use today. For argument's sake, if a T_1-weighted scan and an angiographic scan are needed after contrast agent administration, they may be described as in the following two examples.

If the T_1-weighted images are collected using a 2D spin echo sequence sagittally, a fairly complete description of the sequence could be given as: a 2D, T_1-weighted, velocity compensated, rf spoiled, multi-slice, single-echo spin echo acquisition. In short, taking most of the features for granted, this might be referred to as simply a T_1-weighted multi-slice acquisition.

If the next scan uses a transverse MRA sequence collected post-contrast injection, the description might be as follows: a contrast enhanced, 3D, low flip angle, asymmetric gradient echo, velocity compensated in the read and slice select directions, rf spoiled transverse acquisition. In short form, this could be referred to as a contrast enhanced, time-of-flight, angiographic sequence.

Suggested Reading

The introduction of magnetization preparation in the form of a π-pulse to manipulate contrast (i.e., the concept of inversion recovery) was introduced in the following article:

- G. M. Bydder, R. E. Steiner and I. R. Young, A. S. Hall, D. J. Thomas, J. Marshall, C. A. Pallis and N. J. Legg. Clinical NMR imaging of the brain: 140 cases. *Am. J. Roentgenol.*, 139: 215, 1982.

Two papers dealt with fast imaging using θ-π-π or θ-π pulse trains:

- A. R. Bogdan and P. M. Joseph. RASEE: A rapid spin echo pulse sequence. *Magn. Reson. Imag.*, 8: 13, 1990.

- J. A. Tkach and E. M. Haacke. A comparison of fast spin echo and gradient echo sequences. *Magn. Reson. Imag.*, 6: 374, 1988.

We have only touched on a fraction of sequence designs which are possible; many more are included in this text:

- A. M. Parikh. *Magnetic Resonance Imaging Techniques.* Elsevier, New York, 1992.

There are numerous variants to fast imaging concepts, but two papers deal with eliminating or separating the FID signal from the spin echo signal components:

- H. Bruder, H. Fischer, R. Graumann and M. Deimling. A new steady-state imaging sequence for simultaneous acquisition of two MR images with clearly different contrasts. *Magn. Reson. Med.*, 7: 35, 1988.

- C. T. Moonen, G. Liu, P. van Gelderen and G. Sobering. A fast gradient-recalled MRI technique with increased sensitivity to dynamic susceptibility effects. *Magn. Reson. Med.*, 26: 184, 1992.

Artifacts can be caused by many system and design variables; a large number of these are touched on in the following review:

- R. M. Henkelman and M. J. Bronskill. Artifacts in magnetic resonance imaging. *Rev. Magn. Reson. Med.*, 2: 1, 1987.

Chapter 27

Introduction to MRI Coils and Magnets

Chapter Contents

Summary: Basic electromagnetic equations are introduced to describe the fields produced by and properties of the coils used in MRI. Desirable properties of the various coil systems are discussed. A brief introduction to rf power deposition and specific absorption rate is also given.

Introduction

Heretofore the primary focus has been the effect of magnetic fields on samples. The attention is now directed toward the coils and magnets that produce the requisite MRI fields. The goal of this chapter is to familiarize the reader with a number of basic electromagnetic and mathematical concepts needed to understand the design of the coils that generate the fields used in MRI. Some well-known prototypes of the coils (main magnet, rf, and gradient) are considered in the sections that follow.

The problem of designing field generating coils can be stated very simply. The ideal fields to be used in MRI are very well specified, but the arrangements of wires needed to produce these fields most efficiently are not intuitively obvious. For this reason, the design of coils lies primarily in determining the optimal arrangements of current necessary to produce the magnetic fields used in MRI. These concepts are borne in mind even as the simple designs of coils are discussed.

823

27.1   The Circular Loop as an Example

To understand a number of the magnetic field concepts in this chapter, it is useful to begin with an example. Consider the time-independent field from a circular loop with current I, radius a, coaxial with the z-axis (see Fig. 27.1).

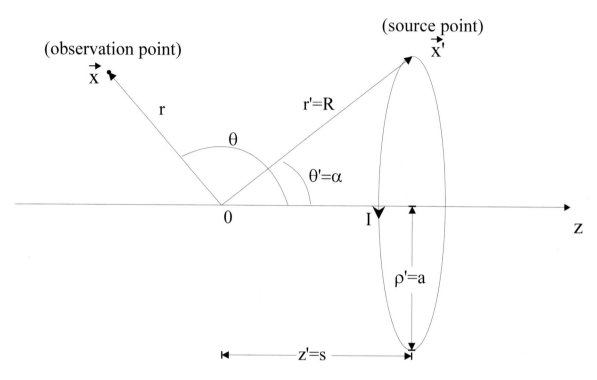

Fig. 27.1: Spherical and cylindrical coordinate systems used to describe the field from a single loop of wire coaxial with the z-axis. The unprimed (primed) coordinates refer to the observation (source) points.

The field from the circular loop can be found from the Biot-Savart Law

$$\vec{B}(\vec{x}) = \frac{\mu_0}{4\pi} \int_{volume} d^3x' \frac{\vec{J}(\vec{x}') \times (\vec{x} - \vec{x}')}{|\vec{x} - \vec{x}'|^3} \tag{27.1}$$

where $\vec{J}(\vec{x}')$ represents an arbitrary time-independent current density (the amount of current moving in a given direction per unit area). In cases involving thin wires (27.1) can be reduced to

$$\vec{B}(\vec{x}) = \frac{\mu_0}{4\pi} \oint_{path} \frac{I d\vec{\ell}' \times (\vec{x} - \vec{x}')}{|\vec{x} - \vec{x}'|^3} \tag{27.2}$$

in which the current in the wire is I and the vector differential along the current path is $d\vec{\ell}'$. This formula is very accurate as long as both the distance $|\vec{x} - \vec{x}'|$ between the wire and the point of observation remain large compared to the cross-sectional diameter of the wire.

The exact form of $\vec{B}$ for a circular loop obtained from the Biot-Savart law (27.2) at a general spatial location is a complicated expression. However, an elementary calculation can be made to find the on-axis field for the circular loop. In terms of the coordinates shown in Fig. 27.1, the current follows the azimuthal $\hat{\phi}'$ direction, and therefore it is easiest to define the problem in terms of cylindrical coordinates

$$
\begin{aligned}
d\vec{\ell}' &= a\,d\phi'\left(-\sin\phi'\hat{x} + \cos\phi'\hat{y}\right) \\
\vec{x} - \vec{x}' &= -a\left(\cos\phi'\hat{x} + \sin\phi'\hat{y}\right) + (z-s)\hat{z}
\end{aligned}
$$

The radius of the loop is a and the loop center is at the axial location s. The integrand of (27.2) becomes

$$
\frac{I\,d\vec{\ell}' \times (\vec{x} - \vec{x}')}{|\vec{x} - \vec{x}'|^3} = \frac{I\,a\,d\phi'\left((z-s)\cos\phi'\hat{x} - (z-s)\sin\phi'\hat{y} + a\hat{z}\right)}{\left(a^2 + (z-s)^2\right)^{3/2}} \tag{27.3}
$$

The integration is performed around the entire loop from 0 to 2π, and the x- and y-components of $\vec{B}$ disappear since the integrals of sine and cosine vanish on that interval. Therefore, the field on the z-axis has only a constant integration for the z component,

$$
B_z(\rho = 0) = \frac{\mu_0 I a^2}{2\left(a^2 + (z-s)^2\right)^{3/2}} \tag{27.4}
$$

A plot of the field for a single wire loop, centered at the origin, as a function of z is shown in Fig. 27.2.

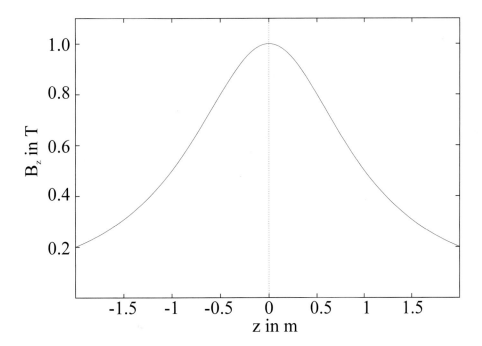

Fig. 27.2: B_z vs z on the axis for a single wire loop centered at the origin ($z' = 0$). The loop radius is 1 m and the current units are chosen for convenience to give $I\mu_0/2 = 1$.

27.1.1   Quality of Field

Both homogeneous and linearly varying fields are used for imaging in MRI, and it is useful to try and understand how homogeneous or linear a given field is. This question is usually answered by decomposing the field in terms of the desired field behavior and contaminating field terms. Consider the field shown in Fig. 27.2 which is not homogeneous, for example, but can be decomposed into a homogeneous term and other terms. The field shown in Fig. 27.2 has been expressed in terms of a power series in z in Fig. 27.3, as an example. The individual lines in Fig. 27.3 represent terms in an expansion of B_z along the axis, and are generally referred to as 'moments.'[1]

This analysis is useful when trying to obtain a homogeneous field, for example, because several coils can be positioned such that their linear and other unwanted moments exactly cancel, leading to a resulting field which is more homogeneous than that of a single coil. The quality of the field produced depends upon how many of the contaminating terms or moments are successfully reduced to zero.

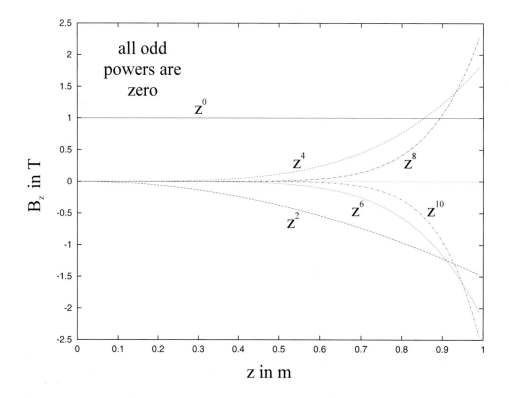

Fig. 27.3: The first six nonzero terms in the series in the expansion of B_z for a single loop centered at the origin as a function of z. This example demonstrates the rapidly decreasing contribution of higher-order moments near the origin.

---

[1]In general, the magnetic field moments used to analyze the fields used in MRI are expressed in terms of spherical harmonics. Spherical harmonics are used because they represent a general solution of Laplace's equation, which the magnetic field must satisfy in free space for a time-independent field. Since most readers may not be familiar with these functions, a Taylor series is used here to introduce the notion of breaking the field down into moments.

One way to obtain an expression for a function as a power series about a particular point is to use a Taylor expansion. Making a Taylor series expansion of the on-axis field from a circular loop (Fig. 27.1) leads to

$$B_z(z) = \frac{\mu_0 I a^2}{2} \left[\frac{1}{R^3} + z \cdot \left(\frac{3s}{R^5} \right) + \frac{1}{2} z^2 \cdot \left(\frac{12s^2 - 3a^2}{R^7} \right) \right. $$
$$\left. + \frac{1}{6} z^3 \cdot \left(\frac{60s^3 - 45sa^2}{R^9} \right) + ... \right] \tag{27.5}$$

where $R = \sqrt{a^2 + s^2}$. If a set of circular loops could be arranged such that the sum of their resulting fields only produced a z^0 term, a perfectly homogeneous field would be found. Unfortunately, it is not possible, practically, to produce a perfectly homogeneous field. However, it might be possible to make sure that the coefficient of moments z^1 to z^{10} are all approximately zero, which, as can be seen from Fig. 27.3, would lead to a very homogeneous field near the origin. In the sections that follow, specific examples of how homogeneous and linearly varying fields are produced will be described.

27.2   The Main Magnet Coil

As mentioned throughout this text the primary job of the main magnet is to cause a population of spins to align parallel to the magnetic field, resulting in a net magnetization of the sample. The magnetization is then manipulated to produce the signal in an MRI experiment. The main magnetic field should be time-independent and very homogeneous.

27.2.1   Classic Designs

There are several main magnet designs that are based on analytic solutions, and they are worth studying to obtain an increased understanding of how field expansions are used to design fields.

Helmholtz Pair

An initial step in producing a magnetic field that is more homogeneous than that shown for the single loop is to combine two coaxial loops symmetrically about the origin, and find the ratio of their separation to radii which gives optimal field homogeneity (see Fig. 27.4). The theoretical tool employed is the Taylor expansion of the field along the axis about $z = 0$ for a pair of coils centered at $z' = \pm s$ with common radius $\rho' = a$ (see (27.4) and (27.5)). The resulting field is the summation of the field from each individual loop. Since the coils have the same radius and current, but different centers, the only difference between their expansions (27.5) is that $s \rightarrow -s$ for the coil at $z' = -s$. The combined series for the symmetric pair of coils has no terms odd in the power z. In general, any current distribution that is symmetric with respect to the $z = 0$ plane will have no odd derivatives in its Taylor series expansion along z.

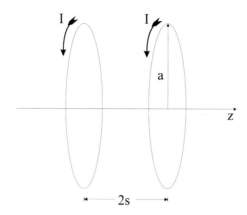

Fig. 27.4: Helmholtz coil pair configuration where the separation of the coils is equal to their radius ($a = 2s$). This choice of spacing leads to a homogeneous field near the origin because the z^2 moment of the field is zero.

It is possible to use a relation between a and s to eliminate the second-order derivative for the two coils which will lead to a more homogeneous field. The second-order term will vanish when

$$a = 2s \qquad (27.6)$$

i.e., the coil radii equals the axial separation of their centers. A single coil set which meets this criterion is referred to as a Helmholtz pair or a Helmholtz coil. The fourth-order term corresponds to the first nonvanishing derivative at the origin for such coils. The resultant field is plotted in Fig. 27.5, showing the uniformity around $z = 0$. The magnetic field remains primarily parallel to z along ρ as well.[2]

Problem 27.1

a) Derive the first two terms shown in (27.5) by an appropriate expansion of (27.4).

b) Write out the z^2 term for the field produced by a Helmholtz coil pair (sum contribution of each coil using (27.4)), and show that this term vanishes under the condition given by (27.6). Make an argument for why all of the terms odd in z are equal to 0.

c) Plot B_z vs z for a symmetric coil pair for two cases. In the first case use the Helmholtz condition (27.6). In the second case, increase a by 10% from this value. Qualitatively comment on the difference in axial homogeneity for these two cases.

---

[2]The variation in the ρ direction is constrained to be small by Maxwell's equations if the variation in the z-direction is small.

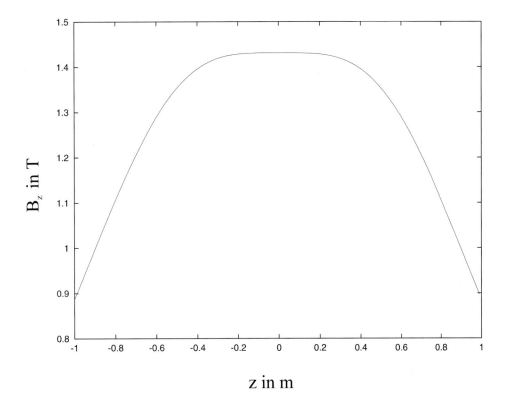

Fig. 27.5: Plot of B_z vs z for a Helmholtz pair. The loop radius is 1 m, the wire separation is therefore also 1 m, and the current units are chosen for convenience to give $I\mu_0/2 = 1$.

Problem 27.2

In an attempt to increase field strength B_0 generated by a Helmholtz pair, an additional coil might be added at the origin. Consider the coil set shown in Fig. 27.6. Assume that z_0, a, b, and I_0 are all given. Find an expression for α in terms of these parameters such that the second derivative of the field produced by all of the coils at the origin is zero. Comment on the potential advantages or disadvantages of this coil set with respect to the simpler Helmholtz coil based upon the discussions presented throughout this section. Some things you may wish to consider include efficiency, overall homogeneity, length, and ease of construction.

Classic Solenoid

An elementary textbook example of a coil which produces a uniform magnetic field near the origin is a long solenoid, coaxial with the z-axis, centered about $z = 0$. A classic uniformly wound solenoid, however, is not the best choice for an MRI main magnet. Good uniformity at the center of such a solenoid requires that its length be large compared to its radius. This is evident from the familiar formula for the z-component of the field along the axis of a solenoid,

$$B_z(z) = \frac{\mu_0 n I}{2}\left(\cos\alpha_1 - \cos\alpha_2\right) \qquad (27.7)$$

where n is the number of turns per unit length, and the angles are described in Fig. 27.7. If $B_z(z)$ is to be approximately constant near the origin, then α_1 and α_2 must also be approximately constant which only occurs if the length of the solenoid is much greater than its radius.

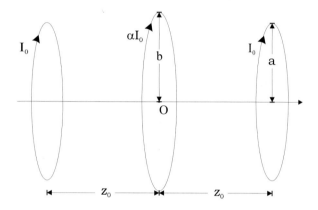

Fig. 27.6: This coil configuration represents a simple addition to the Helmoltz coil pair where a coil has been placed at the center in an attempt to increase the field produced in the imaging region.

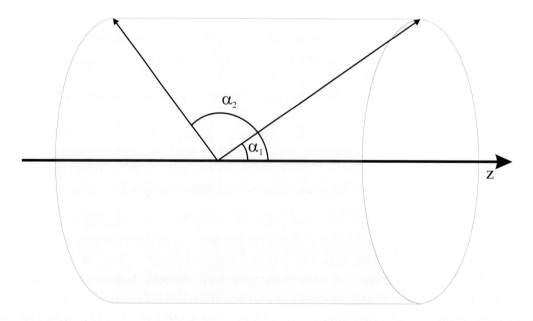

Fig. 27.7: An illustration of a solenoid with radius a. The angles α_1 and α_2 are defined as shown.

Problem 27.3

It is often assumed that a classic solenoid is the simplest choice of coil for generating the static field in MRI. However, sets of bundled coils, such as those shown in Fig. 27.8 are actually the norm. Consider the field generated by a tightly wound solenoid with n turns of wire per unit length as given by (27.7). The angles $\alpha_{1,2}$ are the angles between the z-axis and a line from the origin to the edge of the wires at either end of the solenoid. Using this formula, and assuming the following parameters, $r_{solenoid} = 1.0\,\text{m}$, $n = 1000\,\text{turns/meter}$, an imaging region-of-interest of 50 cm diameter spherical volume, and $I = 1\,\text{amp}$,

a) By an integration using (27.4) show that the field from a solenoid is correctly given by (27.7).

b) Determine the minimum length of the solenoid if the on-axis homogeneity of the magnet must be 5 ppm, i.e., $(B_z(0) - B_z(0.25\,\text{m}))/B_z(0) = 5\,\text{ppm}$.

Hint: This problem is most easily solved by using a numerical analysis, or using a Taylor series expansion of the field.

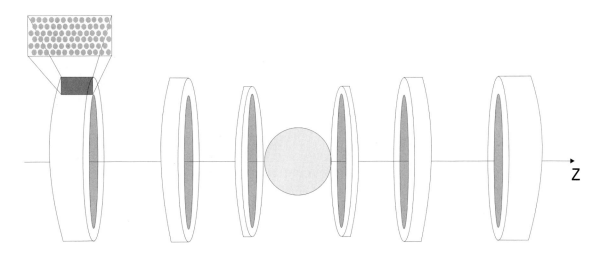

Fig. 27.8: Sketch of a typical set of main magnet coils. The lightly shaded sphere in the center of the figure represents the imaging region. The cutaway of the left-most coil demonstrates that individual superconducting wires are packed together to form the coils.

Further Improving Homogeneity

The Helmholtz pair and solenoid are useful conceptual designs, but are not generally adequate to produce the very homogeneous fields desired in MRI. It is not, in general, possible to obtain the desired field homogeneity by eliminating only the z^2 term from the field, as is the case for the Helmholtz coil. Neither is it reasonable to build a solenoid that is long enough to provide adequate homogeneity over a human whole body imaging region. Advanced designs consist of rectangular bundles of wires centered at axial and radial locations chosen specifically to optimize homogeneity in the imaging volume. A pictorial example of a modern coil configuration is shown in Fig. 27.8.

Problem 27.4

Suppose the technology of superconductivity is not available. Assume that it takes 2 mega-amp turns (current/wire × number of turns or individual wire loops) of wire to generate a 1.0 T field. Assume the following parameters: wire with a 1 mm diameter and a current of 10 amps, average radius, call it a, of the coils to be 1 m, and use $1.7 \times 10^{-8} \,\Omega\text{·m}$ as the resistivity of copper.

a) Find the power required to operate this magnet if copper windings are used. Recall that for a wire

$$\mathcal{R} = \rho \ell / A \tag{27.8}$$

where $\mathcal{R}$ is resistance, ρ is resistivity, ℓ is the total length of the wire, and A is its cross-sectional area. Also, recall that the power dissipated by a resistive wire is given by

$$P = I^2 \mathcal{R} \tag{27.9}$$

b) Imagine for a minute that this power is instead used to heat water. How many liters of water could be heated from $15\,^\circ\text{C}$ to $90\,^\circ\text{C}$ in one minute by the power supplied to this magnet? (This should give the reader some idea of why resistive magnets are not practical for high field magnet use.)

c) Since the quantity which determines the field produced by the magnet is best characterized by amp-turns and copper can not carry very many amps a large number of turns are required to produce a high field. Estimate the weight of both a copper magnet and a superconducting magnet. Assume the density of copper to be 3g/cm^3 and the density of the superconductor to be $2.5\,\text{m/cm}^3$, further assume the superconductor can carry 150 amps of current. Use the amp-turns and average radius figures given above to complete this problem. Qualitatively comment on whether your answer places another restriction on the utility of a resistive magnet at high fields.

d) Patients in MRI often complain of claustrophobic feelings during MR examinations. Consider the effects of increasing the radius of the MRI main magnet in an attempt to give patients more space. Assume that the magnet is constructed of two coils centered at the Helmholtz position ($a = d$ or radius equals separation). Assuming that the same number of amp-turns is used, what would be the relative decrease in $B_0(0)$ if the radius a is taken from 1 m to 2 m. What is the relative increase in the length of wire in this case? Your answers should explain why the radius of the main magnet is not too large.

27.2.2   Desirable Properties of Main Magnets

In order to develop optimal coils, the important operational parameters of the object should be well understood. Several important aspects of the MRI main magnet include: field strength, homogeneity, temporal stability, patient access and comfort, cost effectiveness, minimization of fields generated outside the imaging environment, and access to the patient during scanning for invasive procedures.

Maximizing Field Strength

As mentioned in the introduction the maximum available SNR for an MR experiment is proportional to B_0^α; $(\alpha \geq 1)$ with some variability in the value of the exponent as a function of B_0. Since MRI is an inherently low SNR phenomenon, a primary goal of MRI main magnet design to increase SNR is to maximize B_0 (see Sec. 15.8.2). Maximization of B_0 explains two common aspects of contemporary high field MRI systems. The first is the solenoidal or cylindrical magnet structure. The cylindrical structure of the magnet allows a large amount of field producing wire to be placed close to the imaging environment and is also attractive from an engineering point of view. The second aspect of contemporary machines dictated by increasing B_0 is the use of superconductors to generate B_0. The magnetic field a wire generates is linearly proportional to the current it carries. A copper wire, operating at room temperature, a few millimeters in diameter, can carry approximately 10 amps continuously, and a bundle of such wires must be cooled since the resistance causes a lot of power to be deposited in the wires as heat. A superconducting wire of 1 mm in diameter, however, can support more than a hundred amps of current with no associated heating. The presence of resistance in a room temperature copper wire also means that power must constantly be fed to maintain the field, but a superconducting system will run indefinitely with no additional power, excluding refrigeration, if it is kept superconducting.

Temporal and Spatial Uniformity

As a matter of convention, homogeneity of an MRI magnet is quoted in terms of inhomogeneity or ΔB_0. For example, if a magnet is said to have a homogeneity of 20 ppm, this means that the field varies by 20 millionths of its average value over the region-of-interest. It must be kept in mind that ppm is a relative measure (1 ppm of $x = 1/1,000,000$ of x), but the effect on imaging is a function of the actual field difference. For example, a 1.0 T magnet with a homogeneity of 10 ppm and a 10 T magnet with 10 ppm of homogeneity would have image distortion and signal loss problems due to static field inhomogeneities that differ in magnitude by approximately a factor of ten. An accepted homogeneity level for contemporary whole-body clinical imaging machines might be given as 5 ppm over a 50 cm diameter spherical volume at 1.5 T. All of these figures show that the *static field used in MRI must be very homogeneous*. In order to achieve this level of homogeneity the classic designs described previously are not adequate. In reality, sets of coils such as those shown in Fig. 27.8 are used to obtain ppm homogeneity levels and high field strengths. These coils are developed with an identical philosophy to that described for the Helmholtz coil, except more coils have been added to cancel progressively higher order contaminating moments. The level of accuracy required leads to a unique set of requirements in accuracy of field modeling, and manufacture of coil sets.

The required homogeneity of an MRI magnet is dictated by the desire to avoid the field distortion effects outlined in previous chapters. In order to avoid a majority of field distortion errors, the homogeneity of the magnet should be such that T_2' due to static field inhomogeneities is much longer than an average data acquisition or read gradient period. The spatial frequency of variation in B_0 must also be very low so that ΔB_0 across a pixel is much less than $G_x \Delta x$. In other words, spins are not affected as much by field inhomogeneity as by applied gradient effects. To determine what homogeneity for a magnet is required, however, is difficult because some imaging methodologies require more uniformity than others. The question is also dependent upon the volume being considered, and a magnet with 15 ppm of homogeneity on a 50 cm diameter spherical volume (DSV) may also be able to claim less than 2 ppm on a 30 cm DSV. This is easy to understand from a moment analysis of the magnetic field (see Fig. 27.3) which demonstrates that error contributions are smaller near the origin. This explains why some imaging methods which may be employed on a small volume sample (human head, for example) are much more difficult to use for scanning a larger volume.

The label static implies that the field is independent of time, and in MRI a field which is independent of time would be defined by one which varied by less than a few ppm over the total imaging time, T_T. It is found that for superconducting magnets the fields often vary less than a μT/hour. Therefore, for all practical purposes the time dependence of the main field can be neglected for a superconducting system. This is not the case for a system using resistive wire. In this case variations of the field may occur over times much less than T_T, resulting in image errors due to incorrect demodulation of the signal.

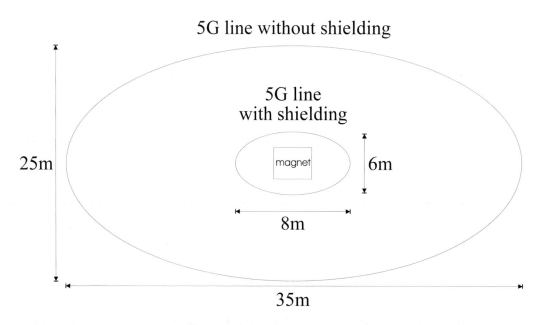

Fig. 27.9: Example of a 1.0 T magnet system with and without active shielding. The two lines circling the magnet represent the 5 G lines before and after shielding is introduced to the system.

Fringe Field Effects

Another concern which must be considered when designing an MRI main magnet is the effect of the field on nearby electronic devices. Fields in excess of $5\,G$ ($5 \times 10^{-4}\,T$) are considered to pose potential risks to people using electronic health aids. Therefore, fields produced outside of the imaging region (fringe fields) must also be considered in the initial design. In fact, unshielded magnets at $0.5\,T$ and above can produce fields in excess of $5\,G$ at distances of 10 to 30 m from the imaging site (see Fig. 27.9), and in hospitals where space is at a premium, shielding of these fields must be one of the primary design concerns.

Problem 27.5

There are really two concerns in the immediate area of MRI main magnets: one is the increased static field level, and the other is the large static field gradients near the magnet. Consider the following situations where a small circular loop will be used to approximate the wires in an electronic device which may be employed near an MRI system.

a) Consider a circular loop of wire that is initially aligned so that its area vector is parallel to the field, and rotates to a position anti-parallel to the field in 1 s (example of time it may take a person to turn quickly). Take the radius of the wire to be 10 cm. Approximate the *emf* induced in the coil in a $5\,G$ field, the earth's magnetic field ($B_{earth} \approx 1\,G$), and a $1.5\,T$ field.

b) Consider moving the same loop from part (a) near the magnet where the magnitude of the field is varying rapidly. Consider a person walking through a region where the field varies linearly from $0\,T$ to $1.0\,T$ in $1.0\,m$. Assume the area vector of the loop is aligned parallel to the field and that the person is walking at a rate of 3 mile/hr. Calculate the *emf* induced in the loop.

c) Based on your answers to the previous parts, would you expect the induced voltages given to be large enough to affect the function of a solid-state device such as a calculator?

Problem 27.6

Answer the following questions about how an iron paper clip would behave in and around an MRI machine.

a) If the paper clip is released from rest in a perfectly uniform field, what will happen?

b) The paper clip is placed on a frictionless imaging table just outside the bore of an MRI machine. Describe what will happen to the paper clip, and estimate the velocity of the paper clip in the center of the magnet. Hint: The dipole moment/mass for iron = 333 A·m^2/kg.

c)   Assume you are placed in a large uniform magnetic field. Can you locate the direction of the field, if your only detection device is a paper clip? Describe how you might do this.

27.2.3   Shielding

As described previously, the static fields produced by the main magnet can present safety risks when electronic devices or metallic objects are brought into the imaging environment. In order to minimize the region where these issues are important most main magnets are shielded to minimize fields produced outside of the imaging environment.

Active Shielding

Active shielding of fringe fields in MRI is generally accomplished by the addition of one coil pair at a larger radius than the interior pairs. The current in the shielding (secondary) coil flows in the opposite direction to the interior coils, and so produces fields which tend to cancel the primary fields. The vector summation of the fields from the primary and shielding coils leads to a large reduction in the overall field outside of the magnet.

Unfortunately shielding in this way also leads to a significant reduction of the interior field. Therefore, to obtain a similar B_0 field, an actively shielded coil must have a significantly larger amount of primary and shielding current than is found in an unshielded magnet. Active shielding more than doubles the amount of total current needed to produce a similar B_0 in most cases.

It appears that active shielding might be overly expensive since the magnet cost is strongly related to the amp-turns used to produce the field. However, this is not the case. Although active shielding does affect the initial magnet cost, since the magnets are superconducting it does not have a significant impact on subsequent operating costs. Also, active shielding simplifies magnet installation. By reducing the external fields, interactions with external magnetic materials are reduced. An actively shielded magnet can be brought to most sites and installed, with little concern for the building structure (iron beams, nearby traffic, etc.).

Ferromagnetic or Passive Shielding

Ferromagnetic shielding in MRI is based upon principles similar to those used in electrical shielding. A magnet designer can make use of the boundary conditions, and properties of materials with large magnetic permeability μ to modify the form of fields local to the magnetic materials.

Ferromagnetic shielding has been used in two primary ways in MRI. In the first case it has simply consisted of iron introduced into the walls of an imaging site where an unshielded magnet has been installed. The distortion of the main field due to the presence of the iron is then corrected on a case-by-case basis. Each new site presents new conditions for the people installing the magnet, and can lead to unique difficulties.

Another way to address ferromagnetic shielding is to include iron in the initial magnet design. The iron material surrounds the primary field producing coils in very close proximity, and its presence is included in the design of the homogeneous field. The effect is included by calculating the fields from the bare coils, and then calculating the contribution to the field from the iron in terms of moments. Advantages of this method are the same as those from active shielding. Disadvantages of this method are that the amount of iron necessary for shielding can lead to very heavy designs which are awkward to transport and install. Also, iron is difficult to treat mathematically, and leads to a large increase in the amount of computational power needed to achieve an initial design.

27.2.4 Shimming

Shimming in magnet technology refers to the process of removing small inhomogeneities which are present in the field after the coil has been wound. It is not possible to consistently produce a set of coils whose homogeneity meets the specifications imposed by the theoretical design. This is due to the large number of variables in the manufacturing process. Some of these variables include machine error in locating coil troughs, wire distribution during winding, contraction of the system when it is cooled to superconducting temperatures ($\approx$ 4 K), shifting of the wires under magnetic (or passive) forces, presence of magnetic impurities in any of the surrounding structures, mechanical stresses during transport, and so forth. As a result when magnets are finally 'brought to field' the homogeneity is typically found to be on the order of several hundred ppm.

It is still necessary to achieve the original design homogeneity for imaging to take place, and a set of corrections must be applied to the field before it is ready for imaging. The process of removing these final inhomogeneities from the magnet is referred to as shimming. There are two primary methods for shimming similar to those employed for shielding. Ferromagnetic (or passive) shimming involves placing pieces of iron in the bore of the magnet close to the imaging region in order to eliminate moments in the field. Active shimming involves adding small amounts of extra current to a set of coils at a slightly larger radius than the primary coil, in order to add or subtract extra field as needed. Analysis of the field inhomogeneities and their corrections are all based upon moment analysis of the field as described in the first section of this chapter. Each piece of shimming iron, or shim coil is designed or positioned to generate specific moments which are used to cancel the unwanted moments present in the manufactured coil.

In order to better understand the need for shims, and how they are employed, an example of a potential field distortion will be discussed. Consider the potential effects of N plastic rods which hold the superconducting coils in place within their refrigerator. Due to their different thermal contraction properties it might be expected that the azimuthal invariance of the coils will be distorted by these rods. In fact it is possible to predict the variation of the field as a function of ϕ they may cause. Their contribution to field distortion may vary as a linear combination of $\cos 2\pi\phi/N$ (each leg causes a distortion), in addition to a $\cos\phi$ distribution of error due to the rods above the magnet being under more tension than the ones below due to gravity. Without any analysis, it is possible to predict that iron placed in the magnet to correct this distortion would have to be similarly distributed.

The field profile is re-evaluated after corrections are added, and another set of shims is added if necessary. This process (measure/shim/evaluate) is repeated until the target field homogeneity for the magnet is achieved. Due to the complexity of the problem, field analysis is generally performed by a computer. The field is measured at a number of points, and the results are fed to the computer which decomposes the field into a sum of moments. The correct currents in shim coils or placement of iron to minimize individual moment contributions are then determined by the computer. Although, distortions can not be predicted in advance, the moment expansion of the field may be used to correct field distortions in a systematic fashion.

27.3   Linearly Varying Field Gradients

The second class of coils employed in MRI are linear magnetic field gradient coils. These coils are used to encode spatially the positions of the spins in MRI by varying the value of the local magnetic field causing spins' Larmor frequencies to vary as a function of their positions. These coils are rapidly switched during MRI sequences to allow the collection of large regions of k-space in a short amount of time.

27.3.1   Classic Designs

There are several gradient coil designs based on analytic solutions that were originally designed to correct field inhomogeneities in spectroscopic magnets. These designs, and simple modifications of them, are still employed in magnets today.

Maxwell Pair (z-Gradient)

The z-gradient coil set is designed to produce a linear variation in the z-component of the field along the axis of the magnet, with a high degree of gradient uniformity in the transverse plane. Circular wire loops are again the most obvious choice since they are azimuthally symmetric and possess reasonable radial uniformity.

As long as a symmetric gradient field is being considered, it is possible to describe the coils in terms of pairs, as was the case for main magnets. However, in the case of the gradient coil pairs their currents will be equal in magnitude, but opposite in direction. Coils on one side of the $z = 0$ plane will generate fields parallel to B_0 while fields due to coils on the other side are anti-parallel to B_0 leading to an overall field variation along z. Linearity is achieved by choosing the relation between the radius of the coils and their axial locations in order to minimize all but the linear z term in (27.5).

For a single coil pair, an analytic solution is available for which the z^3 term from both coils in (27.5) is zero, and the even z powers are all eliminated (see Fig. 27.10). This analysis closely parallels that already presented for the Helmholtz coil. It is found that if

$$d = \sqrt{3}\,a \qquad\qquad (27.10)$$

(see Prob. 27.7) then the lowest order contaminant to the linear field is zero, and a reasonably homogeneous field gradient can be obtained. A coil pair possessing these dimensions is referred to as a *Maxwell pair* or a *Maxwell coil*. Although the Maxwell pair provides reasonably good homogeneity and performance many of today's imaging applications require more

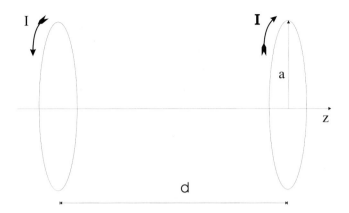

Fig. 27.10: This figure represents a Maxwell coil pair. A set of wire loops coaxial with z are the most efficient choice for producing a z-gradient; however, with only two coils the linearity of the Maxwell pair is limited.

homogeneity over greater distances than can be achieved with the fixed radius-to-length restrictions of this coil.

Improvements to the Maxwell pair are generally achieved by introducing additional coil pairs. The z locations and currents for each coil pair can then be varied to eliminate higher-order moments. This can be accomplished by inspection or with the use of an inverse technique to determine the optimal coil locations and currents.

Problem 27.7

Given a coil pair with radius a, $z' = \pm d/2$, and equal and opposite currents given by I,

a) Show that the even terms in (27.5) are all zero.

b) Derive the Maxwell condition. In other words, find the relation between a and z' such that the z^3 term in (27.5) vanishes.

c) Plot B_z vs z for this coil pair for 2 cases. In the first case use the relation between a and d found in part (b). In the second case, change a or d by approximately 10% from this value. What is the effect on axial linearity?

Golay Pair (x- or y-Gradient)

Producing a transverse gradient is somewhat more complicated than producing a z-gradient. If one is working on a cylindrical geometry, however, the x- and y-gradient coil sets are identical except for a rotation, owing to the azimuthal symmetry of the problem. One of the classic designs for a transverse gradient is the *Golay pair* as depicted in Fig. 27.11.

The variation of B_z along x is primarily due to the innermost azimuthal wires. The two inner wires on the upper coils produce fields parallel to B_0, and the inner wires on the

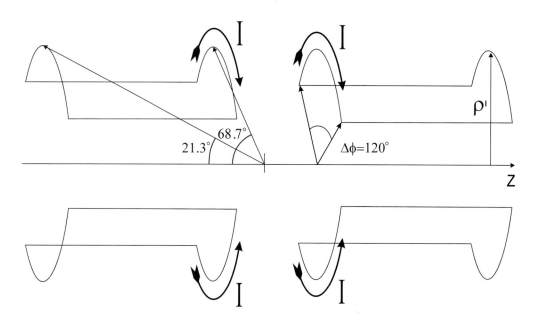

Fig. 27.11: A Golay pair. Notice that only the innermost turns are used to produce the desired field gradient.

lower coil produce fields anti-parallel to B_0. The combination of these fields leads to an overall variation of B_z along the x-axis. If a symmetric gradient is desired along x then the coils can again be chosen with symmetric spatial design and anti-symmetric (with respect to $x = 0$) currents so that all of the even terms in an expansion of B_z along x similar to (27.5) along z vanish. It is obvious that if the coils are to remain on the cylinder, their separation along the x-axis can not be varied, and therefore homogeneity must be optimized by varying the axial location of the azimuthally flowing wire paths. The optimal configuration of the Golay pair is shown in Fig. 27.11. Deriving the optimal configuration for the Golay pair is conceptually the same, but mathematically more difficult, than for the Maxwell and Helmholtz pair (see the papers on coil design in the Suggested Reading). Unfortunately, the Golay pair is found to be a relatively inefficient coil. This should be obvious since it can be seen that only the innermost azimuthal turn of each coil produces the desired variation of the field.

Improvements to the Golay pair have been made by adding more coils with different axial locations and opening angles. These improvements were largely made by inspection. That is, coils were added, and then the system was re-evaluated and modified to eliminate as many higher-order moments from (27.5) as possible.

27.3.2   Calculating Linearly Varying Fields

The Taylor series expansion of the magnetic field is especially useful for studying the gradients produced by a given coil. Analyzing the first derivative terms in Cartesian coordinates gives

$$\vec{x} \cdot \vec{\nabla} B_z(\vec{x})\Big|_{\vec{x}=\vec{0}} = \left(\frac{\partial B_z}{\partial x}\right)\Big|_{\vec{x}=\vec{0}} x + \left(\frac{\partial B_z}{\partial y}\right)\Big|_{\vec{y}=\vec{0}} y + \left(\frac{\partial B_z}{\partial z}\right)\Big|_{\vec{z}=\vec{0}} z$$

$$= G_{0_x} x + G_{0_y} y + G_{0_z} z \qquad (27.11)$$

where only these linear terms have been considered in the previous chapters. It is obvious, however, that the other terms in (27.5) also contribute to the field, and that one of the primary goals in gradient coil design will be to minimize their contribution to the field in the imaging volume.

From the expansion of the field and the Biot-Savart law it is possible to obtain analytic formulas for the gradient at any point due to an arbitrary current distribution.

$$\vec{G}(\vec{x}) = \frac{\mu_0}{4\pi} \vec{\nabla} \int_{volume} d^3 x' \left[\frac{J_x(\vec{x}')(y - y') - J_y(\vec{x}')(x - x')}{|\vec{x} - \vec{x}'|^3} \right] \qquad (27.12)$$

In cases where the current is confined to a two-dimensional surface this expression can often be further reduced by using Maxwell's equations to relate the different components of $\vec{J}$.

In order to obtain the local gradient an alternative to the above formula is often used. This is due to the fact that a large number of programs are available to calculate B_z, and a simple numerical approximation to (27.12) can be obtained by considering the local field gradient to be the slope of B_z between two points separated by some small distance, assuming B_z varies linearly over this distance

$$\begin{aligned}
G_x(\vec{x}) &\approx \frac{B_z(x_2, y, z) - B_z(x_1, y, z)}{x_2 - x_1} \\
G_y(\vec{x}) &\approx \frac{B_z(x, y_2, z) - B_z(x, y_1, z)}{y_2 - y_1} \\
G_z(\vec{x}) &\approx \frac{B_z(x, y, z_2) - B_z(x, y, z_1)}{z_2 - z_1}
\end{aligned} \qquad (27.13)$$

This method of calculation is less efficient, because the field must be calculated at two points, and less accurate. It is often used because a field plot can be generated simultaneously, despite the need to calculate a large number of points in order to get accurate values of the local gradients.

27.3.3 Desirable Properties of Linear Gradient Coils

Gradient coils must satisfy a unique set of performance criteria. Also, much more than main magnets, gradient coils can be designed with a specific imaging application and performance criterion in mind. Some performance criteria universally desirable in gradient coils include: low inductance, high gradient to current ratio, minimal resistance, good gradient uniformity, minimal interaction with conducting shields, absence of torque, high duty cycle, minimum $\partial B/\partial t$, and comfortable patient access (often requires development of coils with novel geometries).

Inductance, Efficiency, and Resistance

For most imaging applications gradient coils are turned on and off as rapidly as possible, but the waveform they follow is not sinusoidal except in specialized EPI applications. Therefore, for the most part resonant circuit theory can not be applied. Instead the only way to attain the rapid switching desired is to minimize the inductance of the coils, or increase the voltage of the amplifiers being used as is illustrated by the basic electromagnetic relationship[3]

$$emf_{applied} = L_{\text{total}} \frac{\partial I}{\partial t} \tag{27.14}$$

Since the voltages which may be safely used in combination with high currents are limited, optimization of rise times (time it takes the gradient to achieve its maximum value) is assumed to be a problem of minimizing the inductance of the gradient system without degrading the quality of the field.

The desirable properties of minimum inductance, high gradient to current ratio, and low resistance are closely related. It is possible to see how achieving any one of these goals is likely to satisfy all three. Consider the electromagnetic energy associated with the gradient coil

$$
\begin{aligned}
\mathcal{E} &= \frac{1}{2} L_{tot} I^2 \\
&= \frac{1}{2} \left[L_{self} + L_{mutual} \right] I^2 \\
&= \frac{1}{2\mu_0} \int_{volume} d^3x \left| \vec{B} \right|^2
\end{aligned}
\tag{27.15}
\tag{27.16}
$$

where L_{self} represents the self inductance of the wires in the gradient coils and L_{mutual} represents the inductance between different wires in the coil set.

L_{self} is proportional to the amount of wire used in the coil which is also proportional to the amount of resistance in the system ($\mathcal{R} = \rho\ell/A_{wire}$). Therefore by minimizing L_{tot}, resistance is also reduced. The resistance of the coils is directly related to the power deposited in the coils, and the amount of heat generated. Heating of the coils is a primary limit on duty cycle.[4]

It can be seen that L_{tot} is also related to the total amount of field produced by the coils. Any fields produced outside of the imaging region reduce the efficiency of the coil, because they require energy for their support, but are not used in the experiments. Reducing L_{tot} while maintaining the desired gradient quality reduces these extraneous fields by decreasing $\int_{volume} d^3x \left| \vec{B} \right|^2$.

27.3.4   Eddy Currents and dB/dt

The rapid switching of the gradients leads to rapidly changing amounts of flux through the rf coils, rf shields, main magnet components, and the person being imaged. This changing

---

[3]The full expression for $emf_{applied}$ is $emf_{applied} = L_{\text{total}}\partial I/\partial t + I \cdot \mathcal{R}$, but when $emf_{applied}/I\mathcal{R} \ll 1$ this term may be neglected. This is generally the case when the gradient coils in MRI are being turned on and off.

[4]Duty cycle is the ratio between amount of time a gradient coil (or any other device) can be on versus the time it must be off. For example, a duty cycle of 50% implies that a gradient may be generating fields half of the time and must be dormant for half of the time. For gradient coils duty cycle often changes with the level of gradient the coil is asked to produce, i.e., a gradient coil with a 50% duty cycle when G_{max} is being generated by the coil may have a duty cycle of 100% when it is only used to produce $G_{max}/2$.

flux leads to voltages and currents being induced in conducting pathways throughout the MRI system. These currents are detrimental to imaging because they produce fields which oppose the applied gradients. They also present potential health risks to patients because, if sufficient voltages are generated in the body, involuntary nerve stimulation might occur.

Rapidly switched gradient coils induce currents in conducting surfaces due to the changing flux associated with the fields being generated. Recall from Ch. 7 that

$$emf = -\frac{\partial \Phi}{\partial t} = \int_{area} \frac{\partial \vec{B}}{\partial t} \cdot d\vec{A} \qquad (27.17)$$

These currents have been referred to as 'eddy currents.' In general the majority of these currents are induced in the rf coils, and in the electromagnetic and thermal shielding surrounding the main magnet. Eddy currents distort gradient response by generating fields of their own which oppose the gradients, reducing the gradient seen by the sample and causing a delay between the time voltages are applied, and fields are seen by the sample. Variations in gradient performance due to eddy currents can lead to phase errors, distortion, and chemical shift artifacts in the resulting images.

As the performance of gradient coils has increased, physiological concerns have also grown. The question arises of whether or not 'eddy currents' can be generated in the body if $\partial B/\partial t$ becomes large enough. Researchers are still determining what levels and duration of $\partial B/\partial t$ the body can be exposed to. In gradient coils there is an important trade-off to be made between maximizing gradient switching rates and reducing $\partial B/\partial t$ effects. The field associated with a gradient along an arbitrary axis ζ is given by

$$B_{z_G}(\zeta) = G_\zeta \zeta \qquad (27.18)$$

If it is assumed that gradients rise linearly from 0 to their maximum value G_{max} then it can be seen that

$$\frac{\partial B_{z_G}(\zeta)}{\partial t} = \frac{G_{max}\zeta}{\text{rise time}} \qquad (27.19)$$

Therefore, the change in B as a function of time is proportional to the distance ζ. In order to decrease the rise time for a coil but avoid an increase in $\partial B/\partial t$ it is necessary to reduce the volume over which the gradient acts.

Volume and Energy

In instances where the volume or size of the gradient coil is reduced, the gains in performance can be impressive, because in addition to reducing $\partial B/\partial t$ effects, the inductance of the coil is reduced. The reduction in inductance is actually greater than the reduction of $\partial B/\partial t$, since it is found that the gradient energy is approximately proportional to

$$\text{energy associated with gradient coil} \propto G^2 r_{DSV}^5 \qquad (27.20)$$

for a spherical imaging region.

All of these considerations lead to the conclusion that whenever possible the gradient homogeneity should only cover the region being imaged in order to maximize gradient performance. This explains the development of gradient coils for various specific imaging applications (biplanar for cardiac, perpendicular cylinder for wrist, etc.). Novel (non-cylindrical) geometries are often employed for specific applications, and therefore gradient coil design methods must be flexible enough to be applied to these differing conditions.

Problem 27.8

In order to understand how the inductance of a gradient coil behaves as a function of both gradient strength and the size of the imaging volume, complete the following calculation to verify (27.20). Assume that $|\vec{B}_{gradient}|$ varies linearly away from the center of the imaging region, and that the field rapidly falls to zero outside of this region

$$|\vec{B}_{gradient}| = \begin{cases} |\vec{B}_{gradient}(r)| = G_0 r & r < r_{DSV} \\ |\vec{B}_{gradient}(r)| = 0 & r > r_{DSV} \end{cases}$$

Calculate $\mathcal{E} = \frac{1}{2\mu_0} \int_{DSV} d^3x |\vec{B}_{gradient}(r)|^2$. How does the energy behave as a function of gradient strength and r_{DSV}? How does the stored energy depend upon G_0? Describe the implications of these results to gradient coil design.

Uniformity

Another question which must be addressed is the uniformity required of the gradient over the imaging volume. In the previous section on main magnets the fields described needed to match ideal conditions to within a few ppm. In gradient coils, however, the accuracy required of the field can range over a much larger set of values. As an example, contemporary gradient coils in use for whole-body human imaging are only accurate to about 5% of their ideal values over the imaging region. Still, for the applications being considered very little image distortion results. The amount of image distortion due to variations in the gradient vary from application to application, and requirements for homogeneity must be determined based upon an investigation of the methods and imaging that will be used.

27.3.5   Active Shielding

In order to minimize eddy currents, gradient coils may be shielded in a manner identical to that described for main magnets. Fields produced outside of the imaging bore can be reduced to a point where eddy currents have little or no effect on the images. However, similar to the case of main magnets, the additional shielding requires additional currents to be applied, and increases the inductance of the gradient coils. The increase in inductance leads to a decrease in switching rate. The only way which this decrease in performance can be compensated is by increasing the applied voltage to the system.

27.3.6   'Linearly Varying' Magnetic Fields

It is found that a linear variation of a single component of the magnetic field can not exist in free space, therefore a more in depth study of the linear field gradient is warranted. Of course, all fields used in MRI must obey Maxwell's equations (A.1). It is possible to show how a linear gradient with only one component is ultimately incompatible with Maxwell's equations. Use the x-gradient as an example

$$\vec{B}_G = G_0 x \hat{z} \tag{27.21}$$

In free space (no sources present) $\vec{B} = \vec{H}$, and $\vec{J} = 0$. The gradient field is constant in time, during data acquisition so all of the time derivatives in (A.1) also vanish. For the given field, then it is seen that $\vec{\nabla} \cdot \vec{B} = 0$ but $\vec{\nabla} \times \vec{B} = \vec{\nabla} \times (G_0 x)\hat{z} = -G_0 \hat{y} \neq 0$. This implies that another component of the field must be present, in order that the linear field variation satisfies Maxwell's equations. In fact, the linear variation of B_z is always accompanied by some variation of B_x or B_y along a direction perpendicular to the gradient.

$$
\begin{aligned}
\vec{B}_{G_x} &= \hat{x} G_0 z + \hat{z} G_0 x \\
\vec{B}_{G_y} &= \hat{y} G_0 z + \hat{z} G_0 y \\
\vec{B}_{G_z} &= \hat{x} a G_0 x + \hat{y} b G_0 y + \hat{z} G_0 z \\
&\quad \text{where} \qquad [a + b = -1]
\end{aligned}
\tag{27.22}
$$

This result is interesting because it implies that although a large amount of work may be done to minimize the moments in the expansion of B_z the linear term itself will be responsible for a set of extraneous field components (referred to as concomitant gradient fields). It is of practical interest to determine the effect of these extra field components on images.

Throughout this book the generic phase relation $\phi(t) = -\gamma B_z t$ has played a central role. However, in Chs. 2 and 3 it was shown that the magnetization really precesses around the axis of the effective field with a frequency that is proportional to the magnitude of effective field. The use of rf radiation to flip the spins away from the z-axis was explained using this concept in Ch. 3. Since, the applied gradients generate B_x and B_y as well as B_z it is necessary to determine how these fields affect the effective field and phase accumulated by the spins. The concern may arise that the additional field component causes the spins to precess about a new axis, but since the gradient fields are approximately two to three orders of magnitude smaller than B_0 the effective rotation axis remains essentially along z, and only phase effects are observed. In order to determine the additional phase accumulation, the x-gradient example will again be considered.

In the presence of a perfectly linear x-gradient the total MRI $\vec{B}$ field is

$$\vec{B}(\vec{x}) = \vec{B}_0 + \vec{B}_{G_x} = G_0 z \hat{x} + G_0 x \hat{z} + B_0 \hat{z} \tag{27.23}$$

therefore

$$
\begin{aligned}
\phi(\vec{x}) &= -\gamma |\vec{B}(\vec{x})| t \\
&= -\gamma |G_0 z \hat{x} + G_0 x \hat{z} + B_0 \hat{z}| t \\
&= -\gamma t \sqrt{(B_0 + G_0 x)^2 + (G_0 z)^2} \\
&\simeq -\gamma \left\{ B_0 + G_0 x + \frac{z^2 G_0^2}{2 B_0} + \mathcal{O}\left(\frac{z^2 G_0^3 x}{B_0^2}\right) \right\} t
\end{aligned}
\tag{27.24}
$$

This expression differs from the usual form $\phi(\vec{x}) = -\gamma(B_0 + \vec{G} \cdot \vec{r})t = -\gamma(B_0 + Gx)t$ for the phase accumulated in the presence of an x-gradient. The additional phase develops along a direction perpendicular to the original gradient (in this case along $\hat{z}$):

$$\Delta\phi_{G_x}(\vec{x}) \simeq -\frac{\gamma z^2 G_0^2 t}{2B_0} \qquad (27.25)$$

The magnitude of this effect is very small at high fields, but can be of concern for imaging at low fields. Determining quantitative values for the amount of extra phase accumulated is left as an exercise.

Problem 27.9

Given the following set of parameters, and assuming a gradient echo experiment is being performed, answer the list of questions. The relevant parameters for proton imaging include $G_{0_x} = 25 \,\text{mT/m}$, $B_0 = 1.5 \,\text{T}$, $T_s = 1 \,\text{ms}$, $\text{FOV}_{x,y,z} = 25 \,\text{cm}$, $\Delta x = \Delta y = \Delta z = 1 \,\text{mm}$, and $\gamma = 2\pi \times 42.58 \times 10^6 \,(\text{rad/s/T})$.

a) Calculate the $\Delta\phi_{G_x}$ at the edge of the imaging volume at the echo.

b) Find the ratio of $\Delta\phi_{G_x}$ to ϕ_{G_x} as a function of sampling time and position. Hence, show that there is a position shift $\Delta x(z)$ given by $G_0 z^2/(2B_0)$.

c) Is the effect large enough that you might expect to see the position of the spins shifted by more than one pixel at the edge of the field-of-view?

d) Repeat parts (a) through (c) for $B_0 = 0.2 \,\text{T}$.

e) Qualitatively discuss whether you would expect this problem to be more or less serious for sodium imaging. Assume you are trying to attain similar resolution for both elements.

27.4   RF Transmit and Receive Coils

The rf coils used in MRI have two purposes. One is to excite the magnetization, and the coils which perform this function are referred to as transmit coils. The second purpose of the rf coils is to receive the signal from the excited spins, and the coils which perform this function are referred to as the receive coils. Some people make the distinction between the coils by referring to transmit coils as rf coils, and receive coils as rf probes. Of course, one coil can be used to both transmit and receive, but often separate coils are used because there are properties that are desirable for each coil to possess to obtain optimal quality images. In this section, some of the desirable properties of both transmit and receive coils are discussed.

Another interesting aspect of rf coils that separates them from gradient and main magnet systems is that they produce and detect time dependent fields. Radiofrequency coils, in fact, fall into an interesting regime. The wavelength of radiofrequencies used for proton imaging is on the order of seven meters for $B_0 \simeq 1.0\,\text{T}$, and finite wavelength effects can mostly be neglected. Therefore, when calculating fields, static solutions present good approximations of the fields produced by the coils, and the time dependence of the fields can be neglected. However, when considering the electronics and other elements that are employed in the systems, understanding the time and frequency responses of the coils and circuits is crucial. In fact, the frequency response of the coils can lead to spatial modulation of the signal in the image.

One consideration of universal importance to rf coils is the issue of quadrature as discussed in Ch. 4. Quadrature refers to the ability of a set of coils to generate or detect the circularly polarized field $\vec{B}_1 = B_1 \hat{x}'$ which involves producing both x- and y-components of the magnetic field in the lab frame. If a coil is only capable of producing a field along one direction in the lab frame ($\vec{B}_1 = B_1 \cos \omega t \, \hat{x}$) then in the rotating frame its effective magnitude after time averaging is reduced by a half ($\vec{B}_1 = \frac{1}{2} B_1 \hat{x}'$). This type of coil has been referred to as linear, and although linear coils are sometimes easier to construct they suffer a $\sqrt{2}$ reduction in their sensitivity.

27.4.1   Transmit Coils

The primary considerations in an rf transmit coil are the homogeneity of the magnetization response, and minimization of the time needed to tip the spins away from the static field. Recall that the time needed to tip the spins is determined by the magnitude of B_1 generated by the rf amplifiers.

In Ch. 16, the flip angle as a function of the applied rf field was given as

$$\theta = \gamma B_1 \tau_{rf} \tag{27.26}$$

For a given flip angle θ, the amount of time needed to generate the desired rotation is inversely proportional to the magnitude of B_1

$$t_{rf_\alpha} \propto \frac{1}{B_1} \propto \frac{1}{\mathcal{B}_1 I} \tag{27.27}$$

where $\mathcal{B}_1$ contains all of the spatial information about B_1, and I is separated to show that B_1 is a linear function of the current. The magnitude of B_1 is determined by the power delivered by the rf amplifier, which is generally fixed,

$$P_{amp} = I^2 Z \tag{27.28}$$

in which I is the current in the coil, and Z is the impedance of the coil circuit at frequency ω

$$Z = \sqrt{R_{eff}^2 + \left(\omega L - \frac{1}{\omega C}\right)^2} \tag{27.29}$$

where L is the inductance of the coil, and C is the capacitance in the coil circuit. It can be seen that if the rf coil is tuned to resonance (i.e., $\omega L - 1/\omega C = 0$), then the time needed to tip the spins depends upon R_{eff} which includes the resistance of the sample, coil, and electronics as well.

27.4.2   Receive Coils or RF Probes

There are two primary properties that are of importance to MRI receive coils or probes: one is to improve the SNR obtained with the coil, and the other is to insure uniformity of the rf receive response over the volume being imaged. Within these two objectives, a number of specific goals can be assessed, but, *in first approximation, a coil which provides high SNR with good homogeneity is desirable.*

There are two factors to be considered in the SNR of a coil: one is the sensitivity of the coil and the other is the noise associated with the coil. In Ch. 7, the signal of an MRI experiment was shown to be proportional to

$$\text{signal} \quad \propto \quad \frac{\partial}{\partial t} \int d^3x \vec{M} \cdot \vec{\mathcal{B}}^{receive} \tag{27.30}$$

An expression for the noise in the coil based upon several thermodynamic principles is given by

$$\text{noise} \quad \propto \quad \sqrt{4kT_{coil}\Delta f \mathcal{R}_{eff}} \tag{27.31}$$

where T_{coil} is the temperature of the coil, Δf is the bandwidth of the experiment, and $\mathcal{R}$ is the resistance of the coil and the body being imaged. The effective resistance, $\mathcal{R}_{eff}$, includes contributions from the coil, electronics, and the sample being imaged

$$\mathcal{R}_{eff} = \mathcal{R}_{coil} + \mathcal{R}_{sample} + \mathcal{R}_{electronics} \tag{27.32}$$

Due to the improvement of electronics, in contemporary imaging experiments ($0.5\,\text{T} \leq B_0 \leq 4.0\,\text{T}$), it is generally seen that $\mathcal{R}_{eff} \approx \mathcal{R}_{sample}$. The resistance which a coil sees from a sample is proportional to the volume of the region of the body from which the coil receives a signal, $V_{sensitive}$ (i.e., $\mathcal{R}_{sample} \propto V_{sensitive}$).

Unlike the case of gradient coils, it is not as easy to develop a simple relation between the imaging volume and the SNR of the associated rf coil, but it is still possible to see the increase of SNR with the decrease of the coil's effective imaging volume. From (27.30) and (27.31), a formula for the SNR associated with a particular coil can be developed

$$\begin{aligned}\text{SNR} \quad &= \quad \frac{\Lambda M_\perp \mathcal{B}_\perp}{\sqrt{4kT_{coil}\Delta f \mathcal{R}_{eff}}}\\[2mm]&\propto \quad \frac{\omega^{7/4}\mathcal{B}_\perp}{\sqrt{T_{coil}\Delta f V_{sensitivity}}}\end{aligned} \tag{27.33}$$

It can be seen from this formula that coils which only cover the imaging region-of-interest are optimal, as was the case with gradient coils. This is due to the increase in SNR from both an increase in $\mathcal{B}_\perp$ obtained by positioning the coil closer to the region-of-interest and by decreasing $V_{sensitivity}$ to the smallest possible volume which reduces $\mathcal{R}_{sample}$.

The above discussion dealing with improvement of SNR for an rf receive coil did not address the issue of field homogeneity. The most serious image artifact associated with any inhomogeneity of the rf receive field is a variation of the intensity profile of the image. The signal from the spins at a given point $\vec{r}$ is proportional to $M_\perp(\vec{r})\mathcal{B}_\perp(\vec{r})$. In most cases, field variations are smooth and relatively slow over the imaging regions so variations in $\mathcal{B}_\perp(\vec{r})$ can be readily identified and taken into account in the interpretation of the images. However, the variations in $\mathcal{B}_\perp(\vec{r})$ become a problem when they reduce the CNR in the image below acceptable levels. The possibility also exists for phase errors to be associated with the rf receive coil. If the coil produces a large amount of both B_y and B_x, phase images will have their phase modulated across the field-of-view.

There is another aspect of rf probe sensitivity that needs to be considered. That is the relation between the region of coil sensitivity and the region of space covered by the gradients. If the region of probe sensitivity is greater than the volume covered by the gradients then objects outside of the imaging region may be misregistered within the imaging volume (see Fig. 27.12). It is necessary that the rf coil not be sensitive to spins outside of the region of gradient homogeneity, since these spins will appear in the image at the same point as fields within the imaging volume at points with identical fields.

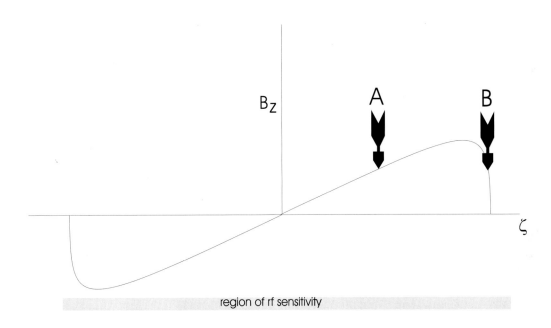

Fig. 27.12: Misregistration in an image can also occur due to a mismatch in the region of rf sensitivity and gradient field homogeneity. Notice that spins at point A and B precess at the same frequency and, therefore, will be encoded at the same location in the image.

27.4.3   Classic Designs

There are a number of coil designs employed in MRI whose widespread use merits individual treatment of their performance characteristics. In this section several coil designs will be investigated in some detail. Their performance and utility will be discussed in general terms.

Saddle Coils

The Helmholtz pair is used to produce a homogeneous $B_0\hat{z}$ field; a similar coil configuration exists for rf coils. A pair of coils is wrapped on a cylindrical surface (See Fig. 27.13) and is referred to as a saddle coil. Remember that for rf coils only the transverse component of the field is of interest; the loops are chosen such that the fields they produce are mainly perpendicular to the axis of the magnet. A power series expansion for the field about the origin can be developed in identical fashion to that described earlier in this chapter, and the x^2, y^2, and z^2 moments can be made to vanish by choosing the appropriate opening angle $\Delta\phi$ and axial length d. In this fashion, the optimal homogeneity over the imaging region may be achieved. Maximum homogeneity is found for these coils when $\Delta\phi = 2\pi/3$ and $d = 4\rho'$.

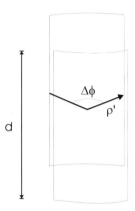

Fig. 27.13: This figure depicts an rf Helmholtz coil pair where $\Delta\phi$ and d have been chosen to minimize the variation of the field over the imaging region. For current directions, see Fig. 27.4.

Birdcage Coil

The birdcage coil is presently the most popular coil configuration for use in MRI since it is a quadrature design, with excellent radial field homogeneity over the imaging volume. Figure 27.14 depicts a birdcage coil. The axial current paths are referred to as the legs of the coil, and the azimuthal paths are referred to as the endrings.

If the current in the legs of the coil is of the form

$$I(t) = I_0 \sin(\omega t + \phi') \tag{27.34}$$

then the field produced in the imaging region is extremely uniform, and rotates its direction with angular frequency ω. In fact, if the length of the birdcage is extended to infinity, and a continuous current distribution is used, the field is perfectly uniform. This also implies that the efficiency of the birdcage is very high since nearly all of the fields produced by the coil are used for imaging.

A limitation of the fields produced by a finite birdcage is that their uniformity decays axially. Besides the finite axial length, the currents in the endrings do not produce uniform

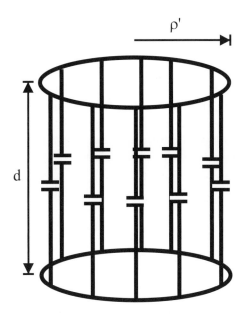

Fig. 27.14: This figure depicts a birdcage coil. Current is distributed as a function of ϕ' in order to optimize the homogeneity of the field in the imaging volume ($I \propto \sin \phi'$).

fields within the imaging volume. It is found, however, that if the coil's length is approximately equal to its diameter, then a roughly spherical volume is found for which the coil has good homogeneity.

Problem 27.10

Verify that the transverse magnetic field as a function of ρ ($\rho < a$) is a constant in an infinitely long birdcage coil. This implies that the current density of the coil is given by $\vec{J}(\vec{r}') = I_0 \sin \phi' \hat{z} \delta(\rho' - a)/a$.

Surface Coils

If the feature to be imaged is localized near the surface of the body, an rf probe coil may be placed directly on the surface of the sample in order to optimize the SNR of the experiment. SNR is maximized because the coil is placed very close to the object being imaged, maximizing $\mathcal{B}$. Further, in general, the $V_{sensitivity}$ for a surface coil is much less than that for a coil surrounding the entire sample. Therefore, $\mathcal{R}_{sample}$ is reduced which reduces noise and further increases the coil's SNR. For imaging small objects near the surface of a body, i.e., the spine, surface coils are an overwhelmingly popular choice of rf probe.

Of course, a single coil placed on the body loses a $1/\sqrt{2}$ factor in SNR because it does not detect quadrature fields. A way around this is to use two surface coils on the body to produce a quadrature field in the desired region. Fig. 27.15 shows an example coil configuration where two surface coils are positioned to produce both x- and y-components of the field in the imaging region. In this way, a surface coil may be used in quadrature to gain back the $\sqrt{2}$ loss in SNR that a single linear surface coil suffers from.

An obvious question to be addressed regarding surface coils is, "What features of a body are near enough to the surface to be imaged with increased SNR by employing a surface coil?" This question is not easy to address directly. In practice, the coil is chosen so that the radius of the coil roughly matches the depth to which imaging is desired.

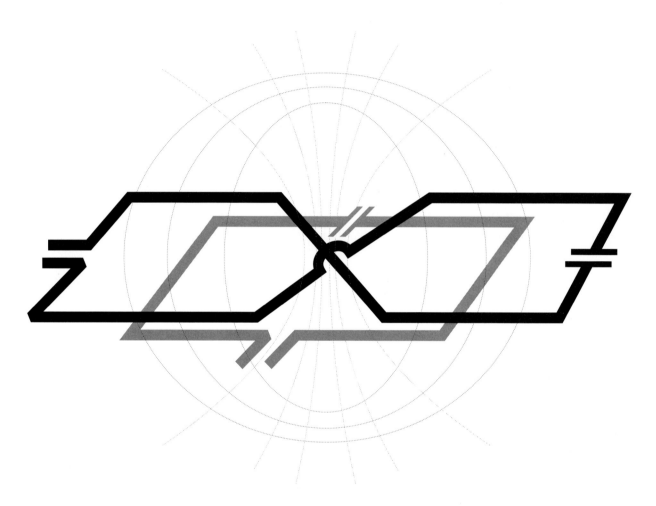

Fig. 27.15: An example of how two surface coils may be combined to produce a circularly polarized field. The dotted lines represent the flux lines produced by each coil. The flux lines from these coils are roughly perpendicular to each other in a region beneath the coil. It is in this region where optimal imaging conditions exist.

Phased Array Coils

In MRI, a phased array coil generally refers to a set of receive coils whose signals are combined to obtain a uniform image over a region larger than any individual coil could cover while taking advantage of the high SNR available from the smaller individual coils. As mentioned previously, smaller coils are used because they have superior SNR individually due to their high B_1/I ratios and their small effective noise volumes. Fig. 27.16a shows an example of

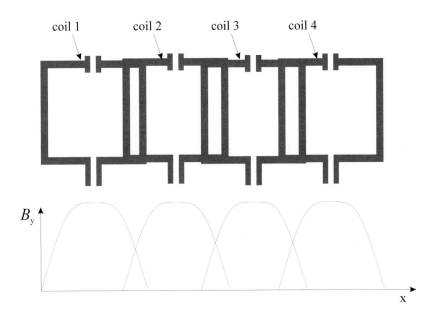

Fig. 27.16: Example of a set of phased array coils is shown in the upper portion of the figure. The coils are overlapped to reduce the electromagnetic coupling between the nearest neighbor coils. The field as a function of x for the individual coils at a given y and z is shown in the bottom of the figure.

four square loops combined in a row. This array could, for example, be used to image the entire spine. Alternatively, it could be wrapped around a person's torso in an attempt to obtain an optimal SNR image of the heart. An example of the sensitivity of the coils as a function of x at a given y and z position is also shown in Fig. 27.16 where the overlap of regions of sensitivity are shown. The signals obtained from the individual coils are combined to give a single image. Methods for combining the signals have been considered in Ch. 15.

In order to obtain optimal SNR from a phased array coil, it is necessary to make sure that the noise from coil to coil is largely uncorrelated. In order to achieve this, each coil should have its own receive circuit so electronic noise is uncorrelated. Also, there should be minimal electromagnetic interaction between the coils to make sure that sample noise is not correlated. Minimizing electromagnetic interaction between the coils is generally achieved in one of two ways. In the first case the coils are simply separated by enough distance that their interaction is minimal. If the coils are in close proximity, however, minimizing the interaction between the coils is not as simple. However, the principle for minimizing the interaction is obvious from the principle of reciprocity and Faraday's law of induction

$$emf_1 = -\frac{d\Phi_{1,2}}{dt} \qquad (27.35)$$

which states that the emf induced in coil 1 is proportional to the change in flux induced in coil 1 by coil 2. The coils should be placed so that the net flux through coil 1 due to coil 2 is zero, and by reciprocity this should also zero the flux through coil 2 due to coil 1. This is generally achieved by overlapping nearest neighbor coils (see Fig. 27.16) such that the flux through the coil and its return flux path sum to zero. An alternative way to describe these conditions is to say that the mutual inductance between the coils is zero.

The possibility of sample noise being correlated from one coil to another still exists, and there are methods for combining the signals from these coils in order to optimize the SNR of the experiment such as those presented in Ch. 15.

Methods for determining the optimal arrangement and number of coils in a phased array are still a subject of research. This is because there are several competing factors to be considered in the design of each coil.

27.4.4   RF Shielding

The alternating fields used to tip the magnetization away from the z-axis in MRI are generally referred to as 'rf' because for hydrogen protons in a field on the order of a tesla or higher, the Larmor frequency is in the bandwidth occupied by FM radio stations. This fact has dual implications for MRI. The first concern is that local sources of signals be shielded from the MR environment. An rf coil designed to receive signals from the body would otherwise indiscriminately receive local signals and integrate them into the MRI data. Both the transmit and receive modes of the rf coils necessitate the shielding of the rf coil system. Fortunately, the rf radiation used is at a high enough frequency that the penetration of the fields into a good conductor is only a few micrometers. Therefore, thin copper shields (solid or even meshed layers) are sufficient to eliminate the transmission of rf fields into, or out of, the MRI environment.

27.4.5   Power Deposition

Another feature of rf transmit fields not discussed previously in detail is the fact that rf energy can be deposited in the body as heat. At field strengths up to 1.5 T, the wavelength of the rf is so long that little energy is absorbed by the body. The move toward higher and higher fields and, hence, larger frequencies, carries with it the safety problem of increased rf power deposition in the body. Contemporary whole-body systems are being made not only at 1.5 T, but also for research purposes from 3.0 T to 7.0 T.

There are government guidelines as to acceptable limits of specific absorption rates (SAR) of radiation deposited into the body to be considered. The human body can only tolerate a few watts per kilogram of tissue before body temperature begins to rise. An average rf amplifier used for human imaging can produce more that 10 kW of power. If all of this power were deposited in the body, MRI of humans would be impossible. Fortunately, little of this power is left in the body and the safety issue revolves around the deposited power, not the electric power, delivered to the body. Still, this figure implies that there is a significant amount of rf power in use, and at higher fields and frequencies, rf power deposition could become a significant problem.

Estimates of the power absorbed by the body can be made by measurements of the quality factor, or Q, of the coil-body system. The Q of the coil is defined to be the resonant frequency[5] times the stored field energy divided by the power loss

$$Q = \omega \frac{\text{stored energy}}{P} \tag{27.36}$$

It can also be considered as the inverse of the fractional energy loss per cycle of the rf. Consequently, at roughly the same frequency and stored energy, the power deposited in the body is

$$P_{body} = P(1 - \frac{Q_{loaded}}{Q_{unloaded}}) \tag{27.37}$$

where

$$P = P_{body} + P_{unloaded} \tag{27.38}$$

When Q is reduced substantially by the loading due to the body, most of the rf power is absorbed in the body. The present guidelines are that the power (or rather the power per unit mass, or watts/kg) deposited should not exceed 1.5 to 3.0 watts/kg over the whole body, or 3 to 8 watts/kg 'locally' (point by point).

To investigate an example, let us derive the first-order formula for the inductive heating caused by a linearly polarized coil with an rf field $\vec{B}_{rf}$ along the z-axis of amplitude $2B_1$ (so that B_1 is the field at rest in the rotating reference frame) for a sphere with radius R. Consider a ring centered at the point $z = r\cos\theta_s$ of an arbitrary radius $r\sin\theta_s$ (where $0 \leq r \leq R$ and θ_s is the usual spherical polar angle). The electric field at this ring can be found from an elementary Faraday line integral around the circumference of the ring, which is related to the rate of change of the magnetic flux through the cross-sectional area via

$$E \equiv |\vec{E}| = \frac{\text{voltage}}{\text{circumference}} = \frac{r\sin\theta_s}{2}\left|\frac{d\vec{B}_{rf}}{dt}\right| = \omega B_1 r\sin\theta_s \tag{27.39}$$

where $\vec{E}$ is the electric field vector and ω the transmit angular frequency.

The local power deposited is then the ohmic power density

$$\frac{dP}{dV} = \frac{1}{2}\sigma E^2 = \frac{1}{2}\sigma\omega^2 B_1^2 r^2 \sin^2\theta_s \tag{27.40}$$

where the conductivity of the sphere is σ. The power deposited in the entire sphere is given by an integral over (27.40), that is, over all rings that make up the sphere,

$$P = \frac{4}{15}\pi\sigma\omega^2 B_1^2 R^5 \tag{27.41}$$

For $\theta = \gamma B_1 \tau_{rf}$, this formula becomes

$$P = \frac{4\pi\sigma\omega^2\theta^2 R^5}{15\gamma^2\tau_{rf}^2} \tag{27.42}$$

The average power (or the energy deposited per unit time) for the sphere is given by

$$\overline{P} = \frac{\text{energy per repetition}}{T_R} = P\frac{\tau_{rf}}{T_R} = \frac{4\pi\sigma\omega^2\theta^2 R^5}{15\gamma^2\tau_{rf}T_R} \tag{27.43}$$

---

[5]The resonant frequency is sometimes referred to as the carrier or base frequency.

For a CP coil (two linearly polarized coils in spatial and temporal quadrature each with amplitude B_1), $\overline{P}$ is one-half that in (27.43).

Problem 27.11

---

a) Carry out the integration over a sphere of radius R for (27.40) to find (27.41).

b) If two linearly polarized coils are used to generate a circularly polarized field, show that $\dfrac{dP}{dV}$ in (27.40) is reduced by a factor of two.

Local power deposition will depend on the local fields. Therefore, the rf penetration will determine, in part, the strength of the local fields and the local SAR (the power deposited per unit mass, usually quoted in watts/kg). The conductivity also plays a key role in the form of the spatial response of the rf penetration and the local power deposition.

Problem 27.12

The rf power deposition is a limiting factor in how many slices can be applied in a spin echo sequence or how short the repeat time can be for a given flip angle for a gradient echo sequence. As an order of magnitude example of how big these effects can be, consider imaging the body at 1.5 T. Assume a coil duty cycle (the fraction of 'on-time') $D = \tau_{rf}/T_R = 0.1$. Take the density of the body to be $1 \, \text{gm/cm}^3$, $\sigma = 0.3 \, \text{S/m}$, and $T_R = 20 \, \text{ms}$ (remember to convert all quantities to SI units). For parts (a) through (c), use $R = 20 \, \text{cm}$.

a) Find the SAR in watts/kg for a circularly polarized coil and $\theta = \pi/2$. Practically, the body is not a uniform conductive material in which large currents can build up. Its structure prevents such currents from forming and, hence, (27.43) significantly overestimates the SAR.

b) When does the local power deposited exceed 8 watts/kg near the surface of the body? Hint: Find an expression for the power deposited in a shell with inner radius 19 cm and outer radius 20 cm.

c) Human eyes contain vitreous humor fluid with conductivity similar to that of CSF (assume that $\sigma_{\text{CSF}} = 1.0 \, \text{S/m}$ at 64 MHz, i.e., $B_0 \simeq 1.5 \, \text{T}$). Take the radius of the eye to be 1 cm. Would you want to be imaged under the above conditions? What about at 7.0 T if $\sigma_{\text{CSF}} = 5.0 \, \text{S/m}$ at a frequency of 300 MHz? How could you modify the imaging experiment to reduce $\overline{P}$?

Suggested Reading

The following are basic electromagnetism references:

- J. D. Jackson. *Classical Electrodynamics.* John Wiley and Sons, 3rd ed., Hoboken, 1999.

- W. Smythe. *Static and Dynamic Electricity.* McGraw-Hill Book Company, New York, 1968.

General signal-to-noise considerations appear in:

- D. G. Gadian. *Nuclear Magnetic Resonance and Its Applications to Living Systems.* 2nd ed., Oxford, University Press, 1995.

The following references provide an introduction to coil design methodology and explanations of the relevant electromagnetic results as they apply to MRI:

- R. W. Brown, H. Fujita, S. Shvartsman, M. Thompson, M. A. Morich, L. S. Petropoulos and V. C. Srivastava. New applications of inverse methods in the design of MRI coils. *Int. J. Appl. Electromagn. Mech.*, 94: 1013, 1997.

- C.-N. Chen and D. I. Hoult. *Biomedical Magnetic Resonance Technology.* Bristol, Philadelphia, 1989.

- F. Romeo and D. I. Hoult. Magnetic field profiling: Analysis and correcting coil design. *Magn. Reson. Med.*, 1: 44, 1984.

- R. Turner. Gradient coil design: A review of methods. *Magn. Reson. Imag.*, 11: 903, 1993.

The effects of higher order field changes on imaging are presented in:

- D. G. Norris and J. M. S. Hutchison. Concomitant magnetic field gradients and their effects on imaging at low magnetic field strengths. *Magn. Reson. Imag.*, 8: 33, 1990.

The role of rf penetration in changing the apparent effective spin density is discussed in these two references:

- G. H. Glover, C. E. Hayes, N. J. Pelc, W. A. Edelstein, O. M. Mueller, H. R. Hart, C. J. Hardy, M. O'Donnell and W. D. Barber. Comparison of linear and circular polarization for magnetic resonance imaging. *J. Magn. Reson.*, 64: 255, 1985.

- L. S. Petropoulos and E. M. Haacke. Higher order frequency dependence of radiofrequency penetration in planar, cylindrical and spherical models. *J. Magn. Reson.*, 91: 466, 1991.

Chapter 28

Parallel Imaging

Chapter Contents

Summary: The basic concepts behind the use of multiple rf coils to reduce the number of phase encoding steps in acquiring spatial information are described. Particular emphasis is placed on the substitution of a portion of phase encoding gradient data with rf data, a procedure that can be used to speed up imaging time. A simple one-dimensional model is employed to compare techniques differing in how the image is reconstructed. Pseudo-inverse matrix methods are introduced and utilized. Also discussed are two important issues where the first is how the signal data may be used to provide indirect information about rf coil sensitivities (i.e., field profiles for the multiple coils in the rf array) that are otherwise hard to measure. The second is the analysis of rf coil noise in parallel imaging, which is complicated by the coupling amongst the multiple coils.

Introduction

Parallel imaging in MRI is the idea of replacing part of the k-space data generated by conventional phase encoding steps (using their associated gradients) with additional rf coil data. The latter are measured with multiple detectors acting in parallel (i.e., simultaneously). Since there are various practical reasons against attempts to replace all the phase encoding data in this manner, including the difficulty of dealing with large numbers of rf channels, the prevalent approach is just to reduce, rather than completely eliminate, the phase encoding steps via simultaneous measurements with multiple rf receive coils. While it might seem appropriate to term this 'partially parallel imaging,' the present convention is to refer to

859

all the different algorithms for reducing phase encoding steps by adding rf measurements as simply 'parallel imaging.'

The primary motivation for replacing phase encoding steps (hereinafter often referred to as gradient steps or gradient data) is to save time, and thus faster imaging has been a mantra for parallel imaging. This technical advance allows us to consider various and possibly combined benefits: more patient comfort, less patient motion artifacts, increased coverage or increased resolution in a region-of-interest, and the economy of increased patient throughput. More generally, there are two prevalent directions, and trade-offs between them, that dominate imaging procedures. The first is collecting images at a given resolution in less time and the second is achieving higher resolution for a fixed time. Given these advantages and new opportunities for applications, parallel imaging has become an important concept in the design of modern rf coils and data acquisition procedures. The key in the simultaneous use of multiple rf coils is either to directly measure the coil 'spatial sensitivities,' or indirectly account for them using the MRI data. The sensitivity of a given coil is its local field profile describing through reciprocity where that coil can efficiently pick up spin signals from that region.

We begin with individual coil signal expressions and their transforms where the focus is on one gradient direction (the phase encoding y-dimension). A simple 'two-step' spin density distribution is introduced for analyzing several parallel imaging algorithms and aliasing issues. The first algorithm is the reconstruction of the image from a complete set of coils followed by a removal of overlapping artifacts using the known coil sensitivities; this is referred to as the x-space method.[1] The second algorithm is the k-space method, where the k-space data lost from the use of fewer gradient steps can be regained as independent data obtained from known coil sensitivities. Important improvements of the k-space approach correspond to using gradient data to determine what are otherwise poorly determined coil sensitivities. Least-squares fits arise from overdetermined problems commonly arising in parallel imaging, and they can be addressed with pseudo-inverse-matrix methods. The manifestation of the noise from individual coils, including the noise coupling throughout the array, on the reconstructed image is an important topic. Finally, we note that, because they are universally used, there are certain well-known acronyms. We return at the relevant junctures to explain the x-space method called 'SENSE,' and three k-space versions called 'SMASH,' 'AUTO-SMASH,' and 'GRAPPA.' A history of this relatively recent development in MRI can be gleaned from the collection of references at the end of this chapter.

28.1 Coil Signals, Their Images, and a One-Dimensional Test Case

In this section, we adapt the signal and reconstruction image formulas from Ch. 7 to individual coil signals and their reconstructed images in order to analyze the different approaches to parallel imaging discussed in the subsequent sections. The formulas may be simplified

---

[1]In general, x-space refers to all three spatial dimensions or image space. In the parallel imaging examples, we restrict ourselves to a single phase encoding dimension along the y-axis and its spatial frequency k_y (shortened to $k_y \equiv k$). Instead of y-space and k_y-space, however, we will refer to x-space and k-space, respectively, throughout this chapter.

to concentrate on one dimension, the phase encoding y-dimension. We review the relationship between the acquired rf data and the reconstructed image, showing where oversampling and more general matrix methods are connected. We introduce a simple one-dimensional spin distribution as a test case to be used in comparing various parallel imaging techniques. Aliasing issues in parallel imaging are also discussed in terms of this simple test case.

28.1.1 Continuous and Discrete Pairs of Transforms for Multiple Coils

Revisiting the demodulated signal (7.30) and adapting it to a y-gradient as in Ch. 9, we neglect the relaxation factors along with the proportionality constants and any additional spatial dependence. The inclusion of additional factors and dimensions is straightforward, and does not alter the conclusions that follow. With a change in notation designed to help us in distinguishing between functions of y (labeled by capitalized letters) and their Fourier transforms (labeled by uncapitalized letters), the signal picked up by the nth rf coil is given by

$$s_n(k) = \int dy \, e^{-i2\pi ky} \mathcal{B}_n(y) M(y), \qquad n = 1, 2, \cdots, N_c \tag{28.1}$$

where the total number of coils is N_c. We let $k_y \equiv k$ for the phase encoding spatial frequency. In complex representation, and with the subscripts and complex conjugation shown in (7.30) left understood, $M(y)$ and $\mathcal{B}_n(y)$ are defined in this chapter to be, respectively, the (two-dimensional transverse) complex magnetization and the (complex conjugate of the) complex receive coil magnetic field

$$\mathcal{B}(y) \equiv \mathcal{B}_x^{receive}(y) - i\mathcal{B}_y^{receive}(y) \tag{28.2}$$

In those examples where we restrict ourselves to real values for $\mathcal{B}_n$, this corresponds to considering only the x-component in (7.29). (This assumes the receive coil produces a field lying predominantly and uniformly along the x-axis in the sample region-of-interest.) We will, however, include both components in some subsequent examples. We often refer to the profile (i.e., spatial dependence) of a component of $\mathcal{B}$ as the coil 'sensitivity' associated with that component. Through the reciprocity discussed first in Ch. 7, 'sensitivity' and 'profile' can be used interchangeably.

With continuous k-space data, the inverse Fourier transform of $s_n(k)$ is

$$S_n(y) = \mathcal{B}_n(y) M(y) = \int dk \, e^{+i2\pi ky} s_n(k), \qquad n = 1, 2, \cdots, N_c \tag{28.3}$$

The extraction of $M(y)$ from (28.3) requires knowledge about $\mathcal{B}_n(y)$, a principal issue to be addressed in all approaches to parallel imaging.[2]

In parallel imaging, the discrete k-space relevant to the discussion of phase encoding steps leads us to the discrete inverse transform in place of (28.3). The discrete transform versions

---

[2]Knowledge of $\mathcal{B}_n(y)$ is important for conventional imaging as well, in order to correct for rf coil inhomogeneities.

of the continuous Fourier transform pair (28.3) and (28.1) are

$$\hat{S}_n(y_j) = \mathcal{B}_n(y_j)\hat{M}(y_j) = \sum_{m=1}^{N_y} \Delta k \, e^{+i2\pi k_m y_j} s_n(k_m), \quad n=1,2,\cdots,N_c, \quad j=1,2,\cdots,N_p$$

$$(28.4)$$

$$s_n(k_m) = \sum_{j=1}^{N_p} \Delta y \, e^{-i2\pi k_m y_j} \mathcal{B}_n(y_j)\hat{M}(y_j), \quad n=1,2,\cdots,N_c, \quad m=1,2,\cdots,N_y \qquad (28.5)$$

for N_p pixels in x-space and N_y steps in k-space (i.e., N_y phase encoding steps). This is the discrete Fourier transform pair found in Ch. 11, but only if $N_p = N_y$.[3] The normalization is also changed to include the Δy and Δk factors.

Referring again to the continuous case, if we know $\mathcal{B}_n(y)$, and, even better, if we know it to be uniform, the traditional approach is to use the discrete inverse Fourier transform (28.4) to reconstruct $\hat{S}_n(y)$, and hence extract the image $\hat{M}(y)$, from sufficiently large coverage of k-space using gradient data. With the $e^{+i2\pi k_m y_j}$ phase factors as a basis set of N_y linearly independent 'vectors,' a sufficient number N_y of k_m values leads to enough different 'vector-components' of $\hat{M}(y)$ to reconstruct it. We expand upon this notion in the following section.

28.1.2   Supplanting Some Gradient Data with RF Coil Data: A Preview

We have noted that parallel imaging refers to taking additional information received through the N_c set of coil signals s_n in order to supplant some gradient k-space information. If a fraction of the N_y gradient data steps (which take time to acquire) can be replaced by rf coil data (which can be acquired simultaneously) then, voilá, we have faster imaging.

The combination of gradient and rf data involves a basis set of $N_y \times N_c$ 'vectors,' which we strive by receive coil design to make sufficiently independent.[4] With the independent and complete set of vectors $e^{-i2\pi k_m y}\mathcal{B}_n(y)\Delta y$, where the jth component is given by $v_{n\times m,\,j} \equiv e^{-i2\pi k_m y_j}\mathcal{B}_n(y_j)\Delta y$, we can invert (28.5) via linear algebra. That is, (28.5) can be written as

$$s_{n\times m} = v_{n\times m,\,j}\hat{M}(y_j) \quad \text{or} \quad s = v\hat{M} \qquad (28.6)$$

with $s_{n\times m} \equiv s_n(k_m)$. If we have enough data to match the desired set of pixels, $N_c N_y = N_p$, the matrix v is square. As long as its determinant is nonzero, we have sufficient and independent data to invert v and the image can be recovered,

$$\hat{M} = v^{-1}s \qquad (28.7)$$

If $N_c N_y > N_p$, the magnetization is overdetermined, corresponding to the fact that v is no longer a square matrix and hence no longer invertible. In this case, a least-squares fit serves as a solution, the basis of inverting (28.6) by way of the pseudo-inverse matrix. We will detail in Sec. 28.2.2 the pseudo-inverse approach when we consider the additional complications due to aliasing.

---

[3]In parallel imaging, N_y has been reduced and is no longer directly related to the final reconstructed image resolution Δy.

[4]The elements of these vectors are the usual data matrix elements connecting the signal to the effective spin density.

28.1.3   A Two-Step Function Example

To compare different approaches in parallel imaging, we will repeatedly reconstruct the image of the simple example of a one-dimensional two-step function $M(y)$. The width of the function is $A = 10$ in arbitrary units, as shown in Fig. 28.1. In all comparisons, the procedure will be to start with 'measured' coil signals, where by this we assume all measurements would be consistent with the calculated integrals in (28.1), if experimental errors are neglected. That is, we pretend we do not know $M(y)$, but we assume we do know a sampling of discrete values of the continuous integrals corresponding to a given number of phase encoding gradient steps; we do not use (28.5). We will compare the discrete image reconstructions (28.4) of the spin density example profile for the different approaches considered in this chapter.

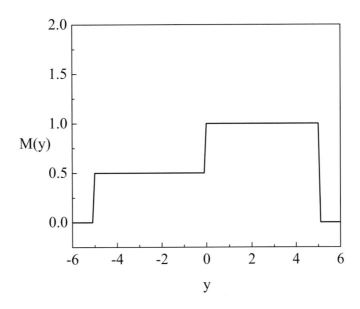

Fig. 28.1: The spin density given by a two-step function: $M(y) = 0.5$ for $-5 < y < 0$ and $M(y) = 1$ for $0 < y < 5$ in arbitrary y units. Thus $A = 10$ for the width of the spin system.

Subsequent reconstructions may be compared to the rf receiving system defined by the single perfect coil ($N_c = 1$) for which $\mathcal{B}_1(y) = 1$ and covers the entire nonzero spin area. Assume that we measure $N_y = 64$ points in 1D k-space ($-n$ to $n - 1$ for $n = 32$ in the MRI sampling convention) with an FOV $L = 12$ in our arbitrary y units. The reconstructed image is shown in Fig. 28.2a, exhibiting the familiar Gibbs ringing effect. In this figure, and others to follow, we have interpolated the reconstructed data to display continuous curves.

28.1.4   Aliasing for the Two-Step Function Example

The aliasing introduced in Ch. 12 is a major issue in parallel imaging. To both remind the reader of this issue and put it in the present context, we change L from the previous no-aliasing case, $L = 12 > A = 10$, to an aliasing example, $L = 6 < A = 10$. The k-space step is doubled accordingly from $\Delta k = 1/12$ to $\Delta k = 1/6$. We also decrease the sampling number (the number of gradient steps) to $N_y = 32$, keeping the k-space range the same. If each of the gradient steps represents a fixed time interval, as for a typical phase encoding gradient, the time of the experiment is halved, but saving imaging time is at the expense of aliasing in this simple example. The result for a single coil with perfect (i.e., uniform) sensitivity is shown in Fig. 28.2b where, for example, the regions $y < -3$ and $y > 3$ (see Fig. 28.2a) are wrapped around to $-3 < y < 3$.

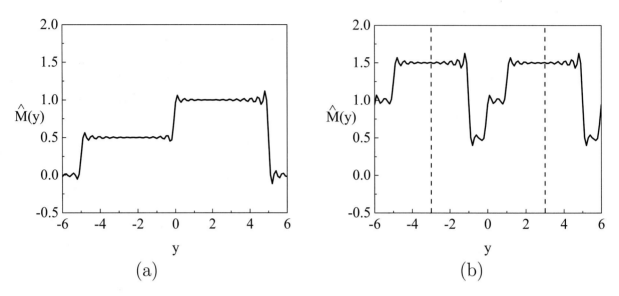

Fig. 28.2: Reconstruction results for the profile in Fig. 28.1 and a single coil with real sensitivity that is constant over the entire y-range. (a) No aliasing occurs for $L = 12 > A = 10$. (b) Aliasing occurs for $L = 6 < A = 10$. Here, a centered FOV is shown by the dashed vertical lines corresponding to the interval $-3 < y < 3$. The result is periodic in L.

It will be useful to consider a formula for aliasing in anticipation of parallel imaging. Consider gradient data acquired for an experiment with a single rf receive coil and an FOV given by L. We consider the rf coil to have a realistic sensitivity profile and the possibility of aliasing even before we undertake any reduction in the number of gradient steps (i.e., $L < A$, with A the sample size). That is, the receive coil sensitivity width R_s may be larger than L such that its data is aliased. For the nth coil, the image product $\hat{S}_n = \mathcal{B}_n \hat{M}$ may be reconstructed from $s_n(k)$ via (28.4), but aliasing corrections must be added to the reconstruction. The folding in of all the spin signals yields a total, aliased image for the region covered by the nth coil with sensitivity $\mathcal{B}_n(y)$. With the object and the original FOV located symmetrically around the origin of the y-axis, the signal is given by

$$\hat{S}_n^{aliased}(y) \;=\; \sum_{p=-\mathcal{N}(A/L)}^{+\mathcal{N}(A/L)} \hat{S}_n(y+pL) \;=\; \sum_{p=-\mathcal{N}(A/L)}^{+\mathcal{N}(A/L)} \mathcal{B}_n(y+pL)\hat{M}(y+pL)$$

$$-L/2 < y < L/2, \quad n = 1, 2, \cdots, N_c \qquad (28.8)$$

where the images $\hat{S}_n$ on the right-hand side are found from (28.4) and $\mathcal{N}(A/L)$ is defined to be the least non-negative integer larger than or equal to $(A/L - 1)/2$. This ceiling function can be written in terms of the floor function denoted by square brackets as the 'largest integer less than or equal to' operation introduced in (10.22)

$$\mathcal{N}(u) = -[(1 - u)/2] \tag{28.9}$$

For a sample that is centered at the nonzero position Y (i.e., not at the center of the middle FOV, which is also considered to be the center of the scanner), we consider the interval in y over which we evaluate (28.8) to be $-L/2 < y - Y < L/2$.

Note, however, that (28.8) is valid for an arbitrary n^{th} coil location because the sensitivity profile $\mathcal{B}_n(y)$ carries that location information, independent of the y-origin, and the profile function will weight the individual terms in the sum accordingly. It is evident in this formula that aliasing from any replicate region is suppressed if the coil has spatially limited sensitivity (see Fig. 12.7c). Simple exercises to gain insight into the connection of multiple coils and aliasing are offered in Prob. 28.1.

Problem 28.1

We are going to put (28.8) to work but with the shortcut of replacing the reconstructed $\hat{M}$ by the exact answer M defined in Fig. 28.1. (Hence, for example, our answers will not exhibit Gibbs ringing.) We consider the possibility of aliasing by assuming the acquired gradient data have an FOV $L = 6$ with one of the replicates centered at $y = 0$. Suppose that we have multiple coils, each with (unphysically) perfectly uniform (boxcar) real sensitivity of unit height.

a) Assume coil n has a boxcar sensitivity, with width exactly matching the range $-6 < y < 6$. Evaluate the sum (28.8) for this coil over that whole range (and not just over the center FOV) and compare the result to Fig. 28.2b.

b) Consider the sum (28.8) for each of three identical coils whose boxcar ranges are now limited to covering exactly the intervals $-6 < y < -2$, $-2 < y < 2$, and $2 < y < 6$, respectively. Do you have aliasing now? Show how you can combine these sums to reconstruct the entire two-step object.

c) Finally, consider three identical coils with the Gaussian profiles shown in Fig. 28.3 and with their functional form given in its caption. The profiles overlap each other, extending beyond the respective interval given in (b). Carry out the sums (28.8) for the three coils and plot their results as functions of y. Is there aliasing present?

It is instructive to keep in mind that the above exercises offer a simple preview to the upcoming section on x-space or image-space parallel imaging.

28.2 Parallel Imaging with an x-Space Approach

We consider now the reconstruction of an image if we are given the gradient data for an FOV smaller than the imaging object and a multiple set of different rf receive coil data. The

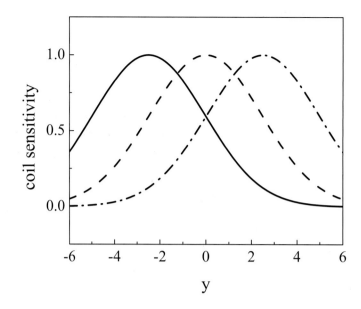

Fig. 28.3: The Gaussian sensitivities $\mathcal{B}_1$(left), $\mathcal{B}_2$(center), and $\mathcal{B}_3$(right) for a three-coil example are shown as solid, dashed, and dot-dashed curves, corresponding to $e^{-(y-y_0)^2/12}$ with centers at $y_0 = -2.5, 0, +2.5$, respectively.

combination of these data is carried out after an inverse Fourier transform has taken us back to the spatial domain. The first discussion in Sec. 28.2.1 is for ideal coils covering the sample without overlap. The more realistic case is analyzed in Sec. 28.2.2 where there is the need to remove the aliasing due to the coil sensitivity extending beyond the FOV. The approach that combines coil images in the spatial domain such that aliasing is removed is called the SENSE (SENSitivity Encoding) method.

28.2.1   Perfect Coil Sensitivities

In general, every coil in a parallel array is localized, meaning the sensitivity is restricted to a finite region of x-space (e.g., the single y-dimension in the 1D modeling carried out in this chapter). For very localized coils, the number of coils must be large enough to cover the whole sample. A simultaneous and straightforward data collection, with each coil's sensitivity corresponding to a different subregion (i.e., very little overlap), leads to a complete image with no aliasing issues. In this unrealistic case (see Sec. 28.2.2 for more practical coil modeling), we can reduce the FOV for each rf coil to its sensitivity range R_s. (This was anticipated by the example in the previous problem.) Comparing to an original image obtained with an FOV equal to the object size A, we could decrease the number of gradient steps by the factor R_s/A, and thereby reduce the imaging time by the same factor.

   The savings in time thus depends on the number of coils and the way we use them to reduce the number of gradient steps. If an original (i.e., full) number of gradient steps $N_{y,full}$ is reduced by parallel imaging to $N_{y,PI}$, the imaging time is reduced by $1/R$ where the so-called acceleration factor R is

$$R \equiv \text{acceleration factor} = \frac{N_{y,full}}{N_{y,PI}} \tag{28.10}$$

for constant time steps. Specifically, $R > 1$ implies a reduction in the number of k-space points and, hence, in the FOV. That is, to keep the total k-space range the same, we require $N_{y,PI}\Delta k_{PI} = N_{y,full}\Delta k_{full}$, in terms of the 'PI' and 'full' step sizes. We observe that $R = \Delta k_{PI}/\Delta k_{full} = \text{FOV}_{full}/\text{FOV}_{PI}$. The FOV has therefore changed in inverse proportion to R.[5]

Consider the special case where the number of combined gradient and rf data points, $N_{y,PI} \times N_c$, is equal to the original data number $N_{y,full}$ obtained with a single coil. The value of the acceleration factor is then given by the number of coils, $R = N_c$. Customarily, however, we have a larger set of (overdetermined) parallel imaging data, $N_{y,PI} \times N_c > N_{y,full}$; therefore, $R < N_c$, under most circumstances.

28.2.2 More Realistic Sensitivities and SENSE

In recapitulation, a $1/R$ decrease in imaging time corresponds to a reduction of the number of gradient steps down to $N_{y,full}/R$. Theoretically, the set N_c of coil signals s_n would lead to this decrease provided that the array of coils completely covered the sample, had zero overlap with each other, and had individual coil sensitivity spreads equal to L/R. However, realistic arrays of coils that completely cover the sample are overlapping. Their sensitivity regions are generally wider than L/R, for R values of interest, so aliasing arises and must be corrected.

Formula for Parallel Imaging with Aliasing

The above fully aliased coil signal (28.8) is easy to 'accelerate,' that is, to adapt to multiple rf coils. For an acceleration factor $R > 1$ such that the FOV is reduced from L to L/R, the reconstructed signal from the nth coil (the object and the central - but now reduced - FOV are still centered on the y origin) is given by

$$\hat{S}_{n,R}^{aliased}(y) = \sum_{p=-\mathcal{N}(AR/L)}^{+\mathcal{N}(AR/L)} \hat{S}_n(y + pL/R) = \sum_{p=-\mathcal{N}(AR/L)}^{+\mathcal{N}(AR/L)} \mathcal{B}_n(y + pL/R)\hat{M}(y + pL/R)$$

$$-L/(2R) < y < L/(2R), \quad n = 1, 2, \cdots, N_c \tag{28.11}$$

As before, (28.11) applies for any coil location, and we shift the interval to $-L/(2R) < y - Y < L/(2R)$ for a sample (and middle FOV) that is centered at the nonzero position Y. The above result is the starting point for an x-space approach to faster imaging: the aforementioned SENSE method. The idea is to have enough signal information to cover the whole object range. This coverage is obtaining by solving for the individual $\hat{M}$ factors, which only provide reduced FOV segments, in the sums of (28.11). Patched together, these factors

---

[5]It may be helpful to note that the data received by each rf coil have the same FOV, which is determined by the size of the phase encoding gradient steps.

yield the image over all y. Thus, in order to extract a faithful image of $\hat{M}(y)$ at a given location y, the set (28.11), for all n, are the ingredients for an inverse matrix calculation, assuming we know the sensitivity factors $\mathcal{B}_n$. If N_r is defined to be the total number of replicates (i.e., the number of terms in the sum over p), including the central FOV L/R, we have $N_r = 2\mathcal{N}(AR/L) + 1$. (Note that $N_r = 1$ refers to no aliasing.) Represent $\hat{S}$ as the $N_c \times 1$ column matrix with elements $\hat{S}_n \equiv \hat{S}_{n,R}^{aliased}(y)$, $\mathcal{B}$ as the $N_c \times N_r$ matrix with $\mathcal{B}_{n,p} \equiv \mathcal{B}_n(y + pL/R)$ elements (one normally maps the index p onto a positive integer, say, $j = 1, 2, ..., N_r$), and $\hat{M}$ as the $N_r \times 1$ column matrix with elements $\hat{M}_p \equiv \hat{M}(y + pL/R)$. The reconstructed signal (28.11) is then given more compactly by

$$\hat{S} = \mathcal{B}\hat{M} \tag{28.12}$$

To solve (28.12) for $\hat{M}$, we encounter the generic matrix inversion problem introduced in Sec. 28.1.2. If $N_r = N_c$, then $\mathcal{B}$ is a square matrix and the extraction of the N_r terms $\hat{M}(y + pL/R)$ for each y is straightforward. It is given by the simple inversion $\hat{M} = \mathcal{B}^{-1}\hat{S}$, provided that the determinant of $\mathcal{B}$ is nonzero.

To address the case $N_r < N_c$, where $\mathcal{B}$ is no longer a square matrix, we can merely throw away the additional $N_c - N_r$ equations, assuming (28.12) involves completely accurate experiments and perfect sensitivity modeling (see Prob. 28.2). However, measurements contain errors such that (28.12) is only approximately satisfied, pixel by pixel and coil by coil. Assuming equal weighting of each measurement (see Sec. 28.4 for a general discussion of weighted errors and noise), we may look for a solution that minimizes $|\hat{S} - \mathcal{B}\hat{M}|^2$, a least-squares solution. This overdetermined problem has a well-known pseudo-inverse solution and is described next.

Pseudo-Inverse Solutions

If $N_r < N_c$, and considering the possibility of errors, we seek the minimum, as a function of $\hat{M}$, of the following functional[6]

$$F \equiv |\hat{S} - \mathcal{B}\hat{M}|^2 = (\hat{S} - \mathcal{B}\hat{M})^\dagger(\hat{S} - \mathcal{B}\hat{M}) = \hat{S}^\dagger\hat{S} - \hat{M}^\dagger\mathcal{B}^\dagger\hat{S} - \hat{S}^\dagger\mathcal{B}\hat{M} + \hat{M}^\dagger\mathcal{B}^\dagger\mathcal{B}\hat{M} \tag{28.13}$$

That is, we ask for the two extremum conditions (which are redundant for the functional considered here in which $\hat{M}$ and $\hat{M}^\dagger$ appear symmetrically)

$$\frac{\partial F}{\partial \hat{M}} = 0, \quad \frac{\partial F}{\partial \hat{M}^\dagger} = 0 \tag{28.14}$$

where the respective partial derivatives are taken with $\hat{M}^\dagger$ and $\hat{M}$ fixed (these are used as the two independent degrees of freedom instead of the real and imaginary parts of $\hat{M}$). From the second condition in (28.14) we obtain

$$-\mathcal{B}^\dagger\hat{S} + \mathcal{B}^\dagger\mathcal{B}\hat{M} = 0 \tag{28.15}$$

---

[6]Recall the Hermitian adjoint of a matrix $\mathcal{M}$, denoted by $\mathcal{M}^\dagger$, corresponds to complex conjugation combined with the transpose operation.

Equation (28.15) can be solved for $\hat{M}$ to give

$$\hat{M} = \mathcal{B}_P^{-1}\hat{S} \tag{28.16}$$

in terms of the so-called pseudo-inverse, or Moore-Penrose, matrix

$$\mathcal{B}_P^{-1} \equiv (\mathcal{B}^\dagger \mathcal{B})^{-1}\mathcal{B}^\dagger \tag{28.17}$$

The first condition in (28.14) is just the adjoint of (28.16) and, as promised, gives nothing new. The key point is that $\mathcal{B}^\dagger \mathcal{B}$ is a square matrix with a garden-variety inverse, even when $\mathcal{B}$ is not square. If $\mathcal{B}$ is a square matrix, $\mathcal{B}_P^{-1}$ reduces to $\mathcal{B}^{-1}(\mathcal{B}^\dagger)^{-1}\mathcal{B}^\dagger = \mathcal{B}^{-1}$, as expected. Throughout this chapter, the pseudo-inverse solution can be employed to find fits involving an excess of data points. In Sec. 28.4, we return to a generalization with weighted errors dominated by coil noise.

For simple illustrations and later reference, we describe how the equations of the above paragraph appear in terms of matrix elements. For instance, (28.13) can be rewritten as the trace

$$F = \sum_{i=1}^{N_c} \left| \hat{S}_i - \sum_{j=1}^{N_r} \mathcal{B}_{ij}\hat{M}_j \right|^2 \tag{28.18}$$

where we have relabeled n by i and we cover the range of N_r replicates by the positive-integer index j. The index j in $\hat{M}_j \equiv \hat{M}(y_j)$ refers, therefore, only to an aliased pixel (all N_r replicates of a given pixel). It does not range over the different N_p physical pixels indicated in (28.4). The first condition in (28.14) corresponds to the N_r equations, $\partial F/\partial \hat{M}_j = 0$, and so forth.

Pixel Aliasing in x-Space

Two trivial but illustrative examples using the indexing labels of (28.18) involve two coils ($i = 1, 2$) with no aliasing and single aliasing ($j = 1$ and $j = 1, 2$) corresponding to acceleration factors, $R = 1$ and $R = 2$, respectively. With real parameters a and b, the $R = 1$ sensitivity (x-component) 2×1 column matrix and its Hermitian conjugate 1×2 row matrix can be taken as

$$\mathcal{B}_{R=1} = \begin{pmatrix} a \\ b \end{pmatrix}, \qquad \mathcal{B}_{R=1}^\dagger = \begin{pmatrix} a & b \end{pmatrix} \tag{28.19}$$

The image reconstruction for a given pixel and the two coils is as follows. From (28.19), the 1×1 matrix is $(\mathcal{B}^\dagger \mathcal{B})_{R=1} = a^2 + b^2$, so the pseudo-inverse solution (28.16) for $R = 1$ is

$$\hat{M}(y_1) = \frac{a}{a^2 + b^2}\hat{S}_1(y_1) + \frac{b}{a^2 + b^2}\hat{S}_2(y_1) \tag{28.20}$$

The feature to be noticed here is the unique sensitivity weighting of the two signals coming out of the least-squares solution.

To simplify the $R = 2$ aliasing example, consider the overlapping coplanar coils shown in Fig. 28.4 along with makeshift but reasonable estimates of their sensitivity profiles. For convenience, choose the two aliased points, y_1 and $y_2 = y_1 + L$, on the left and right edges

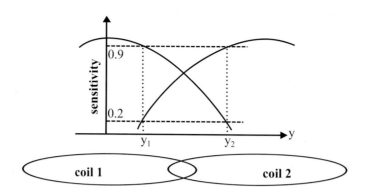

Fig. 28.4: Sampling an aliased spin distribution with coplanar coils and the (reduced) center FOV, $L = y_2 - y_1$. (The sample is not centered at the origin here.) In terms of variables introduced in the text, the measurement of y_1 by the left (right) coil is $a = 0.9$ ($b = 0.2$), in arbitrary units, and vice versa for the measurement of its aliased position, y_2.

of the centered FOV shown in the figure. The square $R = 2$ sensitivity matrix is thus symmetric and given by

$$\mathcal{B}_{R=2} = \begin{pmatrix} a & b \\ b & a \end{pmatrix} \tag{28.21}$$

using the same real parameter notation as in the $R = 1$ case. For the image reconstruction of two aliased pixels, the straightforward matrix inversion of (28.21) for $R = 2$ gives

$$\hat{M}(y_1) = \frac{1}{a^2 - b^2} \left(a\hat{S}_1(y_1) - b\hat{S}_2(y_1) \right)$$

$$\hat{M}(y_2) = \frac{1}{a^2 - b^2} \left(a\hat{S}_2(y_2) - b\hat{S}_1(y_2) \right) \tag{28.22}$$

Here, we note the divergence at $a = b$ signaling our inability in that limit to reconstruct both images with essentially only one independent measurement. Additional features for pixel aliasing in x-space are the subject of Prob. 28.2.

Problem 28.2

A SENSE experiment for two spatial locations (pixels) is performed on our ubiquitous two-step function, Fig. 28.1, where the reconstructed coil signals from y_1 have been aliased into the location y_2, and vice versa. Consider three receive coils (for example, the coils of Fig. 28.4 with a third coplanar coil midway between them) with the sensitivity matrix given by

$$\mathcal{B} = \begin{pmatrix} 0.9 & 0.2 \\ 0.5 & 0.5 \\ 0.2 & 0.9 \end{pmatrix} \tag{28.23}$$

An exact (errorless) but aliased reconstructed signal set for the three coils is the column matrix

$$\hat{S} = \begin{pmatrix} 0.65 \\ 0.75 \\ 1.0 \end{pmatrix} \qquad (28.24)$$

a) What are the least-squares values for the reconstructed magnetization $\hat{M}(y_1)$ and $\hat{M}(y_2)$? Compare this solution to any other solution for the reconstructed magnetization. (One neat way is to simply replace $\mathcal{B}^{\dagger}$ by any arbitrary 2×3 matrix in the pseudo-inverse solution, which still leads to an invertible square matrix.) Explain the (perhaps) surprising result of the comparison.

b) Consider an example with experimental errors in the signals for the three coils. We now take the signal set to be

$$\hat{S} = \begin{pmatrix} 0.6 \\ 0.9 \\ 1.1 \end{pmatrix} \qquad (28.25)$$

Find the pseudo-inverse solution and compare it to your answer in (a). Explain why the answers should, in general, be different.

SENSE Reconstruction over all Pixels

We discuss now an example for reconstructing the spin magnetization $\hat{M}(y)$ over the entire sample. Aliasing is addressed for a given reduction in gradient steps as we return to the two-step function $M(y)$ from Fig. 28.1 and assume three identical coils with real sensitivities. The three overlapping coil sensitivities are chosen to be identical Gaussian field profiles centered over their respective FOVs (Fig. 28.3). The complete x-space reconstruction and the steps taken to obtain it may be understood from the plots in Figs. 28.5 and 28.6. The first step is the 'experimental' acquisition of $s_n(k)$, which means we evaluate (28.1) using the Gaussian sensitivities for (now reduced) $N_{y,PI} = 20$ gradient steps, which are chosen as sufficiently close to one-third of the original number of gradient steps, $N_{y,full} = 64$, yielding $R = 64/20$. (More gradient steps would increase resolution for a fixed FOV but they also increase the time taken for the experiment.) The corresponding FOV_{PI} imaged by each coil is $(20/64)12 = 3.75$ units. Next, their inverse transforms $\hat{S}_n(y+pL/R)$ are found from (28.4). The $p = 0$ (unaliased) terms $\hat{S}_n(y) = \mathcal{B}_n(y)\hat{M}(y)$ are shown as dashed lines and the fully aliased $\hat{S}_{n,R}^{aliased}(y)$ obtained from (28.11) are shown as solid lines in Fig. 28.5 for the three coils.

The reconstructed two-step function $\hat{M}(y)$ is extracted as follows. With three coils and $N_r = 3$, both $\hat{S}$ and $\hat{M}$ in (28.12) are 3×1 matrices, and $\mathcal{B}$ is a 3×3 matrix. A simple square-matrix inversion is all that is required to obtain the solution for $\hat{M}(y)$, the result of which is shown in Fig. 28.6, including the expected Gibbs ringing. Despite the small number of coils, a key is that they cover the object and their sensitivities are assumed to be known exactly, leading to a satisfactory result. For the cases where the coil sensitivities are not well characterized, the k-space methods in Sec. 28.3 are especially useful.

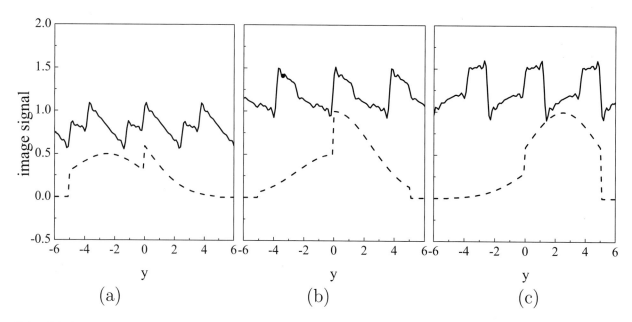

Fig. 28.5: Image intensity plots for the three-coil example described in the text. The dashed lines are the $p = 0$ (unaliased) terms $\mathcal{B}_n(y)\hat{M}(y)$ of (28.11). The solid lines are the total sum $\hat{S}_{n,R}^{aliased}(y)$ from the same equation. (a) Left coil $n = 1$, (b) Center coil $n = 2$, (c) Right coil $n = 3$.

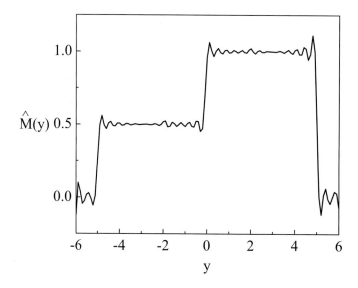

Fig. 28.6: The reconstructed magnetization of the two-step function obtained by square-matrix inversion in the three-coil example discussed in the text. This is a simple SENSE example with exactly known coil sensitivities.

28.3 Parallel Imaging with a k-Space Approach

Instead of combining reconstructed images from coils in different x-space regions, we turn to techniques for combining k-space data from different coils before reconstruction. It is again assumed that the number of gradient steps has been reduced, and the additional rf coils are to take up the slack. As a result of the combination, the k-space data are dense enough to avoid aliasing, and an acceleration $R > 1$ is attained. The set of known coil sensitivity functions in a given rf array can form an expansion basis for approximating complex sinusoids (i.e., phase factors). This approximation can be used to find coil data for additional k-space lines in the method referred to as SMASH (SiMultaneous Acquisition of Spatial Harmonics).

Additionally, there are improved k-space approaches that can cope with uncertainties in the coil sensitivities. The idea is to augment the initially reduced gradient data by 'autocalibrating' gradient data, to gain information about the coils. Fits to combinations of augmented coil signal data lead to formulas for interpolations to new k-space lines in a method called AUTO-SMASH. Further improvement is made by using individual coil signals by themselves for the interpolation in the GRAPPA (GeneRalized Autocalibrating Partially Parallel Acquisitions) method. Examples are described next in order to demonstrate these methods.

28.3.1 Known Sensitivities and SMASH

As before, the 'measured' coil signals corresponding to carrying out the integrations in (28.1) yield a set of data from the combination of $N_{y,PI} \times N_c$ gradient and rf coil measurements

$$
\begin{aligned}
s_n(k_m) &= \int dy\, e^{-i2\pi k_m y} \mathcal{B}_n(y) M(y) \\
&n = 1, 2, \cdots, N_c, \quad m = 1, 2, \cdots, N_{y,PI}
\end{aligned}
\tag{28.26}
$$

Following previous notation, the line spacing for the PI data is $\Delta k_{PI} = \Delta k_m \equiv k_{m+1} - k_m$. ($\Delta k_m$ is assumed to be uniform, so it is actually independent of m.)

How could we find signals for intermediate k values without additional gradient steps and without taking additional time? We can accelerate the experiment by R if we somehow simultaneously add $R - 1$ equally spaced lines between the original lines with individual subspacing given by

$$
\Delta k_{full} = \Delta k_{PI}/R
\tag{28.27}
$$

where, again, 'full' refers to the targeted k-space.[7] In the SENSE approach of Sec. 28.2, it is understood that the entire set of additional k-space lines are provided implicitly by combining additional individual coil signals. Now, however, we explicitly add the lines in the SMASH procedure described next.

Suppose we can find linear combinations of the known N_c coil sensitivities $\mathcal{B}_n$ that, to a good approximation, are equivalent to the additional phase factors $e^{-i2\pi p \Delta k_{full} y}$ for N_{pf}

---

[7]Whether or not there was aliasing with the original FOV$_{PI}$, we consider the final 'full' k-space to be free of aliasing.

different integer values of p.[8] ($N_{pf} = R$ for the scenario described in the previous paragraph.) Specifically, we try to find the weighting coefficients $w_n^{(p)}$ such that

$$\sum_{n=1}^{N_c} w_n^{(p)} \mathcal{B}_n(y) = e^{-i2\pi p \Delta k_{full} y}, \qquad p = 0, 1, 2, \cdots, N_{pf} - 1 \qquad (28.28)$$

where we leave understood that these $2N_{pf} - 1$ real equations can only be approximately satisfied. In practice, the $w_n^{(p)}$ coefficients are found in a least-squares fit via a pseudo-matrix calculation.

If all equations in (28.28) hold, then the same coefficients can be used in a linear combination of coil signals to give

$$
\begin{aligned}
\sum_{n=1}^{N_c} w_n^{(p)} s_n(k_m) &= \int dy \, e^{-i2\pi k_m y} \sum_{n=1}^{N_c} w_n^{(p)} \mathcal{B}_n(y) M(y) \\
&= \int dy \, e^{-i2\pi k_m y} e^{-i2\pi p \Delta k_{full} y} M(y) \\
&\equiv s_{ideal}(k_m + p\Delta k_{full}) \\
&\qquad p = 0, 1, 2, \cdots, N_{pf} - 1, \quad m = 1, 2, \cdots, N_{y,PI} \qquad (28.29)
\end{aligned}
$$

These linear combinations of coil signals have moved us from the set of N_c individual coil signals evaluated at the k-space point k_m to an idealized overall coil signal s_{ideal} evaluated at the set of points $k_m + p\Delta k_{full}$ for each integer $p > 0$. By 'idealized,' we mean a coil signal from a perfectly constant sensitivity $\mathcal{B} = 1$. The $p = 0$ case yields ideal signals for the gradient k-space points $\{k_m\}$.

How many new, or synthetic, k-space points can we generate for our ideal signals? It will depend on the number of harmonics we can accurately construct with our N_c coil basis. The combinations in (28.29) have generated $N_{pf} - 1$ synthetic k-space points for each of the original ones. An immediate consequence is that the $N_{y,PI}$ points are now expanded to $N_{pf} \times N_{y,PI}$ points (playing a role analogous to $N_{y,full}$ in the previous SENSE discussion). Revisiting the way we introduced SMASH, the additional number of data points has been achieved by fewer gradient steps, and thus less time. The corresponding acceleration factor is

$$R = \frac{N_{pf} \times N_{y,PI}}{N_{y,PI}} = N_{pf} \qquad (28.30)$$

as expected. A decrease of $1/N_{pf}$ in imaging time is theoretically possible. Aliasing that may have been present initially in individual coil signals can be eliminated if the final step size Δk_{full} achieved is sufficiently smaller than the original line spacing. The ultimate FOV determined by $1/\Delta k_{full}$ increases in proportion to N_{pf} for a given original FOV $= 1/\Delta k_{PI}$.

Problem 28.3

Suppose that we have three specialized coils with field x-components (real sensitivities) given by $\cos 2\pi y/L$, $\sin 2\pi y/L$, and 1, respectively. The y-components are assumed to be ignorable over the sampling region-of-interest.

---

[8]We thus map the basis of sensitivity functions $\mathcal{B}_n$ to the Fourier basis of phase-space factors $e^{-i2\pi ky}$. We refer the reader back to the discussion in Sec. 28.1.2.

    a) What coil array could you use to generate sensitivities that are approximately the same as these? Hint: Consider the 'butterfly' coil shown in Fig. 27.15.

    b) If we only sample the 'even' points $k_{m+1} = k_m + 2\Delta k_{full}$ for all m, how can we construct the ideal signals at the odd points, $k_{m+1} = k_m + \Delta k_{full}$, using the SMASH method? Assume that $\Delta k_{full} = 1/L$.

    In general, the number of coils required to satisfy (28.28) is larger than the coil number required in the previous x-space method, for a given specific acceleration factor R. This is true even when we generalize to complex values for $\mathcal{B}_n$ (i.e., we include both transverse components of the coil sensitivity). Consider a row of adjacent overlapping coils lying parallel to the y-z plane and with a small offset Δx from the $x = 0$ plane. (We continue to limit ourselves, however, to imaging along the y-axis.) In the reciprocity picture, the spins would experience both transverse field components from the coils (each with unit current). With an argument based on Maxwell's equations, or simply visualizing the field due to a nearby coil loop, and if the real part of the complex conjugate of each coil sensitivity (the x-component) can be approximated by Gaussian behavior, the behavior of the imaginary part (the negative of the y-component) is then approximately proportional to the negative of the derivative of that Gaussian function.[9] Therefore the least-squares fitting as an expansion in sensitivity components is facilitated by the fact that the derivative of the real part of the phase factor, which is the cosine term in (28.28), is proportional to the imaginary part, which has a sine term and an overall minus sign.

    We are ready for the imaging demonstration with the standard two-step function. Three coils with complex sensitivities are used to generate spatial harmonics for $p = 0$ and 1 in (28.28). (The difficulties in obtaining realistic weightings $w_n^{(p)}$ for only two coils is the subject of Prob. 28.4.) The real and imaginary parts of the three coil sensitivities are approximated by the curves in Fig. 28.7a, where the freedom to choose a small coil offset from the x-axis justifies the assumption of a small imaginary part for each coil. The corresponding best fits to (28.28) are determined by a least-squares procedure over $-6 < y < 6$ (we target a final FOV$_{full} = 12$ for all k-space reconstructions of the two-step function). The results for the weights are shown in Table 28.1 and the accuracy of the fits is evident in Fig. 28.7b. The rather poor $p = 0$ fit will be seen to negatively affect the final reconstruction.

	$w_1^{(p)}$	$w_2^{(p)}$	$w_3^{(p)}$
1 $(p=0)$	$1.327 - 0.024i$	-0.658	$1.327 + 0.024i$
$\exp(-i2\pi\Delta k_{full}\, y)$ $(p=1)$	$-1.207 + 0.960i$	2.419	$-1.207 - 0.960i$

Table 28.1: The phase factors for $p = 0$, 1 shown in the left column have been approximated by a series of weighted combinations of the complex sensitivities with the weights shown in each row.

---

    [9]From a Taylor expansion and $\vec{\nabla} \times \vec{B} = 0$, we find $B_y \simeq \Delta x \, \partial B_x/\partial y$ along the $x = \Delta x$ line. See the examples in Fig. 28.7a.

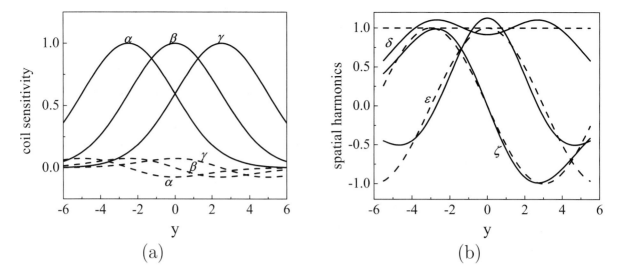

Fig. 28.7: (a) The complex sensitivities of three coils in the y-z plane centered at $y = -2.5$, 0, and 2.5, and labeled by α, β, and γ, respectively. The coils are slightly offset from the x-axis (the offset chosen is $\Delta x = 0.3$). The solid curves are the real parts (x-components) and the dashed curves are the imaginary parts (negative of the y-components, because $\mathcal{B}$ refers to the conjugate in this chapter, and, as explained in a footnote, are thus the negatives of the derivatives of the solid curves multiplied by Δx). The overall normalization is in arbitrary units. (b) The resulting approximations (fits) of the spatial harmonics $\exp(-i2\pi y/L)$, with $L = 12$, for $p = 0$ (horizontal line) and the real (cosine) and imaginary (negative of sine) parts of $p = 1$, and labeled by δ, ϵ, ζ, respectively. The solid lines represent the fits to the dashed lines (exact answers).

Our goal is to find ideal signals for all 64 k-space points: the $p = 0$ and $p = 1$ harmonics give us the ideal signals for the 32 original and 32 augmented points of k-space data, respectively. The acceleration factor therefore equals two, which is less than the number (3) of coils, as forecasted. The discrete inverse Fourier transform leads to the reconstruction of the unaliased two-step image shown in Fig. 28.8. Notice that this reconstruction is inferior to the x-space result of Sec. 28.2. The reason is that we have a limited number of coil sensitivities with which to approximate the harmonic phase factors. In x-space, on the other hand, we only needed to have good coverage of the object. A better result is found for five coils, whose positions are at -5.0, -2.5, 0, 2.5, 5.0, and Gaussian widths are narrower (12 is replaced by 4 in the exponents shown in the caption of Fig. 28.3). Although we use the same offset or $\Delta x = 0.3$, we could just as well use real sensitivities.[10] The improved five-coil result, also shown in Fig. 28.8, corresponds to a better (flatter) fit to the $p = 0$ harmonic and closer fits to the $p = 1$ sinusoids (not included in the plots). The poorer $p = 0$ fit for three coils is largely responsible for the difference in reconstruction.

---

[10]Recall that this corresponds to no y-component for the magnetic field produced by the coil, or zero offset, meaning they are right next to the sample.

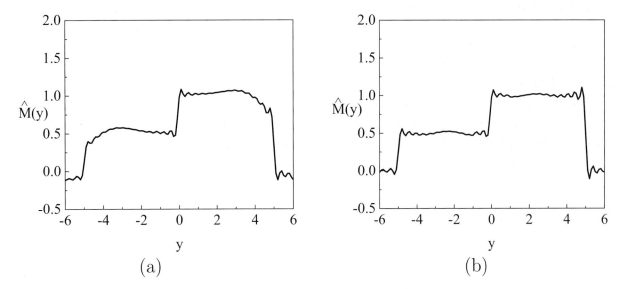

Fig. 28.8: The reconstruction for a two-step function profile from the idealized coil signals (28.29) generated for: (a) Three coils: The weightings have been calculated for the first two harmonics, $p = 0, 1$, and are given in Table 28.1. The resultant 64 k-space points are composed of 32 original coil signals ($p = 0$) and 32 interspersed coil signals ($p = 1$). (b) Five coils: By using more coils and narrower Gaussians, as described in the text, the $p = 0$ harmonic is more accurately approximated and the result is improved. These represent oversimplified SMASH examples with limited coil arrays and data.

Problem 28.4

Consider using two complex coil sensitivities to generate spatial harmonics for $p = 0$ and 1 in (28.28). Assume the real and imaginary parts of the three coils are approximated by Gaussians and derivatives of Gaussians, respectively, with an arbitrary relative normalization between them. Find the corresponding best fits to (28.28) by a least-squares procedure over $-6 < y < 6$ (FOV $= 12$) and show your results as curves analogous to those in Fig. 28.7b. Also, compare your answers for the weights to those in Table 28.1. Is the relative normalization you needed for your result realistic?

28.3.2   Unknown Sensitivities: AUTO-SMASH and GRAPPA

A disadvantage of the methods discussed so far is the need for an *a priori* accurate fit for the sensitivity of each coil. However, in practice, the coil sensitivities are changed under load, and more so at higher frequencies. Even if we could model $B_n(y)$ very well over a phantom, it may have consequential distortions over the heterogeneous human body. In this section we describe an improved method with which we can find weighting coefficients analogous to those in the previous section but without prior knowledge of detailed coil sensitivity.

Additional gradient data beyond the original set are measured to obtain the weights. This is called a 'self-calibrating' technique; it utilizes a limited set of 'autocalibration signal' (ACS) points in k-space to get the weights. In practice, the new data points needed to substitute for the unknown coil information do not represent significant increases in the initial gradient k-space data acquisition.

We remind the reader of the implicit reference to k-space lines in 2D in this chapter. We continue to write $s_n(k)$ instead of $s_n(k_x, k_y)$, leaving k_x understood and using $k_y \equiv k$. Points really are shorthand for phase encoding lines and the tacit 2D signal data play an important role in practical implementations of the methods discussed below.

Composite Coil Signals and AUTO-SMASH

Rather than approximating the harmonic phase factors, we can try to find a good fit for the signal integrals over the phase factors. That is, we can consider global relations such as (28.29) rather than the local equations (28.28), for each k_m point. It is the signal, after all, that is the more directly relevant quantity. In analogy to the ideal signal in SMASH, we define a 'composite' signal for the new points in terms of the weighted sum of individual coil signals.[11] It is given by

$$s_{composite}(k_m + p\Delta k_{full}) \quad = \quad \sum_{n=1}^{N_c} w_n^{(p)} s_n(k_m)$$

$$p = 0, 1, \cdots, R-1, \quad m = 1, 2, \cdots, N_{y,PI} \quad (28.31)$$

with $\Delta k_{full} = \Delta k_{PI}/R$ as before, and interspersed between each of the original $N_{y,PI}$ points in the set $\{k_m\}$ are $R-1$ synthetic points. Thus $N_{y,PI} \times R$ composite signals are constructed via (28.31). Even though the weights will not be determined by a phase-factor fit, the working assumption is that the 'composite' signal will be close to 'ideal.' Aside from an ambiguity in their overall normalization, the goal is to find the weights $w_n^{(p)}$ in order to construct a discrete inverse Fourier transform of the composite signals to obtain image reconstruction.

To obtain the weights without any knowledge of $\mathcal{B}_n(y)$, we will assume all the coils are identical, although at (uniformly displaced) different positions to sufficiently cover the sample. In the absence of additional information about the overall normalization, we make the convenient choice of $w_n^{(0)} = 1$ for all n identical coils. This yields ideal composite signals for the original data corresponding to $p = 0$ in (28.31). To determine the $p = 1$ weights $w_n^{(1)}$, we need the additional ACS data.

We apply gradients to find the coil signals for a small subset of additional points, which serve as ACS data. The ACS data points and a known gradient neighboring setting (some values m' from among the original set of $N_{y,PI}$ values of m) can be used to find the weights through a fitting procedure described in the next paragraph. It is then possible to interpolate other new data from their own neighboring points by using this fit. Define the composite

---

[11]Keep in mind we are always trying to find some kind of k-space function with sufficient coverage to allow good image reconstruction via Fourier inversion.

signal in terms of the ACS individual coil signals

$$s_{composite}(k_{m'} + p\Delta k_{full}) = \sum_{n=1}^{N_c} w_n^{(0)} s_n(k_{m'} + p\Delta k_{full}), \quad p = 1, 2, \cdots, R-1$$

$$\text{for the subset } \{k_{m'} + p\Delta k_{full}\}_{ACS} \quad (28.32)$$

where the ACS subset covers all the points lying between the two gradient points m' and $m' + 1$ for the range of p shown in (28.32). With unit weights at $p = 0$, as explained above, the weightings $w_n^{(p)}$ for $p > 0$ can be determined by requiring (28.32) to be consistent with (28.31) over the ACS subset,

$$\sum_{n=1}^{N_c} w_n^{(0)} s_n(k_{m'} + p\Delta k_{full}) = \sum_{n=1}^{N_c} w_n^{(p)} s_n(k_{m'})$$

$$p = 1, 2, \cdots, R-1 \text{ for } \{k_{m'} + p\Delta k_{full}\}_{ACS} \quad (28.33)$$

Note that the problem in determining any normalization stems from (28.33), with weights homogeneously appearing on both sides of the equation.

We proceed directly to finding the composite signals for the two-step function example using this method. The cartoon illustrates the procedure in Fig. 28.9, but only for a small subset of points. With the same three coils as in Sec. 28.1, the original gradient data is again 'measured' by using their sensitivities to calculate the integrals in (28.1). We assume no direct information about the coils, other than the assumption they are identical in profile. In our illustration, we'll make the by now familiar initial attempt with $\Delta k_{PI} = 2\Delta k_{full}$ (thus, $p = 0$ and 1). As before, we are imaging the two-step function with a target (full) FOV of $L = 12$. But, because we have been considering relatively few points in 1D, we do not have enough k-space data for fits unless we add more ACS points (requiring more initial gradient

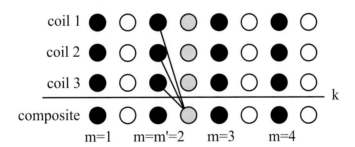

Fig. 28.9: The locations along the vertical axis refer to the signals from the three different coils and the 'composite signal' data. The phase encoding k-space points are marked along the horizontal k-axis with black, white, and gray circles, which refer to measured points (the k_m values), missing points, and the ACS points, respectively. The three lines drawn converging from three measured data points to the ACS composite signal illustrate an example of three coil signals used to obtain a fit to a single ACS composite point. In terms of (28.32), the sum is the composite signal at the point $k_1 + \Delta k_{full}$ (bottom gray circle) constructed from the individual gradient data for all three coils at that same point (top three gray circles), with $R = 2$ ($p = 1$) and $m' = 2$. The four black columns correspond to $N_{y,PI} = 4$.

data and thus a longer experiment). For an improved fit at $p = 1$, therefore, we select and sample a larger number, say, 10 total ACS subsets $k_{m'} + p\Delta k_{full}$ where $m' = 12, 13, ..., 21$ and $\Delta k_{full} = 1/12$. Then the weights $w_n^{(1)}$ are determined by a least-squares procedure fitting the ACS data ($p = 1$) with their 10 (left) adjacent ($p = 0$) subsets $k_{m'}$ according to the recipe illustrated in Fig. 28.9. (Actually, we improve the accuracy of the fits by including all 19 adjacent three-coil subsets, because we can alternate what we call ACS and what we call initial data. The first ACS data column can serve as the initial data for the second original data column, and so forth.) The weights for both harmonics are shown in Table 28.2. The remaining $(32 - 10 = 22)$ interspersed k-space points are then found via (28.31). To take these additional ACS data, the time is only reduced by $42/64 \approx 0.656$ instead of the full reduction factor $1/R = 0.5$.

	$w_1^{(p)}$	$w_2^{(p)}$	$w_3^{(p)}$
$1\ (p=0)$	1	1	1
$\exp(-2\pi i \Delta k_{full}\, y)\ (p=1)$	$-2.181 + 1.724i$	$4.549 - 0.573i$	$-2.097 - 1.097i$

Table 28.2: The weights $w_n^{(p)}$ for two harmonics. The $p = 0$ weights are assumed to be identical for identical coils and their common value could be changed from the convenient value (unity) shown to improve the fit. The $p = 1$ weights are found with an augmented approach explained in the text where the least-squares fit is made for the 19 different adjacent pairings of the ten ACS points and their ten adjacent gradient points.

The composite signals lead to an inverse transform and image reconstruction shown in Fig. 28.10a. This rather poor and inflated result is due principally to the limited number of receive coils. To see the errors made in approximating the phase factors, we have calculated *a posteriori* weighted sums of the (now assumed to be known) $B_n(y)$ factors to examine how well (28.28) is satisfied, for $p = 0, 1$. The results are plotted in Fig. 28.11, where, for $p = 1$, both the real and the imaginary parts are shown. The unsatisfactory zero-harmonic fit is especially evident; its 50–100% overshoot is the principal reason the image reconstruction is too large by the same sort of factor.

To improve the reconstruction, we can get closer to the qualitative two-step profile by using more coils, the results for which are shown in Fig. 28.10b. It would also be possible to utilize the freedom to scale our MRI signals to improve the overall normalization, although we have not carried out that rescaling in the examples pertaining to the figure.

Individual Coil Signals and GRAPPA

We have learned how to use a subset of data to make up for less than adequate information about loaded rf coil profiles, but we also see the need for improvements in this usage. A composite signal approach requires additional sensitivity information, especially about the overall normalization, and, perhaps, more coils to generate better fits. In any case, however, methods in which individual coil signals are summed to form composite signals encounter various practical difficulties. For instance, cancelations due to accumulated errors in the coil sensitivities and in the noise are increasingly serious problems as the number of coils

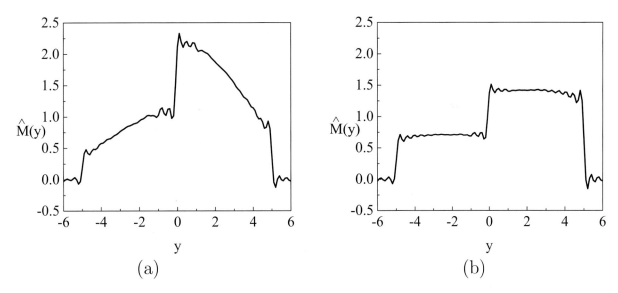

Fig. 28.10: A composite reconstruction for a two-step function profile for (a) three coils with 'unknown' sensitivities. The resultant 64 k-space points are composed of 32 original coil signals ($p = 0$), 10 ACS coil signals ($p = 1$), and 22 interpolated coil signals ($p = 1$). An improved result is shown in (b) by using the five coils introduced in Sec. 28.3.1. These are oversimplified AUTO-SMASH examples with limited coil arrays and data.

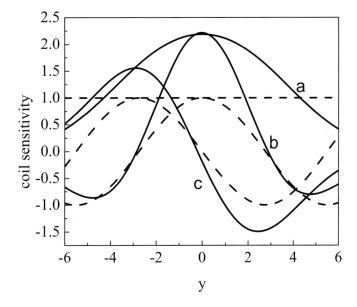

Fig. 28.11: An assessment of the effectiveness in representing the two harmonics, $p = 0, 1$ for the three-coil problem with unknown sensitivities. The curves (a), (b), and (c) refer to constant, cosine, and (negative of) sine fits, respectively. The dashed lines are the corresponding exact results. Improvement in the fits can be achieved by designing different coils and with more information about the overall normalization of their sensitivities.

grows. (A brief discussion on the incorporation of noise into the parallel image reconstruction algorithms is found in Sec. 28.4.)

These difficulties are addressed by an improved usage of data to account for the unknown coil sensitivities. In this approach, the individual coil signals themselves play the role of the composite signal. As previously, additional autocalibration signal points (i.e., lines in 2D) are sampled to generate the weightings in relating unacquired points to acquired points. The weights are introduced in the following sum over known individual coil signals

$$s_n(k_{m'} + p\Delta k_{full}) = \sum_{n'=1}^{N_c} \sum_{q=-N_q^-}^{N_q^+} w_{n,n'}^{(p,q)} s_{n'}(k_{m'} + q\Delta k_{PI})$$

$$p = 1, \cdots, R-1, \quad N_q^- + N_q^+ + 1 = N_q$$

$$\text{for } \{k_{m'} + p\Delta k_{full}\}_{ACS} \tag{28.34}$$

where the ACS subset is defined as in (28.32) and corresponds to a given m' and p. N_q is the total number of gradient data points used in the fit; N_q^- and N_q^+ determine how many are to the left and right of the ACS point, respectively; and recall $\Delta k_{PI} = R\Delta k_{full}$. The goal is to find the weights $w_{n,n'}^{(p,q)}$ for all $N_c \times N_q$ pairs (n', q) for each of the given $N_c \times (R-1)$ pairs (n, p). The method then is to apply those same weights to find the missing points between k_m and k_{m+1}, for $m \neq m'$. To help visualize the fitting procedures, we refer the reader to the corresponding cartoon in Fig. 28.12.

Continuing our pattern of PI study, we demonstrate how to find a reconstructed two-step image with GRAPPA. Again, the gradient and ACS data are acquired with the same three coils of Sec. 28.1, but no direct knowledge of $\mathcal{B}_n(y)$ is assumed. If we follow the schematic of Fig. 28.12, we require 12 weights $w_{n,n'}^{(p,q)}$ for each coil n, but (28.34) yields only one equation for a given set of n, m', and p. Therefore we need (i) more ACS points (i.e., more gradient data points, which will lead to an increase in the time of the experiment) and (ii) a smaller

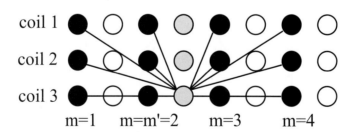

Fig. 28.12: The axes and circles follow the conventions in Fig. 28.9. However, now the lines are drawn from original individual coil data points and connected to an ACS individual coil signal. The lines refer to the action of approximating the ACS signal by a sum of weighted coil signals over the neighboring points, where the weights in this fit are calculated using (28.34). In the cartoon, we see that 12 measured coil signals are fitted to a single ACS point acquired by coil number $n = 3$, for which $R = 2$, $m' = 2$, $N_q^- = 1$, $N_q^+ = 2$ (so the total number of black columns is $N_q = 4$). All unacquired (white) signals for this same coil can be found with these weights applied to an analogous neighborhood.

neighborhood that includes only the adjacent original gradient points. For $p = 1$ (i.e., $R = 2$), and the same 10 total ACS sets (10 columns of three gray circles where the ten m' values are chosen as in the AUTO-SMASH example), (i) leads to a replacement of 10 original white columns by gray columns, and (ii) eliminates the two outside columns of black circles (the total number of original neighborhood gradient points is reduced to $N_q = 2$).

In the above schematic, the 18 weights, $w_{n,n'}^{(1,q)}$, with $q = 0, 1$, are determined by a least-squares procedure over the ACS sets. We repeat the ploy used in the AUTO-SMASH example to increase the number of points available to us for this fit. We alternate between what we call the ACS set and the original set to expand what we call 'ACS' sets from 10 to 19. Each set has three 'ACS' coil signals and its six adjacent coil signals (i.e., two adjacent columns of black or gray circles for this expanded set). The fits give the 18 weights shown in Table 28.3, which can be applied via (28.34) to find the remaining $(32 - 10 = 22)$ points as in the previous composite example, but with one difference.

	$s_1(k_m + \Delta k_{full})$	$s_2(k_m + \Delta k_{full})$	$s_3(k_m + \Delta k_{full})$
$s_1(k_m)$	$-0.382 + 0.371i$	$-0.085 + 0.292i$	$-0.030 + 0.320i$
$s_2(k_m)$	$0.572 + 0.254i$	$0.583 - 0.059i$	$0.591 - 0.423i$
$s_3(k_m)$	$-0.062 - 0.227i$	$-0.114 - 0.231i$	$-0.433 - 0.289i$
$s_1(k_m + 2\Delta k_{full})$	$-0.380 - 0.369i$	$-0.009 - 0.301i$	$0.128 - 0.292i$
$s_2(k_m + 2\Delta k_{full})$	$0.487 - 0.386i$	$0.579 + 0.059i$	$0.462 + 0.554i$
$s_3(k_m + 2\Delta k_{full})$	$0.055 + 0.226i$	$-0.053 + 0.249i$	$-0.430 + 0.288i$

Table 28.3: The 18 weights $w_{n,n'}^{(1,q)}$ for $n, n' = 1, 2, 3$ and $q = 0, 1$ found from the fits of the six adjacent coil signals to the three 'ACS' coil signals with the fitting procedure explained in the text.

The difference is that we are missing the right-most-adjacent column of black circles in attempting to fill in the last column of white circles. We find that the final image reconstruction is not sensitive to how we handle this. That is, whether we just assume the coil signals are zero for $m = 33$ or whether we 'measure' them, the reconstruction is indistinguishable to the eye.

With the above example and handling of the analysis, the 192 (3 sets of 64) individual coil signals $s_n(k_m)$ are at our disposal for the computation of the inverse transforms $\hat{S}_n(y)$ via (28.4). We recall from Sec. 15.1.4 and Prob. 15.3 that SNR may be maximized by taking a sum-of-squares of the individual coil contributions.[12] Hence, for identical noise from each coil and given that we know the coil images $\hat{S}_n(y)$ separately, we may apply the sum-of-squares to obtain the magnitude approximation, defined as $\tilde{S}(y)$, and given by

$$\tilde{S}(y) = \left(\sum_{n=1}^{N_c} \left| \hat{S}_n(y) \right|^2 \right)^{\frac{1}{2}} \qquad (28.35)$$

This leads to the reconstruction of the two-step function shown in Fig. 28.13a for three receive coils. Similar to the SMASH and AUTO-SMASH examples, improvement from the

---

[12]This is also connected to the pseudo-inverse solution for the extremum of the sum-of-squares discussed in Sec. 28.2.2.

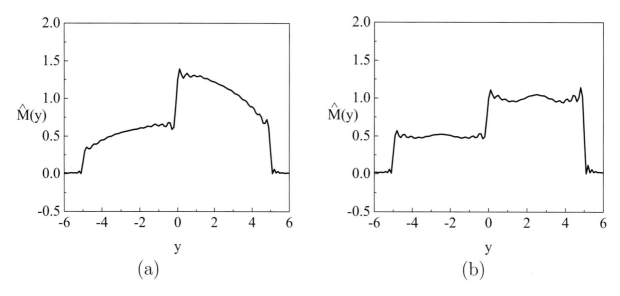

Fig. 28.13: The reconstruction for a two-step function profile for the individual coil fitting procedure generated for (a) a three-coil system with an interpolation based on the adjacent neighborhood
(six coil signals) of one ACS set of three-coil signals. An improved result is shown in (b) by using
the five coils described in Sec. 28.3.1. These are oversimplified GRAPPA examples with limited
coil arrays and data.

employment of five coils is evident in Fig. 28.13b. Even for the small neighborhood (the
adjacent signals in k-space) used in the rather trivial two-step illustration, the method has
proven to be quite effective, especially in achieving a good overall scale. In comparison with
Fig. 28.10, we find improved normalization.

   In the practical imaging world, one can take advantage of good statistics from fits along
the 2D lines of data. Following SMASH and AUTO-SMASH, modern versions of GRAPPA
lead to outstanding advances in fast imaging. With GRAPPA, however, it is important to
note that the discussion has moved from fitting harmonic functions with a series of sensitivity
functions to finding interpolated results for k-space points between the gradient encoding
points.

Problem 28.5

Simple $p = 1$ GRAPPA weights are given below in a table. Using (28.34) and
(28.35), find a formula, in terms of the weights w_{ij} and the coil signals $s_i(k_m)$
and $s_i(k_m + 2\Delta k_{full})$, for the magnitude image $\tilde{S}(y)$, where the operation of the
inverse Fourier transform may be denoted by $\mathcal{F}^{-1}$.

	$s_1(k_m + \Delta k_{full})$	$s_2(k_m + \Delta k_{full})$
$s_1(k_m)$	w_{11}	w_{12}
$s_2(k_m)$	w_{21}	w_{22}
$s_1(k_m + 2\Delta k_{full})$	w_{31}	w_{32}
$s_2(k_m + 2\Delta k_{full})$	w_{41}	w_{42}

28.4   Noise and the g-Factor

In our previous sections, we have reconstructed noiseless images to simplify the explanations and signal processing. Modeling the real world, however, requires the incorporation of noise, which leads to complications in parallel imaging arising from the coupling of the different rf coils to each other. In this section, we address how aliasing and noise affect SNR in x-space followed by remarks concerning noise in k-space.

28.4.1   SNR and g-Factor Derivation

Looking back at Ch. 15, we developed imaging formulas indicating that the signal-to-noise ratio decreases for fewer phase encoding steps at fixed image resolution. Thus parallel imaging typically leads to the reduction, SNR $\propto 1/\sqrt{R}$, for an acceleration factor $R > 1$. In general, there is an additional reduction, due to the interplay of aliasing and the overlapping of the coil sensitivities, that is represented by the so-called g-factor. It is defined in the denominator of the proportionality constant between under-sampled and fully sampled SNRs as follows

$$SNR_R \equiv \frac{SNR_{R=1}}{g\sqrt{R}} \tag{28.36}$$

after separating out the expected $\sqrt{R}$ factor. Because the coil sensitivities generally extend beyond the FOV, aliasing can lead to $g > 1$. In addition, g will depend on coil noise including the secondary noise coming from any significant coupling between coils. We will derive a formula for the g-factor in terms of the coil sensitivities and noise and then discuss simple SENSE examples in the following.

Consider first the case where there is no coupling between coils and the noise from each coil arises only from its own electronics, signal digitization, and sample sensitivity. The generalization of the quadratic function we wish to minimize for an excess of coil data (such as $N_c > N_r$ in Sec. 28.2.2) is (28.18) weighted by the individual coil variances $\sigma_i{}^2$

$$F_{\text{noise weighted}} = \sum_{i=1}^{N_c} \frac{\left| \hat{S}_i - \sum_{j=1}^{N_r} \mathcal{B}_{ij} \hat{M}_j \right|^2}{\sigma_i{}^2} \tag{28.37}$$

To include weighting due to coupling between the coils, we first need to define the general noise matrix.

Define Ψ as the image-space coil noise covariance (square) matrix whose off-diagonal elements give the noise cross-correlation matrix between coils

$$\Psi \equiv \overline{(\eta - \bar{\eta})(\eta - \bar{\eta})^\dagger} \tag{28.38}$$

where, in the present context, the image noise η is defined by[13]

$$\hat{S} = \mathcal{B}\hat{M} + \eta \tag{28.39}$$

---

[13]We refer the reader to Ch. 15 and, for example, (15.18).

The overhead bar in (28.38) indicates the same time average as in the definition of $\bar{\eta}$. (Note that the covariance matrix is Hermitian: $\Psi^\dagger = \Psi$.) We thus seek both $\hat{M}$ and its associated noise η_M in the following.

In matrix form, the generalization of (28.37) is given by

$$F_{\text{noise weighted}} = (\hat{S} - \mathcal{B}\hat{M})^\dagger \Psi^{-1}(\hat{S} - \mathcal{B}\hat{M}) \tag{28.40}$$

In the decoupling limit, the $N_c \times N_c$ noise matrix Ψ is diagonal with elements and inverse

$$\Psi_{\text{no coupling, } ij} = \delta_{ij}\sigma_i^2 \quad \text{or} \quad \Psi^{-1}_{\text{no coupling, } ij} = \delta_{ij}/\sigma_i^2 \tag{28.41}$$

It is thus observed that (28.41) reduces to (28.37) in this limit.

By steps (here and below, we leave some details for the reader to flesh out in Prob. 28.6) similar to those in Sec. 28.2.2, the extremum conditions for (28.40) lead to the pseudo-inverse solution given by

$$\hat{M} = (\mathcal{B}^\dagger \Psi^{-1} \mathcal{B})^{-1} \mathcal{B}^\dagger \Psi^{-1} \hat{S} \tag{28.42}$$

with a second equation for $\hat{M}^\dagger$ merely the adjoint of (28.42) and nothing new. The noise η_M in the reconstructed magnetization $\hat{M}$ is related through (28.42) to the image-space noise in $\hat{S}$

$$\eta_M = (\mathcal{B}^\dagger \Psi^{-1} \mathcal{B})^{-1} \mathcal{B}^\dagger \Psi^{-1} \eta \tag{28.43}$$

For uncoupled white noise, $\bar{\eta} = 0$ and (28.38) reduces to (28.41). The image domain noise column matrix has elements η_i for the ith coil.

To obtain the g-factor, we require the variance σ_M^2 of the reconstructed $\hat{M}$ analogous to (28.38)

$$\sigma_M^2 \equiv \overline{\eta_M \eta_M^\dagger} \tag{28.44}$$

where $\bar{\eta}_M$ is assumed to be zero. Inserting (28.43) into (28.44), noting $\overline{\eta\eta^\dagger} = \Psi$, and using identities such as $A^\dagger B^\dagger = (BA)^\dagger$, we find via Prob. 28.6

$$\sigma_M^2 = (\mathcal{B}^\dagger \Psi^{-1} \mathcal{B})^{-1} \tag{28.45}$$

The covariance matrix (28.45) contains the effects of coil coupling and the overlapping of their sensitivities.

For the SENSE example in Sec. 28.2.2, the signal-to-noise for the ith pixel (with position y_i) in the set of aliased pixels is inversely proportional to the product of the square root of the ith diagonal element of (28.45) times the time-reduction factor $\sqrt{R}$. If we have no aliasing for $R = 1$, $\mathcal{B}$ is reduced to a column matrix such that $(\mathcal{B}^\dagger \Psi^{-1} \mathcal{B})_{R=1}$ is just a number for each pixel i. Hence $[(\mathcal{B}^\dagger \Psi^{-1} \mathcal{B})^{-1}]_{ii, R=1} = [(\mathcal{B}^\dagger \Psi^{-1} \mathcal{B})_{ii, R=1}]^{-1}$. The ratio of the reduced SNR to the full SNR for a given pixel i is therefore

$$\frac{SNR_{i,R}}{SNR_{i,R=1}} = \frac{1}{g_i\sqrt{R}} \tag{28.46}$$

where

$$g_i = \sqrt{[(\mathcal{B}^\dagger \Psi^{-1} \mathcal{B})^{-1}]_{ii,R} \ (\mathcal{B}^\dagger \Psi^{-1} \mathcal{B})_{ii,R=1}} \tag{28.47}$$

The g-factor is independent of the field scale and $\mathcal{B}$ can have arbitrary units in its calculations.

28.4.2   g-Factor Example

We can make use of the earlier example of a pair of overlapping coplanar coils shown in Fig. 28.4. We assume the sampling points to be reduced by one-half, which is to be made up for in parallel imaging by the two rf coils, $R = 2$. Starting with no aliasing in the fully sampled experiment, we only need two replicates for the reduced sampling in (28.11). For convenience, choose the same two aliased points, y_1 and y_2 shown in the figure.

In this example, we shall ignore the noise coupling between the coils (recall from Sec. 27.4 how overlapped coils can be decoupled) and assume the matrix Ψ is diagonal with the same noise variance in each coil. Then Ψ cancels out in the g-factor, and any deviation from unity will be due to aliasing.

The fully sampled and reduced-sampled sensitivities are thereby described by 2×1 column and 2×2 square matrices given in (28.19) and (28.21), respectively. With a and b real, these lead to the matrix products

$$(\mathcal{B}^\dagger\mathcal{B})_{R=1} = a^2 + b^2 \tag{28.48}$$

$$(\mathcal{B}^\dagger\mathcal{B})_{R=2} = \begin{pmatrix} a^2 + b^2 & 2ab \\ 2ab & a^2 + b^2 \end{pmatrix} \tag{28.49}$$

The inverse of the reduced sampling product is

$$(\mathcal{B}^\dagger\mathcal{B})_{R=2}^{-1} = \frac{1}{(a^2 - b^2)^2}\begin{pmatrix} a^2 + b^2 & -2ab \\ -2ab & a^2 + b^2 \end{pmatrix} \tag{28.50}$$

The g-factor for either pixel, $i = 1$ (y_1) or $i = 2$ (y_2) is the same

$$g_{ii} = \sqrt{(\mathcal{B}^\dagger\mathcal{B})_{ii,\,R=2}^{-1}(\mathcal{B}^\dagger\mathcal{B})_{ii,\,R=1}} = \frac{a^2 + b^2}{|a^2 - b^2|} \geq 1 \tag{28.51}$$

For the numbers illustrated in Fig. 28.4, $a = 0.9$, $b = 0.2$, we find $g_{11} = g_{22} = 1.10$, representing a small loss in SNR. For values of b close to a, the g-factor indicates a serious loss of SNR. In general, the g-factor values, and their maxima, are a function of R and range from $g = 1$ for $R = 1$ to $g \approx 1.5$–2.0 for $R = 2$ with typical coil designs. Parallel coils are considered in Prob. 28.6.

Problem 28.6

a) Beginning with their respective preceding equations, derive (28.42) and (28.45). You may want to make use of the steps indicated in the text.

b) Consider the two parallel coils shown in Fig. 28.14. As in the coplanar example, assume $R = 2$, two replicates, and choose two aliased pixel points, $P = (0, -5\,\text{cm}, 0)$, and its alias $Q = (0, 5\,\text{cm}, 0)$, on the opposite edge of the FOV. Again assume the noise is diagonal with the same variance for both coils. Only the single y-component of either sensitivities is nonzero along the y-axis and it is given by the on-axis formula (27.4) for circular loops. If $\mathcal{B}_{coil\,1}(P)$ for the left coil is normalized to unity, show that $\mathcal{B}_{coil\,1}(Q)$ is 0.30. Then show $g_{ii} = 1.20$. Hint: Note g is independent of the overall scale of the sensitivity (so that real numbers can be used in place of imaginary for the y-component). The text example is therefore of immediate use here.

c) By a numerical calculation, test whether the g-factor is changed when the noise variance is different for the two uncoupled coils. Additionally, is it a good approximation to ignore any coupling between the two coils in this example?

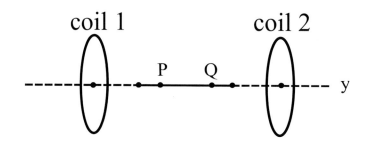

Fig. 28.14: Sampling an aliased uniform spin distribution with two parallel coils and the (reduced) FOV $L = 10$ cm. Each coil has radius 10 cm and they face each other with center positions (0, 20 cm, 0) and (0, −20 cm, 0), respectively. The point P is at (0, −5 cm, 0) with its aliased point Q at (0, 5 cm, 0).

28.5 Additional Topics in Acquisition and Reconstruction

The astute reader may very well ask about the use of multiple coils for the transmit step in MRI and, if experienced in general methods of image processing, she or he may also wonder about the application of 'compressed sensing,' an exciting new development to enable faster imaging for many applications including MRI. In this final section, we very briefly introduce the ideas of parallel transmission and of other methods for utilizing reduced data.

28.5.1 Parallel Transmit Coils

An array of transmit coils can be used to provide new degrees of freedom for rf pulse excitation, analogous to those for an array of receive coils. Two particularly important applications are to use multiple smaller-size transmit coils to 1) 'shim' the B_1 field and/or 2) excite separate ROIs. The first is to compensate for the shorter rf wavelengths required for the higher main magnet field strengths B_0. By adjusting the amplitudes and phases of each coil current, the effective B_1 profile is made more uniform over a larger sampling volume. The second application can be used to speed up imaging or the signal acquisition from a particularly small (localized) region.

How one is to drive the array of small coils is the key to both applications. It is important to map out the B_1 field profile or, simply, to know the flip angle generated locally for a given amplifier power. Comparison of gradient echo signals collected with different flip angles or different repeat times offer several means to solve this problem although there is a variety of similar approaches for B_1 mapping. (For some background on these concepts see Prob. 18.7, Secs. 22.4.2 and 22.5.2, and the references on measuring the actual flip angle in Suggested Reading at the end of this chapter.)

While the treatment of the excitation by a number of overlapping transmit coils has similarities to that of the overlapping receive coils discussed earlier (such as the least-squares calculations in dealing with combinations of sensitivities), we also need to consider the ability to manipulate temporally the rf pulse response using time domain pulse analysis for rf localization (Ch. 16). This is to be integrated into the spatial modeling of each coil in the array. Parallel transmit is a major topic of ultra-high field research in MRI today.

28.5.2 Interpolation, Extrapolation, and Randomization

Certain k-space methods described in this chapter are based on data interpolation concepts (sometimes in a least-squares weighting sense) to fill in missing data with estimated values. In the previous discussion of AUTO-SMASH, for instance, the fleshing out was accomplished by using ACS neighborhoods to estimate a set of weights and then using these weights to help predict nearby missing k-space points. However, this approach may not work well when the points are far from the ACS locations since the weights calculated are not guaranteed to represent the expected k-space behavior far away from the ACS neighborhood. Such differences can arise from the spatial variations of structures in the image itself.

There is another approach to fast imaging, which may be termed 'data extrapolation.' These methods usually collect the center of k-space and attempt to extrapolate the data into regions where there are no data. The partial Fourier methods of Ch. 13 are examples. In some cases, an appropriate change in the basis functions (i.e., generally different from the Fourier transform) is made. After extrapolation, the Fourier image reconstruction can be used again. Initial work in this direction using constrained reconstruction approaches and auto-regressive moving average approaches showed that a 128×128 data set could be used to extrapolate up to at least 256×256 or higher leading to a potential time savings of a factor of 4 or greater. Connecting to both interpolation and extrapolation, we recall zero padding where data are filled out with zeros in order to meet image reconstruction targets. This was also introduced in Ch. 13.

Yet another approach is the widely applied method called 'compressed sensing.' This important development centers on the fact that in MRI, for example, there may be only a small fraction of voxels with significant signal. Such sparsity leads to effective algorithms that randomly undersample k-space, especially for applications such as MR angiography. Scanning time can be very usefully reduced, as shown in a seminal reference given in the Suggested Reading, for 2D and 3D Cartesian Fourier imaging. Accelerations as high as $R = 5$ for MRA were already reported in the initial work. Compressed sensing has since been a major topic of MR research and applications.

Marrying these three ideas may well be feasible where the center of k-space is collected out to something like 128 points, and extra points are then collected to serve as constraints near regions of zero crossings, and then parallel imaging used to save time in the center of k-space. Constraints are used to iterate between the original data collection and applied in the image domain until the missing k-space values are reasonably estimated. Containing the center of k-space is a feature of Cartesian methods but this is not necessarily true for radial or spiral methods. Various combinations of methods will continue to be developed and bode well for the future of fast imaging.

Problem 28.7

Discuss the following:

a) How does partial Fourier imaging compare to the $R = 2$ case of parallel imaging? Consider the case when all data are collected from the origin to after the echo and the case where the data are collected by sampling all the odd data before the echo, at the echo itself, and at the even points after the echo.

b) How could parallel imaging be used in combination with extrapolation methods?

c) How could parallel imaging be used in combination with compressed sensing? Consider both receive and transmit SENSE, for example.

Suggested Reading

The idea of using more rf detector coils to take over the role of the gradient coils has been discussed in work predating the methods described in this chapter:

- J. W. Carlson. An algorithm for NMR imaging reconstruction based on multiple RF receiver coils. *J. Magn. Reson.* 74: 376, 1987.

- M. Hutchinson and U. Raff. Fast MRI data acquisition using multiple detectors. *Magn. Reson. Med.* 6: 87, 1988.

- D. Kwiat, S. Einav and G. Navon. A decoupled coil detector array for fast image acquisition in magnetic resonance imaging. *Med. Phys.* 18: 251, 1991.

The original papers on SENSE, SMASH, AUTO-SMASH, and GRAPPA:

- K. P. Pruessmann, M. Weiger, M. B. Scheidegger and P. Boesiger. SENSE: sensitivity encoding for fast MRI. *Magn. Reson. Med.* 42: 952, 1999.

- D. K. Sodickson and W. J. Manning. Simultaneous acquisition of spatial harmonics (SMASH): Fast imaging with radiofrequency coil arrays. *Magn. Reson. Med.* 38: 591, 1997.

- P. M. Jakob, M. A. Griswold, R. R. Edelman and D. K. Sodickson. AUTO-SMASH: a self-calibrating technique for SMASH imaging. SiMultaneous Acquisition of Spatial Harmonics. *MAGMA* 7: 42, 1998.

- M. A. Griswold, P. M. Jakob, R. M. Heidemann, M. Nittka, V. Jellus, J. Wang, B. Kiefer and A. Haase. Generalized autocalibrating partially parallel acquisitions (GRAPPA). *Magn. Reson. Med.* 47: 1202, 2002.

The following handbook is an impressive addition to the MRI literature and has quite useful sections on parallel imaging:

- M. A. Bernstein, K. F. King and X. J. Zhou. *Handbook of MRI Pulse Sequences.* Elsevier Academic Press, New York, 2004.

Useful references for the last section of this chapter on transmit sense, extrapolation, and compressed sensing:

- U. Katscher, P. Börnert, C. Leussler and J. S. van den Brink. Transmit SENSE. *Magn. Reson. Med.*, 49: 144, 2003.

- E. M. Haacke, Z. P. Liang and S. H. Izen. Constrained Reconstruction: A superresolution optimal signal-to-noise alternative to the Fourier transform in magnetic resonance imaging. *Med. Phys.*, 16: 388, 1989.

- Z. P. Liang, F. E. Boada, R. Todd Constable, E. M. Haacke, P. C. Lauterbur and M. R. Smith. Constrained reconstruction methods in MR imaging. *Rev. Magn. Reson. Med.*, 4: 67, 1992.

- Z. P. Liang and P. C. Lauterbur. An efficient method for dynamic magnetic resonance imaging. *IEEE Trans. Med. Imag.*, 13: 677, 1994.

- M. R. Smith, S. T. Nichols, R. M. Henkelman and M. L. Wood. Application of autoregressive moving average parametric modeling in magnetic resonance image reconstruction. *IEEE Trans. Med. Imag.*, 5: 132, 1986.

- M. Lustig, D. Donoho and J. M. Pauly. Sparse MRI: The application of compressed sensing for rapid MR imaging. *Magn. Reson. Med.*, 58: 1182, 2007.

Appendix A

Electromagnetic Principles: A Brief Overview

Chapter Contents

Introduction

A familiarity with basic electromagnetic properties will assist the reader of this text. A detailed introduction to electromagnetism is beyond the scope of this appendix, but a handful of basic principles and concepts pertinent to MRI are presented, prima facie, in this appendix. The electricity and magnetism sections in introductory college physics texts for engineers and scientists are adequate background for the discussion below.

A.1 Maxwell's Equations

All electromagnetic fields are found to obey Maxwell's equations

$$
(a) \quad \vec{\nabla} \cdot \vec{B} = 0
$$
(no magnetic charges)

$$
(b) \quad \vec{\nabla} \cdot \vec{D} = \rho_q
$$
(Gauss's law)

$$
(c) \quad \vec{\nabla} \times \vec{E} + \frac{\partial \vec{B}}{\partial t} = 0
$$
(Faraday's law)

$$
(d) \quad \vec{\nabla} \times \vec{H} = \vec{J} + \frac{\partial \vec{D}}{\partial t}
$$
(Ampère's law)

$$(A.1)$$

where

$$
\vec{D} = \epsilon \vec{E} \qquad\qquad \vec{B} = \mu \vec{H} \tag{A.2}
$$

with dielectric constant ϵ and permeability μ. The electric charge density is ρ_q and the electric current density (current per unit area) is $\vec{J}$. In theory, all electromagnetic principles applied in this text can be directly derived from these equations but, in practice, it is much easier to work with particular forms and limits of (A.1), some of which will be presented below.

Integral Forms of Maxwell's Equations

Maxwell's equations can also be written in integral form, instead of derivative form. For constant ϵ and μ, we have

$$
\begin{aligned}
(a) &\quad \oint \vec{B} \cdot d\vec{A} = 0 & \text{no magnetic charges}\\
(b) &\quad \epsilon \oint_S \vec{E} \cdot d\vec{A} = \int_V d^3x\, \rho_q(\vec{x}) = q & \text{Gauss's law}\\
(c) &\quad \oint \vec{E} \cdot d\vec{\ell} = -\frac{d}{dt}\left(\int \vec{B} \cdot d\vec{S} \right) & \text{Faraday's law}\\
(d) &\quad \oint \vec{B} \cdot d\vec{\ell} = \mu I + \mu\epsilon \frac{d}{dt}\left(\int \vec{E} \cdot d\vec{S} \right) & \text{Ampère's law}
\end{aligned}
$$
$$(A.3)$$

A key point of Maxwell's equations is that time-varying magnetic fields give rise to electric fields, and vice versa. This is the basis of the detection of the MRI signal (see Secs. A.2 and 7.1).

Another basic notion relevant to MR discussions is that currents (or current densities $\vec{J}$) produce magnetic fields. In MRI, the static field is by definition time independent, the gradient field has mild time dependence, and the rf field is in a relatively low frequency band. Therefore, the time dependence in general can be factored out, and the spatial dependence determined by static methods.

A.2 Faraday's Law of Induction

Faraday's law of induction is

$$
\oint \vec{E} \cdot d\vec{\ell} = -\frac{d}{dt}\left(\int \vec{B} \cdot d\vec{S} \right) \tag{A.4}
$$

Defining the magnetic flux through a surface to be

$$\Phi_B = \int \vec{B} \cdot d\vec{S} \tag{A.5}$$

and considering the case where the surface is bounded by a wire loop, the electromotive force (*emf*) or voltage induced across the ends of the wire is given by

$$emf = \oint \vec{E} \cdot d\vec{\ell} \tag{A.6}$$

When (A.5) and (A.6) are substituted into (A.4), a more familiar form of Faraday's law

$$emf = -\frac{d\Phi_B}{dt} \tag{A.7}$$

is found. Faraday's law states that a time-varying magnetic flux through a loop of wire, or any circuit, generates a voltage whose amplitude is proportional to the (negative of the) time rate of change of the flux. The time-varying magnetic fields associated with the precessing magnetization in MRI induce voltages in the MRI rf receive coil, giving rise to the MRI signal (see Sec. 7.2 for specific details).

A.3   Electromagnetic Forces

Individual electric charges immersed in an electric field or moving through a magnetic field experience electromagnetic forces. The electric force on a charged particle is proportional to, and along the direction of, the electric field. The force generated by a magnetic field on a charged particle is in the direction determined by the right-hand rule perpendicular to the plane defined by the particle's velocity and the direction of the magnetic field. These relations are quantified by the respective Lorentz force and force density equations

$$\vec{F} = q\vec{E} + q\vec{v} \times \vec{B}$$
$$\vec{\mathcal{F}} = \rho\vec{E} + \vec{J} \times \vec{B} \tag{A.8}$$

While a charge at rest in a purely magnetic field experiences no force, a moving charge is deflected by a force perpendicular to its motion. Information about $\vec{B}$ and the charge-to-mass ratio can be determined by measuring such deflections.

Magnetic Charges

There is, at present, no physical evidence for the existence of individual magnetic charges (magnetic monopoles). However, the concept of a magnetic charge can be useful, especially when studying magnetic dipoles which can be modeled as two magnetic charges separated by a fixed distance. The forces on a magnetic charge q_m would be given by

$$\vec{F} = q_m\vec{B} - q_m\vec{v} \times \vec{E} \tag{A.9}$$

A.4   Dipoles in an Electromagnetic Field

The electric dipole moment vector $\vec{d}$ for a system of two opposite charges $\pm q$ separated by a fixed distance d is

$$\vec{d} = qd\hat{n} \qquad (A.10)$$

where $\hat{n}$ points from the negative to the positive charge along the line connecting the two charges. Analogously, the magnetic dipole moment vector $\vec{\mu}_m$ corresponding to two magnetic charges $\pm q_m$ in place of the electric charges is given by

$$\vec{\mu}_m = q_m d\hat{n} \qquad (A.11)$$

In considering the behavior of a magnetic dipole in a magnetic field (the situation of primary interest in MRI), it is useful to continue to keep in mind the analogous behavior of an electric dipole in an electric field.

In a spatially uniform magnetic field, the forces on either charge in a dipole would be equal and opposite so there will be no net force on the dipole. However, there is a net torque on the dipole

$$\vec{N} = \vec{\mu}_m \times \vec{B} \qquad (A.12)$$

Alternatively, if a dipole is placed in a spatially varying field, the force on the two charges are different, giving rise to a net force

$$\vec{F} = \vec{\nabla}(\vec{\mu}_m \cdot \vec{B}) \qquad (A.13)$$

From (A.13), a potential energy associated with an arbitrary orientation of a dipole in a magnetic field may be identified as

$$U = -\vec{\mu}_m \cdot \vec{B} \qquad (A.14)$$

That is, the forces that apply torque to a dipole in a magnetic field, lead to a preferential (lower potential energy) orientation of the dipole parallel to the applied field.

Magnetic Moment Defined by Current Loop

A classical magnetic dipole moment $\vec{\mu}_m$ may also be defined in terms of a current loop. The magnetic moment $\vec{\mu}_m$ associated with a circular loop with radius a carrying a current I is given by

$$\vec{\mu}_m = I\vec{A} = \pi a^2 I \hat{n} \qquad (A.15)$$

where $\hat{n}$ is the normal to the coil. While a current loop and a magnetic charge dipole have fundamentally different internal fields, they have a similar interaction with an external magnetic field through their magnetic dipole moments.

A.5   Formulas for Electromagnetic Energy

In the absence of constraints, groups of electrical charges arrange themselves into a lowest energy state. One way of describing this is that the positive and negative charges move to positions where the electric field is minimized in some way over the volume of the system. Indeed, the electromagnetic energy in free space may be directly associated with the fields according to

$$U = \frac{1}{2\mu_0} \int_V d^3x \left| \vec{B} \right|^2 + \frac{\epsilon_0}{2} \int_V d^3x \left| \vec{E} \right|^2 \tag{A.16}$$

The magnetic field energy in (A.16) may be recast in terms of familiar lumped circuit inductances, which is a form useful for a set of current carrying wires and is given by

$$U = \frac{1}{2} \left(\sum_{i=1}^{N} L I_i^2 + \sum_{j \neq i}^{N} \sum_{i=1}^{N} M_{ij} I_i I_j \right) \tag{A.17}$$

where L_i is the self-inductance of each wire and their mutual inductances, M_{ij}, are

$$M_{ij} = \frac{\mu_0}{4\pi} \int d\vec{\ell_i} \cdot \int d\vec{\ell_j} \frac{1}{|\vec{x}_j - \vec{x}_i|} \tag{A.18}$$

A.6   Static Magnetic Field Calculations

The Maxwell equation $\vec{\nabla} \cdot \vec{B} = 0$ and the vector identity

$$\vec{\nabla} \cdot (\vec{\nabla} \times \vec{A}) = 0 \tag{A.19}$$

imply that $\vec{B}$ can be written as the curl of a magnetic vector potential

$$\vec{B} = \vec{\nabla} \times \vec{A} \tag{A.20}$$

The remaining freedom in choosing $\vec{A}$ (a 'gauge' freedom) allows an additional condition. If it is assumed that

$$\vec{\nabla} \cdot \vec{A} = 0 \tag{A.21}$$

then $\vec{\nabla} \times (\vec{\nabla} \times \vec{A}) = \vec{\nabla}(\vec{\nabla} \cdot \vec{A}) - \nabla^2 \vec{A} = -\nabla^2 \vec{A}$. In the case of time-independent fields, (A.1d) can be rewritten as

$$\nabla^2 \vec{A} = -\mu_0 \vec{J} \tag{A.22}$$

The solution of this equation can be shown to be

$$\vec{A}(\vec{x}) = \frac{\mu_0}{4\pi} \int_{volume} d^3x' \frac{\vec{J}(\vec{x}')}{|\vec{x} - \vec{x}'|} \tag{A.23}$$

$$= \frac{\mu_0}{4\pi} \sum_{loops\ i} I_i \int \frac{d\vec{\ell_i}}{|\vec{x} - \vec{x}_i|} \tag{A.24}$$

with the latter form appropriate for a current distribution $\vec{J}$ corresponding to a sum over a set of discrete current loops.

The Biot-Savart Law

Taking the curl of (A.23) or (A.24), respectively, gives the Biot-Savart law for the magnetic field,

$$\vec{B}(\vec{x}) \;=\; \frac{\mu_0}{4\pi}\int_{volume} d^3x' \frac{\vec{J}(\vec{x}') \times (\vec{x} - \vec{x}')}{|\vec{x} - \vec{x}'|^3} \tag{A.25}$$

$$\;=\; \frac{\mu_0}{4\pi}\sum_{loops\; i} I_i \int \frac{d\vec{\ell}_i \times (\vec{x} - \vec{x}_i)}{|\vec{x} - \vec{x}_i|^3} \tag{A.26}$$

These specifically relate time-independent electric currents to the magnetic fields they produce. Historically, such results were found by Biot and Savart from experiment. As the second formula indicates, they found that the differential magnetic field produced by a current element $I_i d\vec{\ell}_i$ is perpendicular to both the direction of the current element and the direction from the current element to the observation point.

Appendix B

Statistics

Chapter Contents

Introduction

Statistical analysis is important for MR experiments. For measurements of T_1 of a tissue, or any other variable, it is generally necessary to quote both a mean value and a standard deviation. In fact, there may be two or more standard deviations to quote, both the conventional white noise standard deviation and one or more systematic errors caused by motion, geometric variations, or other sources. In this appendix, the normal distribution, the Rayleigh distribution, and type I and type II errors are described.

B.1 Accuracy Versus Precision

The 'accuracy' of a measurement is defined here to be the exactness of the measure of a quantity with a given instrument. For example, measuring the frequency of the MR signal may be limited by the characteristics of the rf circuit such that it can only be measured to an accuracy of 1 Hz. The accuracy of an experiment depends on its design and on the available measuring devices.

The 'precision' of a measurement may be defined to be an estimate of how repeatable it is or how close the measured value is from one experiment to the next. For example, if the MR frequency is measured a second time and the magnetic field has changed or the properties of the rf circuit have changed, then the error associated with these temporal changes limits the precision. The measured standard deviation in a repeated experiment is a representation of the precision of an experiment.

It follows that statements of experimental results should include at least two standard errors: the accuracy of the experiment and the precision of the experiment. It may be that the precision of the experiment is affected by a number of factors, in which case each factor should be separately quoted (see also Sec. B.4.1). While a given experiment may be highly reproducible and have a very low precision (i.e., the noise contribution is very small), it may be the case that an accurate measure of the parameters of interest is still not possible.

B.1.1   Mean and Standard Deviation

The mean or average value of a discrete set of measurements for a random variable x is calculated from

$$\overline{x} = \frac{1}{n} \sum_{i=1}^{n} x_i \qquad 1 \le i \le n \tag{B.1}$$

where x might be T_1, for example. The ith measurement is given by x_i, and n represents the number of measurements made.

The 'biased' variance of these measurements is calculated as a measure of the deviation for all measurements from $\overline{x}$.[1] It is the mean squared measure:

$$\sigma_x^2 = \frac{1}{n} \sum_{i=1}^{n} (x_i - \overline{x})^2 \tag{B.2}$$

The standard deviation is the square root of this variation and is given by σ_x.

Problem B.1

---

a) Show for $y = ax$ where a is a constant that

$$\sigma_y^2 = a^2 \sigma_x^2 \tag{B.3}$$

b) If x_i becomes $x_i + a$, show that σ_x^2 is invariant.

c) Show $\sigma_x^2 = \overline{x^2} - \overline{x}^2$ for a sample of size n.

The unbiased form of the variance is known as the sample variance and is written as

$$s_x^2 = \frac{1}{n-1} \sum_{i=1}^{n} (x_i - \overline{x})^2 \tag{B.4}$$

The unbiased estimate of the variance has an expectation value equal to the actual population variance.

---

[1] The estimate of a random variable is said to be 'biased' if, as the number of measurements n used for generating the estimate of the parameter of interest tends to infinity, the mean of the estimate does not approach the true value of the parameter. Accordingly, the difference between the limiting value of the parameter from its actual value is defined as the 'bias.'

B.2 The Gaussian Probability Distribution

B.2.1 Probability Distribution

The probability distribution $P(x)$ may be defined such that the differential probability for a random variable x to take on a value between x and $x + dx$ is given by $P(x)dx$. For any $P(x)$, the continuous forms of expectation (true mean) and variance are defined by

$$\mu \equiv E(x) \equiv \int_{-\infty}^{\infty} dx \, x P(x) \tag{B.5}$$

and

$$\sigma^2 \equiv E\left((x - \mu)^2\right) \equiv \int_{-\infty}^{\infty} dx \, (x - \mu)^2 P(x) \tag{B.6}$$

The Gaussian or normal distribution, denoted as $N(\mu, \sigma)$, is given by

$$P(x) \equiv \frac{1}{\sigma\sqrt{2\pi}} e^{-(x-\mu)^2/(2\sigma^2)} \tag{B.7}$$

where the following problem assignment is to show that the notation in the definitions (B.5) and (B.6) is consistent with the parameters shown in (B.7). The Gaussian distributed random variable[2] x is said to be $N(\mu, \sigma)$, i.e., normal with mean μ and variance σ^2.

Problem B.2

---

a) Show $\int_{-\infty}^{\infty} dx \, P(x) = 1$, where $P(x)$ is given in (B.7).

b) Show that the mean of the Gaussian distribution $P(x)$ is μ.

c) Show that the variance of the Gaussian distribution $P(x)$ is σ^2.

d) Show $\sigma^2 = E(x^2) - (E(x))^2$ for $P(x)$ in (B.7).

B.2.2 z-Score

The probability of finding an event within some set of values can be expressed in terms of a normalized measure z as follows. Let

$$z \equiv \frac{x - \mu}{\sigma} \tag{B.8}$$

It is convenient to define another distribution $\tilde{P}(z) \equiv \sigma P(x)$ so that the probability that z lies within an interval (z_1, z_2) is given by

$$f(z_1, z_2) \equiv \int_{z_1}^{z_2} \tilde{P}(z)dz \tag{B.9}$$

---

[2]It is often the case that a 'random variable' refers to a Gaussian random variable in the discussions that follow. The function $P(x)$ often represents a Gaussian distribution (B.7).

In particular, the probability that z is smaller than some value z_0 is given by

$$F(z_0) = f(z \leq z_0) \equiv \int_{-\infty}^{z_0} \tilde{P}(z)dz \tag{B.10}$$

where $F(z)$ is the cumulative distribution function. For a Gaussian distribution $N(\mu, \sigma)$, the new distribution is given by

$$\tilde{P}(z) \equiv \frac{1}{\sqrt{2\pi}} e^{-z^2/2} \quad \text{Gaussian distribution} \tag{B.11}$$

B.2.3   Quoting Errors and Confidence Intervals

Once the mean and standard deviation for a distribution are known, it is possible to estimate the precision with which a measurement has been made. For example, the well-known probability of finding a point between $-\sigma$ and σ for an $N(0, \sigma)$ distribution is about 68%.

Problem B.3

---

    a) Show that the probability of finding a point between $(-2\sigma, 2\sigma)$ is approximately 95% and between $(-3\sigma, 3\sigma)$ is approximately 99.7%.

    b) If a set of 100 points is sampled from an $N(0, 1)$ distribution, how many points do you expect to fall between $(-2, 2)$?

B.3   Type I and Type II Errors

The situation of two or more distributions contributing to measurements often arises. A particular hypothesis of interest is whether two measurements have come from either the same or different distributions. Consider the case where two measurements have been made from two normal distributions, $N(0, \sigma)$ and $N(\mu, \sigma)$, as shown in Fig. B.1.

Type I error is the probability $\alpha = 1 - F(z_0)$ that an event which occurs in distribution 1 ($N(0, \sigma)$) is mistaken for an event in distribution 2 ($N(\mu, \sigma)$). It is also referred to as the α-error, p-value, or false positive. It is given by

$$\begin{aligned} \alpha &\equiv p \\ &= 1 - \int_{-\infty}^{z_0} dz\, \tilde{P}(z) \\ &= \frac{1}{2}\text{erfc}(z_0/\sqrt{2}) \end{aligned} \tag{B.12}$$

with the complementary error function $\text{erfc}(y) = 1 - \text{erf}(y)$ where the error function is

$$\text{erf}(y) = \frac{2}{\sqrt{\pi}} \int_0^y du\, e^{-u^2} \tag{B.13}$$

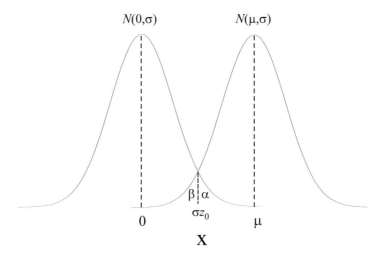

Fig. B.1: Differentiation of two measurements coming from two Gaussian distributions with the same σ. Errors are marked as areas α and β under the respective distributions. For graphical simplicity, z_0 is chosen in the figure such that $\alpha = \beta$.

z_0	1.0	1.5	2.0	2.5	3.0
$F(z_0)$	0.8413	0.9332	0.9773	0.9938	0.9986
α	0.1587	0.0668	0.0227	0.0062	0.0014

Table B.1: Table of type I error values for different z_0.

From standard error function tabulations, it is easy to find a set of common values for α as shown in Table B.1 and to be compared to Prob. B.3.

Type II error is the probability that an event in distribution 2 occurs but is counted as a non-event. This is also referred to as the β-error, q-value, or false negative.

$$
\begin{aligned}
\beta &\equiv q \\
&= \int_{-\infty}^{z_0} dz\, \tilde{P}(z - \mu/\sigma) \\
&= F(z_0 - \mu/\sigma)
\end{aligned}
\tag{B.14}
$$

A receiver operating characteristic curve (usually abbreviated as an ROC curve) can be drawn by plotting the p-values versus the power which is defined in terms of the q-values[3] as $(1 - q)$. The lower the value of p, the more confident one is that the event is not part of distribution 1. The higher $(1 - q)$, the more confident one is that the good events have not been thrown out. The shape of the curve depends on $z_{12} = (\mu_2 - \mu_1)/\sigma$ where μ_1 and μ_2 are the mean values of the two distributions, and $\mu_2 > \mu_1$ (i.e., z_{12} is a sufficient statistic). Figure B.2 shows curves for z_{12} ranging from 1 to 4.

---

[3] A set of ROC curves plotted for different values of p and $(1 - q)$ describes the performance of all observers who use a strictly defined threshold rule to separate the two populations.

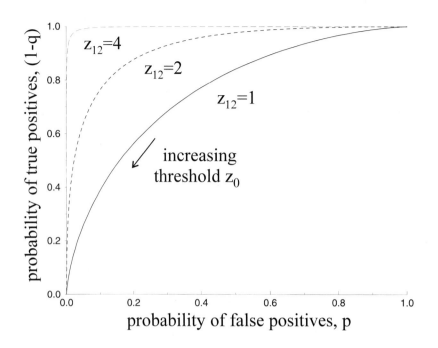

Fig. B.2: An ROC curve for different values of the parameter z_{12}. The larger the value of z_{12}, the farther apart are the two populations, and the easier it is for an observer to classify an observation as belonging to one or the other distribution and, hence, the ROC curve approaches ideality. As z_{12} decreases, the ROC curve approaches that of an observer who is guessing all the time.

B.4   Sum over Several Random Variables

Consider a set of n distributions with random variables x_i from which a set of n measurements (one from each distribution) will be performed. The mean value of the n measurements can be viewed as a normalized sum over n random variables each Gaussian distributed $N(\mu, \sigma)$, i.e., $\overline{x} = (x_1 + x_2 + \cdots + x_n)/n$. The expectation of $\overline{x}$ is then

$$
\begin{aligned}
E(\overline{x}) &= \frac{1}{n} \sum_{i=1}^{n} E(x_i) \\
&= \mu
\end{aligned}
\tag{B.15}
$$

Likewise, since the x_i are all uncorrelated, the variance of $\overline{x}$ is

$$
\begin{aligned}
\mathrm{var}(\overline{x}) &\equiv E\left((\overline{x} - \mu)^2 \right) \\
&= \frac{1}{n^2} E\left(\left(\sum_{i=1}^{n}(x_i - \mu) \right)^2 \right) \\
&= \frac{1}{n^2} \sum_{i=1}^{n} E\left((x_i - \mu)^2 \right) \\
&= \frac{\sigma^2}{n}
\end{aligned}
\tag{B.16}
$$

Hence, the distribution of $\overline{x}$ will also be Gaussian but is distributed $N(\mu, \sigma/\sqrt{n})$, i.e., the standard deviation of the mean is $\sqrt{n}$ times smaller than that from the distribution of the individual random variables themselves. As an example, assume that the noise is measured from 100 points to be 10 units in the center of a uniform phantom and the mean is 1000. The 95% confidence interval for the mean is then (998, 1002).

The use of a histogram can also be a very powerful tool in MRI (see also Sec. B.6.1). If a 3D data set were used to map T_1 values for all the muscles in the leg, for example, and the histogram were Gaussian in nature, then the mean value could be very accurately determined. If the mean were $\overline{x}$ and the number of 3D data points were 2500, then the 99.7% confidence interval for the mean would be $(\overline{x} - 3\sigma/50, \overline{x} + 3\sigma/50)$.

B.4.1 Multiple Noise Sources

For several sources of independent noise, the variance adds in quadrature. Consider three Gaussian distributed random variables x, y, and z. If $z = x + y$, then

$$\text{var}(z) = \text{var}(x) + \text{var}(y) \tag{B.17}$$

when x and y are independent. For the proof of this see Prob. B.4.

Problem B.4

Consider the random variable $z = x + y$ where x and y are uncorrelated (i.e., $E(xy) = 0$) random variables, both $N(0, \sigma)$.

a) Show that $\overline{z} = \overline{x} + \overline{y}$.

b) Show that for uncorrelated data $\text{var}(z) = \text{var}(x) + \text{var}(y)$ or, in alternate notation, $\sigma_z^2 = \sigma_x^2 + \sigma_y^2$.

Consider the case where white noise contributes a variance σ_w^2. Suppose also that ghosting occurs or perhaps there exists some other jitter in the system such as rf power varying in time or from pulse to pulse. These latter sources will be referred to as systematic noise (σ_s^2) even though they may still be white and Gaussian in nature. The total noise variance is

$$\sigma_T^2 = \sigma_w^2 + \sigma_s^2 \tag{B.18}$$

Another simple source for σ_s^2 is from the spatial variation of the sample itself.

Problem B.5

Consider an imperfect rf coil such that it creates a slow linear variation across a uniform phantom. The resulting spin density is

$$\rho(x) = \rho_0 + \lambda x + \eta \tag{B.19}$$

where η is an $N(0, \sigma)$ random variable. You wish to measure the mean and standard deviation at $\rho(0)$ but you must use a region from $x = -x_0$ to $x = x_0$ to get a sufficient number of points for good statistics.

a) Find an expression for σ_T^2 as a function of the geometric factor λ, as well as x_0 and σ^2.

b) If the experiment is repeated N_{acq} times so that σ^2 becomes σ^2/N_{acq} what is the limiting value of σ_T^2? (The remaining variance comes from the shape of $\rho(x)$ in the region $-x_0$ to x_0.) When should N_{acq} be increased no further?

B.5   Rayleigh Distribution

In many instances, the magnitude of the complex image is displayed. The mean and variance must now be calculated for the new random variable

$$z = ((s_R + x)^2 + (s_I + y)^2)^{1/2} \qquad (B.20)$$

where s_R and s_I are the real and imaginary parts of the signal and x and y are $N(0,\sigma)$ random variables. We will consider only the limits where either the noise dominates or the signal dominates.[4] When noise is measured outside an object but within the FOV in a magnitude image, the measured mean $\bar{z}$ and standard deviation σ_z are both proportional to the actual standard deviation of the Gaussian distributed white noise σ in the original complex image. These relationships are found in Prob. B.6. The mean itself is usually used to estimate σ outside the object because spatial variations in the object add to the actual variance. For example, if the mean of the noise measured outside is 125 units, then the actual noise standard deviation σ will be 100 units (see (B.21)). (It should be remembered that the measure $\bar{z}$ is itself an estimate of σ and has an error associated with it.)

Problem B.6 demonstrates that there are two ways to estimate the standard deviation σ of the Gaussian distribution from a Rayleigh distribution. Since the mean of the noise in the Rayleigh distribution is 1.25σ (see (B.21)), then $0.8\bar{z}$ can be used as the estimate for σ. Similarly, $1.5\sigma_z$ can also be used to estimate σ, but variance is a less reliable estimate and, therefore, the former approach is usually used as the estimate for σ.

Problem B.6

Assume $S_R = S_0$ and $S_I = 0$ so that $z = \sqrt{(S_0 + x)^2 + y^2}$.

a) Show that for $S_0 = 0$, the mean of z is

$$\begin{aligned} \bar{z} &= \int\!\!\int dx\, dy\, P(x,y) \cdot z(x,y) \\ &= \sigma\sqrt{\frac{\pi}{2}} \\ &\simeq 1.25\,\sigma \end{aligned} \qquad (B.21)$$

---

[4]The full solution is given by a Rician distribution (see Gudbjartsson and Patz in the Suggested Reading).

where $P(x, y)$ is the joint probability density function for the random variables x and y. Since the random variables x and y are independent, use

$$P(x, y) = P(x) \cdot P(y) \tag{B.22}$$

Hint: Transform from Cartesian coordinates (x, y) to polar coordinates (ρ, θ) to obtain

$$\bar{z} = \frac{1}{2\pi\sigma^2} \int_0^\infty \int_0^{2\pi} d\theta d\rho \, (S_0^2 + 2\rho S_0 \cos\theta + \rho^2)^{1/2} \cdot \rho e^{-\rho^2/2\sigma^2} \tag{B.23}$$

The factor

$$f(\rho) = \frac{1}{\sigma^2} \rho e^{-\rho^2/2\sigma^2} \tag{B.24}$$

represents the Rayleigh distribution.

b) Show that the variance of z is

$$\sigma_z^2 = \int \int dx \, dy \, P(x, y) \cdot ((z(x, y) - \bar{z})^2) \tag{B.25}$$

and for $S_0 = 0$,

$$\begin{aligned} \sigma_z &= (2 - \pi/2)^{1/2}\sigma \\ &\simeq 0.655\,\sigma \end{aligned} \tag{B.26}$$

Note that the Rayleigh distribution is narrower than the Gaussian.

c) Find $\bar{z}$ when $S_0 \gg \sigma$. What do you qualitatively expect it to be?

d) Show $\sigma_z^2 = \sigma^2$ when $S_0 \gg \sigma$.

B.6   Experimental Validation of Noise Distributions

The most straightforward approach used to test the statistical behavior of the system is to run the scan many times. In this section, the images from a single 2D scan run 30 times will be analyzed in a variety of ways to illustrate some of the points discussed in the previous sections.

B.6.1   Histogram Analysis

A very useful construct is to plot a histogram of a region-of-interest. This can lead to a superb measure of a given quantity as the mean $\bar{x}$ will have 95% confidence limits determined by $\bar{x} \pm 2\sigma/\sqrt{n}$ where n is the number of points in the region-of-interest.

The histogram of Gaussian distributed white noise in Fig. B.3d has a measured mean of -0.001 and a standard deviation of 22.53. The region-of-interest contained 15000 pixels. Accordingly, the 95% confidence interval for the mean is -0.001 ± 0.37. An application of this idea would be measuring T_1 of a tissue like gray matter or muscle over a large region-of-interest after a pure T_1 image is obtained (see Ch. 22). Another application is to evaluate whether or not the data follow the expected statistical distributions or are corrupted by other sources of error.

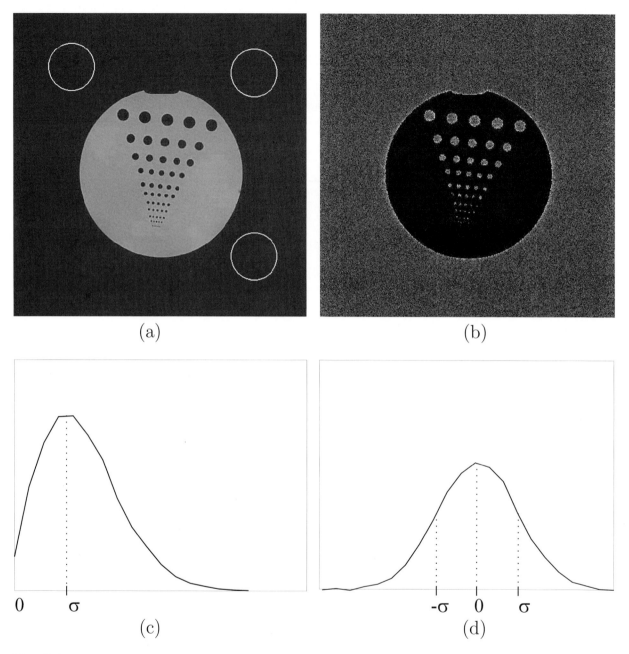

Fig. B.3: White noise distribution from (a) a 2D magnitude image and (b) a real image. The noise is Rayleigh distributed in the magnitude image shown, while it is Gaussian distributed in a real image with the noise highlighted relative to the actual image signal. The magnitude image is shown with three circular regions highlighted. The signal values within these highlighted regions were used to study the statistics of the noise in the respective images. A histogram of the distribution of the approximately 15,000 points is plotted for the three regions shown in (a) for the magnitude image (c) and the real image (d), both reconstructed from the same data set. Both histograms display the expected Rayleigh and Gaussian nature of the respective noise sources.

B.6.2   Mean and Standard Deviation

To demonstrate some of the points discussed in the previous sections, the mean and standard deviation are further evaluated in the same set of 30 images used to create the histogram in Fig. B.3.

The best test of the mean and standard deviation for a single point in an image (magnitude, real, imaginary, or phase) is to repeat the scan many times and measure the same value $\rho(x, y)$ at one coordinate. For one point in the upper right part of the circular phantom in Fig. B.3, the mean $\hat{\rho} = 634$ units and standard deviation $\sigma_\rho = 10$ units.

Problem B.7

The mean and standard deviation measured from the Rayleigh distribution shown in Fig. B.3c are 26.0 and 14.75, respectively. Are these the numbers you would have expected, given the mean and standard deviation of the Gaussian distribution? Give reasons why or why not.

Problem B.8

For a given pixel, what are the 95% confidence intervals for a) the mean over 30 images, and b) the range of values for that pixel from a single image?

Problem B.9

All of the 330 points in the circle shown close to the edge of the phantom in Fig. B.4a are averaged together and give $\hat{\rho} = 626$. The variance of the Gaussian distribution associated with each pixel is 10 units.

a) What is the error in the estimate for the mean?

b) If the measured variance in this region is roughly 10 units, what does this suggest about the spatial variation of the measured signal?

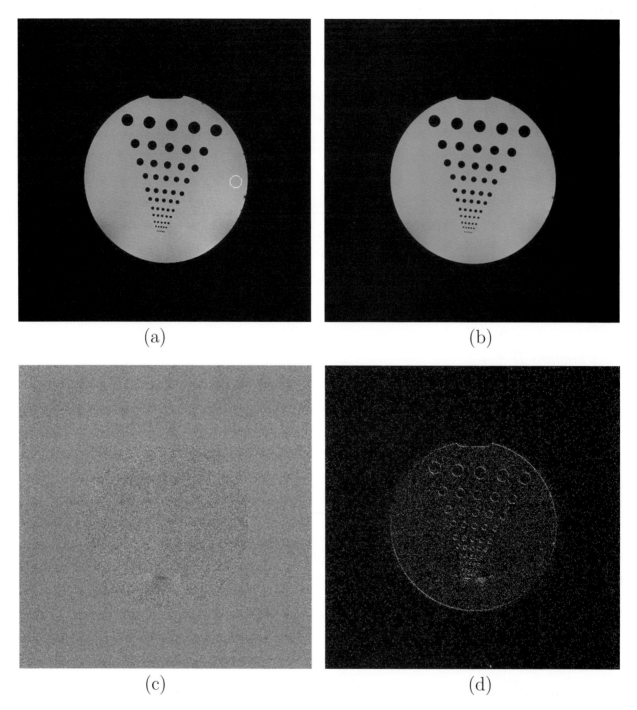

Fig. B.4: Noise behavior of typical MR image acquisitions over multiple acquisitions. (a) One magnitude image from a series of 30 images acquired in a serial manner. (b) Image obtained by averaging the 30 images. As apparent from a comparison of images shown in (a) and (b), the averaged magnitude image has an improved SNR over that of the single image. (c) Image obtained by subtracting two time-adjacent images from the series gives a spatial measure of the temporal stability or variability during the period of acquisition of the 30 images. (d) Image showing the standard deviation of each pixel value over the temporal series. This image again highlights any variability that occurs over the time-period of acquisition of the series of images.

Suggested Reading

- H. Gudbjartsson and S. Patz. The Rician distribution of noisy MRI data. *Magn. Reson. Med.*, 34: 910, 1995.

- R. M. Henkelman. Measurement of signal intensities in the presence of noise in MR images. *Med. Phys.*, 12: 232, 1985. (Erratum: 13: 544, 1986.)

Appendix C

Imaging Parameters to Accompany Figures

On the surface, describing an image may at first sight not appear to be a daunting task, but the devil is in the details. In principle, all information required to reproduce the result being displayed should be given. In practice, it is possible to give a shortened description of the contrast type and sequence design to give a first impression of the origins of the image. Using the appropriate adjectives and the parameters listed here, most images can be well-described. Nevertheless, as new approaches develop, other parameters may be needed to fully describe an image.

Parameter	Symbol (or description)
times	
• field echo time	F_E
• echo time	T_E
• repeat time	T_R
• rf time	τ_{rf}
• sampling interval	Δt
• sampling time	T_s
• inversion or preparation time	T_I or τ_{prep}
gradients	
• read gradient strength	G_R
• slice select gradient	G_{SS}
• flow compensation type	velocity, acceleration, etc.

rf related

- flip angle $\qquad\qquad\qquad\qquad\qquad\qquad\quad$ θ
- rf spoiling $\qquad\qquad\qquad\qquad\qquad$ rf phase increment, ϵ_1
- pulse type $\qquad\qquad\qquad\qquad\quad$ narrowband / broadband
  $\qquad\qquad\qquad\qquad\qquad\qquad\quad$ rectangular / sinc / Gaussian

noise related

- bandwidth/voxel $\qquad\qquad\qquad\qquad\qquad$ $BW/\Delta x$
- number of repetitions (excitations $\qquad\quad$ N_{acq}
  or acquisitions)
- coil type $\qquad\qquad\qquad\qquad$ Helmholtz pair, birdcage, etc.
  $\qquad\qquad\qquad\qquad\qquad\quad$ linearly or circularly polarized

resolution related

- resolution $\qquad\qquad$ Δi for $i = x, y$ or z $(\Delta z = TH$ for 2D)
- field-of-view $\qquad\qquad$ L_i for $i = x, y$ or z (for 3D)
- number of sampled points $\qquad\qquad\qquad$ N_x
- number of phase encoding lines $\qquad\qquad$ N_y
- number of partitions (3D) $\qquad\qquad\qquad$ N_z
- number of slices (multi-slice 2D) $\qquad\quad$ N_s
- matrix display size $\qquad\qquad\qquad\qquad$ N_i^*

reconstruction related

- image reconstruction method $\qquad\quad$ FT, projection reconstruction,
  $\qquad\qquad\qquad\qquad\quad$ partial Fourier reconstruction, etc.
- degree of echo asymmetry $\qquad\qquad$ $(n_+ - n_-)/N_i$
- sampling type $\qquad\qquad\qquad\qquad$ uniform, sinusoidal, etc.
- post-processing method $\qquad\qquad\qquad$ filter type

other

- image slice gap $\qquad\qquad\qquad\qquad$ in multi-slice 2D
- slice order $\qquad\qquad\qquad\qquad$ interleaved, sequential
- gating or triggering $\qquad\qquad\qquad$ respiratory or cardiac
- system specifications $\qquad\qquad\qquad$ gradient rise times
- saturation band $\qquad\qquad\qquad\qquad$ location, thickness
- velocity encoding gradients $\qquad$ critical velocity value, v_c
- diffusion encoding gradient $\qquad\qquad\qquad$ b-value
- k-space order $\qquad\qquad\qquad$ centric, sequential, interleaved

The imaging parameters for the images appearing in all chapters are presented next. The following parameters remain fixed in these images, unless otherwise noted: all rf pulses are Hanning-filtered sinc pulses, images are all reconstructed using DFT image reconstruction, and images are all displayed at the same matrix size as they were collected. If not listed, parameters such as G_R, FOV, and bandwidth/voxel can be calculated from the quoted parameters. In the following list, all imaging parameters are not repeated for each part of a figure. Typically, all imaging parameters are quoted only for the first image. For all other images in that figure, only those parameters that are different from that of the first image are quoted.

Imaging Parameters

19.12 (a), (b) $T_R/T_{E_1}/T_{E_2}/T_{E_3} = 220\,\text{ms}/6.5\,\text{ms}/10.75\,\text{ms}/15.0\,\text{ms}$, $T_s = 1.54\,\text{ms}$, $\Delta x \times \Delta y \times \Delta z = 0.98\,\text{mm} \times 0.98\,\text{mm} \times 4.0\,\text{mm}$, $N_x \times N_y = 256 \times 256$, $\theta = 30°$, $N_{acq} = 1$, $\tau_{rf} = 0.9\,\text{ms}$, $G_{ss} = 7.2\,\text{mT/m}$; (c), (d) $T_E = 5\,\text{ms}$, $T_s = 3.072\,\text{ms}$, $\tau_{rf} = 1.024\,\text{ms}$, $G_{ss} = 5.76\,\text{mT/m}$. 535

19.19 (a) $T_D/T_E = 102.4\,\text{ms}/50\,\text{ms}$, $T_s = 1.54\,\text{ms}$, $\Delta x \times \Delta y \times \Delta z = 1.72\,\text{mm} \times 1.72\,\text{mm} \times 5.0\,\text{mm}$, $N_x \times N_y = 128 \times 128$, $\theta = 90°$, with no fat saturation pre-pulse, $N_{acq} = 1$, $\tau_{rf} = 1.28\,\text{ms}$, $G_{ss} = 10\,\text{mT/m}$; (b) $\theta = 90°$, with fat saturation pre-pulse. 546

19.20 (a), (b) $T_D/T_E = 202\,\text{ms}/52\,\text{ms}$, $T_s = 0.982\,\text{ms}$, $\Delta x \times \Delta y \times \Delta z = 1.95\,\text{mm} \times 2.98\,\text{mm} \times 5.0\,\text{mm}$, $N_x \times N_y = 256 \times 168$, $\theta = 90°$, $N_{acq} = 1$, $\tau_{rf} = 1.28\,\text{ms}$, $G_{ss} = 10\,\text{mT/m}$; (c), (d) $T_R/T_E = 220\,\text{ms}/15\,\text{ms}$, $T_s = 3.072\,\text{ms}$, $\Delta x \times \Delta y \times \Delta z = 1.95\,\text{mm} \times 1.95\,\text{mm} \times 4.0\,\text{mm}$, $N_x \times N_y = 256 \times 256$, $\theta = 30°$, $N_{acq} = 2$, $\tau_{rf} = 1.024\,\text{ms}$, $G_{ss} = 5.76\,\text{mT/m}$. 547

19.21 (a) $T_D/T_E = 230.4\,\text{ms}/68\,\text{ms}$, $T_s = 0.982\,\text{ms}$, $\Delta x \times \Delta y \times \Delta z = 0.96\,\text{mm} \times 1.28\,\text{mm} \times 5.0\,\text{mm}$, $N_x \times N_y = 256 \times 192$, $\theta = 90°$, $N_{acq} = 1$, $\tau_{rf} = 1.28\,\text{ms}$, $G_{ss} = 10\,\text{mT/m}$; (b) $T_R/T_E = 2\,\text{s}/68\,\text{ms}$, $T_s = 12.8\,\text{ms}$, $\tau_{rf} = 2.56\,\text{ms}$, $G_{ss} = 4.8\,\text{mT/m}$. 548

19.27 (a), (b) $T_E = 68\,\text{ms}$, $\Delta x \times \Delta y \times \Delta z = 2.0\,\text{mm} \times 2.0\,\text{mm} \times 6.0\,\text{mm}$, $N_x \times N_y = 256 \times 192$, $\theta = 30°$, $N_{acq} = 1$. (This figure was contributed by Xiaoping Ding.) 557

19.28 (a) $T_E = 98\,\text{ms}$, $\Delta x \times \Delta y \times \Delta z = 2.0\,\text{mm} \times 2.0\,\text{mm} \times 6.0\,\text{mm}$, $N_x \times N_y = 128 \times 128$, $\theta = 90°$, $N_{acq} = 1$; (b) $T_D/T_E = 87\,\text{ms}/29\,\text{ms}$, $T_s = 0.68\,\text{ms}$, $\tau_{rf} = 1.28\,\text{ms}$, $G_{ss} = 4.17\,\text{mT/m}$; (c) $T_D/T_E = 102.4\,\text{ms}/29\,\text{ms}$, $T_s = 0.8\,\text{ms}$, $\tau_{rf} = 1.28\,\text{ms}$, $G_{ss} = 8.33\,\text{mT/m}$; (d) $T_D/T_E = 153.6\,\text{ms}/98\,\text{ms}$, $T_s = 1.2\,\text{ms}$, $\tau_{rf} = 2.56\,\text{ms}$, $G_{ss} = 2\,\text{mT/m}$. 558

19.31 (a) $T_R/T_E = 2.0\,\text{s}/68\,\text{ms}$, $T_s = 12.8\,\text{ms}$, $\Delta x \times \Delta y \times \Delta z = 0.96\,\text{mm} \times 1.28\,\text{mm} \times 5.0\,\text{mm}$, $N_x \times N_y = 256 \times 192$, $\theta = 30°$, $N_{acq} = 1$, $\tau_{rf} = 2.56\,\text{ms}$, $G_{ss} = 4.8\,\text{mT/m}$; (b) $T_D/T_E = 270\,\text{ms}/68\,\text{ms}$, $T_s = 1.2\,\text{ms}$, $\theta = 30°$, $\tau_{rf} = 1.28\,\text{ms}$, $G_{ss} = 10\,\text{mT/m}$; (c) $T_R/T_E = 2\,\text{s}/120\,\text{ms}$, $2\tau = 15\,\text{ms}$, $m = 5$, $T_s = 12.8\,\text{ms}$, $\theta = 90°$, $\tau_{rf} = 5.12\,\text{ms}$, $G_{ss} = 3.6\,\text{mT/m}$; (d) $T_R/T_E = 6\,\text{s}/90\,\text{ms}$, $T_s = 12.8\,\text{ms}$, $\theta = 90°$, $\tau_{rf} = 2.56\,\text{ms}$, $G_{ss} = 4.8\,\text{mT/m}$. 564

20.7 (a), (b) $T_R/T_E = 30\,\text{ms}/5\,\text{ms}$, $T_s = 5.12\,\text{ms}$, $\Delta x \times \Delta y \times \Delta z = 1.0\,\text{mm} \times 1.0\,\text{mm} \times 2.0\,\text{mm}$, $N_x \times N_y \times N_z = 256 \times 256 \times 96$, $\theta = 25°$, $N_{acq} = 1$, $\tau_{rf} = 1.28\,\text{ms}$, $G_{ss} = 1.15\,\text{mT/m}$; (c), (d) $T_E = 15\,\text{ms}$. 582

20.12 (a) $T_R/T_E = 600\,\text{ms}/45\,\text{ms}$, $T_s = 12.8\,\text{ms}$, $\Delta x \times \Delta y \times \Delta z = 0.5\,\text{mm} \times 1.0\,\text{mm} \times 8.0\,\text{mm}$, $N_x \times N_y = 512 \times 192$, $\theta = 65°$, $N_{acq} = 1$, $\tau_{rf} = 5.12\,\text{ms}$, $G_{ss} = 2.16\,\text{mT/m}$; (As usual the image is interpolated to $0.5\,\text{mm} \times 0.5\,\text{mm}$ to maintain the aspect ratio of 1:1 for display purposes.) (b) $T_R = 68\,\text{ms}$, $\theta = 25°$. (Reprinted, with permission, from Fig. 4 in *J. Magn. Reson. Imag.*, 7: 266, 1997.) 593

20.14 Relevant imaging parameters are the same as in Fig. 20.12b. (Reprinted, with permission, from Figs. 4 and 8 in *J. Magn. Reson. Imag.*, 7: 266, 1997.) . . . 595

Index